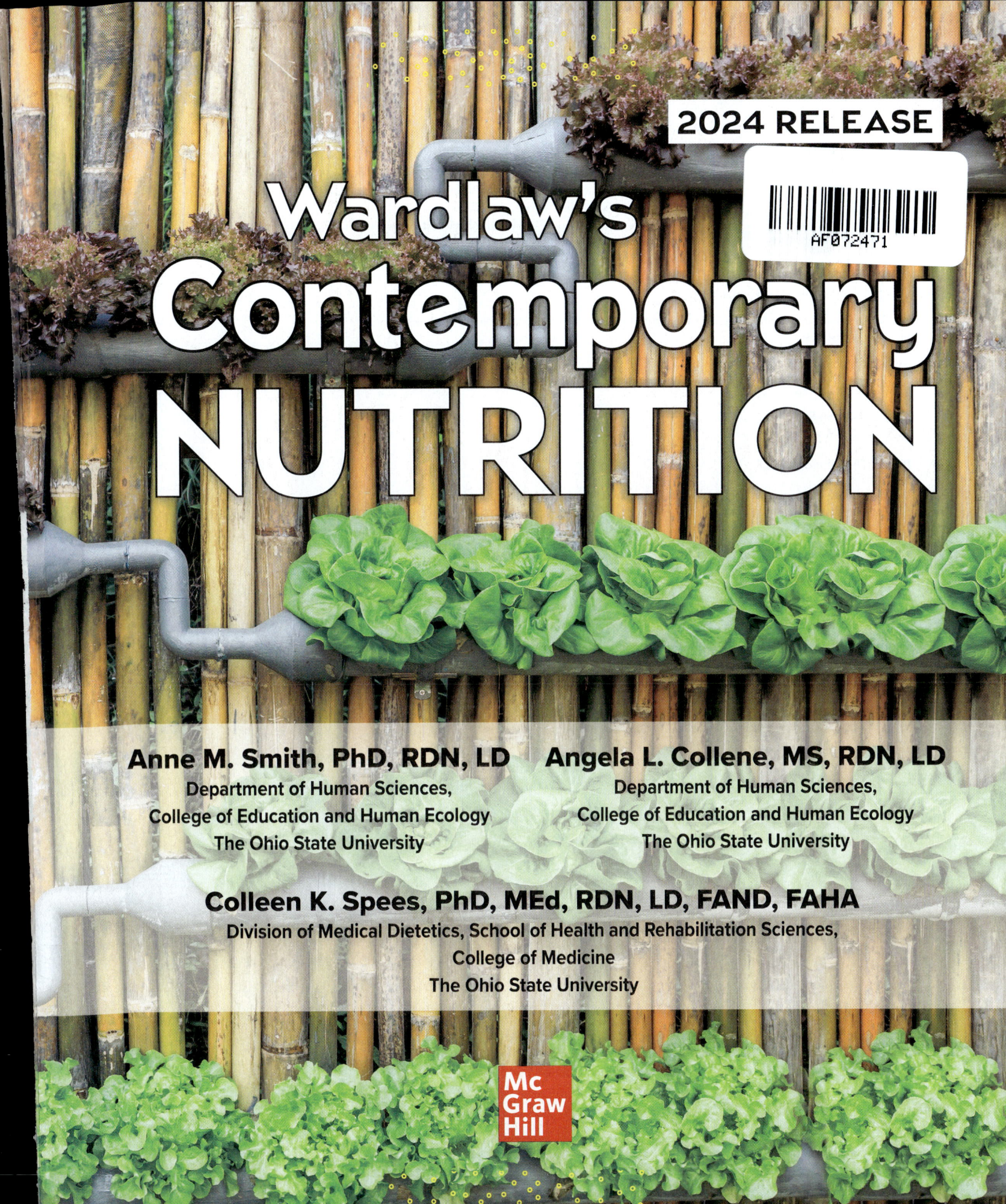

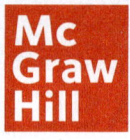

WARDLAW'S CONTEMPORARY NUTRITION

Published by McGraw Hill LLC, 1325 Avenue of the Americas, New York, NY 10019. Copyright ©2024 by McGraw Hill LLC. All rights reserved. Printed in the United States of America. No part of this publication may be reproduced or distributed in any form or by any means, or stored in a database or retrieval system, without the prior written consent of McGraw Hill LLC, including, but not limited to, in any network or other electronic storage or transmission, or broadcast for distance learning.

Some ancillaries, including electronic and print components, may not be available to customers outside the United States.

This book is printed on acid-free paper.

1 2 3 4 5 6 7 8 9 LWI 29 28 27 26 25 24

ISBN 978-1-264-44756-5
MHID 1-264-44756-6

Cover Image: *Thawornmat/123RF*

All credits appearing on page or at the end of the book are considered to be an extension of the copyright page.

The Internet addresses listed in the text were accurate at the time of publication. The inclusion of a website does not indicate an endorsement by the authors or McGraw Hill LLC, and McGraw Hill LLC does not guarantee the accuracy of the information presented at these sites.

mheducation.com/highered

Brief Contents

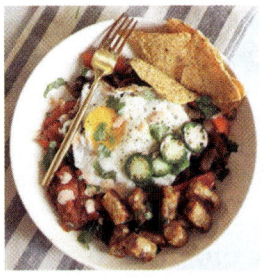 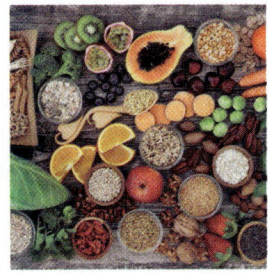 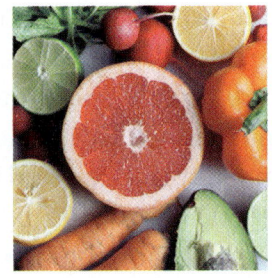 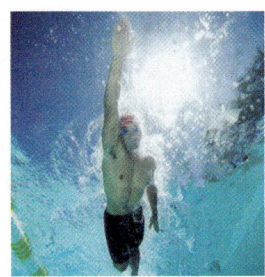 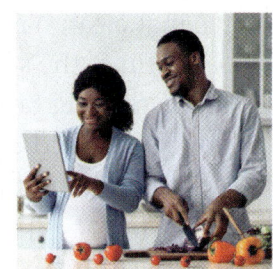

Part One Nutrition: A Key to Health

1. Nutrition, Food Choices, and Health 2
2. Designing a Healthy Eating Pattern 34
3. The Human Body: A Nutrition Perspective 78

Part Two Energy Nutrients and Energy Balance

4. Carbohydrates 124
5. Lipids 164
6. Proteins 206
7. Energy Balance 248

Part Three Vitamins, Minerals, and Water

8. Vitamins and Phytochemicals 292
9. Water and Minerals 362

Part Four Nutrition: Beyond the Nutrients

10. Nutrition: Fitness and Sports 436
11. Eating Disorders 474
12. Protecting Our Food Supply 508
13. Global Nutrition 550

Part Five Nutrition: A Focus on Life Stages

14. Nutrition During Pregnancy and Breastfeeding 580
15. Nutrition from Infancy Through Adolescence 628
16. Nutrition During Adulthood 682

Breakfast bowl: Alexis Joseph/McGraw Hill; dietary fiber health food: Marilyn Barbone/Shutterstock; micronutrients/phytochemicals: Alexis Joseph/McGraw Hill; swimmer: Erik Isakson/Blend Images LLC; couple in kitchen: Prostock-studio/Shutterstock

Dear Students,

Welcome to the fascinating world of nutrition! Because we all eat several times a day and the choices we make can have a dramatic impact on our health, nutrition is our favorite area of science. At the same time, the science of nutrition can seem a bit confusing. The definition of *good nutrition* seems like a moving target; different *nutrition experts* and social media influencers have varying ideas of how we should eat, and often these do not align with the current scientific evidence.

The addition of new products to the marketplace can add to this complexity. Did you know that the average supermarket carries about 47,000 food and beverage products? With so many food manufacturers vying for your attention (and dollars), how can you identify a healthy product? As a nation, we consume many of our meals and snacks away from home. When we eat foods someone else has prepared, we surrender control over what is in our food, where the food came from, and how much of it goes on our plates.

Undoubtedly, you are interested in what you should be eating and how the food you eat affects you. ***Wardlaw's Contemporary Nutrition*** is designed to accurately convey timely and evidence-based nutrition information in a manner that is easy to understand for a diverse group of students. We teach complex scientific concepts at a level that will enable you to apply the material to your own life.

In this 2024 Release of ***Wardlaw's Contemporary Nutrition,*** we have expanded upon several popular features and added a few new features. To help sort fact from fiction, we start each chapter with a new *Fact Check* feature, which calls out common misconceptions about foods and health, then explains what science has to say. We have invited a few of our esteemed colleagues to share their expertise in several new *Ask the RDN* features. Our new *Roots* feature celebrates the culturally diverse origins of our eating patterns and how they impact overall health.

We have written this book to help you make informed choices about dietary patterns that will promote health and wellness throughout all life stages. With this information at your fingertips, you will be well equipped to nourish your body in a way that supports your physical and mental health for a lifetime.

There is much to learn, so let's get started!

Anne Smith
Angela Collene
Colleen Spees

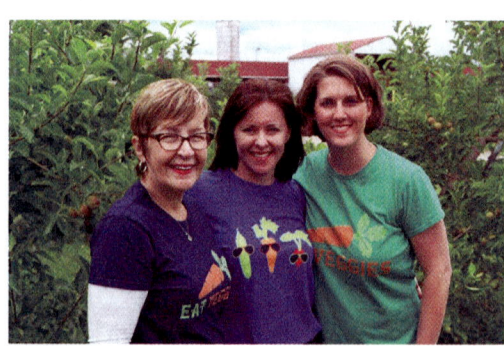

Briana Zabala

Anne Smith, Colleen Spees, and Angela Collene gather at the Hope Garden, a living research, teaching, and service-learning laboratory at The Ohio State University, academic home of the author team.

About the Cover

Growing from the insights shared in our popular *Farm to Fork* and *Sustainable Solutions* features, we are excited to highlight the sustainable practice of hydroponics! As our cover image displays, this alternative agricultural practice involves growing plants in soilless and nutrient-rich root mediums in a variety of controlled environments, including gutters, pipes (as pictured growing vertically on the cover), and other space-saving and inexpensive containers.

About the Authors

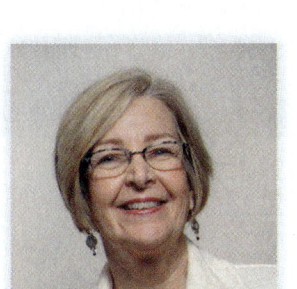

Monty Soungpradith/Open Image Studio LLC

ANNE M. SMITH, PhD, RDN, LD, is an associate professor emeritus at The Ohio State University. She was the recipient of the Outstanding Teacher Award from the College of Human Ecology, the Outstanding Dietetic Educator Award from the Ohio Dietetic Association, the Outstanding Faculty Member Award from the Department of Human Nutrition, and the Distinguished Service Award from the College of Education and Human Ecology for her commitment to undergraduate education in nutrition. Dr. Smith's research in the area of vitamin and mineral metabolism has appeared in prominent nutrition journals, and she was awarded the Research Award from the Ohio Agricultural Research and Development Center. She is a member of the American Society for Nutrition and the Academy of Nutrition and Dietetics.

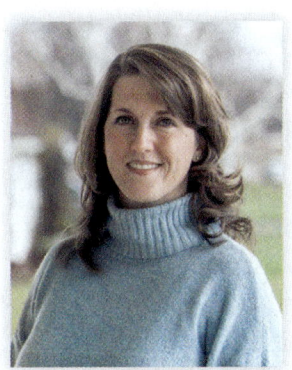

Tim Klontz

ANGELA L. COLLENE, MS, RDN, LD, began her career at her alma mater, The Ohio State University, as a research dietitian for studies related to diabetes and aging. Other professional experiences include community nutrition lecturing and counseling, owner of a personal chef business, and many diverse and rewarding science writing and editing projects. She is currently interested in the intersection between nutrition and mental health and—quite predictably for the mother of three girls—maternal and child nutrition. As a Senior Lecturer, Mrs. Collene teaches introductory nutrition and life cycle nutrition at The Ohio State University, where she received the Provost's Award for Distinguished Teaching by a Lecturer. She is a member of the Academy of Nutrition and Dietetics.

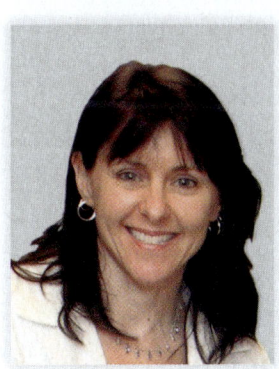

Ralphoto Studio

COLLEEN K. SPEES, PhD, MEd, RDN, LD, FAND, FAHA, is an academic instructor and researcher at The Ohio State University College of Medicine. In addition to teaching Evidence-Based Practice and Nutritional Genomics, Dr. Spees's primary research focus involves conducting biobehavioral clinical interventions aimed at providing optimal nutrition for high-risk populations (see http://go.osu.edu/hope). In addition, Dr. Spees is the recipient of several national awards from the Academy of Nutrition and Dietetics, including the Distinguished Practice Award; Award for Excellence in Oncology Nutrition Research; Outstanding Dietetic Educator Award; Nutrition Informatics Video Challenge Teaching Award; and the Top Innovator in Education Teaching Award. In addition, she serves on the Scientific Panel for the American Cancer Society's Dietary and Physical Activity Guideline. Dr. Spees is also a recognized Fellow of the Academy of Nutrition and Dietetics and the American Heart Association.

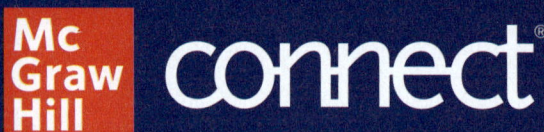

Your complete course platform

Connect enables you to build deeper connections with your students through cohesive digital content and tools, creating engaging learning experiences. We are committed to providing you with the right resources and tools to support all your students along their personal learning journeys.

65%
Less Time Grading

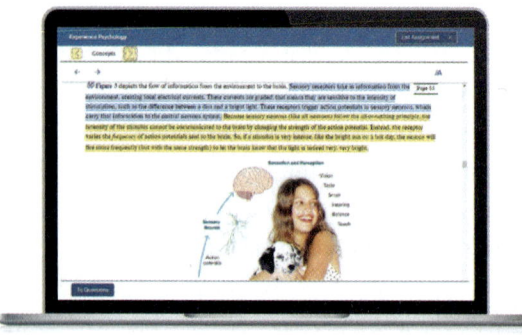

Laptop: Getty Images; Woman/dog: George Doyle/Getty Images

Every learner is unique

In Connect, instructors can assign an adaptive reading experience with SmartBook®. Rooted in advanced learning science principles, SmartBook delivers a personalized experience, focusing students on their learning gaps and ensuring the time they spend studying is time well spent.
mheducation.com/highered/connect/smartbook

Study anytime, anywhere

Encourage your students to download the free ReadAnywhere® app so they can access their online eBook, SmartBook®, or Adaptive Learning Assignments when it's convenient, even when they're offline. Because the app automatically syncs with students' Connect accounts, all their work is available every time they open it.

mheducation.com/readanywhere

"I really liked this app—it made it easy to study when you don't have your textbook in front of you."

Jordan Cunningham, a student at *Eastern Washington University*

Effective tools for efficient studying

Connect is designed to help students be more productive with simple, flexible, intuitive tools that maximize study time and meet students' individual learning needs. Get learning that works for everyone with Connect.

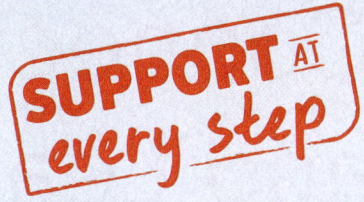

Education for all

McGraw Hill works directly with Accessibility Services departments and faculty to meet the learning needs of all students. Please contact your Accessibility Services Office, and ask them to email **accessibility@mheducation.com**, or visit **mheducation.com/about/accessibility** for more information.

Affordable solutions, added value

Make technology work for you with LMS integration for single sign-on access, mobile access to the digital textbook, and reports to quickly show you how each of your students is doing. And with our Inclusive Access program, you can provide all these tools at the lowest available market price to your students. Ask your McGraw Hill representative for more information.

Solutions for your challenges

A product isn't a solution. Real solutions are affordable, reliable, and come with training and ongoing support when you need it and how you want it. Visit **supportateverystep.com** for videos and resources both you and your students can use throughout the term.

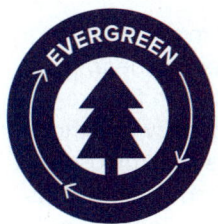

Updated and relevant content

Our Evergreen delivery model provides you with the most relevant and up-to-date content, tools, and accessibility. Engage students and freshen up assignments with up-to-date coverage of select topics and new questions, all without having to switch editions or build a new course.

Connecting Teaching and Learning

McGraw Hill NutritionCalc Plus

NutritionCalc Plus is a **powerful dietary analysis tool** featuring more than 106,000 foods from the reliable and accurate ESHA Research nutrient database, which is comprised of data from the latest USDA Standard Reference database, manufacturer's data, restaurant data, and data from literature sources. NutritionCalc Plus allows users to track food and activities, and then analyze their choices with a robust selection of intuitive reports. The interface was updated to accommodate ADA requirements and modern mobile experience native to today's students.

Virtual Labs

While the sciences are hands-on disciplines, instructors are now often being asked to deliver some of their lab components online, as full online replacements, supplements to prepare for in-person labs, or make-up labs.

These simulations help each student learn the practical and conceptual skills needed, then check for understanding and provide feedback. With adaptive pre-lab and post-lab assessment available, instructors can customize each assignment.

From the instructor's perspective, these simulations may be used in the lecture environment to help students visualize processes, such as digestion of starch and emulsification of lipids.

Dietary Analysis Case Studies in Connect®

One of the challenges instructors face with teaching nutrition classes is having time to grade individual dietary analysis projects. To help overcome this challenge, assign auto-graded dietary analysis case studies. These tools require students to use NutritionCalc Plus to analyze dietary data, generate reports, and answer questions to apply their nutrition knowledge to real-world situations. These assignments were developed and reviewed by faculty who use such assignments in their own teaching. They are designed to be relevant, current, and interesting.

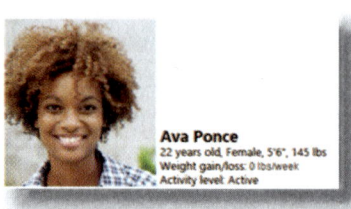

Pkchai/Shutterstock

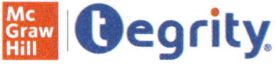

Tegrity: Lectures 24/7
Tegrity in Connect is a tool that makes class time available 24/7 by automatically capturing every lecture. With a simple one-click start-and-stop process, you capture all computer screens and corresponding audio in a format that is easy to search, frame by frame. Students can replay any part of any class with easy-to-use, browser-based viewing on a PC, Mac, or other mobile device.

Educators know that the more students can see, hear, and experience class resources, the better they learn. In fact, studies prove it. Tegrity's unique search feature helps students efficiently find what they need, when they need it, across an entire semester of class recordings. Help turn your students' study time into learning moments immediately supported by your lecture. With Tegrity, you also increase intent listening and class participation by easing students' concerns about note-taking. Using Tegrity in Connect will make it more likely you will see students' faces, not the tops of their heads.

Assess My Diet

AUTO-GRADED PERSONALIZED DIETARY ANALYSIS

Students are using NutritionCalc Plus to analyze their own dietary patterns. But how can instructors integrate that information into a meaningful learning experience? With Assess My Diet, instructors can now assign auto-graded, personalized dietary analysis questions within Connect. These questions refresh their memory on the functions and food sources of each nutrient and prompt the students to evaluate their own eating behaviors. Students can compare their own nutrient intakes to current Dietary Reference Intakes and demonstrate their ability to perform calculations on their own data, such as percentage of calories from saturated fat. They can compare the nutrient density of their own food selections to see which of their food choices provides the most fiber or iron. A benefit of the Assess My Diet question bank is that it offers assignable content that is personalized to the students' data, yet it is still auto-graded. It saves time and keeps all assignments in one place.

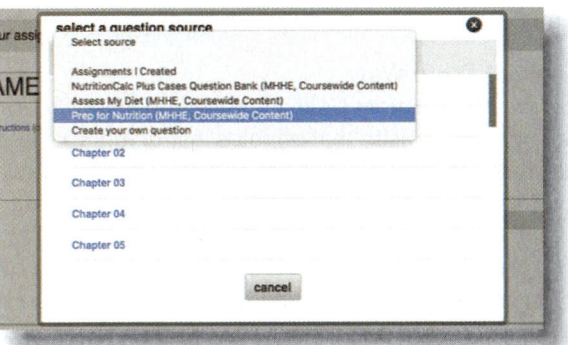

Prep for Nutrition

To help you level-set your classroom, we've created Prep for Nutrition. This question bank highlights a series of questions, including Basic Chemistry, Biology, Dietary Analysis, Mathematics, and Student Success, to give students a refresher on the skills needed to enter and be successful in their course. By having these foundational skills, you will feel more confident your students can begin class, ready to understand more complex concepts and topics. Prep for Nutrition is course-wide for ALL nutrition titles and can be found in the Question Bank dropdown within Connect.

Writing Assignment

Available within Connect and Connect Master, the Writing Assignment tool delivers a learning experience to help students improve their written communication skills and conceptual understanding. As an instructor you can assign, monitor, grade, and provide feedback on writing more efficiently and effectively.

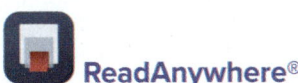 ReadAnywhere®

Read or study when it's convenient for you with McGraw Hill's free ReadAnywhere app. Available for iOS or Android smartphones or tablets, ReadAnywhere gives users access to McGraw Hill tools including the eBook and SmartBook® 2.0 or Adaptive Learning Assignments in Connect. Take notes, highlight, and complete assignments offline—all of your work will sync when you open the app with WiFi access. Log in with your McGraw Hill Connect username and password to start learning—anytime, anywhere!

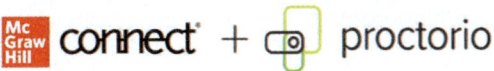

Remote Proctoring & Browser-Locking Capabilities

Remote proctoring and browser-locking capabilities, hosted by Proctorio within Connect, provide control of the assessment environment by enabling security options and verifying the identity of the student.

Seamlessly integrated within Connect, these services allow instructors to control the assessment experience by verifying identification, restricting browser activity, and monitoring student actions.

Instant and detailed reporting gives instructors an at-a-glance view of potential academic integrity concerns, thereby avoiding personal bias and supporting evidence-based claims.

Create

Your Book, Your Way
McGraw Hill's Content Collections Powered by Create® is a self-service website that enables instructors to create custom course materials—print and eBooks—by drawing upon McGraw Hill's comprehensive, cross-disciplinary content. Choose what you want from our high-quality textbooks, articles, and cases. Combine it with your own content quickly and easily, and tap into other rights-secured, third-party content such as readings, cases, and articles. Content can be arranged in a way that makes the most sense for your course, and you can include the course name and information as well. Choose the best format for your course: color print, black-and-white print, or eBook. The eBook can be included in your Connect course and is available on the free ReadAnywhere® app for smartphone or tablet access as well. When you are finished customizing, you will receive a free digital copy to review in just minutes! Visit McGraw Hill Create—www.mcgrawhillcreate.com—today and begin building!

OLC-Aligned Courses

Implementing High-Quality Online Instruction and Assessment through Preconfigured Courseware
In consultation with the Online Learning Consortium (OLC) and our certified Faculty Consultants, McGraw Hill has created pre-configured courseware using OLC's quality scorecard to align with best practices in online course delivery. This turnkey courseware contains a combination of formative assessments, summative assessments, homework, and application activities, and can easily be customized to meet an individual's needs and course outcomes. For more information, visit https://www.mheducation.com/highered/olc.

Polling

Every learner has unique needs. Uncover where and when you're needed with the new Polling tool in McGraw Hill Connect. Polling allows you to discover where students are in real time. Engage students and help them create connections with your course content while gaining valuable insight during lectures. Leverage polling data to deliver personalized instruction when and where it is needed most.

NewsFlash Articles

NewsFlash brings the real world into your classroom. These activities in Connect tie current news stories to key concepts. After interacting with a contemporary news story, students are assessed on their ability to make the connections between real-life events and course content.

Test Builder in Connect

Available within Connect, Test Builder is a cloud-based tool that enables instructors to format tests that can be printed, administered within a Learning Management System, or exported as a Word document. Test Builder offers a modern, streamlined interface for easy content configuration that matches course needs, without requiring a download.

Test Builder allows you to:

- access all test bank content from a particular title.
- easily pinpoint the most relevant content through robust filtering options.
- manipulate the order of questions or scramble questions and/or answers.
- pin questions to a specific location within a test.
- determine your preferred treatment of algorithmic questions.
- choose the layout and spacing.
- add instructions and configure default settings.

Test Builder provides a secure interface for better protection of content and allows for just-in-time updates to flow directly into assessments.

Connecting Students to Today's Nutrition

Understanding Our Audience

We have written *Wardlaw's Contemporary Nutrition* assuming that our students have a limited background in college-level biology, chemistry, or physiology. We have been careful to include the essential science foundation needed to adequately comprehend certain topics in nutrition, such as protein synthesis in Chapter 6. The science in this text has been presented in a simple, straightforward manner so that undergraduate students can master the material and apply it to their own lives. The *Concept Maps* and detailed, annotated figures and infographics bring complex topics into view for students from any major.

Check Out the Functional Approach

An alternative presentation of the contents of this book is available as *Wardlaw's Contemporary Nutrition: A Functional Approach*. The difference, as shown in the tables of contents below, is in Part Three. Instead of describing these nutrients in their traditional categories (e.g., water-soluble vitamins), we discuss them in groups based on their roles in fluid and electrolyte balance, body defenses, bone health, energy metabolism, blood health, and brain health. This format enables students to understand in more detail how these nutrients interact in food and in our bodies to support key functions that sustain our health.

Wardlaw's Contemporary Nutrition

Part One Nutrition: A Key to Health
1. Nutrition, Food Choices, and Health
2. Designing a Healthy Eating Pattern
3. The Human Body: A Nutrition Perspective

Part Two Energy Nutrients and Energy Balance
4. Carbohydrates
5. Lipids
6. Proteins
7. Energy Balance

Part Three Vitamins, Minerals, and Water
8. Vitamins and Phytochemicals
9. Water and Minerals

Part Four Nutrition: Beyond the Nutrients
10. Nutrition: Fitness and Sports
11. Eating Disorders
12. Protecting Our Food Supply
13. Global Nutrition

Part Five Nutrition: A Focus on Life Stages
14. Nutrition During Pregnancy and Breastfeeding
15. Nutrition from Infancy Through Adolescence
16. Nutrition During Adulthood

Wardlaw's Contemporary Nutrition: A Functional Approach

Part One Nutrition: A Key to Health
1. Nutrition, Food Choices, and Health
2. Designing a Healthy Eating Pattern
3. The Human Body: A Nutrition Perspective

Part Two Energy Nutrients and Energy Balance
4. Carbohydrates
5. Lipids
6. Proteins
7. Energy Balance

Part Three Vitamins, Minerals, and Water
8. Overview of Micronutrients and Phytochemicals
9. Fluid and Electrolyte Balance
10. Nutrients Involved in Body Defenses
11. Nutrients Involved in Bone Health
12. Micronutrient Function in Energy Metabolism
13. Nutrients That Support Blood and Brain Health

Part Four Nutrition: Beyond the Nutrients
14. Nutrition: Fitness and Sports
15. Eating Disorders
16. Protecting Our Food Supply
17. Global Nutrition

Part Five Nutrition: A Focus on Life Stages
18. Nutrition During Pregnancy and Breastfeeding
19. Nutrition from Infancy Through Adolescence
20. Nutrition During Adulthood

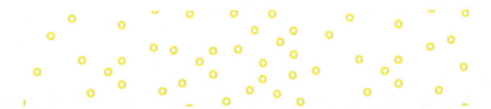

Connecting with Features

Featuring the Lastest Evidence-Based Guidelines and Nutrition Research

Nutrition is a dynamic field. This release has been carefully updated to reflect current scientific understanding, as well as the latest health and nutrition guidelines. And in response to feedback from students and instructors, we are excited to introduce several new and updated features—all designed to engage students and encourage more discussion in the classroom.

Applying Nutrition on a Personal Level

Throughout this release, we reinforce the fact that each person responds differently to nutrients. To further convey the importance of applying nutrition to their personal lives, we include many examples of people and situations that resonate with college students. We also stress the importance of learning to intelligently sort through the seemingly endless range of nutrition messages to recognize reliable information and to sensibly apply it to their own lives. Our goal is to provide students the tools they need to eat healthfully and make informed nutrition decisions after they complete the class. Many of these features can be assigned and graded through Connect to help students learn and apply the information and engage with the text.

The new **Roots** feature digs down to discover the diverse factors that influence our food choices and nutritional status. Cultural traditions, religious observances, and our genetic code impact our dietary patterns.

We continue to build upon our popular **Farm to Fork** feature, presenting a food item and its path to our plates. You will learn where it is grown, how to select the most flavorful and nutritious varieties, and the best methods to store and prepare these foods to maximize their nutritional value. Cashews and olive oil are new in this release.

Roots

Religious Customs Affect Vitamin D Status

In this chapter, you have learned that vitamin D can be synthesized by the skin upon exposure to sunlight. How do religious customs, such as the Quran dress code for Muslim females, affect vitamin D status? The Quran dress code requires Muslim females to cover their bodies except for their hands and face. Some conservative branches of Islam require females to cover the hands and face, as well. Clinical research shows that vitamin D status is significantly lower among Muslim females who wear concealing clothing compared to females who do not follow religious dress codes. Recognizing that vitamin D deficiency may affect not only bone health but also immune function and risk for some chronic diseases, females who are not able to expose skin to natural sunlight must emphasize dietary or supplemental sources of vitamin D to prevent vitamin D deficiency.

Source: Chouraqui J-P, Turck D, Briend A, Darmaun D; Committee on Nutrition of the French Society of Pediatrics. Religious dietary rules and their potential nutritional and health consequences. *Int J Epidemiol*. 2021 Mar 3;50(1):12-26. doi: 10.1093/ije/dyaa182

Considering the continued expansion of the body of research related to the gut microbiome and its impact on human health, we have added several new **Magnificent Microbiome** features that explore relevant interactions between nutrition and the gut microbiota.

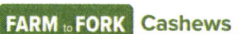

Irritable Bowel Syndrome

An imbalance between beneficial and pathogenic microbes in the gut may play a role in the development of irritable bowel syndrome. Microorganisms influence intestinal function in many ways:
- They stimulate the production of a protective layer of mucus by the intestinal cells.
- They affect the permeability of the intestinal lining, which regulates the movement of substances (both good and bad) from the intestine to the bloodstream.
- They can upregulate or downregulate the inflammatory response.
- They affect nerve signals from the gut to the brain, which may influence the rate of motility in the intestine and the perception of pain.

Researchers are interested in the potential for foods or supplements with probiotics or prebiotics to promote healthier gut function in individuals with IBS.

Source: Simon E, Călinoiu LF, Mitrea L, Vodnar DC. Probiotics, prebiotics, and synbiotics: implications and beneficial effects against irritable bowel syndrome. *Nutrients*. 2021 Jun 20;13(6):2112. doi: 10.3390/nu13062112

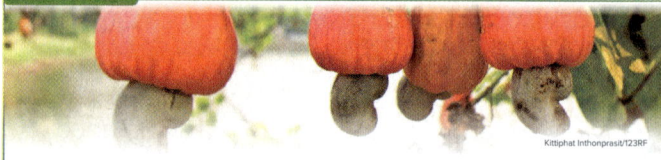

FARM to FORK: Cashews

Kittiphat Inthonprasit/123RF

Cashews are rich in fiber, unsaturated fats, plant protein, and beneficial phytochemicals that may help reduce inflammation and protect us from disease. Cashews are also a good source of copper, a mineral essential for energy production, healthy brain development, and a strong immune system, and magnesium and manganese, important for bone health. They are low in sugar and have been linked to benefits like weight loss, improved blood sugar control to protect against type 2 diabetes, and a healthier heart through lowering blood pressure, triglycerides, and cholesterol. More research is needed, however, to confirm these benefits. Cashews are classified as tree nuts. Therefore, people allergic to tree nuts may have a higher risk of also being allergic to cashews.

Grow
- Cashews are the seeds of a tropical evergreen shrub cultivated in warm, humid climates and related to mango, pistachio, and poison ivy. The cashew seed hangs from the bottom of a cashew apple. Fresh cashew apples taste delicious but are highly perishable.
- The kidney-shaped cashew seed is harvested by hand and is encased in a hard shell with two layers. Between these two layers is a toxic resin, urushiol (also found in poison ivy), which can trigger a skin reaction.
- During processing, the cashew kernels are shelled and cooked to remove the toxic urushiol, and the resulting product is sold as "raw" cashews.

Shop
- Cashews are sold in bags or in bulk bins and may be salted, unsalted, or flavored.
- For the freshest cashews, make sure there is no evidence of moisture or insects and that the cashews are not shriveled. If buying in bulk, smell the cashews to ensure they are not rancid. Cashews sold in vacuum-packed jars or cans will stay fresh longest.
- Cashews sold as "roasted" have been cooked twice—once during the shelling process and then roasted to deepen the color and enhance the flavor, sometimes with salt. Dry-roasted nuts are cooked without any added oil.
- For the most nutritional benefits and to limit excess salt or added fats, consider choosing dry roasted or "raw" unsalted cashew varieties whenever possible.

Store
- Because cashews are high in unsaturated fatty acids, they are susceptible to oxidation and rancidity and should be stored in an airtight container to minimize air exposure.
- Refrigerate or freeze cashews in tightly sealed containers to help them last longer. Cashews can last up to 6 months in the refrigerator and up to 1 year in the freezer.

Prep
- Cashews can be eaten "raw" or roasted and are a portable snack. Whole cashews can be used in stir-fries, soups, salads, and stews. Asian and Indian cuisines frequently include whole or chopped cashews as a stir-fry ingredient and in curries.
- Owing to their creamy texture when blended, cashews are used to make several dairy alternatives. These include cashew milk, cream and cream sauces, cheese, mayonnaise, butter, and pesto.
- To make cashew butter, roast cashews at 330°F/165°C for 10 to 15 minutes, until golden in color and fragrant. After the nuts have cooled, blend them in a food processor until smooth (about 12 to 15 minutes). Cashew butter can be spread on toast, stirred into yogurt or oatmeal, or mixed with oats and dried fruit to make no-bake energy bites.
- To make dairy-free sour cream or cream cheese, soak cashews and blend them with apple cider vinegar or lemon juice. A probiotic can also be used to ferment the cream cheese (https://www.hummusapien.com/vegan-cashew-cream-cheese-recipe/).

Sources: Are cashews good for you? Nutrition, benefits, and downsides. *Healthline*. Updated June 10, 2020. https://www.healthline.com/nutrition/are-cashews-good-for-you Oliveira NN, Mothé CG, Mothé MC, de Oliveira LG. Cashew nut and cashew apple: a scientific and technological monitoring worldwide review. *J Food Sci Technol*. 2020 Jan;57(1):12-21. doi: 10.1007/s13197-019-04051-7

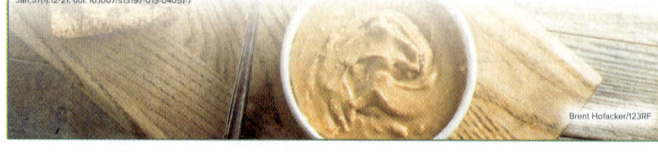

Brent Hofacker/123RF

To counter the steady flow of nutrition misinformation from multiple media outlets, we open each chapter with the ***Fact Check*** feature. The feature highlights a relevant nutrition-related topic, provides a science-based explanation of the current state of the evidence, and points students to the location within each chapter where more details can be found.

FACT CHECK

Should I take collagen for healthy skin?

Collagen accounts for approximately one-third of all the proteins in your body. It has a structural role in bones, joints, muscles, blood vessels, and skin. Many people are interested in the potential for collagen supplements to improve the elasticity, hydration, and firmness of skin to reduce the signs of skin aging. Collagen proteins in food are not absorbed intact but are broken down into small peptides and individual amino acids during digestion. The collagen found in dietary supplements comes from cows, pigs, chickens, and fish and has been hydrolyzed (broken down into small peptides) to promote absorption. Once absorbed, these raw materials can be used to synthesize collagen in cells if it is needed. Other nutrients, such as vitamin C and zinc (sometimes added to collagen supplements), are also required for collagen synthesis. Besides providing the building blocks for protein synthesis, collagen peptides may play a role in regulating the breakdown and synthesis of proteins within the cell. Results of clinical trials show that collagen supplements are well tolerated and can increase skin hydration and elasticity, which decreases the appearance of skin aging. However, further research is underway to determine the best dose and combination of ingredients to support skin health. Should you take a collagen supplement? There is no evidence of adverse effects, and studies do show a benefit for skin outcomes. However, the cost of supplements is a consideration. A varied dietary pattern can provide the building blocks necessary for collagen synthesis at a reasonable cost. In Section 6.6 you will learn more about the structural role of collagen in the body.

Source: de Miranda RB, Weimer P, Rossi RC. Effects of hydrolyzed collagen supplementation on skin aging: a systematic review and meta-analysis. *Int J Dermatol.* 2021;60(12):1449-1461. doi:10.1111/ijd.15518

Ask the RDN continues to appear in every chapter to answer frequently asked questions we hear from our students and colleagues. For many topics, including plant-based eating, sustainability, and child nutrition, we have reached out to experts in their fields to answer questions. This feature highlights the ability of the RDN to translate the latest scientific findings into easy-to-understand, practical, and applicable nutrition information.

ASK THE RDN CBD

Dear RDN: *My friend recently began taking CBD. She said it helps her sleep better and manage her anxiety. What are the pros and cons of taking CBD?*

CBD (cannabidiol) is a cannabinoid found in cannabis and hemp. Many people report that CBD helps manage anxiety, as well as pain, inflammation, muscle spasms, insomnia, seizures, inflammatory bowel disease, IBS, migraines, neurodegenerative disorders, and more. CBD is non-intoxicating. THC (tetrahydrocannabinol), another cannabinoid found in cannabis (and in small amounts in hemp), is known for its intoxicating or "high" effect.

The body processes cannabinoids through a neurotransmitter system *(the endocannabinoid system)* whose function is to promote homeostasis in the body. CBD helps to regulate this system. In fact, our body makes its own cannabinoid, called anandamide, also known as the *bliss molecule.* CBD allows our body to keep more of this *feel good* compound, which may explain why many find relief from anxiety using CBD.

There is pronounced synergy between the cannabinoids, terpenes (responsible for the unique aroma in plants), and flavonoids (that contribute antioxidant and anti-inflammatory effects) in cannabis and hemp. Each individual component of the plant may provide therapeutic benefits on its own, but when combined, the so-called entourage effect is dramatic.

CBD comes in many forms, including sublingual tinctures, water-soluble tinctures, edibles/softgels, topicals, and hemp flower/vape cartridges. There are three types of CBD: full spectrum, broad spectrum, and CBD isolate. Full spectrum products contain all the plant's components, including cannabinoids, terpenes, and flavonoids. Broad-spectrum CBD products contain all these synergistic components, minus the THC. CBD isolate is pure CBD, meaning that it does not contain other synergistic plant compounds, which may decrease efficacy and increase side effects.

Dosing of CBD is very individual, depending on the condition being treated and method of administration. Some people find relief with just 2 milligrams and others may require 50 milligrams or more. It's best to *start low and go slow* to find the minimum effective dose.

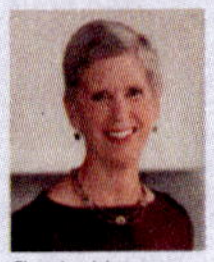

Channing Johnson

Today's market is inundated with CBD products, including many of inferior quality. The Food and Drug Administration found that 70% of CBD products sold online are mislabeled, with some containing zero CBD. It's important to buy CBD products from a trusted and safe source. Look for a certificate of analysis (COA) from an independent lab before buying a product.

A word of caution. Taking orally ingested CBD (i.e., edibles/softgels) with other medications that are contraindicated with grapefruit may result in an adverse event, so it's important to talk with a knowledgeable health care professional.

Including CBD in your self-care routine may be effective for managing anxiety, but it's also important to work on other aspects of your life that may promote wellness: engage in regular physical activity, adhere to a healthy eating pattern, get adequate sleep, practice meditation or yoga, and seek professional help from a licensed mental health provider if symptoms of anxiety are severe.

Yours in health,

Janice Newell Bissex, MS, RDN, FAND

Holistic Cannabis Practitioner

Newsworthy Nutrition, a feature in each chapter, highlights the use of the scientific method in recently published research studies that relate to the chapter topics. In addition, assignable questions in Connect take learning a step further by asking students to read primary literature and apply what they have learned.

Newsworthy Nutrition

Social media use and body dissatisfaction among college-age females

INTRODUCTION: Body dissatisfaction may lead to depression, restrictive dieting, and disordered eating behaviors. Previous research has shown a relationship between body dissatisfaction and exposure to traditional forms of media, such as print and television content. Social media may be especially problematic because it is used frequently and it facilitates social comparisons. However, the relationship between social media use and body dissatisfaction has not been adequately assessed. **OBJECTIVE:** In this cross-sectional study, the researchers aimed to assess the relationships among social media use (e.g., Facebook, Twitter, and Instagram), body dissatisfaction, and negative affect (i.e., depression). **METHODS:** The researchers used a technique called ecological model assessment, in which they contacted subjects in their natural setting on their own schedule. This method has been used to overcome the limitations of retroactive assessments, which may be inaccurate and underestimate social media use. A sample of 30 college students who identified as female at Missouri State University were contacted through their smartphones five times per day for 6 days (1 practice day and 5 test days) to answer a series of questions about social media use (including time spent on social media as well as number of sites visited), mood (the Positive and Negative Affect Schedule-Expanded Form), and body image (the Body Image States Scale). Each assessment took approximately 5 minutes to complete. **RESULTS:** Number of sites visited, but not time spent on social media, was a predictor of body dissatisfaction. Social media use (time spent and number of sites visited) also predicted general negative affect, sadness, and guilt. **CONCLUSION:** This observational study showed that social media use, unlike other forms of media, predicts negative affect and body dissatisfaction. Specifically, consistent messaging about unrealistic body weight or shape across several sites may reinforce body dissatisfaction. This information may assist in the development of media literacy interventions to modify the use of social media and improve and/or develop coping skills. Future studies may employ similar assessment techniques in a larger, more diverse population and should examine the bidirectionality of the relationships between depression or body dissatisfaction and social media use.

Source: Bennett BL, Whisenhunt BL, Hudson DL, et al. Examining the impact of social media on mood and body dissatisfaction using ecological momentary assessment. *J Am Coll Health.* 2020 Jul;68(5):502-508. doi: 10.1080/07448481.2019.1583236

Each chapter presents a relevant ***Case Study***, which presents a real-world scenario and challenges the students to apply their knowledge. This translational application can be used as a teaching strategy in traditional, hybrid, or remote learning. Answers are provided to instructors in Connect.

CASE STUDY Worried About Bone Health

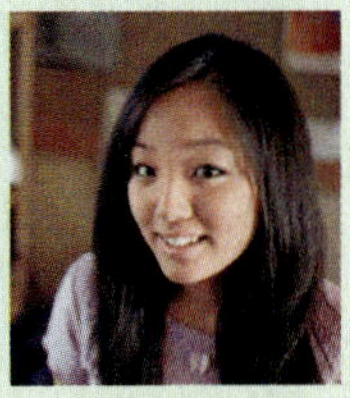

Grace is exploring ways she can decrease her risk for osteoporosis.
Dennis Wise/Digital Vision/Getty Images

Grace, a 23-year-old female of Korean descent, is in her final year of nursing school in Boston. She also works 20 hours per week at a local pharmacy. Grace is worried after a phone call she just received from her father. While out on her walk yesterday, Grace's mother caught her foot on an uneven section of the sidewalk, fell, and broke her hip. The doctor diagnosed Grace's mother with osteoporosis, and the family is worried about the long recovery ahead. As a nursing student, Grace knows how devastating a hip fracture can be. She also knows that osteoporosis can run in families. Grace resolves to do whatever she can to learn about osteoporosis and strengthen her bones now.

She searches online and finds the Osteoporosis Risk Check at https://riskcheck.osteoporosis.foundation. The online tool from the International Osteoporosis Foundation focuses mainly on nonmodifiable risk factors for osteoporosis: age, family history, chronic conditions, and use of medications that can influence bone health. The site also highlights some modifiable risk factors: weight status, exposure to sunlight, physical activity level, intake of good food sources of calcium and vitamin D, and use of alcohol or tobacco products.

Grace is 5′4″ and weighs 105 pounds. Currently, she does not have any chronic health conditions. She does not take any medications or dietary supplements. Grace wonders if her intakes of calcium and vitamin D are adequate. She cooks traditional Korean dishes for half of her meals but eats fast food or sandwiches for the rest. Her go-to beverages are water and unsweetened tea. She admits she has not been able to fit physical activity into her busy schedule lately. On weekends, she goes out with friends and may have a glass or two of wine. Grace does not smoke.

Answer the following questions about Grace's bone health.

1. Go to https://riskcheck.osteoporosis.foundation and fill out the risk assessment using Grace's information. Identify two nonmodifiable risk factors for Grace.
2. Identify two modifiable risk factors for Grace.
3. What are the environmental conditions that inhibit Grace from adequately synthesizing vitamin D? How can she overcome some of them?
4. What are some calcium and vitamin D sources in traditional Korean dishes? (See http://www.pbs.org/hiddenkorea/food.htm for information about traditional Korean food.)
5. Give Grace some tips to increase her calcium and vitamin D intake at fast-food restaurants without significantly increasing costs or calories.
6. Based on her current dietary pattern, do you think Grace should take any dietary supplements? If so, which one(s)?

Complete the Case Study. Responses to these questions can be provided by your instructor.

In response to the drive toward sustainability—including environmental, health, social, and economic issues—we have introduced **Sustainable Solutions**, in which we highlight sustainability topics related to each chapter's content.

Sustainable Solutions
Offal
Does consuming offal sound awful? Offal refers to the entrails and organs, sometimes called *variety meats* or the *odd bits* of animals. Compared to other regions of the world, the United States is one of the lowest consumers of offal. In fact, nearly 60% of U.S. variety meats are exported to Asia. However, if you choose to consume animal products, including offal in your dietary pattern is a sustainable choice. From an agricultural standpoint, consuming everything *from nose to tail* is an efficient use of agricultural resources and cuts down on food waste. From environmental and economic perspectives, consuming these products locally helps to decrease the costs of exporting variety meats to other countries. Furthermore, organ meats are nutrient dense—especially for blood health! They are rich in high-quality protein and provide more iron, zinc, vitamin B-6, and vitamin B-12 than lean muscle meat.

Source: Ratliff E. Offal—health benefits of organ meat. *Today's Dietitian.* 2020 May;22(5):44.

The **Medicine Cabinet** feature presents information on common medications used to treat diseases that have a nutrition connection. These features highlight the ways medications can affect nutritional status, as well as ways food and nutrients can affect how medications work.

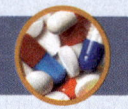
Medicine Cabinet
Anticoagulants
People who are prone to develop blood clots may take anticoagulants or *blood thinners*. One commonly prescribed anticoagulant is Coumadin® (warfarin). This medication inhibits vitamin K–dependent coagulation factors. When taking Coumadin or similar drugs, it is important to keep dietary intake of vitamin K consistent from day to day.

©Peter Dazeley/Photographer's Choice/Getty Images

Source: Hull RD, Garcia DA, Vasquez SR. Patient education: Warfarin (beyond the basics). UpToDate. Updated June 16, 2021. Accessed February 14, 2022. https://www.uptodate.com/contents/warfarin-beyond-the-basics/print

At the end of each chapter, **Nutrition and Your Health** provides an opportunity to explore current nutrition-related health and disease. With topics spanning from nutritional genomics to brain health to healthy aging, this feature provides an opportunity for in-depth classroom or remote discussions on a variety of timely topics.

16.5 Nutrition and Your Health: Lifestyles Linked with Longevity

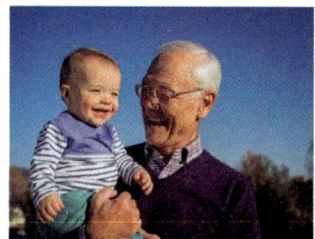
Erik Isakson/Getty Images

The U.S. Census Bureau indicates that the number of adults in the United States who have reached their 100th birthday grew to over 90,000 in 2020. By 2030, it is estimated that there will be over 130,000 centenarians in the U.S.[32] (Fig. 16-11).

However, it would not be desirable to add years to your life without adding life to your years. In other words, we want to know how to extend a healthy life without the burden of chronic diseases. With chronic diseases becoming more and more common in old age, there is increased interest in the behaviors common to people who live exceptionally long lives. Good health and longevity are dependent on numerous factors, including lifestyle and nutrition. Your genetic makeup is also important in determining your lifespan and risk of diseases, but your lifestyle is thought to have an even greater impact.[4]

The Blue Zones
The blue zones are geographic areas whose inhabitants have lived longer and had lower rates of chronic disease than people from other regions of the world. *Blue zones* is a term first used in 2000 by Dan Buettner after leading a *National Geographic* expedition to find the secrets of longevity. The team discovered five regions around the world where people typically live to be over 100 years old.[33,34]

To be considered a certified blue zone, the population lived significantly longer compared to national rates. These populations displayed various behaviors related to their lifestyle, nutrition, genetics, and physical environmental conditions that might be determinants for life quantity and quality. Using epidemiological data, statistics, birth certificates, and other data, five regions on the planet were identified with the highest density of centenarians. These people lived long, healthy, highly active lives and reached age 100 at 10 times greater rates than others in the United States. These regions are described next and in Figure 16-12.[35]

- **Sardinia, Italy:** Some of the oldest men in the world lived in the mountainous Ogliastra region of Sardinia and typically worked on farms and drank one or two glasses of red wine each day.
- **Okinawa, Prefecture of Japan:** The world's oldest females were found in this area, where the dietary pattern was rich in soy-based foods and tai chi, a meditative form of physical activity, was practiced.
- **Ikaria, Greece:** People in this area consumed a Mediterranean diet rich in olive oil, red wine, and homegrown vegetables.
- **Nicoya Peninsula, Costa Rica:** People of this area regularly performed physical jobs into old age. Plant-based foods, such as beans and corn tortillas, formed the base of their dietary pattern.
- **Seventh-day Adventists of Loma Linda, California:** This religious organization followed a strict vegetarian dietary pattern and lived in closely faith-connected communities. In 2020, the Adventist Health system made a commitment to lead the blue zone well-being transformation movement that is the foundation of their 150-year Seventh-day Adventist heritage.

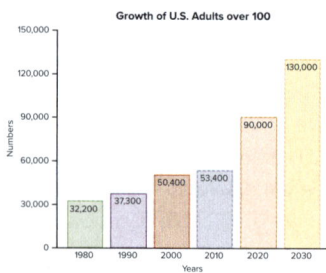
FIGURE 16-11 Estimated growth of U.S. adults living to 100 by the year 2030.
Source: U.S. Census Bureau and Texas A&M.

Connecting to Engaging Visuals

Attractive, Accurate Artwork

Illustrations, photographs, infographics, and tables in the text were created to help students master complex scientific concepts.

- Many illustrations were redesigned or replaced to inspire student inquiry and comprehension and to promote interest and retention of information. Several new infographics have been created to present materials in a more attractive, contemporary style.

- In many figures, color-coding and directional arrows make it easier to follow events and reinforce interrelationships. Process descriptions appear in the body of the figures. This pairing of written explanations and illustrations walks students step-by-step through the process and increases teaching effectiveness.

- Throughout the chapters, every photo and caption has been chosen with the intention to spark critical thinking.

The final result is a striking visual program that holds readers' attention and supports comprehension and critical thinking. The attractive layout and design of this release are clean, bright, and inviting. This creative presentation of the material is geared toward engaging today's visually oriented students.

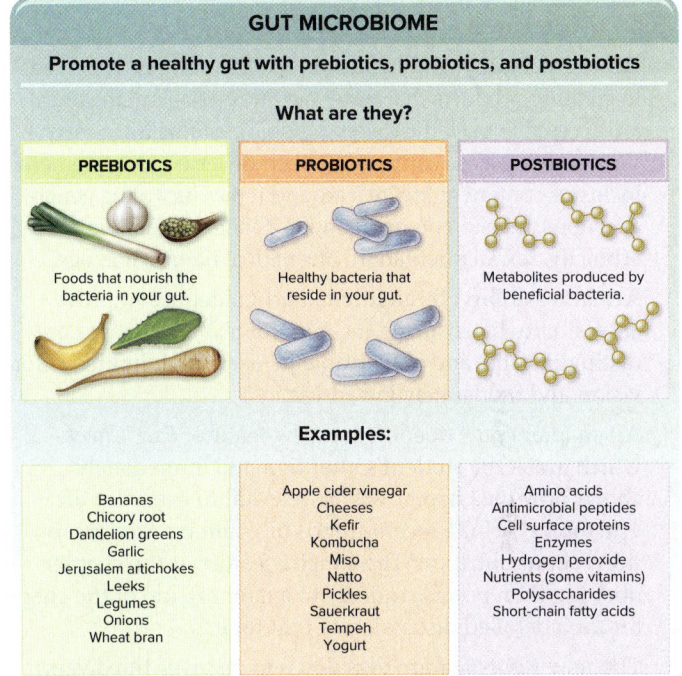

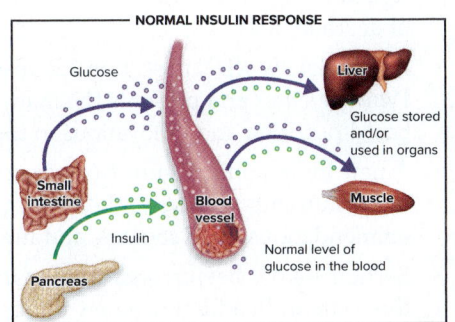

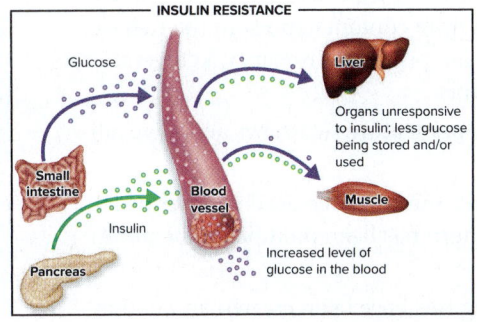

mayonnaise: Iconotec/Alamy Stock Photo; orange juice: Sergei Vinogradov/seralexvi/123RF; broccoli: lynx/iconotec.com/Glow Images; two jars of yogurt: Foodcollection; slice of bread: Ingram Publishing/Age Fotostock; tofu: chengyuzheng/iStock/Getty Images; MyPlate: ChooseMyPlate.gov, U.S. Department of Agriculture

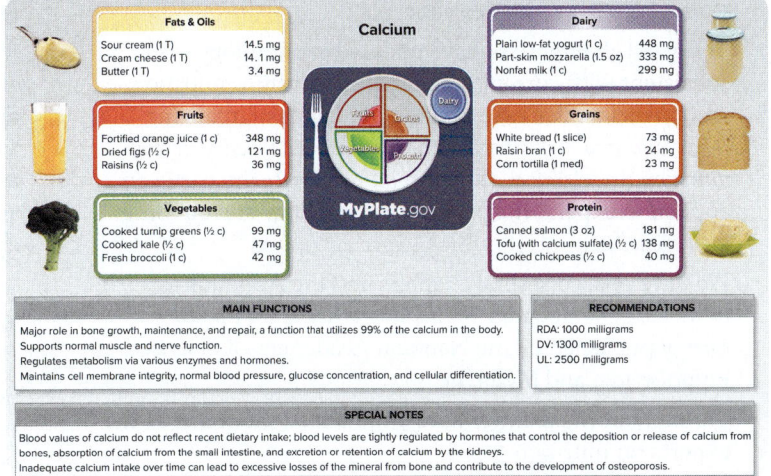

Connecting with the Latest Updates

Global Changes

- **Diversity, Equity, and Inclusion:** McGraw Hill is dedicated to creating products that foster a culture of belonging and are accessible to all the diverse, global customers we serve. Within this release content has been reviewed to implement inclusive content guidelines around topics including generalizations and stereotypes, gender, abilities/disabilities, race/ethnicity, sexual orientation, diversity of names, and age.

- **Art Accessibility:** Strengthened art guidelines improve accessibility by ensuring meaningful text and images are distinguishable and perceivable by users with limited color vision and moderately low vision.

- All chapters now open with a new feature, *Fact Check*, which grabs the student's attention and immediately shows how the chapter will be relevant to everyday life. The topics include recent trends or common misperceptions about nutrition. The concise feature at the chapter opening then points students to a later section of the chapter for a detailed discussion of that topic.

- The new *Roots* feature digs down to discover the diverse factors that influence our food choices and nutritional status.

- Several new *Ask the RDN* features have been included with contributions from content experts in the fields of health disparities, campus food insecurity, ketogenic diets, fertility, and cannabis.

- Two new *Farm to Fork* features (cashews and olive oil) have been added.

- Throughout the text, the language used to describe a healthy dietary pattern has been modified to be more **weight inclusive.**

- Many tables and figures have been created and others transformed into new, **eye-catching infographics** that help students to map complex concepts.

- In several chapters, we have **updated terminology** to be consistent with current usage in public health, nutrition, and medicine. For example, the outdated, stigmatizing term *failure to thrive* has been replaced with *pediatric malnutrition*. In addition, the term *nutrition security* has been applied to expand the previous terminology surrounding *food security*.

- We have revised several chapters and the Appendices to include the updated *2023 Dietary Reference Intakes for Energy* published by the National Academies of Sciences, Engineering, and Medicine.

- Throughout the text, we have emphasized **dietitians as the experts** on nutrition.

- Unlike most nutrition texts on the market, our ancillary materials (Connect test banks and question banks, concept checks, end-of-chapter questions and answer keys, PowerPoint lecture slides, instructor's manual, and teaching strategies) have been reviewed and **revised by the authors!**

Chapter-by-Chapter Revisions

Chapter 1: *Nutrition, Food Choices, and Health*

- The new *Fact Check* in Chapter 1 introduces this new chapter opener feature and highlights the science of nutrition.

- Figure 1-1 has been updated to include food access and genetics as key factors that influence our food choices.

- The section *What Influences Your Food Choices* has been updated with results from the latest Food and Health Survey.

- The *USDA Food Availability and Consumption Data* has been updated (Figs. 1-2 and 1-4) and a new figure (Fig. 1-3) has been included to present food consumption patterns in the U.S.

- The 10 leading causes of death have been updated and presented in Figure 1-5. COVID-19 ranked third for the causes of death in 2021.

- A new *Ask the RDN* in section 1.2 answers the question, *Why Dietetics?* and presents the many facets of evidence-based nutrition and innovations in the field of dietetics.

- A new infographic, Figure 1-6, was created to simplify the macronutrients relative to their energy content, intake recommendations, food sources, and functions.

- Section 1.4 has been reorganized to improve the flow of the content. In addition, a new infographic, Figure 1-8, has been included to simplify metric conversions for students.

- Obesity prevalence rates by U.S. states have been updated and the new data presented in Figure 1-12.

- A new *Newsworthy Nutrition* focusing on the role of diet and lifestyle in early-onset colorectal cancer in Section 1.6. This is a timely feature as the rates of early-onset cancer are growing in the U.S.

- This chapter's *Roots* feature introduces and celebrates global dietary patterns.

- A second and new *Ask the RDN* is featured in Section 1.6 and focuses on *Food is Medicine* initiatives following the *White House Conference on Hunger, Nutrition, and Health*.

- Section 1.7 content has been updated to focus more on healthy lifestyle behaviors instead of the emphasis on body weight.

- The standard alcoholic drink sizes (Fig. 1-13) have been updated to include hard seltzers and flavored malt beverages. The addition of *mocktails* as a growing area of popularity are also presented in this section.
- The *Case Study* on *Choosing a Healthy Breakfast* was expanded to include lifestyle behaviors and now includes recommendations related to alcohol consumption and sleep.

Chapter 2: *Designing a Healthy Eating Pattern*

- This chapter's *Fact Check* helps students understand where beans, peas, and lentils fit in the MyPlate food source categories.
- A new subsection in Section 2.1 describes how food processing affects the nutrient density of foods.
- A new *Magnificent Microbiome* feature explores how dietary patterns—particularly those high in ultraprocessed foods—may influence the gut microbiota.
- The new Figure 2-2 illustrates a simple and relevant way for students to estimate portion sizes.
- An updated Figure 2-4 outlines the key recommendations of the *Dietary Guidelines for Americans*.
- A new *Roots* feature presents the *Latin American Diet Pyramid*.
- An updated *Newsworthy Nutrition* presents a systematic review and meta-analysis of research relating various assessments of dietary quality to health outcomes.
- A narrative description of *Acceptable Macronutrient Distribution Ranges* has been added to the discussion of nutrient recommendations in Section 2.6. Also, a new Table 2-3 summarizes the various types of nutrient recommendations.
- Section 2.8 has been revised to include new content on food labeling policies and clear guidance for interpreting Nutrition Facts labels. Figure 2-16 has been streamlined and updated.
- The *Case Study* on college student eating habits has been revised to stimulate critical thinking about the content presented in Chapter 2.
- A new *Ask the RDN* feature describes the relationship between nutrition and academic performance.
- This chapter includes 13 new references.

Chapter 3: *The Human Body: A Nutrition Perspective*

- The new Figure 3-8 illustrates hormones with nutritional significance, orienting the student to many hormones that will be addressed again in subsequent chapters.
- *Farm to Fork: Onions and Garlic* has moved from Chapter 9 to Chapter 3, near Section 3.7 on the Immune System.
- The new *Roots* feature explains some of the benefits of eating fermented foods.
- A new *Magnificent Microbiome* feature focuses on the role of the microbiome in irritable bowel syndrome.
- *Newsworthy Nutrition* has been updated to present recent research on fecal transplant as a treatment for irritable bowel syndrome.
- This chapter includes 21 new references.

Chapter 4: *Carbohydrates*

- This chapter's *Fact Check* questions the safety and controversies related to artificial sweeteners including the recent carcinogenic claims regarding aspartame.
- A new *Farm to Fork* feature on corn on the cob was added to section 4.1. Corn provides fiber and is a good source of many vitamins and minerals.
- Table 4-1 is new and classifies dietary fibers while providing food sources for each fiber type.
- The new *Sustainable Solutions* features whole grains as a leading source of energy and dietary fiber in global eating patterns.
- Figure 4-11 was added to show common sources of added sugars in typical dietary patterns.
- Two new *Magnificent Microbiome* features, located in sections 4.1 discuss how microbes contribute to metabolism.
- This chapter's new *Roots* feature celebrates the *African Heritage Dietary Pattern* with an accompanying figure (Fig. 4-13) depicting the main dietary components.
- A new *Newsworthy Nutrition* reports the sugar-sweetened beverage consumption in 185 countries.
- A new infographic, Figure 4-18, is now included to provide a simplified graphic detailing the criteria used to diagnose diabetes.
- A new and timely *Ask the RDN* authored by Dr. Carmen Blakely highlights *Nutrition and Health Disparities*.
- Chapter 4 has been updated with seven new references.

Chapter 5: *Lipids*

- Section 5.1 has been renamed as *Lipids: What Are They?*
- Figure 5-4 has been revised to include diglycerides and monoglycerides and annotated to explain the key features of the various forms of lipids.
- Figure 5-11 has been revised and annotated to further describe the absorption of dietary lipids.
- A new Figure 5-13 illustrates the four main lipoproteins in the bloodstream.
- Figure 5-14 has been updated to present a more detailed and accurate view of an adipose cell.
- Table 5-5 has been updated with the latest dietary advice from the *American Heart Association*.
- The new *Roots* feature presents the Nordic diet as a culturally appropriate alternative to the well-known Mediterranean diet.

- The *Case Study* about a heart-healthy eating pattern has been revised to stimulate more critical thinking about the content presented in Chapter 5.
- Dr. Steven Hertzler explains the pros and cons of the keto diet for weight loss in a new *Ask the RDN* feature.
- The *Nutrition and Your Health* section now includes *Life's Essential 8*, emphasizing a more holistic approach to heart health.
- A new *Farm to Fork* investigates the origins and uses of olive oil.
- Chapter 5 has been updated with nine new references.

Chapter 6: *Proteins*

- The chapter opens with a new *Fact Check* feature about collagen supplements.
- Some content within this chapter has been reordered. The discussion of plant-based dietary patterns now appears immediately after the section about protein in foods.
- A new section has been added for *Special Health Concerns Related to Protein Intake*, which includes protein-calorie malnutrition, food allergies, kidney disease, and inborn errors of metabolism.
- All content about nutritional genomics and personalized nutrition has been moved to the revamped *Nutrition and Your Health* section at the end of the chapter.
- A new Figure 6-6 shows examples of denaturation of proteins.
- Figure 6-9 has been updated to include a distinct category for legumes.
- The new *Sustainable Solutions* feature in Section 6.3 examines the role of animal-sourced proteins in planetary health.
- A new *Roots* feature highlights the plant-based dietary patterns of Seventh-day Adventists.
- An updated *Newsworthy Nutrition* feature discusses the influence of plant-based dietary patterns on cardiovascular disease.
- Figure 6-12 has been revised to clearly show how protein status can influence fluid balance in the body.
- The new Figure 6-16 is an infographic that summarizes advice related to protein intake from the *Dietary Guidelines*.
- In the new section about *Special Health Concerns Related to Protein Intake*, the discussion of food allergies and Figure 6-18 now include references to sesame allergy, the ninth most common food allergen and newest addition to the labeling requirements for food allergens.
- Chapter 6 has been updated with 32 new references.

Chapter 7: *Energy Balance*

- Chapter 7 content has been updated with verbiage presenting a more weight-inclusive approach to energy balance and the evidence-based recommendations for those choosing to reduce their body weight.
- This chapter's *Fact Check* helps students understand how weight bias impacts health outcomes.
- Figure 7-1 has been updated with the latest available CDC obesity prevalence data.
- A new infographic, Figure 7-5, provides the percentages of energy use by various organs.
- Section 7.2 and Appendix F have been updated to include the Estimated Energy Requirements aligning with the new 2023 DRIs for energy.
- The American Medical Association's position statement on BMI has been added to Section 7.3.
- Figure 7-16 has been updated to display both upper and lower body fat distribution patterns for both sexes.
- The *Asian Diet Pyramid* is highlighted in this chapter's *Roots* feature with an accompanying figure (Fig. 7-19) presenting the main components.
- The addition of content related to the new World Health Organization's (WHO) position against the use of non-sugar sweeteners to control weight can be found in Section 7.5.
- A new infographic (Fig. 7-20) highlights the CDC guidelines for physical activity for healthy adults.
- Tools for successful weight management and a new *SMART goal worksheet* (Table 7-5) were created to assist students in self-monitoring, goal setting, and other proven behavioral approaches to promote behavior change.
- A section on non-diet strategies to improve health has been added to Section 7.7. These data are based on the recently published systematic literature review by the Academy of Nutrition and Dietetics.
- Table 7-7 presents the latest medications approved for obesity treatment. This now includes the popular GPL-1 agonists (such as Wegovy and Ozempic).
- A weight gain checklist, organized by food groups, has been added in a new Figure 7-28.
- Presentation of the five best overall diet plans has been updated in Table 7-9. The top-rated weight loss plans are further detailed in the text.
- Seven new references have been added to this chapter.

Chapter 8: *Vitamins and Phytochemicals*

- The Chapter 8 *Fact Check* provides details on the vitamin D content of various milk and dairy alternatives.
- A new section (8.2) has been added to this chapter to emphasize phytochemicals including sources, functions, and tips for incorporating more into your dietary pattern.
- This chapter contains several *Roots* features: supertasters describes a genetic variant that can influence acceptability of phytochemical-rich plant sources (section 8.2); religious customs that affect vitamin D status (section 8.4); and nixtamalization, a native method of corn preparation (section 8.10).

- A new infographic (Fig. 8-2) compares water-soluble and fat-soluble vitamins relative to absorption, storage, excretion, toxicity, and deficiencies.
- A new *Farm to Fork* feature on pomegranates is included in section 8.6. These unique fruits are rich in phytochemicals and vitamins.
- A new *Newsworthy Nutrition* details the seminal SELECT trial assessing the impact of selenium and vitamin E supplementation on prostate cancer prevention.
- There are two *Ask the RDN* features in this chapter: one describing the evidence pertaining to detox diets (section 8.8); and one that details the role of nutrition in supporting our immune system (section 8.19).
- Section 8.9 presents a *Case Study* on potential nutrient deficiencies from following a vegan and gluten-free dietary pattern, and section 8.19 presents a case study on choosing dietary and physical activity patterns associated with cancer prevention.
- Choline was relocated to its own section (8.17) given its unique vitamin-like properties.
- A new *Nutrition and Your Health* section has been added to emphasize the state of the science pertaining to dietary supplements.
- A new figure (Fig. 8-35) was created to simplify the three phases of carcinogenesis, and new Figure 8-36 lists the early symptoms of cancer.
- Chapter 8 has been updated with 21 new references.

Chapter 9: *Water and Minerals*
- The new *Fact Check* explains how red meat can fit into a healthy dietary pattern.
- Section 9.1 on Water has been reorganized to be consistent with the presentation of other nutrients.
- The new Figure 9-11 summarizes MyPlate food sources of minerals.
- Section 9.3 now includes a brief explanation of osmosis, solutes, solvents, and concentration to help clarify these important concepts for students with minimal background in science.
- In a new *Ask the RDN* feature, students learn about steps they can take during young adulthood to keep blood pressure in check throughout life.
- In Section 9.6, the narrative explanations of the functions of calcium have been expanded and revised.
- A revised Figure 9-16 illustrates the roles of calcitonin, parathyroid hormone, and vitamin D in the regulation of blood calcium levels.
- The new *Sustainable Solutions* feature evaluates the sustainability of dairy foods.
- A new Figure 9-18 illustrates factors that can increase or decrease calcium absorption from foods.

- The content on osteoporosis has been moved from Section 9.6 and expanded to create a new *Nutrition and Your Health* feature.
- The content on dairy alternatives has been condensed into a new *Ask the RDN* feature.
- A new *Farm to Fork* feature reviews the surprising origin of cashews and highlights the use of cashews as a dairy alternative.
- The new *Roots* feature discusses selenium's role in immunity and the regional differences in the selenium content of food sources.
- Expanded content in Section 9.12 includes a discussion of goitrogens. An updated *Newsworthy Nutrition* feature further explores the impact of goitrogens on iodine status.
- In the *Nutrition and Your Health* section about hypertension, *Newsworthy Nutrition* has been updated with an article that discusses the results of a cross-sectional study about the DASH diet and blood pressure among college students.
- Figure 9-27 has been updated to illustrate the stages of hypertension more clearly.
- A new *Magnificent Microbiome* feature explores the connections among dietary sodium, the gut microbiota, and blood pressure regulation.
- Chapter 9 includes 66 new references.

Chapter 10: *Nutrition: Fitness and Sports*
- The new *Fact Check* answers the question, "If I eat more protein, will I gain more muscle?"
- A new *Roots* features the health of hunter-gatherers, their dietary patterns, and subsequent energy expenditures.
- The FITT equation has been updated to include volume and progression (now FITT-VP).
- Figure 10-2 is a new infographic showing tips to manually measure your own heart rate.
- A new infographic, Figure 10-11, has been added to assist students with understanding the nutritional requirements of athletes.
- Figure 10-13 is a new heat-related illness infographic to help students identify common symptoms and recommended actions to take.
- A new and engaging CDC infographic detailing heat related illnesses appears in Figure 10-12.
- The lists of commonly used sports supplements and illegal substances have been expanded and updated in Table 10-10.

Chapter 11: *Eating Disorders*
- A new *Fact Check* feature explores the demographics of eating disorders.
- In Section 11.1, a new *Roots* feature presents recent research on the genetic underpinnings of eating disorders.

- An updated *Newsworthy Nutrition* feature examines the role of social media in the development of eating disorders.
- In Section 11.2, the discussion of the physical effects of anorexia nervosa has been shortened to improve readability.
- In Section 11.5, two new subsections provide information on rumination disorder and avoidant-restrictive food intake disorder. Also, the explanation of subthreshold eating disorders has been expanded.
- Section 11.6 has been updated to include a recently published consensus statement from a panel of experts on the definition and diagnostic criteria for orthorexia nervosa.
- Chapter 11 includes 37 new references.

Chapter 12: *Protecting Our Food Supply*

- The new *Fact Check* feature highlights the pros and cons of purchasing organic products and points to additional details presented later in the chapter.
- This chapter now begins with the section on food production choices to discuss where our food comes from and how it is produced. Topics include organic food production, biotechnology, and sustainable agriculture.
- A new Figure 12-4 details components of the food production chain and areas presenting risk for contamination.
- Figure 12-5 has been updated with the most recent data on foodborne illness outbreaks across the country.
- A new CDC infographic has been added to show the steps taken in a foodborne outbreak investigation once suspected or detected.
- A new *Newsworthy Nutrition* focuses on foodborne illness outbreaks linked to unpasteurized milk consumption.
- A new CDC Figure 12-8 displays the causes and prevalence of foodborne illness.
- Section 12.4 has been revamped and simplified to present the key bacterial, viral, and parasitic causes of foodborne illnesses (Fig. 12.9, Fig. 12.11, and Fig. 12.13).
- Figure 12-14 is a new infographic showing the amount of caffeine in common beverages.
- The new *Roots* feature discusses global spices and the potential risk for contamination if mishandled.
- Section 12.6 has been reorganized around the CDC's four steps to food safety to simply these concepts and guidelines for keeping your food safe.
- The WHO's golden rules for safe food preparation have been added to emphasize the main recommendations.

Chapter 13: *Global Nutrition*

- The new *Fact Check* explains the difference between malnutrition and hunger. These terms are often used interchangeably with students.
- Figure 13-1 is new and visually presents the prevalence and regions of global hunger.
- Terminology throughout has been updated to reflect the adoption of the term *nutrition security*, with inclusion of diet quality and health equity to food security.
- Figure 13-5 and 13-6 are both new and highlight the main components of nutrition security and its impact on health in the U.S.
- Information on the Farm Bill and resource allocations are now included in Figure 13-5.
- Section 13.2 has been updated and includes a new infographic, Figure 13-5, that displays the Farm Bill resource categories.
- Also in this section, the federal nutrition assistance content has been expanded to include additional details about SNAP, School Breakfast and Lunch Programs, Congregate Meals, and WIC.
- A new *Ask the RDN* on college food and nutrition insecurity is included in Section 13.2.
- This chapter's new *Roots* feature details the practice known as entomophagy, or insect farming, and its contributions towards food and nutrition security.
- Figure 13-9 has been updated and presents the data pertaining to global access to safe water aligning with the Sustainable Development Goal for clean water and sanitation.
- A new *Sustainable Solution* on offal consumption—basically eating everything from nose to tail of an animal. Although not practiced widely in the U.S., this is an efficient use of agricultural resources and cuts down on food waste.
- Chapter 13 has been updated with six new references.

Chapter 14: *Nutrition During Pregnancy and Breastfeeding*

- A new *Fact Check* feature explains the lack of evidence to support maternal dietary restrictions for the prevention of food allergies.
- Section 14.1 has been updated with the latest evidence-based guidelines for the assessment and management of polycystic ovary syndrome.
- Also in Section 14.1, a new *Ask the RDN* feature from Lauren Manaker, MS, RDN, LD, CLEC, author of *Fueling Male Fertility,* describes nutritional strategies to improve male fertility.
- A new Figure 14-3 illustrates important food safety practices for individuals during pregnancy.
- An updated *Newsworthy Nutrition* feature examines the effects of prenatal folic acid supplementation on the cognitive development of the offspring throughout childhood.
- The discussion of energy needs during pregnancy and lactation and Figure 14-9 have been revised to reflect the recently updated DRIs for energy.
- The new *Roots* feature discusses pica, the practice of eating nonfood items, during pregnancy.

- In Section 14.7, use of high-dose vitamin D supplements during breastfeeding is described as an alternative to vitamin D supplementation for infants who are breastfed.
- Chapter 14 includes 38 new references.

Chapter 15: *Nutrition from Infancy Through Adolescence*

- In Section 15.1, we have included additional information about assessing infant and child growth. The term *failure to thrive* has been replaced with *pediatric malnutrition*.
- Information about the calculation of energy needs from infancy through adolescence reflects the latest DRIs for energy.
- Table 15-3 has been updated to include the latest research on the nutrient content of human milk.
- In Section 15.3, we have altered the language in several places to ensure that formula feeding is recognized as a safe and nutritious way to feed an infant when human breast milk is not available.
- The new *Roots* feature reviews the history of wet nursing.
- We present the latest data about the safety of infant foods, including ways to protect infants from exposure to heavy metals and food allergens.
- In Section 15.5, the discussion of childhood obesity has been revised to reflect current evidence from several systematic reviews. Also, a new Figure 15-6 illustrates the consequences of childhood obesity. We have included new content about weight bias.
- Section 15.7 has been updated with new statistics about food allergies and intolerances and new laws that add sesame to the list of common food allergens that must be declared on food labels.
- A new *Ask the RDN* feature discusses the nutrition implications of alpha-gal syndrome, an allergy to red meat that can arise as a result of a tick bite.
- Chapter 15 includes 47 new references.

Chapter 16: *Nutrition During Adulthood*

- This chapter begins with a new *Fact Check* discussing the influence of genetics and environmental exposures on longevity.
- All demographic and prevalence data on aging have been updated in Section 16.1. In addition, the entire chapter has been revised to emphasize healthy aging and active living for this life stage.
- Table 16-1 has been replaced by a new Figure 16-4 and presents the 12 main components of the *Hallmarks of Aging* with accompanying text detailing each component.
- The new *Magnificent Microbiome* focuses on the biological changes that occur with normal aging.
- Essential oils and aromatherapy are highlighted in the new *Sustainable Solutions*.
- A new *Newsworthy Nutrition* presents research on the impact of nutrition on aging.
- A new Figure 16-5 highlights malnutrition risk factors for older adults.
- An *Ask the RDN* authored by Janice Newell Bissex details the pros and cons of taking CBD in this informative new feature.
- Table 16-5 has been replaced by a new Figure 16-10 infographic emphasizing healthy eating tips for older adults.
- We have added a second *Nutrition and Your Health* feature in this chapter to promote healthy lifestyles linked to healthy longevity. This section introduces the popular blue zones phenomenon.
- Global bread intake from the blue zones is highlighted in the new *Roots* feature.
- Chapter 16 has been updated with three new references.

Acknowledgments

It is because of the tireless efforts of a cohesive team of talented professionals that we can bring you the 2024 Release of *Wardlaw's Contemporary Nutrition*. We consider ourselves massively blessed to work with the top-notch staff at McGraw Hill. We thank Lauren Vondra, Portfolio Manager, for her effective leadership of our team. We value the efforts of our Executive Marketing Manager, Tami Hodge, who consistently connects instructors with our work and brings us constructive feedback from the field. We are immensely grateful to our Product Developer, Darlene Schueller, who strategically leads the day-to-day efforts of the entire editorial team. We especially appreciate her longevity over many releases of the *Contemporary Nutrition* products and value her keen eye for detail, strong work ethic, and organizational expertise. We are grateful to our Senior Core Content Project Manager, Diane Nowaczyk, and her staff for their patience and careful coordination of the numerous production efforts needed to create this very appealing and accurate release. We thank Brent dela Cruz, our Lead Assessment Content Project Manager, for his efforts and assistance. We appreciate the meticulous work of our proofreader, Susan Gall, and our Content Licensing Manager, Melissa Homer. We thank our Designer, David Hash, who ensured that every aspect of our work is visually appealing—not just on the printed page but also in a variety of digital formats. We are privileged to work alongside our colleagues Alaa Ilayan, Julia Richardson, and Rachel Williams, whose careful review and creative contributions enhance the quality of the book and digital tools. Finally, we are indebted to our colleagues, friends, and families for their constant encouragement, honest feedback, and shared passion for the science of nutrition.

Ask the RDN Contributors

We are grateful to our reputable and talented RDN colleagues who authored several new *Ask the RDN* features in this release. It was exciting to share the spotlight and include their evidence-based expertise and applicable, down-to-earth recommendations. Many thanks to the following:

Janice Bissex, MS, RDN, FAND
Carmen Blakely, EdD, MEd, RDN, LD
Leslie Bonci, MPH, RDN, CSSD, LDN
Zachari Breeding, MS, RDN, LDN, FAND

Laura Davidson, MS, RDN, LDN
Steven Hertzler, PhD, RD, LD
Alexis Joseph, MS, RDN, LD
Sally Kuzemchak, MS, RDN

Lauren Manaker, MS, RDN, LDN, CLEC, CPT
Chris Vogliano, PhD, RDN

Student-Informed Reviews

We are very pleased to have been able to incorporate real student data points and input, derived from thousands of our SmartBook users, to help guide our revision. *SmartBook heat maps* provided a quick visual snapshot of usage of portions of the text and the relative difficulty students experienced in mastering the content. With these data, we were able to hone not only our text content but also the SmartBook probes.

> With each new release of *Wardlaw's Contemporary Nutrition*, we remember its founding author, Gordon M. Wardlaw. Dr. Wardlaw had a passion for the science of nutrition and the research that supports it and demonstrated an exceptional ability to translate scientific principles into practical knowledge. This skill is what made his book truly "contemporary." It has been a privilege for us to join Dr. Wardlaw as coauthors of this textbook. Like so many other students, colleagues, and friends, we remember Dr. Wardlaw as a source of vast knowledge, good humor, and inspiration. The best way we know to honor our dear friend and mentor is to carry on his legacy of outstanding textbooks in introductory nutrition. *Wardlaw's Contemporary Nutrition* will continue to evolve and reflect current trends and breakthroughs in nutrition science, but Dr. Wardlaw's fingerprints will remain on every page.

Contents

Part One: Nutrition: A Key to Health

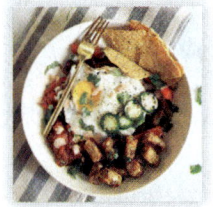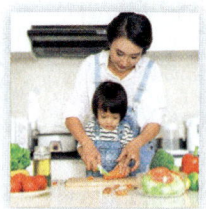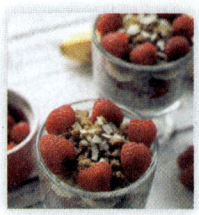

Chapter 1 Nutrition, Food Choices, and Health 2

    FACT CHECK: Is nutrition a science? 3

1.1 Why Do You Choose the Food You Eat? 4

    Sustainable Solutions: Food & Health Survey 7

1.2 How Is Nutrition Connected to Good Health? 8

    Ask the RDN: Why Dietetics? 10

1.3 What Are the Classes and Sources of Nutrients? 10

    Farm to Fork: Tomatoes 14

1.4 What Math Concepts Will Aid Your Study of Nutrition? 14

1.5 How Do We Know What We Know About Nutrition? 18

    Newsworthy Nutrition: Feature introduction 20

1.6 What Is the Current State of North American Eating Patterns and Health? 21

    Newsworthy Nutrition: Role of diet and lifestyle in early-onset colorectal cancer 22

    Roots: Global Dietary Patterns 22

1.7 What Can You Expect from Good Nutrition and a Healthy Lifestyle? 24

    Ask the RDN: Is Food Medicine? 25

1.8 Nutrition and Your Health: Nutrition Implications of Alcohol Consumption 26

    Magnificent Microbiome: Definitions 29

    Case Study: Choosing a Healthy Lifestyle 30

Chapter 2 Designing a Healthy Eating Pattern 34

    FACT CHECK: In MyPlate, do beans, peas, and lentils count as a part of the Protein Foods Group or the Vegetable Group? 35

2.1 A Food Philosophy That Works 36

    Magnificent Microbiome: Dietary Patterns Influence the Gut Microbiota 38

    Farm to Fork: Citrus Fruit 39

2.2 Dietary and Physical Activity Guidelines 41

    Roots: Latin American Diet Pyramid 44

    Newsworthy Nutrition: Impact of diet quality on health outcomes 47

2.3 MyPlate—A Menu-Planning Tool 49

2.4 Nutritional Health 55

2.5 Measuring Nutritional Status 57

2.6 Nutrient Recommendations 59

    Ask the RDN: Transgender Issues 62

2.7 Evaluating Nutrition Information 63

2.8 Food Labels and Dietary Pattern Planning 65

2.9 Nutrition and Your Health: Eating Well as a Student 71

    Case Study: College Student Eating Habits 72

    Sustainable Solutions: Plant-Focused Dietary Pattern 73

    Ask the RDN: Nutrition and Academic Performance 74

Chapter 3 The Human Body: A Nutrition Perspective 78

    FACT CHECK: Does eating spicy foods cause ulcers? 79

3.1 Cells, Tissues, and Organs 80

3.2 Metabolism Is the Chemistry of Life 85

3.3 Cardiovascular System and Lymphatic System 85

3.4 Urinary System 88

    Farm to Fork: Cranberries 89

3.5 Nervous System 89

3.6 Endocrine System 91

3.7 Immune System 93

    Farm to Fork: Onions and Garlic 94

3.8 Digestive System 94

3.9 The Human Microbiota 106

    Roots: Fermented Foods 107

    Newsworthy Nutrition: Fecal microbiota transplant is an effective treatment for irritable bowel syndrome 109

    Magnificent Microbiome: Hygiene Hypothesis 110

3.10 Nutrient Storage Capabilities 111

3.11 Nutrition and Your Health: Common Problems with Digestion 112

    Case Study: Gastroesophageal Reflux Disease 114

    Medicine Cabinet: Controlling Stomach Acid 115

    Magnificent Microbiome: Irritable Bowel Syndrome 117

    Ask the RDN: Gluten-Free Diet 120

Breakfast bowl: Alexis Joseph/McGraw Hill; happy family in the kitchen: Makistock/Shutterstock; chia pudding: Alexis Joseph/McGraw Hill

Part Two: Energy Nutrients and Energy Balance

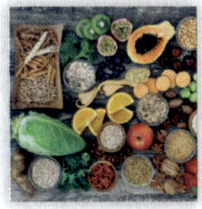 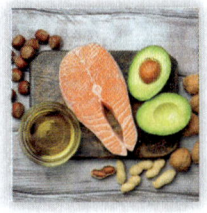 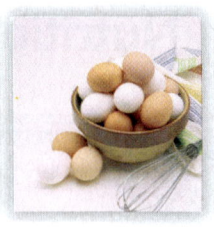 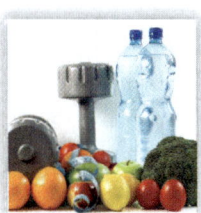

Chapter 4 Carbohydrates 124

FACT CHECK: Are artificial sweeteners safe? **125**
4.1 Carbohydrates—Our Most Important Energy Source 126
    Magnificent Microbiome: Getting Energy from Microbes **126**
4.2 Forms of Carbohydrates 127
    Farm to Fork: Corn on the Cob **127**
4.3 Carbohydrates in Foods 132
    Sustainable Solutions: Whole Grains **137**
    Farm to Fork: Potatoes **137**
4.4 Making Carbohydrates Available for Body Use 142
    Case Study: Problems with Milk Intake **144**
    Magnificent Microbiome: Microbiota-Accessible Carbohydrates **146**
4.5 Putting Carbohydrates to Work in the Body 146
    Roots: African Heritage Dietary Pattern **147**
4.6 Carbohydrate Needs 150
    Newsworthy Nutrition: Sugar-sweetened beverage consumption in 185 countries **154**
4.7 **Nutrition and Your Health: Diabetes—When Blood Glucose Regulation Fails 156**
    Ask the RDN: Nutrition and Health Disparities **160**

Chapter 5 Lipids 164

FACT CHECK: Are eggs bad for your heart? **165**
5.1 Lipids: What Are They? 166
5.2 Fats and Oils in Foods 171
    Farm to Fork: Avocados **173**
    Ask the RDN: Coconut Oil **179**
5.3 Making Lipids Available for Body Use 180
5.4 Carrying Lipids in the Bloodstream 183
    Newsworthy Nutrition: Effects of almond versus cracker snacks among college students **186**
5.5 Roles of Lipids in the Body 187
5.6 Recommendations for Fat Intake 189
    Sustainable Solutions: Aquaculture **191**
    Roots: Nordic Diet **192**
    Case Study: Planning a Heart-Healthy Dietary Pattern **194**
    Ask the RDN: Ketogenic Diet **194**
5.7 **Nutrition and Your Health: Lipids and Cardiovascular Disease 196**
    Farm to Fork: Olive Oil **200**
    Medicine Cabinet: Lipid-Lowering Medications **201**
    Magnificent Microbiome: Heart Health **202**

Chapter 6 Proteins 206

FACT CHECK: Should I take collagen for healthy skin? **207**
6.1 Amino Acids—Building Blocks of Proteins 208
6.2 Protein Synthesis and Organization 209
6.3 Protein in Foods 212
    Farm to Fork: Legumes **217**
    Sustainable Solutions: The Role of Livestock in Planetary Health **218**
6.4 Plant-Based Dietary Patterns 219
    Roots: Vegetarian Dietary Patterns Among Seventh-Day Adventists **221**
    Newsworthy Nutrition: Plant-based dietary patterns linked to lower risk for cardiovascular disease **222**
    Ask the RDN: Plant-Based Eating **225**
6.5 Protein Digestion and Absorption 226
    Magnificent Microbiome: Protein Feeds Microbes **226**
6.6 Putting Proteins to Work in the Body 227
6.7 Protein Needs 232
    Case Study: Planning a Vegetarian Dietary Pattern **236**
6.8 Special Health Concerns Related to Protein Intake 236
6.9 **Nutrition and Your Health: Nutritional Genomics 241**

Chapter 7 Energy Balance 248

FACT CHECK: Does weight bias impact health outcomes? **249**
7.1 Energy Balance and Health Promotion 250
7.2 Determination of Energy Use by the Body 256

Dietary fiber health food: Marilyn Barbone/Shutterstock; healthy fat sources: Julija Dmitrijeva/123RF; eggs: Pixtal/AGE Fotostock; Supermarket, fruit and vegetable: PM78/iStock/Getty Images

7.3	Assessing Body Weight 257	7.7	Behavioral Strategies for Weight Management 271
7.4	Nature Versus Nurture 262	7.8	Management of Overweight and Obesity 276
	Magnificent Microbiome: Appetite **264**	7.9	Professional Help for Weight Loss 279
7.5	Energy Balance Throughout the Life Course 265		**Ask the RDN:** Intermittent Fasting **281**
	Farm to Fork: Stone Fruits **265**	7.10	Treatment of Underweight 284
	Newsworthy Nutrition: Plant-based dietary patterns are associated with improved weight management **266**	**7.11**	**Nutrition and Your Health: Popular Fad Diets—Cause for Concern 286**
	Roots: Asian Diet Pyramid **267**		**Case Study: Choosing a Weight-Management Program 288**
7.6	Physical Activity Promotes Weight Management 269		

Micronutrients/phytochemicals: Alexis Joseph/McGraw Hill; lemon water: Sarah Rusnak; fruit salad: Lew Robertson/Brand Xpictures/Getty Images; cheese: Mitch Hrdlicka/Getty Images; oatmeal with fruit: Alexis Joseph/McGraw Hill; beef and vegetables: Alexis Joseph/McGraw Hill

Part Three: Vitamins, Minerals, and Water

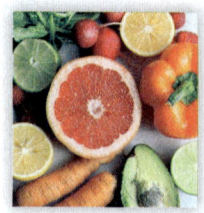
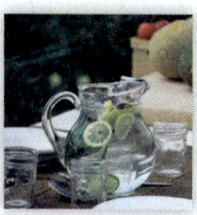

Chapter 8 Vitamins and Phytochemicals 292

   FACT CHECK: What type of milk is the best source of vitamin D? 293

8.1 Vitamins: Vital Dietary Components 294

   Magnificent Microbiome: Vitamin Production 295

8.2 Phytochemicals 298

   Roots: Supertasters 301

   Farm to Fork: Crucifers 301

8.3 Vitamin A (Retinoids) and Carotenoids 302

   Sustainable Solutions: Biofortification 304

   Medicine Cabinet: Vitamin A Derivatives 306

8.4 Vitamin D (Calciferol or Calcitriol) 307

   Farm to Fork: Mushrooms 311

   Roots: Religious Customs Affect Vitamin D Status 312

8.5 Vitamin E (Tocopherols) 312

   Newsworthy Nutrition: Selenium and vitamin E supplements offer no benefit for cancer prevention 315

8.6 Vitamin K (Quinone) 316

   Farm to Fork: Pomegranates 317

   Medicine Cabinet: Anticoagulants 318

8.7 The Water-Soluble Vitamins 319

8.8 Thiamin (Vitamin B-1) 322

   Ask the RDN: Detox Diets 323

8.9 Riboflavin (Vitamin B-2) 324

   Case Study: Deficiency from a Vegan and Gluten-Free Diet? 325

8.10 Niacin (Vitamin B-3) 327

   Roots: Nixtamalization 328

8.11 Pantothenic Acid (Vitamin B-5) 329

8.12 Vitamin B-6 (Pyridoxine) 330

8.13 Biotin (Vitamin B-7) 332

8.14 Folate (Vitamin B-9) 334

8.15 Vitamin B-12 (Cobalamin or Cyanocobalamin) 337

   Medicine Cabinet: Vitamin B-12 339

8.16 Vitamin C (Ascorbic Acid) 340

8.17 Choline: The Newest Vitamin? 343

8.18 Nutrition and Your Health: Dietary Supplements 346

   Newsworthy Nutrition: Increased emergency department visits for dietary supplement users 348

   Case Study: Getting the Most Nutrition from Your Food 350

8.19 Nutrition and Your Health: Nutrition and Cancer 351

   Ask the RDN: Supplements and Immunity 353

   Case Study: Choosing Cancer Prevention Dietary and Physical Activity Patterns 355

Chapter 9 Water and Minerals 362

   FACT CHECK: Can red meat be part of a healthy eating pattern? 363

9.1 Water 364

   Sustainable Solutions: Bottled Water or Tap Water? 372

9.2 Minerals: Essential Elements for Health 373

9.3 Sodium 377

   Ask the RDN: Pass the Salt? 382

9.4 Potassium 383

9.5 Chloride 385

   Farm to Fork: Bananas 385

9.6 Calcium 386

   Ask the RDN: Bone Health Without Dairy 389

   Sustainable Solutions: Sustainability of Dairy 390

   Newsworthy Nutrition: Calcium supplements and cardiovascular disease risk 392

9.7 Phosphorus 394

9.8 Magnesium 396

   Farm to Fork: Cashews 398

9.9 Iron 399

   Magnificent Microbiome: Iron Bioavailability 400

   Case Study: Anemia 403

9.10 Zinc 404

9.11 Selenium 406

   Roots: Selenium 408

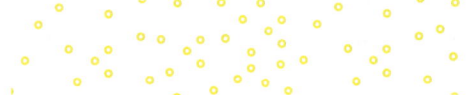

Contents **xxvii**

9.12 Iodine 408

Newsworthy Nutrition: Goitrogens and iodine deficiency 411

9.13 Copper 412

9.14 Fluoride 414

9.15 Chromium 415

9.16 Other Trace Minerals 416

9.17 **Nutrition and Your Health: Minerals and Hypertension** 418

Newsworthy Nutrition: DASH diet is associated with lower blood pressure among college students 419

Magnificent Microbiome: Sodium, Microbiota, and Blood Pressure 420

Medicine Cabinet: Blood Pressure Control 420

9.18 **Nutrition and Your Health: Osteoporosis** 422

Magnificent Microbiome: Gut–Bone Axis 427

Medicine Cabinet: Types of Osteoporosis Medications 428

Case Study: Worried About Bone Health 429

Part Four: Nutrition: Beyond the Nutrients

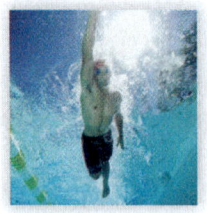
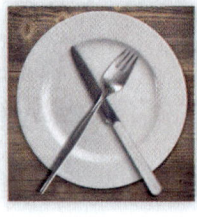
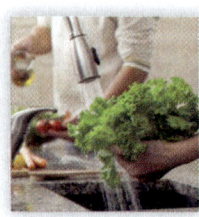
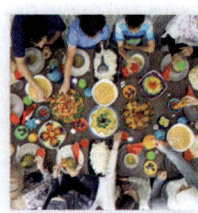

Chapter 10 Nutrition: Fitness and Sports 436

    FACT CHECK: If I eat more protein, will I gain more muscle? 437

10.1 Introduction to Physical Fitness 438

    Roots: Health of Hunter-Gatherers 439

10.2 Achieving and Maintaining Physical Fitness 440

    Magnificent Microbiome: Exercise 444

10.3 Energy Sources for Active Muscles 444

    Newsworthy Nutrition: Branched-chain amino acids impact health and lifespan in mice 448

10.4 Nutrient Recommendations for Active Adults and Athletes 449

    Farm to Fork: Carrots and Beets 453

    Ask the RDN: The No-Meat Athlete 455

10.5 Recommendations for Endurance, Strength, and Power Athletes 461

    Case Study: Planning a Training Diet 467

10.6 Nutrition and Your Health: Ergogenic Aids and Athletic Performance 468

Chapter 11 Eating Disorders 474

    FACT CHECK: Do eating disorders only affect privileged white women? 475

11.1 From Healthy to Disordered Eating Habits 476

    Roots: Genetics and Eating Disorders 478

    Newsworthy Nutrition: Social media use and body dissatisfaction among college-age females 480

11.2 Anorexia Nervosa 481

    Ask the RDN: Not Having a Period is NOT Normal 484

    Magnificent Microbiome: Refeeding the Microbiota 486

11.3 Bulimia Nervosa 487

11.4 Binge Eating Disorder 492

    Case Study: Eating Disorders—Steps to Recovery 495

11.5 Other Eating Disorders 496

11.6 Additional Disordered Eating Patterns 498

11.7 Prevention of Eating Disorders 500

    Farm to Fork: Apples 501

11.8 Nutrition and Your Health: Eating Disorder Reflections 502

Chapter 12 Protecting Our Food Supply 508

    FACT CHECK: Are organic products worth the extra cost? 509

12.1 Food Production Choices 510

    Ask the RDN: Food Waste 515

    Sustainable Solutions: Hydroponics 517

12.2 Environmental Contaminants in Food 518

    Farm to Fork: Melons 523

12.3 Food Preservation and Safety 524

    Magnificent Microbiome: Fermented Foods 528

    Newsworthy Nutrition: Foodborne illness outbreaks linked to unpasteurized milk 529

12.4 Foodborne Illness Caused by Microorganisms 530

    Magnificent Microbiome: Norovirus 533

12.5 Food Additives 534

    Roots: Variety is the SPICE of life 541

12.6 Nutrition and Your Health: Preventing Foodborne Illness 542

    Case Study: Preventing Foodborne Illness at Gatherings 545

Chapter 13 Global Nutrition 550

    FACT CHECK: Is there a difference between *malnutrition* and *hunger?* 551

13.1 World Hunger 552

13.2 Malnutrition in the United States 556

    Ask the RDN: College Food and Nutrition Security 562

13.3 Global Malnutrition 563

    Roots: Insect Farming 564

    Sustainable Solutions: Offal 567

13.4 Global Malnutrition Strategies 568

    Newsworthy Nutrition: Maternal depression and child severe acute malnutrition 570

    Farm to Fork: Pineapples 571

    Magnificent Microbiome: Soil Microbiome 573

13.5 Nutrition and Your Health: Malnutrition at Critical Life Stages 574

    Case Study: Undernutrition During Childhood 575

Swimmer: Erik Isakson/Blend Images LLC; plate and sliverware: grafvision/123RF; washing vegetables for a salad: KatarzynaBialasiewicz/iStock/Getty Images; eating dinner: Zurijeta/Shutterstock

Part Five: Nutrition: A Focus on Life Stages

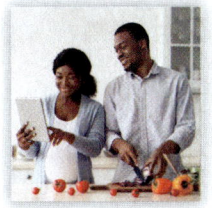
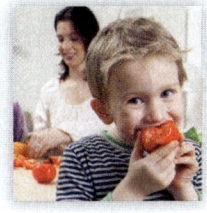
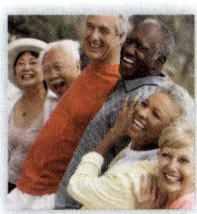

Chapter 14 Nutrition During Pregnancy and Breastfeeding 580

- **FACT CHECK:** Is it necessary to avoid potential food allergens during pregnancy and breastfeeding to reduce the risk for food allergies in the infant? 581
- 14.1 Nutrition and Fertility 582
  - **Ask the RDN:** Male Fertility 585
- 14.2 Prenatal Growth and Development 586
- 14.3 Success in Pregnancy 588
- 14.4 Increased Nutrient Needs to Support Pregnancy 593
  - **Newsworthy Nutrition:** Prenatal folic acid supplementation improves cognitive outcomes in offspring 599
- 14.5 Eating Patterns for Females During Pregnancy 601
  - **Farm to Fork:** Greens 601
  - **Roots:** Cultural Pica 604
  - **Case Study:** Eating for Two 605
- 14.6 Nutrition-Related Concerns During Pregnancy 605
- 14.7 Breastfeeding 609
  - **Magnificent Microbiome:** Colonizing the Infant's GI Tract 611
  - **Sustainable Solutions:** Feeding the Next Generation 615
- **14.8 Nutrition and Your Health: Reducing the Risk of Birth Defects 618**

Chapter 15 Nutrition from Infancy Through Adolescence 628

- **FACT CHECK:** Do toddlers need special toddler drinks to meet nutrient needs? 629
- 15.1 Assessing Growth 630
- 15.2 Infant Nutritional Needs 634
- 15.3 Guidelines for Infant Feeding 638
  - **Roots:** Milk from Another Mother 640
  - **Case Study:** Undernutrition During Infancy 650
- 15.4 Toddlers and Preschool Children: Nutrition Concerns 650
  - **Ask the RDN:** Picky Eating 654
  - **Farm to Fork:** Blueberries 656
  - **Magnificent Microbiome:** Autism Spectrum Disorder 659
- 15.5 School-Age Children: Nutrition Concerns 660
  - **Sustainable Solutions:** Farm to School 666
- 15.6 Teenage Years: Nutrition Concerns 666
  - **Newsworthy Nutrition:** Glycemic load of food choices may influence acne 669
- **15.7 Nutrition and Your Health: Food Allergies and Intolerances 671**
  - **Newsworthy Nutrition:** Early introduction of peanut protein reduces peanut allergy 674
  - **Ask the RDN:** Alpha-Gal Syndrome 675

Chapter 16 Nutrition During Adulthood 682

- **FACT CHECK:** Is longevity mainly determined by your genes? 683
- 16.1 Healthy Aging 684
  - **Magnificent Microbiome:** Aging and Microbiome Diversity 688
  - **Newsworthy Nutrition:** Impact of nutrition on aging 689
  - **Sustainable Solutions:** Essential Oils 690
- 16.2 Nutrient Needs During Adulthood 691
  - **Farm to Fork:** Grapes and Raisins 694
- 16.3 Nutritional Status of Adults 696
  - **Ask the RDN:** CBD 704
- 16.4 Healthful Dietary Patterns for the Adult Years 705
  - **Case Study:** Dietary Assistance for an Older Adult 707
- **16.5 Nutrition and Your Health: Lifestyles Linked with Longevity 709**
  - **Roots:** Bread Intake Across the Blue Zones 712
- **16.6 Nutrition and Your Health: Brain Health 714**
  - **Magnificent Microbiome:** Gut-Brain Axis 716
  - **Newsworthy Nutrition:** Mediterranean-style diet linked to reduced Alzheimer's disease 718

Couple in kitchen: Prostock-studio/Shutterstock; boy eating tomato: Westend61/Getty Images; friends arm in arm: moodboard/Cultura/Getty Images

Appendix A Daily Values Used on Food Labels A-1

Appendix B Diabetes Menu-Planning Tools A-2

Appendix C Dietary Assessment A-16

Appendix D Chemical Structures Important in Nutrition A-23

Appendix E English-Metric Conversions and Metric Units A-28

Appendix F Dietary Reference Intakes A-29

Glossary G-1

Index I-1

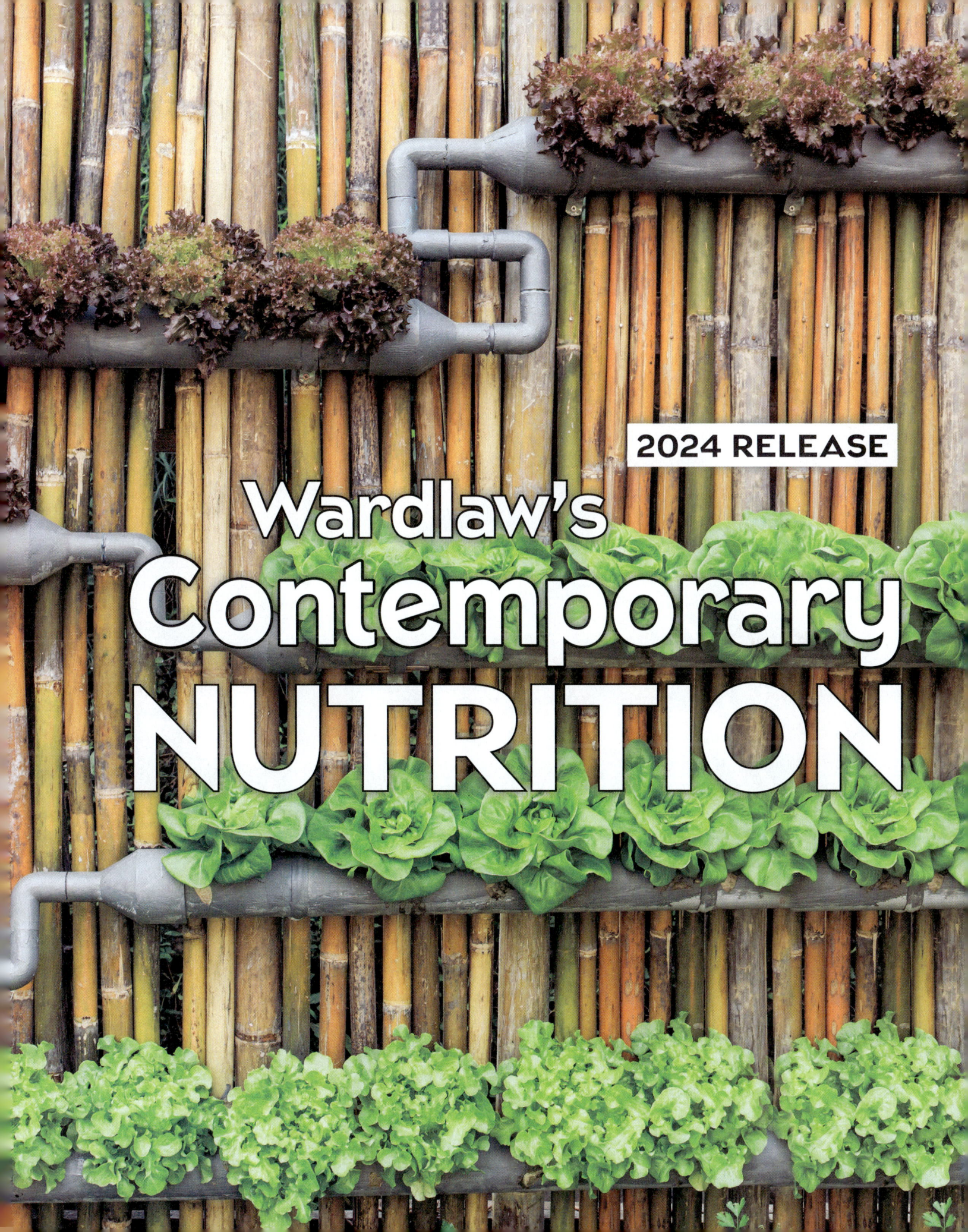

Chapter 1: Nutrition, Food Choices, and Health

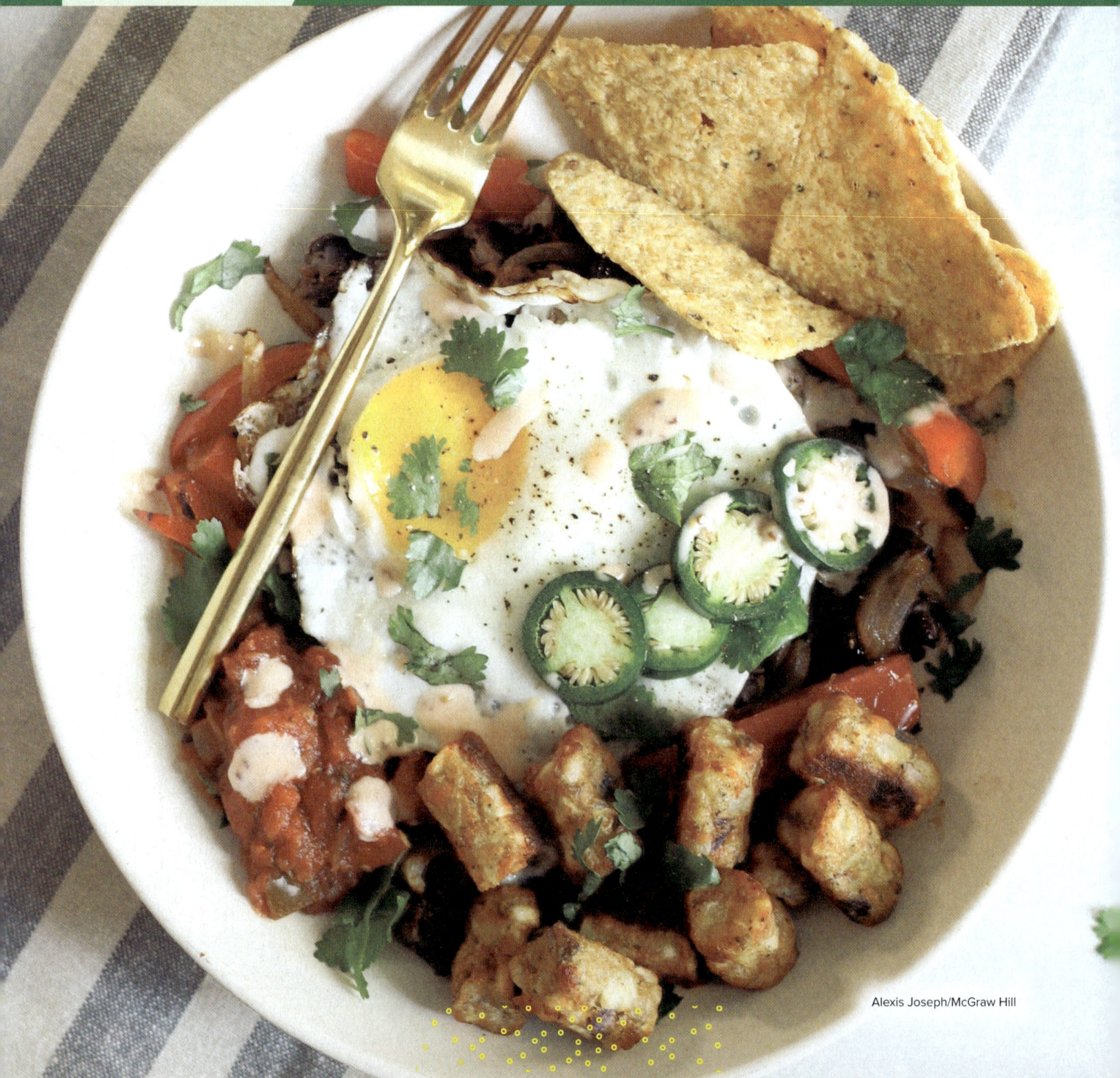

Alexis Joseph/McGraw Hill

Student Learning Outcomes

Chapter 1 is designed to allow you to:

1.1 Describe how our food choices are affected by the flavor, texture, and appearance of food; eating behaviors and food availability; advertising; convenience; cost; sustainability; nutrition; hunger; and appetite.

1.2 Define *nutrition* and identify dietary and lifestyle factors that contribute to the 10 leading causes of death in the United States.

1.3 Define *carbohydrate, protein, lipid, alcohol, vitamin, mineral, water, phytochemical, kilocalorie,* and *fiber*.

1.4 Determine the total calories (kcal) of a food or meal using the weight and calorie content of the energy-yielding nutrients; convert English to metric units; and calculate percentages, such as percent of calories from fat in a meal.

1.5 Understand the scientific method as it is used in forming and testing hypotheses in the field of nutrition; determine the strength of scientific evidence related to nutrition.

1.6 List the major characteristics of a nutritious dietary pattern, the food habits that often need improvement, and the aims of the "Nutrition and Healthy Eating" objectives of *Healthy People 2030*.

1.7 Describe a basic plan for health promotion and disease prevention and what to expect from optimal nutrition and a healthy lifestyle.

1.8 Define current alcohol guidelines and list the risks of excessive alcohol use on both mental and physical health.

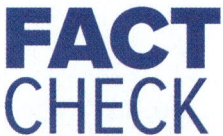

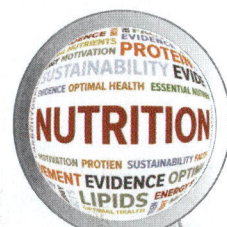

Is nutrition a science?

The answer is a resounding **YES!** Nutrition is a translational science that explores the relationship between dietary patterns and health during all life stages.

This text is your launching point to learn and discover more about nutrition. We will give you the tools you need to fully understand the basics and then will introduce more complex topics and resources for those wishing to dig a bit deeper.

The ultimate goal is to help you obtain the facts and the best path to optimal nutrition and sustained health. The information presented within is based on emerging science that is translated into everyday actions and is grounded in the evidence and shown to promote lifelong health.

Nutrition research has clearly shown that a lifestyle that includes a **dietary pattern** rich in vegetables; fruits; whole grains; seafood; eggs; beans, peas, and lentils; unsalted nuts and seeds; fat-free and low-fat dairy products; and lean meats and poultry—when prepared with no or little added sugars, saturated fat, and sodium—coupled with regular physical activity, can enhance our current quality of life and keep us healthy for many years to come. Unfortunately, this healthy lifestyle is not always easy to follow. When it comes to *nutrition*, it is clear that some of our dietary patterns are out of balance with our metabolism, physiology, and **physical activity** level.

For more details on each chapter's *Fact Check*, look for the magnifying glass icon (🔍) in the left margin of each chapter. In this chapter, you will find it in Section 1.5. There, you can read more about the science of nutrition and the scientific method.

And, after completion of this course, you should understand the science behind the food choices and lifestyle behaviors you make that impact your mental and physical health throughout life. We call this achievement of making food choices that are healthy for you **nutrition literacy.**

dietary pattern The quantity, proportion, variety, or combination of different foods, drinks, and nutrients in diets, and the frequency with which they are habitually consumed.

physical activity Any movement of skeletal muscles that requires energy.

nutrition literacy Degree to which individuals obtain, process, and understand nutrition information and the skills needed in order to make appropriate nutrition-related decisions.

alcohol Ethyl alcohol or ethanol (CH_3CH_2OH) is the compound in alcoholic beverages.

1.1 Why Do You Choose the Food You Eat?

In your lifetime, you will likely consume about 85,000 meals and 40 tons of food. Although this consumption pattern is based on American dietary patterns, keep in mind that food consumption varies around the world based on different cultures, traditions, availability, local customs, and dietary preferences. Many factors—some internal, some external—influence our food choices and behaviors. This chapter begins with a discussion of these factors and ends with current information about **alcohol** consumption and its relationship to our health. In between, we examine the powerful effect of dietary patterns in determining overall health and take a close look at the general classes of nutrients—as well as the calories—supplied by what we eat and drink. We also present the major characteristics of the *Dietary Guidelines for Americans* and our progress toward meeting nutrition-related objectives of *Healthy People 2030*. A review of the scientific process behind nutrition recommendations is also included, along with an introduction to our timely features that appear in each chapter: *Fact Check*, *Farm to Fork*, *Newsworthy Nutrition*, *Magnificent Microbiome*, *Sustainable Solutions*, *Case Studies*, and *Ask the RDN*. Our newest feature, *Roots,* celebrates the various cultures, customs, and lifestyles specific to nutrition and health.

Identifying what drives us to eat and what affects our food choices will help us understand the complexity of factors that influence eating, especially the effects of our routines and food advertising (Fig. 1-1). You can then appreciate why foods may have different meanings to various individuals and cultures and thus why others' dietary patterns and preferences may differ from yours.

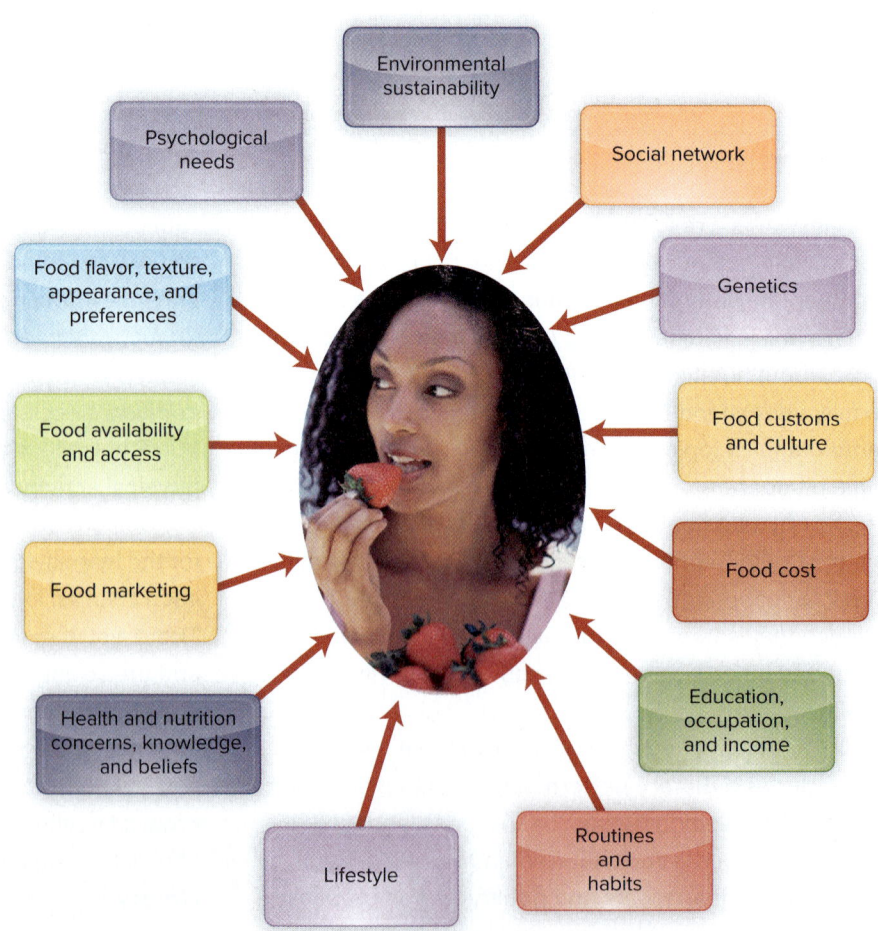

FIGURE 1-1 Food choices are affected by many factors. Florian Franke/Purestock/SuperStock

WHAT INFLUENCES YOUR FOOD CHOICES?

North American adults spent almost 75 minutes a day eating and drinking.[1] If we live to be 80 years old, we will have spent over 4 years eating and drinking! Overall, our daily food choices stem from a complicated mix of biological and social influences. The *Food and Health Survey* found that, from a list of key factors, the majority (87%) said that taste influenced their food and beverage purchases, followed by price (76%), healthfulness (62%), convenience (61%), and environmental sustainability (34%).[2] In addition, 68% of respondents reported that familiarity was another important factor in making purchasing decisions. Now, let's examine some of the key reasons we choose what we eat and drink.

Flavor, texture, and appearance, also known as *taste,* are some of the most important factors determining our food choices. Creating more flavorful foods that are both healthy and profitable is a major focus of the food industry. The challenge is to combine the taste of the foods we prefer with the most nutritious and healthy characteristics. The good news is that chefs and food bloggers are dedicating themselves to creating nutritious food that is also delicious.

Early influences related to various people, places, and events have a continuing impact on our food choices. Many food customs, including ethnic eating patterns, begin as we are introduced to foods during childhood. Parents can lay a strong foundation knowing that exposure to food choices during early childhood is important in influencing later health behaviors. Developing healthy patterns during childhood will help ensure healthy preferences and choices when we are teenagers and adults.

Eating behaviors and food availability strongly influence choices. Food Availability and Consumption Data from the U.S. Department of Agriculture (USDA) show that adults consume more than the recommended amounts from the proteins and the grains group. Potatoes and tomatoes are the most commonly consumed vegetables (Fig. 1-2), with French fries and pizza contributing to their popularity. Apples and oranges are the most commonly consumed fruits, but they are consumed mostly in juice form (Fig. 1-3). Milk and cheese, especially mozzarella cheese, comprise most of the dairy consumption; milk consumption has shown a big decline, while cheese consumption has doubled and yogurt consumption increased (Fig. 1-4).

Marketing and advertising are major tools for capturing the food interest of the consumer. Consumers have more food choices than ever, and the food industry in the United States spends billions on advertising. Some of this advertising is helpful, as it promotes the importance of healthy food components such as calcium and fiber. However, the food industry also advertises highly sweetened cereals, cookies, snacks, and soft drinks because they bring in the greatest profits. Studies have shown an association between TV advertising of foods and drinks and childhood **obesity** in the United States.[3] These findings suggest that exposure to food advertisements may encourage eating behaviors that do not align with healthy dietary recommendations for our youth. Research also indicates that mass media influences the onset of eating disorders through its depiction of extremely thin models as stereotypes of attractive bodies.[4]

Restaurant dining plays a significant role in our food choices. Americans eat and drink about one-third of their calories from foods prepared away from home. Restaurant food is often calorie dense, served in larger portions, and of poorer nutritional quality compared to foods made at home. To help individuals make informed and more healthy decisions, many eating establishments and chain restaurants list the calorie content of foods and beverages on their menus or menu boards and include additional nutrition information upon request. More information can be found at fda.gov/CaloriesOnTheMenu.

Time and convenience have become significant influences affecting food choices. Current lifestyles limit the time available for food preparation. Restaurants, supermarkets, and meal delivery services have responded to our demanding work schedules and long hours away from home by supplying prepared meals, microwavable entrees, online grocery shopping and curbside pick-up, and quick-prep meals delivered to your door.

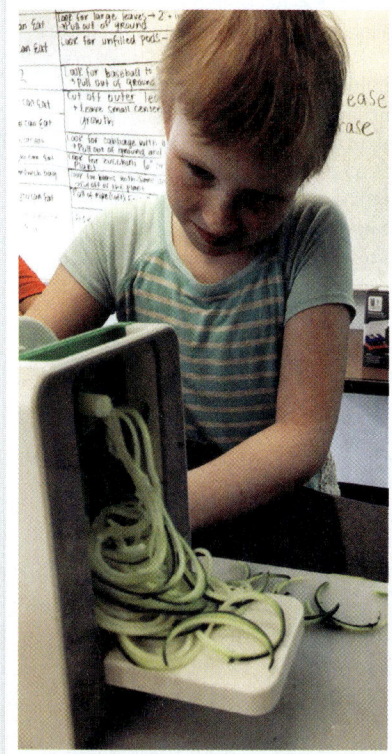

This beautiful child, a survivor of brain cancer, is participating in a garden-based program for families designed to improve dietary and physical activity patterns. Here, she is making *zoodles,* or zucchini noodles.

Exposing children to growing, preparing, and eating healthy foods, such as this veggie pasta, lays a strong foundation for healthful choices throughout life. Indeed, children become more *adventurous eaters* and are willing to try new foods when they participate in the growing, harvesting, and preparation of foods. **Can you think of other ways to encourage children to become more adventurous eaters?** Jeff Laubert

obesity Ratio of weight to height that is significantly higher than what is associated with optimal health, usually due to excessive body fat. For adults, this is most often defined as BMI of 30 or higher. For children, this is often defined as BMI-for-age at the 95th percentile or higher.

FIGURE 1-2 According to food availability data, the favorite vegetables of individuals in the United States are potatoes and tomatoes. North Americans consumed 49 pounds of potatoes per person and 31 pounds of tomatoes, with 60% as canned tomatoes. Onions were the third highest consumed vegetable at 9 pounds per person.

Source: USDA, Economic Research Service, Loss-Adjusted Food Availability Data, 2019

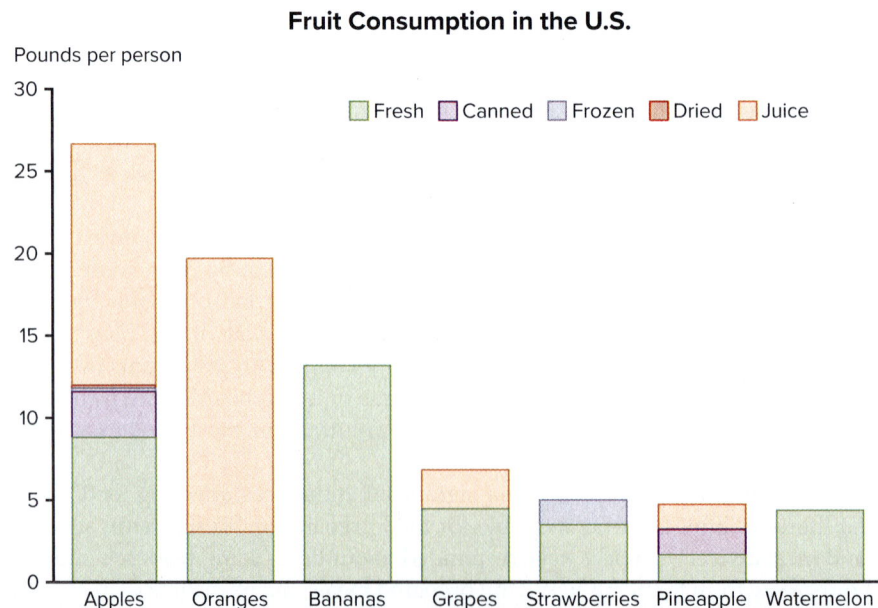

Note: Loss-adjusted food availability data are proxies for consumption.

Cost and economics play a role in our food choices. After taste, cost is the number-two reason why people choose the food they do.[2] While the average adult now spends less on groceries than in the past, young adults and those with higher incomes spend the most on food. As income increases, so do meals eaten away from home, and as calorie intake increases, so does the food bill.

Sustainability also affects your food choices. With future generations in mind, many consumers are becoming more socially responsible to care for the environment. College students have become a big part of the movement to purchase local, seasonal, and sustainable food and to spread awareness that the way we produce and eat food can

FIGURE 1-3 Apples held the top spot for total fruit available for consumption in 2021 with loss-adjusted apple juice availability at 14.7 pounds (1.7 gallons) per person; fresh apples at roughly 9 pounds per person; and canned, dried, and frozen apples totaling to 3.1 pounds per person. Bananas (13.2 pounds per person) topped the list of most popular fresh fruits, while orange juice (16.6 pounds or 1.9 gallons) remained the top fruit juice available for consumption in the United States.

Source: USDA, Economic Research Service, Loss-Adjusted Food Availability Data, 2021. https://www.ers.usda.gov/data-products/ag-and-food-statistics-charting-the-essentials/food-availability-and-consumption/?topicId=080e8d1d-e61e-4bd8-beac-51f0f1d1f0fe

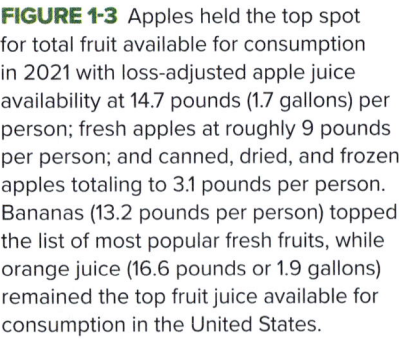

Note: Loss-adjusted food availability data are adjusted for food spoilage, plate waste, and other losses to more closely approximate actual consumption.

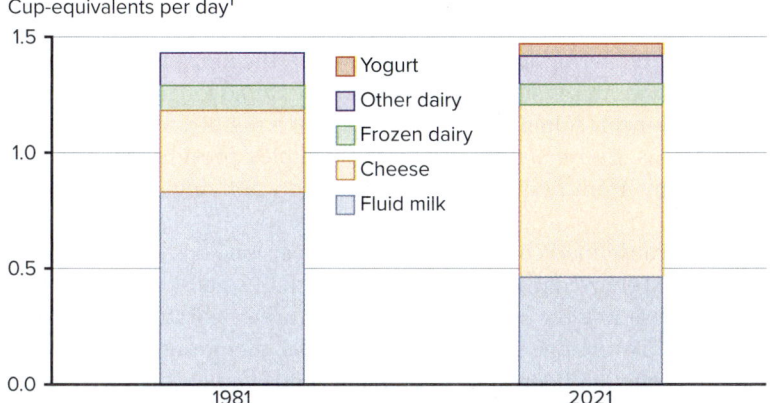

FIGURE 1-4 According to food availability data from the USDA, adults consumed a similar amount of dairy products (1.5 cup-equivalents of dairy products per person per day in 2021). This is half the recommended amount for a 2000 kcal per day diet. Although the overall quantity is slightly higher in 2021 compared to 1981, the types of dairy products consumed have changed. Milk consumption has decreased from 0.8 to 0.5 cups per person per day, while cheese consumption has doubled and yogurt consumption has increased.

Source: USDA, Economic Research Service, Loss-Adjusted Food Availability Data, 2021, https://www.ers.usda.gov/data-products/ag-and-food-statistics-charting-the-essentials/food-availability-and-consumption/?topicId=080e8d1d-e61e-4bd8-beac-51f0f1d1f0fe

[1]Based on a 2000-calorie-per-day diet. Loss-adjusted food availability data are adjusted for food spoilage, plate waste, and other losses to approximate actual intake. "Other dairy" includes evaporated milk, condensed milk, dry milk products, cottage cheese, and half and half.

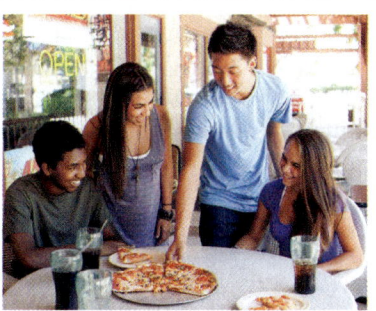

Jacob is majoring in nutrition and is well aware of the importance of a healthy dietary pattern. He has recently been attentive to his meals and is confused. He notices that he eats a great deal of high-fat foods, such as chicken wings, cheese, chips, ice cream, and chocolate, and few fruits, vegetables, and whole grains. He also has a daily cappuccino with lots of whipped cream. **What three factors may be influencing Jacob's food choices? What advice would you give him on how to have his dietary pattern match his needs?**
Sarah Casillas/DigitalVision/Getty Images

Sustainable Solutions

Food & Health Survey

More than half of the respondents to the *Food & Health Survey* stated the top three indicators of products being sourced in an environmentally sustainable way were: (1) recyclable packaging; (2) labeled as sustainably sourced; and (3) reusable packaging. Other indicators included being labeled as locally grown, sustainably sourced, non-GMO/non-bioengineered, and organic.

Source: International Food Information Council Foundation (IFIC). *2023 Food & Health Survey.* https://foodinsight.org/2023-food-and-health-survey/

slow the rate of global warming, build strong communities, and improve our health. While the *Food & Health Survey* found that environmental sustainability was an important driver of food purchasing, most consumers continue to find it hard to know whether the food choices they make are environmentally sustainable. These consumers agreed that environmental sustainability would have a greater influence on food choices if it was easier to know which choices were in fact environmentally sustainable. For instance, when making environmentally sustainable animal protein purchases, consumers surveyed looked for labels such as "no added **hormones**," "grass-fed animals," and "locally raised."[5]

Nutrition—or what we think of as *healthy foods*—also directs our food purchases. Adults who tend to make health-related food choices are often well-educated, middle-class professionals who are generally health oriented, have active lifestyles, and focus on weight control. The survey found that a subset of consumers report they actively seek out foods or follow a dietary pattern for specific health benefits such as weight loss, energy, digestive health, and heart health.[2] Nutrition and health information on food package labels has also been shown to affect food choices.

WHY ARE YOU SO HUNGRY?

Both **hunger** and **appetite** influence our desire to eat. These drives differ dramatically. Hunger is primarily our physical, biological drive to eat and is controlled by internal body mechanisms. For example, as foods are digested and absorbed, the stomach and small intestine send signals to the liver and brain telling us to reduce further food intake.

Appetite, our primarily psychological drive to eat, is affected by many of the external factors we discussed earlier, such as environmental and psychological factors and social cues and customs (Fig. 1-1). Appetite can be triggered simply by seeing a tempting dessert or smelling popcorn at the movie theater. Fulfilling either or both drives by eating sufficient food normally brings a state of **satiety,** a feeling of satisfaction that temporarily halts our desire to continue eating.

hormone A chemical messenger produced by a gland and released into the blood to travel to target tissues at distant sites throughout the body.

hunger The primarily physiological (internal) drive to find and eat food.

appetite The primarily psychological (external) influences that encourage us to find and eat food, often in the absence of obvious hunger.

satiety A state in which there is no longer a desire to eat; a feeling of satisfaction.

hypothalamus A region of the forebrain that controls body temperature, thirst, and hunger.

The *feeding center* and the *satiety center* are in the **hypothalamus,** a region of the brain that helps regulate satiety. They work in opposite ways, like a tug-of-war, to promote adequate availability of nutrients at all times. When we haven't eaten for a while, stimulation of the feeding center signals us to eat. As we eat, the nutrient content in the blood rises, and the satiety center is stimulated. This is why we no longer have a strong desire to seek food after a meal. Admittedly, this concept of a tug-of-war between the feeding and satiety centers is an oversimplification of a complex process. The various feeding and satiety messages from body cells to the brain do not single-handedly determine what we eat.

We often eat because food comforts us. Almost everyone has encountered a mouth-watering dessert and enjoyed it, even on a full stomach. It smells, tastes, and looks good. We might eat because it is the right time of day, we are celebrating, or we are seeking emotional comfort to overcome the blues. After a meal, memories of pleasant tastes and feelings reinforce appetite. If stress or depression sends you to the refrigerator, you are mostly seeking comfort, not food fuel. Appetite may not be a physical process, but it certainly can influence food intake.

When food is abundant, appetite—not hunger—more frequently triggers eating. Satiety associated with consuming a meal may reside primarily in our psychological frame of mind. Also, because satiety regulation is not perfect, body weight can fluctuate. We become accustomed to a certain amount of food at a meal. Providing less than that amount leaves us wanting more. One way to use this observation for weight management purposes is to train your eye to expect less food by slowly decreasing serving sizes to more appropriate amounts. Your appetite then readjusts as you expect less food. You should now understand that daily food consumption is a complicated mix of biological and social influences. Try keeping track of what triggers your eating for a few days. Is it primarily hunger or appetite?

✓ CONCEPT CHECK 1.1

1. What are the factors that influence our food choices?
2. Which two vegetables are the most consumed in the U.S., and why?
3. How do *hunger* and *appetite* differ in the way they influence our desire to eat?
4. What factors influence satiety?

1.2 How Is Nutrition Connected to Good Health?

Fortunately, our dietary patterns can support good health in many ways, depending on their components. You just learned, however, that lifestyle habits and other factors may have a bigger impact on our food choices than the food components themselves. Unfortunately, many individuals have diseases that could have been prevented if they had known more about the foods and, more importantly, had applied this knowledge to plan meals and design their eating pattern. We will now look at the effect these choices are having on our health both today and in the future.

WHAT IS NUTRITION?

As you learned in the *Fact Check*, nutrition is the science that links foods to health. It includes the processes by which the human organism ingests, digests, absorbs, transports, uses, and excretes food substances.

WHERE DO WE FIND NUTRIENTS?

nutrients Chemical substances in food that contribute to health, many of which are essential parts of a dietary pattern. Nutrients nourish us by providing calories to fulfill energy needs, materials for building body parts, and factors to regulate necessary chemical processes in the body.

What is the difference between food and **nutrients?** Food provides the energy (in the form of calories) as well as the compounds needed to build and maintain all body cells. Nutrients are the substances obtained from food that are vital for growth and maintenance of a healthy body throughout life. For a substance to be considered an **essential nutrient,** three characteristics are needed:

1. At least one specific biological function of the nutrient must be identified in the body.
2. Omission of the nutrient from the dietary pattern must lead to a decline in certain biological functions, such as production of blood cells.
3. Replacing the omitted nutrient in the dietary pattern before permanent damage occurs will restore those normal biological functions.

WHY STUDY NUTRITION?

We all may feel like nutrition experts because we all eat several times a day. Nutrition knowledge can be confusing, however, and seem like a moving target. You just learned that nutrition is only one of many factors that influence our eating patterns. Studying nutrition will help you erase any misconceptions you have about food and nutrition and will assist you in making informed choices about the foods you eat and their relationship to health.

Nutrition is a lifestyle factor that is a key to developing and maintaining an optimal state of health. A poor dietary pattern and a sedentary lifestyle are known to be **risk factors** for life-threatening **chronic diseases** such as **cardiovascular disease (i.e., heart disease), hypertension,** type 2 **diabetes,** and some forms of **cancer.** Together, these and related disorders account for two-thirds of all deaths in the United States (Fig. 1-5). Not meeting nutrient needs in our younger years makes us more likely to suffer health consequences, such as bone fractures from the disease **osteoporosis,** in later years.

The combination of a suboptimal eating patterns and inadequate physical activity contributes to hundreds of thousands of fatal cases of cardiovascular disease, cancers, and diabetes each year. In addition, obesity is considered the second-leading cause of preventable death in North America after tobacco-related deaths. Obesity and other chronic diseases are often preventable, and the cost of prevention, usually when we are children and young adults, is small compared to the cost of treating these diseases when we are older.

The good news is that an increased interest in health, fitness, and nutrition has been associated with decreasing trends for heart disease, cancers, and **stroke.** Mortality from heart disease, the leading cause of death, has been declining steadily since 1980. As you gain an understanding about your lifestyle behaviors and increase your knowledge about nutrition, you will have the opportunity to significantly reduce your risk for many common health problems.

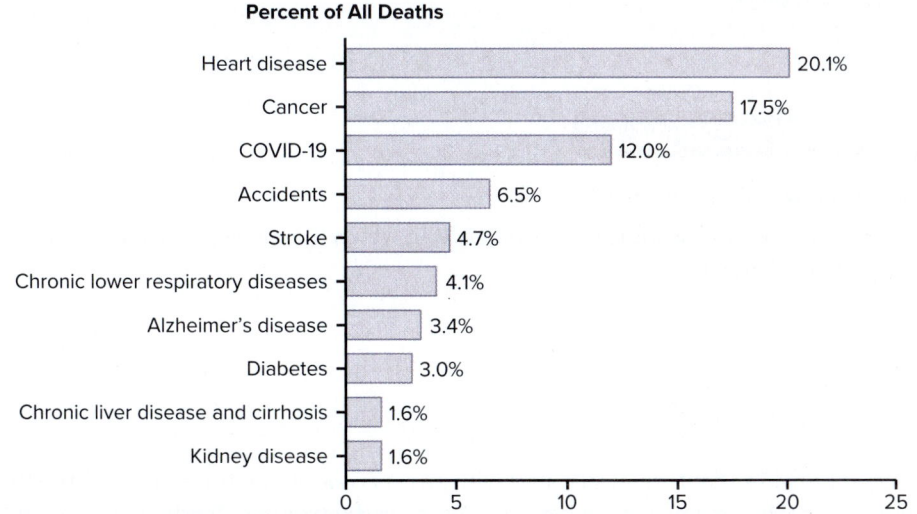

FIGURE 1-5 Ten leading causes of death in the United States.
Source: Centers for Disease Control and Prevention *National Vital Statistics Report, Deaths: Leading Causes for 2021.*

essential nutrient In nutritional terms, a substance that, when left out of a dietary pattern, leads to signs of poor health. The body either cannot produce this nutrient or cannot produce enough of it to meet its needs. If added back to a dietary pattern before permanent damage occurs, the affected aspects of health are restored.

risk factors A term used frequently when discussing the factors contributing to the development of a disease. A risk factor is an aspect of our lives, such as heredity, lifestyle choices (e.g., use of tobacco products), or nutritional habits.

chronic disease The result of a combination of genetic, physiological, environmental, and behavioral factors leading to diseases of long duration. Also referred to as *noncommunicable diseases (NCDs)*.

cardiovascular disease A general term that refers to any disease of the heart and circulatory system. This disease is generally characterized by the deposition of fatty material in the blood vessels (hardening of the arteries), which in turn can lead to organ damage and death. Also termed *coronary heart disease (CHD)* or simply, *heart disease,* as the vessels of the heart are the primary sites of the disease.

hypertension A condition in which blood pressure remains persistently elevated. Obesity, inactivity, alcohol intake, excess salt intake, and genetics may each contribute to the problem.

diabetes A group of diseases characterized by high blood glucose. Type 1 diabetes involves insufficient or no release of the hormone insulin by the pancreas and therefore requires daily insulin therapy. Type 2 diabetes results from either insufficient release of insulin or general inability of insulin to act on certain body cells, such as muscle cells. Persons with type 2 diabetes may or may not require insulin therapy.

cancer A condition characterized by uncontrolled growth of abnormal cells.

osteoporosis The presence of a stress-induced fracture or a T-score of −2.5 or lower. The bones are porous and fragile due to low mineral density.

stroke A decrease or loss in blood flow to the brain that results from a blood clot or other change in arteries in the brain. This in turn causes the death of brain tissue. Also called a *cerebrovascular accident.*

registered dietitian nutritionist (RDN) A person who has completed a degree program approved by the Accreditation Council for Education in Nutrition and Dietetics (ACEND), performed at least 1200 hours of supervised professional practice, passed a national registration examination, and complies with continuing education requirements.

ASK THE RDN: Why Dietetics?

Dear RDN: Why did you become a **registered dietitian nutritionist**?

Growing up in the 1980s and 1990s, it seemed like the important people in my life were always "on a diet." My family members, caregivers, and teachers latched onto every passing fad, turning away from their favorite foods in order to lose weight. Watching my role models follow various diet trends and fitness gurus, I formed a belief that calories were something to be controlled and that dieting was virtuous.

Throughout my adolescent years, my interest in nutrition and fitness grew. I immersed myself in nutrition and fitness and even experimented with many popular trends. At that point in my life, I didn't know enough to discern nutrition fact from fiction, but I certainly thought I was an expert!

In high school, I was drawn to the science linking foods to health and found my way to the field of dietetics. I was interested in helping others (and myself) use foods on a path to achieving their weight and fitness goals. Once I got to college, I began learning the *science* of nutrition and realized that nutrition is about SO MUCH MORE than calories and body weight. I was amazed to learn how the chemical compounds (i.e., nutrients) in the foods we eat become part of us: these are the building blocks of every single cell that help to form chemical messengers involved in regulating body processes and providing the fuel that powers us. Although I was still preoccupied with weight management, I slowly gained an appreciation for the role of nutrition in every aspect of physical and mental health.

What I love most about nutrition is that there is always something new to learn. The science of nutrition is only about 100 years old, and new evidence about the role of nutrition in health and disease continues to unfold. These days, the aspect of nutrition that fascinates me most is nutritional psychiatry—the connections between nutrition and mental health. This field didn't even exist when I was in school!

So, although I first chose dietetics due to an early interest in fitness and weight management, I stuck with it because I love food, science, and learning. In this text, our goal is to equip you and your classmates to separate facts from fads. Also, we want students to have a positive relationship with food and explore dietary patterns that promote and optimize your physical and mental health!

Keeping the *new* in nutrition!

Angela Collene, MS, RDN, LD

Senior Lecturer, The Ohio State University, Author of *Wardlaw's Contemporary Nutrition* and *Wardlaw's Contemporary Nutrition: A Functional Approach*

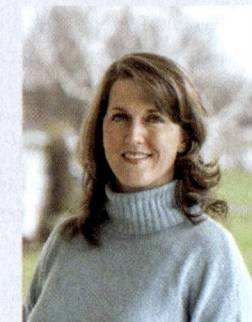
Tim Klontz

carbohydrate A compound containing carbon, hydrogen, and oxygen atoms. Most are known as *sugars, starches,* and *fibers*.

lipid A compound containing much carbon and hydrogen, little oxygen, and sometimes other atoms. Lipids do not dissolve in water and include fats, oils, and cholesterol.

protein Food and body compounds made of more than 100 amino acids; proteins contain carbon, hydrogen, oxygen, nitrogen, and sometimes other atoms in a specific configuration. Proteins contain the form of nitrogen most easily used by the human body.

vitamin An essential organic (carbon-containing) compound needed in small amounts in the dietary pattern to help regulate and support chemical reactions and processes in the body.

mineral Element used in the body to promote chemical reactions and to form body structures.

water The universal solvent; chemically, H_2O. The body is composed of about 60% water. Water (fluid) needs are about 9 (females) or 13 (males) cups per day; needs are greater if one exercises heavily.

✓ CONCEPT CHECK 1.2

1. How do we define *nutrition*?
2. What are the three leading causes of death in which the dietary pattern plays a part in the United States?

1.3 What Are the Classes and Sources of Nutrients?

To begin the study of nutrition, let's start with an overview of the six classes of nutrients. You are probably already familiar with the terms **carbohydrates, lipids** (fats and oils), **proteins, vitamins,** and **minerals.** These nutrients, plus **water,** make up the six classes of nutrients found in food.

Macronutrients			
	Carbohydrates	**Lipids**	**Proteins**
Energy Content	4 kcal/gram	9 kcal/gram	4 kcal/gram
Recommendations	45–65% of total energy needs	20–35% of total energy needs	10–35% of total energy needs
Sources	Grains, vegetables, fruits, and dairy	Oils, dairy, fatty fish, nuts and seeds	Meat, poultry, fish, dairy, nuts and seeds, beans, peas, lentils, and soy
Functions	Provides energy to all cells in the body, spares protein breakdown, and promotes digestive health	Contributes to the structure and function of cell membranes, aids in fat-soluble vitamin absorption, and serves as the primary energy storage	Provides the main structural material for all cells and an important component of hormones and enzymes

FIGURE 1-6 Comparison of macronutrients. Carbohydrates: Elena Schweitzer/Shutterstock; Lipids: tinalarsson/iStock/Getty Images; Proteins: Image Source/Glow Images

Nutrients can be assigned to three functional categories: (1) those that primarily provide us with calories to meet energy needs (expressed in **kilocalories [kcal]**); (2) those important for growth, development, and maintenance; and (3) those that act to keep body functions running smoothly. Some overlap in function exists among these categories. The energy-yielding nutrients (carbohydrates, lipids, and protein) along with water are needed in relatively large amounts, so they are called **macronutrients**. Vitamins and minerals are needed in such small amounts in the dietary pattern that they are called **micronutrients**. See Figure 1-6 for a summary of the energy-yielding nutrients.

CARBOHYDRATES

Chemically, carbohydrates can exist in foods as **simple sugars** and **complex carbohydrates**. Simple sugars, frequently referred to as *sugars* or *simple carbohydrates,* are relatively small molecules. These sugars are found naturally in fruits, vegetables, and dairy products. Table sugar, known as sucrose, is a simple sugar that is added to many foods we eat. Glucose, also known as blood sugar, is a simple sugar in your blood. Complex carbohydrates are formed when many simple sugars are joined together. Plants store carbohydrates in the form of **starch,** a complex carbohydrate made up of hundreds of glucose units. Breads, cereals, grains, and starchy vegetables are the main sources of complex carbohydrates.

During digestion, complex carbohydrates are broken down into single sugar molecules (such as glucose) and absorbed into the bloodstream via **cells** lining the small intestine. However, the **bonds** between the sugar molecules in certain complex carbohydrates, called **fiber,** cannot be broken down by human digestive processes. Fiber passes through the small intestine undigested to provide bulk for the stool (feces) formed in the large intestine (colon).

Aside from enjoying their taste, we need sugars and other carbohydrates in our dietary patterns primarily to help satisfy the calorie needs of our body cells. Carbohydrates

kilocalorie (kcal) Heat energy needed to raise the temperature of 1000 grams (1 L) of water 1 degree Celsius.

macronutrient A nutrient needed in gram quantities in a dietary pattern.

micronutrient A nutrient needed in milligram or microgram quantities in a dietary pattern.

simple sugar Monosaccharide or disaccharide in the dietary pattern. Also referred to as *sugars* or *simple carbohydrates*.

complex carbohydrate Carbohydrate composed of many monosaccharide molecules. Examples include glycogen, starch, and fiber.

starch A carbohydrate made of multiple units of glucose attached together in a form the body can digest; also known as *complex carbohydrate*.

cell The structural basis of plant and animal organization. In animals it is bounded by a cell membrane. Cells have the ability to take up compounds from and excrete compounds into their surroundings.

bond A linkage between two atoms formed by the sharing of electrons, or attractions.

fiber Substances in plant foods not digested in the human stomach or small intestine. These add bulk to feces. Fiber naturally found in foods is also called *dietary fiber*.

phytochemical A chemical found in plants. Some phytochemicals may contribute to a reduced risk of cancer or cardiovascular disease in people who consume them regularly.

essential fatty acids Fatty acids that must be supplied by the diet to maintain health. Currently, only linoleic acid and alpha-linolenic acid are classified as essential.

enzyme A compound that speeds up the rate of a chemical reaction but is not altered by the reaction. Almost all enzymes are proteins (some are made of genetic material).

amino acid The building block for proteins containing a central carbon atom with nitrogen and other atoms attached.

chemical reaction An interaction between two chemicals that changes both chemicals.

organic compounds In chemistry, any chemical compounds that contain carbon.

fat-soluble A group of vitamins that are soluble in dietary fats and are absorbed along with fats in the small intestine. There are four fat-soluble vitamins: Vitamins A, D, E, and K.

water-soluble A group of vitamins that dissolve in water and are easily absorbed into the bloodstream. These vitamins are not stored in large amounts in the body and are excreted in the urine. There are nine water-soluble vitamins: vitamin C and eight B vitamins.

provide a major source of calories for the body, 4 kcal per gram on average. Glucose, a simple sugar that the body can derive from most carbohydrates, is a major source of calories for most cells. When insufficient carbohydrate is consumed, the body is forced to make glucose from proteins, and this is not a healthy alternative. Most foods high in carbohydrates, such as fruits, vegetables, and whole grains, are also excellent sources of vitamins, minerals, and **phytochemicals.**

LIPIDS

Lipids (mostly fats and oils) in the foods we eat also provide energy. Lipids yield more calories per gram than do carbohydrates, 9 kcal per gram on average, because of differences in their chemical composition. They are also the main form for energy (calorie) storage in the body.

In this book, the more familiar terms *fats* and *oils* will generally be used, rather than *lipids*. Lipids do not dissolve in water. Generally, fats are lipids that are solid at room temperature, and oils are lipids that are liquid at room temperature. We obtain fats and oils from animal and plant sources. Animal fats, such as butter or lard, are solid at room temperature. Plant oils, such as corn or olive oil, tend to be liquid at room temperature. To promote heart health, most people would benefit from using more plant oils in place of solid fats.

Certain fats are essential nutrients that must come from our dietary pattern. These key fats that the body cannot produce, called **essential fatty acids,** perform several important functions in the body. They help regulate blood pressure and play a role in the synthesis and repair of vital cell parts. However, we need only about 4 tablespoons of a common plant oil (such as olive or soybean oil) each day to supply our essential fatty acids. A serving of fatty fish, such as salmon or tuna, at least twice a week is another healthy source of fats. The unique fatty acids in these fish complement the healthy aspects of common plant oils.

PROTEINS

Proteins are the main structural material in the body. For example, proteins constitute a major part of bone and muscle; they are also important components in blood, body cells, **enzymes,** and immune factors. Proteins can also provide calories for the body, 4 kcal per gram on average. Typically, however, the body uses little protein for the purpose of meeting daily calorie needs. Proteins are formed when **amino acids** are bonded together. Some amino acids are essential nutrients.

Protein comes from animal and plant sources. Animal products such as meat, poultry, fish, dairy, and eggs are significant sources of protein in most dietary patterns. Beans, peas, lentils, nuts, seeds, and soy products are good plant protein sources. If protein consumption is greater than what is needed for body functions, the excess is used for calorie needs and carbohydrate production but ultimately can be converted to and stored as fat.

VITAMINS

The main function of vitamins is to enable many **chemical reactions** to occur in the body. Some of these reactions help release the energy trapped in carbohydrates, lipids, and proteins. Remember, however, that vitamins themselves contain no usable calories for the body.

The 13 vitamins are **organic compounds** that can be divided into two groups: Four are **fat-soluble** because they dissolve in fat (vitamins A, D, E, and K); nine are **water-soluble** because they dissolve in water (the B vitamins and vitamin C). These two groups of vitamins have different sources, functions, and characteristics. Water-soluble vitamins are found mainly in fruits and vegetables, whereas dairy products, nuts,

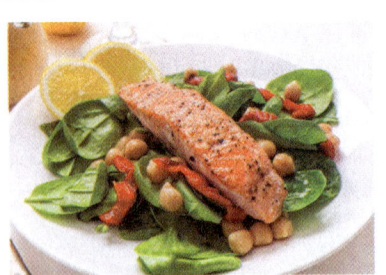

Salmon is a fatty fish that is a healthy source of essential fatty acids. **How many times per week is fatty fish recommended for most adults?** Olga Nayashkova/Shutterstock

seeds, oils, and fortified breakfast cereals are good sources of fat-soluble vitamins. Cooking destroys water-soluble vitamins much more readily than it does fat-soluble vitamins. Water-soluble vitamins are also excreted from the body much more readily than are fat-soluble vitamins. Thus, the fat-soluble vitamins, especially vitamin A, have the ability to accumulate in excessive amounts in the body, which then can lead to **toxicity.**

MINERALS

Minerals are structurally simple, **inorganic** substances that do not contain carbon **atoms.** Minerals such as sodium and potassium typically function independently in the body, whereas minerals such as calcium and phosphorus function together in tissue, such as bone. Because of their simple structure, minerals are not destroyed during cooking, but they can still be lost if they dissolve in the water used for cooking and that water is then discarded. Minerals provide no calories for the body but are critical players in nervous system functioning, water balance, structural (e.g., skeletal) systems, and many other cellular processes.

The essential minerals required in the dietary pattern are divided into two groups—**major minerals** and **trace minerals**—because dietary needs and concentrations in the body vary enormously. If daily needs are less than 100 milligrams, the mineral is classified as a trace mineral; if more, it is a major mineral. Minerals that function based on their electrical charge when dissolved in water are also called **electrolytes.** These include sodium, potassium, and chloride. Many major minerals are found naturally in dairy products and fruits, whereas many trace minerals are found in meats, poultry, fish, and nuts.

WATER

Water makes up the sixth class of nutrients. Although sometimes overlooked as a nutrient, water (H_2O) has numerous vital functions in the body. It acts as a **solvent** and lubricant, as a vehicle for transporting nutrients and waste, and as a medium for temperature regulation and chemical processes. For these reasons, and because the human body is approximately 60% water, the average adult male should consume about 3 liters (about 13 cups) of water and/or other fluids every day; adult females need closer to 2.2 liters (about 9 cups) per day. Fluid needs vary widely, however, based on differences in body mass and environmental conditions.

Water is obviously available from all beverages and is also the major component in some foods, such as many fruits and vegetables (e.g., lettuce, grapes, and melons). The body even makes some water as a by-product of **metabolism.**

OTHER IMPORTANT COMPONENTS IN FOOD

Another group of compounds called phytochemicals are found in foods from plant sources, especially within the fruit and vegetable groups. Although these phytochemicals are not considered essential nutrients, they provide significant health benefits. For example, evidence from animal and laboratory studies indicates that compounds such as polyphenols in many berries prevent the growth of certain cancer cells. Research also suggests that the health benefits of phytochemicals are best obtained through the consumption of whole foods rather than dietary supplements.

Foods with high phytochemical content are sometimes called *superfoods* because of the health benefits they are thought to confer. Yet there is no legal definition for this term, and it is often overused in marketing certain foods. Although there is not enough evidence to link individual phytochemicals with specific health benefits, there is enough proof to suggest that consuming phytochemical-rich foods and beverages may help prevent disease.

---

toxicity Capacity of a substance to produce injury or illness at some dosage.

inorganic Any substance lacking carbon atoms bonded to hydrogen atoms in the chemical structure.

atom Smallest combining unit of an element, such as iron or calcium. Atoms consist of protons, neutrons, and electrons.

major mineral Vital to health, a mineral that is required in the dietary pattern in amounts greater than 100 milligrams per day.

trace mineral Vital to health, a mineral that is required in the dietary pattern in amounts less than 100 milligrams per day.

electrolyte A mineral that separates into positively or negatively charged ions in water. Electrolytes are able to transmit an electrical current.

solvent A liquid substance in which other substances dissolve.

metabolism Chemical processes in the body by which energy is provided in useful forms and vital activities are sustained.

FARM to FORK: Tomatoes

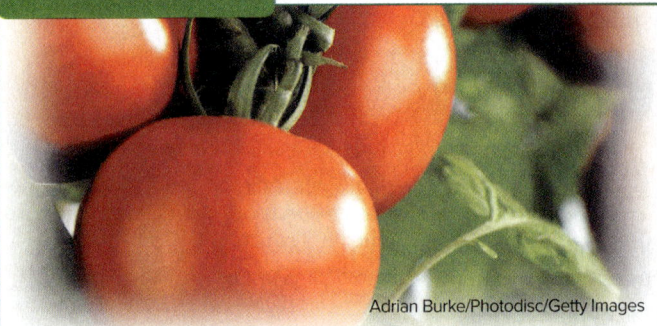

Adrian Burke/Photodisc/Getty Images

Tomatoes are very good sources of the antioxidants lycopene and vitamin C and are also rich in beta-carotene, manganese, and vitamin E.

Grow
- Naturally ripened tomatoes are more nutritious and flavorful than the artificially ripened tomatoes sold in supermarkets. If you can, purchase local tomatoes, including heirloom varieties, at nearby farmers' markets.
- Consider growing your own tomatoes, even in containers, to enjoy nutritious varieties harvested at the peak of ripeness.

Shop
- Choose tomatoes with the darkest red color to obtain the most nutrients and the greatest amount of the phytochemical lycopene.
- Purchase smaller tomatoes for their sweetness and flavor, and enjoy the most lycopene and vitamin C.
- Buy processed tomato products, including jars or cans of tomato paste and sauce, for their highly bioavailable lycopene.

Store
- To preserve the flavor of fresh tomatoes, store them stem side up at room temperature. Flavor and aroma quickly decrease when tomatoes are stored in the refrigerator.
- Grape tomatoes should be stored in plastic clamshells (i.e., original packaging) to prevent them from drying out.
- Tomatoes are ripe and ready to eat when they are a deep color but still firm. Eat ripe tomatoes within 2 or 3 days.

Prep
- Use the whole tomato. The juice contains the flavor enhancer glutamate, and the skin and seeds provide vitamin C and lycopene.
- Snack on nutrition-packed grape tomatoes, and slice or chop them for salads, omelets, sandwiches, or tacos.
- Cooking tomatoes increases the **bioavailability** of nutrients and phytochemicals.
- Add tomato paste to recipes as a concentrated source of flavor, color, nutrients, and phytochemicals, with no added sugar or salt.

Source: Robinson J. Tomatoes: bringing back their flavor and nutrients. In *Eating on the Wild Side*. New York: Little, Brown and Company; 2013.

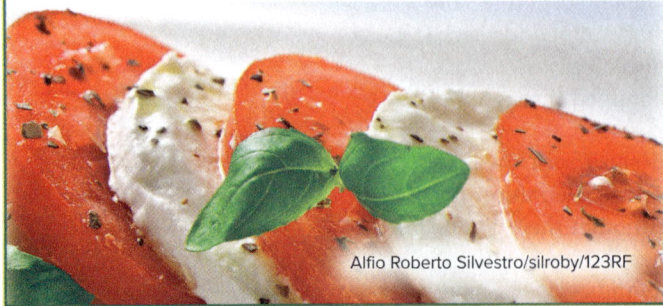

Alfio Roberto Silvestro/silroby/123RF

bioavailability The degree to which an ingested nutrient is digested and absorbed and thus is available to the body.

More information about phytochemicals will be covered in Chapter 8. In addition, our *Farm to Fork* feature appears in every chapter and presents practical information on how to grow, shop, store, and prepare various fruits and vegetables to obtain and preserve their flavor and nutrients. Tomatoes are an important source of phytochemicals and are discussed in this chapter's *Farm to Fork* feature.

SOURCES OF NUTRIENTS

Now that you know the six classes of nutrients, it is important to understand the quantities of the various nutrients that people consume. On a daily basis, we consume about 500 grams (about 1 pound), of protein, fat, and carbohydrate combined. In contrast, the typical daily mineral intake totals about 20 grams (about 4 teaspoons), and the daily vitamin intake totals less than 300 milligrams (about 1/15 of a teaspoon). Although we require a gram or so of some minerals, such as calcium and phosphorus, we need only a few milligrams or less of other minerals, such as zinc, each day.

The nutrient content of the foods we eat also differs from the nutrient composition of the human body. This is because growth, development, and maintenance of the human body are directed by the genetic material (DNA) inside body cells. This genetic blueprint determines how each cell uses the essential nutrients to perform body functions. These nutrients can come from a variety of sources. Cells are not concerned about whether available amino acids come from animal or plant sources. The food that you eat provides cells with basic materials to function according to the directions supplied by the genetic material (genes) housed in body cells.

✓ CONCEPT CHECK 1.3

1. What are the six classes of nutrients?
2. What are the three general functions of nutrients in the body?
3. What are phytochemicals?

1.4 What Math Concepts Will Aid Your Study of Nutrition?

CALCULATING PERCENTAGES

You will use a few mathematical concepts in studying nutrition. Besides performing addition, subtraction, multiplication, and division, you need to know how to calculate percentages and convert English units of measurement to metric units.

The term *percent* (%) refers to a part of the total when the total represents 100 parts. For example, if you earn 80%

on your first nutrition exam, you will have answered the equivalent of 80 out of 100 questions correctly. This equivalent also could be 8 correct answers out of 10; 80% also describes 16 of 20 (16/20 = 0.80 or 80%). The decimal form of percent is based on 100% being equal to 1.00. Percentages are used frequently when referring to menus and nutrient composition, as we saw in the previous calculation of the percentage of total calorie intake from each nutrient. The best way to master this concept is to calculate some percentages. Some examples follow:

Question	Answer
What is 6% of 45?	6% = 0.06, so 0.06 × 45 = 2.7
What percent of 99 is 3?	3/99 = 0.03 or 3% (0.03 × 100)
Joe ate 15% of the adult Recommended Dietary Allowance for iron (RDA = 8 milligrams) at lunch. How many milligrams did he eat?	
	0.15 × 8 milligrams = 1.2 milligrams

CALORIES

We obtain the energy we need for body functions and physical activity from various calorie sources: carbohydrates (4 kcal per gram), fats (9 kcal per gram), and proteins (4 kcal per gram). Foods generally provide more than one calorie source. Plant oils, such as soybean or olive oil, are one exception; these are 100% fat at 9 kcal per gram (Fig. 1-7).

Alcohol is also a potential source of calories, supplying about 7 kcal per gram. It is not considered an essential nutrient, however, because it is not required for human function. Still, alcoholic beverages contribute calories to the eating patterns of many adults. The nutritional implications of alcohol consumption are discussed in Section 1.8.

The body releases energy (measured in calories) from the chemical bonds in carbohydrate, protein, and fat (and alcohol) in order to:

- Build new compounds.
- Perform muscular movements.
- Promote nerve transmission.
- Maintain electrolyte balance within cells.

A calorie is the amount of heat energy it takes to raise the temperature of 1 gram of water 1 degree Celsius (1°C, centigrade scale). A calorie is a tiny measure of heat relative to the amount of calories we eat and use. Food energy is more conveniently expressed in terms of the kilocalorie (kcal), which equals 1000 calories. Note that if the "c" in calories is capitalized, this also signifies kilocalories.

A kilocalorie is the amount of heat energy it takes to raise the temperature of 1000 grams (1 liter) of water by 1°C. The abbreviation *kcal* is used throughout this book. Any values given on food labels in calories are actually in kilocalories. For instance, a suggested intake of 2000 calories per day on a food label is technically 2000 kcal.

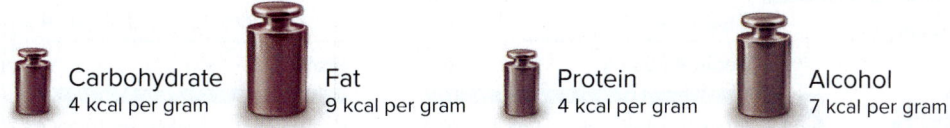

FIGURE 1-7 Calorie content of energy nutrients and alcohol. The weights illustrate their relative energy potential per gram.

CALCULATING CALORIES

The calorie estimates for carbohydrate (4 kcal/g), fat (9 kcal/g), protein (4 kcal/g), and alcohol (7 kcal/g) can be used to determine the calorie content of a food.

Let's practice by calculating the calories in these items:

8-Ounce Piña Colada

Carbohydrate	57 grams × 4 =	228 kcal
Fat	5 grams × 9 =	45 kcal
Protein	1 gram × 4 =	4 kcal
Alcohol	23 grams × 7 =	161 kcal
Total		438 kcal

1 Grilled Chicken Sandwich

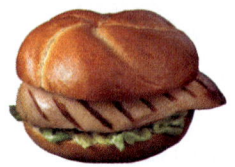
Burke/Triolo/Getty Images

Carbohydrate	46 grams × 4 =	184 kcal
Fat	14 grams × 9 =	126 kcal
Protein	45 grams × 4 =	180 kcal
Alcohol	0 gram × 7 =	0 kcal
Total		490 kcal

You can also use the calories per gram estimates to determine what portion of total calorie intake is contributed by the various calorie-yielding nutrients. Assume that one day you consume 290 grams of carbohydrates, 60 grams of fat, and 70 grams of protein: (290 g carb × 4 kcal/g) + (60 g fat × 9 kcal/g) + (70 g protein × 4 kcal/g) = 1980 total kcal. The percentage of your total calorie intake derived from each nutrient can then be determined:

% of kcal as carbohydrate = (290 × 4) ÷ 1980 = 0.59 (× 100 = 59%)
% of kcal as fat = (60 × 9) ÷ 1980 = 0.27 (× 100 = 27%)
% of kcal as protein = (70 × 4) ÷ 1980 = 0.14 (× 100 = 14%)

Check your calculations by adding the percentages together. Do they total 100%?

NUTRITION FACT LABEL CALCULATION

Use the nutrient values on the Nutrition Facts label above to determine the exact calories from one slice of this whole wheat bread:

(15 g carbohydrate × 4 kcal/g) + (1 g total fat × 9 kcal/g) + (3 g protein × 4 kcal/g) = 81 total kcal. Note the label lists 80 kcal, suggesting that the calorie value was rounded down.

Whole Wheat Bread

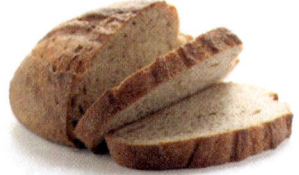
Fullerene/iStock/Getty Images

Nutrition Facts

19 servings per container

Serving size　　　1 slice (36g)

Amount per serving

Calories　80

	% Daily Value*
Total Fat 1g	2%
Saturated Fat 0g	0%
Trans Fat less than 1g	**
Cholesterol 0mg	0%
Sodium 200mg	8%

	% Daily Value*
Total Carbohydrate 15g	5%
Dietary Fiber 2g	8%
Total Sugars 3g	
Includes 2g Added Sugars	4%
Protein 3g	

Vitamin D 0mcg 0% • Calcium 30mg 3% • Iron 1mg 5% • Potassium 70mg 2%

* The % Daily Value (DV) tells you how much a nutrient in a serving of food contributes to a daily diet. 2,000 calories a day is used for general nutrition advice.

THE METRIC SYSTEM

The basic units of the metric system are the meter, which indicates length; the gram, which indicates weight; and the liter, which indicates volume (Fig. 1-8). Appendix E in this textbook lists conversions from the metric system to the English system (feet, pounds, and cups) and vice versa.

METRIC CONVERSION
Converting U.S. Customary and Metric Measurements

U.S. Measurement	Metric Conversion	Measurement	Conversion
1 inch	= 2.54 centimeters	1 millimeter	= 0.04 inch
1 foot	= 0.3048 meter	1 centimeter	= 0.39 inch
1 yard	= 0.914 meter	1 meter	= 39.37 inches
1 mile	= 1.609 kilometers	1 kilometer	= 0.62 mile
1 acre	= 0.405 hectare	1 hectare	= 2.47 acres
1 (fluid) ounce	= 29.573 milliliters		
1 (fluid) pint	= 0.473 liter		
1 (fluid) quart	= 0.946 liter	1 liter (fluid)	= 1.057 quarts
1 gallon	= 3.785 liters		
1 (dry) pint	= 0.550 liter		
1 (dry) quart	= 1.101 liters	1 liter (dry)	= 0.908 quart
1 ounce	= 28.349 grams	1 gram	= 0.035 ounce
1 pound	= 0.453 kilogram	1 kilogram	= 2.2046 pounds
1 ton (2,000 lbs.)	= 0.907 metric ton		
1 square inch	= 6.45 sq. cm	1 square cm	= 0.155 sq. inch
1 square foot	= 0.0929 sq. meters	1 square meter	= 1.2 sq. yards
1 square yard	= 0.836 sq. meters	1 square km	= 0.4 sq. mile

FIGURE 1-8 Metric conversion reference chart.

Let's Practice!

The label of a 5.3-ounce container of Greek yogurt contains 15 grams of sugar. How many teaspoons of sugar does this equal?

$$1 \text{ teaspoon} = 5 \text{ grams of sugar}$$

$$15 \text{ grams} \div 5 \text{ grams/teaspoon} = 3 \text{ teaspoons of sugar}$$

How many ounces are in 8 cups of water?

$$8 \text{ cups of water} = 64 \text{ ounces (or 2 quarts)}$$

Your water bottle holds 500 milliliters. How many milliliters or liters should you drink to equal 8 cups?

$$8 \text{ cups} \times 240 \text{ millileters/cup} = 1920 \text{ millileters} = 1.92 \text{ liters (almost four 500 millileter bottles)}$$

In the field of nutrition, it is important to remember:

- 1 kilogram = 2.2 pounds
- 1 ounce weighs 28 grams
- 2.54 centimeters = 1 inch
- 1 liter almost equals 1 quart
- micro = 1/1,000,000
- milli = 1/1000
- centi = 1/100
- kilo = 1000

> ✓ **CONCEPT CHECK 1.4**
>
> 1. What are the energy (calorie) values for each of the *energy nutrients*?
> 2. Convert 154 pounds of body weight into kilograms.

1.5 How Do We Know What We Know About Nutrition?

The knowledge we have about nutrition and nutrient needs comes from research. Like other sciences, the research that sets the foundation for nutrition knowledge has been developed using the *scientific method,* a testing procedure designed to detect and eliminate error. In other words, the scientific method functions as a truth finder.

THE SCIENTIFIC METHOD

The first step of the scientific method is the observation of a natural phenomenon (Fig. 1-9). Scientists then suggest possible explanations, called **hypotheses,** for the phenomenon. At times, historical events have provided clues to important relationships in nutrition science, such as the link between the need for vitamin C and the development of the disease **scurvy.** Another approach is for scientists to study dietary and disease patterns among various populations, a research method called **epidemiology.**

Thus, hypotheses about the role of the dietary pattern in various health problems can be suggested by historical and epidemiological findings. *Proving* the role of particular dietary components, however, requires controlled experiments. The data gathered from experiments may either support or refute each hypothesis. If the

hypotheses Tentative explanations by a scientist to explain a phenomenon.

scurvy The vitamin C deficiency disease characterized by weakness, fatigue, slow wound healing, bone pain, fractures, sore and bleeding gums, diarrhea, and pinpoint hemorrhages on the skin.

epidemiology The study of how disease rates vary among different population groups.

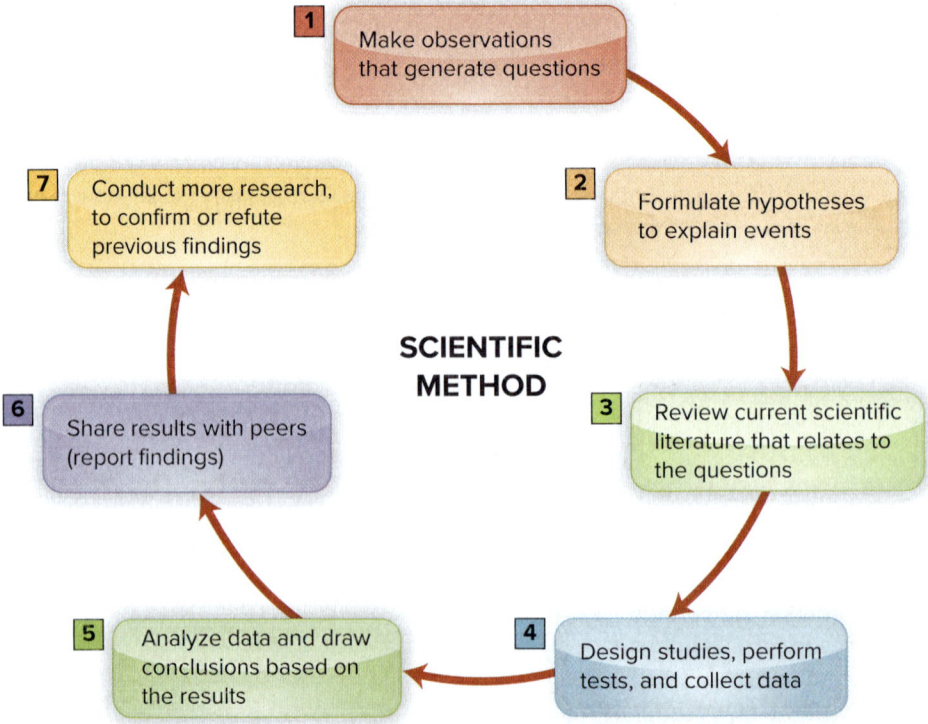

FIGURE 1-9 The scientific method. Scientists consistently follow these steps when testing hypotheses. Scientists do not accept a nutrition or other scientific hypothesis until it has been thoroughly tested using the scientific method.

results of many experiments support a hypothesis, scientists accept the hypothesis as a **theory**.

Once an experiment is complete, scientists summarize the findings and seek to publish the results in scientific journals. Generally, before articles are published in scientific journals, they undergo a critical **peer review** by other scientists familiar with the subject, which helps to ensure that only high-quality, objective research findings are published. Peer review occurs between steps 5 and 6 in Figure 1-9.

Keep in mind that one experiment is never enough to prove a particular hypothesis or provide a basis for nutritional recommendations. Rather, through follow-up studies, the results obtained in one laboratory must be confirmed by similar experiments conducted in other laboratories and, possibly, under varying circumstances. Only then can we really trust and use the results.

STRENGTH OF SCIENTIFIC EVIDENCE

When answering questions about nutrition needs, we look for the best available evidence. The hierarchy of evidence (Fig. 1-10) is based on the rigor (strength and precision) of the research methods used and provides a framework to help us locate the best evidence. The first step is to search for a recent well-conducted **systematic review**. A systematic review is a thorough analysis of the results of all available studies in a particular area. If the studies have the same outcome measures, a systematic review may include a **meta-analysis** of the statistical results of the studies.

If a current systematic review is not available, we move down to the next level of evidence, the primary studies. The most rigorous type of controlled experiment, a **randomized controlled trial,** follows a study design that is **double-blind** and **placebo** controlled. In this type of study, a group of participants (called the experimental group) follows a specific protocol (e.g., consuming a certain food or nutrient),

theory An explanation for a phenomenon that has numerous lines of evidence to support it.

peer review Evaluation of work by professionals of similar competence (peers) to the producers of the work to maintain standards of quality and credibility. Scholarly peer review is used to determine if a scientific study is suitable for publication.

systematic review A thorough summary of the results of available carefully designed health care studies (controlled trials) in a particular area.

meta-analysis A statistical examination of data from multiple scientific studies of the same subject in order to determine overall trends.

randomized controlled trial An experimental design that is double-blind and placebo controlled.

double-blind A study or trial in which any information that may influence the behavior of the tester or the subject is withheld until after the test.

placebo Generally, an inactive medicine or treatment used to disguise the treatments given to the participants in an experiment.

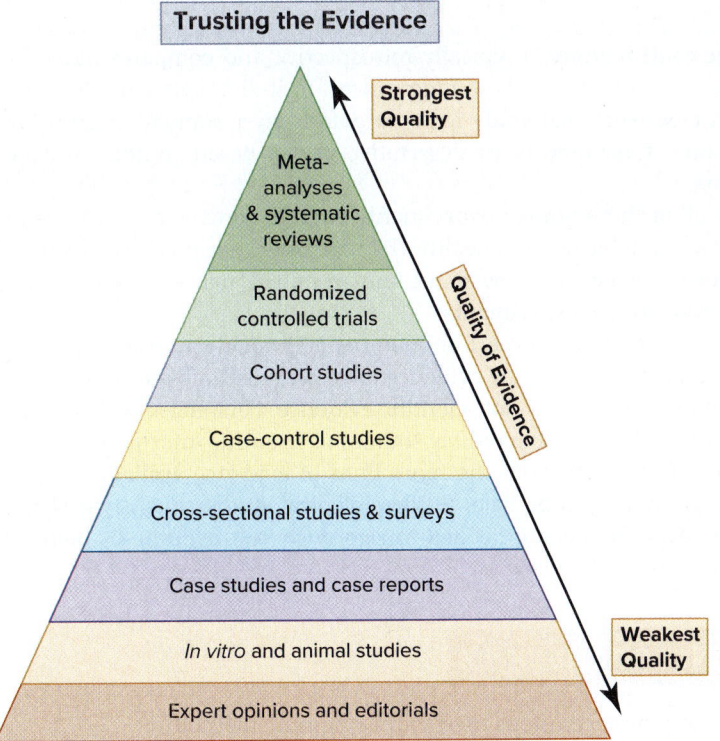

FIGURE 1-10 Hierarchy of scientific evidence with the strongest types of evidence at the top progressing to the weakest types of evidence at the bottom.
Source: thelogicofscience.com.

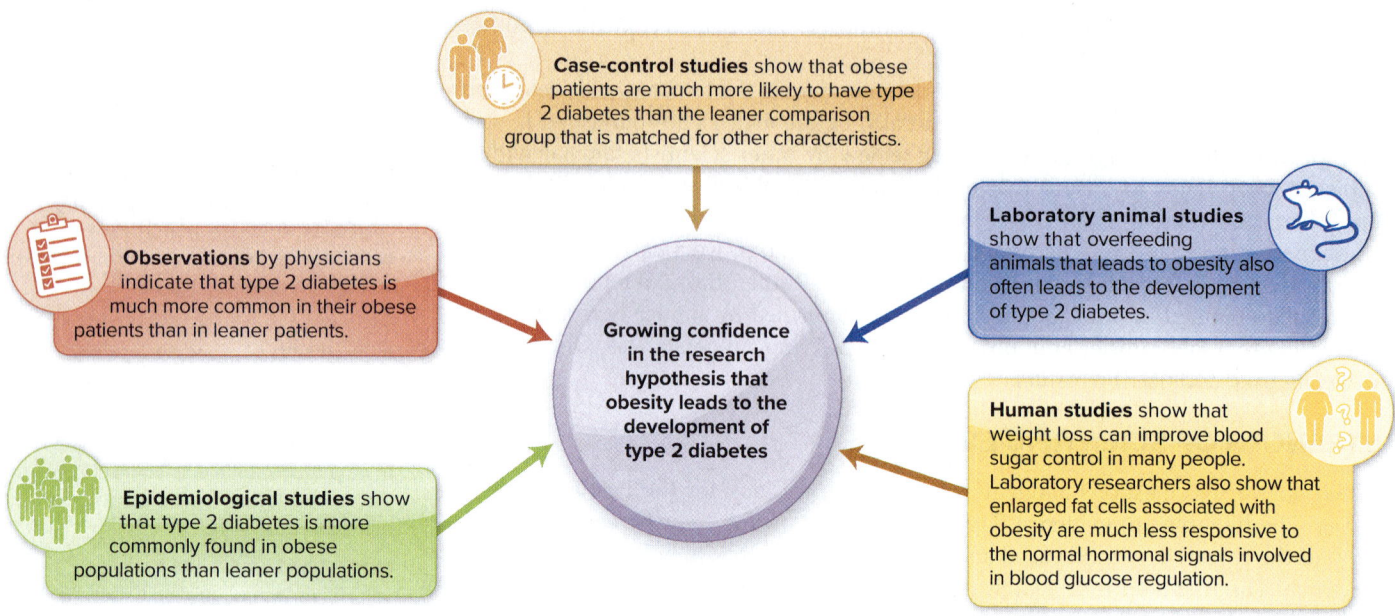

FIGURE 1-11 Data from a variety of sources can come together to support a research hypothesis. This diagram shows how various types of research data support the hypothesis that obesity leads to the development of type 2 diabetes.

cohort studies Observational studies that look at large groups of people, prospectively or retrospectively, studying their exposure to certain risk factors for disease.

case-control study A study in which individuals who have a disease or condition, such as lung cancer, are compared with individuals who do not have the condition.

cross-sectional study Type of observational study that analyzes data from a population group at one specific point in time and based on particular variables of interest.

case reports Descriptive studies based on uncontrolled observations of individual patients.

animal experiments Use of animals to study disease to understand more about human disease.

Newsworthy Nutrition

Feature introduction

In each chapter, we have highlighted the use of the scientific method in research studies in the feature *Newsworthy Nutrition*. These are recently published or landmark studies that relate to chapter topics and that have made a significant impact on our nutrition knowledge. We have selected articles that have used a variety of study designs from the hierarchy of scientific evidence. Enjoy!

and participants in a corresponding control group follow their normal habits or consume a placebo. People are randomly assigned to each group. Scientists then observe the experimental group over time to see if there is any effect not found in the control group.

Cohort studies are further down the evidence hierarchy because they are observational studies that look at large groups of people and examine their exposure to certain risk factors for disease. If data are gathered going forward, they are called prospective studies; if data that are already collected are assessed, they are considered retrospective studies.

A **case-control study** is typically retrospective and compares individuals who have a disease or condition, such as lung cancer, to individuals who do not have the condition. A **cross-sectional study** looks at data from a population group at one specific point in time. **Case reports** are descriptive studies based on uncontrolled observations of patients.

While all of these human experiments provide convincing evidence about relationships between nutrients and health, they are often not practical or ethical to conduct. Thus, much of what we know about human nutritional needs and functions has been gleaned from **animal experiments**.

Finally, editorials and expert opinion papers provide an overview of a specific topic but do not qualify as adequate evidence to answer research questions. It is just as important to understand what is not scientific evidence. Personal anecdotes, YouTube videos, and many websites are not credible sources of scientific information.

As shown in Figure 1-11, the more lines of evidence available to support an idea, the more likely it is to be true. Epidemiological studies may suggest hypotheses, but controlled experiments are needed to rigorously test hypotheses before nutrition recommendations can be made.

✓ CONCEPT CHECK 1.5

1. What are the seven steps used in the scientific method?
2. Name the various types of research studies that can be done to test a hypothesis.
3. List the two strongest types of scientific evidence.

1.6 What Is the Current State of North American Eating Patterns and Health?

DO OBESITY-RELATED DISEASES THREATEN OUR FUTURE?

Over 70% of adults are currently affected by **overweight** or obesity. Where you live is also a factor, with obesity rates varying by state. State by state, obesity data from the CDC (Fig. 1-12) indicate that most states with the lowest obesity rates were in the Northeast or the West, and the South and the Midwest had the highest prevalence of obesity.[6] Three states (Oklahoma, Louisiana, and West Virginia) have 40% or more adults with obesity. Overall, obesity prevalence decreased by level of education. Adults without a high school degree or equivalent had the highest obesity rates and young adults were half as likely to have obesity as middle-aged adults.

On a global scale, obesity has nearly tripled since 1975. What was once considered a problem for high-income countries, obesity has expanded to include middle- and low-income countries. The World Health Organization (WHO) attributes the rising global obesity rates to changes in dietary and physical activity patterns due to societal and environmental changes in the health, agriculture, transport, urban planning, environment, food processing, distribution, marketing, and education sectors. This chapter's *Newsorthy Nutrition* addresses diet and lifestyle factors that are associated with the increasing incidence of colorectal cancer.

Obesity plays a role in chronic illness, including heart disease, stroke, high blood pressure, high cholesterol, diabetes, arthritis, and certain cancers. Obesity is also an expensive disease, with more than $173 billion spent annually on health care related to obesity in the United States.[7] Medical costs for adults who had obesity were over $1850 higher than medical costs for people with healthy weight. Although obesity is complex, dietary patterns and physical activity are modifiable in most cases and certainly play a role.

ASSESSING CURRENT EATING PATTERNS

With the aim of finding out what adults eat, federal agencies conduct surveys to collect data about food and nutrient consumption and the connections between dietary patterns

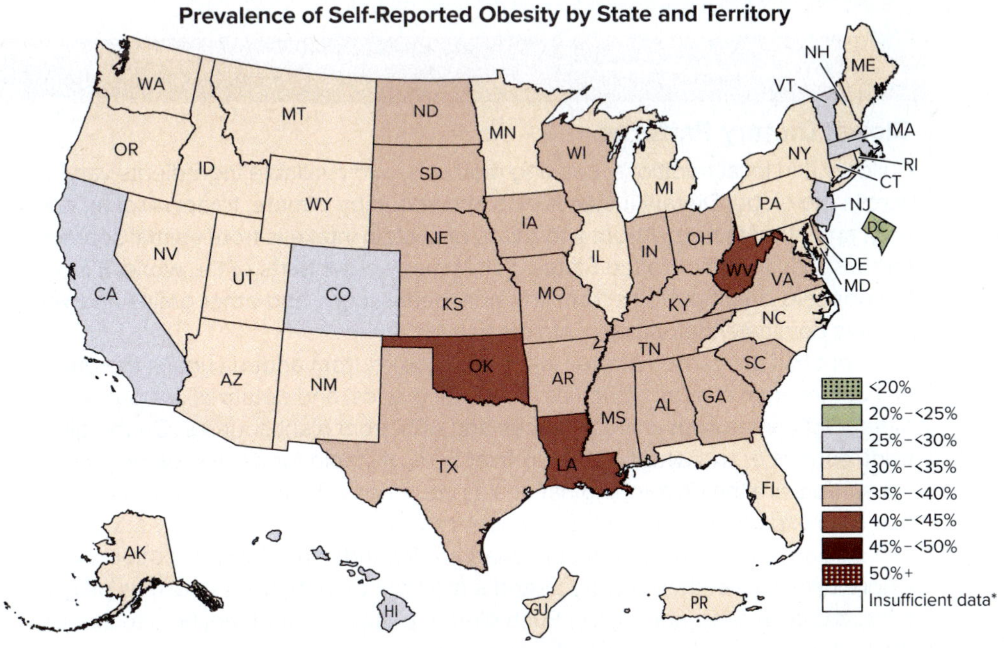

overweight A ratio of weight to height that is moderately higher than what is associated with optimal health. For adults, this is typically defined as BMI within the range of 25.0 up to 30. For children, this is typically defined as BMI-for-age from the 85th up to the 95th percentile.

FIGURE 1-12 The CDC 2022 adult obesity prevalence maps for 50 states, the District of Columbia, and 3 U.S. territories displaying the proportion of adults with a body mass index (BMI) equal to or greater than 30 (≥ 30 kg/m^2) based on self-reported weight and height.

Source: CDC, Prevalence of Self-Reported Obesity by State and Territory, BRFSS, 2020-22.

Newsworthy Nutrition

Role of diet and lifestyle in early-onset colorectal cancer

INTRODUCTION: An alarming increase in cases of early-onset colorectal cancer (CRC) has been documented across the globe. These cancers are defined by a diagnosis in patients younger than 50 years of age. This review summarizes the current evidence on the role of diet and lifestyle as CRC risk factors. **METHODS:** In this *systematic review*, the authors searched research databases according to the Preferred Reporting Items for Systematic Reviews and Meta-Analyses (PRISMA) to identify original studies evaluating diet, alcohol, physical activity, BMI, and smoking in CRC. Twenty-six studies met the seach criteria and were included in the final analysis. **RESULTS:** Protective and deleterious effects of diet and lifestyle in early-onset colorectal cancer are presented in each figure throughout the review. Recent, high-quality studies demonstrated alcohol and obesity have the strongest association with early-onset CRC. Additional risk factors include low levels of physical activity, cigarette smoking, consumption of sugary drinks and processed meat, and a diet low in fruits and vegetables. **CONCLUSION:** Given the growing burden of early-onset colorectal cancer and its globally increasing trends, the authors advocate for including dietary and lifestyle modifications to complement colorectal screening for early-onset colorectal cancer prevention.

Source: Puzzono M, Mannucci A, Grannò S, Zuppardo RA, Galli A, Danese S, Cavestro GM. The role of diet and lifestyle in early-onset colorectal cancer: a systematic review. *Cancers*. 2021; 13(23):5933. https://doi.org/10.3390/cancers13235933

and health. In the United States, the U.S. Department of Health and Human Services monitors food consumption with the National Health and Nutrition Examination Survey (NHANES). The Food and Nutrition Board of the National Academy of Sciences advocates that:

- 10% to 35% of calories come from protein
- 45% to 65% from carbohydrate
- 20% to 35% from fat

Roots

Global Dietary Patterns

Culinary and local traditions, cooking methods, and available ingredients vary across the globe. Dietary intake is also influenced by climate, trade, religion, economy, and other factors. About two-thirds of protein intake is from animal sources for most adults in the United States. Yet, in many other parts of the world, it is just the opposite. Plant proteins from soy, rice, beans, corn, and other grains and vegetables dominate their protein intakes.

About half the carbohydrates in the U.S. comes from added sugars; the other half comes from starches (such as in pastas, breads, and potatoes). About 60% of dietary fat comes from animal sources and 40% from plant sources. On the global front, corn, rice, and wheat make up over 50% of staple foods. Top carbohydrate consumers are the developing nations as countries with lower incomes and limited crop exports often rely on staple low-cost foods that are primarily starchy and carbohydrate-rich. Topping the chart are Rwanda and Burundi, both in Africa, where over 80% of their dietary patterns are from carbohydrates such as plantains, cassava, peas, and maize. Such dietary patterns, over time, help to explain the high rates of malnutrition in these countries.

Sources: World Atlas, FAO

Adult dietary patterns show that U.S. adults consume about 15% of their calorie intake as proteins, 46% as carbohydrates, and 35% as fats.[8]

HEALTH OBJECTIVES FOR THE UNITED STATES

Health promotion and disease prevention have been public health strategies for the past several decades. Every 10 years, the U.S. Department of Health and Human Services (HHS) issues a collection of health objectives for the nation. These objectives are developed by experts in federal agencies, target major public health concerns, and set goals for the coming decade.

In 2020, the HHS's Office of Disease Prevention and Health Promotion released *Healthy People 2030,* the nation's 10-year plan for addressing our most critical public health priorities and challenges that includes 355 core, measurable objectives with 10-year targets.[9] Objectives are organized under five topics: (1) health conditions; (2) health behaviors; (3) populations; (4) settings and systems; and, for the first time, (5) social determinants of health. There are also new objectives related to opioid use disorder and youth e-cigarette use, and resources for adapting *Healthy People 2030* to emerging public health threats like COVID-19.

The overarching goals of *Healthy People 2030* are to:

- Attain healthy, thriving lives and well-being free of preventable disease, disability, injury, and premature death.
- Eliminate health disparities, achieve health equity, and attain health literacy to improve the health and well-being of all.
- Create social, physical, and economic environments that promote attaining the full potential for health and well-being for all.
- Promote healthy development, healthy behaviors, and well-being across all life stages.
- Engage leadership, key constituents, and the public across multiple sectors to take action and design policies that improve the health and well-being of all.

Healthy People 2030 includes a specific nutrition topic area called *Nutrition and Healthy Eating,* and its overall goal is to improve health by promoting healthy eating and making nutritious foods available. These nutrition-related objectives aim to encourage public health interventions:

- Reduce household food insecurity and hunger.
- Eliminate very low food security in children.
- Reduce iron deficiency in children aged 1 to 2 years.
- Increase the proportion of schools that don't sell less healthy foods and drinks.
- Increase consumption of fruits (especially whole fruit), vegetables (particularly dark green; red and orange; beans, peas, and lentils; starchy; and other vegetables), whole grains, calcium, potassium, and vitamin D.
- Reduce consumption of **added sugars,** saturated fat, and sodium.

added sugars Nutritive sweeteners (e.g., sugars and syrups) that are not naturally present in foods but are added during processing for the purpose of flavoring and/or preserving foods.

In addition to these general nutrition objectives, there are others that relate to nutrition issues specific to different life stages and diseases, including obesity, as well as objectives that focus on physical activity as well as food safety.

In the next section, we discuss recommendations to consume a variety of nutrient-dense foods within and across the food groups, especially vegetables; fruits; whole grains; seafood; eggs; beans, peas, and lentils; unsalted nuts and seeds; fat-free and low-fat dairy products; and lean meats and poultry—when prepared with no or little added sugars, saturated fat, and sodium. These foods will provide nutrients that are often overlooked, including various vitamins, minerals, fiber, and phytochemicals.

> ### ✓ CONCEPT CHECK 1.6
>
> 1. List the major characteristics of dietary patterns in the United States.
> 2. List three health objectives that could improve the health of adults.

1.7 What Can You Expect from Good Nutrition and a Healthy Lifestyle?

The obesity epidemic and prevalence of chronic diseases are evidence that many of our eating patterns and lifestyles are suboptimal. The strong association between obesity and poor health is clear. The reverse is also well documented. Yet the National Institutes of Health reports that when a person who is overweight or obese loses just 5% to 10% of body weight, that person's risks of many chronic diseases are greatly reduced.[10]

HEALTHY LIFESTYLE BEHAVIORS

Many aspects of our environment make it difficult to obtain and maintain healthy lifestyle behaviors and a healthy body composition. In Chapter 16, you will learn about the Blue Zones. These are regions across the globe where individuals tend to live to 100 years of age and prosper. These regions have been studied and are shown to engage in positive lifestyle behaviors that are linked to their healthy longevity. It's never too late to start!

THE TOTAL DIETARY PATTERN

Fortunately, we have more opportunities than ever before to make healthy choices! Today, we can choose from a wide variety of nutritious food products due to continual food innovations by manufacturers. We can enjoy our personal preferences, explore cultural diversity, celebrate varied cuisines, and become more adventurous eaters while maintaining diet quality.

Affluence, however, has also led to sedentary lifestyles and high intakes of added sugars, saturated fat, sodium, and alcohol. This lifestyle pattern has led to increases in cardiovascular disease, hypertension, diabetes, cancers, and obesity. Greater efforts are needed by the general public to improve variety in our dietary patterns, especially from fruits, vegetables, whole grains, legumes, seeds, and nuts. With better technology and greater choices, we can have a much healthier eating pattern today than ever before—if we know what choices to make!

Nutrition experts generally agree that there are no *good* or *bad* foods, but some foods provide relatively few nutrients in comparison to their calorie content. As you reexamine your lifestyle behaviors, remember your health is largely your responsibility. Your body has a natural ability to heal itself. Our current health is a byproduct of our behaviors over our lifespan. You can't change the past, but you certainly can impact your future.

Prevention of disease is an important investment. These recommendations will help promote health and prevent chronic diseases:

1. Consume enough essential nutrients, including fiber, while moderating calories, solid fat, and added sugars.
2. Minimize alcohol intake.
3. Consume sufficient water (9 to 13 cups per day).
4. Move more and sit less! Engage in adequate, regular physical activity (aim for at least 150 minutes throughout the week).
5. Identify effective (and healthy) coping mechanisms to manage stress.
6. Strive to get adequate sleep (7 to 9 hours per night).
7. Do not use tobacco products, e-cigarettes, vaping products, or illicit drugs.
8. Use prescribed medications prudently.

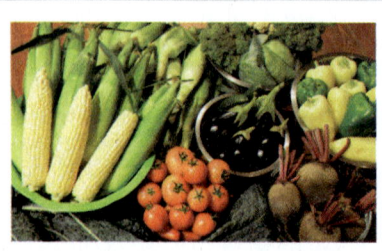

Access to fresh fruits and vegetables through farmers' markets and community gardens is important to a healthy lifestyle. **Do you know where your local farmers' market is located?** Visit the National Farmers Market Directory to find markets near you! Mary-Jon Ludy/McGraw Hill

ASK THE RDN: Is Food Medicine?

Dear RDN: *Social media posts have been promoting Food is Medicine or Food as Medicine. Can food replace medicine?*

The *White House Conference on Hunger, Nutrition, and Health* propelled the *Food is Medicine* platform to new heights in 2022. *Food is Medicine* (or *Food as Medicine*, according to some organizations) initiatives do not advocate that food should replace medicine or pharmaceuticals. Instead, it acknowledges that food plays a central role in supporting our health and well-being. Indeed, some nutrients and bioactive compounds found in whole foods have therapeutic effects on the body and contribute to disease prevention, management, and treatment.

Throughout the course, you will be provided with many examples of how specific nutrients support key physiological processes such as energy production, growth, repair, and immune function. For example, in terms of disease prevention, high-quality dietary patterns are associated with reduced risk of diet-related chronic diseases, including heart disease, type 2 diabetes, obesity, certain cancers, and neurological disorders. Furthermore, dietary strategies can help some people manage existing diseases.

Here are just a few examples of the ways food is medicine:

- It is well established that individuals with type 2 diabetes benefit from modifying their dietary patterns to manage blood sugar levels.
- Many foods possess anti-inflammatory properties to support a healthy immune system. Omega-3 fatty acids, walnuts, and flaxseeds are examples of anti-inflammatory food sources. Antioxidant-rich foods, such as leafy greens, berries, nuts, and seeds can also help protect against oxidative stress and support the immune system.
- Studies are now confirming that the gut microbiome can have a critical role in digestion, nutrient absorption, and immune function. Consuming a diverse range of fiber-rich foods like fruits, vegetables, legumes, and whole grains can promote a healthy gut microbiome, which in turn positively impacts overall health.
- Emerging research is now pointing to a link between dietary patterns and mental health. Certain nutrients, such as omega-3 fatty acids, B vitamins, and antioxidants, contribute to brain health and help manage conditions like depression and anxiety. Additionally, adopting a balanced diet and maintaining stable blood sugar levels can support stable mood and energy levels.

In sum, although food cannot replace medical treatments, it can significantly contribute to overall health and play a supportive role in preventing and managing various health conditions. When in doubt, consult with your primary care provider or a registered dietitian to develop personalized dietary approaches based on individual needs and health conditions.

Food is health,

Colleen Spees, PhD, MEd, RDN, LD, FAND

Associate Professor, The Ohio State University College of Medicine, Author of *Wardlaw's Contemporary Nutrition* and *Wardlaw's Contemporary Nutrition: A Functional Approach*

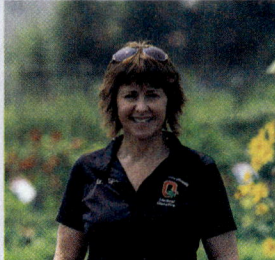

Wendy Pramik/The Ohio State University

✓ CONCEPT CHECK 1.7

1. What lifestyle patterns have led to increases in cardiovascular disease, hypertension, diabetes, cancers, and obesity?
2. What are the main dietary and lifestyle recommendations for health promotion and disease prevention?

1.8 Nutrition and Your Health: Nutrition Implications of Alcohol Consumption

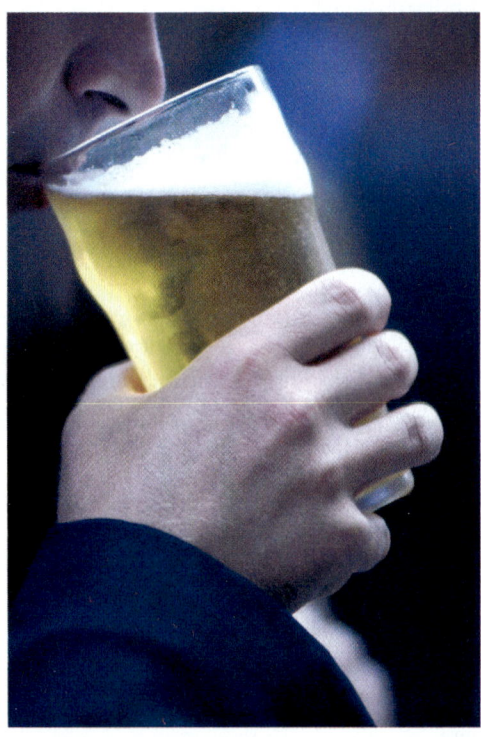

UK Stock Images Ltd/Grantly Lynch/Alamy Stock Photo

Given the wide spectrum of alcohol use and abuse, knowledge of alcohol consumption and its relationship to overall health is essential to the study of nutrition. Excessive alcohol intake results in over 95,000 deaths and costs our economy approximately $250 billion per year in the United States.[11]

Alcoholic beverages contain the chemical form of alcohol known as **ethanol.** Although not a nutrient, alcohol is a source of calories (about 7 kcal per gram). Over half of American adults drink alcohol. On average, alcohol accounts for about 5% of total calories in the average dietary pattern.

The *Dietary Guidelines for Americans* defines an alcoholic drink equivalent as 14 grams of alcohol.[12] Most cans or bottles of beer are 12 fluid ounces, but some may contain as much as 40 fluid ounces. Malt liquor and most craft beers have a slightly higher alcohol content than regular beer, so the equivalent drink size is 8 fluid ounces. For wine, a 5-fluid-ounce glass is the equivalent. The alcohol, carbohydrate, and calorie contents of standard drink sizes are depicted in Figure 1-13.

Moderate drinking is defined by the CDC as up to two drinks per day for adult males and up to one drink per day for adult females. **Heavy drinking** is usually defined as consuming 15 or more drinks per week for males and 8 or more drinks per week for females. **Binge drinking** is characterized by a pattern of drinking within a short period of time (usually within a few hours) causing blood alcohol concentration (BAC) to rise above the legal limit of 0.08%. It is defined as five or more drinks for adult males or four or more drinks for adult females in about 2 hours.

Moderate consumption of alcohol is viewed by most adults as an acceptable behavior with mixed health benefits. However, only about half of alcohol consumed is done so in moderation. One in six U.S. adults binge drinks, consuming about eight drinks per binge, about four times a month. Binge drinking is most common among younger adults ages 18 to 34 and is about twice as prevalent among males as among females. Problem drinking that becomes severe is given the medical diagnosis of **alcohol use disorder.** Over 16 million people in the United States have alcohol use disorder (often referred to as alcohol dependence or alcoholism). By far, alcohol is the most commonly abused drug in the U.S.

How Are Alcoholic Beverages Produced?

The basis of alcohol production is fermentation, a process by which microorganisms break down simple sugars (e.g., glucose or maltose) to alcohol, carbon dioxide, and water in the absence of oxygen. Wine is formed by the fermentation of grape or other fruit juices. Beer is made from malted cereal grain. Distilled spirits, such as vodka, gin, and whiskey, are made from any number of fruits, vegetables, and grains. The final characteristics of a product are determined by production temperatures, the composition of the food used for fermentation, and aging techniques. Alcohol *proof* represents twice the volume of alcohol in percentage terms. Thus, an 80 proof vodka contains 40% alcohol.

> **Rethink Your Drink**
> Have you ever wondered how much alcohol is in your drink? How many calories are in it? What is your cost per week, month, or year to drink? Visit the National Institutes of Health alcohol calculator at https://www.rethinkingdrinking.niaaa.nih.gov.
>
> Thankfully, mocktails and nonalcoholic cocktail options continue to grow in popularity, especially among younger consumers. See https://ific.org/media-information/press-releases/food-trends-for-2023/ for more info!

ethanol Chemical term for the form of alcohol found in alcoholic beverages.

moderate drinking For males, consuming no more than two drinks per day, and for females, consuming no more than one drink per day.

heavy drinking Any pattern of alcohol consumption defined as consuming 15 drinks or more per week for males and 8 drinks or more per week for females.

binge drinking Drinking sufficient alcohol within a 2-hour period to increase blood alcohol content to 0.08% or higher; for males, consuming five or more drinks in a row; for females, consuming four or more drinks in a row.

alcohol use disorder Problem drinking characterized by a compulsive pattern of alcohol use that leads to significant impairment or distress.

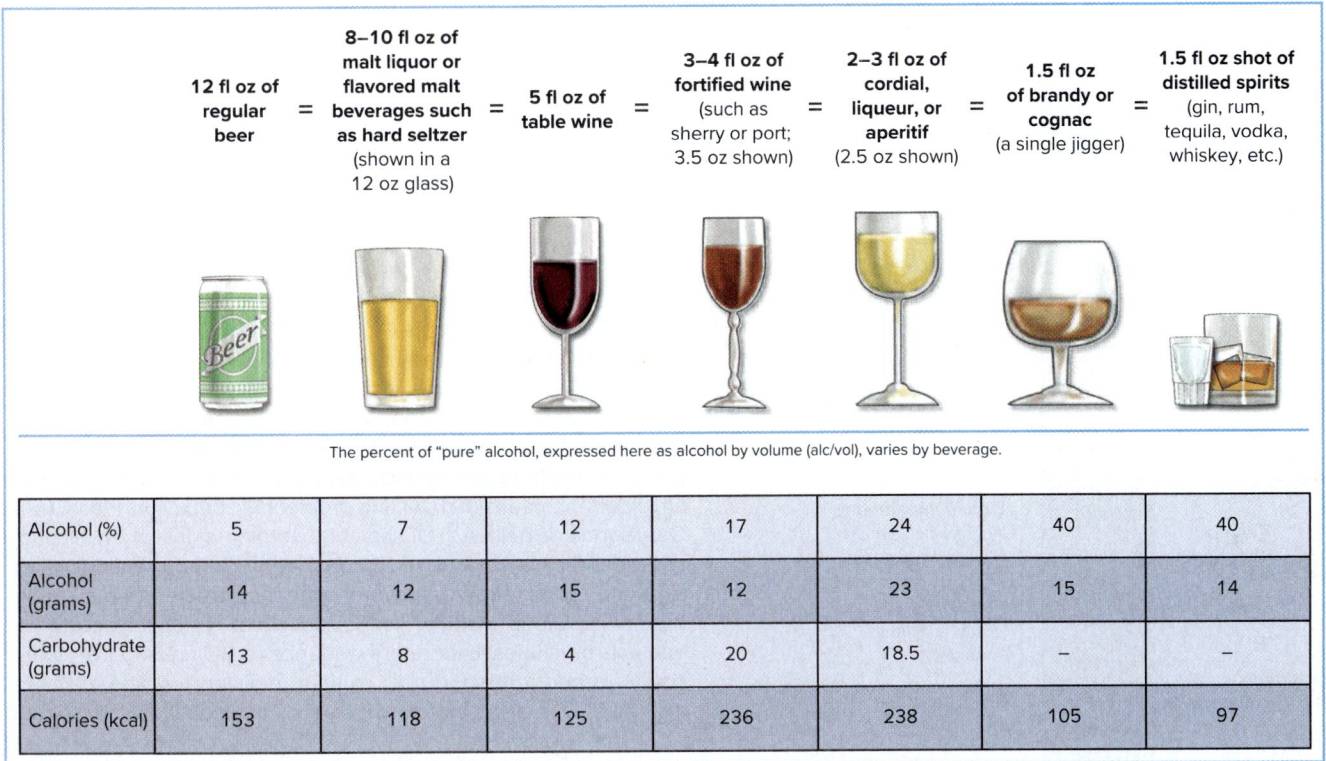

FIGURE 1-13 The standard drink sizes shown provide about 14 grams of alcohol. Keep in mind that alcoholic beverages served in bars and restaurants can be 20% to 45% larger than a standard drink.

Source: National Institute on Alcohol Abuse and Alcoholism

Absorption and Metabolism of Alcohol

Alcohol requires no digestion. It is absorbed rapidly from the GI tract by **passive diffusion,** making it the most efficiently absorbed of all calorie sources. Once absorbed, alcohol is freely distributed into all the fluid compartments within the body. About 1% to 3% of alcohol is excreted via urine, and about 1% to 5% evaporates via the breath, the basis for the breathalyzer test. Most alcohol (90% to 98%), however, is metabolized. The liver is the primary site for alcohol metabolism, and some may also be metabolized by the cells lining the stomach. The main pathway of alcohol metabolism involves the enzymes **alcohol dehydrogenase** and **acetaldehyde dehydrogenase.**

As a person's alcohol consumption exceeds the body's capacity to metabolize it, blood alcohol concentration rises, the brain is exposed to alcohol, and symptoms of impairment appear (Fig. 1-14). Absorption and metabolism of alcohol depend on numerous factors: genetics, sex, body size, physical condition, meal composition, gastric emptying rate, alcohol content of the beverage, certain drugs, chronic alcohol use, and level of fatigue. Females absorb and metabolize alcohol less efficiently than males. The amount of alcohol metabolized by the cells lining the stomach is greater in males than in females. Females also have less body water in which to dilute the alcohol than do males. Overall, females develop chronic alcohol-related ailments, such as cirrhosis of the liver, more rapidly than males do with the same alcohol-consumption habits.

Moderate Alcohol Use

The risks and benefits of moderate alcohol use remain controversial. The associated benefits with intakes of no more than two drinks per day for males and no more than one drink per day for females are linked to socialization and relaxation by people of legal drinking age. In terms of physiological benefits, moderate drinkers experience lower risk of developing cardiovascular diseases and type 2 diabetes. However, the National Cancer Institute documents that there is strong scientific consensus that alcohol consumption can cause several types of cancer.

Heavy Alcohol Use

Alcohol use disorder (AUD) is a medical diagnosis defined as a problematic pattern of alcohol use leading to significant impairment or distress. This definition integrates both alcohol abuse and alcohol dependence into a single disorder with mild, moderate, and severe subclassifications. According to the *DSM-5,* diagnosis

passive diffusion Movement of a substance across a semipermeable membrane from an area of higher solute concentration to an area of lower solute concentration. This type of transport does not require a carrier and does not require energy.

alcohol dehydrogenase An enzyme used in alcohol (ethanol) metabolism that converts alcohol into acetaldehyde.

acetaldehyde dehydrogenase An enzyme used in ethanol metabolism that eventually converts acetaldehyde into carbon dioxide and water.

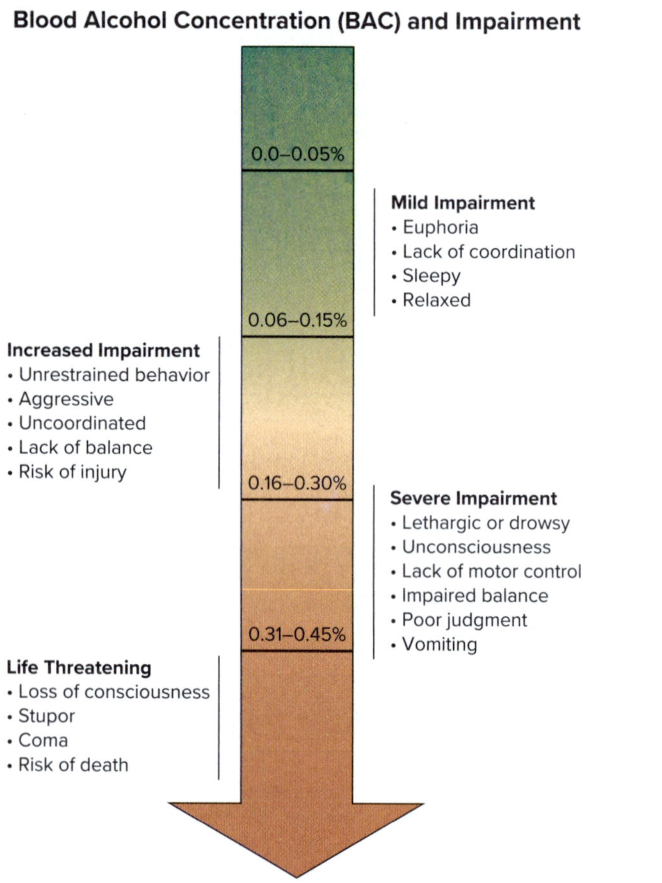

Blood Alcohol Concentration (BAC) and Impairment

- 0.0–0.05%

Mild Impairment
- Euphoria
- Lack of coordination
- Sleepy
- Relaxed

- 0.06–0.15%

Increased Impairment
- Unrestrained behavior
- Aggressive
- Uncoordinated
- Lack of balance
- Risk of injury

- 0.16–0.30%

Severe Impairment
- Lethargic or drowsy
- Unconsciousness
- Lack of motor control
- Impaired balance
- Poor judgment
- Vomiting

- 0.31–0.45%

Life Threatening
- Loss of consciousness
- Stupor
- Coma
- Risk of death

FIGURE 1-14 Signs and symptoms of alcohol overdose. It is important to recognize the observable signs of alcohol overdose. If you notice some signs of an overdose, do not hesitate to call 911 or wait for all symptoms to be present. Be alert and stay safe.
Source: Understanding the Dangers of Alcohol Overdose, https://www.niaaa.nih.gov/publications/brochures-and-fact-sheets/understanding-dangers-of-alcohol-overdose

depends on meeting two or more of the following criteria within the past year.[13] In the past year, have you:

- Had times when you ended up drinking more, or longer, than you intended?
- More than once wanted to reduce or stop drinking, or tried to, but couldn't?
- Spent a lot of time drinking? Or being sick or hungover?
- Wanted a drink so badly you couldn't think of anything else?
- Found that drinking—or being sick from drinking—often interfered with taking care of your home or family? Or caused issue at work or school?
- Continued to drink even though it was causing trouble with your family or friends?
- Quit or cut back on activities that were important or interesting to you, or gave you pleasure, in order to drink?
- Gotten into situations while or after drinking that increased your chances of getting hurt (such as driving, swimming, using machinery, walking in a dangerous area, or having unsafe sex)?
- Continued to drink even though it was making you feel depressed or anxious or adding to other health problems? Or after having had a memory blackout?

- Had to drink much more than you once did to get the effect you want? Or found that your usual number of drinks had much less effect than before?
- Found that when the effects of alcohol were wearing off, you had withdrawal symptoms, such as trouble sleeping, shakiness, restlessness, nausea, sweating, a racing heart, or a seizure? Or sensed things that were not there?

Alcohol use disorders affect about 17% of adult males and about 8% of adult females at some point in their lives. Studies suggest over half of a person's risk for developing these disorders is genetic.[14] Therefore, people with a family history of heavy drinking, particularly children of parents with alcohol use disorders, should be especially aware of their alcohol consumption.

Early diagnosis of alcohol use disorders can prevent multiple health problems and save millions in health care costs. Asking a person about the quantity and frequency of alcohol consumption is an important means of detecting problematic behaviors (see CAGE Questionnaire below).[15] Observable warning signs of an alcohol use disorder may include an alcohol odor on the breath, flushed face and reddened skin, nervous system disorders (such as tremors), unexplained work or school absences, frequent accidents, and falls or injuries. Laboratory evidence (e.g., impaired liver function, enlarged red blood cells, nutrient deficiencies, and elevated triglycerides) is also helpful for diagnosis of alcohol use disorders.

> **CAGE Questionnaire**
>
> The CAGE Questionnaire is used to identify alcohol use disorders. More than one positive response suggests an alcohol problem.
>
> **C:** Have you ever felt you ought to _cut_ down on drinking?
> **A:** Have people _annoyed_ you by criticizing your drinking?
> **G:** Have you ever felt bad or _guilty_ about your drinking?
> **E:** Have you ever had a drink first thing in the morning to steady your nerves or get rid of a hangover (an _eye-opener_)?
>
> Source: https://pubs.niaaa.nih.gov/publications/arh28-2/78-79.htm

Although it is one of the most preventable health problems, alcohol use disorders typically reduce a person's life expectancy by up to 30 years. It is most damaging to the liver. **Cirrhosis** develops in up to 20% of cases of alcohol use disorders and is a leading reason for liver transplants, affecting about 2 million people in the U.S.[16] This chronic and usually relentlessly progressive disease is characterized by fatty infiltration of the liver. Fatty liver occurs in response to increased synthesis of fat and decreased use of it for energy by the liver. Eventually, the enlarged fat deposits choke off the blood supply, depriving the liver cells of oxygen and nutrients. Liver cells eventually accumulate so much fat that they burst, die, and are replaced by connective (scar) tissue. At this stage, the liver is deemed cirrhotic (Fig. 1-15). Early stages of alcoholic liver injury are reversible, but advanced stages are not. Once a person has cirrhosis, there is a 50% chance of death within 4 years, a far worse prognosis than

cirrhosis A loss of functioning liver cells, which are replaced by nonfunctioning connective tissue. Any substance that poisons liver cells can lead to cirrhosis. The most common cause is chronic, excessive alcohol intake. Exposure to certain industrial chemicals also can lead to cirrhosis.

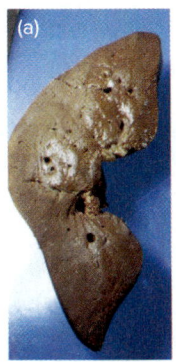 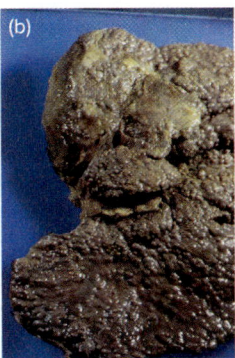

FIGURE 1-15 Effects of alcohol on the liver. Alcohol is particularly damaging to this organ. Pictured are: (a) a healthy liver and (b) a liver with cirrhosis. There is no cure for this disease except a liver transplant. Arthur Glauberman/Science Source

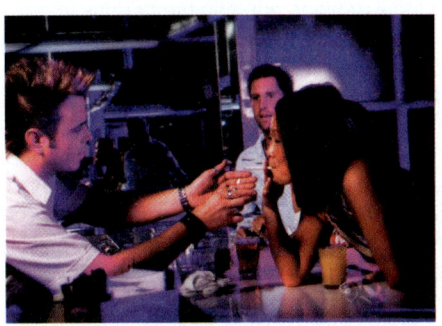

For many people, drinking and smoking go hand in hand. **What health problems arise from the combination of these behaviors?** Ingram Publishing/Getty Images

for many cancers. Although no specific level of alcohol consumption guarantees cirrhosis, some evidence suggests that damage is caused by a dose as low as 25 grams per day (less than 2 beers).

Alcoholic beverages have little nutritional value, and thus nutrient deficiencies are a common result of alcohol use disorders. The protein and vitamin contents are extremely low to marginal. Iron content varies widely between drinks, with red wine ranking higher in iron. Deficiencies arise mainly from poor nutrient intakes, but increased urinary losses and fat malabsorption (linked to poor pancreatic function) also contribute. Vitamins most susceptible to depletion from heavy drinking include thiamin, vitamins A, D, E, and K; niacin; folate; vitamins B-6 and B-12; and vitamin C. Mineral deficiencies of calcium, phosphorus, potassium, magnesium, zinc, and iron are also possible. Conversely, vitamin and mineral toxicity is also of concern with heavy drinking. Damage to the GI tract and liver, as well as high levels of some minerals in alcoholic beverages, may lead to toxicity of vitamin A, iron, lead, or cobalt. In nutritional treatment of alcohol use disorders, the immediate aim is eliminating alcohol intake, followed by restoration of nutrient stores.

Older adults are uniquely vulnerable to alcohol use disorders, perhaps due to an abundance of free time, social events involving drinking, interactions with medications, loneliness, or depression. Common symptoms of alcohol use disorders—trembling hands, slurred speech, sleep problems, memory loss, and unsteady gait—can be easily overlooked as signs of aging. Slower alcohol metabolism and decreased body water allow older adults to become intoxicated from a smaller amount of alcohol than their younger counterparts. Even moderate alcohol consumption can exacerbate some chronic health conditions, such as diabetes and osteoporosis. As well, small amounts of alcohol can react negatively with various medications used by older persons. The adverse health effects of drinking may be amplified in older adults, so the National Institute of Alcohol Abuse and Alcoholism (NIAAA) recommends people over the age of 65 limit alcohol consumption to no more than seven drinks in one week.

Once a diagnosis of an alcohol use disorder is established, a primary care provider can arrange appropriate treatment and counseling for the person and their family. Treatment often includes the use of targeted medications, counseling, and social support. *Alcoholics Anonymous* or other reputable therapy programs can support those struggling with alcohol use disorders and their families as they recover from this devastating disease.

Guidance Regarding Alcohol Use

The following are guidelines regarding the use of alcoholic beverages:

- The *Dietary Guidelines* do not recommend that individuals who do not currently drink alcohol start drinking for any reason.
- Replace alcohol with mocktails and nonalcoholic drink options. These trends continue to grow in popularity—especially for younger consumers.

magnificent microbiome

Definitions
Some fermented foods contain live microorganisms, called *probiotics*. During processing, live organisms and any microbiota benefits are removed from beer and wine. *Microbiota* refers to the entire population of microorganisms (bacteria, fungi, viruses, and parasites) living in a specific environment. *Microbiome* includes the microbiota, their genetic code, and their immediate environment. Look for interesting facts about the magnificent microbiome in every chapter.

probiotics Live microorganisms that, when administered in adequate amounts, confer health benefits on the host.

microbiota Community of microorganisms living in a particular region; with regard to our discussion of probiotics, the community of microorganisms coexisting on and within the human body.

microbiome Entire collection of microorganisms, their genes, and their environment.

- If adults of legal drinking age choose to drink in moderation, they should limit intake to two drinks or less in a day for males and one drink or less in a day for females. Drinking less is better for health than drinking more.
- Alcoholic beverages are not a component of the USDA Dietary Patterns. The amount of alcohol and calories in beverages varies and should be accounted for within the limits of healthy dietary patterns, so that calorie limits are not exceeded.
- Individuals should not drink if they are driving, are planning to drive or operate machinery, or are participating in other activities requiring skill, coordination, and alertness.
- There are also some people who should not drink at all, such as if they are pregnant or might be pregnant, are breastfeeding, or are under the legal age for drinking; if they have certain medical conditions or are taking certain medications that can interact with alcohol; and if they are recovering from an alcohol use disorder or are unable to control the amount they drink.

To learn more about alcohol, visit these websites:

- National Institute on Alcohol Abuse and Alcoholism: www.niaaa.nih.gov
- American Society of Addiction Medicine: www.asam.org
- Centers for Disease Control and Prevention: www.cdc.gov/alcohol

✓ CONCEPT CHECK 1.8

1. Describe two risks of alcohol consumption.
2. What are four criteria used to diagnose alcohol use disorder?
3. The *Dietary Guidelines* recommend that which groups of individuals completely refrain from alcohol consumption?

CASE STUDY: Choosing a Healthy Lifestyle

Harrison is a 20-year-old college student that often finds himself feeling stressed and fatigued. His dietary pattern primarily consists of quick, grab-and-go convenience foods and alcohol to unwind after a long day of classes and studying. Lately, he's been pulling all-nighters, neglecting regular meals, and opting for sugary snacks and caffeinated drinks to keep him going.

Harrison's unhealthy behaviors have begun to take a toll on his physical and mental well-being. His academic performance is suffering, and he frequently experiences mood swings and low energy levels. Answer the questions below to determine the healthiest yet time-saving options for Harrison.

1. Would a low-fat granola bar and iced coffee from the grab-and-go be a good source of calories and nutrients for Harrison? Would this choice satisfy his hunger for very long?
2. Harrison could also pick up a ham, egg, and cheese bagel to eat during class. How do the calorie, fat, and sodium contents of this breakfast sandwich compare to the granola and iced coffee option? Would this be a healthy breakfast choice every day?
3. What steps can Harrison take to establish a balanced routine that prioritizes both academics and self-care? How can Harrison manage stress and relax without relying on alcohol?

Complete the Case Study. Responses to these questions can be provided by your instructor.

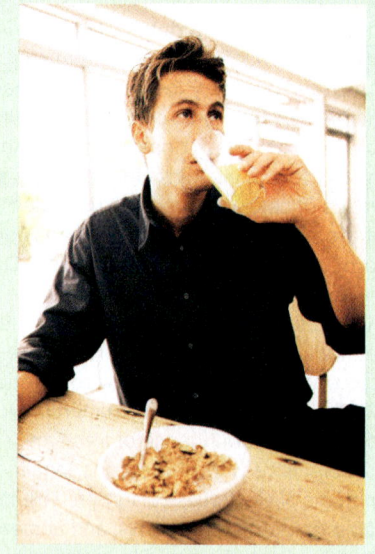

With a little bit of planning, healthy choices can be both quick and healthy. Stockbyte/Getty Images

Summary (Numbers refer to numbered sections in the chapter)

1.1 The taste, flavor, texture, and appearance of foods primarily influence our food choices. Several other factors also help determine eating patterns and choices: food availability and convenience, early childhood experiences and ethnic customs, nutrition and health concerns, advertising, restaurants, environmental sustainability, genetics, and economics. A variety of external (appetite-related) forces affect satiety (feeling of satisfaction that halts our desire to continue eating). Hunger cues combine with appetite cues, such as easy availability of food, to promote food intake.

1.2 Nutrition is a lifestyle factor that is a key to developing and maintaining an optimal state of health. Food provides the energy (in the form of calories) as compounds needed to build and maintain all body cells. Nutrients are the substances obtained from food that are vital for growth and maintenance of a healthy body throughout life. A suboptimal eating pattern and a sedentary lifestyle are known to be risk factors for life-threatening chronic diseases such as heart disease, hypertension, diabetes, and cancer. Failing to meet nutrient needs in younger years makes us more likely to suffer poor health consequences in later years.

1.3 Nutrition is the study of how the body uses food substances to promote and support growth, maintenance, and reproduction of cells. Essential nutrients in foods fall into six classes: (1) carbohydrates; (2) lipids (mostly fats and oils); (3) proteins; (4) vitamins; (5) minerals; and (6) water. The first three are macronutrients and, along with alcohol, provide calories for the body to use. Vitamins and minerals are micronutrients. Phytochemicals are plant chemicals that may contribute to a reduced risk of disease in people who consume them.

1.4 The body transforms the energy contained in carbohydrate, protein, and fat into other forms of energy that in turn allow the body to function. Fat provides, on average, 9 kcal per gram, whereas both protein and carbohydrate provide, on average, 4 kcal per gram. Alcohol also supplies about 7 kcal per gram. Calculating percentages and converting English units to metric units are important skills needed for the study of nutrition.

1.5 The scientific method is the process for testing the validity of possible explanations of a phenomenon, called hypotheses. Experiments are conducted to either support or refute a specific hypothesis. Once we have enough experimental information to support a specific hypothesis, it then can be called a theory. All of us need to be skeptical of new ideas in the nutrition field, waiting until many lines of experimental evidence support a concept before adopting any suggested dietary practice. Systematic reviews, randomized controlled trials, and cohort studies provide the most reliable scientific evidence.

1.6 Although complex, eating larger portions of calorie-dense foods and beverages and not engaging in enough physical activity are thought to contribute to the growing obesity crisis. Results from large nutrition surveys suggest that more of us need to focus on consuming dietary patterns that supply healthier options rich in vitamins, minerals, and fiber. The *Dietary Guidelines for Americans* and *Healthy People 2030* are national initiatives that include specific objectives related to healthful dietary patterns. These objectives aim to help encourage people to consume the recommended amounts of healthy foods and nutrients—like fruits, vegetables, whole grains, legumes, seeds, and nuts—to reduce their risk for chronic diseases and improve their health.

1.7 A basic plan for health promotion and disease prevention includes following a varied dietary pattern, performing regular physical activity, not using tobacco products, consuming adequate water and other fluids, getting enough sleep, limiting alcohol intake (if consumed), and appropriately coping with stress. The primary focus of nutrition planning should be on food, not on dietary supplements.

1.8 Alcohol contributes approximately 7 kcal per gram, requires no digestion, and is metabolized primarily in the liver. The risks of alcohol use far exceed any potential benefits. If alcohol is consumed, it should only be consumed in moderation and preferably with meals. Females (and older adults, in general) are advised to drink no more than one drink per day; males should drink no more than two drinks per day.

Check Your Knowledge (Answers are available at the end of this question set)

1. Our primary psychological drive to eat that is affected by many external food-choice mechanisms is called
   a. hunger.
   b. appetite.
   c. satiety.
   d. feeding.

2. Energy-yielding nutrients include
   a. vitamins, minerals, and water.
   b. carbohydrates, proteins, and fats.
   c. trace minerals and fat-soluble vitamins.
   d. iron, vitamin C, and potassium.

3. The essential nutrients
   a. must be consumed at every meal.
   b. are required for infants but not adults.
   c. can be made in the body when they are needed.
   d. cannot be made by the body and therefore must be consumed to maintain health.

4. Sugars, starches, and dietary fibers are examples of
   a. proteins.
   b. vitamins.
   c. carbohydrates.
   d. minerals.

5. Which nutrient classes are most important in the regulation of body processes?
   a. Vitamins
   b. Carbohydrates
   c. Minerals
   d. Both a and c

6. A food that contains 10 grams of fat would yield _____ kcal.
   a. 40   b. 70   c. 90   d. 120

7. A kcal is a
   a. measure of heat energy.
   b. measure of fat in food.
   c. heating device.
   d. term used to describe the amount of sugar and fat in foods.

8. If you consume 300 grams of carbohydrate in a day that you consume 2400 kcal, the carbohydrates will provide _____ % of your total energy intake.
   a. 12.5   b. 30   c. 50   d. 60

9. Which of the following is true about dietary patterns in the United States?
   a. Most of our protein comes from plant sources.
   b. About half of our carbohydrates come from simple sugars.
   c. Most of our fats come from plant sources.
   d. Most of our carbohydrates come from starches.

10. Alcohol is most damaging to the
    a. brain cells because alcohol can be used as an energy source even before glucose.
    b. kidney cells because this is where alcohol is excreted.
    c. gallbladder because this is where alcohol is stored.
    d. liver cells because this is where alcohol is metabolized.

Answer Key: 1. b (LO 1.1), 2. b (LO 1.3), 3. d (LO 1.3), 4. c (LO 1.3), 5. d (LO 1.3), 6. c (LO 1.4), 7. a (LO 1.4), 8. c (LO 1.4), 9. c (LO 1.5), 10. d (LO 1.8)

Study Questions (Numbers refer to Learning Outcomes)

1. What part of the brain controls hunger and satiety in the body? List other factors that influence our food choices. **(LO 1.1)**

2. Describe how your food preferences have been shaped by the following factors:
   a. Exposure to foods at an early age
   b. Advertising
   c. Dining out
   d. Peer pressure
   e. Economic factors **(LO 1.1)**

3. What products in your supermarket reflect the consumer demand for healthier foods? For convenience? **(LO 1.1)**

4. Name one chronic disease associated with poor diet quality. Now list a few corresponding risk factors. **(LO 1.2)**

5. Describe two sources of fat, and explain why the differences are important in terms of overall health. **(LO 1.3)**

6. Identify three ways that water is used in the body. **(LO 1.3)**

7. Explain the concept of calories as it relates to foods. What are the values used to calculate calories from grams of carbohydrate, fat, protein, and alcohol? **(LO 1.4)**

8. A bowl of broccoli cheddar soup contains 21 grams of carbohydrate, 13 grams of fat, and 12 grams of protein. Calculate the percentage of calories derived from fat. **(LO 1.4)**

9. List the steps of the scientific method used to test a hypothesis. **(LO 1.5)**

10. According to national nutrition surveys, which nutrients tend to be underconsumed by many adults? Why do you think this is the case? **(LO 1.6)**

11. List recommendations that can promote your health and prevent chronic diseases. **(LO 1.7)**

12. List two risks of heavy drinking. Should a nondrinker take up drinking for the health benefits? **(LO 1.8)**

References

1. U.S. Bureau of Labor Statistics. *American Time Use Survey.* Table A-1 (Time spent in detailed primary activities and percent of the civilian population engaging in each activity, averages per day by sex, 2022 anual averages). https://www.bls.gov/tus/a1-2022.pdf

2. International Food Information Council Foundation (IFIC). *2023 Food & Health Survey.* Sept 19, 2023. https://foodinsight.org/2023-food-and-health-survey/

3. The impact of food advertising on childhood obesity. American Psychological Association. Accessed Sept 21, 2023. https://www.apa.org/topics/obesity/food-advertising-children

4. Media & eating disorders. National Eating Disorders Association. Accessed Sept 14, 2023. https://www.nationaleatingdisorders.org/media-eating-disorders

5. Sims T. Where do sustainable and healthy food choices intersect? *Food Insight.* July 25, 2019. Accessed Sept 12, 2023. https://foodinsight.org/healthy-diets-environmental-sustainability

6. Overweight & obesity: adult obesity prevalence maps. Centers for Disease Control and Prevention. Accessed Sept 19, 2023. https://www.cdc.gov/obesity/data/prevalence-maps.html

7. Overweight & obesity: adult obesity facts. Centers for Disease Control and Prevention. June 2021. Accessed October 12, 2021. https://www.cdc.gov/obesity/data/adult.html

8. Centers for Disease Control and Prevention, National Center for Health Statistics. May 17, 2023. Accessed Sept 19, 2023. https://www.cdc.gov/nchs/fastats/diet.htm

9. U.S. Department of Health and Human Services, Office of Disease Prevention and Health Promotion. April 26, 2022. Accessed Sept 21, 2023. https://health.gov/healthypeople

10. Magkos F, Fraterrigo G, Yoshino J, et al. Effects of moderate and subsequent progressive weight loss on metabolic function and adipose tissue biology in humans with obesity. *Cell Metab*. 2016 Feb 22. pii: S1550-4131(16)30053-5. doi: 10.1016/j.cmet.2016.02.005. [Epub ahead of print]. PMID: 26916363.

11. Excessive alcohol use. Centers for Disease Control and Prevention, National Center for Chronic Disease Prevention and Health Promotion (NCCDPHP). September 2020. Accessed October 12, 2021. https://www.cdc.gov/chronicdisease/resources/publications/factsheets/alcohol.htm

12. U.S. Department of Agriculture, U.S. Department of Health and Human Services. *Dietary Guidelines for Americans, 2020–2025*. 9th ed. December 2020. http://DietaryGuidelines.gov

13. Alcohol use disorder. National Institutes of Health, National Institute on Alcohol Abuse and Alcoholism. Accessed October 17, 2021. https://www.niaaa.nih.gov/publications/brochures-and-fact-sheets/alcohol-use-disorder-comparison-between-dsm

14. Understanding alcohol use disorder. National Institutes of Health, National Institute on Alcohol Abuse and Alcoholism. Accessed October 12, 2021. https://www.niaaa.nih.gov/publications/brochures-and-fact-sheets/understanding-alcohol-use-disorder

15. National Institutes of Health, National Institute on Alcohol Abuse and Alcoholism. *Assessing Alcohol Problems: A Guide for Clinicians and Researchers*. 2nd ed. NIH Pub. No. 03–3745. U.S. Dept. of Health and Human Services, Public Health Service; revised 2003. http://pubs.niaaa.nih.gov/publications/AssessingAlcohol/index.htm

16. Cholankeril G, Ahmed A. Alcoholic liver disease replaces hepatitis C virus infection as the leading indication for liver transplantation in the United States. *Clin Gastroenterol Hepatol*. 2018 Aug;16(8):1356-1358. doi: 10.1016/j.cgh.2017.11.045

Design Element Credits: Fact Check/magnifying glass icon: McGraw Hill; Magnificent Microbiome background image: Alena Ohneva/Shutterstock; Sustainable Solutions icon: McGraw Hill; Roots icon: McGraw Hill; Medicine Cabinet icon: Peter Dazeley/Photographer's Choice/Getty Images

Chapter 2: Designing a Healthy Eating Pattern

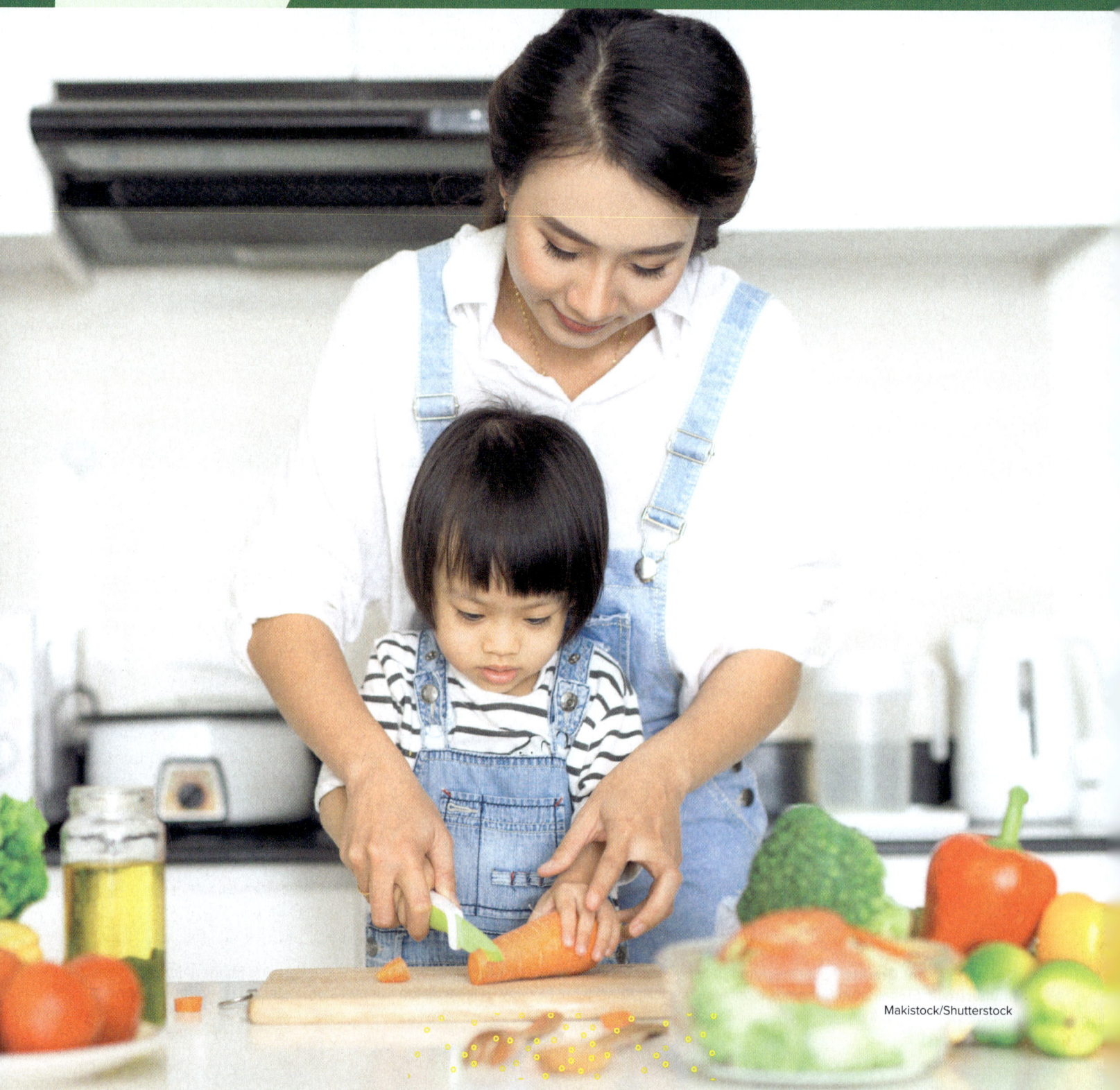

Makistock/Shutterstock

Student Learning Outcomes

Chapter 2 is designed to allow you to:

2.1 Outline the basic principles of a healthy dietary pattern using the concepts of nutrient density and energy density.

2.2 List the purpose and key recommendations of the *Dietary Guidelines* and the *Physical Activity Guidelines for Americans*.

2.3 Design a meal that conforms to MyPlate recommendations.

2.4 Describe the two forms of malnutrition.

2.5 Outline the **A**nthropometric, **B**iochemical, **C**linical, **D**ietary, and **E**nvironmental (ABCDE) measurements used in nutritional assessment.

2.6 Describe the specific categories of nutrient recommendations within the Dietary Reference Intakes.

2.7 Identify reliable sources of nutrition information.

2.8 Use the Nutrition Facts label, list of ingredients, and health and nutrient claims on food labels to choose nutrient-dense foods.

2.9 Identify food and nutrition issues relevant to college students.

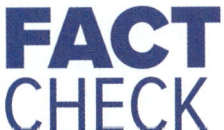
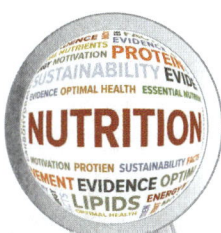

In MyPlate, do beans, peas, and lentils count as a part of the Protein Foods Group or the Vegetable Group?

This chapter is designed to provide you with the tools you need to craft a healthy and sustainable dietary pattern to promote optimal health and wellness. The *Dietary Guidelines for Americans* will guide you on this journey as we explore the components of healthy eating and lifestyle patterns—an approach that will minimize your risks of developing nutrition-related diseases. The goal is to gain a firm understanding of these concepts before you study the key nutrients in detail. Just like in the captivating photograph on the previous page, lifelong dietary patterns can be fostered from an early age, and the joy of consuming nutritious foods and beverages can be passed through generations.

MyPlate was developed to help consumers adopt the *Dietary Guidelines* and empower consumers to make better food choices. Overall, there are five MyPlate food groups: fruits, vegetables, grains, dairy, and protein foods. In this chapter, we will explore the nutritional benefits of each food group.

Collectively, beans, peas, and lentils are known as *pulses*. Pulses are the edible seeds found in the pods of legumes (a type of plant that bears its seeds in pods). Specific examples of pulses include kidney beans, pinto beans, black beans, pink beans, black-eyed peas, garbanzo beans (chickpeas), split peas, pigeon peas, mung beans, and lentils of various colors. You may find them dry, canned, or frozen. They are all excellent sources of protein, dietary fiber, and many vitamins and minerals. These nutritional properties are similar to both vegetables and protein foods, so they may be classified into either food group!

Visit Section 2.3 in this chapter to decide where beans, peas, and lentils fit into your MyPlate plan.

2.1 A Food Philosophy That Works

Does a healthy lifestyle mean you have to give up your favorite foods? Absolutely not! A healthy eating pattern should not be restrictive, monotonous, or overpriced. There are no inherently *good* or *bad* foods. Most nutrition experts agree that all foods can fit. Eating well to optimize health and minimize your risk for nutrition-related diseases involves three core dietary principles:

- Meet your nutritional needs primarily from foods and beverages.
- Choose a variety of options from each food group.
- Pay attention to portion size.

Let's describe these principles in more detail and identify ways you can apply them in your own life.

MEET NUTRITIONAL NEEDS PRIMARILY FROM FOODS AND BEVERAGES

You learned in Chapter 1 that foods and beverages provide the nutrients that serve as fuel, building blocks, and regulators for a healthy body. The quality and quantity of the foods and beverages you choose can have an important impact on your health outcomes.

Each person requires a certain amount of energy (i.e., calories) to maintain vital functions and support physical activity. A mismatch between your usual energy intake and your daily calorie requirements can lead to changes in body weight, which may be undesirable and/or accompanied by health risks.

What Is Nutrient Density? To meet our daily nutrient needs within our calorie limits, we must choose nutrient-dense foods and beverages most of the time. The **nutrient density** of a food or beverage is a comparison of its nutrient content with the amount of calories it provides. Foods and beverages are characterized as nutrient dense if they provide a large amount of a nutrient (or nutrients) relative to calories. To summarize the concept:

nutrient density The ratio derived by dividing a food's nutrient content by its calorie content. When the food's overall nutrient contribution exceeds its contribution to our calorie needs, the food is considered to have a favorable nutrient density.

$$\text{Nutrient density} = \frac{\text{Amount of nutrient per serving}}{\text{Amount of calories per serving}}$$

Generally, nutrient density is evaluated with respect to individual nutrients. For example, let's compare a whole, fresh orange to a serving of orange juice. Like many fruits and vegetables, both of these options are sources of vitamin C. One medium orange provides 70 milligrams (mg) of vitamin C and 60 kcal. One cup of orange juice provides 85 milligrams of vitamin C and 120 kcal.

1 medium orange
$$\frac{70 \text{ mg of vitamin C}}{60 \text{ kcal}} = 1.2 \text{ mg/kcal}$$

1 cup of orange juice
$$\frac{85 \text{ mg of vitamin C}}{120 \text{ kcal}} = 0.7 \text{ mg/kcal}$$

This example shows that the whole, fresh fruit is a more nutrient-dense source of vitamin C than the fruit juice. You are more likely to meet your nutrient needs without exceeding your daily calorie needs if you choose whole fruits instead of fruit juice. This is just one example of a simple swap you can use to make more nutrient-dense choices in your eating pattern. Figure 2-1 also shows other ways you can apply nutrient-dense swaps to improve your overall dietary pattern.

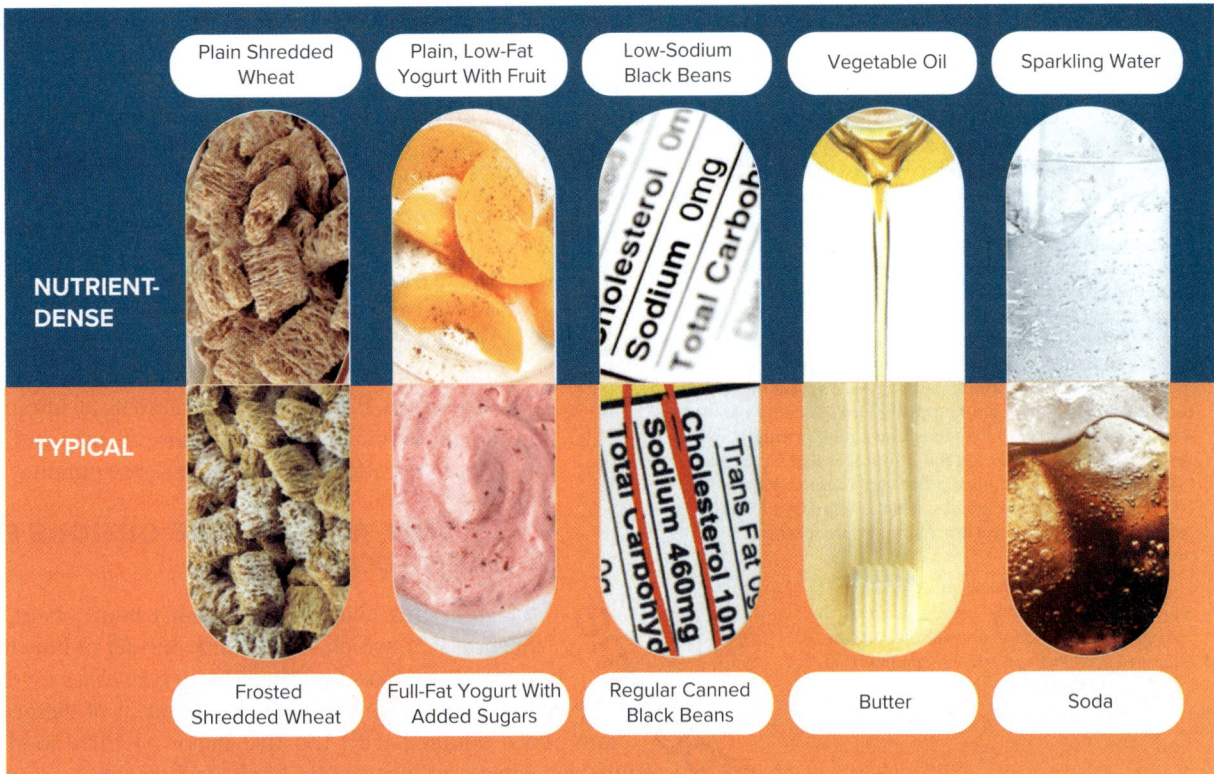

FIGURE 2-1 The *Dietary Guidelines* promotes simple swaps to increase the nutrient density of your dietary pattern. Every food and beverage choice is an opportunity to move toward a healthy dietary pattern. These are just a few examples of small, realistic dietary modifications you can make throughout the day. Several small changes can add up to a big difference in the nutrient density of your dietary pattern.

U. S. Department of Agriculture and U. S. Department of Health and Human Services. *Dietary Guidelines for Americans, 2020–2025*. 9th Edition. December 2020. Available at DietaryGuidelines.gov

How Does Food Processing Impact the Nutrient Density of Foods? Recently, researchers have been exploring the impact of food processing on diet quality and health outcomes. Food processing can affect the nutrient density of foods (and overall dietary patterns) in either positive or negative ways. There are several ways to define and categorize processed foods, but the most popular one is the Nova classification.[1] In the Nova classification, foods are separated into four categories:

- Group 1: Unprocessed or minimally processed foods. This group includes fresh, frozen, or dried fruits or vegetables; grains; legumes; meat; fish; and milk that have undergone no processing or have only been processed by grinding, roasting, pasteurization, or freezing. Examples: frozen vegetables, dried herbs, dried lentils, fresh eggs, oatmeal, milk, or plain yogurt.
- Group 2: Processed culinary ingredients. This group includes substances that have been extracted, pressed, or centrifuged from Group 1 foods or from nature to be used in culinary preparations. Examples: table sugar, maple syrup, plant oils, butter, and table salt.
- Group 3: Processed foods. This group includes foods that are manufactured using unprocessed or minimally processed foods (from Group 1) along with some processed culinary ingredients (from Group 2). Examples: canned fruits; artisinal breads; cheeses; salted nuts; salted, smoked, or cured meat or fish.
- Group 4: **Ultraprocessed foods.** This group includes foods that are industrial formulations of several ingredients, including Group 2 ingredients and small or no amounts of whole foods. These foods typically contain a variety of additives such as flavors, colors, sweeteners, and emulsifiers. Examples: commercially prepared baked goods, candies, packaged snacks, sausage, chicken nuggets, soft drinks, artificial sweeteners, enriched bread and pasta, frozen meals, and ready-to-eat breakfast cereals.

ultraprocessed foods Edible products made with industrial formulations of several ingredients that are derived from whole foods or synthesized by food manufacturers, typically including additives such as flavors, colors, sweeteners, or emulsifiers.

magnificent microbiome

Dietary Patterns Influence the Gut Microbiota

Dietary patterns are associated with risks for various noncommunicable diseases, such as cardiovascular diseases, type 2 diabetes, cancer, and depression. Although the nutrient contributions of dietary patterns certainly play a role, researchers are increasingly interested in the role of the gut microbiota as a mediator of the link between dietary patterns and disease. The foods and beverages we consume provide energy and nutrients for human cells, of course, but they also provide sustenance for the vast community of microorganisms that live inside the gastrointestinal tract. The gut microbiota, in turn, produces many compounds that influence human health. Recently, researchers have observed a relationship between intakes of highly processed (or ultraprocessed) foods and human health. Indeed, ultra-processed foods influence the composition of the microbiota, which likely plays a role in the relationship between the intake of ultraprocessed foods and health outcomes.

Source: Cuevas-Sierra A, Milagro FI, Aranaz P, Martínez JA, Riezu-Boj JI. Gut microbiota differences according to ultra-processed food consumption in a Spanish population. *Nutrients.* 2021;13(8):2710. Published 2021 Aug 6. doi:10.3390/nu13082710

Food processing has both pros and cons. A dietary pattern dominated by foods processed with added sugars, salt, and fat may make it difficult to meet nutrient needs within calorie limits and may contribute to risks for heart disease and hypertension. On the other hand, some food processing makes foods safer to eat. For example, the addition of salt or sugar to foods can inhibit bacterial growth. With prolonged shelf life, some processed foods are more affordable and accessible. Also, processes such as fortification add nutrients to certain foods. In fact, enriched wheat flour, yogurt, and fortified, ready-to-eat breakfast cereals—categorized as ultraprocessed foods by the Nova classification—make important contributions to meeting daily nutrient needs for many Americans. If we attempt to eliminate all ultraprocessed foods from our dietary patterns, we may end up omitting many affordable, nutrient-dense options.[2]

CHOOSE A VARIETY OF OPTIONS FROM EACH FOOD GROUP

Later in this chapter, you'll learn more about MyPlate (Section 2.3), which is a visual reminder of how to build a balanced meal based on the *Dietary Guidelines for Americans* (Section 2.2). As we introduce the concept of dietary variety, familiarize yourself with the five major MyPlate food groups: fruits, vegetables, grains, protein foods, and dairy.

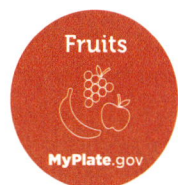 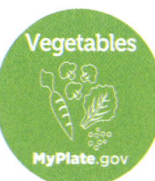 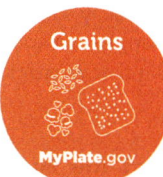 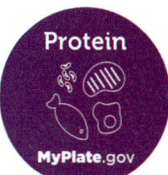 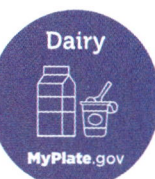

U.S. Department of Agriculture or USDA

Dietary variety means two things: (1) choosing foods from all the food groups and (2) mixing up your selections within each food group. This concept is important for achieving nutrient adequacy because each food provides some nutrients, but no single food provides all the essential nutrients.

In our discussion of nutrient density in the last section, we focused on oranges. Citrus fruits, which are highlighted in the *Farm to Fork* feature in this chapter, are good sources of carbohydrates, vitamin C, and potassium. Although citrus fruits are rich in phytochemicals and several essential nutrients, other choices within the fruits group—strawberries, mangoes, and bananas—provide different nutrients. You should strive to include a variety of colorful fruits and vegetables over the course of each day and throughout each week.

However, even if you consume a huge variety of fruits, you will still miss out on some nutrients. You'll need to include foods from other food groups, as well. Go for the grains to get some B vitamins. Vary your veggies to get some vitamin K and folate. Pack in some protein foods for iron, zinc, and vitamin B-12. Dairy delivers your calcium and vitamin D.

An added bonus of dietary variety, especially within the fruit and vegetable groups, is the inclusion of a rich supply of phytochemicals.[3] In Chapter 1 we introduced phytochemicals. More details will be presented on phytochemicals in Chapter 8. To obtain the health benefits of these plant compounds, it is important to consume a variety of fruits, vegetables, whole grains, beans, peas, lentils, nuts, and seeds. Keep in mind that all forms of foods—fresh, canned, dried, frozen, and 100% juices—can be included in your healthy dietary pattern. Evidence from research studies links the regular consumption of fruits and vegetables with reduced risks for cancers and other chronic diseases.[4]

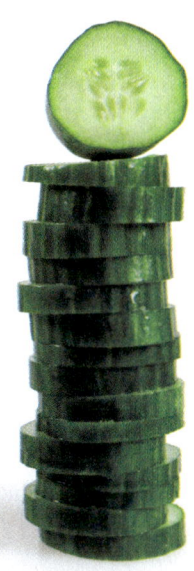

Vegetables, such as sliced cucumbers, avocados, artichokes, and more can be added to salads, sandwiches, pizza, burritos, soups, stews, and grain bowls to increase your nutrient density and phytochemical intake. Jupiterimages/Polka Dot/Getty Images

Carrots, which provide a pigment that forms vitamin A, may be your favorite vegetable. However, if you consume carrots every day as your only vegetable source, you may miss out on other vitamins, such as folate. You will need to include some other vegetables, such as broccoli and asparagus, to get some folate. Importantly, recent data suggest that it is better to focus on whole foods and overall eating patterns rather than trying to isolate individual nutrients or phytochemicals to successfully reduce disease risk.[5]

Are you beginning to get a sense of how different foods and food groups contribute to your health in unique ways? Strive for diversity among the food groups and within each food group to obtain all your essential nutrients, plus an array of phytochemicals!

PAY ATTENTION TO PORTION SIZE

The term *portion size* is used to describe the amount of a food or beverage consumed or served on one eating occasion. The term *serving size*, included on the Nutrition Facts label, can be used to help you choose appropriate portion sizes. Both of these terms are relevant to the concept of moderation. Eating in moderation requires you to pay attention to portion sizes and plan your daily eating pattern to avoid excessive intakes of any individual nutrients.

Figure 2-2 illustrates a convenient way to estimate portion size using the parts of your hand. You can compare your portion sizes of foods to the serving sizes recommended on food labels to gain a better understanding of your own calorie and nutrient intake. Common household units are also listed in Appendix E with their metric equivalents. Note that ounces and fluid ounces differ: ounces are a measure of weight (used for solid foods), whereas fluid ounces are a measure of volume (used for liquids).

What Is Energy Density? **Energy density** is a measurement that best describes the calorie content of a food. The energy density of a food is determined by comparing the calorie (kilocalorie) content with the weight of food. A food that is rich in calories but weighs relatively little is considered *energy dense*. Some examples of foods with high energy density include sugar-sweetened beverages, cookies, fried foods, and even some fat-free snacks. Sometimes these are called "empty calories" because they supply lots of energy but few essential nutrients. Foods with low energy density include fruits, vegetables, and any food that incorporates lots of water during cooking, such as oatmeal (Fig. 2-3).

$$\text{Energy density} = \frac{\text{Amount of energy (kcal) per serving}}{\text{Weight or volume of serving}}$$

energy density A comparison of the calorie (kcal) content of a food with the weight of the food. An energy-dense food is high in calories but weighs very little (e.g., potato chips), whereas a food low in energy density has few calories but weighs a lot (e.g., an orange).

FARM to FORK — Citrus Fruit

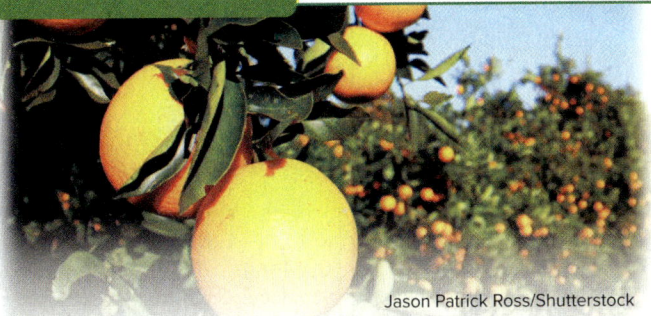
Jason Patrick Ross/Shutterstock

Oranges, tangelos, grapefruit, lemons, and limes make up the glorious and sunny citrus fruit family. The most popular citrus is the navel orange, easily identified by its belly button on the blossom end of the fruit. Indeed, more than 11 million tons of oranges are grown in the United States each year. Yet few know that the most nutrient-dense part of citrus is the white inner membrane found just below the skin. Called the pith, this spongy substance contains the phytochemicals naringenin, hesperidin, and others that have known antioxidant, antibacterial, antiviral, anti-inflammatory, and anti-allergenic properties!

Grow
- Most citrus is grown in California, Arizona, and Texas, while most orange juice and grapefruit are produced in Florida.
- To grow an indoor citrus tree, buy premixed potting soil formulated specifically for citrus trees. Most citrus trees require 8 to 12 hours of sunlight each day in a south-facing window.

Shop
- The first crop of U.S. oranges typically hits the supermarket shelves in October each year.
- When purchasing citrus, look for the largest fruits with the deepest colors; these have had more time to ripen on the tree.
- Instead of purchasing bottled orange juice, select juice concentrate to boost your flavonoid intake by 45%.

Store
- Citrus fruits do not continue to ripen after they have been picked, so it is best to enjoy them soon after purchase.
- If you can't enjoy citrus fruits within a few days of purchasing, refrigerate them. Do not place them in a plastic bag as this will increase moisture and mold.
- If you cannot eat your oranges within a few weeks, squeeze them and make orange juice!

Prep
- Many recipes call for citrus peels or zest to add a splash of exotic flavor to favorite dishes.
- Sliced citrus makes a perfect addition to salads and adds an ample dose of phytochemicals to any meal.
- Citrus juice is also a component of many recipes and dressings.
- And let's not forget the simple pleasure of adding citrus slices to enhance the flavor of ice water.

Source: Robinson J. Citrus fruits: beyond vitamin C. In: *Eating on the Wild Side: The Missing Link in Optimum Health.* New York, NY: Little, Brown & Co.; 2013.

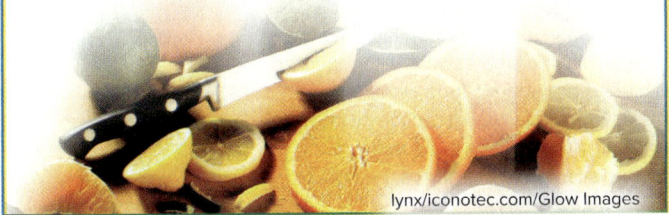
lynx/iconotec.com/Glow Images

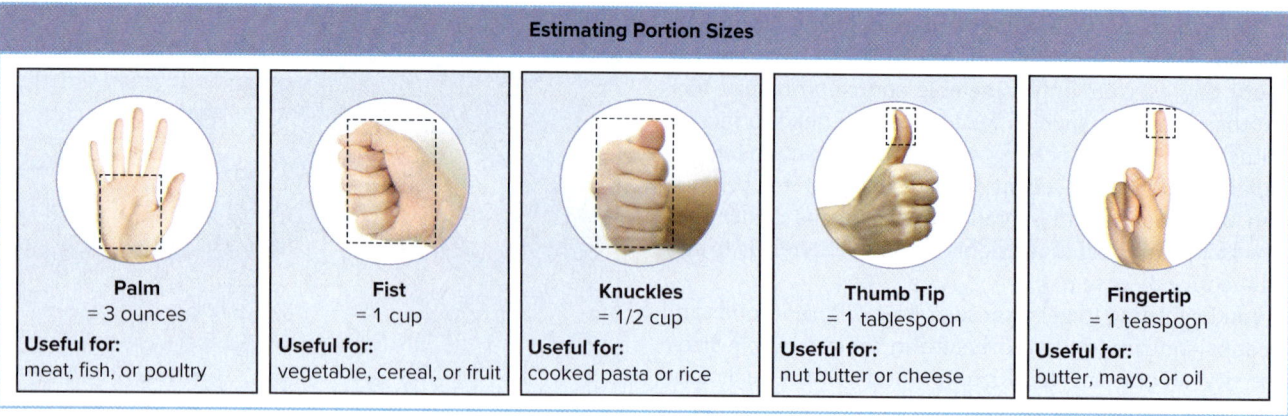

FIGURE 2-2 A "handy" tool to estimate portion sizes of foods.
Palm: McGraw Hill; Fist, Knuckles: Mark Dierker/McGraw Hill; Thumb Tip: AFTERDAY/Shutterstock; Fingertip: Holly Hildreth/McGraw Hill

Overall, foods with lots of water and fiber are low in energy density: they help you feel full but provide few calories.[6] Alternatively, foods with high energy density pack a lot of calories into a small space, so it's easy to consume several hundred kilocalories before feeling satiated.

Many foods, such as peanut butter, nuts, and seeds, are both energy dense and nutrient dense. Energy-dense foods can have a place in your dietary pattern, but you will have to plan for them. For example, chocolate is a very energy-dense food, but a small portion at the end of a meal can supply a satisfying finale. In addition, foods with high energy density can help individuals with poor appetites, such as some older adults, to maintain or gain weight.

As you will see in Section 2.2, you can use your knowledge about nutrient density, energy density, variety, and portion sizes to plan a healthy dietary pattern. Choose smaller portions of energy-dense foods (especially sources of saturated fat, added sugars, and alcohol). For example, if you plan to eat a bacon cheeseburger (relatively high in fat, salt, and calories) at lunch, you should select more nutrient-dense foods, such as fruits and vegetables, at other meals that day.[3] If you prefer whole milk to low-fat or fat-free milk, try to reduce the fat elsewhere throughout your day. Remember that dietary patterns, over time, correlate with many health outcomes. Occasional treats, eaten in moderation, are fine for most individuals. Plan for these occasions and balance them out with nutrient-dense foods throughout the rest of your week.

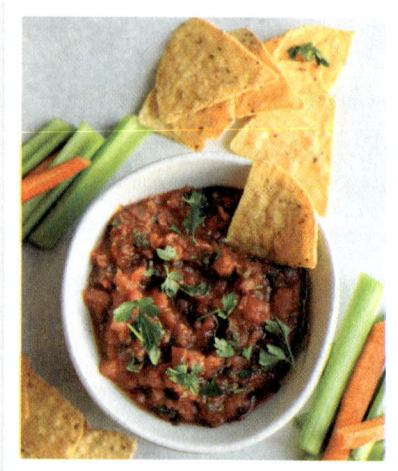

Instead of serving tortilla chips with queso, choose salsa. With its low energy density, salsa helps to balance out the high-energy-dense tortilla chips. In addition, salsa provides a variety of phytochemicals from its fresh vegetables and herbs. **What is the difference between energy density and nutrient density?** Alexis Joseph/McGraw Hill

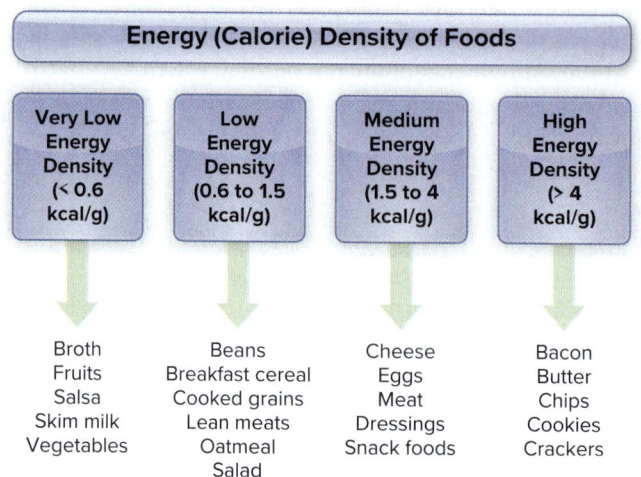

FIGURE 2-3 Low-energy-dense foods are often better sources of nutrients than high-energy-dense foods. Energy-dense foods tend to be highly processed, high in added sugars and saturated fats, and low in fiber. Making smart swaps, like replacing a high-energy-dense food with a low-energy-dense food, will reduce calories and will often provide more nutrients.
Source: data adapted from Rolls B. *The Ultimate Volumetrics Diet.* New York: HarperCollins; 2012.

✓ CONCEPT CHECK 2.1

1. List three benefits of eating plenty of fruits and vegetables.
2. How would you express the concepts of nutrient density and energy density as equations?
3. Describe one change you could make to improve the nutrient density of your typical dietary pattern.

2.2 Dietary and Physical Activity Guidelines

For more than a century, nutrition experts have been translating the science of nutrition into practical dietary advice. The earliest food guidance systems were designed to reduce the risk of nutrient deficiencies. Today, although many people have insufficient intakes of dietary fiber, vitamin D, calcium, and potassium, severe nutrient deficiency diseases are uncommon in industrialized countries. In the present day, major health problems frequently stem from overconsumption of calories, added sugars, saturated fat, alcohol, and sodium.

The following sections of this chapter describe guidelines and tools for planning healthy lifestyles. You will notice how those core concepts of nutrient density, variety, and portion control keep showing up throughout our discussions of the *Dietary Guidelines*, the *Physical Activity Guidelines*, and MyPlate.

DIETARY GUIDELINES—THE BASIS FOR MENU PLANNING

Since 1980, the U.S. Departments of Agriculture (USDA) and Health and Human Services (HHS) have jointly published the *Dietary Guidelines for Americans*.[7] Updated at least every 5 years, these science-based public health guidelines aim to improve dietary patterns to promote health, reduce risk of chronic disease, and meet nutrient needs. Notably, the current edition of the *Dietary Guidelines* is the first to include specific recommendations for all stages of life, including infants, toddlers, and pregnant and breastfeeding females.

In the next few pages, we will explore the four foundational guidelines of the latest edition of the *Dietary Guidelines* (see Fig. 2.4). Briefly, they are:

1. Follow a healthy dietary pattern at every life stage.
2. Customize and enjoy nutrient-dense food and beverage choices to reflect personal preferences, cultural traditions, and budgetary considerations.
3. Focus on meeting food group needs with nutrient-dense foods and beverages and stay within calorie limits.
4. Limit foods and beverages higher in added sugars, saturated fat, and sodium, and limit alcoholic beverages.

The goals of a nutritious dietary pattern are to meet nutrient needs, achieve and maintain a healthy body weight, and minimize the risk of chronic diseases. The *Dietary Guidelines* uses the Healthy U.S.-Style Dietary Pattern to exemplify the specific amounts of foods from each food group (and other components) that make up healthy eating patterns. It shows how many servings from each food group are recommended at various calorie levels and is based on foods individuals typically consume (in nutrient-dense forms and appropriate amounts). The *Dietary Guidelines* also includes the Healthy Mediterranean-Style Dietary Pattern and the Healthy Vegetarian Dietary Pattern as alternatives to the Healthy U.S.-Style Dietary Pattern. More information about healthy eating patterns will be presented in Section 2.3.

The *Dietary Guidelines* serves as the foundation of federal food, nutrition, and health policies and programs. In addition, it is used to develop nutrition education materials for the public, such as the MyPlate resources (http://myplate.gov).[8]

Dietary Guidelines for Americans, 2020–2025
Key Recommendations

1. Follow a healthy dietary pattern at every life stage.

At every life stage—infancy, toddlerhood, childhood, adolescence, adulthood, pregnancy, lactation, and older adulthood—it is never too early or too late to eat healthfully.

- **For about the first 6 months of life,** exclusively feed infants human milk. Continue to feed infants human milk through at least the first year of life, and longer if desired. Feed infants iron-fortified infant formula during the first year of life when human milk is unavailable. Provide infants with supplemental vitamin D beginning soon after birth.
- **At about 6 months,** introduce infants to nutrient-dense complementary foods. Introduce infants to potentially allergenic foods along with other complementary foods. Encourage infants and toddlers to consume a variety of foods from all food groups. Include foods rich in iron and zinc, particularly for infants fed human milk.
- **From 12 months through older adulthood,** follow a healthy dietary pattern across the lifespan to meet nutrient needs, help achieve a healthy body weight, and reduce the risk of chronic disease.

2. Customize and enjoy nutrient-dense food and beverage choices to reflect personal preferences, cultural traditions, and budgetary considerations.

A healthy dietary pattern can benefit all individuals regardless of age, race, or ethnicity, or current health status. The *Dietary Guidelines* provides a framework intended to be customized to individual needs and preferences, as well as the foodways of the diverse cultures in the United States.

3. Focus on meeting food group needs with nutrient-dense foods and beverages and stay within calorie limits.

An underlying premise of the *Dietary Guidelines* is that nutritional needs should be met primarily from foods and beverages—specifically, nutrient-dense foods and beverages. Nutrient-dense foods provide vitamins, minerals, and other health-promoting components and have no or little added sugars, saturated fat, and sodium. A healthy dietary pattern consists of nutrient-dense forms of foods and beverages across all food groups, in recommended amounts, and within calorie limits.

The core elements that make up a healthy dietary pattern include:

- **Vegetables** of all types—dark green; red and orange; beans, peas, and lentils; starchy; and other vegetables
- **Fruits,** especially whole fruit
- **Grains,** at least half of which are whole grain
- **Dairy,** including fat-free or low-fat milk, yogurt, and cheese, and/or lactose-free versions and fortified soy beverages and yogurt as alternatives
- **Protein foods,** including lean meats, poultry, and eggs; seafood; beans, peas, and lentils; and nuts, seeds, and soy products
- **Oils,** including vegetable oils and oils in food, such as seafood and nuts

4. Limit foods and beverages higher in added sugars, saturated fat, and sodium, and limit alcoholic beverages.

At every life stage, meeting food group recommendations—even with nutrient-dense choices—requires most of a person's daily calorie needs and sodium limits. A healthy dietary pattern doesn't have much room for extra added sugars, saturated fat, or sodium—or for alcoholic beverages. A small amount of added sugars, saturated fat, or sodium can be added to nutrient-dense foods and beverages to help meet food group recommendations, but foods and beverages high in these components should be limited. **Limits are:**

- **Added sugars**—Less than 10% of calories per day starting at age 2. Avoid foods and beverages with added sugars for those younger than age 2.
- **Saturated fat**—Less than 10% of calories per day starting at age 2.
- **Sodium**—Less than 2300 milligrams per day—and even less for children younger than age 14.
- **Alcoholic beverages**—Adult of legal drinking age can choose not to drink or to drink in moderation by limiting intake to 2 drinks or less in a day for males and 1 drink or less in a day for females, when alcohol is consumed. Drinking less is better for health than drinking more. There are some adults who should not drink alcohol, such as females who are pregnant.

FIGURE 2-4 Key Recommendations from the *Dietary Guidelines for Americans*.

Source: U.S. Department of Agriculture and U.S. Department of Health and Human Services. *Dietary Guidelines for Americans, 2020–2025*. 9th Edition. December 2020. Available at DietaryGuidelines.gov

However, because the *Dietary Guidelines* has a public health orientation, it is not intended to serve as clinical recommendations for treating disease. As you learned in Chapter 1, chronic diseases result from genetic, biological, behavioral, socioeconomic, and environmental factors. Those with chronic conditions have complex health care needs that should be addressed by a primary care provider.

Guideline 1: Follow a healthy dietary pattern at every life stage. Previous editions of the *Dietary Guidelines* have focused primarily on adults, but this edition takes a life-stage approach. Indeed, each life stage has unique nutritional requirements and distinct feeding challenges. The hope is that healthy behaviors beginning in infancy and early childhood will positively impact health throughout life, but it is never too late to start incorporating the *Dietary Guidelines* into your lifestyle.

From birth through adolescence, the *Dietary Guidelines* focuses on strategies that will meet the relatively high energy and nutrient needs of infants and children to support optimal growth and development and maintain a healthy body weight. For the first 6 months of life, infants should receive human milk or iron-fortified infant formula. Around 6 months of age, we can introduce age-appropriate solid foods, building up to a varied repertoire of nutrient-dense foods from all food groups. Throughout childhood and adolescence, focus on meeting energy and nutrient needs from nutrient-dense foods and beverages to support continued growth and development and prevent childhood obesity.

Moving into adulthood, the focus of dietary recommendations shifts to achieving and maintaining a healthy body weight and minimizing risks for nutrition-related chronic diseases. Adhering to the Healthy U.S.-Style Dietary Pattern will help adults meet their nutrient needs while not exceeding their daily energy requirements.

For pregnant and breastfeeding females, the *Dietary Guidelines* now provides recommendations to meet the increased energy and nutrient demands to support reproduction.

For older adults, nutrient density becomes increasingly important because daily calorie needs naturally decline whereas protein and micronutrient requirements remain high. In some cases, dietary supplements are recommended, but nutrient-dense foods and beverages are emphasized for all life stages. See Chapters 14, 15, and 16 for additional details on nutrition across these life stages.

Guideline 2: Customize and enjoy nutrient-dense food and beverage choices to reflect personal preferences, cultural traditions, and budgetary considerations. Take note of the fundamental message that all individuals, no matter their age, sex, race, ethnicity, economic circumstances, or health status, can benefit from adopting healthy dietary patterns.[8] The eating patterns promoted by the *Dietary Guidelines* are flexible, so individuals can customize their choices to meet their personal preferences, cultural traditions, and budget. This edition of the *Dietary Guidelines* includes food examples that represent diverse cultures. The dietary patterns proposed within the *Dietary Guidelines* are not prescriptive; they provide a framework for healthy eating that can be populated by foods to please each person's palate and align with cultural traditions. Healthy eating does not have to break your budget, either. The *Dietary Guidelines* suggests healthful, yet affordable options, such as canned and frozen foods when fresh produce is not accessible.

Guideline 3: Focus on meeting food group needs with nutrient-dense foods and beverages and stay within calorie limits. In light of the high prevalence of overweight and obesity, the *Dietary Guidelines* encourages all Americans to meet their nutrient needs within calorie limits. As you will study in Chapter 7, the balance between calories consumed (from foods and beverages) and calories expended (through physical

Roots

Latin American Diet Pyramid

Our dietary patterns have been shaped by many forces, including personal preferences, family traditions, religious observances, economics, climate, terrain, war, trade, and immigration. One vibrant example is the traditional dietary pattern of Latin America.

Latin America encompasses Mexico, Central America, South America, and the Caribbean. Dietary choices in this area have been shaped by the traditional eating patterns of the region's indigenous populations (e.g., Aztecs, Incas, Mayans, and Native Americans) as well as those of immigrants who settled there from Spain, Portugal, and Africa. Traditional eating patterns in Latin America were primarily plant-based, including abundant whole grains, fruits, vegetables, legumes, nuts, and seeds. Along with a physically active lifestyle, this eating pattern—nutrient dense, rich in dietary fiber, and low in saturated fat and added sugars—supported health and longevity.

More recently, however, the typical food choices among populations of Latin American descent have shifted to include more highly processed and animal-based foods. Individuals have become increasingly reliant on foods prepared outside the home. Physical activity has declined. These shifts have led to some adverse health trends in Hispanic/Latino communities: increased prevalence of obesity, diabetes, and cardiovascular disease.

By promoting a return to the traditional foodways of the region, the Latin American Heritage Diet (Fig. 2-5), aims to address lifestyle factors that have contributed to these health concerns. The majority of foods that form the basis of every meal are plants raised in Latin America. Citrus fruits, plantains, avocados, chard (leafy greens), peppers, yams, maize, quinoa, frijoles (beans), pepitas (pumpkin seeds), and olive oil are a few of the plant-based foods pictured on the pyramid. Many of the protein sources are plant-based, but fish, other seafood, poultry, eggs, and dairy products may be included several times per week. Meats and sweets are infrequent treats in the Latin American Diet Pyramid. Water is recommended as the beverage of choice. Beyond the foods themselves, the Latin American Heritage Diet emphasizes the prime importance of the family: families cook together, eat together, and exercise together.

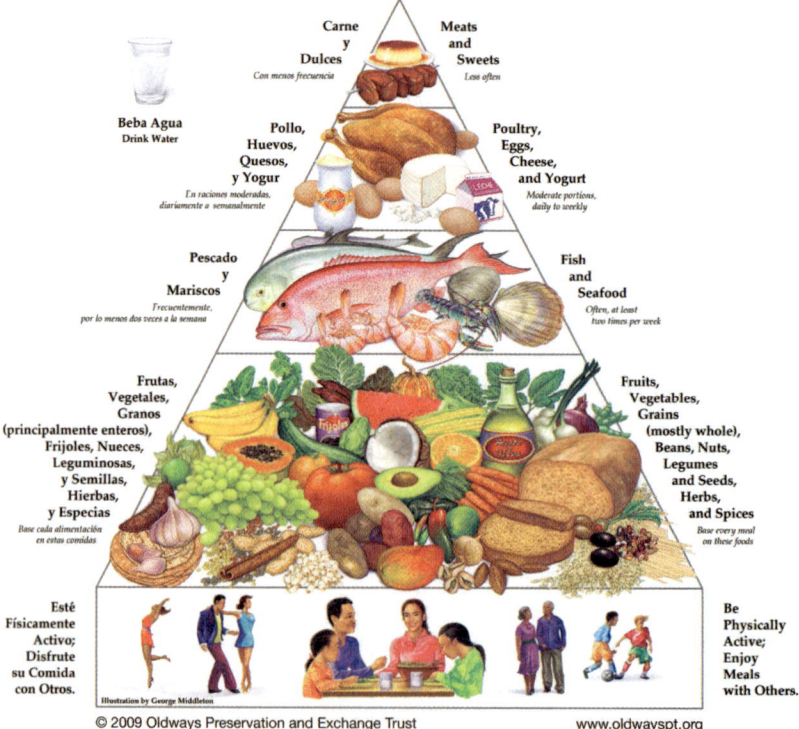

FIGURE 2-5 The Latin American Diet Pyramid is based on a foundation of whole, plant-based foods that represent the flavors and traditions of Mexico, South America, Central America, and the Caribbean. The Latin American Diet Pyramid features fish and other seafood at least two times per week, along with moderate portions of poultry, eggs, cheese, and yogurt. Meats and sweets are to be consumed infrequently. Water is the beverage of choice.
Source: Oldways Latin American Diet Pyramid: https://oldwayspt.org/resources/oldways-latin-american-diet-pyramid

Source: A Taste of Latin American Heritage webinar. Oldways. July 14, 2020. https://youtu.be/bRfHx4OZEok?si=imVGkKW2o7pAks_p

activity and metabolic processes) ultimately determines an individual's body weight. The total number of calories you need each day to maintain your current body weight varies according to age, sex assigned at birth, body size (i.e., height and weight), physical activity patterns, as well as life stage (e.g., pregnancy). Furthermore, individuals who desire to gain or lose weight will need to adjust their calorie intake.

How many calories do you need each day? Refer to Figure 2-6 or use an online calculator (e.g., NutritionCalc Plus in Connect) as a starting point. Keep in mind, however, these tools only provide estimates. Many factors, including genetic variations, can influence an individual's calorie requirements. The best way to tell if you are consuming enough calories is to monitor changes in body weight over time—if your calorie intake exceeds your calorie needs, weight gain will occur. Conversely, if your calorie intake is too low, weight loss will occur.

The latest guidelines include a resounding call to action—*Make Every Bite Count with the Dietary Guidelines*. In other words, aim to meet your essential nutrient needs with nutrient-dense foods and beverages rather than wasting calories on food choices that provide unnecessary added sugars and saturated fats. Build your eating pattern on a foundation of vegetables; fruits; whole grains; lean meats; poultry; seafood; eggs; beans, peas, and lentils; unsalted nuts and seeds; and fat-free or low-fat dairy products. This type of dietary pattern will (1) contribute to overall nutrient adequacy, (2) support healthy gastrointestinal function, (3) aid in weight management, and (4) decrease the risk for nutrition-related chronic diseases, especially cardiovascular disease, type 2 diabetes, cancers, and osteoporosis.[9]

	Calorie (kcal) Level	
Children	Sedentary →	Active
2–3 years	1000 →	1400
Females		
4–8 years	1200 →	1800
9–13	1400 →	2200
14–18	1800 →	2400
19–30	1800 →	2400
31–50	1800 →	2200
51+	1600 →	2200
Males		
4–8 years	1200 →	2000
9–13	1600 →	2600
14–18	2000 →	3200
19–30	2400 →	3000
31–50	2200 →	3000
51+	2000 →	2800

FIGURE 2-6 Estimates of calorie (kcal) needs based on activity levels.

Source: U.S. Department of Agriculture and U.S. Department of Health and Human Services. *Dietary Guidelines for Americans, 2020–2025*. 9th Edition. December 2020. Available at DietaryGuidelines.gov.

Guideline 4: Limit foods and beverages higher in added sugars, saturated fat, and sodium, and limit alcoholic beverages. High intakes of added sugars, saturated fats, and sodium are linked to excessive weight gain and an increased risk for type 2 diabetes, hypertension, cardiovascular disease, and some types of cancer. Foods with added sugars and saturated fats often have high energy density but low nutrient density. In other words, they are high in calories but provide few essential nutrients. The *Dietary Guidelines* recommends limiting intakes of these food components.

Added sugars refer to sugars and other sweeteners that are added during food processing or preparation. The *Dietary Guidelines* recommends limiting the intake of added sugars to less than 10% of total calories for those over age 2. For infants and toddlers younger than 2 years of age, the *Dietary Guidelines* recommends avoiding added sugars. Infants and toddlers have high nutrient needs, but they can only consume a small volume of food at one time. Therefore, food choices must be nutrient dense! You will learn about the differences between added sugars and natural sugars in Chapter 4.

Saturated fats are found mostly in animal sources (e.g., butter and beef fat) and tropical oils (e.g., palm oil and coconut oil). They may also be added during food processing and cooking. High intakes of saturated fats are linked to increased risk for cardiovascular disease. Thus, the *Dietary Guidelines* recommends limiting the intake of saturated fats to less than 10% of total calories per day for those age 2 and older. In practice, this means opting for plant oils, fatty fish, nuts, and seeds in place of some animal sources of fat. Chapter 5 explores the differences between saturated and unsaturated fats in more detail.

Sodium should be limited to less than 2300 milligrams per day for those 14 years and older. Individuals vary, but in general, high intakes of sodium are linked to increased risk for hypertension, which is the most common chronic disease among adults. Sodium is naturally present in foods in small amounts, but highly processed foods and restaurant foods are sources of excessive sodium. Choosing whole, unprocessed foods in place of highly processed foods and preparing most meals at home are good ways to cut back on sodium. You will learn more about the link between sodium and hypertension in Chapter 9.

When consumed in moderation, alcohol may have some health benefits, such as reduced risk for cardiovascular disease. However, excessive use of alcohol contributes to many health problems, including hypertension, some types of cancer, and liver disease. If adults of legal drinking age choose to drink alcohol, they should do so in moderation, which is defined as up to two drinks per day for males or up to one drink per day for females. The health implications of alcohol consumption are described in greater detail in Chapter 1.

How well do Americans comply with the *Dietary Guidelines*? As shown in Figure 2-7, many Americans fall short of getting their recommended daily servings of vegetables, fruits, and dairy. Although Americans meet the recommendations for intake of total grains and total protein foods, typical choices within these food groups do not align with recommendations. In Chapter 4, you will learn about the differences between whole and refined grains. To reap the unique health benefits of both, the *Dietary Guidelines* recommends making half your grains whole. However, current American dietary patterns rely too heavily on refined grains. Within the protein foods group, many Americans would benefit from selecting leaner meats and choosing seafood and plant sources of protein in place of meats, poultry, and eggs sometimes.

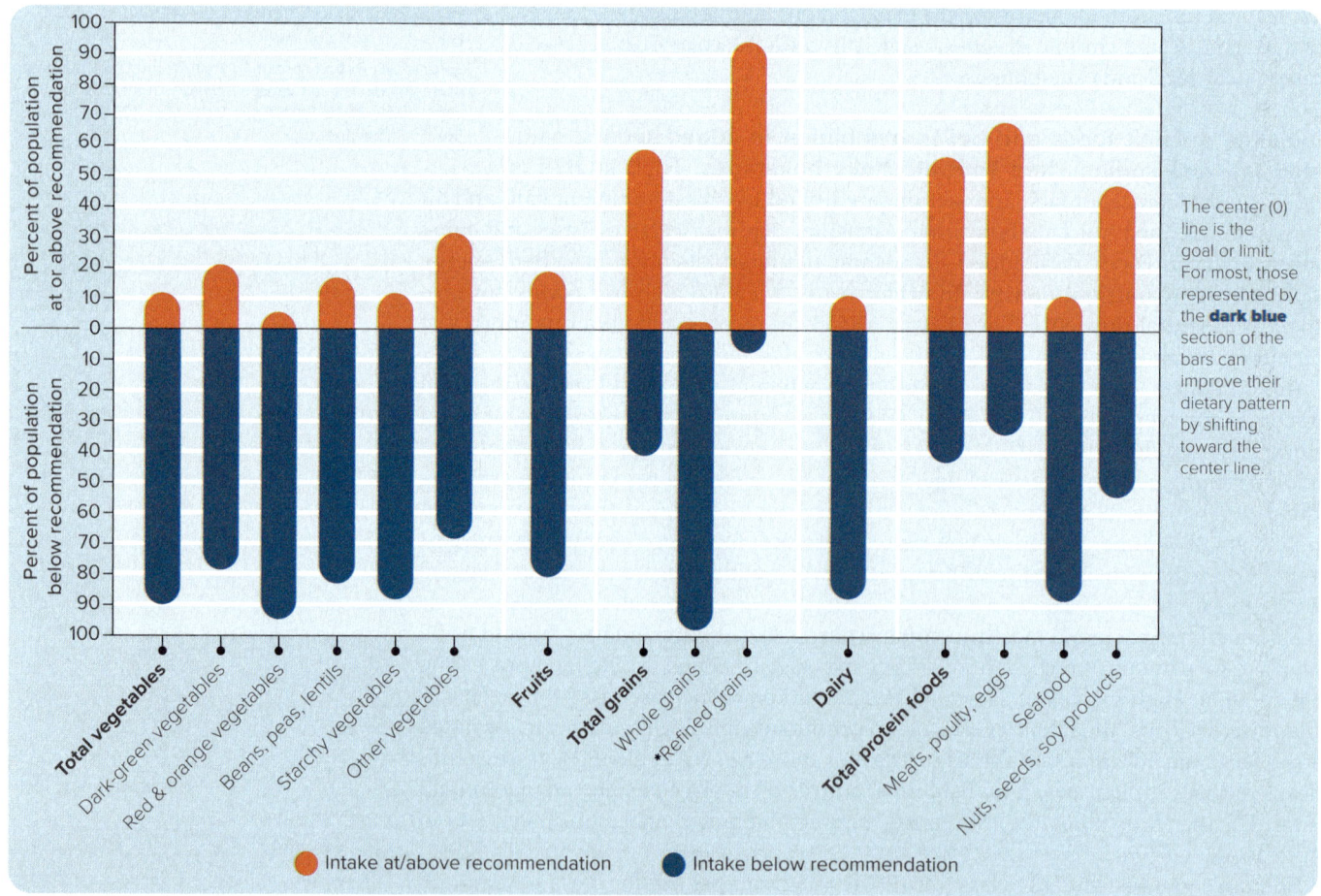

FIGURE 2-7 Percent of the U.S. population ages 1 and older who are below and at or above each dietary goal. Note: Recommended daily intake of whole grains is to be at least half of total grain consumption, and the limit for refined grains is to be no more than half of total grain consumption.

Source: Analysis of *What We Eat in America*, NHANES 2013-2016, ages 1 and older, 2 days dietary intake data, weighted. Recommended Intake Ranges: Healthy U.S.-Style Dietary Patterns

Newsworthy Nutrition

Impact of diet quality on health outcomes

INTRODUCTION: Improving dietary patterns and quality is a modifiable behavior that has been shown to improve health outcomes in previous studies. **OBJECTIVE:** To determine if diet quality, measured in terms of the Healthy Eating Index, the Alternate Healthy Eating Index, and the Dietary Approaches to Stop Hypertension score, influenced health status for U.S. adults. The authors hypothesized that diets of the highest quality would be associated with lower risk of noncommunicable disease. **METHODS:** A literature search was performed to identify studies published from 2014 to 2020 using electronic databases PubMed, Scopus, and Embase. Summary risk ratios (RRs) and confidence intervals were analyzed for over 3.2 million participants from 113 reports and stratified by high versus low adherence categories. **RESULTS:** Higher dietary pattern scores were associated with a significant reduction in the risk of all-cause mortality (22%), cardiovascular disease (20%), cancer (14%), type 2 diabetes (19%), and neurodegenerative disease (18%). High-quality diets were also associated with a significant reduction in the risk of overall mortality (17%) and cancer mortality (18%) among cancer survivors. **CONCLUSION:** Diets of the highest quality, as assessed by the HEI, AHEI, and DASH scores, resulted in a significant risk reduction for disease and all-cause mortality. These data support adherence to the Dietary Guidelines for the prevention of disease.

Source: Morze J, Danielewicz A, Hoffmann G, Schwingshackl L. Diet quality as assessed by the Healthy Eating Index, Alternate Healthy Eating Index, Dietary Approaches to Stop Hypertension score, and health outcomes: a second update of a systematic review and meta-analysis of cohort studies. *J Acad Nutr Diet.* 2020;120(12):1998-2031.e15. doi: 10.1016/j.jand.2020.08.076

Evidently, typical American eating patterns need some improvement! As you progress through this course, you will gather lots of practical strategies to reach better health through better food choices. This chapter's *Newsworthy Nutrition* feature highlights the positive health impacts associated with high-quality dietary patterns.

Healthy Eating Patterns. The ultimate goal of a nutritious dietary pattern is to support a healthy body weight and help reduce the risk of chronic disease. The *Dietary Guidelines* use the Healthy U.S.-Style Dietary Pattern to exemplify the specific amounts of food groups and other components that make up healthy eating patterns. It is based on foods Americans typically consume, but in nutrient-dense forms and appropriate amounts. The **Healthy Eating Index (HEI)** is an objective measure of concordance with the *Dietary Guidelines*. The current HEI score in the U.S. is 58 (out of 100).[10] Clearly, there is much room for improvement in the dietary patterns of Americans.

Healthy Eating Index (HEI) A measure of diet quality that can be used to assess compliance with the *Dietary Guidelines*.

PHYSICAL ACTIVITY GUIDELINES FOR AMERICANS

In line with its goal to enhance the health and well-being of all Americans, the U.S. Department of Health and Human Services updated and published the second *Physical Activity Guidelines for Americans* as a complement to the *Dietary Guidelines*.[11] The overarching idea continues to be that regular physical activity for people of all ages, races, ethnicities, and physical abilities produces immediate health benefits.

The key physical activity guidelines provide measurable physical activity standards for individuals ages 3 and older. Specific recommendations also apply to special population groups, including pregnant and postpartum females, adults with disabilities, and people with chronic medical conditions. The adult guidelines are presented in Table 2-1. You will learn more about specific physical activity guidelines for children, adolescents, and older adults in subsequent chapters. Overall, the main message is to *move more and sit less.* For adults, major health benefits occur with at least 150 to 300 minutes per

TABLE 2-1 ■ Types of Physical Activity and Adult Recommendations of the *Physical Activity Guidelines for Americans*

Type	Description
Aerobic	Includes forms of activity that are intense enough and performed long enough to maintain or improve an individual's cardiorespiratory fitness.
Anaerobic	Refers to high-intensity activity that exceeds the capacity of the cardiovascular system to provide oxygen to muscle cells for the usual oxygen-consuming metabolic pathways.
Muscle-strengthening	Activities that maintain or improve muscular strength, endurance, or power.
Bone-strengthening	Movements that create impact and muscle-loading forces on bone.
Balance training	Training activities and movements that safely challenge postural control.
Flexibility training	Also called stretching, these activities improve the range and ease of movement around a joint.
Mind-body	Typically combines muscle strengthening, balance training, light-intensity aerobic activity, and flexibility in one package.
Age	**Description**
Adults	Adults who sit less and do any amount of moderate to vigorous physical activity gain health benefits. • For substantial health benefits, adults should do at least 150 to 300 minutes a week of moderate-intensity, or 75 to 150 minutes a week of vigorous-intensity, aerobic physical activity, or an equivalent combination of moderate and vigorous-intensity aerobic activity. Preferably, aerobic activity should be spread throughout the week. • Additional health benefits are gained by engaging in physical activity beyond 300 minutes of moderate-intensity physical activity each week. • Adults should also do muscle-strengthening activities of moderate or greater intensity that involve all major muscle groups on 2 or more days each week.
Guidelines for safe physical activity	To do physical activity safely and reduce risk of injuries and other adverse events, people should: • Understand the risks, yet be confident that physical activity can be safe for almost everyone. • Choose types of physical activity that are appropriate for their current fitness level and health goals because some activities are safer than others. • Increase physical activity gradually over time to meet key guidelines or health goals. Inactive people should "start low and go slow" by starting with lower-intensity activities and gradually increasing how often and for how long activities are done. • Protect themselves by using appropriate gear and sports equipment, choosing safe environments, following rules and policies, and making sensible choices about when, where, and how to be active. • Be under the care of a health care provider if they have chronic conditions or symptoms. People with chronic conditions and symptoms can consult a health care professional or physical activity specialist about the types and amounts of activity appropriate for them.

Source: U.S. Department of Health and Human Services. *Physical Activity Guidelines for Americans.* 2nd ed. 2018. https://health.gov/paguidelines/second-edition

aerobic Requiring oxygen; with reference to physical activity, all forms of activity that are intense enough and performed long enough to maintain or improve an individual's cardiorespiratory fitness.

anaerobic Not requiring oxygen; with reference to physical activity, high intensity activity that exceeds the capacity of the cardiovascular system to provide oxygen to muscle cells for the usual oxygen-consuming metabolic pathways.

week of moderate-intensity aerobic activity. Ideally, adults should also engage in muscle-strengthening activities at least 2 days each week. Children and adolescents should strive to include 60 minutes of physical activity per day. For optimum benefits, include both aerobic and muscle-strengthening activities. Overall, physical activity should be enjoyable and safe for each individual.

✓ CONCEPT CHECK 2.2

1. What are the four key guidelines of the *Dietary Guidelines for Americans*?
2. Which life stages are addressed in the *Dietary Guidelines*?
3. How many minutes of moderate-intensity physical activity are advised per week in the *Physical Activity Guidelines* for adults?

2.3 MyPlate—A Menu-Planning Tool

The titles, food groupings, and shapes of food guides have evolved since the first edition published by the USDA a century ago. The most recent food-guidance systems have provided a means for individualization of dietary advice via interactive tools available online. MyPlate shapes the key recommendations from the *Dietary Guidelines* into an easily recognizable and extremely applicable visual: a meal place setting.

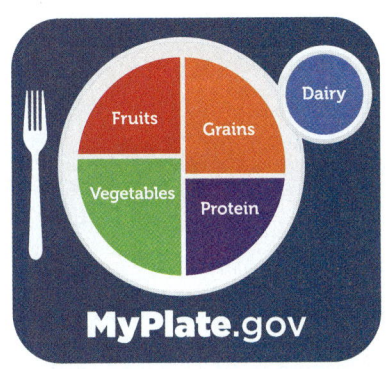

DISHING UP MYPLATE

Although it is not intended to stand alone as a source of dietary advice, MyPlate serves as a reminder of how to build a healthy plate at mealtimes. It emphasizes important areas of the dietary pattern that are in need of improvement. Recall from the discussion of the *Dietary Guidelines* that most individuals need to increase their proportions of fruits, vegetables, whole grains, and fat-free or low-fat dairy products while decreasing consumption of refined grains and high-fat meats.

MyPlate does not display a separate group for fats and oils, as they are mostly incorporated into other foods. The MyPlate food guide recommends limiting solid fats and focusing instead on plant oils, which are sources of essential fatty acids and vitamin E.

The MyPlate icon includes five food groups:
- **Vegetables** should include a variety of colors. This nutrient-dense food group includes all fresh, frozen, canned, dried, and cooked vegetables.
- **Fruits** include all fresh, frozen, canned, dried, and 100% fruit juices. Fruits and vegetables should cover half of your plate.
- **Grains** should cover just over 25% of your plate with a goal of eating at least 50% of all grains as whole grains.
- **Dairy** and fortified soy alternatives choices should be fat-free or low-fat. Aim for 2 to 3 cups per day.
- **Protein** foods include meats, poultry, eggs, seafood, nuts, seeds, and soy products. Try to focus on lean and plant-based proteins in your dietary pattern.

U.S. Department of Agriculture

MAKE EVERY BITE COUNT WHEN BUILDING A HEALTHY EATING PATTERN

A healthy dietary pattern is essential at every stage of life and has a profound impact on both physical and mental health. The MyPlate.gov website provides ideas and tips to help you personalize an eating pattern that meets your individual needs and promotes lifelong health.

Think about how you can put the following guidelines into action, over the course of your day or week, to create a healthy and sustainable eating routine.

Choices Matter—Focus on Those That Work for You!
- Focus on making healthy food and beverage choices from all five food groups, including fruits, vegetables, grains, protein foods, and dairy, to get the nutrients you need.
- Eat the appropriate amount of calories for you based on your age, gender, height, weight, and physical activity level to achieve and maintain a healthy weight and reduce your risk of many chronic diseases.

Choose an Eating Style Low in Saturated Fat, Sodium, and Added Sugars.
- Use Nutrition Facts labels and ingredient lists to locate the amounts of saturated fat, sodium, and added sugars in the foods and beverages you choose.
- Incorporate food and beverage choices that are lower in saturated fat, sodium, and added sugars.

Make Small Changes to Create a Healthier Eating Pattern.
- Think of each positive change as a personal "win" on your path to living healthier. Create little victories that fit into your lifestyle and celebrate them!
- Start with a few of these small changes:
  - Make half your plate fruits and vegetables.
    - Focus on whole fruits.
    - Vary your veggies to consume a rainbow of colors.
  - Make half your grains whole grains.
  - Move to low-fat and fat-free dairy or alternatives.
  - Vary your lean protein routine.
  - Eat and drink the right amount to support a healthy weight.

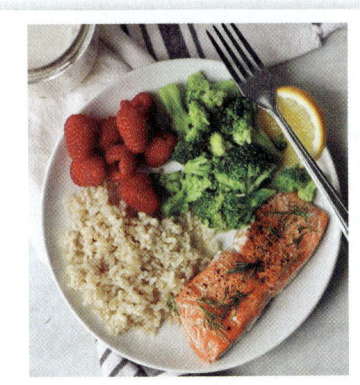

MyPlate is a visual representation of the advice contained in the *Dietary Guidelines for Americans.* Use MyPlate to assist with meal planning **How many MyPlate food groups are represented in this meal?** Alexis Joseph/McGraw Hill

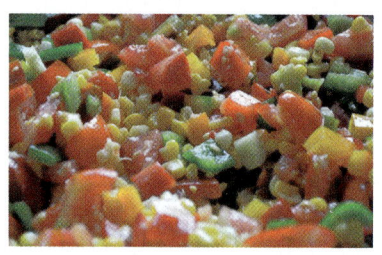

Focus on nutrient-rich foods as you strive to meet your nutrient needs. The more colorful the food on your plate, the greater the content of nutrients and phytochemicals. **Can you name the MyPlate sources of phytochemicals?** Mary-Jon Ludy, Bowling Green State University, Garden of Hope image

MYPLATE DAILY PLAN

On the MyPlate.gov website, you will find an interactive tool, *MyPlate Plan,* that estimates your calorie needs and suggests a food pattern based on your age, gender, height, and weight (Table 2-2). These daily food plans provide useful information for each food group, including recommended daily amounts in common household measures. Modified daily food plans are also available for children (starting at 2 years of age), pregnant or breastfeeding females, and those interested in losing weight. Be sure to visit the site to generate your own daily food plan. If you prefer to use apps, try the *Start Simple with MyPlate App.*

The recommended serving sizes are provided in cups for vegetables, fruits, and dairy and fortified soy alternatives. Grains and protein foods are listed in ounces. Figure 2-8 shows what equals a serving for each of the MyPlate food groups.

After daily food group recommendations have been met, some calories are left over for foods and beverages rich in saturated fats, added sugars, and alcohol, which are typically low in essential nutrients. These are sometimes called *discretionary calories* or *empty calories.* Saturated fats are solid at room temperature and include many animal fats (e.g., butter and beef fat) and tropical plant oils (e.g., coconut oil). Some saturated fats, such as the white marbling in a ribeye steak and the fat contained in milk, are naturally present in foods (Fig. 2-9). Others, such as the shortening or butter used to make frosting for a cake, are added during food processing or preparation. Added sugars include sugars and syrups that are added to foods during processing or preparation. Examples of foods that are major contributors of these discretionary calories in the American dietary pattern are cakes, cookies, pastries, soft drinks, energy drinks, cheese, pizza, ice cream, and processed meats. The MyPlate Plan makes some allowance for discretionary calories throughout the day. About 85% of the calories you consume daily are needed to meet the nutrient-dense food group recommendations. The remaining 15% of calories are discretionary calories that may be used for added sugars or saturated fat intake. For most individuals, this equates to 250 to 350 discretionary calories per day.

TABLE 2-2 ■ Healthy U.S.-Style Dietary Pattern for Adults Ages 19 through 59 from MyPlate Food Groups

- A "cup" of **Fruit** is equivalent to 1 cup of whole fruit, 1 cup of fruit juice, or ½ cup of dried fruit.
- A "cup" of **Vegetables** is equivalent to 1 cup of raw or cooked vegetables, 1 cup of vegetable juice, or 2 cups of raw, leafy greens.
- An "ounce-equivalent" of **Grains** is equal to 1 slice of bread, 1 cup of ready-to-eat breakfast cereal, or ½ cup of cooked pasta, rice, or cereal.
- An "ounce-equivalent" of **Protein** refers to 1 ounce of meat, fish, or poultry; 1 egg; 1 tablespoon of nut butter; ¼ cup of cooked legumes; or ½ ounce of nuts or seeds. NOTE: Dry beans and peas can count either as vegetables or protein foods.
- A "cup" of **Dairy** is equivalent to 1 cup of milk, soy milk, or yogurt; 1.5 ounces of natural cheese; or 1 ounce of processed cheese.
- **Oils** refer to nontropical plant oils, such as canola, corn, olive, peanut, safflower, soybean, and sunflower oils.
- **Calories for Other Uses** include added sugars and rich sources of saturated fat, such as butter, shortening, lard, or tropic plant oils (e.g., coconut oil).

Daily Amount of Food from Each Group Based on Calorie Level

Calories	1200	1600	2000	2400	2800	3200
Fruits	1 cup	1.5 cups	2 cups	2 cups	2.5 cups	2.5 cups
Vegetables	1.5 cups	2 cups	2.5 cups	3 cups	3.5 cups	4 cups
Grains	4 oz-eq	5 oz-eq	6 oz-eq	8 oz-eq	10 oz-eq	10 oz-eq
Protein	3 oz-eq	5 oz-eq	5.5 oz-eq	6.5 oz-eq	7 oz-eq	7 oz-eq
Dairy	2 cups	3 cups	3 cups	3 cups	3 cups	3 cups
Oils	17 grams	22 grams	27 grams	31 grams	36 grams	51 grams

Limit on Calories for Other Uses

Calories for Other Uses	80	100	240	320	370	580

Note: oz-eq stands for ounce equivalent.

MyPlate Build-a-Meal

Vegetables	Fruits	Grains	Protein	Dairy
1 c raw, cooked, canned; 2 c leafy greens; 1 c 100% vegetable juice	1 c raw, frozen, canned; ½ c dried; 1 c 100% fruit juice	1 slice bread; 1 oz dry cereal; ½ c cooked rice/pasta/cereal	1 oz lean meat, poultry, fish; ¼ c cooked beans; 1 egg; 1 tbsp nut butter; ½ oz nuts or seeds	1 c milk, yogurt, or soymilk; 1½ oz natural cheese; 1 oz processed cheese
Broccoli Cabbage Leafy greens Mushrooms Onions Peas Peppers Sweet potatoes Yellow squash Zucchini	Apple Banana Berries Grapes Kiwi Mango Orange Peach Pineapple Raisins	Barley Bread Brown rice Cereal Farro Freekah Millet Oats Pasta Quinoa	Beans Eggs Fish Lean beef Nut butters Peanuts Poultry Soybeans Tofu	Almond milk Cheese Cottage cheese Cow's milk Greek yogurt Kefir Ricotta Soymilk Yogurt

FIGURE 2-8 This build-a-meal guide can help you through creating nutritious meals using the MyPlate food groups. Aim to incorporate 4 or 5 foods from each different food group for each meal. The serving sizes listed (in the white boxes above) will assist with portion control.
Source: Adapted from USDA https://www.myplate.gov/eat-healthy/healthy-eating-budget/make-plan (my plate) Source: USDA

MENU PLANNING WITH MYPLATE

Overall, MyPlate exemplifies the foundations of a healthy eating pattern you have already learned. To achieve optimal nutrition, remember the following points when using MyPlate to plan your daily menus:

- Start with a few small changes and think of each positive change as a personal "win" on your path to living healthier.

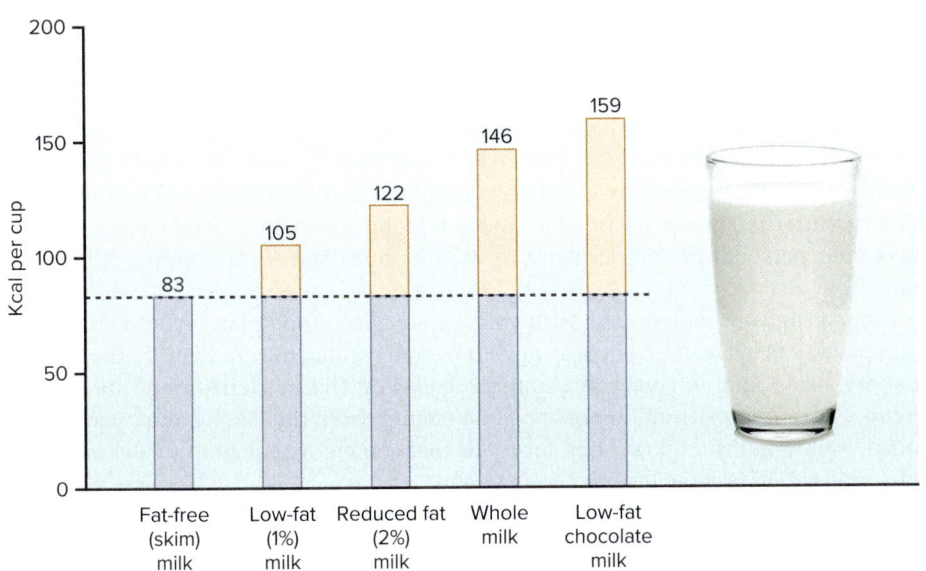

FIGURE 2-9 Not all dairy is the same. This bar graph compares the difference in calories from various types of milk. The yellow bars represent the added calories from fat and sugar in various milks compared to fat-free milk. Note that milk also contains some natural sugars.
(Milk) Nipaporn Panyacharoen/Shutterstock
Source: USDA Food and Nutrient Database.

- Eat the appropriate amount of calories for you based on your age, sex assigned at birth, height, weight, and physical activity level to achieve and maintain a healthy weight and reduce your risk of many chronic diseases.
- Use a nutrient-dense, whole-food philosophy to build your own plate.
- Variety is vital for the successful implementation of MyPlate. There is no single, perfect food. Likewise, no food group is more important than another; each food group makes an important, distinctive contribution to nutrient intake.
- Choose a variety of healthy foods and beverages from each food group. For a sample meal plan, visit MyPlate.gov to find your MyPlate Plan or download the *Start Simple with MyPlate* app. The foods within a group may vary widely with respect to nutrients and calories. For example, the calorie content of 3 ounces of baked potato is 79 kcal, whereas 3 ounces of potato chips are 452 kcal.
- Choose primarily low-fat or fat-free dairy or fortified soy alternatives. By reducing calorie intake in this way, you can select more items from other food groups. If milk causes intestinal gas and bloating, consider fortified soy alternatives, yogurt, or cheese.
- Use Nutrition Facts labels and ingredient lists to increase your awareness of the amounts of saturated fat, sodium, and added sugars in the foods and beverages you choose.
- Include plant foods that are good sources of protein, such as nuts, seeds, soy products, beans, peas, and lentils, at least several times a week because many are rich in vitamins (such as vitamin E), minerals (such as magnesium), and fiber.
- Make half your plate vegetables and fruits and try to include a dark green or orange vegetable for vitamin A and a vitamin C–rich fruit, such as an orange, every day. Try not to focus primarily on starchy vegetables for your main vegetable choice. According to the Centers for Disease Control and Prevention (CDC), only 12% of American adults meet the guidelines for fruit, and 10% meet the standard for vegetables.[12] Increased consumption of these foods is important because they contribute vitamins, minerals, fiber, and phytochemicals. Focus on whole fruits and vary your veggies to consume a rainbow of colors.
- Choose whole grain varieties of breads, cereals, rice, and pasta because they contribute nutrients such as vitamin E and fiber. A daily serving of a whole grain, ready-to-eat breakfast cereal is an excellent choice because the vitamins (such as vitamin B-6) and minerals (such as zinc), along with fiber, help fill in common nutritional gaps.
- Include some unsaturated plant oils on a daily basis, such as those in salad dressing, nuts, and seeds, and try to eat fish at least twice a week. These sources of fat promote heart health and brain health.

HOW DOES YOUR PLATE RATE?

The *Dietary Guidelines* emphasizes the totality of your eating patterns over all life stages. In other words, a dietary pattern is more than the sum of its individual parts. Healthy eating patterns should not be rigid plans that are difficult to follow. Rather, dietary patterns should be flexible and adaptable to include foods you enjoy that meet your personal preferences and fit within your lifestyle, traditions, culture, and budget.

Comparing your daily intake with your personalized food plan recommendations is a simple way to evaluate the quality of your overall eating pattern. Identify the nutrients that are suboptimal in your eating pattern based on the nutrients found in each food group. For example, if you do not consume enough from the dairy group, your calcium intake is most likely too low. Look for foods that you enjoy that supply calcium, such as calcium-fortified orange juice or Greek yogurt.

The Protein Foods Group includes animal-based proteins such as meat, poultry, seafood, and eggs. Yet beans and peas, soy products, nuts, and seeds are also considered part of the Protein Foods Group. MyPlate food groups are classified based on their overall nutrient profile. Protein foods are also sources of B vitamins, vitamin E, iron, zinc, and magnesium.

Recall from the *Fact Check* at the beginning of the chapter, beans, peas, and lentils are unique vegetables that can count in your MyPlate plan in either the Vegetable Group or the Protein Foods Group. To decide which group is the best fit for you, reflect on your overall dietary pattern. If you regularly consume meat, poultry, and seafood, then you would count your beans, peas, and lentils in the Vegetable Group. If you rarely eat animal proteins or are vegan or vegetarian, you would count some of your beans, peas, and lentils in the Protein Foods Group. Yet do not be confused by green peas, green lima beans, and green (string) beans. These vegetables are not part of the beans, peas, and lentils subgroup because their nutrient composition is similar to other vegetable subgroups. For example, green peas and lima beans are in the Starchy Vegetable subgroup and green beans are grouped with Other Vegetables.

Food quality is just as important as food quantity when it comes to good nutrition. Review the simple meal and snack swaps leading to simple and more nutrient-dense dietary patterns (Fig. 2-10). For a more detailed analysis of your current eating pattern, use the NutritionCalc Plus function in Connect to compare your food choices to MyPlate. With a detailed dietary analysis, you can compare your intakes

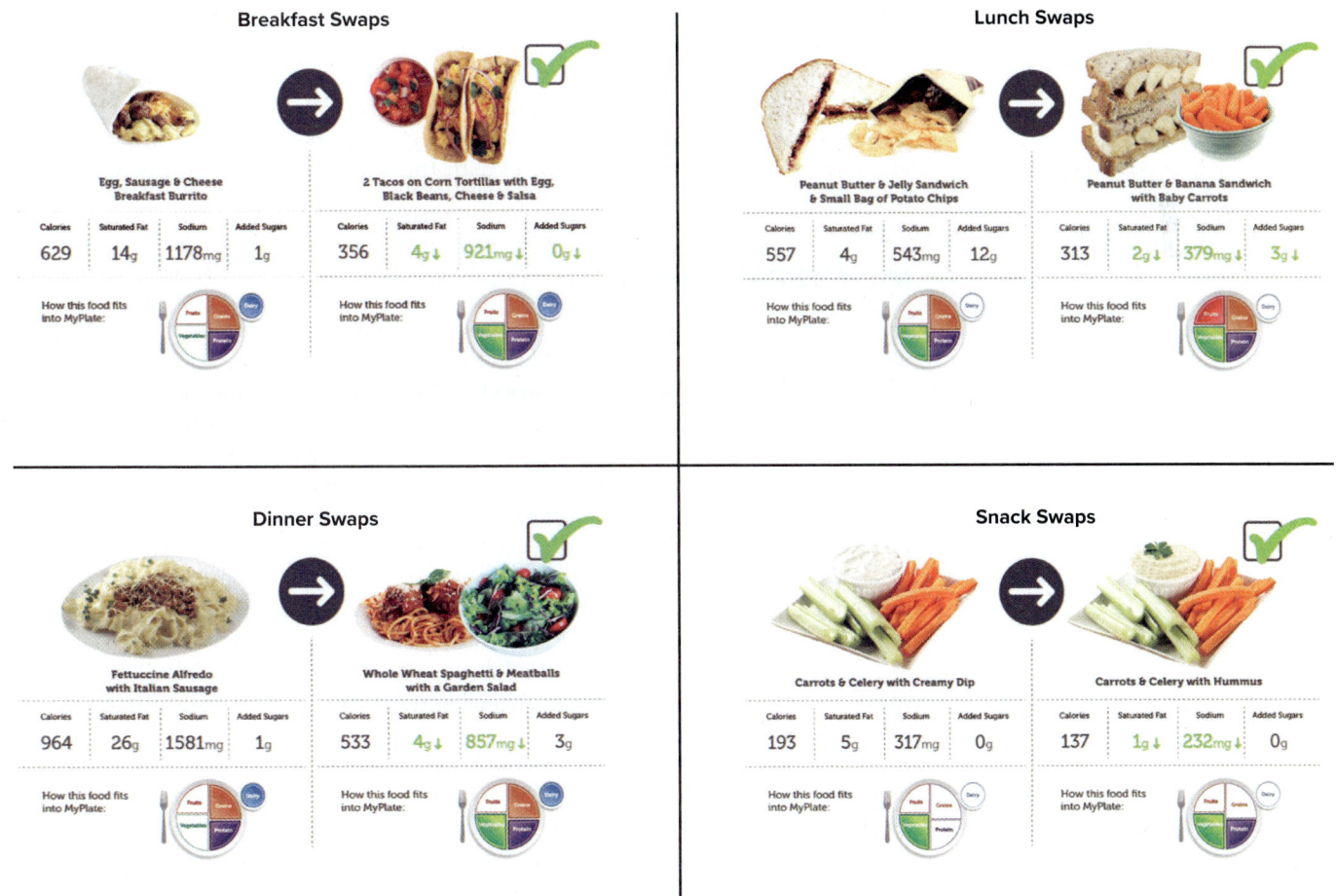

FIGURE 2-10 These quick and simple meal swaps will result in a more nutrient-dense dietary pattern. Note the nutrient comparisons under each meal and the colored MyPlate icons depicting the food groups represented in each meal. U.S. Department of Agriculture (USDA)

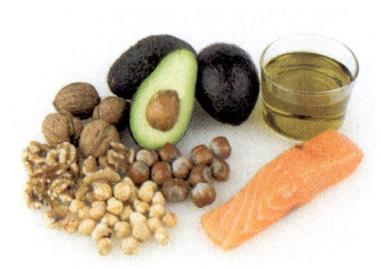

Solid fats contribute over 15% of total calories in the typical American's dietary pattern, but they have little to offer in terms of essential nutrients and dietary fiber. Instead of solid fats, choose plant oils, nuts, and seeds. **What types of fats are naturally found in salmon, avocado, olives, almonds, and plant-based oils?** tinalarsson/iStock/Getty Images

of individual nutrients to recommendations and clearly see the areas that need improvement. Even small changes to your dietary and physical activity patterns can have positive results.

LIMITATIONS OF MYPLATE

Although MyPlate will promote important changes in eating patterns, it has certain limitations. Some critics say that the icon is too simple. For example, it does not immediately provide information about overall calories, serving sizes, or number of servings to choose from each food group. However, many of these details will vary by person. Users can access the accompanying materials available on the MyPlate.gov website to obtain a personally tailored daily food plan.

The MyPlate icon does not address the types of foods to choose within each food group. Making appropriate food choices for weight management and prevention of diet-related chronic diseases requires consumers to have some nutrition knowledge. Fortunately, public health messages and online content related to MyPlate are available to educate Americans.

MyPlate shows how to build a healthy plate at mealtimes, but it does not adequately address the total diet, which in reality includes many snacks between meals. Meal and snack patterns are available in the MyPlate Plan for children but not for adults.

As with any public health campaign, it is possible that the people who need it most will overlook the MyPlate message. Educated consumers with access to interactive MyPlate tools likely already comply with many of the *Dietary Guidelines*. Populations with poor diets may be unlikely or unable to access online materials to find their personalized MyPlate Plan.

Overall, the MyPlate icon is a relevant and recognizable tool that immediately shows us how to build a healthy plate at mealtimes. The strength of MyPlate lies in its simplicity. It conveys the major messages that are needed when shopping, cooking, and eating and can be enhanced with the details provided on the MyPlate.gov website.

MEDITERRANEAN DIET

The Mediterranean Diet Pyramid is a useful alternative to MyPlate. It is based on the dietary patterns of the Southern Mediterranean region, which has enjoyed low rates of chronic diseases and long life expectancies.[13,14] As shown on the pyramid in Figure 2-11, foods from plant sources form the foundation of this plan. The foundation of this plan includes eating 5 to 10 servings of fruits and nonstarchy vegetables a day. For most produce, each serving is ½ cup cooked or 1 cup raw. In this plan, olives, olive oil, and avocados are considered healthy sources of fat. You also can include a handful of nuts or seeds daily as good sources of healthy fats, fiber, and protein. Legumes (beans, peas, and lentils) are also plant sources of fiber and protein. Eat ½ cup of cooked legumes, including hummus, at least twice a week. Up to four (1-ounce) portions of whole grain bread, pasta, or quinoa are included each day. A serving of grains is 1 slice of bread or ½ cup of cooked pasta, rice, or cereal. The abundant herbs and spices used in the Mediterranean dietary pattern have known antioxidant and anti-inflammatory properties.

As you make your way up the pyramid, eat a 4-ounce serving of fish two to three times a week. Moderate portions (3 or 4 ounces) of lean meat and poultry or 2 eggs are recommended once a week or every few days. Choose low-fat dairy (up to three 1-cup servings a day) from cultured sources such as yogurt or kefir. These are easier to digest and supply beneficial bacteria.

Water is always the beverage of choice. Very moderate drinking of wine (one to two 5-ounce glasses of red wine per day) may have limited health benefits—but proceed with caution. Finally, remember that regular physical activity is an important aspect of the Mediterranean lifestyle, as is eating meals with family and friends.

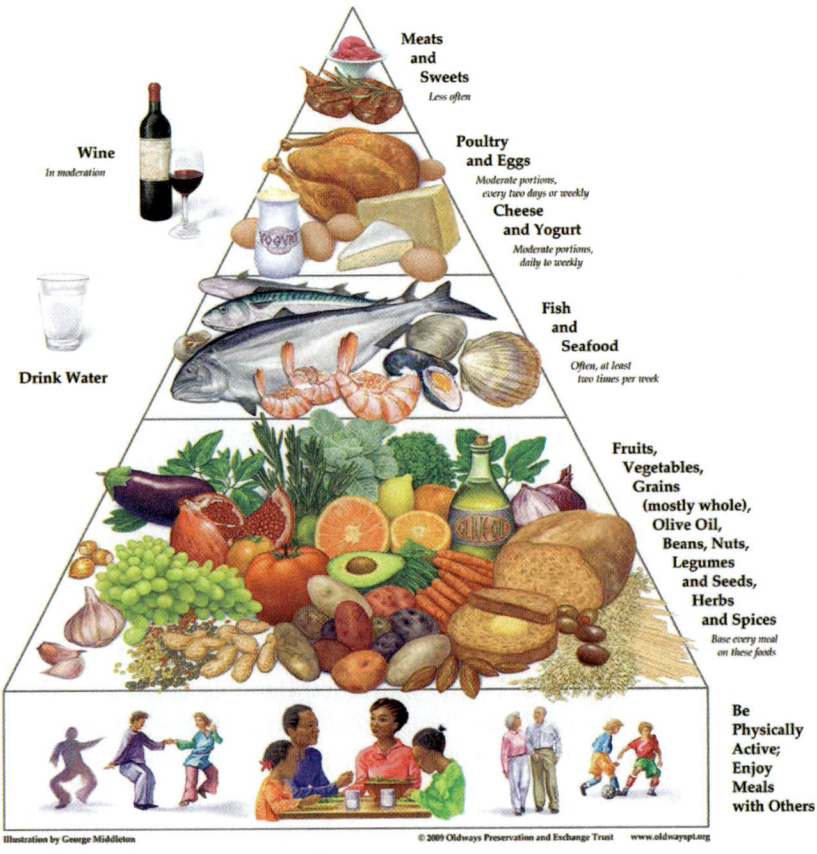

FIGURE 2-11 The Mediterranean Diet Pyramid is based on dietary patterns from the Mediterranean region. Base every meal on fruits, vegetables, whole grains, olive oil, beans, nuts, legumes, and seeds; eat fish and seafood at least two times per week; eat poultry and eggs every 2 days or weekly; eat cheese and yogurt daily to weekly; eat meats and sweets less often; drink water; drink red wine in moderation; be physically active; and enjoy meals with others.
2009 Oldways Preservation & Exchange Trust, www.oldwayspt.org. Used by permission

✓ CONCEPT CHECK 2.3

1. What is the website where you can find all of the tools associated with MyPlate?
2. What are the five major food groups represented on MyPlate?
3. List the main components of the Mediterranean Diet.

2.4 Nutritional Health

The ultimate intent of the sound nutrition advice found in the *Dietary Guidelines* and the MyPlate food guide is to promote optimal **nutritional status** for individuals. The amount of each nutrient needed to achieve this goal is the basis for published dietary intake recommendations. We have already discussed general dietary guidelines and will cover more specific nutrient recommendations later in this chapter. Adequate nutritional status is needed to ensure body tissues have enough of each nutrient to support normal metabolic functions and surplus stores that can be used in times of increased nutritional need. An optimal nutritional state can be achieved by obtaining essential nutrients from a variety of foods and adhering to the *Dietary Guidelines*. On the other end of the spectrum, **malnutrition** refers to both **overnutrition** and **undernutrition.** Neither state is conducive to good health. Furthermore, it is possible to be both over-nourished (e.g., consume excess calories) and undernourished (e.g., consume too few essential vitamins and minerals) at the same time.

nutritional status The nutritional health of a person as determined by anthropometric measurements (height, weight, circumferences, and so on), biochemical measurements of nutrients or their by-products in blood and urine, a clinical (physical) examination, a dietary analysis, and economic evaluation; also called *nutritional state*.

malnutrition Failing health that results from chronic eating practices that do not coincide with nutritional needs.

overnutrition A state in which nutritional intake greatly exceeds the body's needs.

undernutrition Failing health that results from a long-standing dietary intake that is suboptimal and does not meet nutritional needs.

UNDERNUTRITION

Undernutrition occurs when nutrient intake does not meet nutrient needs. At first, any surpluses are put to use; then, as stores are exhausted, nutritional status begins to decline. Many nutrients are in high demand due to constant cell loss and regeneration in the body, such as in the gastrointestinal (GI) tract. For this reason, the stores of certain nutrients, including many of the B vitamins, are exhausted rapidly and therefore must be replenished regularly. In addition, some females in North America do not consume sufficient iron to compensate for monthly menstrual losses and eventually deplete their iron stores (Fig. 2-12).

Hidden hunger describes a state of micronutrient deficiency, when the quality of food consumed does not meet the nutrient requirements for normal metabolic functions and maintenance. Once the availability of a nutrient falls too low, the body's metabolic processes slow down or stop. At this state of nutrient deficiency, there are often no observable **symptoms;** thus, it is termed a **subclinical** deficiency. A subclinical deficiency can go on for some time before individuals suffer detectable nutrient deficiency symptoms. Eventually, clinical symptoms will develop. Clinical evidence of a nutritional deficiency—perhaps in the skin, hair, nails, tongue, or eyes—can occur within months, but overt symptoms may take years to develop. Often, clinicians do not detect a problem until a deficiency produces observable symptoms, such as excessive bruising from a vitamin C deficiency.

OVERNUTRITION

Prolonged consumption of more nutrients than the body needs can lead to overnutrition. In the short term (e.g., 1 to 2 weeks), overnutrition may cause only a few symptoms, such as stomach distress from excess iron intake. If an excess intake continues, however, some nutrients may accumulate to toxic amounts, which can lead to serious consequences. For example, too much vitamin A during pregnancy can cause birth defects.

The most common form of overnutrition in developed nations is an excess intake of calories that leads to overweight and obesity. In the long run, obesity contributes to other serious diseases, such as type 2 diabetes and certain forms of cancer. The USDA's

hidden hunger A lack of vitamins and minerals that occurs when the quality of foods people eat does not meet their nutrient requirements.

symptom A change in health status noted by the person with the problem, such as stomach pain.

subclinical Stage of a disease or disorder not severe enough to produce symptoms that can be detected or diagnosed.

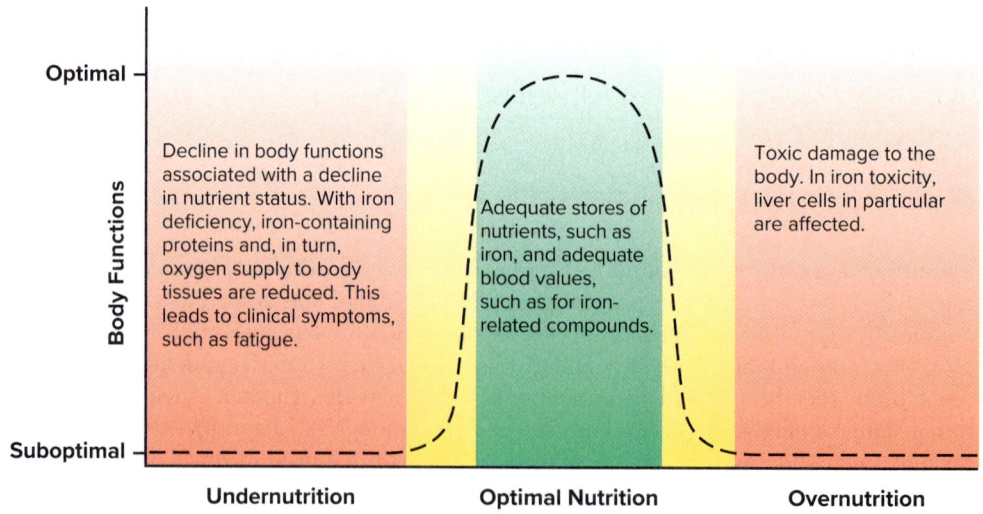

FIGURE 2-12 The general scheme of nutritional status. Green reflects optimal nutritional status, yellow indicates a marginal nutritional status, and red reflects a poor nutritional status (undernutrition or overnutrition). This general concept can be applied to all nutrients. Iron was chosen as an example because iron deficiency is the most common nutrient deficiency worldwide.

Food and Nutrition Information Service (www.nal.usda.gov/fnic) has many useful resources about weight control. Energy balance and body composition will be covered in Chapter 7.

> ✓ **CONCEPT CHECK 2.4**
>
> 1. What are the main differences between an optimal nutritional state and a state of malnutrition?
> 2. What are the two categories of malnutrition and main characteristics of each?
> 3. Describe the characteristics of hidden hunger.

2.5 Measuring Nutritional Status

To find out how nutritionally fit you are, a nutritional assessment needs to be performed. Generally, this is performed by a primary care provider, often with the aid of a registered dietitian nutritionist (RDN).

ANALYZING BACKGROUND FACTORS

Because your health history plays an important role in determining nutritional and health status, it must be carefully recorded and critically analyzed as part of a nutritional assessment. Other related information includes (1) a medical history, especially for any disease states or treatments that could affect nutrient absorption or use; (2) a list of medications; (3) social history (e.g., marital status and living conditions); (4) health literacy level; and (5) economic status to determine the ability to access and prepare food.

ASSESSING NUTRITIONAL STATUS USING THE ABCDES

In addition to background factors, five elements of nutritional assessment help to provide a comprehensive profile of nutritional status. **Anthropometric assessment** is used to assess the size, shape, and composition of the human body. These measurements often include body mass index (height, weight), circumference measures, bioelectrical impedance, and skinfold measures. Most measures of body composition are easy to obtain and are generally reliable. However, an in-depth examination of nutritional health is inadequate without the more expensive process of **biochemical assessment.** This involves the measurement of nutrients; by-products of nutrients; or factors known to affect the digestion, absorption, and/or metabolism of nutrients. A **clinical assessment** is often necessary to determine physical evidence (e.g., hypertension) of diet-related diseases or deficiencies. Then, a close look at the person's eating pattern (**dietary assessment**), including a record of previous dietary intake or food frequency, would help to determine any possible problem areas. Finally, adding the **environmental assessment** (from the background information) provides further details about the living conditions, education level, and ability to access and prepare foods needed to maintain optimal health. Taken together, these five assessments form the ABCDEs of nutritional assessment (Fig. 2-13).

anthropometric assessment Measurement of body weight and the lengths and proportions of parts of the body.

biochemical assessment Measurement of biochemical functions (e.g., concentrations of nutrient by-products or biologic activities in the blood, feces, or urine) related to a nutrient's function.

clinical assessment Examination of general appearance of skin, eyes, and tongue; sense of touch; ability to cough and walk; and evidence of rapid hair loss.

dietary assessment Estimation of typical food choices relying mostly on the recounting of one's usual intake or a record of one's previous days' intake.

environmental assessment Includes details about living conditions, education level, and the ability of the person to purchase, transport, and prepare food. The person's weekly budget for food purchases is also a key factor to consider.

LIMITATIONS OF NUTRITIONAL ASSESSMENT

A long time may elapse between the initial development of suboptimal nutritional status and the first clinical evidence of a problem. For instance, an eating pattern high in saturated fats often increases blood cholesterol without producing any clinical evidence for years. However, when the blood vessels become sufficiently blocked

FIGURE 2-13 A complete nutritional assessment includes anthropometric, biochemical, clinical, dietary, and environmental information. This information comes from a combination of patient report and history, physical assessment, and evaluation of other objective indicators (e.g., lab values).
DNY59/E+/Getty Images; TippaPatt/Shutterstock; Rick Brady/McGraw Hill; Rob Mattingley/E+/Getty Images; Hannamariah/Shutterstock

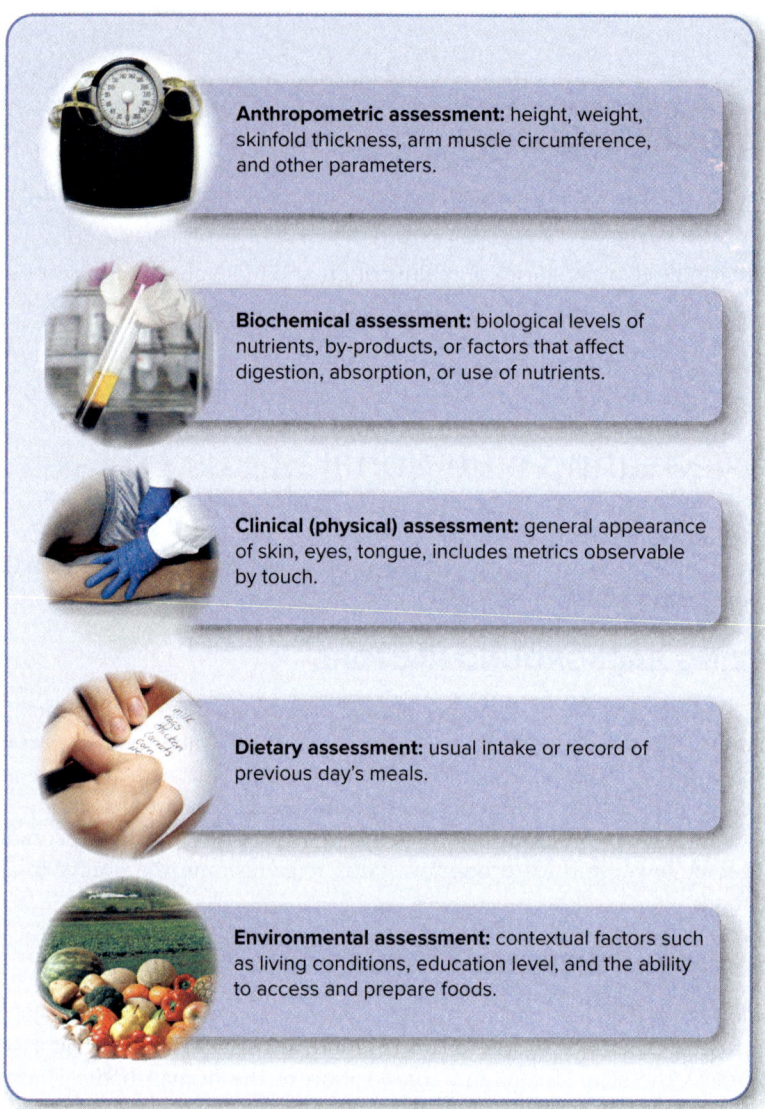

heart attack Rapid fall in heart function caused by reduced blood flow through the heart's blood vessels. Often part of the heart dies in the process. Technically called a *myocardial infarction*.

by cholesterol and other substances, chest pain or a **heart attack** may occur. Another example of a serious health condition with delayed symptoms is low bone density resulting from a calcium deficiency—a particularly relevant issue for adolescent and young adult females. Many young females do not consume the needed amount of calcium but suffer no obvious effects in their younger years; however, the bone structures of these females with low calcium intakes do not reach full potential during the years of growth, increasing the risk for osteoporosis later in life. Furthermore, clinical symptoms of some nutritional deficiencies (e.g., diarrhea, inability to walk normally, and facial sores) are not very specific. These may have causes other than poor nutrition.

✓ CONCEPT CHECK 2.5

1. What are the ABCDE categories used in assessing nutritional status?
2. Describe two limitations of nutritional assessment.

2.6 Nutrient Recommendations

The overarching goal of any healthy eating plan is to meet nutrient needs. To begin, we must determine what amount of each essential nutrient is necessary to maintain health. Most of the terms that describe nutrient needs fall under one umbrella term: **Dietary Reference Intakes (DRIs)** (Table 2-3). The development of DRIs is an ongoing, collaborative effort between the National Academies of Sciences, Engineering, and Medicine in the United States and Health Canada. Included under the DRI umbrella are **Recommended Dietary Allowances (RDAs), Adequate Intakes (AIs), Estimated Energy Requirements (EERs), Tolerable Upper Intake Levels (Upper Levels or ULs), Chronic Disease Risk Reduction Intakes (CDRRs)**, and **Acceptable Macronutrient Distribution Ranges (AMDRs).**

RECOMMENDED DIETARY ALLOWANCE

A Recommended Dietary Allowance (RDA) is the daily amount of a nutrient that will meet the needs of nearly all individuals (about 98%) of a particular age and sex. Individuals can compare their daily intake of specific nutrients to the RDA. Although slight deviations in nutrient intakes above or below the RDA for a particular nutrient are typically no reason for concern, a significant deviation below (about 70%) or above (about 300% for some nutrients) the RDA for an extended time can result in a deficiency or toxicity of that nutrient, respectively.

ADEQUATE INTAKE

An RDA can be set for a nutrient only if there is sufficient information about the human needs for that particular nutrient. Today, there is not enough information on some

Dietary Reference Intakes (DRIs) Term used to encompass nutrient recommendations made by the Food and Nutrition Board of the National Academies of Sciences, Engineering, and Medicine. These include RDAs, AIs, EERs, CDRRs, and ULs.

Recommended Dietary Allowance (RDA) Nutrient intake amount sufficient to meet the needs of 97% to 98% of the individuals in a specific life stage.

Adequate Intake (AI) Nutrient intake amount set for any nutrient for which insufficient research is available to establish an RDA. AIs are based on estimates of intakes that appear to maintain a defined nutritional state in a specific life stage.

Estimated Energy Requirement (EER) The average dietary energy intake that is predicted to maintain energy balance in an adult of a defined age, sex, weight, height, and level of physical activity.

Tolerable Upper Intake Level (UL) Maximum chronic daily intake level of a nutrient that is unlikely to cause adverse health effects in almost all people in a specific life stage.

Chronic Disease Risk Reduction Intake (CDRR) Category of DRIs based upon chronic disease risk.

Acceptable Macronutrient Distribution Range (AMDR) Range of carbohydrate, protein, or fat intake (as a percentage of total calories) that is associated with reduced risk of chronic disease, yet provides adequate amounts of essential nutrients.

TABLE 2-3 ■ Dietary Reference Intakes and Daily Value

RDA	**Recommended Dietary Allowance.** Use to evaluate your current intake for a specific nutrient. The further you stray above or below this value, the greater your chances of developing nutritional problems.
AI	**Adequate Intake.** Use to evaluate your current intake of nutrients but realize that an AI designation implies that further research is required before scientists can establish a more definitive recommendation.
EER	**Estimated Energy Requirement.** Use to estimate calorie needs of the average person within a specific height, weight, sex, age, and physical activity pattern.
UL	**Tolerable Upper Intake Level.** Use to evaluate the highest amount of daily nutrient intake unlikely to cause adverse health effects in the long run in almost all people in a population. This number applies to chronic use and is set to protect even very susceptible people in the healthy general population. As intake increases above the Upper Level, the potential for adverse effects generally increases.
CDRR	**Chronic Disease Risk Reduction Intake.** Based upon scientific evidence, the CDRR intake recommendations were developed to specifically address chronic disease risk. CDRRs have been set for sodium to reduce the risk of cardiovascular disease.
AMDR	**Acceptable Macronutrient Distribution Range.** Use to estimate or evaluate the macronutrient distribution (i.e., percentage of total calories from carbohydrates, proteins, or fats) of a dietary pattern. If energy intake is matched with energy requirements, macronutrient intakes within the AMDRs typically provide adequate nutrients and are associated with the lowest risks for chronic diseases.
DV	**Daily Value.** Use as a rough guide for comparing the nutrient content of a food to approximate human needs. Typically, the Daily Value used on food labels refers to age 4 years through adulthood. It is based on a 2000 kcal diet. Some Daily Values also increase slightly with higher calorie intakes (see Fig. 2-16 in Section 2.8 on food labeling).

nutrients, such as chromium, to set such a precise standard as an RDA. For these nutrients, the DRIs include a category called an Adequate Intake (AI). This standard is based on the dietary intakes of people who appear to be maintaining nutritional health. That amount of intake is assumed to be adequate, as no evidence of a nutritional deficiency is apparent.

ESTIMATED ENERGY REQUIREMENT

For calorie needs, we use the Estimated Energy Requirement (EER) instead of an RDA or AI. In contrast to the RDAs, which are set somewhat higher than the average requirements for nutrients, the EER is set for the average person. While a slight excess of vitamins and minerals is not harmful, a long-term excess of even a small amount of calories will lead to weight gain. Therefore, the calculation of EER needs to be more specific, taking into account age, sex, height, weight, and physical activity level. In some cases, the additional calorie needs for growth and lactation are also included. Remember, the EER is based on the average person. Thus, it can only serve as a starting point for estimating calorie needs.

TOLERABLE UPPER INTAKE LEVEL

A Tolerable Upper Intake Level (Upper Level or UL) has been set for some vitamins and minerals (Appendix F). The UL is the highest amount of a nutrient unlikely to cause adverse health effects in the long run. As intake exceeds the UL, the risk of ill effects increases. These amounts generally should not be exceeded day after day, as toxicity could develop. For people eating a variety of foods and/or using a balanced multivitamin and mineral supplement, exceeding the UL is unusual. Problems are more likely to arise with eating patterns that promote excessive intakes of a limited variety of foods, with the use of many fortified foods, or with excessive doses of individual vitamins or minerals.

CHRONIC DISEASE RISK REDUCTION INTAKES

DRIs are reference values that provide recommendations for adequate and safe intakes in apparently healthy individuals. Yet after reviewing the body of scientific evidence, the National Academies of Sciences, Engineering, and Medicine established the new Chronic Disease Risk Reduction Intakes (CDRR) DRI category. These are the first DRIs that are disease-specific and target risk reduction for chronic disease. The CDRR value for sodium was set after it was found to be linked to the risk of cardiovascular disease.

ACCEPTABLE MACRONUTRIENT DISTRIBUTION RANGE

An Acceptable Macronutrient Distribution Range (AMDR) is the range of intake of carbohydrates, protein, or fats (as a percentage of total calorie intake) that is associated with a reduced risk of chronic disease while providing essential nutrients. If an individual's usual macronutrient distribution falls outside the AMDRs, the risks of chronic diseases or insufficient intakes of essential nutrients are higher. These vary somewhat across life stages, but the AMDRs for adults are as follows:

- Carbohydrates: 45% to 65% of total calories
- Protein: 10% to 35% of total calories
- Fat: 20% to 35% of total calories

DAILY VALUE

A nutrition standard more relevant to everyday life is the **Daily Value (DV).** The DVs do not fall under the umbrella of Dietary Reference Intakes, which are specific to age, sex assigned at birth, and life stage. Instead, the DV is a more generic standard used on food labels. It serves as a general reference for anyone from 4 years of age through adulthood and is based on consuming a 2000 kcal diet. DVs are mostly set at or close to

Daily Value (DV) Quantity (expressed in percentage) of a specific nutrient that corresponds to the total percentage of the daily requirements for a particular nutrient based on a 2000 kcal diet.

the highest RDA value or related nutrient standard seen in the various age and gender categories for a specific nutrient and are listed in Appendix A. DVs have been set for vitamins, minerals, total fat and carbohydrate, and other dietary components. For fat and cholesterol, the DVs represent a maximum level, not a goal one should strive to reach. DVs allow consumers to easily compare their intake from a specific food to desirable (or maximum) intakes.

APPLICATION OF NUTRIENT STANDARDS

As nutrient intake increases, the RDA for the nutrient, if set, is eventually met and a deficient state is no longer present (Fig. 2-14). An individual's needs most likely will be met because RDAs are set high to include almost all people. Related to the RDA concept of meeting an individual's needs are the standards of AI and the EER. These can be used to estimate an individual's needs for some nutrients and calories, respectively. Still, keep in mind that these standards do not share the same degree of accuracy as the RDA. For example, EER may have to be adjusted upward if the individual is very physically active. See *Ask the RDN* in this section to learn how recommendations may vary for transgender individuals. Finally, as nutrient intake increases above the UL, poor nutritional health is again likely. However, this poor health is due now to the toxic effects of a nutrient rather than those of a deficiency.

The type of standard set for nutrients depends on the quality of available evidence. A nutrient recommendation backed by lots of experimental research will be expressed as an RDA. For a nutrient that still requires more research, only an AI is presented. We use the EER as a starting point for determining calorie needs. Some nutrients also have a UL if information on toxicity or adverse health effects is available. Periodically, new DRIs or categories of values become available as expert committees review and interpret the available research. As mentioned, a new DRI category, called Chronic Disease

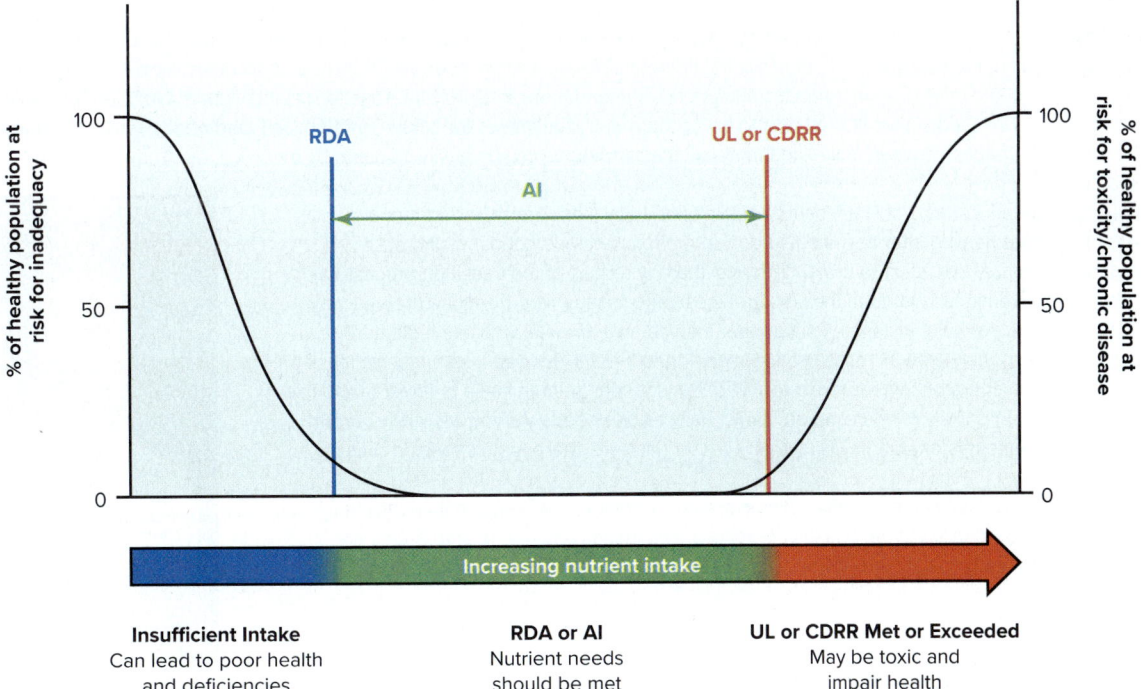

FIGURE 2-14 This figure shows the relationship of the Dietary Reference Intakes (DRIs) to each other and the percentage of the population covered by each. At intakes between the RDA and the UL or CDRR, the risk of either an inadequate diet or adverse effects from the nutrient in question is close to zero. The UL is the highest level of nutrient intake likely to pose no risks of adverse health effects to almost all individuals in the general population. The CDRR is the level above which risk for chronic disease (e.g., hypertension) increases. At intakes above the UL or CDRR, there is risk of possible adverse effects. The AI is set for some nutrients instead of an RDA. There is no established benefit for healthy individuals if they consume nutrient intakes above the RDA or AI.

Risk Reduction Intake (CDRR) was established for sodium based upon scientific evidence linking it to cardiovascular disease.

RDAs and related standards are intended mainly for diet planning. Specifically, an eating pattern should aim to meet the RDA or AI as appropriate and not to exceed the UL or CDRR over the long term. Specific RDA, AI, EER, UL, CDRR, and AMDR standards are found in Appendix F. To learn more about these nutrient standards, visit Dietary Guidance at the Food and Nutrition Information Center's website (www.nal.usda.gov/fnic).

ASK THE RDN | Transgender Issues

Dear RDN: What are the main considerations for providing informed nutrition care for transgender individuals?

To better understand potential differences in nutrient requirements for transgender individuals, let us start with defining important terms. The term *transgender* refers to someone's expression of gender. *Gender expression* (or *gender identity*) is unrelated to the physical attributes of a person (i.e., *sex*). For transgender individuals, the sex they were assigned at birth and their own gender identity do not match. On the other hand, *cisgender* individuals share the same gender as their birth-assigned *sex*. Because most people identify as cisgender, we use this term less often. Sexual orientation, or the gender to which one is attracted, is not related to gender identity.

In the medical field, understanding an individual's gender identity is sometimes complicated because an individual's birth-assigned sex is often listed as *gender* on medical documentation regardless of the person's gender identity. In fact, many medical institutions and insurance companies do not accept transgender identity as an option on medical charts.

Simply asking about and acknowledging a person's gender expression and preferred pronoun are important first steps to improving the overall health care experience for transgender individuals. According to a survey of over 6000 transgender individuals, almost 30% of participants reported postponing medical care due to perceived discrimination from their health care providers, while 19% reported being refused medical care completely. By establishing a climate of respect and rapport, the provider will be better positioned to help an individual make changes to improve health.

In this chapter, you learned about many Dietary Reference Intakes, including Estimated Energy Requirements, which are different for males and females. Should we rely on the nutrient recommendations for the transgender individual's birth-assigned sex or the individual's gender identity?

Calorie, protein, and fluid requirements are typically no different between transgender and cisgender individuals. However, we don't have enough research data to know for sure how specific nutrient recommendations may vary for transgender individuals. Nutrition professionals who work with transgender clients have started relying on gender-neutral estimates for calorie, protein, and fluid needs, which are based on body weight. Slight differences between male and female recommendations can be easily adjusted by a registered dietitian nutritionist.

Nutritional requirements certainly do change as a result of physical (i.e., surgical) or hormonal interventions. To promote healing after transition surgery, protein and calorie needs will increase. Transgender individuals may also elect to utilize hormonal therapy as part of the transition process (with or without surgical interventions). Although the timing of these effects may vary, hormone therapy may alter a person's metabolic rate. For instance, transgender men (female to male) who use testosterone hormone therapy can experience an increase in muscle and bone mass. Changes in lean muscle mass will certainly increase calorie and protein needs long term. For transgender women (male to female) who use progesterone, weight gain is likely, which can also impact daily calorie needs. As you will learn, current recommendations for some micronutrients also vary by sex. At this time, there are no specific DRIs for transgender individuals.

In order to ensure consistent and supportive care, close collaboration and honest communication between transgender individuals and the health care team are essential. As more research data are gathered, we will have greater insight into the specific nutrient requirements for this community.

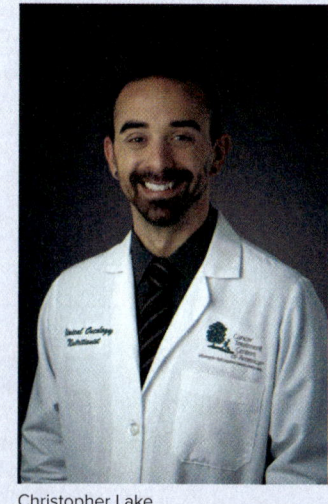

Christopher Lake

Cheers,

Zachari Breeding, MS, RDN, LDN, FAND

Clinical dietitian, professional chef, and owner of Sage Nutritious Solutions

Sources: Grant JM, Mottet LA, Tanis J, Harrison J, Herman JL, Keisling M. *Injustice at Every Turn: A Report of the National Transgender Discrimination Survey.* Washington, DC: National Center for Transgender Equality and National Gay and Lesbian Task Force; 2011.

Weinand JD, Safer JD. Hormone therapy in transgender adults is safe with provider supervision; a review of hormone therapy sequelae for transgender individuals. *J Clin Transl Endocrinol.* 2015 Jun;2(2):55-60. doi: 10.1016/j.jcte.2015.02.003

✓ CONCEPT CHECK 2.6

1. How do the definitions of RDA and AI differ? Can a nutrient have both an RDA and an AI?
2. Which DRI category includes the highest amounts of a nutrient unlikely to cause adverse health effects?
3. Chronic Disease Risk Reduction Intakes (CDRRs) have been established for what nutrient?

2.7 Evaluating Nutrition Information

Each day, you encounter nutrition information from multiple sources: from your friends and family, through your earbuds, on the screens of your devices. . . . Some of this nutrition information is shocking. Some of it seems too good to be true. Some sources of nutrition information conflict with others. It cannot all be true! How can you separate nutrition fact from fiction?

Here are a few guidelines to help you evaluate nutrition information:

1. Apply the basic principles of nutrition along with the *Dietary Guidelines* to any nutrition claim, including those on websites. Do you note any inconsistencies? Do reliable references support the claims? Beware of the following:
   - Testimonials about personal experience
   - Nonreputable publications without peer review
   - Promises of dramatic and often rapid results
   - Lack of evidence from other scientific studies
2. Examine the background and scientific credentials of the individual, organization, or authors making the nutritional claim. Usually, a reputable author is one with a nationally recognized university or medical center that offers programs or courses in the field of nutrition, medicine, or other health-related specialty.
3. Be wary if the answer is *Yes* to any of the following questions about a nutrition claim:
   - Are only advantages discussed and possible disadvantages ignored?
   - Are claims made about *curing* disease? Do they sound too good to be true?
   - Is extreme bias against the medical community or traditional medical treatments evident?
   - Is the claim touted as a *new* or *secret* scientific breakthrough?
4. Note the size and duration of any study cited in support of a nutrition claim. The larger it is and the longer it went on, the more dependable its findings. Also consider the type of study. Investigate the group studies. Are they relevant to you? Also keep in mind that *contributes to, is linked to,* or *is associated with* does not mean *causes.*
5. Beware of news conferences and social media hype regarding the latest findings. Much of this will not survive more detailed scientific evaluation.
6. When you meet with a nutrition professional, you should expect that professional will do the following:
   - Ask questions about your medical history, lifestyle, and current eating patterns.
   - Formulate a dietary pattern tailored to your specific needs.
   - Schedule follow-up visits to track your progress, answer any questions, and help keep you motivated.
   - Involve family members in the conversation when appropriate.
7. Avoid individuals who prescribe **megadoses** of vitamin and mineral supplements for everyone, especially those who profit from these products.
8. Examine product labels carefully. Be skeptical of any promotional information about a product that is not clearly stated on the label.

megadose Large intake of a nutrient well beyond estimates of needs or what would be found in a balanced diet; 2 to 10 times above human needs is typically a starting point.

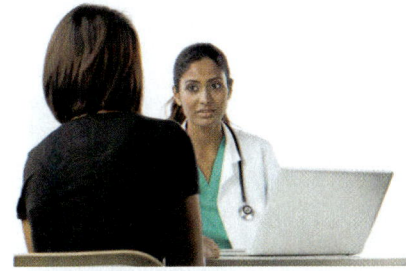

Many individuals use the terms *dietitian* and *nutritionist* interchangeably, but they are not the same! ALL registered dietitian nutritionists (RDN) are nutritionists, but not all nutritionists are dietitians. That's right—anyone can claim to be a "nutritionist"! To learn more about this important distinction, visit https://www.healthline.com/nutrition/dietitian-vs-nutritionist. Stuart Jenner/Shutterstock

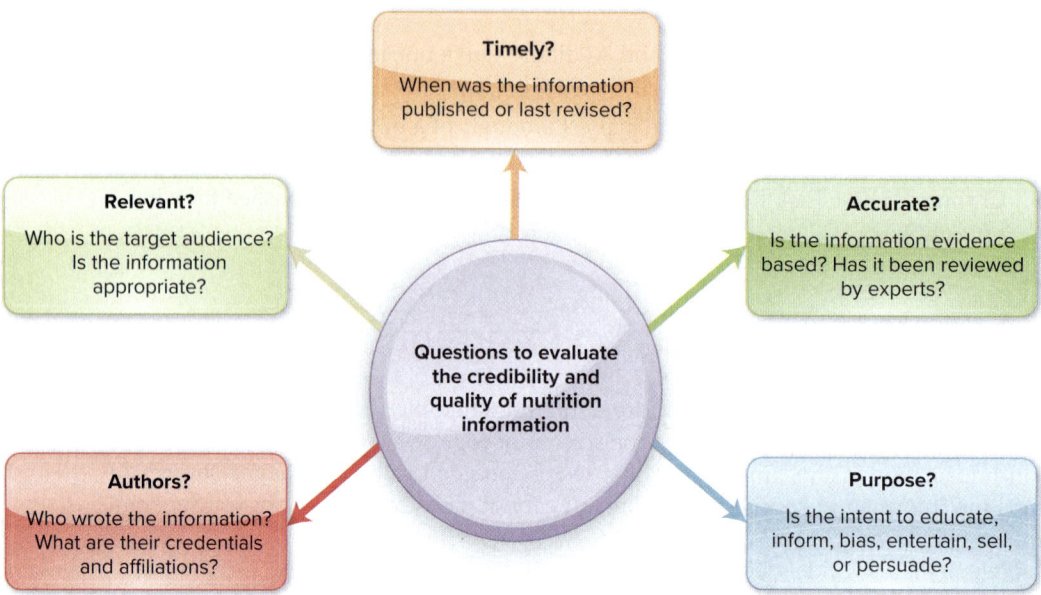

FIGURE 2-15 Adapted from the CRAAP Test, used to evaluate information and its quality.
Source: Adapted from https://library.csuchico.edu/help/source-or-information-good.

Figure 2-15 summarizes five simple inquiries that will give you some clues about the credibility of nutrition information.

Overall, nutrition is a rapidly advancing field, and there are always new findings. If it seems overwhelming or you need help applying nutrition information to your own life, consult your primary care provider or registered dietitian nutritionist first. Registered dietitian nutritionists specialize in translating complex nutrition information into practical advice that can fit into your lifestyle![15]

NUTRITION AND FITNESS APPS

Over the last decade, there has been a significant increase in mobile phone app development related to nutrition and physical activity. Numerous options have entered the marketplace, including those that provide nutrition education, enable tracking of dietary and physical activity patterns, or provide feedback and accountability. Specific to MyPlate, there are many apps to help get you started toward making healthier choices. The *Start Simple with MyPlate* app can help you set simple daily food goals and make positive changes. The *Shop Simple with MyPlate* app will help you find budget-friendly and cost-saving opportunities in your area.

With thousands to choose from, navigating these apps can be an overwhelming experience for consumers. It is important to pick an app based on the underlying nutrition-related concern as research shows some have little basis in behavioral theory and may not assist in behavior change.[16] Others, however, have been found to be motivating and encouraging. Working with nutrition professionals to gauge the most appropriate options is a good place to start, and as options continue to emerge, they are regularly reviewed by the Academy of Nutrition and Dietetics.[17]

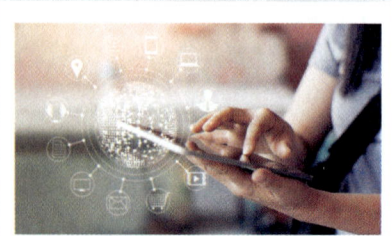

In recent years, use of diet, fitness, and other health apps has skyrocketed. **What benefits have you found from tracking your nutrition and fitness? Are there any potential drawbacks?** Pop Nukoonrat/ipopba/123RF

✓ CONCEPT CHECK 2.7

1. What are three characteristics that suggest a nutrition claim is unreliable?
2. What should your expectations be when meeting with a nutrition professional?

2.8 Food Labels and Dietary Pattern Planning

Today, nearly all foods sold in stores must bear a label with the following information: the product name, name and address of the manufacturer, amount of product in the package, a Nutrition Facts label, and the ingredients listed in descending order by weight. Food and beverage labeling is monitored by the Food and Drug Administration (FDA) in the United States.[18]

NUTRITION FACTS LABELS

Beginning in the 1960s, food manufacturers were voluntarily including information about nutrient content on the labels of some foods, but it wasn't until the 1970s that the FDA started to develop what would later become the Nutrition Facts label. In 1990, Congress passed the Nutrition Labeling and Education Act, which put the FDA in charge of which foods would need to be labeled and what information would appear on the label. Over the next few years, the FDA designed a user-friendly layout for the Nutrition Facts label and established Daily Values to help consumers compare the nutrient content of foods to their daily requirements for certain nutrients. By 1993, standardized nutrition labeling was mandated for most packaged foods.[19]

Over the years, advances in nutrition knowledge have prompted several updates to the Nutrition Facts label. For example, in 2003, after scientific evidence showed that *trans* fats contributed to unhealthy changes in blood lipids, food manufacturers were required to include *trans* fats on the Nutrition Facts label. More recently, in 2020, the layout and content of the Nutrition Facts label were updated to promote healthier eating and combat obesity. Several changes, such as increasing the type size for "Calories," "Servings per container," and the "Serving size" declaration, and bolding the number of calories and the "Serving size" declaration, were aimed at making it easier for individuals to know how many calories they are consuming. The standard serving sizes for some foods were updated to more accurately represent the portions typically consumed by individuals. To eliminate confusion about the number of servings in a container and calories in a serving, larger packages, such as a pint of ice cream, have two columns on the labels: one for "per serving" and one for "per package." The Daily Values were updated to reflect the latest Dietary Reference Intakes. The nutrients required to be listed on the Nutrition Facts label have also changed: added sugars, potassium, and vitamin D were added to the label, whereas "Calories from fat" was eliminated. All these changes were based on the latest scientific data about nutrients of public health concern.[18]

Currently, the following components must be listed on the Nutrition Facts label (Fig. 2-16):

- Total calories (kcal)
- Total fat
- Saturated fat
- *Trans* fat
- Cholesterol
- Sodium
- Total carbohydrate
- Fiber
- Total sugars
- Added sugars
- Protein
- Vitamin D
- Calcium
- Iron
- Potassium

In addition to these required components, manufacturers may choose to list polyunsaturated and monounsaturated fat, additional vitamins and minerals, and others. Listing an additional nutrient becomes *required* if the food is fortified with that nutrient or if a claim is made about the health benefits of the specific nutrient. More information about the Nutrition Facts label is available at www.fda.gov/food/nutrition-education-resources-materials/new-nutrition-facts-label.[18]

Using the Daily Values. In Section 2.6, you learned that DVs are generic nutrient intake standards used on food labels. The DVs are set at or close to the highest RDA or related nutrient standard across life stages and, where calorie requirements make a difference, they reflect the amounts of nutrients needed for a 2000 kcal diet. (If the

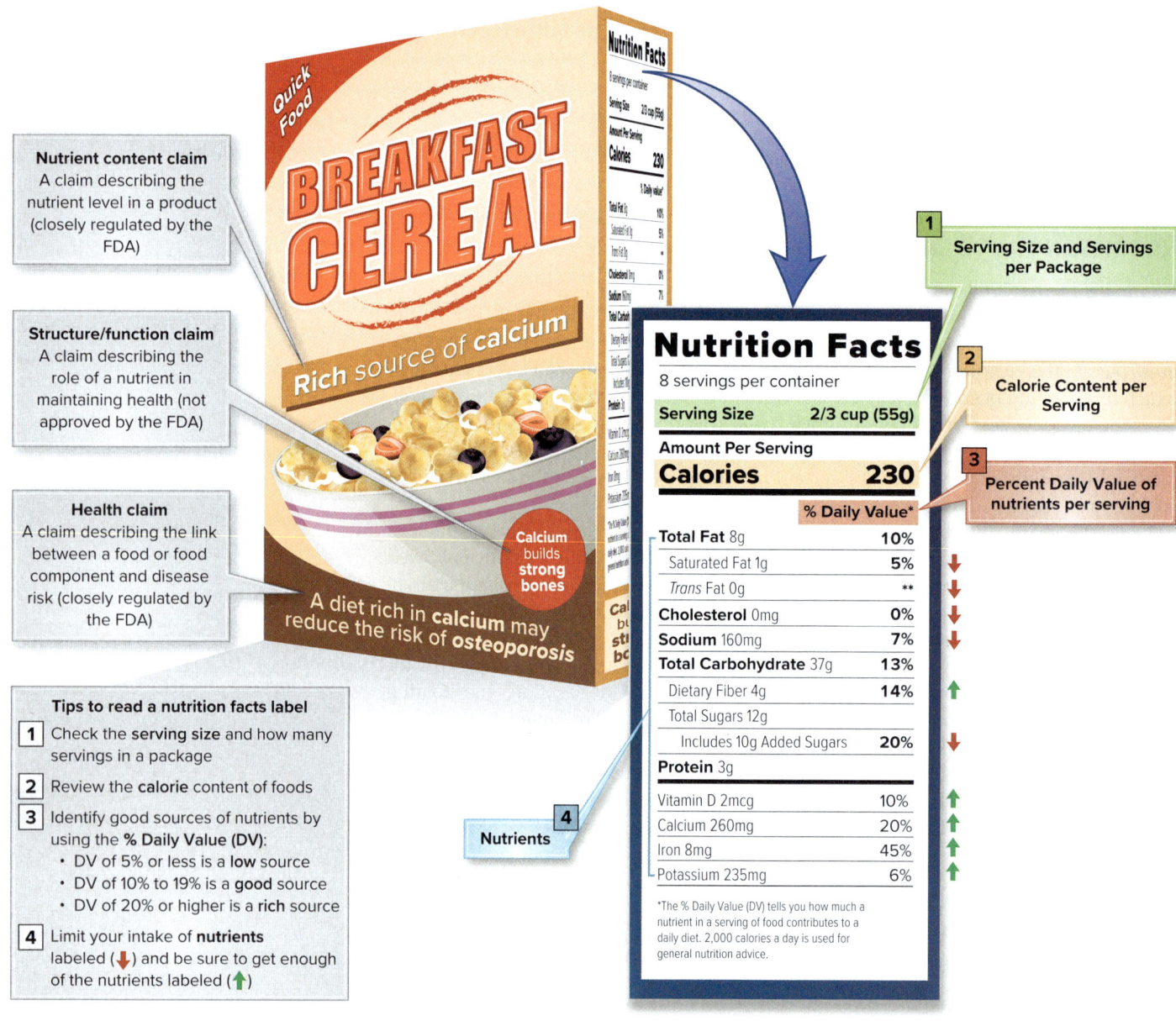

FIGURE 2-16 Food labels must list product name, name and address of the manufacturer, amount of product in the package, and ingredients. The Nutrition Facts label is required on virtually all packaged food products. The % Daily Value listed on the label represents the proportion of approximate daily nutrient needs provided by a single serving of the food product. Next to the Nutrition Facts label, the downward arrows indicate nutrients that should be reduced in the typical American dietary pattern. The upward arrows indicate nutrients that should be increased in the typical American dietary pattern.

label is large enough, the DVs for a 2500 kcal diet may be listed as well.) The percentage of the Daily Value (% Daily Value or % DV) shown for each nutrient indicates approximately how well one serving of the food meets your total daily requirement for that nutrient. For example, a serving of yogurt provides 10% of the DV for calcium. Currently, the DV for calcium is set at 1300 milligrams (which is the RDA for calcium during adolescence—the highest RDA of all life stages). Depending on your age and life stage, the DV may not exactly match your specific nutrient requirements, but in general, a serving of yogurt provides about 10% of all the calcium you need in one day.

You will see a % DV for most nutrients listed on the Nutrition Facts label. However, the % DV for protein is not mandatory on foods because protein deficiency is not a public health concern in the United States. If the % Daily Value for protein is given on a label, FDA requires that the product be analyzed for protein quality. This procedure is expensive and time-consuming, so many companies opt not to list a % Daily Value for protein. However, labels on foods for infants and children under 4 years of age must include the % Daily Value for protein, as must the labels on any food carrying a claim about protein content.

Please note for some nutrients, the DV represents a *limit* rather than a target to be reached. For example, the DV for saturated fat is 20 grams for a 2000 kcal dietary pattern. The *Dietary Guidelines* advises us to limit saturated fat intake to less than 10% of total calories; 20 grams of saturated fat would provide just under 10% of 2000 kcal. Similarly, the DV for added sugars is 50 grams (approximately 10% of 2000 kcal), the DV for cholesterol is 300 milligrams, and the DV for sodium is 2300 mg. Excessive intakes of these nutrients may contribute to the development of chronic diseases.

As shown in Figure 2-16, you can use the DVs to select foods that meet your nutrient goals. If a food provides at least 10% of the DV for a particular nutrient, it is considered a *good* source of the nutrient. If a food provides at least 20% of a nutrient, it is considered a *high* or *rich* source of that nutrient. Conversely, if a food provides less than 5% of a given nutrient, it is a *low* or *poor* source of that nutrient. How can you put this information into practice? If you have been diagnosed with iron-deficiency anemia and you need to incorporate more food sources of iron in your dietary pattern, you can use the DVs on the Nutrition Facts label to select foods that are good or rich sources of iron.

Overall, the DVs on Nutrition Facts labels allow consumers to quickly compare their intakes of nutrients from a specific food to recommended nutrient intakes for the day.

Exceptions to Food Labeling. Foods such as fresh fruits, vegetables, and fish currently are not required to have Nutrition Facts labels. However, many grocers have voluntarily chosen to provide their customers with information about these products on posters or pamphlets that may contain recipes that can assist you in your endeavor to improve your eating pattern.

LABELING CLAIMS ON FOOD PACKAGES

Food manufacturers are not allowed to make label claims about the use of foods for the prevention or treatment of disease, yet consumers are very interested in the evidence linking foods and nutrients to health. The FDA regulates the use of various claims that appear on food labels. There are three main types of label claims: nutrient content claims, health claims, and structure/function claims.

Nutrient Content Claims. Nutrient content claims can help consumers identify foods that are high or low sources of various nutrients. Nutrient content claims must follow very specific legal definitions. For example, if a product claims to be "low sodium," it must have 140 milligrams of sodium or less per serving. A list of definitions for nutrient claims allowed on food labels is given in Table 2-4.

Health Claims. Carefully worded health claims may also appear on food labels. Health claims describe the relationship between a food, food component, or ingredient and the risk for a disease or health condition. Based on the quality of the evidence, there are a few different categories of health claims, but in general, they allow food manufacturers to market their products to health-conscious consumers.

Before a health claim can be made for a food product, it must meet two general requirements. First, the food must be a "good source" (before any fortification) of fiber, protein, vitamin A, vitamin C, calcium, or iron. Second, a single serving of the food product cannot contain more than 13 grams of fat, 4 grams of saturated fat, 60 milligrams of cholesterol, or 480 milligrams of sodium. If a food exceeds any one of these requirements, no health claim can be made for it, despite its other nutritional qualities. For example, even though whole milk is high in calcium, its label can't make a health

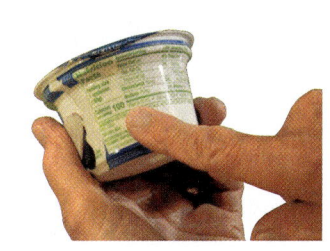

Use the Nutrition Facts label to learn more about the nutrient content of the foods you eat. Nutrient content is expressed as a percent of Daily Value (DV). **How can you use the % DV information on a food label to identify foods that are *rich* sources of a nutrient (e.g., calcium)?** Mary-Jon Ludy/McGraw Hill

TABLE 2-4 ■ Common Nutrient Claims Allowed on Food Labels

Sugar	
Sugar free: less than 0.5 gram (g) per serving	
No added sugars; without added sugars: no sugar or sugar-containing ingredient added	
Reduced sugar: at least 25% less sugar per serving than reference food	
Calories	
Calorie free: less than 5 kcal per serving	
Low calorie: 40 kcal or less per serving	
Fiber	
High fiber: 5 grams or more per serving	
Good source of fiber: 2.5 to 4.9 grams per serving	
More or added fiber: at least 2.5 grams more per serving than reference food	
Fat	
Fat free: less than 0.5 gram of fat per serving	
Low fat: 3 grams or less per serving	
Sodium	
Sodium free: less than 5 milligrams per serving	
Low sodium: 140 milligrams or less per serving	
Other Terms	
Enriched: replacing nutrients lost in processing	
Fortified: adding nutrients not originally present in the food	
Healthy: an individual food that is low fat and low saturated fat and has no more than 360 to 480 mg sodium or 60 mg cholesterol per serving and provides at least 10% of the Daily Value for vitamin A, vitamin C, protein, calcium, iron, or fiber	

Light or lite: contains ⅓ fewer calories or ½ less fat than the reference food; also can describe characteristics such as texture and color	
Good source: provides at least 10% to 19% of the Daily Value for a particular nutrient	
High: provides 20% or more of the Daily Value for a particular nutrient	

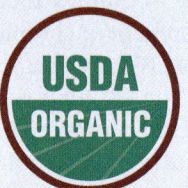
U.S. Department of Agriculture

Organic: grown without the use of pesticides, synthetic fertilizers, sewage sludge, genetically modified organisms, or ionizing radiation; meat, poultry, eggs, and dairy products from animals free of antibiotics or growth hormones; at least 95% of ingredients (by weight) must meet guidelines to be labeled "organic" on the front of the package. If the front label instead says "made with organic ingredients," only 70% of the ingredients must be organic

Natural: free of food colors, synthetic flavors, or any other synthetic substance

Meat and Poultry Products

Extra lean: less than 5 grams of fat, 2 grams of saturated fat, and 95 milligrams of cholesterol per serving (or 100 grams of an individual food)

Lean: less than 10 grams of fat, 4.5 grams of saturated fat, and 95 milligrams of cholesterol per serving (or 100 grams of an individual food)

Reduced: at least 25% less than the usual product

Low cholesterol: 20 milligrams or less and 2 grams or less of saturated fat per serving

Many definitions are from FDA's *Dictionary of Terms,* as established in conjunction with the 1990 Nutrition Labeling and Education Act (NLEA).
Source of USDA Organic seal: https://www.ams.usda.gov/rules-regulations/organic/organic-seal. U.S. Department of Agriculture

claim about calcium and osteoporosis because whole milk contains 5 grams of saturated fat per serving.

Currently, the FDA limits the use of health messages to specific instances in which there is significant scientific agreement that a relationship exists between a nutrient, food, or food constituent and the disease. Table 2-5 lists some approved health claims that may appear on food labels.

Structure/Function Claims. A third type of label claim is a structure/function claim. These claims describe the role of a nutrient or ingredient in the normal structure or function of the human body. For example, a food manufacturer may include a statement such as "calcium builds strong bones" on the label for yogurt. Structure/function claims are not as tightly regulated as nutrient claims or health claims. Although they may appear on conventional foods, structure/function claims are most commonly used on dietary supplements (Section 8.18).

TABLE 2-5 ■ Approved Health Claims on Food Labels

Health Condition	Food, Food Component, or Ingredient
Osteoporosis	Calcium and vitamin D
Cancer	Total fat, whole grains, fibers, fruits, and vegetables
Neural tube defects	Folate
Coronary heart disease	Saturated fat, soluble fiber, soy protein, stanols/sterols
Hypertension	Sodium
Dental caries	Noncariogenic sweeteners

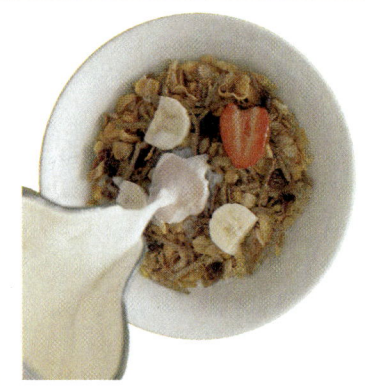

Breakfast is a great time to start the day off right. Check the Nutrition Facts label to be sure your cereal meets these criteria:

- Go for whole grains. Look for whole grain or bran among the first two ingredients in the list of ingredients.
- Check the serving sizes, which range from 30 grams (1 oz) for light cereals to 55 grams (2 oz) for heavy cereals.
- Choose cereals that do not have more than 1.2 teaspoons (7 grams) of total sugar for light cereals and 2.5 teaspoons (11 grams) for heavy cereals.
- Get enough unprocessed fiber, such as wheat bran, whole grain wheat, and oats.
- Look for cereals with less than 2.5 grams of saturated fat.

List some examples of breakfast cereals that provide at least 3 grams of fiber per serving. Peter Cade/Photodisc/Getty Images

Source: Five things to check before you buy breakfast cereal. Center for Science in the Public Interest. https://cspinet.org/tip/five-things-check-you-buy-breakfast-cereal

allergen A foreign protein, or antigen, that induces excess production of certain immune system antibodies; subsequent exposure to the same protein leads to allergic symptoms. Whereas all allergens are antigens, not all antigens are allergens.

Top Food Allergens	
Eggs	Soybeans
Fish	Tree nuts
Milk	Wheat
Peanuts	Sesame
Shellfish	

LABELING OF FOOD ALLERGENS

The Food Allergen Labeling and Consumer Protection Act (FALCPA) requires manufacturers to label food products that contain an ingredient that is or contains protein from a major food **allergen.** According to the FDA, there are nine allergens that have to be labeled: milk, eggs, fish, crustacean shellfish, tree nuts, peanuts, sesame, wheat, and soybeans. This information can be stated in one of two ways. The first option is to include the name of the food source in parentheses following the common or usual name of the major food allergen in the list of ingredients if the name of the food source of the major allergen does not appear elsewhere in the ingredients list. The second option is to put the word *Contains* followed by the name of the food source from which the major food allergen is derived immediately after or adjacent to the list of ingredients in type size that is no smaller than the ingredient type size (e.g., Contains Wheat, Milk, Eggs, and Soy).

MENU NUTRITION LABELING

Adults consume about 30% of their total calories from food and beverages prepared away from home. Dining out often increases the intake of calories, saturated fats, and sodium as compared with home-prepared meals. For the average person, consuming just one meal away from home each week equates to approximately 2 additional pounds each year. Over a 5-year period, that would translate to 10 extra pounds! To guide consumers to make informed and healthier decisions, many restaurants now list the calories of menu items on their menu boards and provide additional nutritional information online or by request.

The FDA provides these tips for dining out:

- Compare calorie and nutrition information to select the most nutrient-dense options.
- Be cautious with side dishes. Look for steamed, grilled, or broiled options.
- Many restaurant meals are quite large. Consider boxing up half to take home and enjoy later.
- Request sauces and salad dressings on the side to control the amount used.
- As with side dishes, focus on dishes that are baked, roasted, steamed, grilled, or broiled. Dishes described as creamy, fried, breaded, battered, or buttered are often much higher in calories.

For more information about restaurant menu labeling, visit https://www.fda.gov/food/nutrition-education-resources-materials/calories-menu.

MENU PLANNING WITH LABELS

All of the tools discussed in this chapter greatly aid in menu planning. Menu planning can start with MyPlate. The totality of choices made within the groups can then be evaluated using the *Dietary Guidelines.* Individual foods that make up a dietary pattern can be examined more closely using the Daily Values listed on the Nutrition Facts label of the product. For the most part, these Daily Values are in line with the Recommended Dietary Allowances and related nutrient standards. The Nutrition Facts label is especially useful in identifying nutrient-dense foods (foods high in a specific nutrient, such as vitamin D, but low in the relative amount of calories provided) and energy-dense foods (foods that provide a lot of calories for a relatively small serving size). Research has shown that individuals who read the Nutrition Facts when shopping for food report healthier nutrient consumption compared to nonusers.[20] Calorie labeling, in isolation, will not likely impact the obesity epidemic, as research has documented that many consumers do not alter their calorie intake based upon this information. Yet, it is plausible that subsequent changes may follow, thus setting the stage for ultimate success. For instance, raising public awareness may improve consumer behaviors and understanding. Consumers may then demand lower-calorie or lower-sodium alternatives in both grocery outlets and restaurants. Food manufacturers and industry may respond by modifying their formulations with public health in mind.[21]

✓ CONCEPT CHECK 2.8

1. What calorie level is used to determine the % Daily Value on a food label?
2. What are the two general requirements that must be met for a health claim on a food label?

2.9 Nutrition and Your Health: Eating Well as a Student

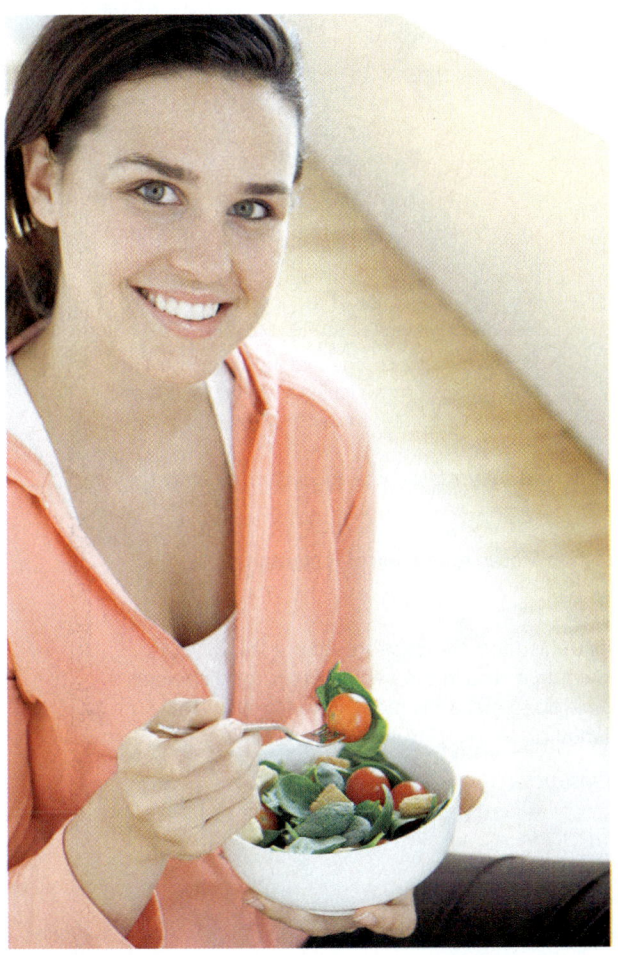

Laura Doss/Fancy Collection/SuperStock

Whether you are a traditional college student or a returning student balancing school, work, and family, studies show that the eating patterns of college students are not optimal. Typically, students fall short of nutrition recommendations for whole grains, vegetables, fruits, milk, and meat, opting instead to max out on fats, sweets, and alcohol. This information is disturbing because students are forming many health behaviors that will persist throughout life.

What is it about the student lifestyle that makes it so difficult to build healthy habits? In this section, we discuss several topics and provide possible solutions.

Food Choices

For traditional college students, these years are often a time for independence and a chance to make personal lifestyle decisions. Yet these years also pose some challenges that impact behaviors. For example, when you are writing papers and cramming for exams, balanced meals are all too easily replaced by high-fat and high-calorie fast foods, convenience items, and sugary, caffeinated beverages. Physical activity is often sacrificed in favor of study time. In a recent study of college students living on and off campus, two-thirds of the students reported skipping meals, with *no time to prepare* the major reason for this behavior.[22]

Also consider that campuses have a wide variety of dining choices. Dining halls, food trucks, fast-food establishments, bars, and vending machines combine to offer food 24 hours per day. While it is certainly possible to make wise food choices at each of these outlets, the temptations of convenience, taste, and value (i.e., inexpensive, oversized portions) may persuade the college student to select unhealthy options.

Meals and snacks are also times to socialize. You may unintentionally eat a big lunch at noon without regard to hunger if your classmates are meeting in the dining hall or food court to catch up. While chatting, it is easy to lose track of portions and to overeat. In addition, food may be a source of familiarity and comfort in a new and stressful place.

Weight Management

Studies show that many college students gain weight during their first year.[23] The *freshman 15* is a term used to describe the weight gained by students during their first year of college. Although it is becoming evident that most new students actually do not gain 15 pounds, it is common for students' dietary patterns to vary widely and result in weight loss or gain. Two lifestyle factors that made a difference in weight gain among the students include heavy drinking and working during college.

There are several reasons to maintain a healthy weight. Research clearly demonstrates that setting several small, achievable goals can spur motivation. Body weight is a balancing act between calories in and calories out. Try keeping track of your calorie consumption for several days and comparing that to your energy needs, based on your age, sex, and activity level. You can use the NutritionCalc Plus application in Connect to estimate your energy needs.

For those electing to lose weight, a healthy rate of weight loss is 1 to 2 pounds per week. Greater rates of weight loss will not likely be sustained over time. Remember that the numbers on the scale are not as important as your body composition—the amount of fat in relation to lean mass. In order to lose weight, you must create an energy deficit, either by restricting energy intake below what you need to maintain your current weight or by increasing your physical activity. For an adult with excess weight, an energy deficit of approximately

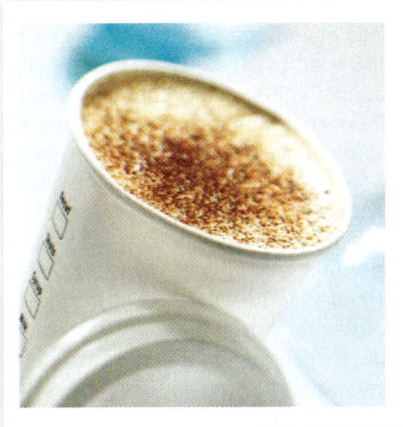

Fancy coffee beverages, such as lattes and cappuccinos, are often expensive and can increase calorie consumption by 200 kcal or more per serving. **What would be an appropriate substitution for these energy-dense drinks?**
Andrew Bret Wallis/BananaStock/PunchStock/Getty Images

CASE STUDY: College Student Eating Habits

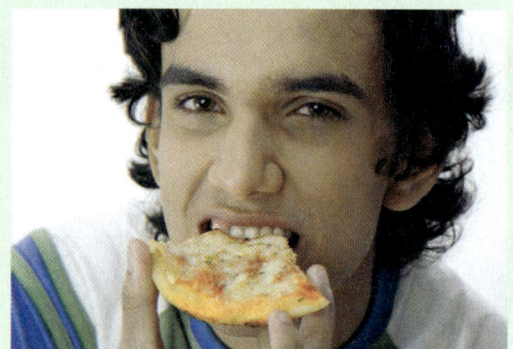

Mateo is like many other college students. He grew up on a quick bowl of cereal and milk for breakfast and a hamburger, French fries, and cola for lunch, either in the school cafeteria or at a local fast-food restaurant. At dinner, he generally avoided eating any of his vegetables, and by 9:00 P.M. he was deep into chips and cookies. Mateo has taken most of these habits to college. He prefers coffee for breakfast and possibly a chocolate donut. Lunch is still mainly a hamburger, French fries, and cola, but pizza and tacos now alternate more frequently than when he was in high school. One thing Mateo really likes about the restaurants on campus is that, for a few cents more, he can make his hamburger a double or get extra cheese and pepperoni on his pizza. This helps him stretch his food dollar; searching out large-portion value meals for lunch and dinner has become part of a typical day. Now that he is in college, some of Mateo's calories also come from alcohol. He will often have a beer with dinner a couple nights a week and will binge on a six-pack or more while tailgating before Saturday football games.

Now that he is a college student, Mateo could use some advice on developing a healthy, adult eating pattern. Dinodia Photos/Alamy Stock Photo

Provide Mateo some advice about his eating pattern. Start with his positive habits and then provide some constructive criticism, based on what you now know.

Answer the following questions, and as you make suggestions for Mateo, think about your favorite food choices, why they are your favorites, and whether these are positive choices.

1. Start with Mateo's positive habits: What healthy choices are being made when Mateo eats at local restaurants?
2. Now provide some constructive feedback:
   a. Why is ordering the "value meals" a potential problem over time?
   b. Give three examples of ways Mateo could improve the nutrient density of his food choices throughout the day.
   c. Why is variety important in dietary planning? Suggest two ways Mateo could increase the variety of his food choices.
   d. Consider Mateo's typical lunch of a burger, fries, and cola. What could he do to make his meal more like MyPlate?
   e. What concerns would you share with Mateo about his weekly alcohol intake?

Complete the Case Study. Responses to these questions can be provided by your instructor.

---

500 kcal per day will result in weight loss of about 25 pounds over a year's time. As weight is lost, energy needs gradually decrease, such that further deficits will be required to lose additional weight.

Although it may be tempting to skip, consuming a nutritious breakfast sets the stage for a healthy eating pattern. Starting the day off with a serving of lean protein (e.g., egg, Greek yogurt, or protein shake), a fortified whole grain breakfast cereal, low-fat milk, and a serving of fruit puts you on the right path for meeting recommendations for fiber, calcium, and fruit. Studies also show that eating breakfast may prevent overeating later in the day.

One of the biggest contributors to weight gain for college students is consuming several hundred calories per day in the form of sugar-sweetened or alcoholic beverages. One 12-ounce can of regular cola contains about 156 kcal.[24] A 12-ounce can of regular beer has 155 kcal. Popular gourmet coffee drinks contribute many liquid calories over time. A 12-ounce caffe mocha boasts approximately 238 kcal, and frozen coffee drinks typically contribute about 246 kcal. Even fruit juices have at least 100 kcal per 8-ounce glass. A convenient stash of water is the best way to quench your thirst.

Physical activity is very important to any weight loss and weight maintenance plan, but sticking with it is hard to do. When you find yourself short on time, physical fitness is often the first thing that goes. To ensure your success at boosting daily activity, choose activities you enjoy, such as working out with friends at the campus recreation center, participating in intramural sports, or taking an activity class like dancing. Don't forget to include brisk walking to and from classes.

Tips to Avoid Weight Gain

- **Eat a nutritious breakfast.** Rev up your metabolism with a lean protein source such as an egg or Greek yogurt, a serving of whole grains such as a fiber-rich breakfast cereal, and a fruit.
- **Plan ahead.** Eat a nutrient-dense meal or snack every few hours.
- **Limit liquid calories.** Drink water instead of high-calorie soft drinks, fruit juice, alcohol, or flavored coffee drinks. If you drink alcohol, limit it to no more than two drinks per day for men and one drink per day for women.
- **Stock the fridge and pantry.** Keep a stash of nutrient-dense snacks such as string cheese, popcorn, nuts, and fruit (fresh, canned, or dried).
- **Move more and sit less.** Engage in regular physical activity whenever possible.

Alcohol and Binge Drinking

Excessive alcohol consumption is a big problem on college campuses and in general for many young adults. Many college students consider drinking alcohol, legally or not, to be a rite of passage into adulthood. On campuses, binge drinking—consuming five or more drinks in about 2 hours for males or four drinks or more for females—has become an epidemic. A new level of extreme drinking goes far beyond binge drinking. Drinking games contribute to extreme drinking during many parties and 21st birthday celebrations.

The statistics on the impact of binge drinking on college campuses are sobering. It is estimated that about 40% of students on college campuses participate in binge drinking. Each year, over 600,000 college students between the ages of 18 and 24 suffer from unintentional injuries related to alcohol use. In addition to deaths and injuries, other problems stemming from binge drinking include unsafe sexual behavior, long-term health problems, suicides, academic issues, legal troubles, and alcohol abuse or dependence. Twenty percent of college students meet the criteria for alcohol use disorders.[23]

In addition, alcohol consumption definitely contributes to weight gain—by virtue of its own calories and the increased food consumption at events where drinking occurs. If you choose to drink alcohol, do so in moderation—no more than two drinks per day for males and one drink per day for females. Be aware of the warning signs and dangers of alcohol poisoning shown here.[25]

The warning signs and symptoms of alcohol poisoning:
- Cold, clammy, pale, or bluish skin
- Semi-consciousness or unconsciousness
- Slow respiration of 8 or fewer breaths per minute or lapses between breaths of more than 8 seconds
- Strong odor of alcohol, which usually accompanies these symptoms

Source: CDC

Eating Disorders

As many as 30% of college students are at risk of developing an eating disorder. **Disordered eating** is a short-term change in eating patterns. Sometimes, disordered eating habits may lead to an eating disorder, such as anorexia nervosa, bulimia nervosa, or binge eating disorder. Advice on what to do if you suspect that someone you know is suffering from an eating disorder will be discussed later in the text.

Starving the body also starves the brain, which limits performance in academics and beyond. The negative consequences of disordered eating may last a lifetime. Frequently, what begins as a weight-loss fad diet spirals into a much larger problem. Eating disorders are not just diets gone bad: they require professional intervention. Left unchecked, eating disorders can lead to serious adverse effects, such as loss of menstrual periods, bone disorders, gastrointestinal problems, kidney issues, heart abnormalities, and even death.

Choosing a Plant-Forward Lifestyle

Many young adults experiment with or adopt a vegetarian or **vegan** eating pattern. Plant-focused dietary patterns can meet nutrition needs and decrease risk of many chronic diseases, but they require appropriate planning at all life stages.

Protein is not typically deficient in vegetarian eating patterns, even with a vegan diet, which contains no animal products.

disordered eating Mild and short-term changes in eating patterns that occur in relation to a stressful event, an illness, or a desire to modify one's dietary pattern for a variety of health and personal appearance reasons.

 Sustainable Solutions

Plant-Focused Dietary Pattern

Plant-forward or plant-focused dietary patterns celebrate, but are not limited to, plant-based foods. Plant food sources include fruits and vegetables (produce); whole grains; beans, other legumes (pulses), and soy foods; nuts and seeds; plant oils; and herbs and spices. Dietary patterns rich in plant foods reflect evidence-based principles supporting personal and environmental health and sustainability.

However, vegetarians, and especially vegans, may be at risk for deficiencies of several vitamins and minerals. Consuming a fortified ready-to-eat breakfast cereal is an easy and inexpensive way to obtain these nutrients.

Restaurants and campus dining services have responded to the growing interest in plant-forward meals by offering a variety of vegetarian options. For optimal health benefits, choose foods that are baked, steamed, or stir-fried rather than deep-fried; select whole grains rather than refined carbohydrates; and consume foods fortified with vitamins and minerals. Even if you do not follow a plant-based eating pattern all the time, choosing several plant-focused meals each week can help with weight control and boost intake of fiber and beneficial phytochemicals. The MyPlate Plan recommends that the largest portion of your plate be filled with plant foods, including grains, fruits, and vegetables.

Fuel for Competition: Student Athletes

Students who compete in sports, such as intramural and intercollegiate athletics, need to consume more calories and nutrients. Despite an emphasis on a lean physique, athletes at all levels must take care not to severely restrict calories, as this could negatively impact performance and health. Muscles require adequate carbohydrates for fuel

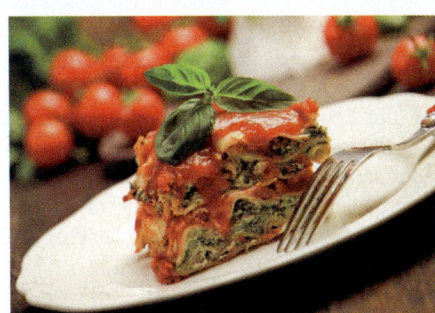

Many students adopt a vegetarian eating pattern during college. Guidelines for planning a nutritious vegetarian eating pattern with items such as this veggie-stuffed lasagna dish are presented in Chapter 6. **Which plant-based meals do you enjoy?** Francesco83/Shutterstock

vegan Referring to a dietary pattern that only includes foods of plant origin.

ASK THE RDN: Nutrition and Academic Performance

Dear RDN: *Could dietary changes help me get better grades?*

Surprisingly, there are just a few studies that have examined the effects of nutrition on academic performance. Most of those studies were conducted with school-age children, and they are all observational studies, which means we can't say for certain that one dietary factor *causes* better academic performance; we can just see that certain behaviors are *related to* better performance.

One observation about the impact of nutrition on academic performance among college students is that eating breakfast is associated with better academic performance. Why might this be true? It is possible that the benefits of breakfast on academic performance have nothing to do with nutrition. Eating breakfast might just be a marker of a better student—one who gets up early, leaving enough time to eat breakfast before getting to class. Eating breakfast may also be an indicator of better socioeconomic status. Indeed, there are many reasons why better socioeconomic status is related to success in school. But there are several nutritional reasons why eating breakfast may improve academic performance.

Eating carbohydrates will provide some much-needed energy for your brain cells. Whereas most cells can use carbohydrates, fats, or proteins for fuel, your brain relies on glucose under most conditions. When blood sugar levels are low, we usually feel hungry and a bit irritable. Indeed, studies show that skipping breakfast is linked to decreased cognitive function and negative mood.

The quality of your breakfast matters, too! A systematic review of many studies of breakfast composition and cognition showed that a breakfast with a lower glycemic load is associated with better performance on cognitive tasks. In other words, foods with a lot of simple sugars provide glucose to your brain *in a hurry*, but it may be better to choose meals with a combination of complex carbohydrates, protein, and fat to *maintain a steady supply* of glucose and other nutrients to the brain over several hours.

Besides supplying energy, eating breakfast is also associated with better nutrient intakes. People who eat breakfast tend to have better diet quality, in general. Breakfast cereals are typically fortified with a variety of micronutrients. Among children, fortified breakfast cereal is the leading source of vitamin A, iron, and B vitamins, such as folic acid. Iron is needed for healthy red blood cells, which bring oxygen to your brain. Iron and B vitamins are involved in other brain functions, as well: nerve myelination, neurotransmitter synthesis, and energy metabolism. Even marginal deficiencies of iron and B vitamins have been related to decreased academic achievement.

Besides breakfast, several studies show that intake of fruit is positively correlated with academic achievement. According to NHANES data, fruit and vegetable consumption decline during early adulthood. The majority of adults in their 20s consume less than 1 serving of fruit per day. Like breakfast, eating fruit may also simply be a marker of better overall dietary quality or better socioeconomic status. Perhaps higher-achieving students have higher levels of health knowledge that lead to higher fruit intake. Or perhaps higher micronutrient intake among students who regularly consume fruit improves brain function.

A few studies have linked higher fast-food intake with lower academic achievement. Frequent fast-food consumption is probably a marker of poor health habits overall. Fast-food meals are higher in calories, saturated fat, and sodium but lower in fiber and many micronutrients compared to home-prepared meals. Perhaps students who frequently consume fast food have lower intakes of micronutrients that support optimal brain function.

In Chapter 2 and throughout the pages of this book, you will notice that we're big fans of the Mediterranean diet. It protects heart health, it's useful for weight management, and it may prevent Alzheimer's disease. Well, guess what! Young adults who adhere to a Mediterranean diet also perform better in school. We don't know the mechanisms for sure, but the Mediterranean diet is based on whole, unprocessed fruits, vegetables, and grains, which supply complex carbohydrates—a sustained source of energy for your brain throughout the day. There is also evidence that higher intakes of seafood (a source of omega-3 fatty acids) may improve mood and cognitive function.

To put it all together, I'd recommend starting your day with breakfast to give that busy brain of yours some fuel! A fortified, whole-grain breakfast cereal with milk is an excellent choice. Try a breakfast burrito with scrambled eggs and chopped veggies wrapped in a tortilla. Top a cup of Greek yogurt with some diced fruit and granola. Throughout the rest of the day, try to eat regular meals—complex carbohydrates along with some protein and fats—to provide a steady supply of energy to your brain.

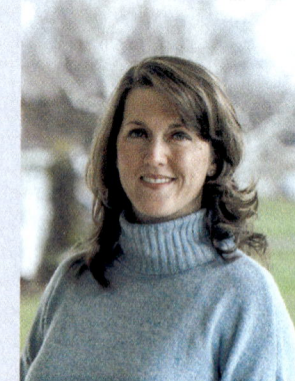
Tim Klontz

Eating well to make the grade,

Angela Collene, MS, RDN, LD

Senior Lecturer, The Ohio State University, Author of *Wardlaw's Contemporary Nutrition* and *Wardlaw's Contemporary Nutrition: A Functional Approach*

Sources: Antonopoulou M, Mantzorou M, Serdari A, et al. Evaluating Mediterranean diet adherence in university student populations: does this dietary pattern affect students' academic performance and mental health? *Int J Health Plan Manage*. 2020 Jan;35(1):5-21. doi: 10.1002/hpm.2881

Burrows TL, Whatnall MC, Patterson AJ, Hutchesson MJ. Associations between dietary intake and academic achievement in college students: a systematic review. *Healthcare (Basel)*. 2017 Sep 25;5(4):60. doi: 10.3390/healthcare5040060

Reuter PR, Forster BL, Brister SR. The influence of eating habits on the academic performance of university students. *J Am Coll Health*. Nov-Dec 2021;69(8):921-927. doi: 10.1080/07448481.2020.1715986

and protein for growth and repair. Fat, as well, is an important source of stored energy for use during physical activity. In addition to the calories needed to fuel the body, fluids are essential for health and performance. Water is adequate to replenish losses for most activities.

Athletes also should take care not to be wooed by the supplement industry. Simply increasing food intake to meet the energy demands of athletic training should be sufficient to meet most vitamin and mineral needs. Individual vitamin, mineral, amino acid, or herbal supplements are rarely advised, in spite of the hype of supplement makers. More about sports nutrition will be discussed in Chapter 10.

Tips for Eating Well on a Student's Budget

Because higher education can be hard on the wallet, it is good to know that it is possible to eat well on campus on a budget. Over 30% of college students experience some food insecurity, including disruptions in eating patterns and reduced food intake.[26] If you live on campus, try to participate in a prepaid campus meal plan if possible. These plans are generally designed to offer great food value with a variety of nutritious foods. If you live off campus or have your own kitchen, try to plan ahead. Packing a lunch from home rather than grabbing lunch on the run will save you money and put you in control of healthy choices. Some campuses now have food pantries for students. This is an excellent resource when food access issues arise.

Avoid shopping on an empty stomach: everything will look good, and you'll likely buy more. Instead, stock your fridge and pantry with healthy foods so they are the first things on hand when you get hungry. Try to have a list in hand and stick to it because impulse buys tend to drain your wallet. Try store-brand rather than name-brand items. Keep healthy snacks around and limit junk food. Eat more fruits and vegetables. Make use of canned and frozen fruits and vegetables; they are just as nutritious, particularly if you choose low-sodium and low-sugar options. Canned (fruits, tuna) and dry (oatmeal) foods can be nutritious and last a long time, so you can avoid waste. Drink water and limit sugary, alcoholic, and highly caffeinated beverages. Finally, avoid using food to combat stress and try working out instead.

✓ CONCEPT CHECK 2.9

1. Name three aspects of the student lifestyle that make it difficult to build nutritious eating habits.
2. Specify three tips for eating well on a student's budget.

Summary (Numbers refer to numbered sections in the chapter)

2.1 A healthy dietary pattern includes a variety of nutrient-dense foods to meet nutrient needs within calorie limits. Such an eating pattern helps to minimize the risk of developing nutrition-related diseases.

Nutrient density reflects the nutrient content of a food in relation to its calorie content. Nutrient-dense foods are relatively rich in nutrients in comparison with calorie content.

The energy density of a food is determined by comparing calorie content with the weight of food. A food rich in calories but weighing relatively very little, such as cookies, fried foods in general, and most snack foods (including fat-free brands), is considered energy dense. Foods with low energy density include fruits, vegetables, and any food that incorporates lots of water during cooking, such as oatmeal.

2.2 *Dietary Guidelines for Americans* has been issued to help improve the health of all individuals throughout every life stage from birth through older adulthood. The *Dietary Guidelines* emphasizes a healthy eating pattern that includes a variety of vegetables from all of the subgroups, whole fruits, whole grains, fat-free or low-fat dairy, and a variety of lean and plant-based protein foods, and it limits saturated fats, added sugars, sodium, and alcohol. According to the *Physical Activity Guidelines*, Americans should aim for 150 to 300 minutes per week of moderate-intensity physical activity.

2.3 MyPlate and accompanying online tools are designed to translate nutrient recommendations into a food plan at every stage of life. It emphasizes eating a variety of fruits, vegetables, grains, dairy or fortified soy alternatives, and protein foods. When deciding what to eat or drink, make every bite count.

2.4 A person's nutritional status can be categorized as optimal when the body has adequate nutrient stores for times of increased needs. Malnutrition encompasses both undernutrition, which may be present with or without clinical symptoms, and overnutrition, which can lead to vitamin and mineral toxicities and various obesity-related chronic diseases.

2.5 Evaluation of nutritional status involves analyzing background factors, as well as anthropometric, biochemical, clinical, dietary, and environmental assessments. It is not always possible to detect nutritional inadequacies via nutritional assessment because symptoms of deficiencies are often nonspecific and may not appear for many years.

2.6 Dietary Reference Intakes (DRIs) are a set of energy and nutrient intake standards established for the United States and Canada. Recommended Dietary Allowances (RDAs) are set for many nutrients. These amounts yield enough of each nutrient to meet the needs of healthy individuals within specific sex and age categories. Adequate Intake (AI) is the standard used when not enough information is available to set a more specific RDA. Estimated Energy Requirements (EERs) set calorie needs for both sexes at various ages and physical activity patterns. Tolerable Upper Intake Levels (Upper Levels or ULs) for nutrient intake have been set for some vitamins and minerals. Chronic Disease Risk Reduction Intakes (CDRRs) are set for sodium and are the only Dietary Reference Intakes (DRIs) specific to disease risk. An Acceptable Macronutrient Distribution Range (AMDR) is the range of intake of carbohydrates, protein, or fats (as a percentage of total calorie intake) that is associated with a reduced risk of chronic disease while providing essential nutrients. All of these dietary standards fall under the term DRIs.

Daily Values are used as a basis for expressing the nutrient content of foods on the Nutrition Facts label and are based for the most part on the RDAs.

2.7 Apply the basic principles of nutrition to evaluate any nutrition claim. Several indicators of nutrition misinformation include insufficient scientific evidence to support a product claim, lack of credible sources, promises of unbelievable results, or distrust of the medical community. To sort nutrition fact from fiction, seek the advice of a registered dietitian nutritionist.

2.8 Food labels are useful tools to track your nutrient intake and learn more about the nutritional characteristics of the foods you eat. Most packaged foods (mandated) and some whole, fresh foods (voluntary) display food labels. Nutrition Facts labels must include information about serving size, calories, lipids (total fat, saturated fat, *trans* fat, and cholesterol), sodium, carbohydrates (total carbohydrates, dietary fiber, total sugars, and added sugars), protein, vitamin D, calcium, iron, and potassium. Any health claims listed must follow FDA-set criteria.

2.9 Eating patterns and other health habits of college students often fail to align with the *Dietary Guidelines*. This information is disturbing from a public health standpoint because young adulthood is the time when many health behaviors are formed and will likely persist throughout life. Issues of particular importance for students in college are weight management, alcohol consumption, food security, and eating disorders.

Check Your Knowledge (Answers are available at the end of this question set)

1. Anthropometric measurements include
   a. height, weight, skinfolds, and body circumferences.
   b. blood concentrations of nutrients.
   c. a diet history of the previous days' intake.
   d. blood levels of enzyme activities.

2. Foods with *high* nutrient density offer the _____ nutrients for the _____ calories.
   a. least, lowest
   b. least, most
   c. most, lowest
   d. most, most

3. A meal of a bean burrito, cucumber salad, and glass of milk represents foods from all MyPlate food groups except
   a. dairy.
   b. protein.
   c. vegetables.
   d. fruits.

4. The *Dietary Guidelines* recommend that we increase which of the following foods?
   a. Refined grains
   b. Whole milk products
   c. Seafood
   d. Added sugars

5. How many minutes of moderate-intensity physical activity are recommended for adults in the *Physical Activity Guidelines for Americans*?
   a. 150 to 300 minutes per week
   b. 30 to 60 minutes every day
   c. 50 to 150 minutes every day
   d. 30 to 60 minutes three days a week

6. The term *Daily Value* is used on
   a. restaurant menus.
   b. food labels.
   c. medical charts.
   d. health claims.

7. The Tolerable Upper Intake Level, or UL, is used to
   a. estimate calorie needs of the average person.
   b. evaluate the highest amount of daily nutrient intake unlikely to cause adverse health effects.
   c. evaluate your current intake for a specific nutrient.
   d. compare the nutrient content of a food to approximate human needs.

8. The current food label must list
   a. a picture of the product.
   b. a uniform and realistic serving size.
   c. the RDA for each age group.
   d. ingredients alphabetically.

9. The most common type of undernutrition worldwide is
   a. anorexia.
   b. protein deficiency.
   c. obesity.
   d. iron deficiency.

10. A behavior that will decrease the risk of weight gain in college is to
    a. skip breakfast.
    b. drink more liquid calories.
    c. stock your fridge with nutritious snacks.
    d. move less and sit more.

Answer Key: 1. a (LO 2.5), 2. c (LO 2.1), 3. d (LO 2.3), 4. c (LO 2.2), 5. a (LO 2.2), 6. b (LO 2.8), 7. b (LO 2.6), 8. b (LO 2.8), 9. d (LO 2.4), 10. c (LO 2.9)

Study Questions (Numbers refer to Learning Outcomes)

1. How would you explain the concepts of nutrient density and energy density to a fourth-grade class? **(LO 2.1)**

2. Describe the intent of the *Dietary Guidelines for Americans*. Based on the discussion of the *Dietary Guidelines*, suggest two key dietary changes the typical adult should consider making. **(LO 2.2)**

3. What changes to your eating pattern would you need to make to comply with the healthy eating guidelines exemplified by MyPlate on a regular basis? **(LO 2.3)**

4. Can a person have both undernutrition and overnutrition at the same time? Explain your response. **(LO 2.4)**

5. What steps would you follow to evaluate the nutritional state of an undernourished person? **(LO 2.5)**
6. How do RDAs and AIs differ from Daily Values in intention and application? **(LO 2.6)**
7. What would you list as the top five sources of reliable nutrition information? What makes these sources reliable? **(LO 2.7)**
8. Dietitians encourage all people to read labels on food packages to learn more about what they eat. What four nutrients could easily be tracked in your diet if you read the Nutrition Facts labels regularly on food products? **(LO 2.8)**
9. Define the USDA definition for the term *good source.* **(LO 2.8)**
10. List some specific health claims that can be made on food labels. **(LO 2.8)**
11. List five strategies to avoid weight gain during college. **(LO 2.9)**

References

1. Steele EM, O'Connor LE, Juul F, et al. Identifying and estimating ultraprocessed food intake in the US NHANES according to the Nova Classification System of Food Processing. *J Nutr.* 2023;153(1):225-241. doi:10.1016/j.tjnut.2022.09.001
2. Hess JM, Comeau ME, Casperson S, et al. Dietary Guidelines meet NOVA: developing a menu for a healthy dietary pattern using ultra-processed foods. *J Nutr.* 2023;153(8):2472-2481. doi:10.1016/j.tjnut.2023.06.028
3. Hingle MD, Kandiah J, Maggi A. Practice paper of the Academy of Nutrition and Dietetics: selecting nutrient-dense foods for good health. *J Acad Nutr Diet.* 2016 Sep;116(9):1473-1479. doi: 10.1016/j.jand.2016.06.375
4. Wallace TC, Bailey RL, Blumberg JB, et al. Fruits, vegetables, and health: a comprehensive narrative, umbrella review of the science and recommendations for enhanced public policy to improve intake. *Crit Rev Food Sci Nutr.* 2020;60(13):2174-2211. doi: 10.1080/10408398.2019.1632258
5. Alissa EM, Ferns GA. Dietary fruits and vegetables and cardiovascular diseases risk. *Crit Rev Food Sci Nutr.* 2017 Jun 12;57(9):1950-1962. doi: 10.1080/10408398.2015.1040487
6. Rolls BJ. Dietary energy density: applying behavioural science to weight management. *Nutr Bull.* 2017 Sep;42(3):246-253. doi: 10.1111/nbu.12280
7. U.S. Department of Agriculture; U.S. Department of Health and Human Services. *Dietary Guidelines for Americans, 2020–2025.* 9th ed. December 2020. Accessed October 14, 2023. http://DietaryGuidelines.gov
8. Snetselaar LG, de Jesus JM, DeSilva DM, Stoody EE. Dietary Guidelines for Americans, 2020–2025: understanding the scientific process, guidelines, and key recommendations. *Nutr Today.* 2021;56(6):287-295. doi:10.1097/NT.0000000000000512
9. Schwingshackl L, Bogensberger B, Hoffmann G. Diet quality as assessed by the Healthy Eating Index, Alternate Healthy Eating Index, Dietary Approaches to Stop Hypertension score, and health outcomes: an updated systematic review and meta-analysis of cohort studies. *J Acad Nutr Diet.* 2018 Jan;118(1):74-100.e11. doi: 10.1016/j.jand.2017.08.024
10. HEI Scores for Americans. USDA Food and Nutrition Service. July 14, 2023. Accessed October 14, 2023. https://www.fns.usda.gov/cnpp/hei-scores-americans
11. Physical activity guidelines for Americans. U.S. Department of Health and Human Services. 2018. Accessed October 17, 2021. https://www.health.gov/PAGuidelines
12. Lee SH, Moore LV, Park S, Harris DM, Blanck HM. Adults meeting fruit and vegetable intake recommendations — United States, 2019. *MMWR Morb Mortal Wkly Rep.* 2022;71(1):1-9. Published 2022 Jan 7. doi:10.15585/mmwr.mm7101a1
13. Mediterranean diet. Oldways Preservation Trust. Accessed October 17, 2023. https://oldwayspt.org/traditional-diets/mediterranean-diet
14. What is the Mediterranean Diet? American Heart Association. April 18, 2018. Accessed October 17, 2023. https://www.heart.org/en/healthy-living/healthy-eating/eat-smart/nutrition-basics/mediterranean-diet
15. Diekman C, Ryan CD, Oliver TL. Misinformation and disinformation in food science and nutrition: impact on practice. *J Nutr.* 2023;153(1):3-9. doi:10.1016/j.tjnut.2022.10.001
16. El Khoury CF, Karavetian M, Halfens RJG, Crutzen R, Khoja L, Schols JMGA. The effects of dietary mobile apps on nutritional outcomes in adults with chronic diseases: a systematic review and meta-analysis. *J Acad Nutr Diet.* 2019 Apr;119(4):626-651. doi: 10.1016/j.jand.2018.11.010
17. Academy of Nutrition and Dietetics. *Food and Nutrition Magazine.* Accessed October 15, 2023. https://foodandnutrition.org/tag/apps/
18. Industry resources on the changes to the Nutrition Facts label. U.S. Food & Drug Administration. Accessed October 15, 2023. https://www.fda.gov/food/food-labeling-nutrition/industry-resources-changes-nutrition-facts-label
19. Institute of Medicine. *Examination of Front-of-Package Nutrition Rating Systems and Symbols: Phase I Report.* Washington, DC: The National Academies Press; 2010.
20. Ollberding NJ, Wolf RL, Contento I. Food label use and its relation to dietary intake among US adults. *J Am Diet Assoc.* 2010;110(8):1233-1237. doi:10.1016/j.jada.2010.05.007
21. Miller LMS, Cassady DL, Applegate EA, et al. Relationships among food label use, motivation, and dietary quality. *Nutrients.* 2015 Feb 5;7(2):1068-1080. doi: 10.3390/nu7021068
22. Choi S, Lee Y. Relationship of college students' residence to frequency of meal skipping and snacking pattern. *J Acad Nutr Diet.* 2012 Sep 1;112(9 Suppl):A24. doi: 10.1016/j.jand.2012.06.082
23. College alcoholism. Alcohol Rehab Guide. Accessed October 17, 2023. https://www.alcoholrehabguide.org/resources/college-alcohol-abuse
24. USDA Food and Nutrient Database for Dietary Studies and USDA Food Patterns Equivalents Database 2017–2018. U.S. Department of Agriculture, Agricultural Research Service, Food Surveys Research Group. https://ars.usda.gov/nea/bhnrc/fsrg
25. Alcohol poisoning deaths. Centers for Disease Control and Prevention. January 2015. Accessed October 17, 2023. https://www.cdc.gov/vitalsigns/pdf/2015-01-vitalsigns.pdf
26. Nikolaus CJ, An R, Ellison B, Nickols-Richardson SM. Food insecurity among college students in the United States: a scoping review. *Adv Nutr.* 2020;11(2):327–348. doi:10.1093/advances/nmz111

Design Element Credits: Fact Check/magnifying glass icon: McGraw Hill; Magnificent Microbiome background image: Alena Ohneva/Shutterstock; Sustainable Solutions icon: McGraw Hill; Roots icon: McGraw Hill; Medicine Cabinet icon: Peter Dazeley/Photographer's Choice/Getty Images

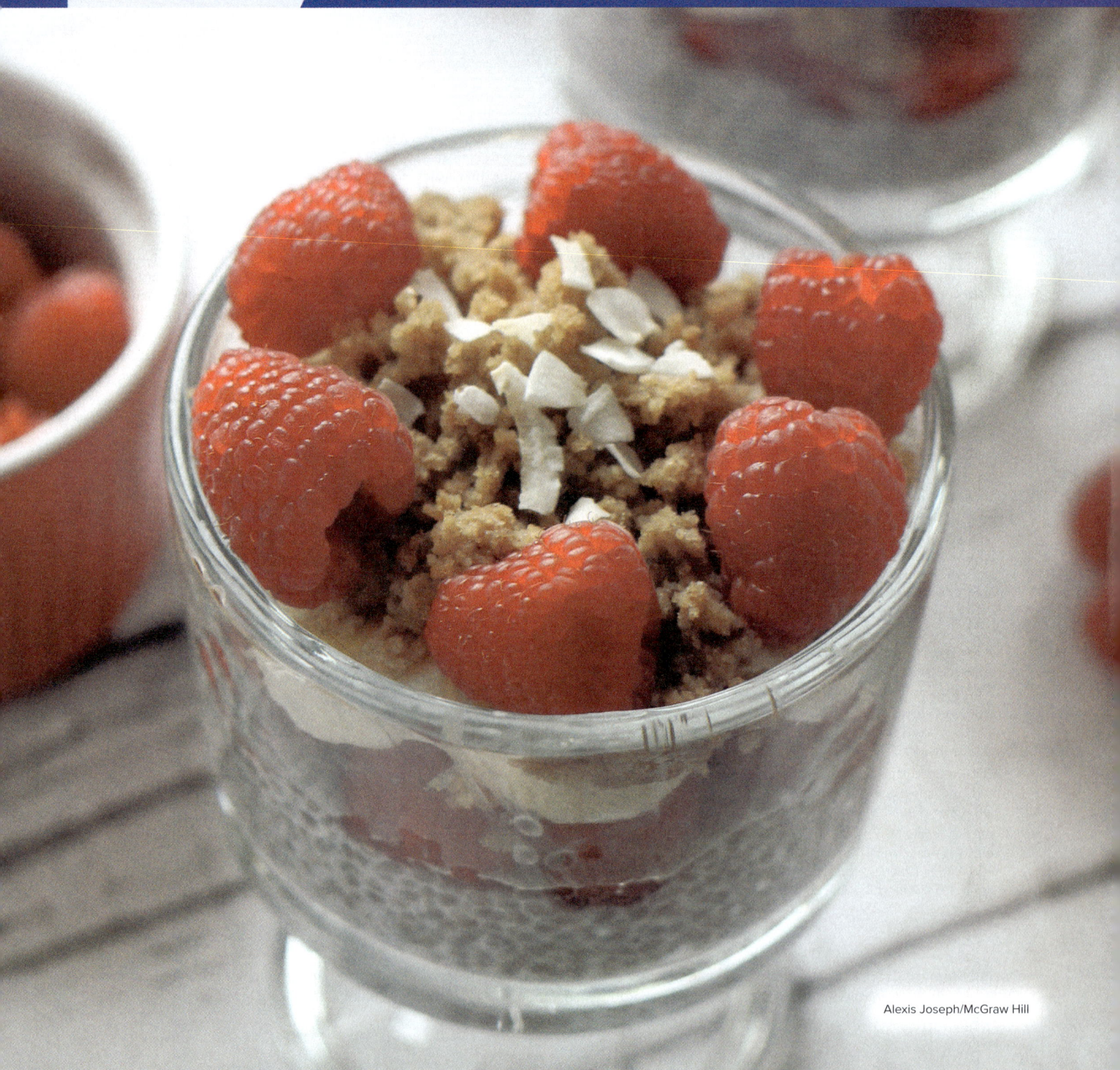

Chapter 3

The Human Body: A Nutrition Perspective

Alexis Joseph/McGraw Hill

Student Learning Outcomes

Chapter 3 is designed to allow you to:

3.1 Identify some basic roles of nutrients in human physiology.

3.2 Outline the functions of cell components and how cells work.

3.3 Define *metabolism* and differentiate between anabolic and catabolic reactions.

3.4 Identify the roles of the cardiovascular and lymphatic systems in nutrition.

3.5 List basic characteristics of the urinary system and its role in nutrition.

3.6 List basic characteristics of the nervous system and its role in nutrition.

3.7 List basic characteristics of the endocrine system, especially the pancreas, and its role in nutrition.

3.8 List basic characteristics of the immune system and its role in nutrition.

3.9 Describe the roles of the mouth, stomach, small intestine, large intestine, liver, gallbladder, and pancreas in digestion and absorption of nutrients.

3.10 Discuss the importance of the microbiota for human health.

3.11 Summarize how nutrients are stored in the body.

3.12 Identify the major nutrition-related gastrointestinal health problems and approaches to treatment.

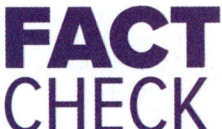
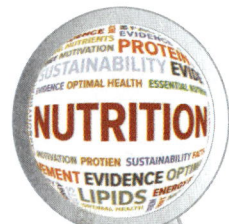

FACT CHECK

Does eating spicy foods cause ulcers?

Medical experts once thought that peptic ulcers were caused by stress or by eating spicy or acidic foods. However, in 1982, an internist named Barry Marshall and a pathologist named Robin Warren discovered that most cases of peptic ulcers are caused by an infection with the acid-resistant bacterium *Helicobacter pylori*. (If you're fascinated by stomach-churning medical dramas, look up the story of Barry Marshall, who purposely infected himself with a ghastly brew of *H. pylori* to prove to his colleagues that these spiral-shaped bacteria can cause ulcers!)

It is estimated that about half of the world's population are carriers of *H. pylori,* but it only causes problems in about 10% to 15% of infected individuals. These bacteria disrupt the thick layer of mucus that lines the stomach, allowing acids and enzymes that normally digest foods inside the stomach to irritate and erode the stomach lining. Great news: a course of antibiotics can cure *H. pylori* infection. This discovery was such a big deal that Marshall and Warren were awarded the Nobel Prize in 2005 for their work.

While spicy or acidic foods may irritate an existing ulcer, they do not cause ulcers. Read more about causes of ulcers and options for treatment in Section 3.11.

3.1 Cells, Tissues, and Organs

CELLS

A cell is the basic structural and functional component of life—and your body has trillions of them! Each cell is a self-contained, living entity, specialized to perform particular functions. In the human body, all cells have a few common features: membranes, cytoplasm, and **organelles** that perform specialized functions (Fig. 3-1).

Cell (Plasma) Membrane. The fluid and organelles inside the cell are separated from the fluid outside the cell by a cell (plasma) membrane. (Please note that cell membranes are not the same as cell walls, which are found in plant cells.) The cell membrane itself is not an organelle, but it holds the cellular contents (cytoplasm and organelles) together and regulates the flow of substances into and out of the cell. Cell-to-cell communication also occurs by way of the cell membrane.

The cell membrane, illustrated in Figure 3-2, is a lipid bilayer. It consists of a double layer of **phospholipids**. A phospholipid is a unique type of lipid that has a water-soluble head and a fat-soluble tail. In a lipid bilayer, the water-soluble heads of many phospholipids face the watery environments that exist both inside and outside the cell. The fat-soluble tails are tucked into the interior of the cell membrane. Molecules of **cholesterol**, another type of lipid, are also embedded within the lipid bilayer. Cholesterol adds some rigidity and stability to the cell membrane. You will learn more about phospholipids and cholesterol in Chapter 5.

organelles Compartments, particles, or filaments that perform specialized functions within a cell.

phospholipid Any of a class of fat-related substances that contain phosphorus, fatty acids, and a nitrogen-containing component. Phospholipids are an essential part of every cell.

cholesterol A waxy lipid found in all body cells. It has a structure containing multiple chemical rings. Cholesterol is found only in food ingredients of animal origin.

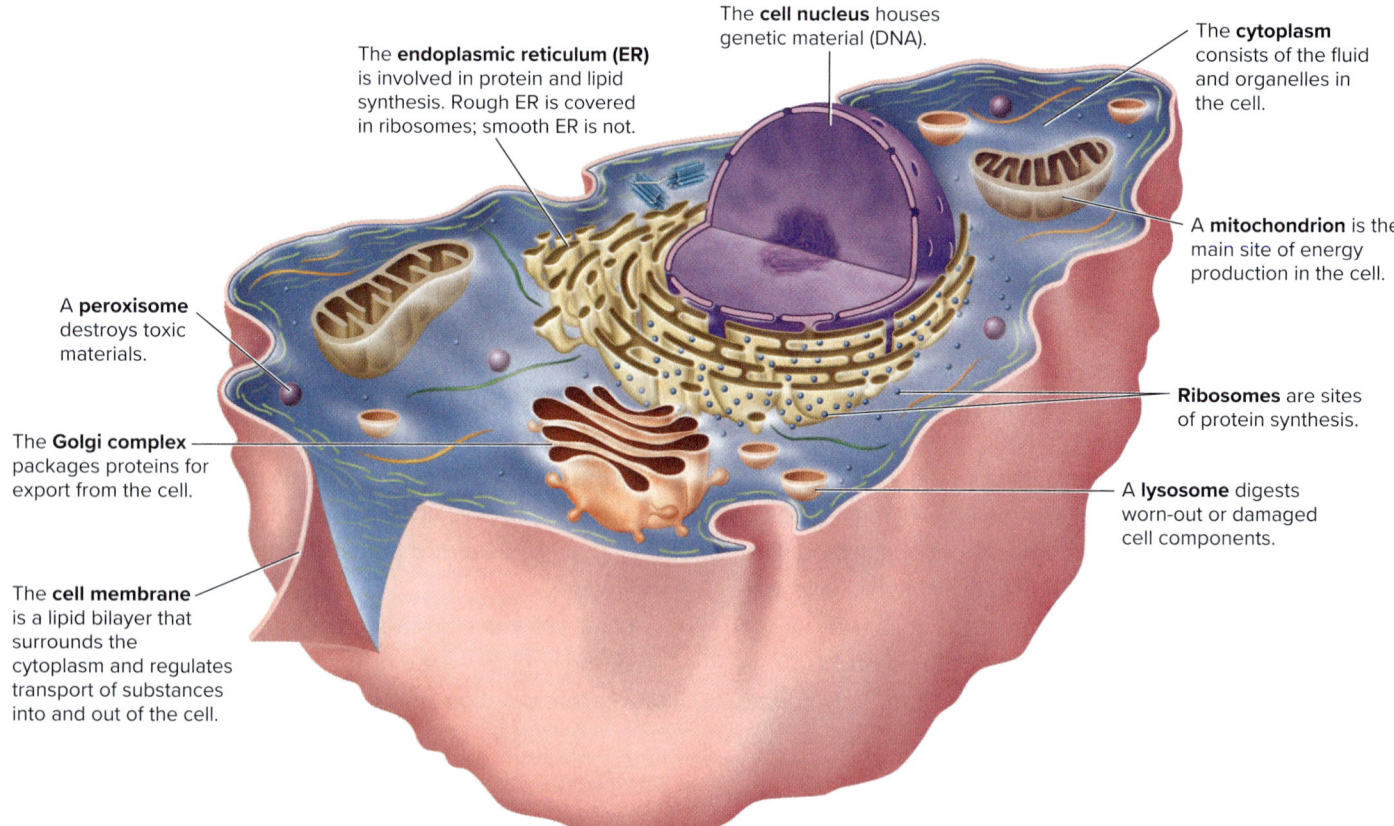

FIGURE 3-1 An animal cell. Almost all human cells contain the organelles described above. Shown here, but not discussed in the text, are the nucleolus, nuclear envelope, and centrioles. The nucleolus participates in genetic-related functions. The nuclear envelope encloses the nucleus. The centrioles participate in cell division.

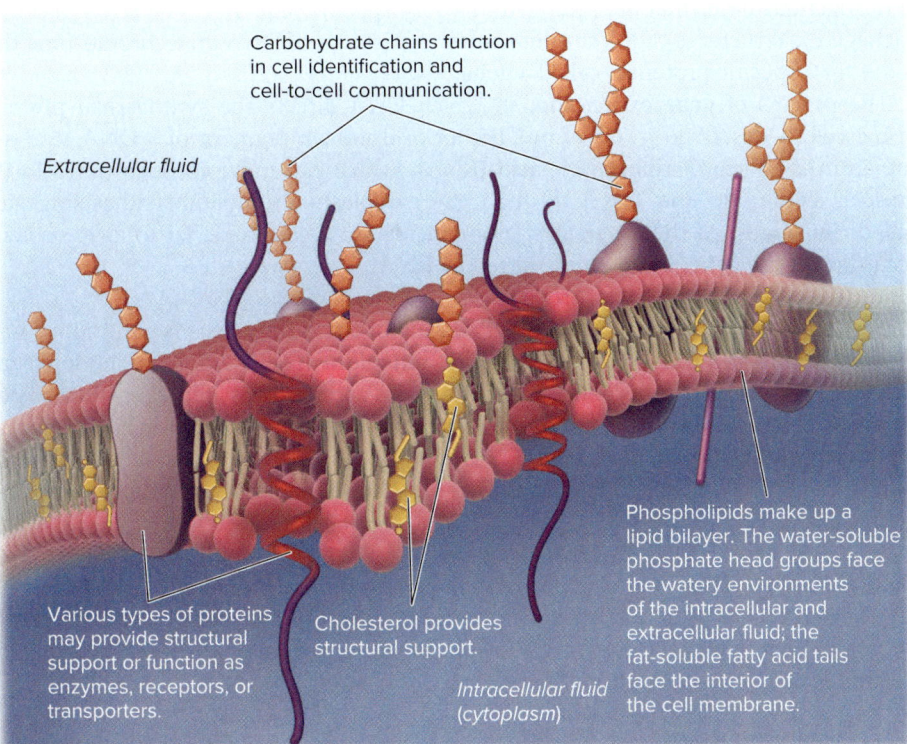

FIGURE 3-2 Cell membrane. The cell membrane is composed of a lipid bilayer. Carbohydrates and proteins serve important roles in the cell membrane, too.

A variety of proteins are part of the cell membrane. Some proteins provide structural support. Others function as enzymes, which regulate chemical reactions (see Section 3.8). Some proteins serve as gates or transporters to move substances across the cell membrane. Still other proteins on the outside surface of the cell membrane act as receptors, binding to essential substances that the cell needs and drawing them into the cell. Proteins are discussed in more detail in Chapter 6.

Besides lipids and proteins, the membrane also contains carbohydrates that mark the exterior of the cell. These carbohydrates are combined with either protein or fat, and they help to send messages to the cell's organelles and serve as identification markers for the cell. In the immune response, these carbohydrate tags help the immune system to detect invaders and initiate defensive actions. You will learn more about carbohydrates in Chapter 4.

Cytoplasm. The **cytoplasm** (also known as *cytosol*) is the combination of fluid material and organelles within the cell, not including the nucleus. A small amount of the energy used by the cell can be produced by chemical processes that occur in the cytoplasm. At least 15 different organelles can be found within the cytoplasm; the nutritional relevance of just six of the organelles will be discussed in the next few subsections.

Mitochondria. Mitochondria (singular: mitochondrion) are sometimes called the "power plants" or the "powerhouse" of the cell. These organelles are largely responsible for converting the chemical energy in carbohydrates, lipids, proteins, and alcohol from foods and drinks into a form of energy that cells can use. Except for red blood cells, all cells contain mitochondria.

Nucleus. With the exception of red blood cells, all cells have one or more nuclei (singular: nucleus). The **nucleus** is surrounded by its own double membrane, similar to the cell membrane. The role of the nucleus is to store and protect the cell's "code book" of directions for making the substances (i.e., proteins) the cell needs. These directions exist in the form of **deoxyribonucleic acid (DNA)**, which is a double strand

cytoplasm The fluid and organelles (except the nucleus) in a cell; also called *cytosol*.

mitochondria (singular: mitochondrion) Organelles that are the main sites of energy production in a cell. They contain the pathway for oxidizing fat for fuel, among other metabolic pathways.

nucleus (plural: nuclei) Membrane-bound organelle that contains the genetic information (DNA) for cell protein synthesis and cell replication.

deoxyribonucleic acid (DNA) Double strand of nucleic acids that carries hereditary information in cells; DNA directs the synthesis of cell proteins.

chromosome A single, large DNA molecule and its associated proteins; contains many genes to store and transmit genetic information.

gene A specific segment on a chromosome. Genes provide the blueprint for the production of cell proteins.

gene expression Use of DNA information on a gene to produce a protein.

ribonucleic acid (RNA) The single-stranded nucleic acid involved in the transcription of genetic information and translation of that information into protein structure.

ribosomes Cytoplasmic particles that mediate the linking together of amino acids to form proteins; may exist freely in the cytoplasm or attached to endoplasmic reticulum.

endoplasmic reticulum (ER) An organelle composed of a network of canals running through the cytoplasm. Part of the endoplasmic reticulum contains ribosomes.

Golgi complex The cell organelle near the nucleus that packages proteins and lipids for secretion or distribution to other organelles.

secretory vesicles Membrane-bound vesicles produced by the Golgi complex; contain protein and other compounds to be secreted by the cell.

lysosome A cellular organelle that contains digestive enzymes for use inside the cell for turnover of cell parts.

peroxisome A cell organelle that destroys toxic products within the cell.

catalase Enzyme that catalyzes the decomposition of hydrogen peroxide into water and oxygen.

epithelial tissue The surface cells that line the outside of the body and all external passages within it.

connective tissue Protein tissue that holds different structures in the body together. Some body structures are made up of connective tissue—notably, tendons and cartilage. Connective tissue also forms part of bone and the nonmuscular structures of arteries and veins.

muscle tissue A type of tissue adapted to contract to cause movement.

nervous tissue Tissue composed of highly branched, elongated cells that transport nerve impulses from one part of the body to another.

of nitrogenous bases that are arranged in a very specific sequence. The DNA in cells is packaged as structures called **chromosomes**. A segment of DNA on a chromosome that codes for a specific protein is called a **gene**.

The process of **gene expression,** in which DNA directs the synthesis of proteins in the cell, is described in detail in Chapter 6. Briefly, a segment of a DNA strand is copied in the form of **ribonucleic acid (RNA),** which can move through pores in the nuclear membrane and travel through the cytoplasm to protein-synthesizing sites called **ribosomes**. At the ribosomes, amino acids are linked together to form proteins according to the genetic code transmitted by RNA.

Endoplasmic Reticulum. The outer membrane of the cell nucleus is continuous with a network of tubes called the **endoplasmic reticulum (ER)**. Part of the endoplasmic reticulum is covered in ribosomes, where the RNA code is translated to synthesize new proteins. The sections of the endoplasmic reticulum that are covered in ribosomes are called *rough* (as opposed to *smooth*) ER. Other parts of the endoplasmic reticulum are involved in lipid synthesis, detoxification of harmful substances, and storage of calcium in the cell.

Golgi Complex. The **Golgi complex** (also known as the *Golgi apparatus* or *Golgi body*) is a packaging site for proteins and lipids produced in the cell. It consists of sacs within the cytoplasm, where proteins and lipids are packaged into **secretory vesicles** for transport within the cell or secretion from the cell.

Lysosomes. Lysosomes are the cell's digestive system. They are sacs that contain enzymes for the digestion of foreign material. Sometimes known as "suicide bags," they are responsible for digesting worn-out or damaged cell components. Certain cells associated with immune function contain many lysosomes.

Peroxisomes. Peroxisomes contain enzymes that detoxify harmful chemicals. Peroxisomes get their name from the fact that hydrogen peroxide (H_2O_2) is formed as a result of some detoxification reactions inside this organelle. To counter the damaging effects of hydrogen peroxide within the cell, peroxisomes also contain a protective enzyme called **catalase,** which breaks down hydrogen peroxide into water and oxygen. Peroxisomes also have a minor role in metabolizing alcohol.

TISSUES

When groups of similar cells work together to accomplish a specialized task, the arrangement is referred to as a tissue. Humans are composed of four primary types of tissue: epithelial, connective, muscle, and nervous tissue.

- **Epithelial tissue** is composed of cells that cover surfaces both inside and outside the body. For example, epithelial cells make up the lining of the respiratory tract. Epithelial cells secrete important substances, absorb nutrients, and excrete waste.
- **Connective tissue** supports and protects the body, stores fat, and produces blood cells.
- **Muscle tissue** is designed for movement.
- **Nervous tissue,** which is found in the brain and spinal cord, is designed for communication.

ORGANS

One, two, or more types of tissue combine to form more complex structures called **organs**. At a still higher level of organization, several organs that work together form an **organ system,** such as the digestive system. All organs contribute to nutritional health, and a person's overall nutritional state determines how well each organ functions. Examine Figure 3-3 to learn about the nutritional relevance of the 12 organ systems.

Cardiovascular System

Major components
heart, blood vessels, and blood

Functions
Carries blood and regulates blood supply

Transports nutrients, waste products, hormones, and gases (oxygen and carbon dioxide) throughout the body

Regulates blood pressure

Lymphatic and Immune Systems

Major lymphatic components
lymph, lymphocytes, lymphatic vessels, and lymph nodes

Major immune components
white blood cells, lymph vessels and nodes, spleen, thymus gland, and other lymph tissues

Lymphatic functions
Removes foreign substances from blood and lymph

Maintains tissue fluid balance

Aids fat absorption

Immune functions
Provides defense against pathogens

Formation of white blood cells

Urinary System

Major components
kidneys, urinary bladder, and the ducts that carry urine

Functions
Removes waste products from the blood and forms urine

Regulates blood acid–base (pH) balance, overall chemical balance, and water balance

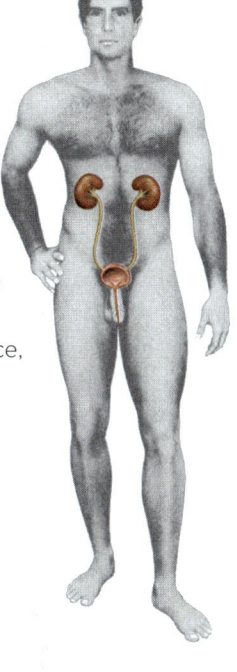

Nervous System

Major components
brain, spinal cord, nerves, and sensory receptors

Functions
Detects and interprets sensation

Controls movements, physiological, and intellectual functions

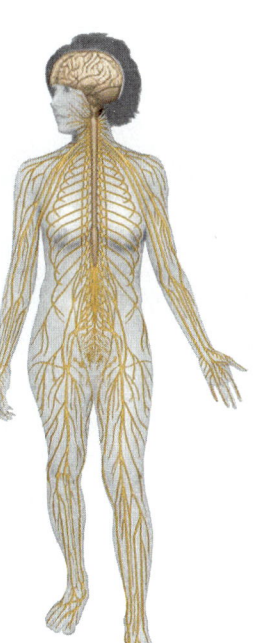

Endocrine System

Major components
hypothalamus, pituitary gland, thyroid gland, thymus gland, pancreas, adrenal glands, and gonads (ovaries in females; testes in males)

Functions
Regulates metabolism, growth, reproduction, and many other functions by producing and releasing hormones

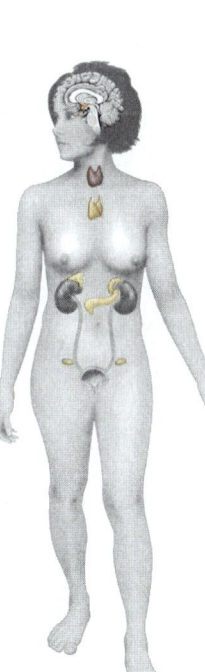

Digestive System

Major components
mouth, esophagus, stomach, intestines, and accessory organs (liver, gallbladder, and pancreas)

Functions
Performs the mechanical and chemical processes of digestion of food, absorption of nutrients, and elimination of wastes

Assists the immune system by destroying some pathogens and forming a barrier against foreign materials

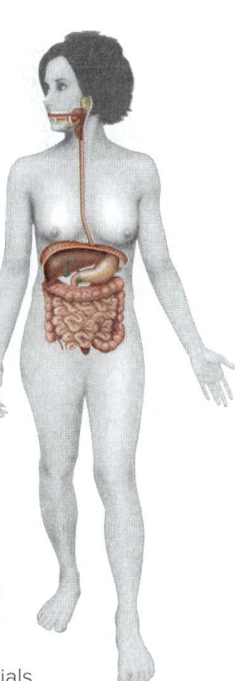

FIGURE 3-3 Organ systems of the body.

84 Wardlaw's Contemporary Nutrition

Integumentary System

Major components
skin, hair, nails, and sweat glands

Functions
Protects the body

Regulates body temperature

Prevents water loss

Produces vitamin D

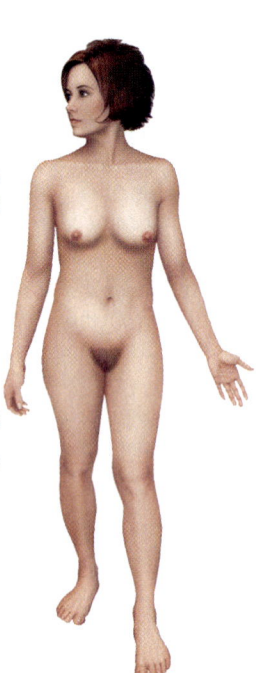

Skeletal System

Major components
bones, cartilage, ligaments, and joints

Functions
Protects organs

Supports body weight

Allows body movement

Produces blood cells

Stores minerals

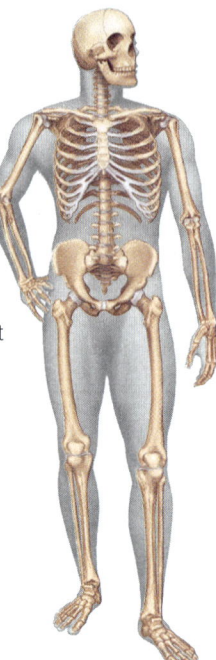

Muscular System

Major components
smooth, cardiac, and skeletal muscle

Functions
Produces body movement, heartbeat, and body heat

Propels food in the digestive tract

Maintains posture

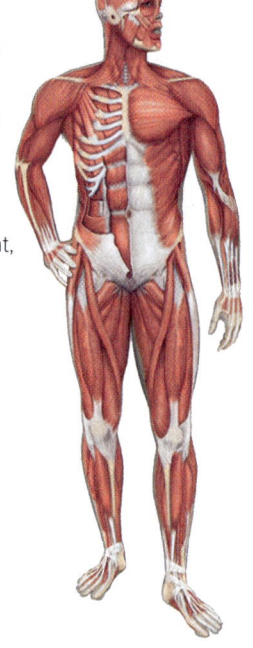

Respiratory System

Major components
lungs and respiratory passages

Functions
Exchanges gases (oxygen and carbon dioxide) between the blood and the air

Regulates blood acid–base (pH) balance

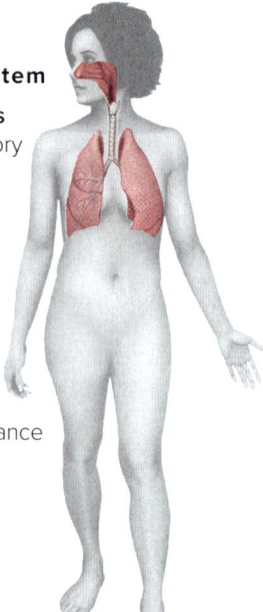

Reproductive System

Major components
gonads (ovaries and testes), genitals, and breasts

Functions
Performs the processes of sexual maturation and reproduction

Influences sexual functions and behaviors

Produces human milk to nourish an infant

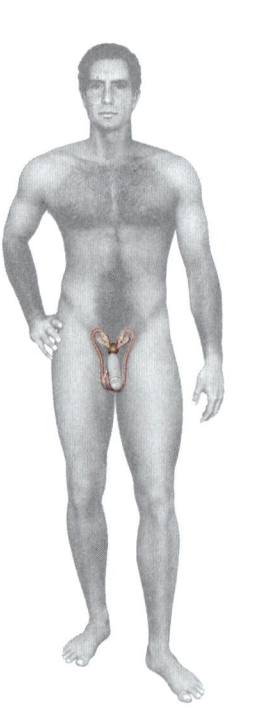 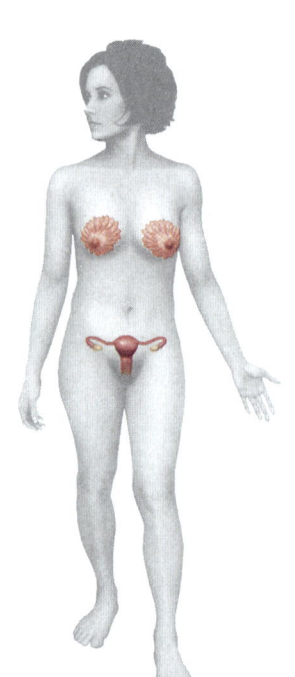

FIGURE 3-3 Organ systems of the body (*continued*).

organ A group of tissues designed to perform a specific function; for example, the heart, which contains muscle tissue, nervous tissue, and so on.

organ system A collection of organs that work together to perform an overall function.

There are lots of interactions among the various organ systems. Sometimes organs within a system can serve another system. For example, the basic function of the digestive system is to convert the food we eat into absorbable nutrients. At the same time, the digestive system serves the immune system by preventing dangerous pathogens from invading and causing illness in the body. As you study nutrition, you will note the multiple roles played by many organs.

The main objective of this chapter is to understand the actions of nutrients as they affect different cells, tissues, organs, and organ systems. As we explore several key organ systems—cardiovascular, lymphatic, urinary, nervous, endocrine, immune, and digestive—look for the ways each system both *affects* and *is affected by* nutrition.

✓ CONCEPT CHECK 3.1

1. Choose three organelles and explain their relevance to human nutrition.
2. List the four types of tissues and give an example of where you could find each in the body.
3. Examine Figure 3-3. Provide three examples of ways the organs of one system support the functions of another system.

3.2 Metabolism Is the Chemistry of Life

Metabolism refers to the entire collection of chemical processes (reactions) involved in maintaining life. It encompasses all of the sequences of chemical reactions that occur in the body's cells. Some of these reactions take place in the cytoplasm and organelles we have just discussed. They enable us to release and use energy from foods, store sources of fuel for later use, convert toxic substances into less harmful products, and prepare waste products for excretion.

Metabolic reactions can be categorized as either anabolic or catabolic. In **anabolic** reactions, molecules are joined together to synthesize new, larger products. Anabolic reactions require energy. Other reactions are **catabolic,** in which larger materials are broken down into smaller molecules. Catabolic reactions release energy. The catabolism of carbohydrates, fats, and proteins yields energy. Energy metabolism begins in the cytoplasm with the initial breakdown of glucose. The remaining steps of energy metabolism take place in the mitochondria. Ultimately, these reactions harness the chemical energy in food to make the high-energy compound **adenosine triphosphate (ATP),** which our cells can use to do work.

Chemical reactions occur constantly in every living cell; the production of new substances (anabolism) is balanced by the breakdown of older ones (catabolism). An example is the constant formation and breakdown of bone. For bone turnover to occur, cells require a continuous supply of energy derived from dietary carbohydrates, lipids, and proteins. Cells also need water, building materials (e.g., protein and minerals), and chemical regulators (e.g., hormones, enzymes, vitamins, and minerals). Almost all cells also need a steady supply of oxygen from the lungs.

Are you beginning to see how important nutrition is to all the functions of the human body?

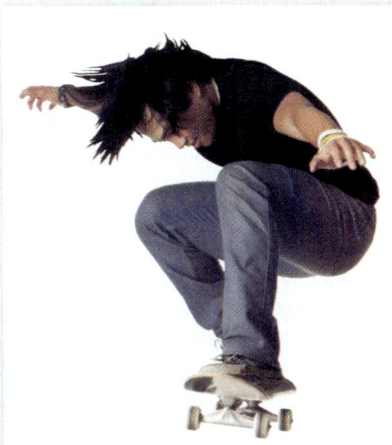

Where do you get the energy to work and play? Your cells use the energy stored in the chemical bonds of carbohydrates, fats, and proteins to generate ATP. RubberBall Productions/Photodisc/Getty Images

anabolic Relating to pathways that use small, simple compounds to build larger, more complex compounds.

catabolic Relating to pathways that break down large compounds into smaller compounds.

adenosine triphosphate (ATP) The main energy currency for cells. ATP energy is used to promote ion pumping, enzyme activity, and muscular contraction.

✓ CONCEPT CHECK 3.2

1. What are the differences between anabolic and catabolic reactions?
2. What is the purpose of ATP?
3. Describe three ways essential nutrients support cell functions.

3.3 Cardiovascular System and Lymphatic System

The body has two separate organ systems that circulate fluids in the body: the **cardiovascular system** and the **lymphatic system.** Some texts group these two systems together as the *circulatory system,* but each system has distinct components and functions. The cardiovascular system consists of the heart and blood vessels. The lymphatic system consists of lymphatic vessels and a number of lymph tissues. Blood flows through the cardiovascular system, while **lymph** flows through the lymphatic system.

cardiovascular system The body system consisting of the heart, blood vessels, and blood. This system transports nutrients, waste products, gases, and hormones throughout the body and plays an important role in immune responses and regulation of body temperature.

lymphatic system A system of vessels and lymph that accepts fluid surrounding cells and large particles, such as products of fat absorption. Lymph eventually passes into the bloodstream from the lymphatic system.

lymph A clear fluid that flows through lymph vessels; carries most forms of fat after their absorption by the small intestine.

plasma The fluid, extracellular portion of blood.

red blood cells Cells that transport oxygen and carbon dioxide through the blood; also called *erythrocytes*.

white blood cells Variety of immune cells that circulate in the lymph and blood and work to neutralize, detoxify, and/or destroy pathogens and other foreign proteins; also called *leukocytes*.

platelets Protoplasmic disks in the blood that promote coagulation; also called *thrombocytes*.

artery A blood vessel that carries blood away from the heart.

capillary A microscopic blood vessel that connects the smallest arteries and veins; site of nutrient, oxygen, and waste exchange between body cells and the blood.

CARDIOVASCULAR SYSTEM

The heart is a muscular pump that normally contracts and relaxes 50 to 90 times per minute when the body is at rest. This continual pumping, measured by taking your pulse, keeps blood moving through the blood vessels. The blood that flows through the cardiovascular system is composed of **plasma, red blood cells, white blood cells, platelets,** and many other substances. It travels two basic routes. In the first route, blood circulates from the right side of the heart, through the lungs, and then back to the heart. In the lungs, blood picks up oxygen and releases carbon dioxide. After this exchange of gases has taken place, blood is *oxygenated* and returns to the left side of the heart. In the second route, the oxygenated blood circulates from the left side of the heart to all other body cells, eventually returning back to the right side of the heart (Fig. 3-4). After blood has circulated throughout the body, it is *deoxygenated*. (As you review anatomy diagrams in this book, recognize that *left* and *right* designations refer to the left and right sides of your body, not of the diagram in front of you.)

In the cardiovascular system, blood leaves the heart via **arteries,** which branch into **capillaries,** a network of tiny blood vessels that are just one cell layer thick. The exchange

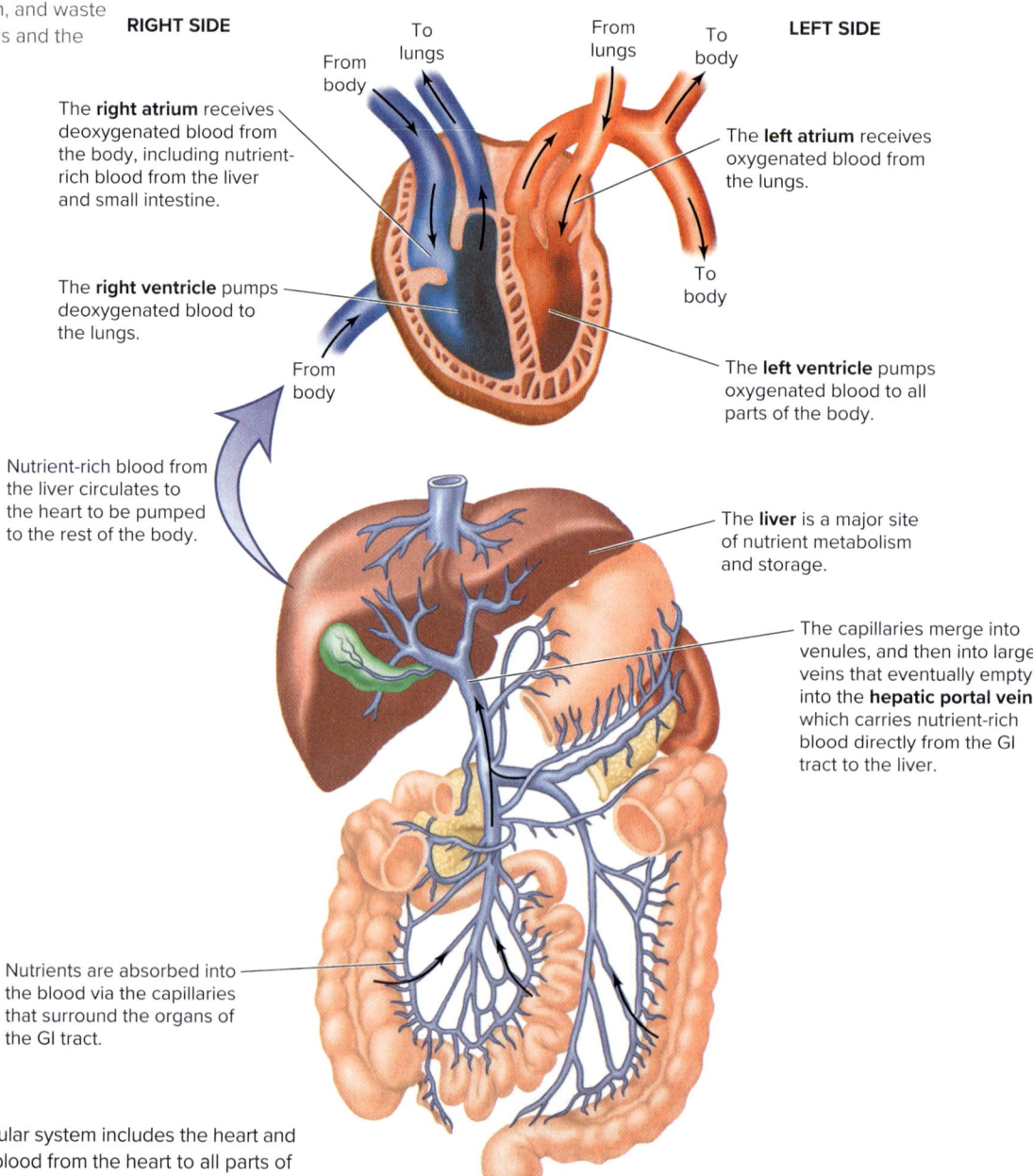

FIGURE 3-4 The cardiovascular system includes the heart and blood vessels. Arteries carry blood from the heart to all parts of the body, including the digestive system. Blood that leaves the gastrointestinal (GI) tract is rich in nutrients.

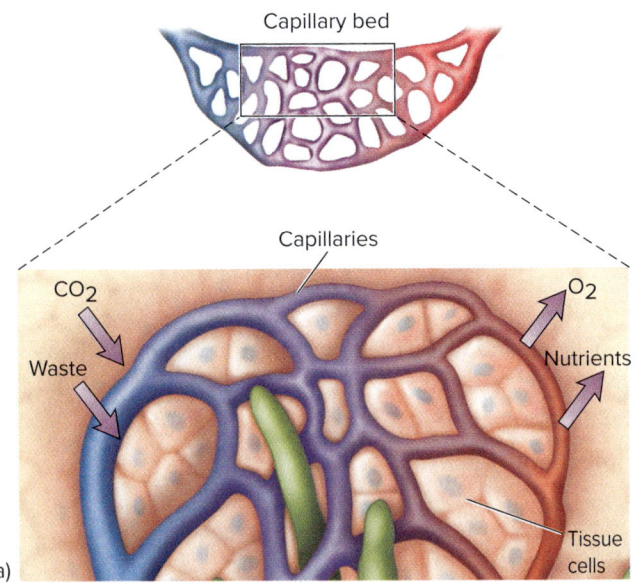 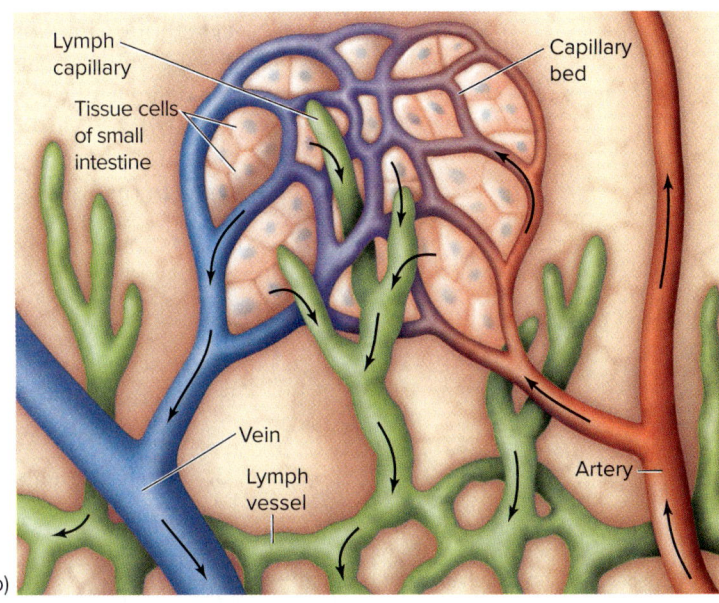

FIGURE 3-5 Blood vessels and lymph vessels. (a) The exchange of oxygen (O_2) and nutrients for carbon dioxide (CO_2) and other waste products occurs between the capillaries and the surrounding tissues. (b) Lymph vessels are also present in capillary beds, such as in the small intestine. Lymph vessels in the small intestine are also called *lacteals*. The lymph vessels have closed ends and are important for the absorption of fat and fat-soluble vitamins.

of nutrients, oxygen, and waste products between the blood and cells occurs through the tiny, weblike pores of the capillaries (Fig. 3-5). The blood then returns to the heart via the **veins.**

The cardiovascular system facilitates the exchange of oxygen, nutrients, and wastes between the body's internal and external environments. Other functions include the delivery of hormones to their target cells, maintenance of a constant body temperature, and distribution of white blood cells throughout the body.

vein A blood vessel that carries blood to the heart.

Portal Circulation in the Gastrointestinal Tract. Once absorbed through the stomach or intestinal wall, nutrients reach one of two destinations. Some nutrients are taken up by the cells that line the gastrointestinal (GI) tract to nourish those tissues. Most of these water-soluble nutrients from recently eaten foods, however, are transferred into the **hepatic portal circulation.** (The term *hepatic* refers to the liver. There are other portal systems in physiology, but the simpler terms *portal circulation* or *portal vein* usually refer to hepatic portal circulation.) To enter portal circulation, the nutrients pass from the intestinal capillaries into veins that eventually merge into a very large vein called the **hepatic portal vein.** Unlike most veins in the body—which carry blood back to the heart—this portal vein leads directly to the liver (Fig. 3-4). This enables the liver to process absorbed nutrients before they enter the general circulation of the bloodstream. Overall, hepatic portal circulation represents a special form of circulation in the cardiovascular system.

hepatic portal circulation The portion of the cardiovascular system that uses a large vein (portal vein) to carry nutrient-rich blood from capillaries in the intestines and portions of the stomach to the liver.

hepatic portal vein Large vein that carries absorbed nutrients from the gastrointestinal tract to the liver.

LYMPHATIC SYSTEM

The lymphatic system consists of a network of lymphatic vessels and the fluid (lymph) that moves through them. The lymph vessels take up excess fluid that collects between cells and return it to the bloodstream. Lymph is similar to blood, consisting largely of plasma (fluid portion of the blood) that has found its way out of capillaries and into the spaces between cells. Lymph also contains white blood cells, which support immune function, as well as dietary fats that have been absorbed from the small intestine. However, neither red blood cells nor platelets are present. Lymph is collected in tiny lymph vessels all over the body and moves through even larger vessels until it eventually empties into the cardiovascular system through a duct near the heart. The lymphatic system does not have a pump (like the heart); its flow is driven by muscle contractions arising from normal body movements.

lacteal Lymphatic vessel that absorbs fats from the small intestine.

Lymphatic Circulation in the Gastrointestinal Tract. The lymphatic vessels that serve the gastrointestinal tract are specifically known as **lacteals**. Besides contributing to the defense of the body against invading pathogens, lacteals play an important role in nutrition. Most dietary fats are too large to enter the capillaries that surround the cardiovascular system. Instead, most dietary fats enter the lacteals and travel through the lymphatic system until lymph is emptied into the bloodstream by a duct near the heart.

✓ CONCEPT CHECK 3.3

1. Describe how nutrients, oxygen, and wastes are exchanged between the body's internal and external environments.
2. What is hepatic portal circulation?
3. Which nutrients are absorbed into the lymph?

3.4 Urinary System

urinary system The body system consisting of the kidneys, urinary bladder, and the ducts that carry urine. This system removes waste products from the blood and regulates blood acid–base balance, overall chemical balance, and water balance in the body.

ureter Tube that transports urine from the kidney to the urinary bladder.

urethra Tube that transports urine from the urinary bladder to the outside of the body.

urea Nitrogenous waste product of protein metabolism; major source of nitrogen in the urine.

pH A measure of relative acidity or alkalinity of a solution. The pH scale is 0 to 14. A pH of 7 is neutral; a pH below 7 is acidic; a pH above 7 is alkaline.

The **urinary system** is composed of two kidneys, one on each side of the spinal column. Each kidney is connected to the bladder by a **ureter.** The bladder is emptied by way of the **urethra** (Fig. 3-6). The main function of the kidneys is to remove waste from the body. The kidneys are constantly filtering blood to control its composition.

This results in the formation of urine, which is composed of water, dissolved waste products of metabolism (e.g., **urea**), and excess or unneeded water-soluble vitamins and various minerals.

Together with the lungs, the kidneys help to maintain the acid–base balance **(pH)** of the blood. The kidneys contribute to bone health because they convert a form of vitamin D into its active hormone form. The kidneys also produce a hormone that stimulates red blood cell synthesis. During times of fasting, the kidneys even produce glucose from certain amino acids. Thus, the kidneys perform many important functions related to nutrition.

The proper function of the kidneys is closely tied to the strength of the cardiovascular system, particularly its ability to maintain adequate blood pressure, and the consumption

FIGURE 3-6 Organs of the urinary system. The urinary system of the female is shown. The male's urinary system is the same, except that the urethra extends through the penis.

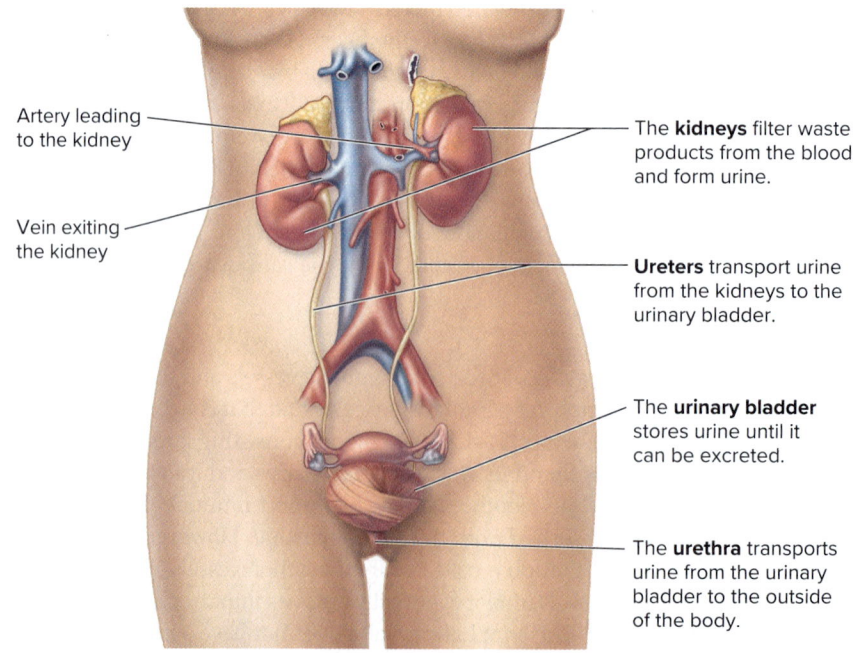

of sufficient fluid. Uncontrolled diabetes, hypertension, and drug abuse are harmful to the kidneys. *Farm to Fork* in this section highlights cranberries, which may be helpful for preventing infections in the GI and urinary tracts.

✓ CONCEPT CHECK 3.4

1. List three functions of the kidneys.
2. Trace the path of waste products out of the body.

3.5 Nervous System

The **nervous system** is a regulatory system that centrally controls most body functions. The nervous system can detect changes occurring in various organs and the external environment and initiate corrective action when needed to maintain a constant internal body environment. The nervous system also regulates activities that change almost instantly, such as voluntary muscle contractions and the body's response to stress or danger. The body has many receptors that receive information about what is happening within the body and in the outside environment. For the most part, these receptors are found in our eyes, ears, skin, nose, and stomach. We act on information from these receptors via the nervous system.

The basic structural and functional unit of the nervous system is the **neuron.** Neurons are elongated, highly branched cells. The body contains about 100 billion neurons. Neurons respond to electrical and chemical signals, conduct electrical impulses, and release chemical regulators. Overall, neurons allow us to perceive what is occurring in our environment, engage in learning, store vital information in memory, and control the body's voluntary (and involuntary) actions.

The brain stores information, reacts to incoming information, solves problems, and generates thoughts. In addition, the brain plans a course of action based on the other sensory inputs. Responses to the stimuli are carried out mostly through the rest of the nervous system.

How are nutrients involved in the function of the nervous system? Transmission of a signal (nerve impulse) occurs by way of a change in the concentrations of two minerals, sodium and potassium, across the cell membrane of a neuron. As you will learn in Chapter 9, sodium and potassium can conduct an electrical current when they are dissolved in water. As a

nervous system The body system consisting of the brain, spinal cord, nerves, and sensory receptors. This system detects sensations, directs movements, and controls physiological and intellectual functions.

neuron The structural and functional unit of the nervous system. Consists of a cell body, dendrites, and an axon.

FARM to FORK Cranberries

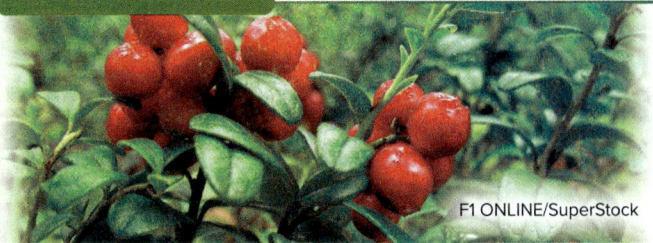

F1 ONLINE/SuperStock

Phytochemicals in cranberries may impede the ability of some bacteria to clump together and adhere to epithelial tissue. In addition, prebiotic compounds in cranberries may favorably alter the gut microbiota. Thus, cranberries may be beneficial for preventing infections of the GI and urinary tracts, which could reduce the need for antibiotics.

Grow
- Cranberries grow in wet, mossy areas known as bogs. To harvest cranberries, growers flood the bogs, knock them off their vines with mechanized beaters, then quickly collect the berries when they float to the surface.
- Cold growing temperatures actually increase the sugar content of the berries, making them less tart.
- Enjoy fresh cranberries during the winter months. Frozen or dried varieties, which are quite nutritious, are available anytime of the year.

Shop
- Look for firm berries with the deepest red color. The red pigments (anthocyanins and proanthocyanidins) are powerful cancer-fighting phytochemicals! As mentioned above, the phytochemicals in cranberries may impede the ability of some bacteria to adhere to and grow on epithelial tissue (e.g., in the urinary tract).
- Food manufacturers add sugars to dried cranberries. Choose varieties that are made with less sugar.
- Although it doesn't pack quite the same disease-fighting punch as fresh cranberries, cranberry juice may be useful for fending off GI and urinary tract infections. Look for brands with less added sugar.

Store
- Fresh cranberries can be stored in the refrigerator for 1 week. They should be kept in the crisper drawer in a perforated bag (i.e., the original packaging) to maintain optimal water content and exposure to air.
- If you don't plan to eat fresh cranberries within 1 week of purchase, freezing the berries is the best option to preserve nutrients.

Prep
- Add dried cranberries to salads or trail mix to add a dose of antioxidants as well as flavor. In recipes, pairing cranberries with sweeter fruits, such as apples and pears, can strike a nice balance between sweet and tart.
- Fresh, frozen, or dried cranberries make a colorful addition to baked goods, but for maximum health benefits, enjoy cranberries raw. Cooking the berries greatly reduces their antioxidant content.

Sources: Blumberg JB, Basu A, Krueger CG, et al. Impact of cranberries on gut microbiota and cardiometabolic health: proceedings of the Cranberry Health Research Conference 2015. *Adv. Nutr.* 2016 Jul;7(4):759S-770S. doi: 10.3945/an.116.012583

Robinson J. Strawberries, cranberries, and raspberries: three of our most nutritious fruits. In: *Eating on the Wild Side: The Missing Link to Optimum Health.* New York: Little, Brown & Co.; 2013.

Williams G, Hahn D, Stephens JH, Craig JC, Hodson EM. Cranberries for preventing urinary tract infections. *Cochrane Database Syst Rev.* 2023;4(4):CD001321. Published 2023 Apr 17. doi:10.1002/14651858.CD001321.pub6

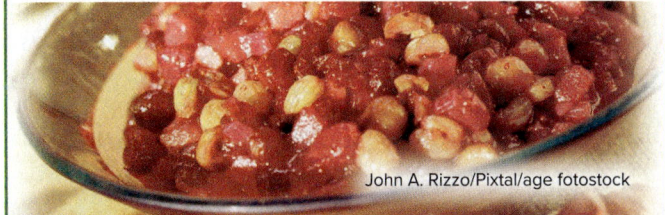

John A. Rizzo/Pixtal/age fotostock

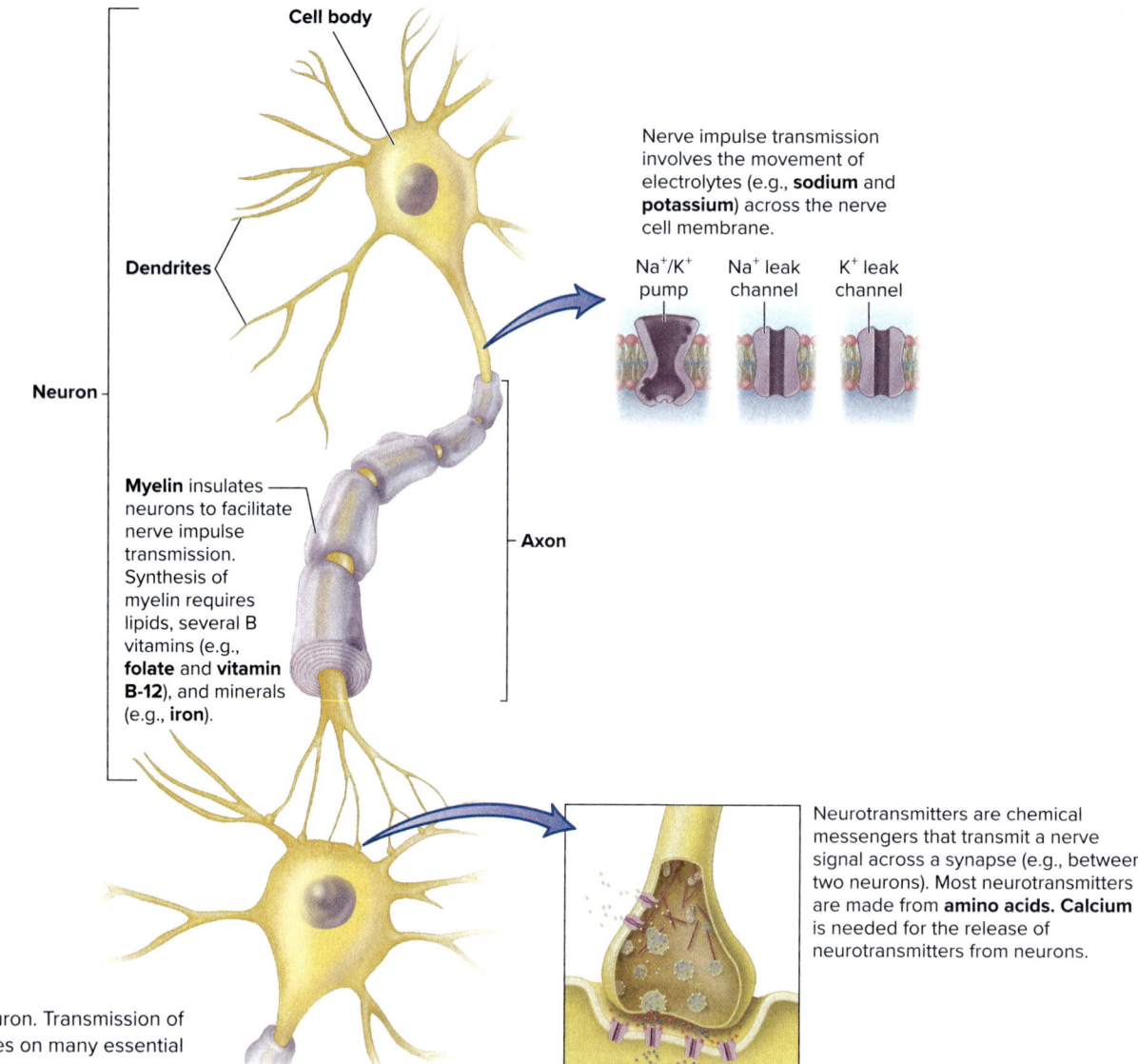

FIGURE 3-7 A neuron. Transmission of nerve impulses relies on many essential nutrients.

synapse The space between one neuron and another neuron (or cell).

neurotransmitter A compound made by a nerve cell that allows for communication between it and other cells.

serotonin A neurotransmitter involved in the regulation of mood, sleep, and appetite.

norepinephrine A neurotransmitter from nerve endings and a hormone from the adrenal gland. It is released in times of stress and is involved in hunger regulation, blood glucose regulation, and other body processes.

epinephrine A hormone that is released by the adrenal glands (located on each kidney) at times of stress. It acts to increase glycogen breakdown in the liver, among other functions. Also known as *adrenaline*.

myelin A combination of lipids and proteins that covers nerve fibers.

neuron responds to a stimulus, these minerals facilitate the transmission of an electrical impulse along the neuron.

When the signal must bridge a gap **(synapse)** from one neuron to the next or between a neuron and its target tissue (e.g., muscle), the electrical message can be converted into a chemical signal called a **neurotransmitter** (Fig. 3-7). Most neurotransmitters are made from amino acids, derived from the protein in foods. For example, the amino acid tryptophan is used to make **serotonin,** a neurotransmitter involved in the regulation of mood, sleep, and many other body functions. The amino acid tyrosine is used to make the neurotransmitters **norepinephrine** and **epinephrine** (also called adrenaline), which are involved in our body's response to stress.

Other nutrients also play a role in the nervous system. Calcium is needed for the release of neurotransmitters from neurons. Lipids and several B vitamins (e.g., folate and vitamin B-12) and minerals (e.g., iron) play a role in the formation of the **myelin** sheath, which provides insulation around specific parts of most neurons. Finally, a regular supply of carbohydrate in the form of glucose is important for supplying fuel for the brain. The brain can use other energy sources but generally relies on glucose.

CONCEPT CHECK 3.5

1. Why are sodium and potassium important for the work of the nervous system?
2. How are signals transmitted between one neuron and the next? Why are amino acids important in this process?
3. Which nutrient is the brain's preferred source of energy?

3.6 Endocrine System

The **endocrine system** plays a major role in the regulation of metabolism, reproduction, water balance, and many other functions through the action of hormones (Fig. 3-8). Think of hormones as the chemical messengers of the body. They are produced in the **endocrine glands,** released into the blood, and eventually cause changes in target tissues throughout the body. A particular hormone does not affect all cells in the body; it only affects cells with the correct **receptor** protein. These binding sites, which generally are found on cell membranes of target tissues, are highly specific for a certain hormone. Often, binding of a hormone to a receptor on the cell membrane activates additional compounds called second messengers within the cell to carry out the assigned task. A few hormones can penetrate the cell membrane and eventually bind to receptors on the DNA in the nucleus.

There are at least 50 different hormones at work in the body. Throughout this text, you will learn about the nutritional relevance of just a few.

- Several hormones assist in the regulation of food intake and digestion. **Leptin** and **ghrelin** are two hormones that regulate appetite. **Cholecystokinin** sends a signal to

endocrine system The body system consisting of the various glands and the hormones these glands secrete. This system has major regulatory functions in the body, such as reproduction and cell metabolism.

endocrine gland A hormone-producing gland.

receptor A site in a cell at which compounds (such as hormones) bind. Cells that contain receptors for a specific compound are partially controlled by that compound.

leptin A hormone made by adipose tissue in proportion to total fat stores in the body that influences long-term regulation of fat mass. Leptin also influences appetite and the release of insulin.

ghrelin A hormone produced by stomach cells and the brain that stimulates appetite.

cholecystokinin A hormone produced by the small intestinal cells that stimulates enzyme release from the pancreas and bile release from the gallbladder.

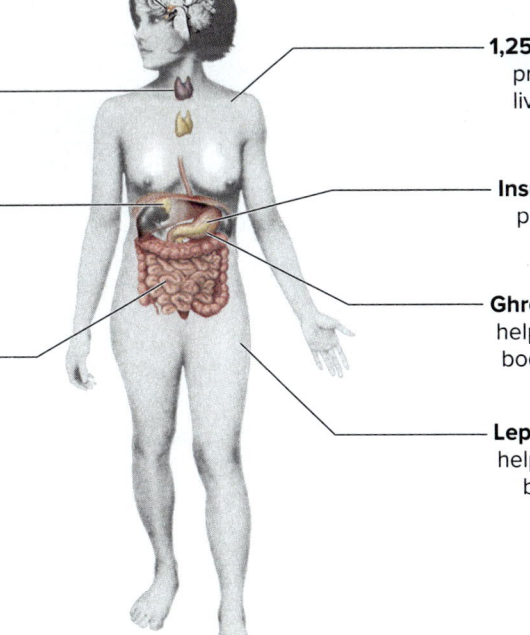

Growth hormone (produced by pituitary gland) promotes protein synthesis and growth; increases use of fat as fuel.

Thyroid hormone (produced by thyroid gland) regulates metabolic rate, growth, and development.

Epinephrine and **norepinephrine** (produced by adrenal glands) increase blood glucose and increase metabolic rate during times of stress.

Cholecystokinin (produced by small intestine and brain) regulates the movement of food through the GI tract and stimulates the release of bile and pancreatic juice into the small intestine.

1,25-dihydroxyvitamin D_3 (calcitriol; produced by skin and activated in liver and kidneys) regulates blood calcium level.

Insulin and **glucagon** (produced by pancreas) regulate blood glucose level.

Ghrelin (produced by stomach cells) helps to regulate energy intake and body weight by stimulating hunger.

Leptin (produced by adipose tissue) helps to regulate energy intake and body weight by reducing hunger.

FIGURE 3-8 Some hormones with nutritional significance.

insulin A hormone produced by the pancreas. Insulin allows for the movement of glucose from the blood into body cells and signals the synthesis of glycogen.

glucagon A hormone made by the pancreas that stimulates the breakdown of glycogen in the liver into glucose; this ends up increasing blood glucose. Glucagon also increases the generation of glucose from noncarbohydrate substances.

prohormone Inactive precursor to a hormone.

1,25-dihydroxyvitamin D₃ Biologically active form of vitamin D; also called *calcitriol*; sometimes shortened to *1,25(OH)D₃*.

digestive organs to secrete bile and digestive enzymes. Other hormones regulate how quickly food moves along the gastrointestinal tract.[1]

- **Insulin** and **glucagon** are two hormones that are synthesized in and released from the pancreas to control the amount of glucose in the blood (Fig. 3-9). When blood glucose rises above normal (usually after a meal), insulin is released from the pancreas and travels through the bloodstream to the muscle, adipose, and liver cells of the body. Among its many functions, insulin allows cells to take up and store glucose. Glucagon has the opposite effect on blood glucose. When blood glucose levels are lower than normal, glucagon triggers the release of stored glucose and the conversion of certain amino acids into glucose, which causes blood glucose to increase.

- Vitamin D is a **prohormone,** meaning that it can be converted into an active hormone in the body. When you consume foods that contain vitamin D, it is in an inactive form. Chemical reactions in the liver and kidneys convert vitamin D into its active form, **1,25-dihydroxyvitamin D₃**, also called *calcitriol*. The active vitamin D hormone regulates a variety of body processes, including

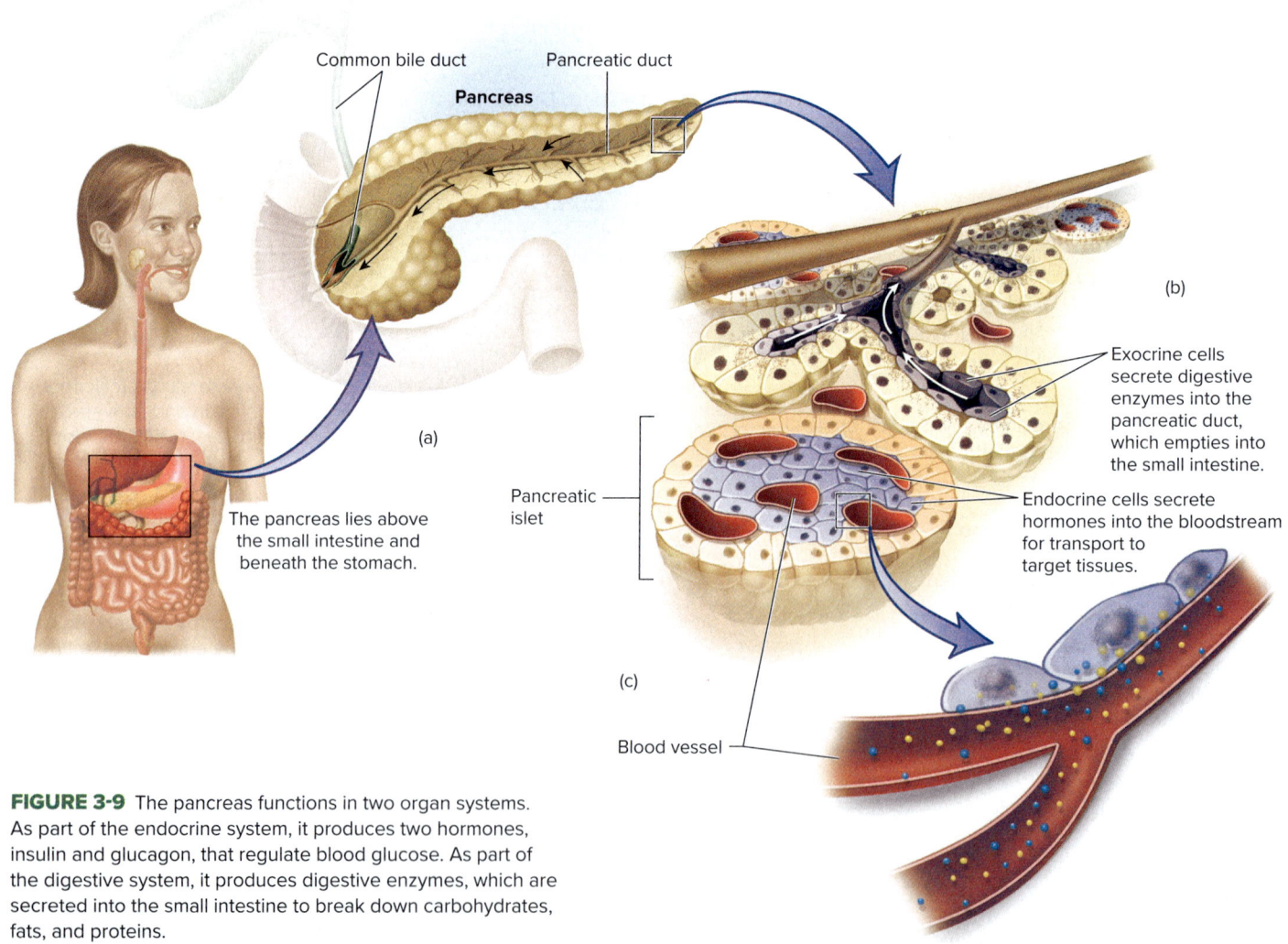

FIGURE 3-9 The pancreas functions in two organ systems. As part of the endocrine system, it produces two hormones, insulin and glucagon, that regulate blood glucose. As part of the digestive system, it produces digestive enzymes, which are secreted into the small intestine to break down carbohydrates, fats, and proteins.

maintenance of blood calcium levels, nerve and muscle development, and immune function.
- Iodine (an essential mineral) is important for thyroid hormone function. **Thyroid hormones,** synthesized in and released from the thyroid gland, help to control the body's metabolic rate—the rate at which you break down carbohydrates, fats, and proteins to make ATP.

thyroid hormones Hormones produced by the thyroid gland that regulate growth and metabolic rate.

✓ CONCEPT CHECK 3.6

1. Examine Figure 3-9. What are the *endocrine* roles of the pancreas? What are the *exocrine* roles of the pancreas?
2. What effect does insulin have on the storage of nutrients?
3. If a person has hypothyroidism, the thyroid gland produces low levels of thyroid hormone. Will a person with hypothyroidism tend to lose weight or gain weight? Explain your answer.

3.7 Immune System

Cells that form a protective barrier—skin and intestinal cells—work in concert with the cells and tissues of the immune system to defend the body against infection. The immune system is a collection of diverse tissues that work together to prevent infection, break down aged and dying cells, and remove abnormal cells. Lymphoid tissue and white blood cells are specific to the immune system, but other body systems also support the immune system: the skin and GI tract provide physical and chemical barriers against invading **pathogens.** In addition, specialized **gut-associated lymphoid tissues (GALT)** are scattered throughout the intestinal tract. GALT assists the cells of the GI tract in keeping pathogens from entering the bloodstream. The lymphatic system is another major site of immune activity: the **lymph nodes** trap pathogens, and the lymph itself transports white blood cells through the body.

We are born with some aspects of immune function, such as physical and chemical barriers against infection, the inflammatory response, and the ability of some white blood cells to engulf microorganisms by **phagocytosis.** These are termed **nonspecific (innate) immunity** because they protect the body against invasion by any microorganism. The skin and the intestinal cells support the immune system by forming an important barrier against invading microorganisms. If the integrity of either one of these barriers is compromised, microorganisms can invade the body and cause illness. Substances secreted by the skin and intestinal cells can also destroy pathogens.

If the body's nonspecific immune defenses are unable to block a microorganism's entry into the bloodstream, cells and chemicals involved in **specific (adaptive) immunity** will identify and destroy the invading pathogen. Specific immunity involves the process by which some types of white blood cells produce **antibodies** (also called *immunoglobulins*) that target specific microorganisms or foreign proteins (known as **antigens**). After initial exposure to an antigen, a "memory" is created such that a second exposure to the substance will produce a more vigorous and rapid response.

The immune system provides a very clear example of the interrelationship between nutrition status and organ system function. In developing nations, where food shortages are common, malnutrition increases susceptibility to infectious diseases, such as

pathogen A microorganism that can cause disease.

gut-associated lymphoid tissues (GALT) Clusters of lymphoid cells located throughout the gastrointestinal tract that destroy pathogens.

lymph nodes Clusters of lymphoid tissue, situated along the lymph vessels, that trap and destroy pathogens.

phagocytosis A process in which a cell forms an indentation, and solid particles enter the indentation and are engulfed by the cell.

nonspecific immunity Defenses that stop the invasion of pathogens; requires no previous encounter with a pathogen; also called *innate immunity*.

specific immunity Function of white blood cells directed at specific antigens; also called *adaptive immunity*.

antibody Blood protein that binds foreign proteins found in the body; also called *immunoglobulin*.

antigen Any substance that induces a state of sensitivity and/or resistance to microorganisms or toxic substances after a lag period; a foreign substance that stimulates a specific aspect of the immune system.

FARM to FORK: Onions and Garlic

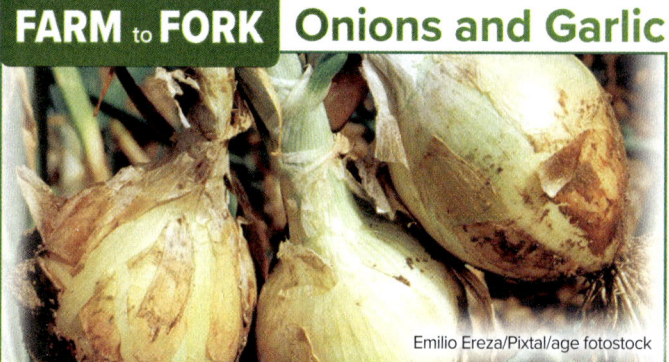

Emilio Ereza/Pixtal/age fotostock

Recall that prebiotics are foods that nourish the bacteria in your gut. Onions and garlic, along with shallots, scallions, chives, and leeks, are part of the allium family and serve as excellent prebiotics. The alliums have long been associated with health and medicinal properties. The hot, pungent flavor of alliums comes from thiosulfinates, compounds that contain the mineral sulfur. Some of these compounds have been shown to have antiviral and antibacterial properties.

Grow
- The most common garlic grown in America, the California silverskin, is very productive. Plant one clove and a new head grows with 16 cloves.
- Several varieties of onions are grown, including white, yellow, red, pearl, and the sweet onions, such as Vidalia.
- Farmers have cultivated larger and sweeter varieties of onions that are popular but have much lower health benefits than wild varieties.
- Green onions, or scallions, are one of the most nutritious alliums and are easy to grow even in small gardens.

Shop
- Buy garlic bulbs that are plump and tightly encased in their papery outer wrapping. If the outer skin is loose or frayed, the bulbs may be dried or moldy.
- Purchase onions with their papery skin intact; this outer skin preserves the juiciness of the onion and protects it from mold and fungal infections.

Store
- Garlic can be stored for 1 or 2 months but becomes more pungent the longer it is stored.
- Store sweet onions and garlic on a shelf in the refrigerator to keep them freshest. Keep them out of the crisper drawer where the high humidity will cause them to sprout. Other onions can be stored in a net bag in a cool, dark location such as an unheated room or basement.

Prep
- Before cooking, garlic should be sliced, chopped, or minced, and then allowed to rest for 10 minutes. This will maximize the production of allicin (a phytochemical) before heat destroys the enzyme that creates it.
- Onions can be cooked as soon as you slice or chop them without losing any health benefits. All cooking methods, except boiling, increase the quercetin content of onions. Cooking also makes the hottest onions taste mild and sweet.

Source: Robinson J. Alliums: all things to all people. In: *Eating on the Wild Side: The Missing Link to Optimum Health*. New York: Little, Brown & Co.; 2013.

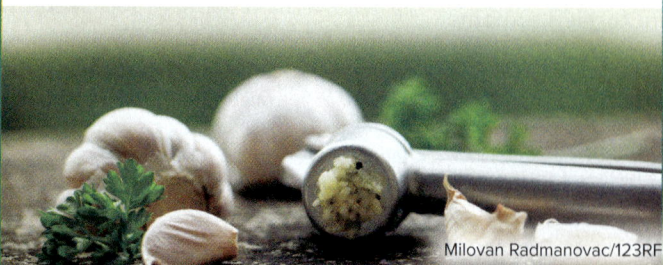

Milovan Radmanovac/123RF

---

diarrheal disease. The turnover of many cells of the immune system is quite rapid—only a few hours or days. The constant synthesis of new cells requires steady nutrient intake. Nutrients that are important for the health of the immune system include essential fatty acids; protein; vitamins A, C, D, E, and some B vitamins; and the minerals iron, copper, and zinc.[2] Chapters 8 and 9 further explore the functions of micronutrients. *Farm to Fork* in this section explores the impact of some phytochemicals from the allium family on immune function.

✓ CONCEPT CHECK 3.7

1. Contrast nonspecific (innate) and specific (adaptive) immunity.
2. What are the roles of antigens and antibodies in the immune response?
3. List three nutrients that support the immune system.

3.8 Digestive System

The foods and beverages we consume, for the most part, must undergo extensive alteration by the **digestive system** to provide us with usable nutrients. The digestive system is composed of six hollow organs that make up the **gastrointestinal (GI) tract** as well as three accessory organs that secrete important substances into the GI tract. The processes of **digestion** and **absorption** take place inside the GI tract (Fig. 3-10). The open space inside the GI tract is called the **lumen.** Nutrients from the food we eat must pass through the walls of the GI tract—from the lumen through the cells lining the GI tract—to be absorbed into the bloodstream.

There are two ways food is broken down in the GI tract: *mechanical* digestion and *chemical* digestion. Mechanical digestion takes place as soon as you begin chewing your

---

digestive system System consisting of the gastrointestinal tract and accessory structures (liver, gallbladder, and pancreas). This system performs the mechanical and chemical processes of digestion, absorption of nutrients, and elimination of wastes.

gastrointestinal (GI) tract The main sites in the body used for digestion and absorption of nutrients. It consists of the mouth, esophagus, stomach, small intestine, large intestine, rectum, and anus. Also called the *digestive tract*.

digestion Process by which large ingested molecules are mechanically and chemically broken down to produce basic nutrients that can be absorbed across the wall of the GI tract.

absorption The process by which substances are taken up from the GI tract and enter the bloodstream or the lymph.

lumen The hollow opening inside a tube, such as the GI tract.

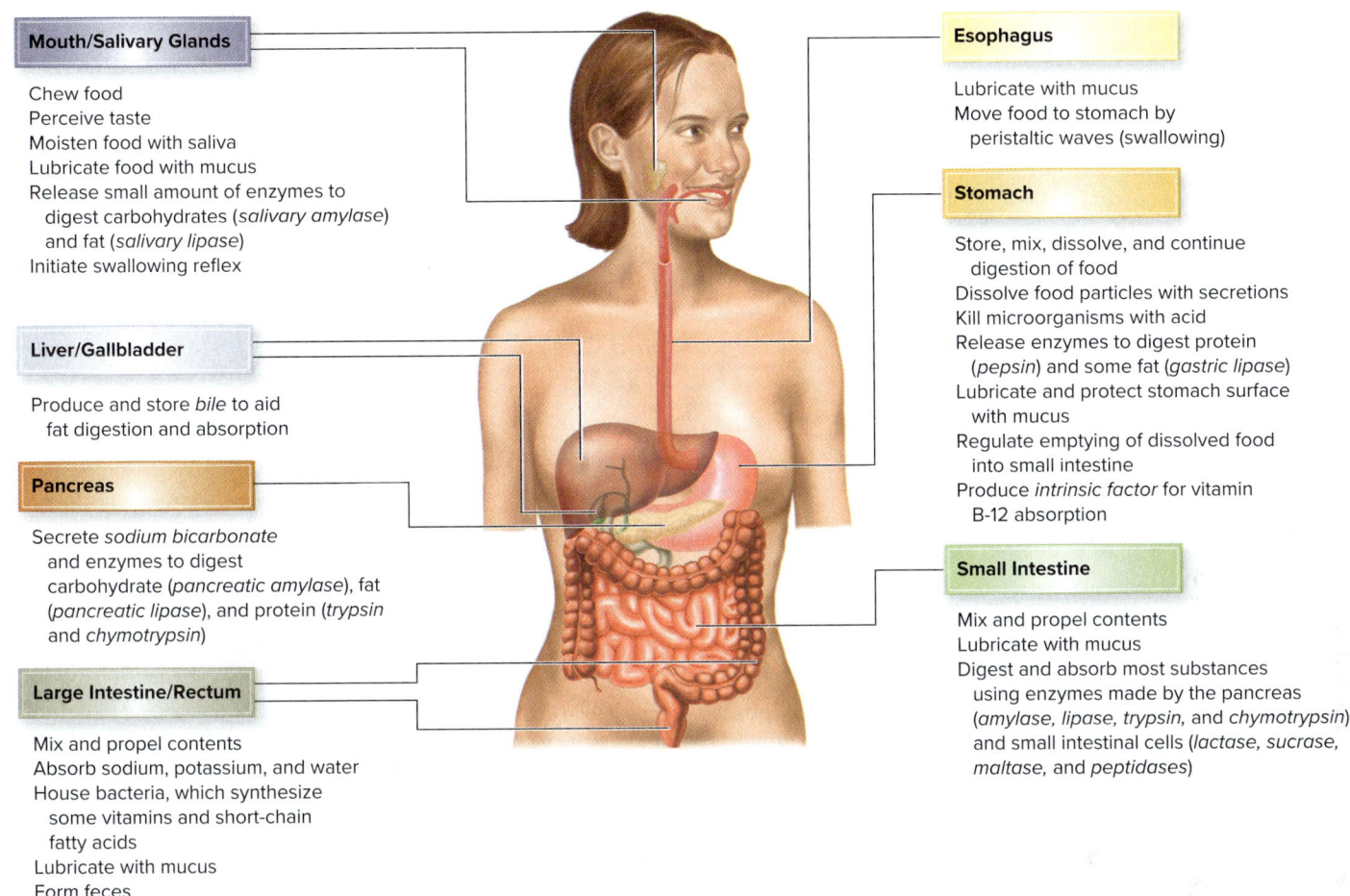

FIGURE 3-10 Digestive system. The digestive system consists of the organs of the GI tract and the accessory organs. Partially digested food spends about 2 to 3 hours in the stomach (longer for large meals). Passage through the small intestine takes 3 to 10 hours, followed by up to 72 hours in the large intestine. On average, digestion and absorption of a meal take about 2 days. Food matter tends to pass more quickly through the GI tract of males than females.

food and continues as muscular contractions simultaneously mix and move food through the length of the GI tract. Chemical digestion refers to the chemical breakdown of foods by acid and enzymes secreted into the GI tract. Enzymes are a key part of chemical digestion. Each enzyme is specific to one type of chemical process. For example, the enzyme that recognizes and digests table sugar (sucrose) ignores milk sugar (lactose). Besides working on only specific types of chemicals, enzymes are sensitive to acidic and alkaline conditions, temperature, and the types of vitamins and minerals they require to function. Digestive enzymes that work in the acidic environment of the stomach do not work well in the alkaline environment of the small intestine. The pancreas and small intestine produce most of the digestive enzymes; however, the mouth and the stomach also contribute their own enzymes to the process of digestion. The organs of the digestive system are able to fine-tune the production of each type of digestive enzyme in response to the nutritional makeup and amount of food consumed. Overall, the enzymes of the digestive system work together to hasten the breakdown of ingested food into absorbable nutrients (Fig. 3-11).

As food moves along the GI tract, nutrients are absorbed. The primary site of nutrient absorption is the small intestine. By the time the meal contents reach the large intestine, most of the usable nutrients have been absorbed. What remains is waste. The final role of the digestive system is elimination of wastes.

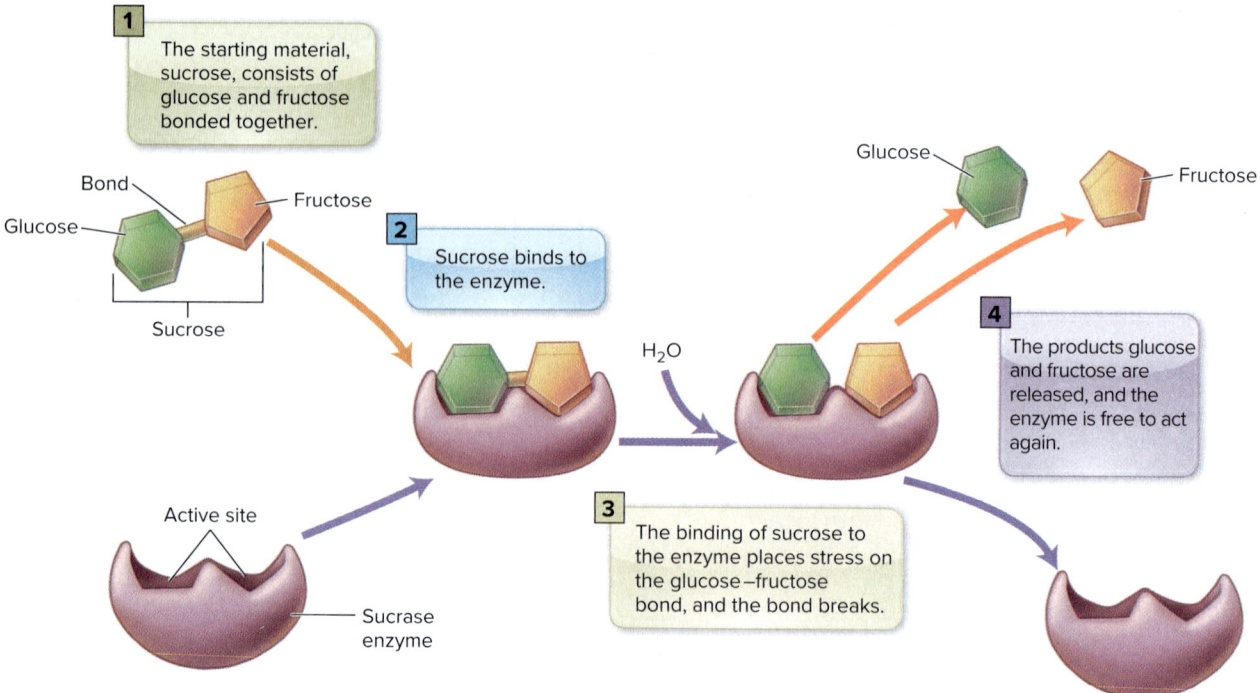

FIGURE 3-11 A model of enzyme action. The enzyme sucrase splits the sugar sucrose into two simpler sugars, glucose and fructose. Energy (in the form of ATP) is needed to make some reactions occur. The activity of some enzymes depends on the presence of specific vitamin or mineral cofactors.

Most of the processes of digestion and absorption are under *autonomic* (i.e., involuntary) control. The functions involved in digestion and absorption are controlled by signals from the nervous system, hormones from the endocrine system, and hormone-like compounds.

Take a moment to study Figure 3-10. In the next few subsections, we will examine the functions of each organ in detail. Can you label each organ on a diagram? Can you briefly describe the role of each organ in digestion and absorption?

MOUTH

The mouth has the unique ability to sense the taste of the foods we consume. By interacting with chemical compounds in foods, taste receptors (located on the tongue and other areas of the mouth) identify specific flavor(s). The sense of taste is important for survival! Taste sensations help us to recognize foods that provide the energy and nutrients we need (e.g., carbohydrates, protein, and sodium). They also help us to detect potential toxins. The taste of food (or the anticipation of it) signals the rest of the GI tract to prepare for the digestion of food.

Most sources simply describe five basic taste sensations: sweet, sour, salty, bitter, and **umami**, but research on the science of taste is ongoing. In 2015, researchers confirmed humans have a specific taste receptor for fat, which they called **oleogustus**,[3] and in 2023, researchers discovered a specific mechanism by which we detect the flavor of ammonia, which is toxic in large amounts.[4]

Surprisingly, the nose and our sense of smell greatly contribute to our ability to sense the taste of food. When you chew a food, chemicals are released that stimulate the nasal passages. Thus, it makes perfect sense that when your nose is congested, even your favorite foods will not taste as good as they normally do.

umami A brothy, meaty, savory flavor in some foods. Monosodium glutamate enhances this flavor when added to foods.

oleogustus A taste for fat. The presence of fatty acids in foods stimulates taste receptors in the mouth; this sensation is unpleasant.

TABLE 3-1 ■ Important Secretions of the Digestive System

Secretion	Site of Production	Purpose
Saliva	Mouth	Contains enzymes that make a minor contribution to starch and fat digestion Lubrication of food for swallowing
Mucus	Mouth, esophagus, stomach, small intestine, large intestine	Protects GI tract cells Lubricates food as it travels through the GI tract
Enzymes	Mouth, stomach, small intestine, pancreas	Promote digestion of carbohydrates, fats, and proteins into forms small enough for absorption (examples: amylases, lipases, proteases)
Acid	Stomach	Promotes digestion of protein Destroys pathogens Solubilizes some minerals Activates some enzymes
Bile	Liver (stored in gallbladder)	Aids fat digestion in the small intestine by suspending fat in water using **bile acids,** cholesterol, and phospholipids
Bicarbonate	Pancreas, small intestine	Neutralizes stomach acid when it reaches the small intestine
Hormones	Stomach, small intestine, pancreas	Stimulate production and/or release of acid, enzymes, bile, and bicarbonate Regulate movement of food matter through the GI tract
Intrinsic factor	Stomach	Facilitates absorption of vitamin B-12 in the small intestine

Digestion begins in the mouth. The chewing action of the teeth contributes to the mechanical digestion of foods. Chemical digestion begins with **saliva,** produced by the salivary glands. Saliva functions as a solvent so that food particles can be further separated and tasted. In addition, saliva contains a starch-digesting enzyme, salivary **amylase,** and a fat-digesting enzyme, **lipase. Mucus,** another component of saliva, is a lubricant that makes it easier to swallow a mouthful of food. The food then travels to the esophagus. The important secretions of digestion are listed in Table 3-1.

ESOPHAGUS

The **esophagus** is a long tube that connects the **pharynx** with the stomach. Near the pharynx is a flap of tissue (called the **epiglottis**) that prevents a **bolus** of swallowed food from entering the **trachea** (windpipe) (Fig. 3-12). During swallowing, food lands on the epiglottis, folding it down to cover the opening of the trachea. Breathing also stops automatically. These responses ensure that swallowed food will only travel down the esophagus. If food becomes lodged in the trachea, choking will occur (the victim will not be able to speak, cough, or breathe).

At the top of the esophagus, nerve fibers release signals to tell the GI tract that food has been consumed. This results in an increase in GI muscle action, called **peristalsis.** These waves of muscular contractions force the food in one direction along the digestive tract from the mouth toward the anus (Fig. 3-13).

At the end of the esophagus is the **lower esophageal sphincter,** a ring of muscle that constricts (closes) after food enters the stomach. In general, the function of sphincters is to prevent the backflow of the contents of the GI tract. Sphincters respond to various stimuli, such as signals from the nervous system, hormones, acidic conditions, and pressure that builds up around the sphincter. The primary

bile acid A compound produced by the liver. Bile acids are the main component of bile, which aids in emulsification of fat during digestion in the small intestine.

saliva Watery fluid, produced by the salivary glands in the mouth, which contains lubricants, enzymes, and other substances.

amylase Starch-digesting enzyme produced by the salivary glands and the pancreas.

lipase Fat-digesting enzyme produced by the salivary glands, stomach, and pancreas.

mucus A thick fluid secreted by many cells throughout the body. It contains a compound that has both carbohydrate and protein parts. It acts as a lubricant and means of protection for cells.

esophagus A tube in the GI tract that connects the pharynx with the stomach.

pharynx A cavity located at the back of the oral and nasal cavities, commonly known as the *throat*. It is part of the digestive tract and the respiratory tract.

epiglottis The flap that folds down over the trachea during swallowing.

bolus A moistened mass of food swallowed from the oral cavity into the pharynx.

trachea The airway that extends from the throat, down the neck, to the lungs; also called the *windpipe*.

peristalsis A coordinated muscular contraction used to propel food down the gastrointestinal tract.

lower esophageal sphincter A circular muscle that constricts the opening of the esophagus to the stomach. Also called the *gastroesophageal sphincter* or the *cardiac sphincter.*

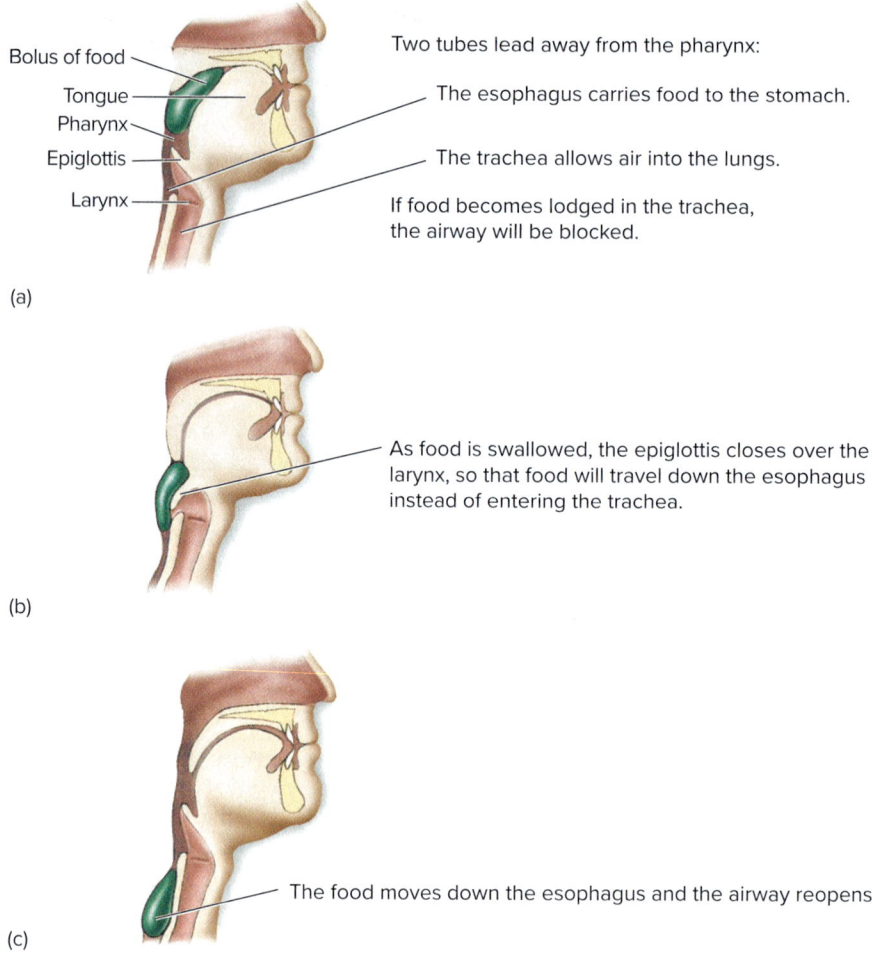

FIGURE 3-12 The process of swallowing.

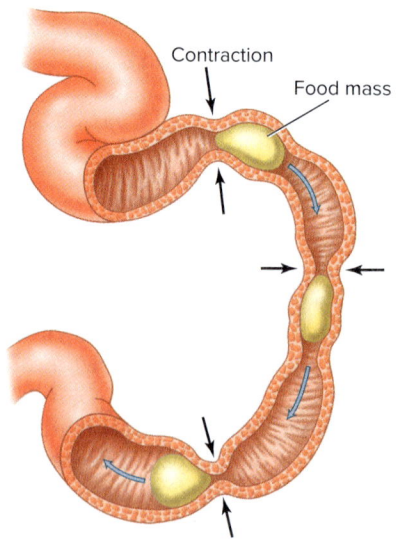

FIGURE 3-13 Peristalsis. Peristalsis is a progressive type of muscular movement, propelling material from point to point along the GI tract. To begin this, a ring of contraction occurs where the GI wall is stretched, passing the food mass forward. The moving food mass triggers a ring of contraction in the next region, which pushes the food mass even farther along. The result is a ring of contraction that moves like a wave along the GI tract, pushing the food mass down the tract.

function of the lower esophageal sphincter is to prevent the acidic contents of the stomach from flowing back up into the esophagus. Dysfunction of this sphincter can cause heartburn (Section 3.11).

No digestion or absorption occurs in the esophagus; it serves merely to transport food from the mouth to the stomach. The cells of the esophagus secrete mucus to lubricate the passage of food, but no digestive enzymes are produced.

STOMACH

The stomach is a large sac that can hold up to 4 cups (or 1 quart) of food for several hours until all of the food has been moved into the small intestine. Stomach size varies from person to person and can be reduced surgically as a radical treatment for obesity (more on this in Section 7.9). While in the stomach, the food is mixed with gastric juice, which contains water, hydrochloric acid, and enzymes. (*Gastric* is a term pertaining to the stomach.) The acid in the gastric juice halts the biological activity of proteins, converts some inactive digestive enzymes into their active forms, partially digests food protein, and makes dietary minerals soluble so that they can be absorbed. The mixing that takes place in the stomach produces a watery food mixture, called **chyme,** which slowly leaves the stomach a teaspoon (5 milliliters) at a time and enters the small intestine. Following a meal, the stomach contents are emptied into the small intestine over the course of 1 to 4 hours. The **pyloric sphincter,** located at the base of the stomach, controls the rate at which the chyme is released into the small intestine (Fig. 3-14). Some water and alcohol are absorbed from the stomach into the bloodstream, but most nutrient absorption will occur in the small intestine.

If the acid and enzymes in the stomach are strong enough to break apart food proteins and kill pathogens, how does the stomach tissue itself withstand destruction by these harsh chemicals? First, the production of acid and enzymes in the stomach is regulated by hormones (e.g., gastrin) that are released when we are eating or thinking

chyme A mixture of stomach secretions and partially digested food.

pyloric sphincter Ring of smooth muscle between the stomach and the small intestine.

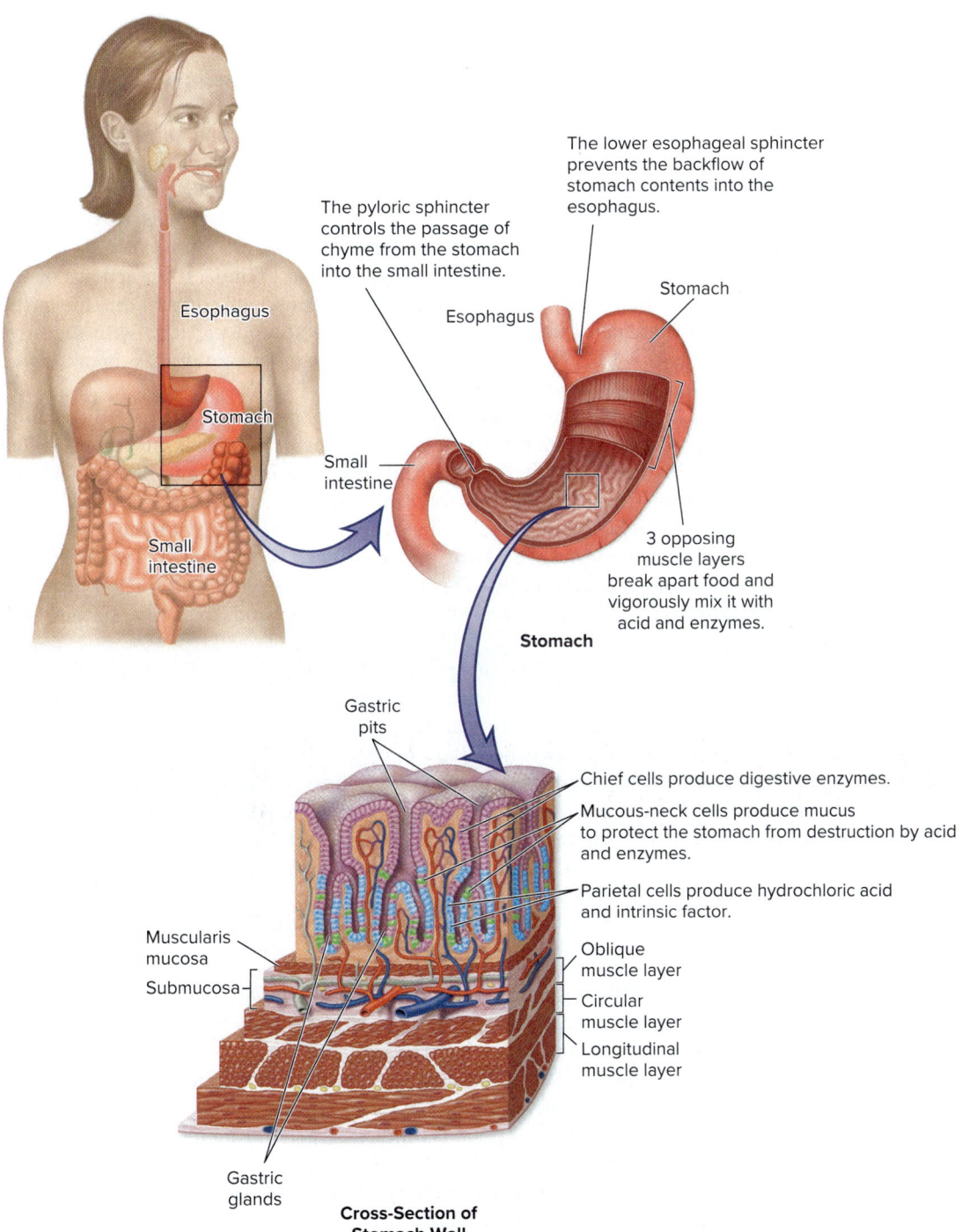

FIGURE 3-14 Physiology of the stomach.

about eating. Between meals, the stomach cells do not produce much acid and enzymes. Second, the stomach produces a thick layer of mucus that forms a protective barrier over the stomach lining.

One other important function of the stomach is the production of a substance called **intrinsic factor.** This vital protein-like compound is essential for the absorption of vitamin B-12. You will learn about the digestion and absorption of vitamin B-12 in Section 8.15.

intrinsic factor A protein-like compound produced by the stomach that enhances vitamin B-12 absorption in the ileum.

SMALL INTESTINE

The small intestine is considered "small" because its diameter is only 1 inch (2.5 centimeters). It is actually quite long—about 10 feet (3 meters), beginning at the stomach and extending to the large intestine (Fig. 3-15). The three parts of the small intestine are the **duodenum** (first 10 inches), the **jejunum** (second 4 feet), and the **ileum** (last 5 feet).

Most of the digestion and absorption of food occurs in the small intestine. As chyme moves from the stomach into the first part of the small intestine, it is still very acidic. You just learned that the stomach secretes a thick layer of mucus to protect itself from the strong acid. However, if the small intestine were coated with mucus, digestion and absorption would be very limited. Instead, the pancreas and intestinal cells secrete **bicarbonate** to neutralize the acid. The neutral pH also optimizes the activity of the digestive enzymes that work in the small intestine. Muscular contractions move the chyme through the small intestine and thoroughly mix food particles with digestive juices (review Fig. 3-13). The digestive juices contain enzymes that break down carbohydrates, protein, and fat into absorbable units.

The physical structure of the small intestine is very important to the body's ability to digest and absorb the nutrients it needs. The lining of the small intestine is called the mucosa and is folded many times; within these folds are fingerlike projections called **villi.** These "fingers" are constantly moving, which helps them trap food to enhance absorption. Each individual villus (singular) is made up of many **absorptive cells** (also called *enterocytes*), and the mucosal surface of each of these cells is folded even further into **microvilli.** The combined folds, villi, and microvilli in the small intestine increase its surface area 600 times beyond that of a simple tube (Fig. 3-15)!

The absorptive cells have a short lifespan of only 3 to 5 days.[5] In fact, before this time next week, all the cells making up your intestinal lining today will have been shed and replaced by new cells, which are constantly produced in the crypts between the villi (Fig. 3-15). Rapid cell turnover is necessary to cope with the damage caused by continuous exposure to acid, enzymes, bacteria, and toxins. Such rapid cell turnover leads to high nutrient needs for the small intestine. Fortunately, many of the old cells can be broken down and their parts can be absorbed and reused. The health of the cells is further enhanced by various hormones and other substances that participate in or are produced as part of the digestive process.

The small intestine absorbs nutrients through the intestinal wall through various means and processes, as illustrated in Figure 3-16.

- **Passive diffusion:** When the nutrient concentration is higher in the lumen of the small intestine than in the absorptive cells, the difference in nutrient concentration drives the nutrient into the absorptive cells by diffusion. Fats, water, and some minerals are examples of nutrients that move down a concentration gradient to be absorbed by passive diffusion.
- **Facilitated diffusion:** Some compounds require a carrier protein to follow a concentration gradient into absorptive cells. This type of absorption is called facilitated diffusion. Fructose is one example of a compound that makes use of such a carrier to allow for facilitated diffusion.
- **Active absorption:** In addition to the need for a carrier protein, some nutrients also require energy input to move from the lumen of the small intestine into

duodenum First segment of the small intestine that receives chyme from the stomach and digestive juices from the pancreas and gallbladder. This is the site of most chemical digestion of nutrients; approximately 10 inches in length.

jejunum Middle segment of the small intestine; approximately 4 feet in length.

ileum Last segment of the small intestine; approximately 5 feet in length.

bicarbonate Alkaline compound produced as part of the body's buffer systems. For example, the pancreas secretes bicarbonate to neutralize the hydrochloric acid in chyme in the small intestine.

villi (singular: villus) The fingerlike protrusions into the small intestine that participate in digestion and absorption of food.

absorptive cells The intestinal cells that line the villi and participate in nutrient absorption; also known as *enterocytes*.

microvilli Extensive folds on the mucosal surface of the absorptive cells.

passive diffusion Movement of a substance across a semipermeable membrane from an area of higher solute concentration to an area of lower solute concentration. This type of transport does not require a carrier and does not require energy.

facilitated diffusion Movement of a substance across a semipermeable membrane from an area of higher solute concentration to an area of lower solute concentration. This type of transport does not require energy, but it does require a carrier.

active absorption Movement of a substance across a semipermeable membrane from an area of lower solute concentration to an area of higher solute concentration. This type of transport requires energy and a carrier.

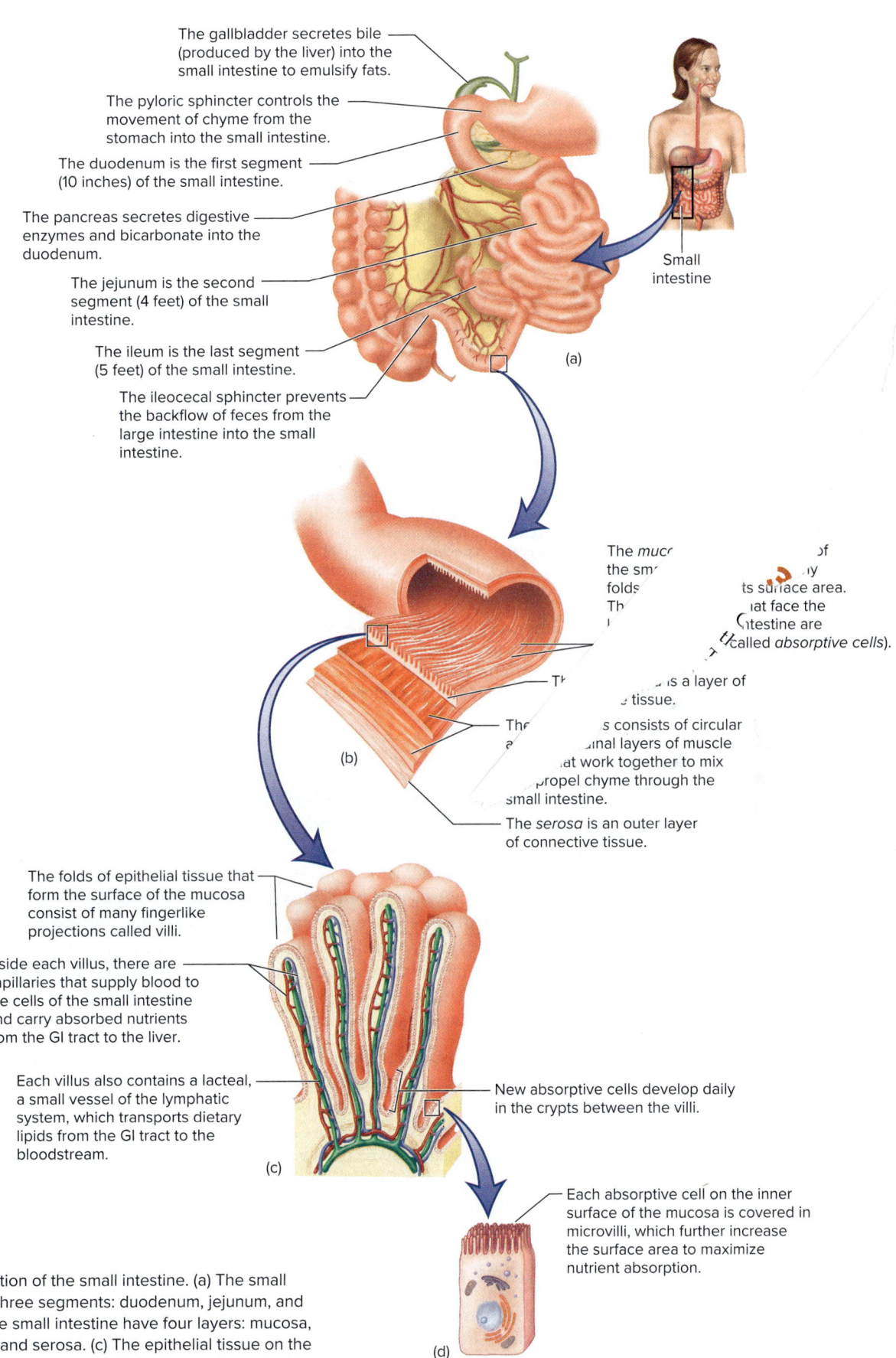

FIGURE 3-15 Organization of the small intestine. (a) The small intestine is divided into three segments: duodenum, jejunum, and ileum. (b) The walls of the small intestine have four layers: mucosa, submucosa, muscularis, and serosa. (c) The epithelial tissue on the inner surface of the mucosa has many villi. (d) The surface of each villus is covered in many absorptive cells with microvilli.

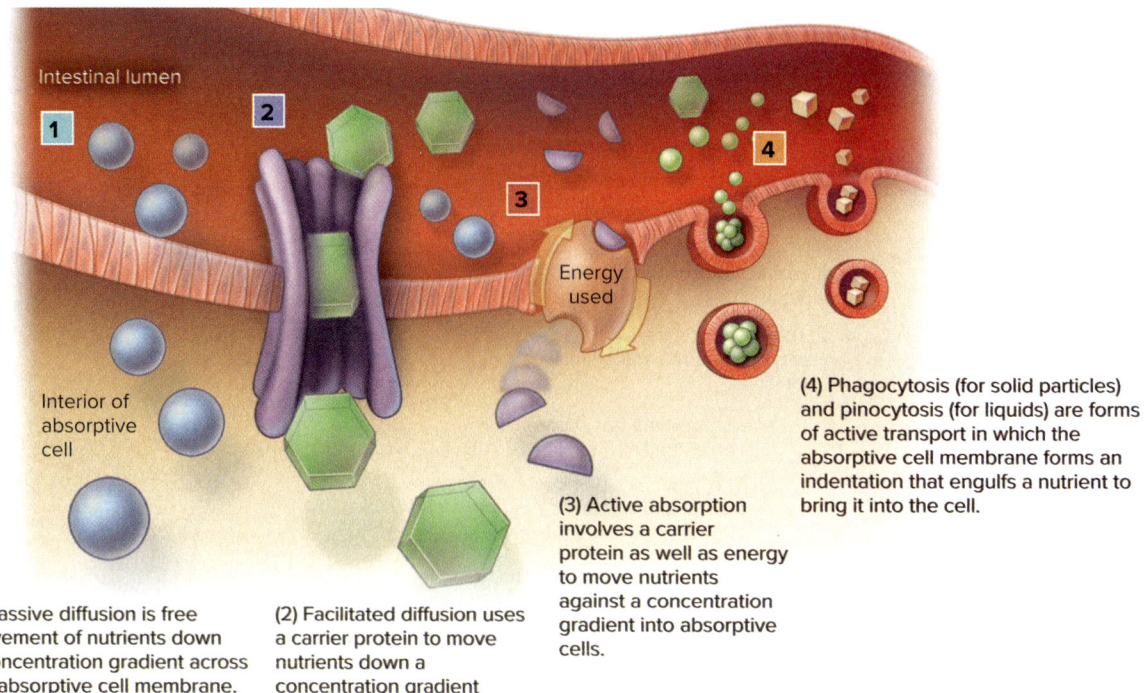

FIGURE 3-16 Nutrient absorption relies on four major absorptive processes. Passive diffusion (1) and facilitated diffusion (2) move solutes *down a concentration gradient* (i.e., from an area of high nutrient concentration to an area of low nutrient concentration), so they do not require energy. Active absorption (3) and phagocytosis (4) move solutes *against a concentration gradient* (i.e., from an area of low nutrient concentration to an area of high nutrient concentration), so they do require energy.

pinocytosis A process in which a cell forms an indentation, and fluid enters the indentation and is engulfed by the cell.

ileocecal sphincter The ring of smooth muscle between the end of the small intestine and the beginning of the large intestine.

feces Mass of water, fiber, tough connective tissues, bacterial cells, and sloughed intestinal cells that passes through the large intestine and is excreted through the anus; also called *stool*.

the absorptive cells. This mechanism makes it possible for cells to take up nutrients even when they are consumed in low concentrations (i.e., against a concentration gradient). Some sugars, such as glucose, are actively absorbed, as are amino acids.

- Phagocytosis and **pinocytosis:** In a further means of active absorption, absorptive cells literally engulf solid particles (phagocytosis) or liquids (pinocytosis). A cell membrane forms an indentation, and when particles or fluids move into the indentation, the cell membrane surrounds and engulfs them. This process is used when an infant absorbs immune substances from human milk (see Section 14.7).

Once absorbed, water-soluble compounds such as glucose and amino acids are transported by the capillaries to the hepatic portal vein, which leads directly to the liver. Most fats are absorbed into the lymph vessels, which eventually empty into the bloodstream (review Figs. 3-4 and 3-5).

Undigested food cannot be absorbed into cells of the small intestine. Any undigested food that reaches the end of the small intestine passes through the **ileocecal sphincter** and moves into the large intestine. The ileocecal sphincter prevents the contents of the large intestine from backing up and reentering the small intestine.

LARGE INTESTINE

By the time undigested food matter (now called **feces**) makes it to the large intestine, it bears little resemblance to the food that was originally eaten. If the previous steps of digestion and absorption have worked properly, only a minor amount (5%) of carbohydrate, protein, and fat escapes absorption to reach the large intestine.

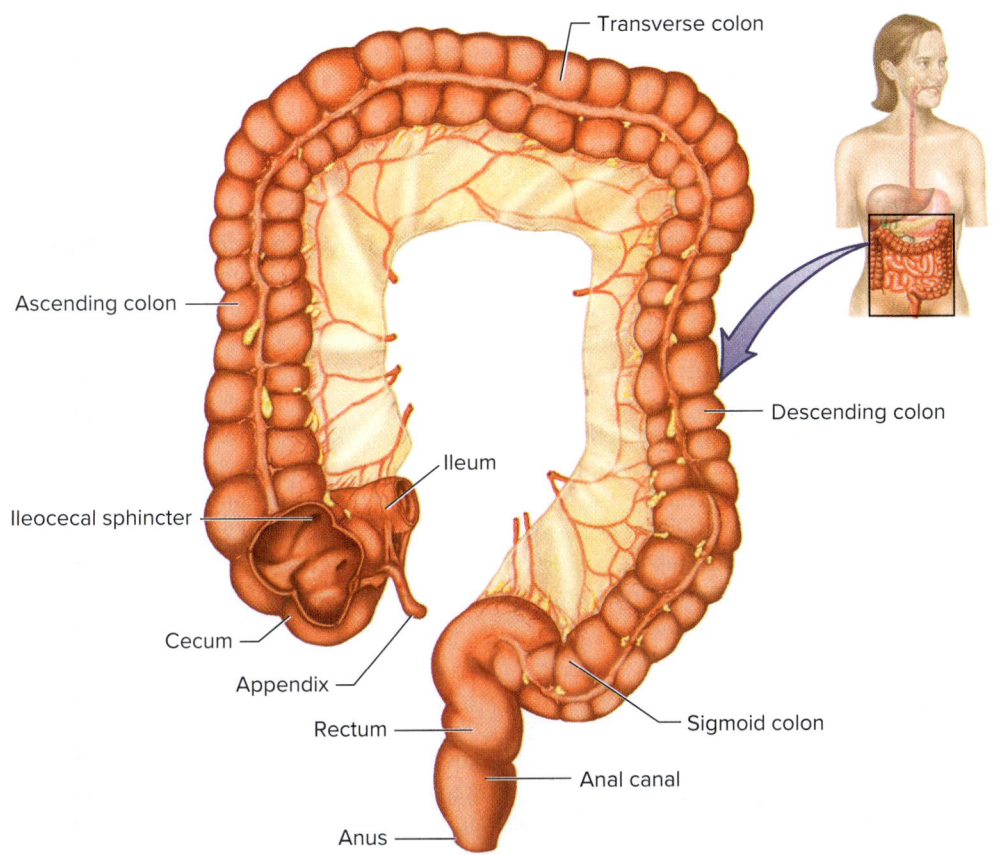

FIGURE 3-17 The parts of the large intestine include the cecum, ascending colon, transverse colon, descending colon, and sigmoid colon. Overall, the large intestine is about 3.5 feet (1.1 meters) long.

The large intestine (sometimes called the *colon*) can be subdivided into five main segments: the **cecum, ascending colon, transverse colon, descending colon,** and **sigmoid colon** (Fig. 3-17). Unlike the small intestine, the large intestine has no villi and no digestive enzymes. Also, the cells of the large intestine produce more mucus than the cells of the small intestine. The mucus secreted by these cells functions to hold the feces together, facilitate the movement of feces through the large intestine, and protect the cells of the large intestine from the bacterial activity within it. Despite the thicker layer of mucus and the absence of villi, a few nutrients can be absorbed from the large intestine: water, a few vitamins, some fatty acids, and the minerals sodium and potassium (Table 3-2).

cecum A pouch at the first part of the large intestine that houses many bacteria.

ascending colon Segment of the large intestine that carries feces from the cecum, up the right side of the abdomen, to the transverse colon.

transverse colon Segment of the large intestine that carries feces from the ascending colon, from right to left across the top of the abdomen, to the descending colon.

descending colon Segment of the large intestine that carries feces from the transverse colon, down the left side of the abdomen, to the sigmoid colon.

sigmoid colon Last segment of the large intestine that carries feces from the descending colon to the rectum.

TABLE 3-2 ■ A Summary of Absorption Along the GI Tract

Organ	Primary Nutrients Absorbed
Stomach	Alcohol (20% of total)
	Water (minor amount)
Small intestine	All minerals (e.g., calcium, magnesium, and iron)
	Glucose
	Amino acids
	Fats
	Vitamins
	Water (70% to 90% of total)
	Alcohol (80% of total)
	Bile acids
Large intestine	A few minerals (sodium and potassium)
	Some fatty acids
	Gases
	Water (10% to 30% of total)

The large intestine is home to a large population of bacteria (over 500 different species[6]), which are collectively called the microbiota. Bacteria in the large intestine are able to break down some of the remaining food products that enter the large intestine, such as the milk sugar lactose (in lactose-intolerant people) and some components of fiber. Also, the bacteria that live in the large intestine produce some vitamins (e.g., vitamin K and biotin) that can be absorbed. Some of the products of bacterial metabolism in the large intestine, which include various fatty acids and gases, can be absorbed and exert health effects in other areas of the body. A growing body of research shows that intestinal bacteria play a significant role in the maintenance of health, not just for the colon, but throughout the body! See Section 3.9 for more information about the importance of the gut microbiota for human health.

Some water remains in the material that enters the large intestine because the small intestine absorbs only 70% to 90% of the fluid it receives, which includes large amounts of secretions produced during digestion (review Table 3-1). The remnants of a meal also contain some minerals and some fiber. As water is gradually absorbed from feces by the cells of the large intestine, the feces change from liquid to semisolid as they pass through the organ. By the time it is expelled from the body, what remains in the feces is undigested carbohydrates (i.e., fiber); tough connective tissues (from animal foods); bacteria from the large intestine; some body wastes (e.g., parts of dead intestinal cells); and a small amount of water.

RECTUM

The feces (also known as *stool*) remains in the last portion of the large intestine, the **rectum,** until muscular movements push it into the **anus** to be eliminated. The presence of feces in the rectum stimulates elimination. The anus contains two **anal sphincters** (internal and external), one of which is under voluntary control (external sphincter). Relaxation of this sphincter allows for elimination.

ACCESSORY ORGANS

The liver, **gallbladder,** and pancreas work with the GI tract and are considered accessory organs to the process of digestion (review Fig. 3-10). These accessory organs are not part of the GI tract (i.e., food never touches the accessory organs), but they play necessary roles in the process of digestion. These organs secrete digestive fluids into the GI tract and facilitate the digestion of food into absorbable nutrients.

Liver and Gallbladder. The liver produces a substance called **bile.** The bile is stored and concentrated in the gallbladder until the gallbladder receives a hormonal signal to release bile into the small intestine. This signal is induced by the presence of fat in the small intestine. Bile is released and delivered to the first segment of the small intestine (i.e., the duodenum) via a tube called the bile duct (Fig. 3-18).

Bile is an emulsifier. During digestion, bile enables large portions of fat in the chyme to separate into smaller bits so that lipase enzymes can do the work of fat digestion (Chapter 5 will cover this process in detail). Interestingly, some of the bile constituents can be "recycled" in a process known as **enterohepatic circulation:** components of bile are reabsorbed from the small intestine, returned to the liver via the portal vein, and reused.

The liver also releases some waste products (e.g., excess minerals, breakdown products from cell metabolism) into the bile. These wastes will eventually end up in the large intestine and will be excreted as part of the feces. The liver functions in this manner to remove unwanted substances from the blood. (The kidneys also remove waste products from the blood and excrete these wastes as part of urine. However, the kidneys are part of the urinary system, not the digestive system.)

---

rectum Terminal section of the large intestine where feces are held prior to expulsion.

anus Last portion of the GI tract; serves as an outlet for the digestive system.

anal sphincters A group of two sphincters (inner and outer) that help control expulsion of feces from the body.

gallbladder An organ attached to the underside of the liver; site of bile storage, concentration, and eventual secretion.

bile A liver secretion stored in the gallbladder and released through the common bile duct into the first segment of the small intestine. It is essential for the digestion and absorption of fat.

enterohepatic circulation A continual recycling of compounds such as bile acids between the small intestine and the liver.

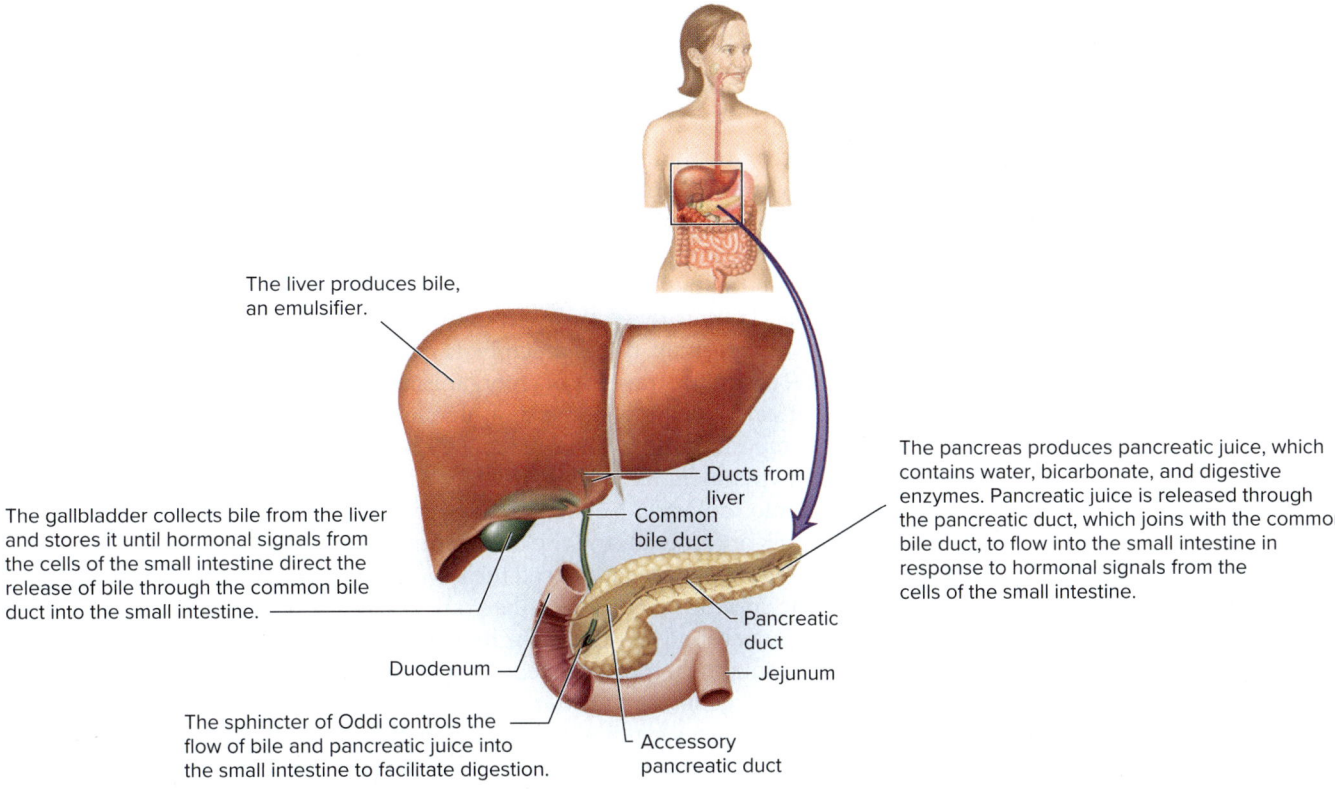

FIGURE 3-18 Although food does not come into contact with these accessory organs, the liver, gallbladder, and pancreas are important for digestion.

Pancreas. The pancreas has both endocrine and digestive functions. As a gland of the endocrine system, the pancreas manufactures hormones—insulin and glucagon—that are secreted into the blood to regulate blood glucose levels (review Fig. 3-9). As an organ of the digestive system, it produces "pancreatic juice," a mixture of water, bicarbonate, and a variety of digestive enzymes capable of breaking apart carbohydrates, proteins, and fats into small fragments. The role of bicarbonate is to neutralize chyme, which is quite acidic as it moves from the stomach into the duodenum. As noted earlier, the small intestine does not have a thick, protective layer of mucus because mucus would impede nutrient absorption. Instead, the neutralizing capacity of bicarbonate from the pancreas protects the walls of the small intestine from erosion by acid, which could otherwise lead to the formation of an ulcer (see Section 3.11).

✓ CONCEPT CHECK 3.8

1. Choose three secretions of the digestive system. Where is each secreted? What is the role of each in the process of digestion?
2. What are enzymes? Is bile an enzyme?
3. How do mucus and surface area affect absorption?
4. Which absorptive processes use energy? How does the *concentration gradient* factor into this?
5. What did you have for lunch today? Trace the path of your meal through the digestive system. Where is each macronutrient broken down as it passes through the GI tract? Where is each absorbed?

3.9 The Human Microbiota

As soon as we are born (and perhaps before birth!), we are exposed to a vast array of microorganisms from the world around us. Some of these microorganisms take up residence in and on the human body—the skin, the respiratory tract, the genitourinary tract, and the gastrointestinal tract. Over the first few years of life, a fairly stable community of microorganisms colonizes the human host. This community of more than 100 trillion microorganisms is known as the human microbiota. Scientists have come to recognize the human microbiota as a human organ, given its high metabolic activity and impact on nearly every aspect of human health.

The precise composition of the microbiota varies from person to person. So far, more than 2300 different strains of microorganisms have been identified in the human microbiota, but each person is home to a unique community of only a few hundred species. The composition of bacteria in your GI tract depends on a variety of factors: genetics, age, environmental exposures, dietary pattern, and other lifestyle factors.[7] The way you came into the world (vaginal or Cesarean birth), the way you were fed as an infant (breast milk or formula), and the use of antibiotics to treat acute infections were a few of the variables that have influenced the development of your gut microbiota.

Whatever the specific composition, there are at least as many microbial cells living in and on the human body as there are human cells. Also consider that all of these microbial cells contain their own genes. As a whole, the microbiome contains about 150 times as many genes as the human genome![8] Pathogenic (i.e., disease-causing) strains of microorganisms synthesize compounds that can make us sick. For example, there is evidence that certain patterns in the microbiome are linked to the occurrence of cardiovascular disease, type 2 diabetes, and chronic liver diseases. Some bacteria produce toxins that are linked to the development of colon cancer. However, many microbial genes code for proteins that affect human health in beneficial ways. Some affect the integrity of the epithelial tissue that lines the large intestine. Some may enhance the absorption of minerals, such as iron and calcium. Others may affect cholesterol synthesis. Many of these microbes, including lactic acid bacteria and *bifidobacteria*, enhance immune function.

By far, the community of microorganisms living in the gastrointestinal tract—the *gut microbiota*—has been the most studied area of the human microbiota. Microbes live all along the GI tract, but the large intestine is the organ most heavily colonized with bacteria (Fig. 3-19). As we continue to look at the human body from a nutrition perspective, let's see how the gut microbiota specifically influences human health.

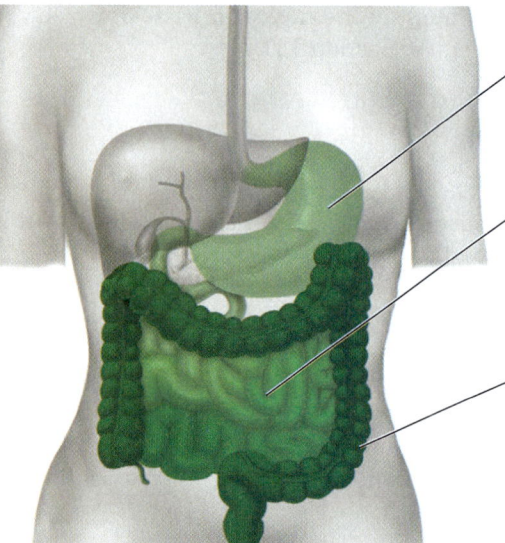

FIGURE 3-19 Bacteria and other microorganisms reside throughout the entire gastrointestinal tract, but the large intestine is the most heavily colonized organ. The shading represents the relative population density of microbes along the length of the GI tract.

The stomach is sparsely populated by about 1000 colony-forming units (CFU) per gram of contents. The low pH limits growth of most microorganisms.

As the pH of the small intestine increases through the duodenum, jejunum, and ileum, microorganisms begin to flourish. There are at least 1 million CFU per gram of contents inside the ileum.

The large intestine houses more than 100,000,000,000 CFU per gram of contents.

PROBIOTICS, PREBIOTICS, SYNBIOTICS, AND POSTBIOTICS

Probiotics are live microorganisms that have positive effects on human health if they are consumed in sufficient quantities. These live microorganisms can be ingested as part of foods (e.g., yogurt and kefir), or they can be administered as supplements (e.g., pills, powders, or suppositories). Common probiotic bacteria used in foods and supplements include species of *Lactobacillus, Lactococcus,* and *Streptococcus* (frequently grouped together as lactic acid bacteria because they produce lactic acid when they are used to ferment dairy foods), as well as some species of the *Bifidobacterium* genus. Notice that the definition of probiotics is not limited to bacteria; although many probiotic microorganisms are bacteria, *Saccharomyces boulardii* is a strain of yeast that can also promote human health.[9]

Prebiotics, on the other hand, are not living microorganisms. Prebiotics are ingredients (typically carbohydrates) that are not well digested by human enzymes but serve as fuel for beneficial bacteria in the gut.[10] For example, **fructooligosaccharides (FOS)** and **galactooligosaccharides (GOS)** are short chains of carbohydrates that can be fermented (i.e., broken down) and used for energy by probiotic bacteria. Human milk, as you will read in Chapter 14, contains prebiotics that selectively promote the growth of beneficial bifidobacteria in the digestive tracts of infants.

Synbiotics are food products or dietary supplements that contain both probiotics and prebiotics. The two components may work in the same or different parts of the GI tract, but they both work to improve human health.

Now researchers are focusing on **postbiotics** and **paraprobiotics**.[11] Postbiotics are the metabolic products of probiotic microorganisms. When probiotic microorganisms colonize the body, they produce compounds that can influence the health of their human hosts. For example, when bifidobacteria and lactobacilli ferment undigested carbohydrates in the colon, they produce short-chain fatty acids that can serve as an energy source for the cells of the GI tract. Furthermore, some postbiotics can be absorbed and transported through the blood to have diverse and far-reaching effects throughout the body. Paraprobiotics are inactivated probiotic microorganisms that may provide some of the health benefits of probiotics. See Figure 3-20 for a summary of prebiotics, probiotics, and postbiotics.

prebiotic Selectively fermented ingredient that results in specific changes in the composition and/or activity of the gastrointestinal microbiota, thus conferring benefits upon the host.

fructooligosaccharides (FOS) Small, poorly digested carbohydrates made of glucose and fructose; a type of prebiotic found in onion, garlic, leeks, chicory, artichokes, asparagus, and bananas.

galactooligosaccharides (GOS) Small, poorly digested carbohydrates made of glucose and galactose; a type of prebiotic found in legumes, pistachios, and cashews.

synbiotic Combination of pro- and prebiotics taken to confer health benefits on the host.

postbiotics Metabolic by-products of the microorganisms that colonize the human body.

paraprobiotics Inactivated cells or cell extracts of probiotic microorganisms that may confer health benefits when consumed by humans.

Roots

Fermented Foods

Fermented foods are produced by controlled microbial growth to yield desirable end products that improve food safety, flavor, and nutritional value. Some fermented foods are revered for their medicinal properties, mainly in the treatment of gastrointestinal conditions. A variety of microorganisms may be used in fermentation, but the most common are the lactic acid bacteria. Base materials include grains, milk, fruits, vegetables, legumes, or meats.

Traditional Indian cuisines prominently feature a vast array of fermented foods. *Dahi* is a popular fermented dairy food made from the milk of cow, buffalo, or yak. *Idli* is a fermented food made from rice and lentils. Fermented meats and fish are an economical source of protein for populations without access to refrigeration or other methods of food preservation.

If they are eaten daily, fermented foods do impact the human gut microbiota. However, even if the microbes in fermented foods do not colonize the gut, they can still have a positive effect on health by improving the digestibility of foods, enhancing the bioavailability of minerals, and producing bioactive compounds, such as B vitamins. In fact, the *Dietary Guidelines for Indians* promotes the use of fermented foods for their nutritional value.

Source: Satish Kumar R, Kanmani P, Yuvaraj N, Paari KA, Pattukumar V, Arul V. Traditional Indian fermented foods: a rich source of lactic acid bacteria. *Int J Food Sci Nutr.* 2013 Jun;64(4):415-428. doi: 10.3109/09637486.2012.746288

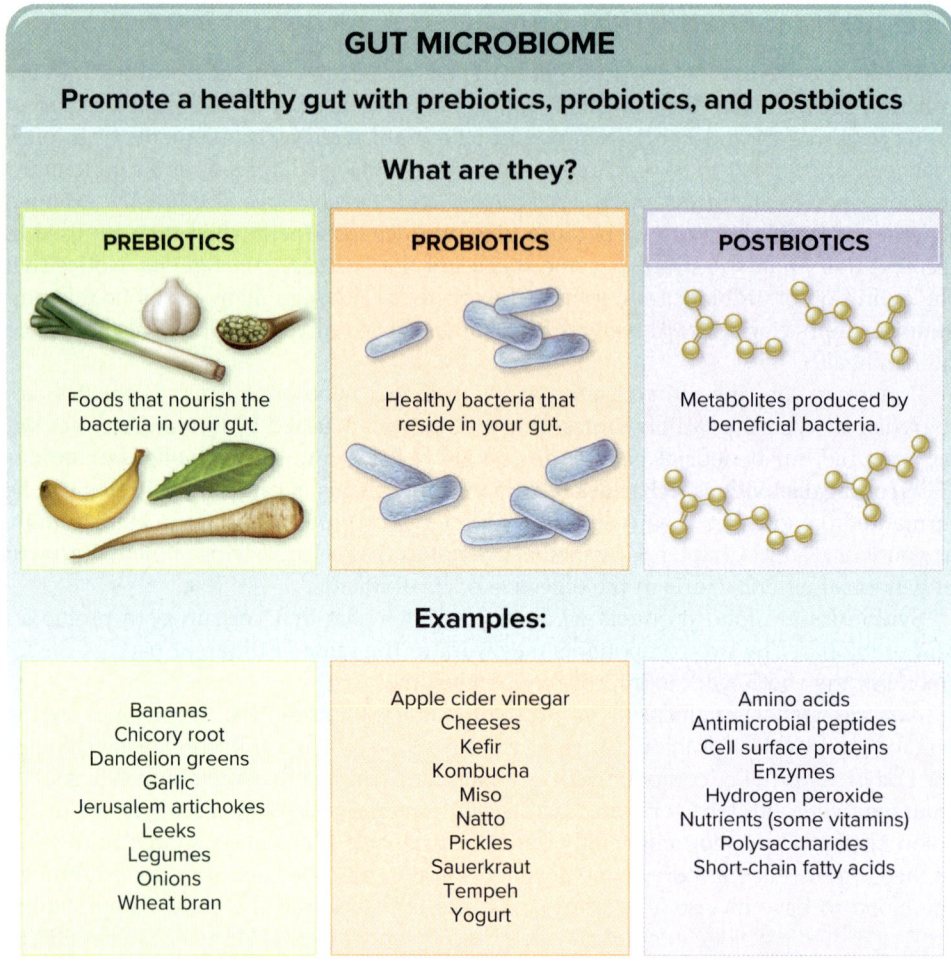

FIGURE 3-20 The gut microbiome can be influenced by our dietary patterns. In turn, the microorganisms that inhabit the GI tract influence human health in a variety of ways.

GASTROINTESTINAL HEALTH

In healthy humans, the GI tract is home to some pathogenic microbes as well as beneficial microbes. The beneficial species keep the pathogenic species in check by competing with them for living space and food and by producing some antimicrobial compounds. The activity of microorganisms in the gut stimulates the maturation of the epithelial tissue that lines the gastrointestinal tract. Picture the thin layer of cells that line the intestine. There are tiny spaces between these cells that allow some materials to pass through but keep other materials in the lumen of the intestine and out of the blood supply. The junctions between these cells are normally stitched together tightly by proteins. Some compounds produced by the microbiota influence the synthesis of these tight junction proteins, which affects the integrity of the intestine's epithelial tissue. This is important for nutrient absorption and immune protection.

Dysbiosis is a term that refers to an imbalance of *good* and *bad* microbes in the gut. Sometimes, such a disruption is short-lived, such as a viral infection that leads to diarrhea. The immune system works to destroy the pathogen, and beneficial microbes also play a role in restoring balance (see *Newsworthy Nutrition* in this section). However, research evidence suggests that gut dysbiosis is at the root of many long-term gastrointestinal diseases, including irritable bowel syndrome and inflammatory bowel diseases (see Section 3.11).[12] Researchers are actively looking for ways to manipulate the gut microbiota as a way to prevent or treat these diseases.

dysbiosis A harmful disturbance in the balance of beneficial and pathogenic microorganisms in the microbiota.

Newsworthy Nutrition

Fecal microbiota transplant is an effective treatment for irritable bowel syndrome

INTRODUCTION: Irritable bowel syndrome (IBS) is a common GI disorder that significantly diminishes quality of life. Researchers have not yet pinpointed a cause for IBS, but there is evidence of disturbances in the gut microbiota among patients with IBS. **OBJECTIVES:** In this *double-blind, randomized, placebo-controlled trial*, the researchers wanted to determine if a fecal microbiota transplant (FMT) from a healthy donor could improve IBS symptoms. **METHODS:** 165 patients with IBS were randomized to receive one of three treatments: FMT of 60 grams of healthy donor stool, 30 grams of healthy donor stool, or placebo (the patient's own feces). Patients were followed for 3 months after FMT to assess IBS symptoms and other aspects of quality of life using a variety of questionnaires. Changes in intestinal bacterial profile were assessed using 16S rRNA gene sequencing. **RESULTS:** After 3 months, FMT from a healthy donor significantly improved IBS symptoms, fatigue, quality of life, and intestinal bacterial profiles. **CONCLUSION:** This study demonstrated with a randomized, controlled, double-blind trial that a fecal microbiota transplant from a healthy donor is an effective treatment for IBS. Importantly, this study demonstrated the feasibility of using previously frozen samples from a healthy donor and administering FMT with a gastroscope via the upper tract.

Source: El-Salhy M, Hatlebakk JG, Gilja OH, Kristoffersen AB, Hausken T. Efficacy of faecal microbiota transplantation for patients with irritable bowel syndrome in a randomised, double-blind, placebo-controlled study. *Gut.* 2020 May;69(5):859-867. doi: 10.1136/gutjnl-2019-319630

NUTRITIONAL STATUS

Some strains of bacteria contribute to human nutritional status as well. Although human enzymes cannot break down dietary fiber, bacterial enzymes can metabolize some of those carbohydrates. As they do so, they effectively harvest additional energy from these foods for us. The short-chain fatty acids produced as a by-product of microbial metabolism of fiber serve as fuel for the cells that line the intestine. In addition, bacteria in the GI tract synthesize several vitamins. Although the majority of vitamins are absorbed in the small intestine, some of the vitamin K and several B vitamins produced by microbes in the large intestine may contribute to human nutritional status.[8]

IMMUNE FUNCTION

The gut microbiota profoundly influences immune function. In laboratory animals that are born and raised in a sterile environment, the immune system is underdeveloped and the organisms are more susceptible to autoimmune diseases and allergies. It is evident that a healthy gut microbiota is crucial for proper immune system development and maintenance.

During infancy and childhood, beneficial organisms support the proper development of the immune system. Exposure of GALT to microorganisms promotes the maturation of the immune cells. GALT makes up about 70% of all immune tissue in the body, and much of the GALT is situated in the large intestine, where the microbiota flourishes. Through early interactions with microorganisms in the gut, the cells of the immune system "learn" to recognize and differentiate between what is harmful and what is not. Production of certain antibodies by the mucosal cells is increased.

As mentioned, normal microbial activity in the gut stimulates the proper development of the epithelial tissue that lines the gastrointestinal tract, which serves as a barrier against pathogenic organisms. The cells that line the intestines are knitted

magnificent microbiome

Hygiene Hypothesis
According to the hygiene hypothesis, our tendency to sanitize every surface and treat every infection with antibiotics reduces exposure of the immune system to a diverse community of microorganisms. The understimulated immune system becomes sensitized to harmless proteins, such as food proteins, beneficial bacteria, or the body's own cells. Being *too* clean might make us more likely to develop allergies and autoimmune diseases.

hygiene hypothesis Assumption that reduced exposure to microorganisms in the environment (e.g., as a result of overuse of antibacterial soaps and antibiotics) impairs proper development of the immune system, making a person more susceptible to allergies and autoimmune diseases.

together by tight junctions, which are a network of tiny strands of protein that regulate the absorption of nutrients and block the entry of large molecules and pathogens. If the integrity of these tight junctions is compromised, the intestinal lining becomes more permeable. Increased gut permeability might allow large molecules, including microorganisms, to move from the lumen of the GI tract into body tissues, leading to infections. Some researchers wonder if increased gut permeability is involved in the development of allergies and autoimmune diseases. Genetics alone cannot explain the increased rates of these disorders in recent years, leading researchers to suspect that environmental factors are at work. Blame may rest with changes in eating patterns, infectious disease rates, use of antibiotics, or the makeup of the microbiota.[13]

Beneficial strains of microorganisms may also directly compete with and reduce the activity of disease-causing organisms in the GI tract.[14,15] This occurs by several mechanisms. The metabolic activity of beneficial microorganisms changes the acidity of the environment in the gut, which makes it less hospitable to the pathogenic microorganisms. Increasing loads of beneficial bacteria will compete with pathogenic bacteria for binding sites and sources of food. Finally, some probiotic microorganisms directly bind to pathogens or secrete substances that kill them.

Beyond these direct interactions, the gut microbiota also produces compounds that can be absorbed into the blood and regulate immune function. For example, the amino acids and short-chain fatty acids produced by the gut microbiota can influence the synthesis of inflammatory compounds, not just in the gut but throughout the body.[16]

MUCH MORE TO LEARN

In this section, you have learned about a few of the many health effects of the human microbiota. Researchers are interested in how the microbiota and their metabolites may influence a variety of other health outcomes, including weight control,[17] cardiovascular disease,[18] blood glucose,[8] and even mental health.[19] In later chapters, you will see additional information about the microbiota and human health in the *Magnificent Microbiome* features.

Continued study of the microbial genome will help researchers to understand how microorganisms exert their influences on human health. The Integrative Human Microbiome Project in the United States and the Human Microbiome Action project in Europe are two large-scale efforts to map the microbial genome and understand the interactions between human and microbial genes. We have come a long way in our understanding of the ways probiotics and prebiotics can influence human health, especially gastrointestinal health and body defenses. Even so, there are many things left to uncover.

✓ CONCEPT CHECK 3.9

1. In simple terms, explain the differences among *probiotics, prebiotics,* and *postbiotics.*
2. Other than yogurt, list two food sources of probiotic microorganisms.
3. Describe two ways the gut microbiota may work to support human health.

3.10 Nutrient Storage Capabilities

The human body must maintain reserves of nutrients. Otherwise, we would need to eat continuously! Storage capacities vary for each different nutrient.

Where do our cells get energy? Carbohydrates are a quick energy source. To meet immediate energy needs, the blood maintains a small reserve of glucose. If blood glucose gets too low, we can tap into a supply of glycogen—the storage form of glucose. Most healthy adults store enough glycogen in the liver and muscle tissues to fuel us for about 1 day. For longer-term energy needs, fats are the most efficient way to store energy. They yield the most energy per gram (9 kcal per gram, compared to just 4 kcal per gram for carbohydrates or protein), and they take up less space (because they are not stored with water). Our **adipose tissue** houses enough stored triglycerides for us to survive several weeks without food (provided we have access to adequate water).

Vitamins and minerals are stored in the liver, glands, and bones. When people do not meet their needs for certain nutrients, blood levels of these nutrients can be maintained by breaking down body tissues. For example, if dietary calcium intake is inadequate, calcium will be withdrawn from bone to maintain blood calcium levels within a normal range. If you do not eat enough protein to replace daily losses, eventually muscles and organs will be broken down to supply amino acids for essential body functions. Over the long term, nutrient deficiencies weaken tissues and disrupt the body's functions.

Many people believe that if too much of a nutrient is obtained—for example, from a vitamin or mineral supplement—only what is needed is stored and the rest will be excreted by the body. Though true for some nutrients, such as vitamin C, the large dosages of other nutrients frequently found in supplements, such as vitamin A and iron, can cause harmful side effects because they are not readily excreted. This is one reason why obtaining your nutrients primarily (or exclusively) from a balanced diet is the safest means to acquire the building blocks you need to maintain the good health of all organ systems.

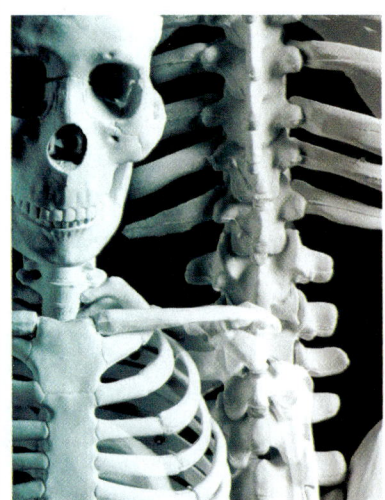

The skeletal system provides a reserve of calcium for day-to-day needs. **If your dietary intake of calcium is inadequate, what happens to your bones?** Jason Reed/Ryan McVay/Photodisc/Getty Images

adipose tissue Connective tissue made up of cells that store fat; also cushions and insulates the body.

✓ CONCEPT CHECK 3.10

1. What is the body's most efficient form of energy storage?
2. Why is it important to consume nutrients daily?
3. When it comes to vitamins and minerals, is consuming more than the RDA or AI a good way to ensure optimal nutrition status? Why or why not?

3.11 Nutrition and Your Health: Common Problems with Digestion

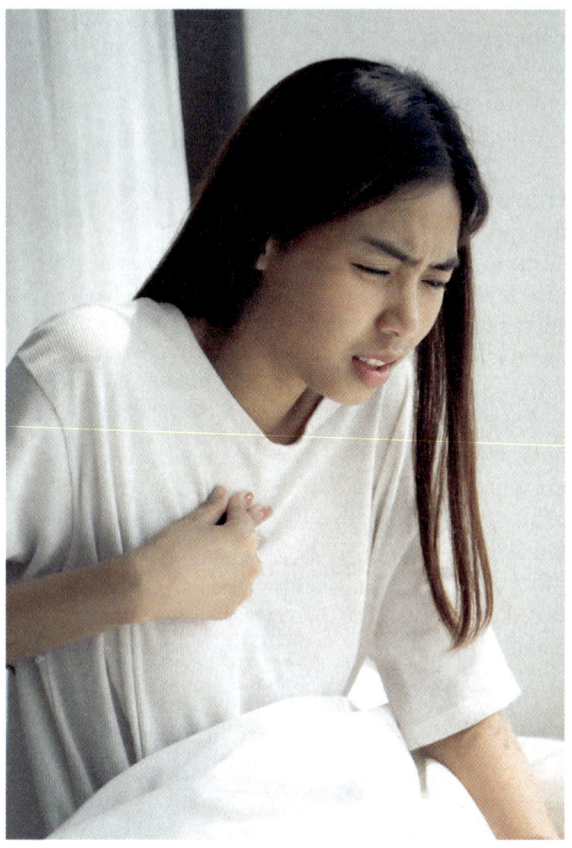
9nong/123RF

When suffering from persistent heartburn or GERD, see a doctor if you have

- difficulty swallowing or pain when swallowing.
- lack of appetite.
- persistent vomiting.
- heartburn that resists treatment with medications.
- unexplained weight loss.
- chest pain.
- blood loss or anemia.
- blood in stool or vomit.

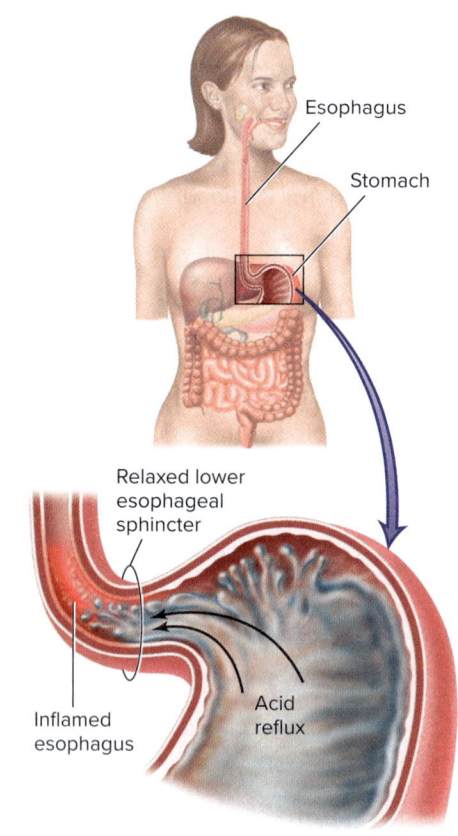

FIGURE 3-21 Heartburn is a sign of reflux of stomach acid into the esophagus.

Without fanfare, the digestive system does the important work of extracting nutrients from the food you eat to supply the needs of your body's trillions of cells. It is not until something goes awry that you notice digestion at all. In this section, you will learn about nutritional strategies to cope with heartburn, ulcers, constipation, diverticulosis and diverticulitis, hemorrhoids, diarrhea, irritable bowel syndrome (IBS), gallstones, and celiac disease.

Heartburn

An estimated 60 million Americans experience heartburn, also known as acid reflux, at least once per month[20] (Fig. 3-21). This gnawing pain in the upper chest is caused by the movement of acid from the stomach into the esophagus. Unlike the stomach, the esophagus has very little mucus to protect it, so acid quickly erodes the lining of this organ. Acid reflux symptoms may include pain, nausea, gagging, cough, or hoarseness. The recurrent and therefore more serious form of the problem is called **gastroesophageal reflux disease (GERD).** GERD is diagnosed when symptoms occur two or more times per week.

gastroesophageal reflux disease (GERD) Disease that results from stomach acid backing up into the esophagus. The acid irritates the lining of the esophagus, causing pain.

112 Wardlaw's Contemporary Nutrition

Heartburn is caused by relaxation of the lower esophageal sphincter. Typically, it should be relaxed only during swallowing, but in individuals with GERD, it is relaxed at other times as well. Increased pressure against the lower esophageal sphincter (e.g., as a result of pregnancy or obesity) heightens risk for heartburn. The hormonal changes of pregnancy also tend to relax the lower esophageal sphincter. For some people, slow movement of gastric contents from the stomach to the small intestine complicates the problem.

If left untreated, heartburn can damage the lining of the esophagus, leading to chronic esophageal inflammation and an increased risk of esophageal cancer. Heartburn sufferers should follow the general recommendations given in Table 3-3. For occasional heartburn, quick relief can be found with over-the-counter antacids. Taking antacids will reduce the acid in the stomach but will not stop the acid reflux. For more persistent symptoms (i.e., a few days per week or every day), H₂ blockers or **proton pump inhibitors (PPIs)** may be needed (see the *Medicine Cabinet* feature in this section). PPIs provide long-lasting relief by reducing stomach acid production and should be taken before the first meal of the day because they take longer to work. Medications that improve GI **motility** may also be useful. If the proper medications are not effective at controlling GERD, surgery may be needed to strengthen the weakened lower esophageal sphincter.[21]

Peptic Ulcers

A **peptic ulcer** occurs when the lining of the esophagus, stomach, or small intestine is eroded by the acid secreted by stomach cells (Fig. 3-22). A disruption of the layer of mucus that usually protects the stomach allows acid and protein-digesting enzymes to damage the stomach lining. Acid can also erode the lining of the esophagus and the first part of the small intestine, the duodenum. This can cause pain, blood loss, and **perforation**. An estimated 4.6 million people in the United States are affected by peptic ulcers.[22] In young people, most ulcers occur in the

proton pump inhibitor (PPI) A medication that inhibits the ability of gastric cells to produce acid.

motility Generally, the ability to move spontaneously. In this context, it refers to movement of food through the GI tract.

peptic ulcer Erosion of the tissue lining, usually in the stomach or the upper small intestine.

perforation A hole made by boring or piercing. With reference to the gastrointestinal tract, the hole is in the wall of the esophagus, stomach, intestine, rectum, or gallbladder. Complications include bleeding and infection.

TABLE 3-3 ■ Nutrition and Lifestyle Recommendations for Care of Heartburn and Peptic Ulcers

	Heartburn	Peptic Ulcers
Avoid smoking.	✓	✓
Avoid large doses of aspirin, ibuprofen, and other NSAID compounds unless a physician advises otherwise.[a]	✓	✓
Achieve or maintain a healthy body weight.	✓	✓
Eat small, low-fat meals.	✓	✓
Limit alcohol consumption.	✓	✓
Limit consumption of caffeine (e.g., coffee, some soft drinks).	✓	✓
Consume a nutritionally complete diet with adequate fiber.	✓	✓
Avoid foods that worsen symptoms:[b]		
• Acidic foods (e.g., orange juice, tomato products)	✓	✓
• Highly spiced foods (e.g., chili, cayenne, and black pepper)	✓	✓
• Carbonated beverages	✓	✓
• Foods that relax the lower esophageal sphincter (e.g., peppermint, spearmint, chocolate)	✓	
• Onions and garlic	✓	
Avoid tight-fitting clothing.	✓	
Elevate the head of the bed 6 to 8 inches.	✓	
Avoid eating at least 3 to 4 hours before lying down.	✓	
Wash hands often and follow food safety guidelines.		✓

[a] For people who must use these medications, FDA has approved an NSAID combined with a medication to reduce gastric damage. The medication reduces gastric acid production and enhances mucus secretion.

[b] These foods do not *cause* heartburn or ulcers, but some may irritate sites of existing damage in the esophagus or stomach.

CASE STUDY: Gastroesophageal Reflux Disease

Caitlin is a 20-year-old college sophomore. Over the last few months, she has been experiencing regular bouts of heartburn. This usually happens after a large lunch or dinner. Occasionally, she has even bent down after dinner to pick up something and had some stomach contents travel back up her esophagus and into her mouth. This especially frightened Caitlin, so she visited the University Health Center.

The nurse practitioner at the center told Caitlin it was good that she came in for a checkup because she suspects Caitlin has gastroesophageal reflux disease. She tells Caitlin that this can lead to serious problems if left untreated. She provides Caitlin with a pamphlet describing GERD and schedules an appointment with a physician for further evaluation.

1. What is the difference between heartburn and GERD?
2. What dietary and lifestyle habits may have contributed to Caitlin's symptoms of GERD?
3. The nurse practitioner mentioned that GERD can lead to serious consequences if left untreated. List three negative consequences of untreated GERD.
4. Summarize three dietary strategies that may help Caitlin cope with this health problem.
5. What types of medications have been especially useful for treating GERD?

Complete the Case Study. Responses to these questions can be provided by your instructor.

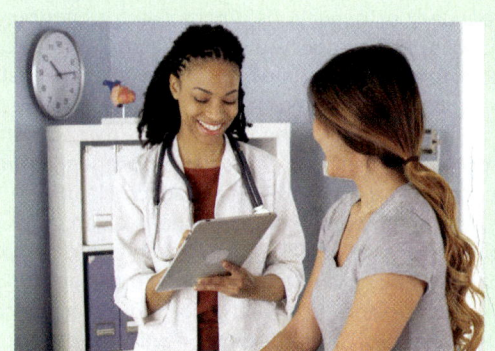

Caitlin was wise to see a health professional about her persistent heartburn.
Rocketclips, Inc./Shutterstock

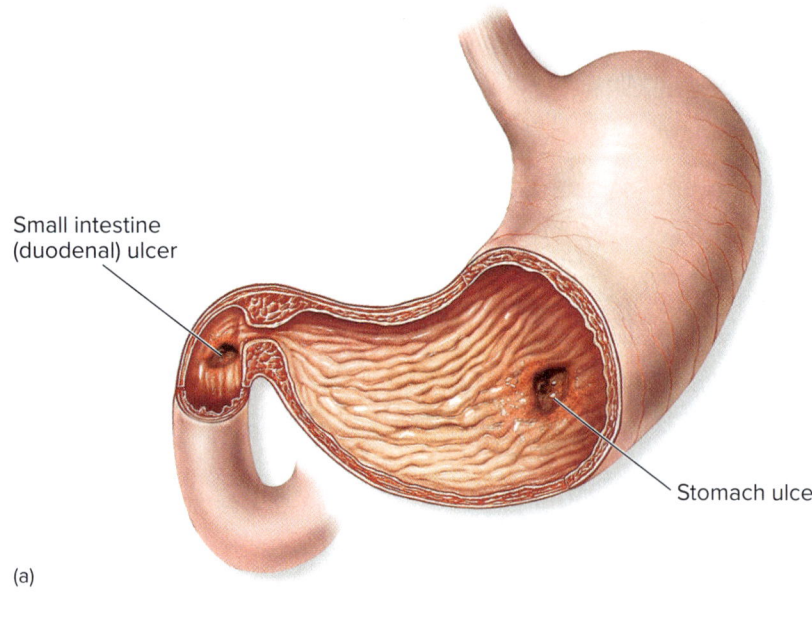

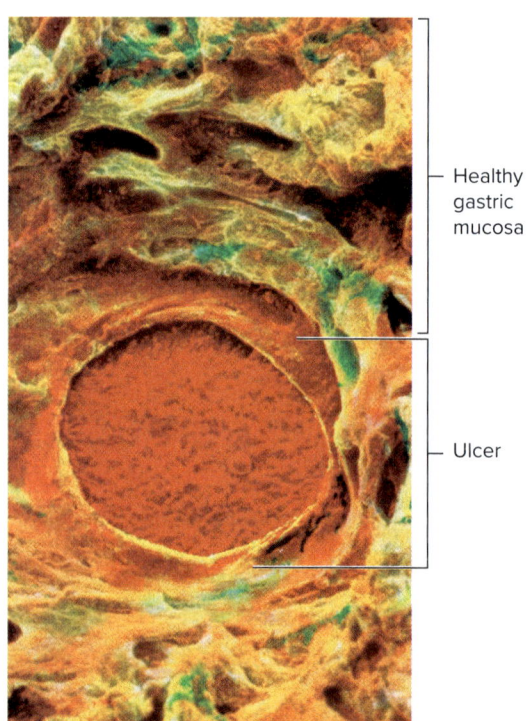

FIGURE 3-22 (a) A peptic ulcer in the stomach or small intestine. *H. pylori* bacteria and NSAIDs (e.g., ibuprofen) cause ulcers by impairing mucosal defense, especially in the stomach. Smoking, genetics, and stress also can impair mucosal defense or cause an increase in the release of pepsin and stomach acid. (b) Close-up of a stomach ulcer. This needs to be treated or eventual perforation of the stomach is possible.
(b) J. James/Science Source

small intestine, whereas in older people, they are most common in the stomach.

How do you know if you have a peptic ulcer? Some people experience no symptoms at all, but most notice stomach pain about 2 hours after eating. Stomach acid acting on a meal irritates the ulcer after most of the meal has moved from the site of the ulcer. Other symptoms may include weight loss, lack of appetite, nausea and vomiting, or bloating. Vomiting blood or what looks like coffee grounds and the appearance of black, tarry stools are signs of bleeding in the GI tract. Any evidence of GI bleeding warrants immediate medical attention.

The two chief culprits of peptic ulcer disease are infection of the stomach by the acid-resistant bacterium *Helicobacter pylori* (70% to 90% of peptic ulcers) and heavy use of **nonsteroidal anti-inflammatory drugs (NSAIDs)**.[22] Both *H. pylori* and NSAIDs disrupt the thick layer of mucus that normally protects the stomach from the action of acids and enzymes. Conditions that cause excessive stomach acid production also play a role. In addition, cigarette smoking is known to cause ulcers, increase ulcer complications such as bleeding, and lead to ulcer treatment failure.

The primary risk associated with an ulcer is the possibility that it will erode entirely through the stomach or intestinal wall. The GI contents could then spill into the body cavities, causing a massive infection. In addition, an ulcer may damage a blood vessel, leading to substantial blood loss. Never ignore the early warning signs of ulcer development, which include a persistent gnawing or burning near the stomach that may occur immediately following a meal or awaken you at night.

Today, a combination approach is used for ulcer therapy.[23] People infected with *H. pylori* are given antibiotics and stomach acid–blocking medications (see the *Medicine Cabinet* feature in this section). There is a 90% cure rate for *H. pylori* infections in the first week of this treatment. Recurrence is unlikely if the infection is cured, but an incomplete cure almost certainly leads to repeated ulcer formation.

Are dietary changes effective for prevention or treatment of peptic ulcers? Many people think that eating spicy or acidic foods can cause ulcers. Contrary to popular belief, these foods do not cause ulcers. However, once an ulcer has developed, these foods may irritate damaged tissues. Thus, for some people, avoidance of spicy or acidic foods may help to relieve symptoms.

In the past, milk and cream were thought to help cure ulcers. Clinicians now know that milk and cream are two of the worst foods for a person with ulcers because the calcium in these foods stimulates acid secretion and actually inhibits ulcer healing.

Overall, medical treatment of *H. pylori* infection has so revolutionized ulcer therapy that dietary changes are of minor importance. People with ulcers should refrain from smoking and minimize the use of NSAIDs. Current dietary therapy approaches simply recommend avoidance of foods that tend to worsen ulcer symptoms (see Table 3-3).

Constipation

What does it mean to be "regular" when it comes to bowel function? Individuals vary, but in general, normal bowel frequency ranges from three times per day to three times per week. **Constipation**, a condition characterized by difficult or infrequent evacuation of the bowels, is common. About 16% of adults report symptoms of constipation.[24] As you learned in Section 3.8, the primary role of the large intestine is to absorb fluid. If fecal material moves too slowly through the large intestine, so much fluid is absorbed that the feces become dry, hard, and difficult to pass.

There are many possible causes for constipation. The muscular movement of feces through the GI tract is regulated by neurological and hormonal signals, so disorders of the nervous system or muscular function could alter bowel motility. A physical obstruction in the GI tract could also be to blame. Constipation may be a side effect of certain medications (e.g., antacids) or dietary supplements (e.g., iron or calcium). More often, however, constipation arises due to inadequate dietary fiber and/or fluid intake or poor toileting habits.

Increasing dietary intakes of fiber and fluid are usually safe and effective strategies for treating mild cases of constipation.[24] Whole grain breads and cereals, beans, and dried fruits are excellent sources of fiber. Fiber stimulates peristalsis by drawing water into the large intestine and helping to form a bulky, soft fecal output. Additional fluid should be consumed to facilitate fiber's action in the large intestine. Also, people with constipation may need to develop more regular bowel habits. When people regularly ignore their normal bowel reflexes (e.g., because it is inconvenient to interrupt occupational or social activities), feces can become hard and dry. Allowing the same time each day for a bowel movement can help to train the large intestine to respond routinely. Regular physical activity can also stimulate the GI tract to function normally.[25]

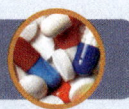

Medicine Cabinet

Controlling Stomach Acid

Proton pump inhibitors (PPIs) are medications that inhibit the ability of gastric cells to secrete hydrogen ions and thus reduce acid production. Low doses of this class of medications may be available without a prescription. Although excess acid production can cause problems, stomach acid is important for the digestion and absorption of many nutrients. Prolonged use of PPIs could decrease vitamin B-12, vitamin C, calcium, iron, and magnesium status.

Examples:
- Omeprazole (Prilosec®)
- Lansoprazole (Prevacid®)
- Rabeprazole (Aciphex®)
- Esomeprazole (Nexium®)

H₂ blockers impede the stimulating effect of histamine on acid-producing cells in the stomach.

Examples:
- Cimetidine (Tagamet®)
- Nizatidine (Axid®)
- Famotidine (Pepcid®)

---

nonsteroidal anti-inflammatory drugs (NSAIDs) Medications used to treat painful inflammatory conditions, such as arthritis. Examples: aspirin, ibuprofen (Advil®), and naproxen (Aleve®).

constipation A condition characterized by difficult and/or infrequent bowel movements (i.e., fewer than three bowel movements per week).

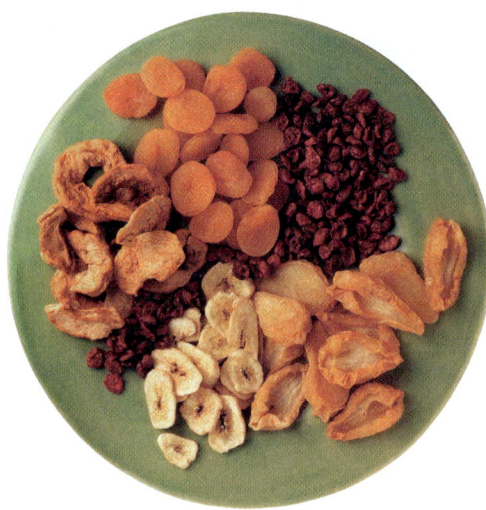

Dried fruits are a natural source of fiber and can help prevent constipation when consumed with an adequate amount of fluid.
C Squared Studios/Photodisc/Getty Images

In more severe cases, **laxatives** can alleviate constipation. Some laxatives work by irritating the intestinal nerve junctions to stimulate peristalsis, while others that contain fiber draw water into the intestine to enlarge fecal output. The larger output stretches the peristaltic muscles, making them rebound and then constrict. Regular use of laxatives, however, should be supervised by a primary care provider. Overall, if laxatives are necessary, the bulk-forming fiber laxatives, such as **psyllium** husk, are the safest to use.[25]

Hemorrhoids

Hemorrhoids, also called *piles,* are swollen veins of the rectum and anus. The blood vessels in this area are subject to intense pressure, especially during bowel movements. Added stress to the vessels from pregnancy, obesity, prolonged sitting, violent coughing or sneezing, or straining during bowel movements (particularly with constipation) can lead to a hemorrhoid.

Hemorrhoids can develop unnoticed until a strained bowel movement precipitates symptoms. Itching (caused by moisture in the anal canal), swelling, and irritation are the most common symptoms. Pain, if present, is usually aching and steady. Bleeding may result from a hemorrhoid and appear in the toilet as a bright red streak in the feces. The sensation of a mass in the anal canal after a bowel movement is a symptom of an internal hemorrhoid that protrudes through the anus.

laxative A medication or other substance that stimulates evacuation of the intestinal tract.

psyllium Mostly soluble type of dietary fiber found in the seeds of the plantago plant; common ingredient in bulk-forming laxatives, such as Metamucil®.

hemorrhoid A swollen vein in the rectum or anus.

Anyone can develop a hemorrhoid, and about half of adults over age 50 do.[26] Diet, lifestyle, and heredity may contribute to the problem. For example, a low-fiber diet can lead to hemorrhoids as a result of straining during bowel movements. If you think you have a hemorrhoid, you should consult your primary care provider. Rectal bleeding, although usually caused by hemorrhoids, may also indicate other problems, such as cancer.

A physician may suggest a variety of self-care measures for hemorrhoids. Pain can be lessened by applying warm, soft compresses or sitting in a tub of warm water for 15 to 20 minutes. Dietary recommendations are the same as those for treating constipation, emphasizing the need to consume adequate fiber and fluid. Over-the-counter remedies, such as Preparation H®, can also offer relief from symptoms.

Diverticular Disease

Diverticulosis is a common GI problem. In the United States, at least 30% of adults over the age of 50 have diverticulosis, and its prevalence increases with age.[27] Diverticulosis occurs when parts of the inner layer (mucosa) of the intestinal wall (usually in the large intestine) protrude outward between the surrounding bands of muscle, forming small pouches called **diverticula** (Fig. 3-23). The presence of diverticula is called diverticulosis. The exact cause of diverticulosis is unknown. Scientists used to think that a low-fiber diet led to diverticulosis, but recent studies demonstrate that dietary fiber intake is not consistently related to the development of the condition. Genetics play a role. Modifiable risk factors include obesity, inactivity, excessive use of alcohol, smoking, and use of certain medications. Current research on the role of the gut microbiota in the development of diverticular disease is inconclusive.[28]

diverticulosis The condition of having many diverticula in the large intestine.

diverticula Pouches that protrude through the exterior wall of the large intestine.

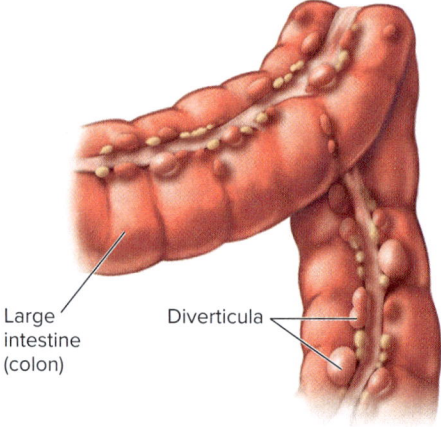

FIGURE 3-23 Diverticulosis is a condition in which small pouches (diverticula) form in the wall of the intestine. When diverticula become inflamed or infected, the condition is called diverticulitis.

Although many adults have diverticulosis, it usually does not cause any noticeable symptoms. Among a small proportion of individuals with diverticulosis, the diverticula become inflamed or infected. This condition is known as **diverticulitis.** If diverticulitis develops, it is characterized by intense abdominal pain, sometimes accompanied by bowel irregularities (constipation is most common), nausea, vomiting, and fever. Rarely, inflamed diverticula may rupture, leading to bleeding, formation of an abscess, or leakage of intestinal contents into the abdominal cavity.[27]

During flare-ups of diverticulitis, a low-fiber, liquid diet may be helpful to promote healing. Antibiotics may be prescribed. However, once the inflammation subsides, a high-fiber dietary pattern is generally recommended to maintain intestinal health. Advice to avoid certain foods, such as popcorn, nuts, or seeds, is outdated. Health care providers used to recommend that individuals with diverticulosis should avoid nuts, seeds, and other foods with tough, indigestible hulls based on the premise that these small bits of food matter could get stuck in the diverticula and lead to increased bacterial activity, inflammation, and infection. However, evidence shows no relationship between intake of popcorn, nuts, or seeds and occurrence of diverticulitis. Thus, it is not necessary for people with diverticulosis to restrict these nutrient-rich foods from their dietary patterns.[29]

diverticulitis Inflammation of the diverticula, which may be related to bacterial activity inside the diverticula.

FODMAPs **F**ermentable **o**ligosaccharides, **d**isaccharides, **m**onosaccharides, **a**nd **p**olyols. These carbohydrates may be poorly digested and lead to GI symptoms such as bloating, gas, and diarrhea in some people.

Irritable Bowel Syndrome
An imbalance between beneficial and pathogenic microbes in the gut may play a role in the development of irritable bowel syndrome. Microorganisms influence intestinal function in many ways:
- They stimulate the production of a protective layer of mucus by the intestinal cells.
- They affect the permeability of the intestinal lining, which regulates the movement of substances (both good and bad) from the intestine to the bloodstream.
- They can upregulate or downregulate the inflammatory response.
- They affect nerve signals from the gut to the brain, which may influence the rate of motility in the intestine and the perception of pain.

Researchers are interested in the potential for foods or supplements with probiotics or prebiotics to promote healthier gut function in individuals with IBS.

Source: Simon E, Călinoiu LF, Mitrea L, Vodnar DC. Probiotics, prebiotics, and synbiotics: implications and beneficial effects against irritable bowel syndrome. *Nutrients.* 2021 Jun 20;13(6):2112. doi: 10.3390/nu13062112

Irritable Bowel Syndrome

An estimated 12% of adults have irritable bowel syndrome (IBS), characterized by a combination of bloating, abdominal pain, and irregular bowel function (diarrhea, constipation, or alternating episodes of both[30]). It is about twice as common in females as it is in males. The disease leads to about 3.5 million visits to primary care providers in the United States each year. Although it does not lead to cancer or other serious digestive problems, the physical discomfort and anxiety of IBS can significantly impact quality of life.

It is difficult to pinpoint an exact cause for IBS. Alterations in some of the hormones that regulate the movement of food matter through the GI tract may be to blame. Also, inflammatory responses in the GI tract could be involved for some people with IBS. Recent studies demonstrate alterations in the activity of gut microorganisms in people with IBS. Gut microorganisms produce compounds that affect many body systems. Perhaps IBS leads to changes in the microbiota, or perhaps imbalances in the gut microbiota trigger the range of problems that plague people with IBS.

Most people who suffer from IBS perceive that their symptoms are related to food, but there is little evidence of true food allergies or intolerances. When it comes to specific foods, poorly digested carbohydrates are a prime suspect (see the discussion of **FODMAPs** in Chapter 4).[31] Fructose, sugar alcohols, and other carbohydrates may lead to diarrhea or excessive gas if they reach the large intestine undigested. Depression and stress are also associated with IBS; up to 50% of sufferers report a history of verbal or sexual abuse.

Given the diversity of symptoms and possible causes, therapy must be individualized. Medications that target nerves or alter the bacterial population in the GI tract may help people who suffer from frequent diarrhea. For IBS patients whose primary complaint is constipation, medications are available to stimulate peristalsis or block abdominal pain.

Medications may be expensive, and some have side effects. Therefore, dietary strategies to cope with IBS are of great interest. Some, but not all, patients with IBS experience improvements with a low-FODMAP dietary pattern. For several weeks, they eliminate (or greatly reduce) their intake of foods containing FODMAPs, including wheat, onions, legumes, and dairy products. Then, foods are gradually added back to the dietary pattern to determine which can be tolerated and which should be avoided over the long term.[31] Probiotics and peppermint oil have been shown to decrease symptoms of IBS and improve overall quality of life.[30] The patient should limit or eliminate caffeine-containing foods and beverages. Low-fat and more frequent, small meals may help because large meals can trigger contractions of the large intestine. Other strategies include a reduction in stress, psychological counseling, and antidepressant medications. Hypnosis has been shown to relieve symptoms in severe cases.

Beware that following an eating pattern that eliminates certain foods or entire food groups can limit nutritional adequacy. Indeed, research indicates that intakes of some nutrients, including calcium and vitamin A, are inadequate among people with IBS. An experienced registered dietitian nutritionist is a valuable resource to help a person with IBS identify problem foods and plan a nutritionally adequate dietary pattern.

Diarrhea

Diarrhea is defined as increased fluidity, frequency, or amount of bowel movements compared to a person's usual pattern. Most cases of diarrhea are of short duration and result from viral or bacterial infections. These microorganisms produce substances that cause the intestinal cells to secrete fluid rather than absorb fluid. Another form of diarrhea can be caused by consumption of substances that are not readily absorbed, such as **sorbitol**, a sugar alcohol found in sugarless gum (see Section 4.3). When consumed in large amounts, the unabsorbed substance draws water into the intestines, leading to diarrhea.

The goal of nutrition therapy for any form of diarrhea is to prevent dehydration. Increasing intake of water and electrolytes is the first line of defense against dehydration. Prompt treatment of dehydration—within 24 to 48 hours—is critical, especially for infants and older adults. Diarrhea that lasts more than 7 days in adults should be investigated by a primary care provider as it can be a sign of a more serious intestinal disease, especially if there is also blood in the stool.

For diarrhea caused by infection, dietary changes (besides increased fluid intake) are usually not necessary. Some health care providers recommend temporarily decreasing intake of caffeine, fat, fiber, and poorly absorbed carbohydrates, but other sources show that maintaining a regular diet speeds recovery. Foods containing probiotics may assist recovery. For diarrhea caused by a poorly absorbed substance, such as excess sugar alcohols or lactose, avoidance of the offending substance is the key to relief.[32]

Gallstones

Gallstones are a major cause of illness and surgery, affecting 10% to 20% of U.S. adults.[33] Gallstones are pieces of solid material that develop in the gallbladder when substances in the bile—primarily cholesterol (80% of gallstones)—form crystal-like particles. They may be as small as a grain of sand or as large as a golf ball (Fig. 3-24). These stones are caused by a combination of factors, with excess weight being the primary modifiable risk factor, especially among females. Other factors include genetic background (e.g., Native Americans), advanced age (> 60 years), pregnancy, reduced activity of the gallbladder (contracts less than normal), altered bile composition (e.g., too much cholesterol or not enough bile salts), diabetes, and eating pattern (e.g., low-fiber diets). In addition, gallstones may develop during rapid weight loss or prolonged fasting (as the liver metabolizes more fat, it secretes more cholesterol into the bile).

Gallstones may cause intermittent pain in the upper right abdomen, gas and bloating, nausea or vomiting, or other health problems. Medications are available to dissolve gallstones, but these take a long time to work, and the recurrence of gallstones after therapy is common. Therefore, surgical removal of the gallbladder is the most common method for treating gallstones (500,000 surgeries per year in the United States[33]).

The best prevention strategy is to maintain a healthy body weight, especially for females. Avoiding rapid weight loss (> 3 pounds per week), limiting animal protein and focusing more on plant protein intake (especially nuts), and following a high-fiber diet can help as well. Regular physical activity is also recommended, as are moderate to no caffeine and alcohol intake.[33]

Celiac Disease and Gluten Sensitivity

Celiac disease (sometimes called *celiac sprue*) affects an estimated 0.7% of the U.S. population.[34] Development of celiac disease depends on two factors: a genetic predisposition and dietary exposure to a protein called **gluten**. Gluten is a type of protein found in certain grains: wheat, rye, and barley. Protein-digesting enzymes in the GI tract break down some of the bonds in gluten, but digestion is incomplete. These partially digested proteins can be absorbed into the cells lining the small intestine. When people with a genetic predisposition for celiac disease are exposed to these small proteins from gluten, they experience an inflammatory reaction. Although many people think celiac disease is a **food allergy**, it is actually an *autoimmune* response: the immune system attacks and destroys its own cells. (You will learn more about food allergies in Section 6.8 and Section 15.7.)

The autoimmune response that occurs after exposure to gluten targets the cells of the small intestine, causing a flattening of the villi, which thereby reduces the absorptive surface (Fig. 3-25). The production of some digestive enzymes is decreased, and the ability of the small intestine to absorb nutrients is impaired. Malabsorption leads to a variety of GI complaints: diarrhea, bloating, cramps, and flatulence. In fact, it is common for celiac disease to be misdiagnosed as IBS. However, the pathology underlying celiac disease has far worse

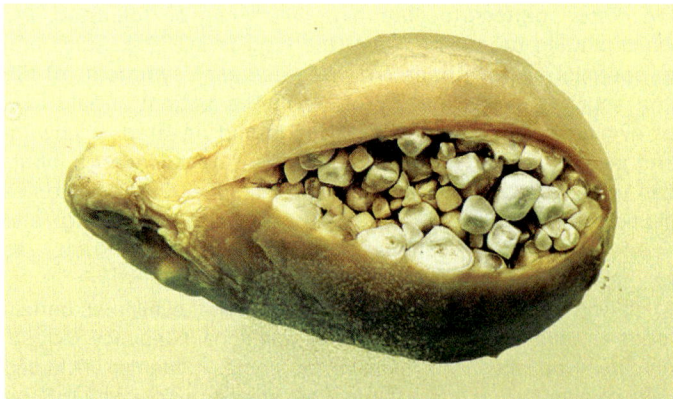

FIGURE 3-24 Gallbladder and gallstones seen after surgical removal from the body. Size and composition of the stones vary from one case to another.
The Sydney Morning Herald/Fairfax Media/Getty Images

diarrhea Increased fluidity, frequency, or amount of bowel movements (i.e., three or more loose stools per day).

sorbitol Alcohol derivative of glucose that yields about 3 kcal/g but is slowly absorbed from the small intestine; used in some sugarless gums and dietetic foods.

celiac disease Chronic, immune-mediated disease precipitated by exposure to dietary gluten in genetically predisposed people.

gluten Poorly digested protein found in wheat, barley, and rye.

food allergy An adverse reaction to food that involves an immune response; also called *food hypersensitivity*.

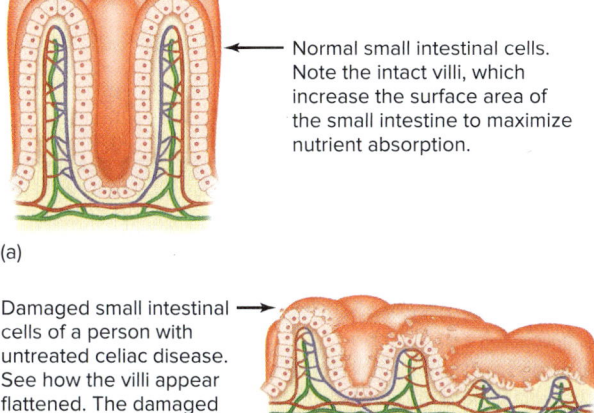

FIGURE 3-25 Cross-section of the lining of (a) a normal small intestine and (b) the small intestine of an individual with untreated celiac disease.

consequences than IBS. Over time, malabsorption of nutrients can lead to fatigue, weight loss (or poor growth in children), anemia, infertility, and bone loss.[35]

If celiac disease is suspected, the first step in making a formal diagnosis is a blood test for the presence of antibodies to gluten. This may be followed by one or more biopsies of the small intestine to confirm the pathological defects. There is also a genetic test for celiac disease, but having the gene does not always predict development of the disease.

Strict dietary avoidance of food products containing wheat, rye, and barley is the only proven way to manage the disease.[35] On food labels, food manufacturers must identify the presence of wheat (one of nine major food allergens). However, rye and barley are not as easy to spot. Therefore, people following a gluten-free diet must learn to carefully interpret the list of ingredients to identify sources of gluten. Within the grains group, rice, potato flour, cornmeal, buckwheat, arrowroot, and soy are gluten free, but ingredients such as wheat, rye, barley, bran, graham flour, semolina, spelt, and malt are sources of gluten and must be avoided. Oats do not traditionally contain gluten, but contamination in the field or during food processing could introduce gluten into this grain as well.

People with celiac disease quickly learn that wheat, barley, and rye can be hidden ingredients in any food group. Wheat and its derivatives are used to thicken sauces and condiments, as flavoring agents in dairy products and many other processed foods, and in breading for deep-fried vegetables and meats. It is helpful that many food manufacturers now voluntarily disclose the presence or absence of gluten in their products. However, not all products clearly identify gluten. Dining out is yet another challenge: Even a dusting of wheat flour can have adverse effects for a person with celiac disease.

After several weeks on a gluten-free diet, the small intestine lining regenerates, GI symptoms subside, and nutrient absorption improves. So far, the gluten-free diet is the only proven way to manage celiac disease, but research on other treatments is underway. Food scientists are working toward developing strains of wheat, barley, and rye that do not contain gluten. From a gastroenterological perspective, other approaches are to supply digestive enzymes that will break down the gluten proteins before they stimulate an autoimmune response and to use polymers that will bind to gluten in the GI tract and prevent it from being absorbed. From an immunological perspective, researchers are looking at medications that could block immune responses that damage the small intestine.

A related issue is **nonceliac wheat sensitivity (NCWS)**, sometimes called *gluten sensitivity* or *gluten intolerance*. Some people experience symptoms of celiac disease after ingestion of gluten, but they do not have the small intestine pathology of celiac disease, nor do they express the antibodies typical of celiac disease. Some reports indicate that for each person who is diagnosed with celiac disease, as many as six others have NCWS. Aside from GI symptoms, patients with NCWS may also report fatigue, headache, muscle and joint pain, and/or sleep disorders. Symptoms subside with a gluten-free diet but reappear when gluten is reintroduced. The medical community recognizes NCWS as a verifiable condition, but the mechanism that causes it is not well understood. There is no diagnostic test for the condition at this time—only the effectiveness of the gluten-free diet in alleviating symptoms. Many questions remain: Is NCWS a permanent condition? Is there a level of gluten intake that would not trigger symptoms? Could components of wheat other than gluten (e.g., FODMAPs) be responsible for triggering symptoms?[36]

Overall, the prevalence and awareness of celiac disease and NCWS seem to be on the rise. A cause for the increased prevalence has not been pinpointed, but some scientists speculate that changes in wheat production or widespread use of wheat in the food supply may be to blame. Others suspect that an infection or exposure to some environmental toxin could lead to gluten sensitization.

Summary

The conditions discussed here can be very serious, possibly leading to malnutrition, internal bleeding, and life-threatening infections. It is important to seek competent medical advice if you or someone you know suspects a GI disorder. However, you should feel empowered to know that you can control some risks and complement medical treatment with nutrition and other lifestyle changes. Overall, keeping body weight within a healthy range, meeting recommendations for fiber and fluid intake, and avoiding tobacco and overuse of NSAID medications are useful strategies that can help you cope with several common disorders of the GI tract.

nonceliac wheat sensitivity (NCWS) One or more of a variety of immune-related conditions with symptoms similar to celiac disease that are precipitated by the ingestion of gluten in people who do not have celiac disease.

ASK THE RDN: Gluten-Free Diet

Dear RDN: Will a gluten-free diet help me lose weight?

The media are brimming with popular advice to eliminate wheat and other grains from your eating pattern, promising everything from a clear mind to a trim waistline. For individuals with celiac disease and nonceliac wheat sensitivity, avoiding gluten is a health priority. It will likely correct gastrointestinal complications and a range of other symptoms such as fatigue and body pain. Weight loss, however, is not one of the benefits of a gluten-free diet.

The only reason a gluten-free diet might induce weight loss is because it can be restrictive. For the person who regularly overconsumes bread, pasta, pizza, and baked goods, eliminating all sources of gluten could limit these food choices, thus leading to weight loss. Important point: Weight loss is the result of a calorie deficit, not the lack of gluten. Now, with the increased availability of gluten-free options in grocery stores and restaurants, you will soon realize that a gluten-free diet may not be that restrictive after all.

In fact, you may actually *gain* weight on a gluten-free diet. For a person with celiac disease, as the small intestine heals, nutrient absorption will increase and appetite will likely improve. In addition, many gluten-free products contain more calories than their wheat-based counterparts. To compensate for losses of taste and texture, some gluten-free products incorporate extra fat or sugar. For example, a typical slice of whole-grain wheat bread is about 80 kcal; some brands of gluten-free bread provide as many as 140 kcal per slice. Keep in mind that the "Gluten-Free" claim does not make a food healthy!

Lastly, grains are an important part of a balanced eating pattern. They provide calories, but they also supply dietary fiber and essential vitamins and minerals. Wheat flour is fortified with thiamin, niacin, riboflavin, folic acid, and iron. So, if you are planning to try a gluten-free diet, work with a registered dietitian nutritionist to ensure that your eating pattern meets your nutrient needs. Choose whole gluten-free grains and unprocessed fruits and vegetables to replace wheat and balance calories to avoid weight gain.

With a grain of truth,

Angela Collene, MS, RDN, LD
Senior Lecturer, The Ohio State University, Author of *Wardlaw's Contemporary Nutrition* and *Wardlaw's Contemporary Nutrition: A Functional Approach*

Tim Klontz

✓ CONCEPT CHECK 3.11

1. What is the leading cause of peptic ulcers?
2. Describe the relationship between spicy foods and ulcers: Do spicy foods cause ulcers? Should a person with an ulcer eat spicy foods?
3. What are the two best dietary strategies to prevent or treat constipation?
4. What is the most important nutritional concern for a person experiencing diarrhea?
5. Based on what you have learned about digestion and absorption of nutrients, is taking laxatives an effective way to prevent fat gain from excess calorie intake? Why or why not?

Summary (Numbers refer to numbered sections in the chapter)

3.1 Cells join together to make up tissues, tissues unite to form organs, and organs work together in organ systems. Cells are the basic structural units of the human body. Almost all cells contain the same organelles, but cell structure varies according to the type of job that cells must perform. Epithelial, connective, muscle, and nervous tissues are the four primary types of tissues in the human body. Each organ system both affects and is affected by nutrient intake.

3.2 Metabolism refers to all the chemical reactions involved in maintaining life, including the synthesis (anabolism) of new compounds and the breakdown (catabolism) of carbohydrates, fats, and proteins to yield energy in the form of adenosine triphosphate (ATP). Some nutrients (e.g., vitamins and minerals) are important regulators of metabolic reactions.

3.3 From the cells of the GI tract, water-soluble nutrients are absorbed into capillaries and fat-soluble nutrients are absorbed into lymph vessels, which eventually connect to the bloodstream. Blood delivers nutrients and oxygen to cells and picks up waste products as it circulates around the body.

3.4 In the urinary system, the kidneys are responsible for filtering the blood, removing body waste, and maintaining the chemical composition of the blood.

3.5 The nervous system allows for communication and regulation. Vitamin B-12 is part of the insulation that surrounds neurons. Transmission of nerve impulses relies on sodium and potassium. Neurotransmitters are made from amino acids.

3.6 The endocrine system produces hormones—protein-based chemical messengers—to regulate metabolic reactions and the levels of nutrients in the blood.

3.7 With assistance from the skin and the gastrointestinal tract, the immune system protects the body from pathogens. Optimal immune system function relies on protein; essential fatty acids; vitamins A, C, and D; some B vitamins; and the minerals iron, zinc, and copper.

3.8 The GI tract consists of the mouth, esophagus, stomach, small intestine, large intestine (colon), rectum, and anus. The liver, gallbladder, and pancreas are accessory organs that participate in digestion and absorption.

Spaced along the GI tract are sphincters that regulate the flow of food matter. Peristalsis is the movement of food matter along the GI tract. Nerves, hormones, and other substances control the activity of sphincters and peristaltic muscles.

Digestive enzymes are secreted by the mouth, stomach, small intestine, and pancreas. Bile from the liver aids the digestion of fat. Some protein and fat are digested in the stomach, but most digestion occurs in the small intestine. In the large intestine, no further digestion by human enzymes takes place, but bacterial enzymes break down some dietary components.

Most absorption occurs through the cells of the villi, which line the small intestine. Absorptive processes include passive diffusion, facilitated diffusion, active transport, phagocytosis, and pinocytosis. The large intestine absorbs water, a few minerals, and some products of microbial fermentation. Any remaining undigested materials are eliminated in the feces.

3.9 The community of microorganisms living in and on the human body is called the human microbiota. The microbiome includes the microbiota and its genome. Gut dysbiosis, or a harmful imbalance between beneficial and pathogenic strains of microorganisms in the gut, may contribute to many common health conditions. Probiotics are beneficial bacteria that can be consumed as part of food or supplements, colonize the gut, and confer health benefits on the host. Prebiotics are food substances (usually carbohydrates) that serve as fuel for the probiotic microorganisms. Postbiotics are the by-products of microbial metabolism. Some postbiotics affect the GI tract locally and others can be absorbed. The gut microbiota is now recognized to influence human health, not only in the GI tract, but throughout the body.

3.10 Limited stores of nutrients are present in the blood for immediate use. Some nutrients, such as minerals and fat-soluble vitamins, can be stored extensively in bone, adipose, and liver tissues. Excessive storage of nutrients can be toxic. Conversely, breakdown of vital tissues can supply nutrients in times of need, but continued breakdown eventually leads to ill health.

3.11 Common GI tract diseases, such as heartburn, constipation, and irritable bowel syndrome, can be treated with a combination of medications, dietary changes, and other lifestyle modifications.

Check Your Knowledge (Answers are available at the end of this question set)

1. Which of these nutrients is (are) important for the proper function of cell membranes?
   a. Lipids
   b. Proteins
   c. Carbohydrates
   d. All of these

2. The chemical reactions that break down carbohydrates, fats, and proteins to yield energy are _____ reactions.
   a. anabolic
   b. catabolic

3. The stomach is protected from digesting itself by producing
   a. bile.
   b. a thick layer of mucus.
   c. hydroxyl ions to neutralize acid.
   d. antipepsin that destroys enzymes.

4. The lower esophageal sphincter is located between the
   a. esophagus and stomach.
   b. stomach and duodenum.
   c. ileum and cecum.
   d. colon and anus.

5. A muscular contraction that propels food along the GI tract is called
   a. a sphincter.
   b. enterohepatic circulation.
   c. centrifugation.
   d. peristalsis.

6. Bicarbonate ions (HCO_3^-) from the pancreas
   a. neutralize acid in the esophagus.
   b. are synthesized in the pyloric sphincter.
   c. neutralize bile in the duodenum.
   d. neutralize acid in the duodenum.

7. Most chemical digestion occurs in the
   a. mouth.
   b. stomach.
   c. small intestine.
   d. large intestine.
   e. liver.

8. Bile is formed in the _____ and stored in the _____.
   a. stomach, pancreas
   b. duodenum, kidney
   c. liver, gallbladder
   d. gallbladder, liver
9. Which of the following terms refers to the entire collection of microorganisms, their genes, and their environment?
   a. Microbiota
   b. Microbiome
   c. Probiotic
   d. Dysbiosis
10. Treatment of ulcers may include
    a. H_2 blockers.
    b. proton pump inhibitors.
    c. antibiotics.
    d. all of these.

Answer Key: 1. d (LO 3.1), 2. b (LO 3.3), 3. b (LO 3.9), 4. a (LO 3.9), 5. d (LO 3.9), 6. d (LO 3.9), 7. c (LO 3.9), 8. c (LO 3.9), 9. b (LO 3.10), 10. d (LO 3.12).

Study Questions (Numbers refer to Learning Outcomes)

1. Draw and label parts of the cell, and explain the function of each organelle as it relates to human nutrition. **(LO 3.2)**
2. Identify at least one nutrition-related function of each of the 12 organ systems. **(LO 3.4)**
3. How is blood routed to and from the small intestine? Which classes of nutrients enter the body via the blood? Via the lymph? **(LO 3.4)**
4. How are neurotransmitters and hormones different? How are they the same? Give one example of each. **(LO 3.6, LO 3.7)**
5. Explain why the small intestine is better suited than the other GI tract organs to absorb nutrients. **(LO 3.9)**
6. What is one role of acid in the process of digestion? Where is it secreted? **(LO 3.9)**
7. Contrast the processes of active absorption and passive diffusion of nutrients. **(LO 3.9)**
8. Identify two accessory organs that secrete digestive substances into the small intestine. How do the substances secreted by these organs contribute to the digestion of food? **(LO 3.9)**
9. In which organ systems would the following substances be found? chyme **(LO 3.9)**, plasma **(LO 3.4)**, lymph **(LO 3.4)**, urine **(LO 3.5)**
10. Choose one common digestive disorder and explain how dietary modifications can be used to prevent or treat the disorder. **(LO 3.12)**

References

1. McCulloch M. Appetite hormones. *Today's Dietitian.* 2015 Jul;17(7):26.
2. Calder PC. Nutrition and immunity: lessons for COVID-19. *Eur J Clin Nutr.* 2021 Sep;75(9):1309-1318. doi: 10.1038/s41430-021-00949-8
3. Running CA, Craig BA, Mattes RD. Oleogustus: the unique taste of fat. *Chem Senses.* 2015;40(7):507-516. doi:10.1093/chemse/bjv036
4. Liang Z, Wilson CE, Teng B, Kinnamon SC, Liman ER. The proton channel OTOP1 is a sensor for the taste of ammonium chloride. *Nat Commun.* 2023;14(1):6194. Published 2023 Oct 5. doi:10.1038/s41467-023-41637-4
5. Sender R, Milo R. The distribution of cellular turnover in the human body. *Nat Med.* 2021 Jan;27(1):45-48. doi: 10.1038/s41591-020-01182-9
6. Canny GO, McCormick BA. Bacteria in the intestine, helpful residents or enemies from within? *Infect Immun.* 2008 Aug;76(8):3360-3373. doi: 10.1128/IAI.00187-08
7. Perler BK, Friedman ES, Wu GD. The role of the gut microbiota in the relationship between diet and human health. *Annu Rev Physiol.* 2023;85:449-468. doi:10.1146/annurev-physiol-031522-092054
8. Wang B, Yao M, Lv L, Ling Z, Li L. The human microbiota in health and disease. *Engineering.* 2017 Feb;3(1):71-82. doi: 10.1016/J.ENG/2017.01.008
9. Effects of probiotics and prebiotics on our microbiota. International Scientific Association for Prebiotics and Probiotics. 2017. Accessed November 28, 2019. https://isappscience.org
10. Davani-Davari D, Negahdaripour M, Karimzadeh I, et al. Prebiotics: definitions, types, sources, mechanisms, and clinical applications. *Foods.* 2019 Mar 9;8(3):92. doi: 10.3390/foods8030092
11. Monteiro SS, Schnorr CE, Pasquali MAB. Paraprobiotics and postbiotics—current state of scientific research and future trends toward the development of functional foods. *Foods.* 2023;12(12):2394. Published 2023 Jun 16. doi:10.3390/foods12122394
12. Wu R, Xiong R, Li Y, Chen J, Yan R. Gut microbiome, metabolome, host immunity associated with inflammatory bowel disease and intervention of fecal microbiota transplantation [published online ahead of print, 2023 May 26]. *J Autoimmun.* 2023;103062. doi:10.1016/j.jaut.2023.103062
13. Bach JF. Revisiting the hygiene hypothesis in the context of autoimmunity. *Front Immunol.* 2021;11:615192. Published 2021 Jan 28. doi:10.3389/fimmu.2020.615192
14. Liang D, Leung RK-K, Guan W, Au WW. Involvement of gut microbiome in human health and disease: brief overview, knowledge gaps and research opportunities. *Gut Pathog.* 2018 Jan 25;10:3. doi: 10.1186/s13099-018-0230-4
15. Ximenez C, Torres J. Development of microbiota in infants and its role in maturation of gut mucosa and immune system. *Arch Med Res.* 2017 Nov;48(8):666-680. doi: 10.1016/j.arcmed.2017.11.007
16. Danneskiold-Samsøe NB, Dias de Freitas Queiroz Barros H, Santos R, et al. Interplay between food and gut microbiota in health and disease. *Food Res Int.* 2019 Jan;115:23-31. doi: 10.1016/j.foodres.2018.07.043
17. Moran-Ramos S, López-Contreras BE, Canizales-Quinteros S. Gut microbiota in obesity and metabolic abnormalities: a matter of composition or functionality? *Arch Med Res.* 2017 Nov;48(8):735-753. doi: 10.1016/j.arcmed.2017.11.003

18. Jie Z, Xia H, Z S-L, et al. The gut microbiome in atherosclerotic cardiovascular disease. *Nat Commun.* 2017 Oct;8(1):845. doi: 10.1038/s41467-017-00900-1

19. Xiong RG, Li J, Cheng J, et al. The role of gut microbiota in anxiety, depression, and other mental disorders as well as the protective effects of dietary components. *Nutrients.* 2023;15(14):3258. Published 2023 Jul 23. doi:10.3390/nu15143258

20. Heartburn: what you need to know. *NIH MedlinePlus Magazine.* January 21, 2020. Accessed October 21, 2023. https://magazine.medlineplus.gov/article/heartburn-what-you-need-to-know

21. Acid reflux (GER & GERD) in adults. U.S. Department of Health and Human Services, National Institutes of Health, National Institute of Diabetes and Digestive and Kidney Diseases. 2020. Accessed October 21, 2023. https://www.niddk.nih.gov/health-information/digestive-diseases/acid-reflux-ger-gerd-adults

22. Anand BS. Peptic ulcer disease. Medscape. Updated April 26, 2021. Accessed October 21, 2023. https://emedicine.medscape.com/article/181753-overview#a7

23. Peptic ulcers (stomach ulcers). U.S. Department of Health and Human Services, National Institutes of Health, National Institute of Diabetes and Digestive and Kidney Diseases. September 2022. Accessed October 21, 2023. https://www.niddk.nih.gov/health-information/digestive-diseases/peptic-ulcers-stomach-ulcers

24. Constipation. U.S. Department of Health and Human Services, National Institutes of Health, National Institute of Diabetes and Digestive and Kidney Diseases. 2018. Accessed October 21, 2023. https://www.niddk.nih.gov/health-information/digestive-diseases/constipation

25. Scarlata K. Digestive wellness: get things moving—a dietitian's guide to relieving constipation. *Today's Dietitian.* 2016 July;18(7):10.

26. Hemorrhoids. U.S. Department of Health and Human Services, National Institutes of Health, National Institute of Diabetes and Digestive and Kidney Diseases. 2016. Accessed October 22, 2023. https://www.niddk.nih.gov/health-information/digestive-diseases/hemorrhoids

27. Diverticular disease. U.S. Department of Health and Human Services, National Institutes of Health, National Institute of Diabetes and Digestive and Kidney Diseases. 2021. Accessed October 22, 2023. https://www.niddk.nih.gov/health-information/digestive-diseases/diverticulosis-diverticulitis

28. Cameron R, Duncanson K, Hoedt EC, et al. Does the microbiome play a role in the pathogenesis of colonic diverticular disease? A systematic review. *J Gastroenterol Hepatol.* 2023;38(7):1028-1039. doi:10.1111/jgh.16142

29. Peery AF, Shaukat A, Strate LL. AGA clinical practice update on medical management of colonic diverticulitis: expert review. *Gastroenterology.* 2021;160(3):906-911.e1. doi:10.1053/j.gastro.2020.09.059

30. Irritable bowel syndrome (IBS). U.S. Department of Health and Human Services, National Institutes of Health, National Institute of Diabetes and Digestive and Kidney Diseases. 2017. Accessed October 22, 2023. https://www.niddk.nih.gov/health-information/digestive-diseases/irritable-bowel-syndrome

31. Lacy BE, Pimentel M, Brenner DM, et al. ACG clinical guideline: management of irritable bowel syndrome. *Am J Gastroenterol.* 2021;116(1):17-44. doi:10.14309/ajg.0000000000001036

32. Diarrhea. U.S. Department of Health and Human Services, National Institutes of Health, National Institute of Diabetes and Digestive and Kidney Diseases. 2016. Accessed October 22, 2023. https://www.niddk.nih.gov/health-information/digestive-diseases/diarrhea

33. Bloom AA. Cholecystitis. Medscape. Updated July 13, 2022. Accessed October 23, 2023. https://emedicine.medscape.com/article/171886-overview

34. Rubin JE, Crowe SE. Celiac disease. *Ann Intern Med.* 2020 Jan;172(1):ITC1-ITC16. doi: 10.7326/AITC202001070

35. Shiha MG, Chetcuti Zammit S, Elli L, Sanders DS, Sidhu R. Updates in the diagnosis and management of coeliac disease. *Best Pract Res Clin Gastroenterol.* 2023 Jun-Aug; 64-65:101843. doi:10.1016/j.bpg.2023.101843

36. Catassi C, Catassi G, Naspi L. Nonceliac gluten sensitivity. *Curr Opin Clin Nutr Metab Care.* 2023;26(5):490-494. doi:10.1097/MCO.0000000000000925

Design Element Credits: Fact Check/magnifying glass icon: McGraw Hill; Magnificent Microbiome background image: Alena Ohneva/Shutterstock; Sustainable Solutions icon: McGraw Hill; Roots icon: McGraw Hill; Medicine Cabinet icon: Peter Dazeley/Photographer's Choice/Getty Images

Chapter 4: Carbohydrates

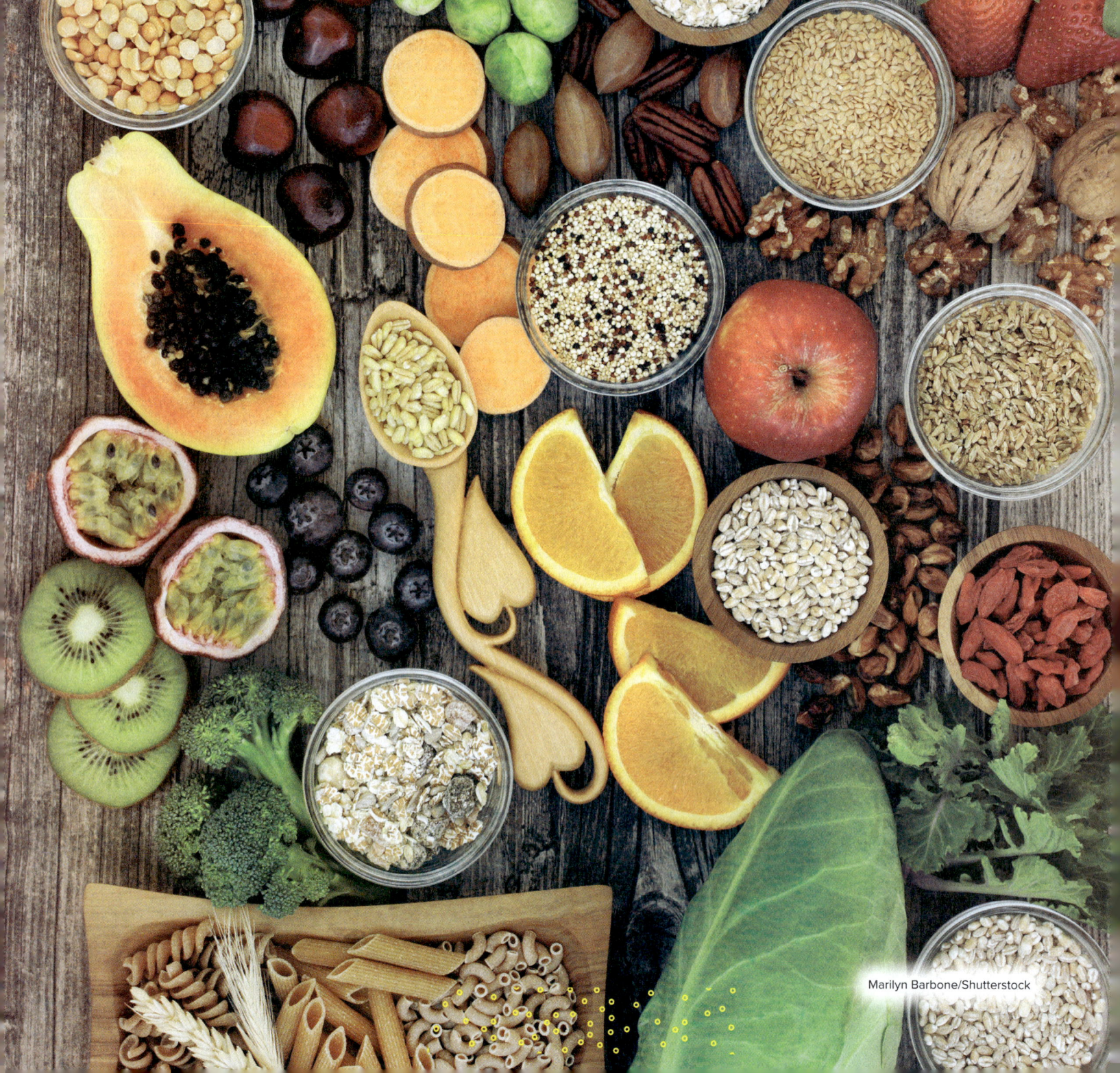

Marilyn Barbone/Shutterstock

Student Learning Outcomes

Chapter 4 is designed to allow you to:

4.1 Explain how carbohydrates are synthesized and their role in a healthy dietary pattern.

4.2 Identify the basic structures of the major carbohydrates: monosaccharides, disaccharides, and polysaccharides.

4.3 Describe food sources of carbohydrates and list some artificial sweeteners.

4.4 Explain carbohydrate digestion, absorption, metabolism, and glucose regulation.

4.5 List the functions of carbohydrates in the body, the results of inadequate carbohydrate intake, and the beneficial effects of fiber.

4.6 State the RDA for carbohydrate and guidelines for carbohydrate intake.

4.7 Identify the consequences of diabetes, and explain appropriate lifestyle behaviors that will reduce the adverse effects of this chronic disease.

FACT CHECK

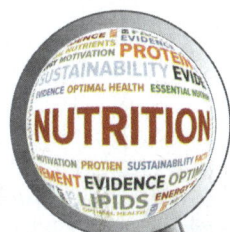

Are artificial sweeteners safe?

Artificial sweeteners are growing in popularity and often referred to as high-intensity sweeteners, nonnutritive sweeteners, and sugar substitutes. They are found in a wide variety of foods and beverages and are typically marketed as "sugar-free" or "diet" products. They are many times sweeter than sugar but contribute only a few or no calories when added to food.

Artificial sweeteners are regulated by the Food and Drug Administration (FDA) as food additives. Each sweetener must be reviewed and approved by the FDA before being marketed for sale, yet much controversy remains regarding the safety of artificial sweeteners.

In 2023, the artificial sweetener **aspartame** was categorized as "possibly carcinogenic to humans," by the International Agency for Research on Cancer (IARC). The scientific cancer community was quick to remind aspartame consumers that the acceptable daily intake (0 to 40 mg/kg body weight) has not changed. Keep in mind this is equivalent to drinking between 9 and 14 cans of diet soda pop per day!

The evidence-based cancer prevention guidelines also have not changed. These continue to recommend limiting consumption of sugar-sweetened beverages and encourage drinking mainly water and unsweetened drinks (unsweetened tea or coffee; infused water with fruits, lemon or herbs).[1] Visit Section 4.3 to learn more about consumption trends, safety, and the latest scientific evidence surrounding the most commonly used artificial sweeteners.

Source: FDA

artificial sweetener Synthetic types of sugar substitutes that can be used instead of cane sugar or sucrose.

aspartame Artificial sweetener made of two amino acids and methanol; about 200 times sweeter than sucrose.

magnificent microbiome

Getting Energy from Microbes

In Chapter 3, you learned that the small intestine is the primary site of digestion and absorption. Although no further digestion occurs in the large intestine by human enzymes, the gut microbiota is able to metabolize some food components that make it to the large intestine. Fermentation of dietary fiber by microorganisms in the large intestine yields short-chain fatty acids, some of which can be absorbed by the cells lining the large intestine. Researchers estimate that these products of fermentation may supply up to 10% of human energy needs.

Source: McNeil NI. The contribution of the large intestine to energy supplies in man. *Am J Clin Nutr.* 1984;39(2):338-342. doi: 10.1093/ajcn/39.2.338

glycogen A carbohydrate made of multiple units of glucose with a highly branched structure. It is the storage form of glucose in humans and is synthesized (and stored) in the liver and muscles.

photosynthesis Process by which plants use energy from the sun to synthesize energy-yielding compounds, such as glucose.

4.1 Carbohydrates—Our Most Important Energy Source

Carbohydrates are a main fuel source for some cells, especially those in the brain, nervous system, and red blood cells. Muscles also rely on a dependable supply of carbohydrates to fuel intense physical activity. As mentioned, carbohydrates provide approximately 4 kcal per gram and are a readily available fuel for cells, in the form of both blood glucose and **glycogen** stored in the liver and muscles. The glycogen stored in the liver can be used to maintain blood glucose concentrations when you have not eaten for several hours or the food you eat does not supply enough carbohydrates. Regular intake of carbohydrates is important because liver glycogen stores can be depleted in about 18 hours if no carbohydrates are consumed. After that point, the body is forced to produce alternative fuel sources, from the breakdown of either protein or fat stores, depending on dietary patterns. To obtain adequate energy, the recommendation is that 45% to 65% of the calories we consume each day come from carbohydrates.[2]

As you will see in this chapter, whole grain products have greater overall health benefits than refined and highly processed forms of carbohydrate. Let's explore this concept further as we learn about carbohydrates in detail.

Green plants synthesize most of the carbohydrates in our foods. Plant leaves capture the sun's solar energy in their cells and transform it into chemical energy. This energy is then stored in the chemical bonds of the carbohydrate glucose as it is produced from carbon dioxide in the air and water in the soil. This complex process is called **photosynthesis** (Fig. 4-1). Translated into chemical terms, 6 molecules of carbon dioxide combine with 6 molecules of water using energy from the sun to form 1 molecule of glucose and release 6 molecules of oxygen into the air. Converting solar energy into chemical bonds in the sugar is a key part of the process.

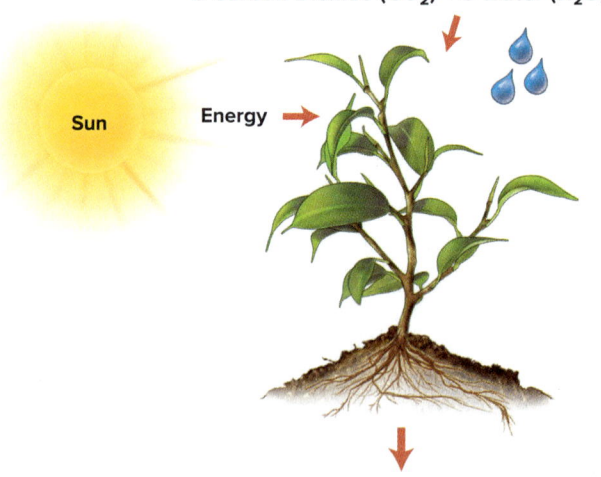

6 Carbon Dioxide (CO_2) + 6 Water (H_2O)

Sun → Energy →

Glucose ($C_6H_{12}O_6$) + 6 Oxygen (O_2)

Photosynthesis Equation
6 carbon dioxide + 6 water + solar energy → glucose + 6 oxygen

FIGURE 4-1 A summary of photosynthesis. Plants use carbon dioxide, water, and the sun's energy to produce glucose (sugar). Glucose is then stored in the plant and can undergo further metabolism to form starch and fiber in the plant.

✓ CONCEPT CHECK 4.1

1. Why are carbohydrates considered our most valuable energy source?
2. What are the main components needed for photosynthesis?

4.2 Forms of Carbohydrates

As the name suggests, most carbohydrate molecules are composed of carbon, hydrogen, and oxygen atoms. The simplest forms of carbohydrates are sugars. Simple sugars include **monosaccharides** and **disaccharides.** Larger, more complex forms of carbohydrates, the **polysaccharides,** are primarily called starches or fibers, depending on their digestibility. Starches, like corn featured in this chapter's *Farm to Fork*, are digestible, whereas fibers are not. Polysaccharides will be discussed later in this chapter.

Simple carbohydrates (also called simple sugars) contain only one (single) or two (double) sugar units and are called monosaccharides and disaccharides, respectively. These carbohydrates are quickly digested and absorbed. This rapid increase in blood sugar can result in a burst of energy that may be followed by fatigue as energy is depleted. Simple sugars are found in refined sugars, such as table sugar. These types of added sugars provide calories but lack vitamins, minerals, and fiber. This is why excessive added sugars contribute to weight gain. Recall that not all simple sugars are alike. On the other hand, naturally occurring simple sugars, found in fruit and milk, contribute key nutrients to our dietary pattern and should not be avoided. On the Nutrition Facts label, sugars are labeled as *Total Sugars*, with *Added Sugars* listed as a subcategory.

MONOSACCHARIDES: GLUCOSE, FRUCTOSE, AND GALACTOSE

Monosaccharides are the simple sugar units (*mono* means "one") that serve as the basic unit of all carbohydrate structures. The most common monosaccharides in foods are glucose, fructose, and galactose (Fig. 4-2). Although the structures vary between the monosaccharides, the chemical composition ($C_6H_{12}O_6$) remains the same in each.

Glucose. **Glucose** is the major monosaccharide found in the body. Glucose is also known as dextrose, and glucose in the bloodstream may be called blood sugar. Glucose is an important source of energy for human cells, although few foods contain glucose as their primary carbohydrate source. Most glucose comes from the digestion of starches and **sucrose** (common table sugar). Sucrose is made up of the monosaccharides glucose and fructose. For the most part, sugars and other carbohydrates in foods are eventually converted into glucose in the liver. This glucose then becomes available to serve as a source of fuel for cells.

Fructose. Also called fruit sugar, **fructose** is found naturally in fruits and forms half of each sucrose molecule. After it is consumed, fructose is absorbed by the small intestine and then transported to the liver, where it is quickly metabolized. Much is converted to glucose, but excess fructose may form other compounds, such as fat. Most of the free fructose in the food we eat comes from the use of **high-fructose corn syrup (HFCS)** in highly processed foods, including soft drinks, canned foods, cereals and baked goods, desserts, sweetened and flavored products (yogurt, condiments, jams, and jellies), candies, and many fast-food items.

FARM to FORK Corn on the Cob

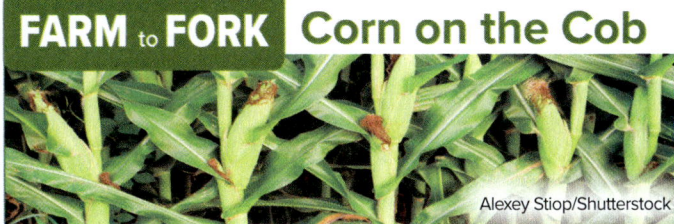
Alexey Stiop/Shutterstock

Each ear of corn has about 800 succulent, supersweet kernels in 16 rows. Corn provides fiber and about 25% of the world's calories, and it is a good source of many B vitamins, phosphorus, vitamin C, and magnesium. Compared to earlier varieties, however, modern corn has been transformed to be supersweet with up to 40% sugar and is much lower in phytochemicals. In contrast, blue corn, which is sacred to southwestern American Indians, is extremely high in the antioxidant anthocyanins. White and yellow corn contain no anthocyanins. Corn has long been the staple crop in south-central Mexico, and the American-Indian population introduced it to the first colonists in North America.

Grow
- Most corn varieties available from seed catalogs are supersweet cultivars.
- If growing a supersweet corn, choose the most colorful variety for the greatest phytochemical content. White corn varieties have lost the beta-carotene.
- For corn that is lower in sugar, choose seeds that are labeled *old fashioned*, *heritage*, or *heirloom*.

Shop
- Buy the freshest corn at a farmers' market or a U-pick farm.
- Choose varieties that are deep yellow—or even red, blue, black, or purple—to get the most phytochemicals. Compared to white corn, deep-yellow varieties contain over 50 times more beta-carotene, as well as lutein and zeaxanthin that reduce the risk of macular degeneration and cataracts. Supersweet varieties will be low in nutrients but will be extra sweet and tender.

Store
- Because old-fashioned or heirloom corn will not be extra sweet, ears should be chilled as soon as you pick them, and cooked and eaten within hours of harvesting to keep their sugar from turning to starch. Supersweet varieties, however, if chilled, retain their sweetness for days.
- Canned and frozen corn can be stored much longer and is typically as nutritious as fresh corn, although canning corn does lower its vitamin C content.

Prep
- Valuable nutrients are lost in the cooking water if you boil corn. Steam, grill, or microwave ears of corn before shucking them because corn husks help preserve nutrients during cooking.
- For microwaving, cut off the silks extending outside the husks, arrange the ears evenly in the microwave, and cook on high. Allow 3 to 4 minutes for a single ear, and add 1 to 2 minutes for each additional ear. Let corn cool for 5 minutes before husking and removing silk. Prepare corn similarly for grilling and grill for about 5 minutes, turning frequently. Corn is sweet enough to eat as is, and it is delicious drizzled with butter or lime juice and sprinkled with Parmesan cheese.

Source: Robinson J. Corn on the cob: how supersweet it is. In: *Eating on the Wild Side: The Missing Link to Optimum Health.* New York: Little, Brown & Co.; 2013.

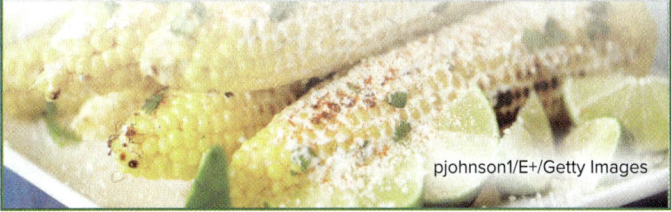
pjohnson1/E+/Getty Images

FIGURE 4-2 Chemical structure of monosaccharides.

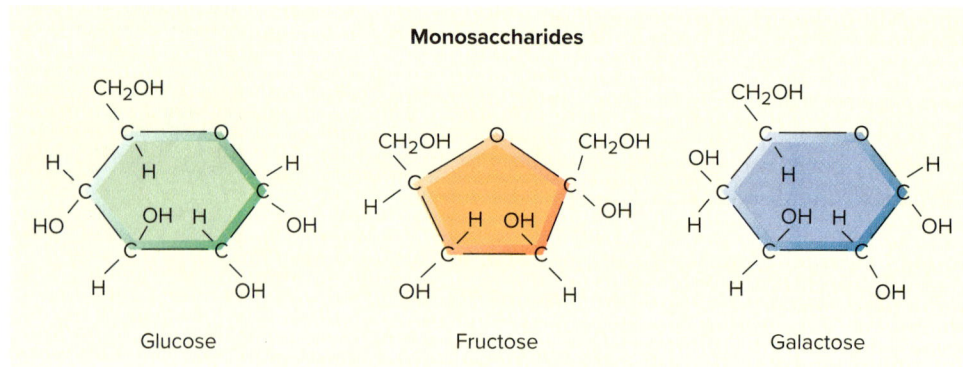

monosaccharide Simple sugar, such as glucose, that is not broken down further during digestion.

disaccharide Class of sugars formed by the chemical bonding of two monosaccharides.

polysaccharides Complex carbohydrates containing many glucose units, from 10 to 1000 or more. Also called *complex carbohydrates*.

glucose A six-carbon sugar that exists in a ring form; found as such in blood and in table sugar bound to fructose; also known as *dextrose*, it is one of the simple sugars.

sucrose Disaccharide composed of fructose bonded to glucose; also known as *table sugar*.

fructose A six-carbon monosaccharide that usually exists in a ring form; found in fruits and honey; also known as *fruit sugar*.

high-fructose corn syrup (HFCS) Corn syrup that has been manufactured to contain between 42% and 55% fructose.

galactose A six-carbon monosaccharide that usually exists in a ring form; closely related to glucose.

lactose A disaccharide consisting of glucose bonded to galactose; also known as *milk sugar*.

maltose A disaccharide consisting of glucose bonded to glucose; also known as *malt sugar*.

fermentation The conversion of carbohydrates to alcohols, acids, and carbon dioxide without the use of oxygen.

Galactose. The sugar **galactose** has nearly the same structure as glucose. Large quantities of pure galactose do not exist in nature. Instead, galactose is usually found bonded to glucose in **lactose,** a sugar found in milk products. During digestion, lactose is broken down to galactose and glucose and then absorbed. When galactose arrives at the liver, it is either transformed into glucose or further metabolized into glycogen, depending on the body's energy needs at the time. When required for milk production in the mammary gland of females while lactating, galactose is resynthesized from glucose to help form the milk sugar lactose. Although milk consumption is recommended for lactating females, this amazing process produces milk for the baby even if no milk is consumed!

DISACCHARIDES: SUCROSE, LACTOSE, AND MALTOSE

Disaccharides are formed when two monosaccharides combine (*di* means "two"). The disaccharides in food are sucrose, lactose, and **maltose.** All contain glucose (Fig. 4-3).

Sucrose. Sucrose forms when the two sugars, glucose and fructose, bond together (Fig. 4-3). Sucrose is found naturally in sugarcane, sugar beets, honey, and maple sugar. These products are processed to varying degrees to make brown, white, and powdered sugars.

Lactose. Lactose forms when glucose bonds with galactose during the synthesis of milk. Therefore, our major food source for lactose is milk products. Section 4.4 on lactose maldigestion and lactose intolerance discusses the issues that result when a person can't readily digest lactose.

Maltose. Maltose results when starch is broken down to just two glucose molecules bonded together. Maltose plays an important role in the beer and liquor industry. In the production of these alcoholic beverages, starches are converted to simpler carbohydrates by enzymes present in the grains. The breakdown products are then mixed with yeast cells in the absence of oxygen (anaerobic environment). The yeast cells convert most of the sugars to alcohol (ethanol) and carbon dioxide through a process called **fermentation.** Very little maltose remains in the final product. Small amounts of maltose can be found in some foods, including fruits, vegetables, and breads. Most maltose that we digest (in the small intestine) is produced during our own digestion of starch.

POLYSACCHARIDES: STARCH, GLYCOGEN, AND FIBER

Complex carbohydrates are digested more slowly than simple carbohydrates and supply a consistent and steady release of sugar (glucose) into the bloodstream. As with simple sugars, some complex carbohydrates are better choices than others. Let's explore more about complex carbohydrates next.

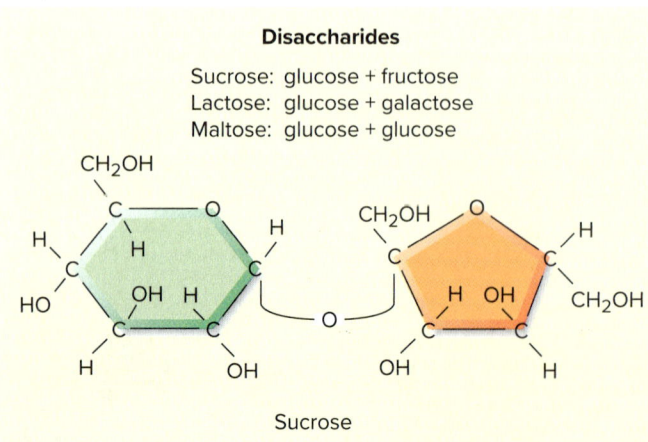

FIGURE 4-3 Chemical structure of the disaccharide sucrose.

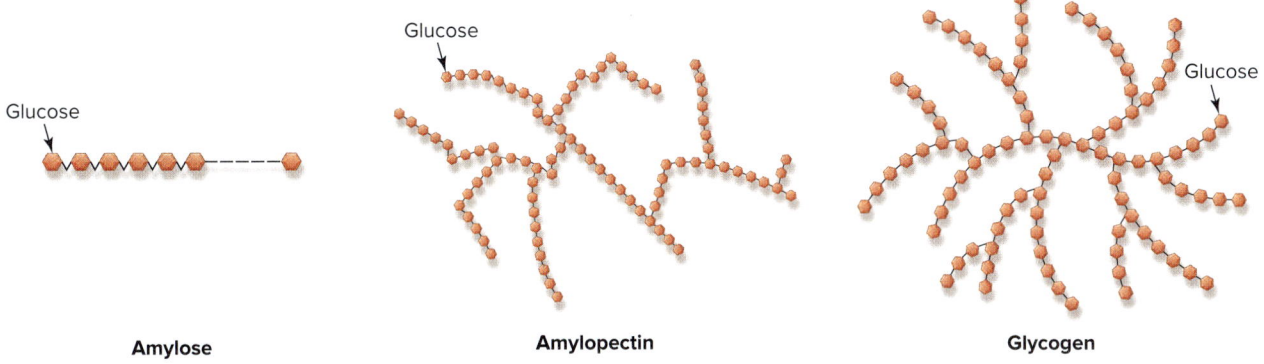

FIGURE 4-4 Comparison of common starch (amylose and amylopectin) structures compared to the highly branched structure of glycogen. Mainly stored in the liver and the skeletal muscles, glycogen serves as the body's storage form of glucose.

Starch. In many foods, numerous single-sugar units are bonded together to form a chain known as starch, which is a type of polysaccharide (*poly* means "many"). Polysaccharides, also called complex carbohydrates, may contain 1000 or more glucose units and are found chiefly in grains, vegetables, and fruits. When the Nutrition Facts label on food products lists Other Carbohydrates, this primarily refers to the starch content.

Plants store carbohydrates in two forms of starch digestible by humans: **amylose** and amylopectin. Amylose, a long, straight chain of glucose units, comprises about 20% of the digestible starch found in vegetables, beans, breads, pasta, and rice (Fig. 4-4). **Amylopectin** has a highly branched-chain structure and makes up the remaining 80% of digestible starches in the food we eat.

The enzymes that break down starches to glucose and other related sugars act only at the end of a glucose chain. Amylopectin, because it is branched, provides many more sites (exposed ends) for action. Therefore, amylopectin is digested more rapidly and raises blood glucose much more readily than amylose.

As we learn more about the microbiome, we are learning more about **resistant starch.** In several ways, the behavior of resistant starch is similar to soluble fiber with some benefits of insoluble fibers. For example, starch is typically digested and absorbed rapidly, resulting in a more rapid rise in blood glucose over a short period of time. Because resistant starch is not digested, it does not provide us energy or cause a surge in blood glucose. Yet it does act as a prebiotic to feed our helpful gut bacteria. Food sources of resistant starches include legumes, seeds, and raw foods (potatoes, green bananas). In addition, cooking and then cooling starchy foods (potatoes, rice, pasta) can increase the resistant starch content of otherwise starchy foods.

Glycogen. Animals, including humans, store glucose in the form of glycogen. Glycogen consists of a chain of glucose units with many branches, providing even more sites for enzyme action than amylopectin (Fig. 4-4). Because of its highly branched structure that can be broken down quickly, glycogen is an ideal storage form of carbohydrate in the body.

The liver and muscles are the major storage sites for glycogen. Because the amount of glucose immediately available in body fluids can provide only about 80 to 120 kcal, the carbohydrate energy stored as glycogen—amounting to about 1800 kcal—is extremely important.[3] Of this 1800 kcal, liver glycogen (about 400 kcal) can readily contribute to blood glucose. Muscle glycogen stores (about 1400 kcal) cannot raise blood glucose but instead supply glucose for muscle use, especially during high-intensity and endurance exercise. Although animals store glycogen in their muscles, animal products such as meats, fish, and poultry are not good sources of carbohydrates because glycogen stores quickly degrade after the animal dies.

Fiber. Plant fibers differ from starches because the chemical bonds that join the individual sugar units together cannot be digested by enzymes in the gastrointestinal (GI) tract. Fiber is not a single substance but a group of substances with similar characteristics. The group is composed of the carbohydrates **cellulose, hemicelluloses, pectins, gums,**

amylose A digestible straight-chain type of starch composed of glucose units.

amylopectin A digestible branched-chain type of starch composed of glucose units.

resistant starch Indigestible dietary fiber sequestered in plant walls. Bananas and legumes are rich sources.

cellulose An indigestible, insoluble, straight-chain polysaccharide made of glucose molecules and found in plant cell walls.

hemicellulose An insoluble fiber containing xylose, galactose, glucose, and other monosaccharides bonded together.

pectin A soluble viscous fiber containing chains of monosaccharides and characteristically found between plant cell walls.

gums Polysaccharides occurring naturally that cause an increase in viscosity; used as thickeners, gels, emulsifiers, and stabilizers.

FIGURE 4-5 Soluble and insoluble fiber. (a) The skin of an apple consists of the insoluble fiber cellulose, which provides structure for the fruit. The soluble fiber pectin glues together the fruit cells. (b) The outside layer of a wheat kernel is made of layers of bran—primarily hemicellulose, an insoluble nonfermentable fiber—making this whole grain a good source of fiber. Overall, fruits, vegetables, whole grains, and beans are rich in fiber.

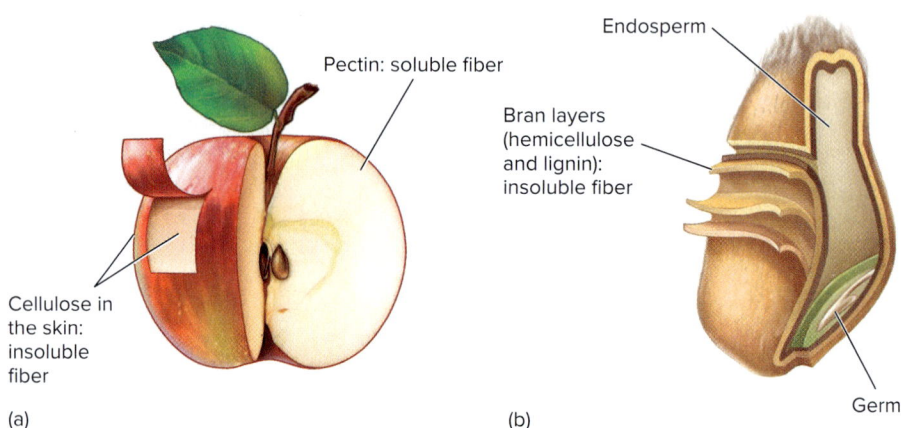

β-glucan Oats and barley are rich sources of these glucose polymers.

inulin A mixture of fructose chains that vary in length and occur naturally in plants.

lignin An insoluble noncarbohydrate dietary fiber found in cell walls of woody plants and seeds.

dietary fiber Indigestible fiber found in food.

whole grains Grains containing the entire seed of the plant, including the bran, germ, and endosperm (starchy interior). Examples are whole wheat bread and brown rice.

insoluble fiber A fiber that is not easily metabolized by intestinal bacteria; also called *nonfermentable fiber.*

mucilage A gelatinous substance of plants that contains protein and polysaccharides and is similar to plant gums.

soluble fiber A fiber that is readily fermented by bacteria in the large intestine; also called *viscous fiber.*

β-glucans, inulin, and resistant starch, as well as the noncarbohydrate **lignin**. In total, these constitute all the nonstarch polysaccharides in foods. Nutrition Facts labels combine the individual forms of fiber together under the term **dietary fiber**. Naturally occurring dietary fiber is found in beans, peas, lentils, fruits, nuts, seeds, vegetables, wheat bran, and whole grains (including whole oats, brown rice, popcorn, and quinoa) and foods made with whole grain ingredients (including breads, cereals, crackers, and pasta).

Cellulose, hemicelluloses, and lignin form the structural parts of plants. Bran layers form the outer covering of all grains and are rich in hemicelluloses and lignin. **Whole (unrefined) grains** are good sources of bran fiber (Fig. 4-5). Because the majority of these fibers neither readily dissolve in water nor are easily metabolized by intestinal bacteria, they are called *insoluble*. **Insoluble fiber,** or *roughage,* is found in wheat bran, nuts, fruit skins, and some vegetables. This type of fiber acts as a natural laxative because it speeds up the transit time of food through the GI tract.

Pectins, gums, and **mucilages** are contained around and inside plant cells. These fibers either dissolve or absorb water and are therefore called **soluble.** They also are readily fermented by bacteria in the large intestine. These fibers are primarily found in beans, oats, oat bran, and some fruits and vegetables. Soluble fiber slows the rate of absorption by attracting water into the GI tract, reduces blood cholesterol, promotes satiety, and controls blood glucose (Table 4-1).

The main types of fiber include: (1) dietary fiber, which describes the indigestible carbohydrates and lignin that are naturally occurring and intact in plants; and

TABLE 4-1 ■ Classification of Dietary Fibers

Fiber Type	Food Source					
	Whole Grains	Vegetables	Fruits	Legumes/Dried Beans and Peas	Nuts and Seeds	Added Functional Fiber
Viscous: Soluble Dissolves in water Forms viscous gels	Barley Oatmeal Oat bran Flaxseed	Eggplant Okra Sweet potato Brussels sprouts	Apples Oranges Pears Many other fruits	Chickpeas Dried beans (black, kidney, navy) Lentils Split peas	Chia seeds Flaxseeds	β-glucan Guar gum (raw, but not partially hydrolyzed) Pectin Psyllium
Fermentable: Mainly soluble Dissolves in water Forms very viscous or visco-elastic gels	Barley Oatmeal Oat bran	Artichokes Asparagus Mushrooms Onions Seaweed	Bananas (unripe)	Chickpeas Dried beans (black, kidney, navy) Lentils Split peas	N/A	β-glucan Chicory root fiber Inulin Resistant starch Wheat dextrin
Insoluble or Nonfermentable "Bulking": Does not dissolve in water Does not trap water Poorly fermented	Popcorn Quinoa Wheat bran Whole wheat Whole rye	Most vegetables	Apples Avocado Berries Guava Pears	Chickpeas Dried beans (black, kidney, navy) Lentils Split peas	Most nuts and seeds	Cellulose Methylcellulose

Adapted from Karen Collins, Today's Dietitian. https://www.todaysdietitian.com/newarchives/images/pdf/Dietary_Table.pdf

(2) **functional fiber,** which consists of isolated indigestible carbohydrates that have beneficial physiological effects in humans. More specifically, fiber is classified based on *solubility* (soluble vs insoluble), *viscosity* (viscous vs non-viscous) and *fermentability* (fermentable vs non-fermentable). Food labels do not generally distinguish between soluble and insoluble fibers, and most foods contain mixtures of both soluble and insoluble fibers.

Functional fibers can either be extracted from natural plant or animal sources or synthetically manufactured. The commercially produced functional, or isolated, fibers include resistant starch, polydextrose, indigestible dextrins, and inulin in supplements or added to foods such as yogurt, cereal, bars, and bread. The health benefits of many of these fibers are still unclear and are therefore a hot discussion topic.[4] Figure 4-6 will help you visually display the connectedness of all carbohydrates.

functional fiber Indigestible carbohydrates that have beneficial physiological effects in humans.

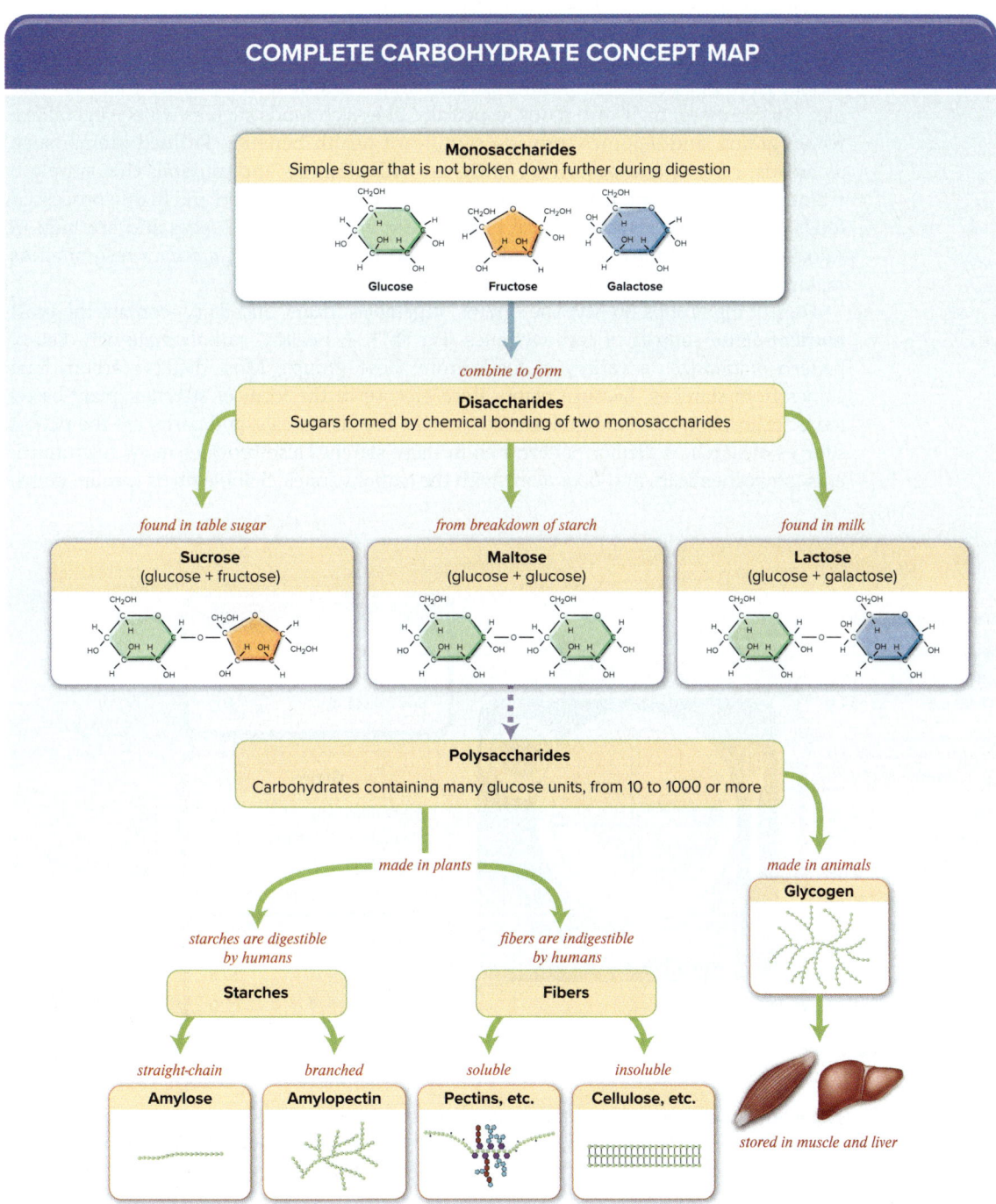

FIGURE 4-6 This Complete Carbohydrate Concept Map summarizes the various forms, characteristics, and basic structures of the simple and complex carbohydrates.

✓ CONCEPT CHECK 4.2

1. What are the specific names and definitions of the monosaccharides and disaccharides, and what happens to them when they are digested and absorbed?
2. What is a polysaccharide, and what are the differences between the plant polysaccharides?
3. What is the name of the storage form of glucose? Where is this compound located in the body?
4. What is the difference between soluble, insoluble, and functional fiber?

4.3 Carbohydrates in Foods

All carbs are not created equal. Many people think carbohydrate-rich foods cause weight gain, but pound for pound, carbohydrates supply fewer calories than fats and oils. Furthermore, high-carb foods, especially fiber-rich foods such as fruits, vegetables, whole grains, and legumes, provide significant health benefits. Refined grains, such as breads, cereals, and pastas, are enriched with vitamins and minerals that supply B vitamins, folic acid, and iron to our dietary patterns. Other refined and highly processed foods, such as cookies, cakes, and pastries, are energy-dense choices and are high in calories but contain few nutrients. For this reason, the *Dietary Guidelines* recommends making at least half of the grains you eat whole grains.

Four of the groups on MyPlate—grains, vegetables, fruits, and dairy—contain the most nutrient-dense sources of carbohydrates (Fig. 4-7). A healthy, carbohydrate-rich dietary pattern emphasizes a variety of foods from these groups. Most dietary carbohydrate comes from starches. Because plants store glucose in the form of starches, plant-based foods (beans, potatoes, and grains used to make breads, cereals, and pasta) are the richest sources of starch. A dietary pattern rich in these starches also provides many micronutrients, phytochemicals, and fiber along with the carbohydrates. Soluble fibers (pectin, gums,

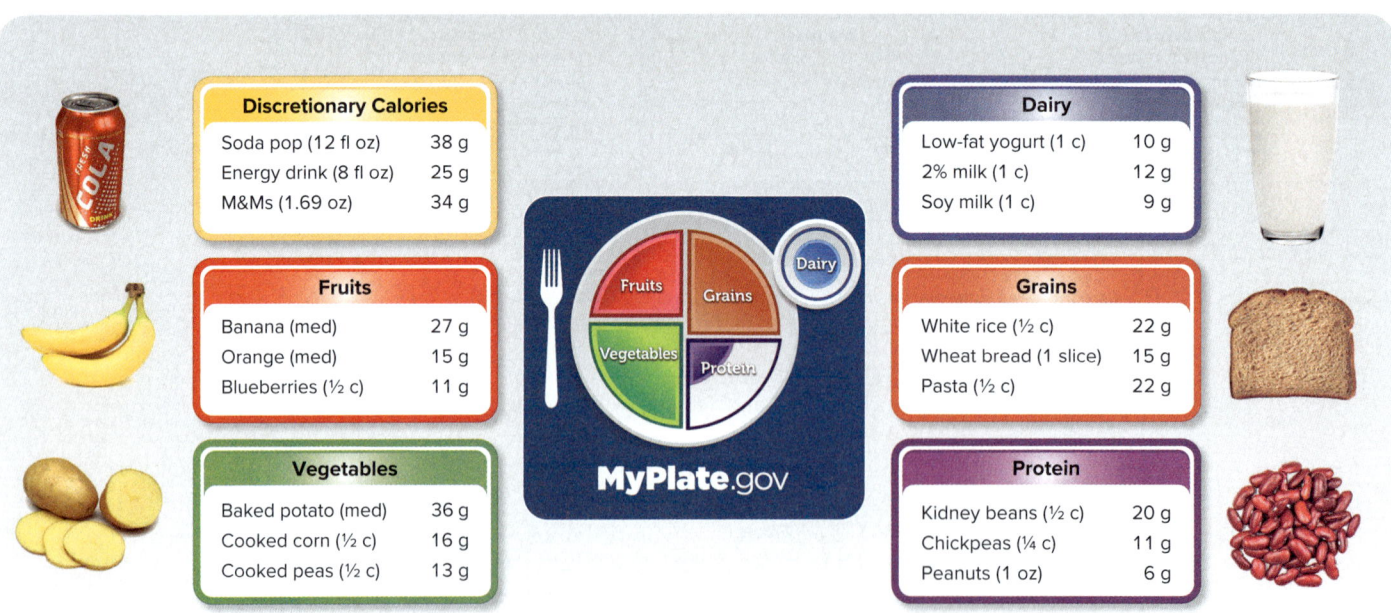

FIGURE 4-7 Food sources of carbohydrates. Overall, the richest sources of carbohydrates are discretionary calories (sugar-sweetened beverages), starchy vegetables (potatoes), and fruits (bananas). (MyPlate) U.S. Department of Agriculture; cola drink: Oleksiy Mark/scanrail/iStockphoto/Getty Images; bananas: Holly Hildreth/McGraw Hill; potato: Kaan Ates/E+/Getty Images; milk: Nipaporn Panyacharoen/Shutterstock; wheat bread: Alex Cao/Photodisc/Getty Images; kidney beans: zerbor/123RF

Source: U.S. Department of Agriculture, Agricultural Research Service. FoodData Central, 2019. fdc.nal.usda.gov.

Make Smart Beverage Choices

During the Day
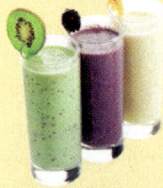
Keep a water bottle with you at all times.

Limit sugar-sweetened beverages. Try sugar-free sparkling or mineral water.

Drink water throughout the day and at meals.

Add lemon, cucumbers, oranges, strawberries, or herbs to vary the flavor.

Download an app to keep track of your water intake.

Smoothie Smarts
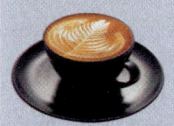
Know your smoothie! Be sure you know all ingredients and amounts used to craft your smoothie.

Divide homemade smoothies into 2 servings and store one for later.

Check the calorie count and added sugars of smoothies before you buy.

Request a no-sugar-added smoothie.

Coffee Shop Options
Opt for low-fat milk or soy milk.

Always order the smallest size to save both calories and money.

Skip the cream and extra flavorings or consider sugar-free syrups.

Limit blended coffee drinks or select a light version.

FIGURE 4-8 Smart beverage choices. Each day we make beverage choices that impact overall dietary patterns. Smoothies, energy drinks, sports beverages, and coffee-based gourmet drinks often contribute excess calories, added sugars, and sometimes fat to our dietary patterns. You can improve beverage choices by following these tips. Sven Kahns/McGraw Hill (top); Nenad Aksic/nesharm/iStockphoto/Getty Images (middle); Cathy Yeulet/amenic181/123RF (bottom)

and mucilage) are found in the skins and flesh of many fruits and berries; as thickeners and stabilizers in jams, yogurts, sauces, and fillings; and in products that contain psyllium and seaweed. Fiber is also available as a supplement or as an additive to certain foods (functional fiber) such that individuals with relatively low intakes of natural dietary fiber can obtain the health benefits of fiber. Be sure to discuss the pros and cons of fiber supplementation with your primary care provider or registered dietitian nutritionist (RDN).

Unfortunately, the top carbohydrate sources for U.S. adults include sugar-sweetened beverages, followed by desserts and sweet snacks. Sugar-sweetened beverages are typically sweetened with added sugars such as brown sugar, corn sweetener, corn syrup, dextrose, fructose, glucose, high-fructose corn syrup, honey, lactose, malt syrup, maltose, molasses, raw sugar, and sucrose. Examples of sugar-sweetened beverages include regular soda, fruit drinks, sports drinks, energy drinks, sweetened waters, and coffee and tea with added sugars. Remember that these sources provide many calories and few nutrients. This is why the *Dietary Guidelines* recommends limiting added sugars to less than 10% of total calories per day.

Many individuals are paying more attention to carbohydrate intake and including more whole grain versions of breads, pasta, rice, and cereals, as well as fruits and vegetables, in their dietary patterns. The decline in soft drink consumption is particularly encouraging, with consumers turning to water and unsweetened tea and coffee instead. More tips for making smart beverage choices can be found in Figure 4-8.

It is important to understand the percentage of calories from carbohydrates when planning a healthy dietary pattern. The food sources that yield the highest percentage of calories from carbohydrates are table sugar, honey, jam, jelly, fruit, and plain baked potatoes. Cornflakes, rice, bread, and noodles are next, all containing at least 74% of calories as carbohydrates. Foods with moderate amounts of carbohydrate calories are peas, broccoli, oatmeal, dry beans and other legumes, cream pies, French fries, and fat-free milk. In these foods, the carbohydrate content is diluted either by protein, as in the case of fat-free milk, or by fat, as in the case of cream pies. Foods with essentially no carbohydrates include beef, eggs, chicken, fish, vegetable oils, butter, and margarine (Fig. 4-7).

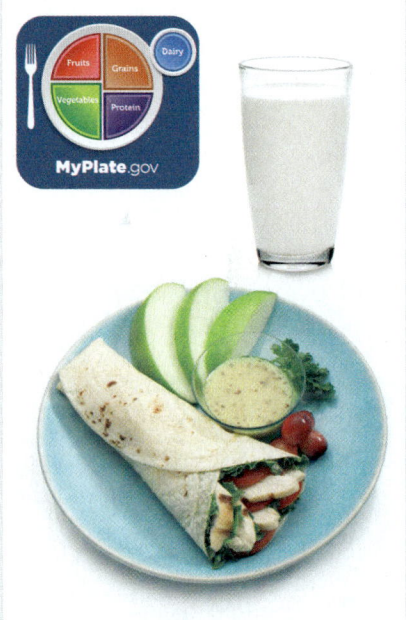

A typical American lunch is shown here with the MyPlate icon. Think about how many food groups are represented by this meal of a baked chicken and veggie burrito on a whole grain tortilla with an apple, grapes, and glass of low-fat milk. **How does this lunch compare to MyPlate? Can you think of a dinner meal that has items from all of the MyPlate food groups?** (MyPlate) U.S. Department of Agriculture; chicken wrap: Lew Robertson/Brand X Pictures/Stockbyte/Getty Images; glass of milk: Nipaporn Panyacharoen/Shutterstock

TABLE 4-2 ■ **Characteristics of Refined and Whole Grains**

Refined Grains	Whole Grains
Contains endosperm only	Contains all components of grain seed or kernel (bran, germ, and endosperm)
Increased blood glucose response	Complex carbohydrate with slower glucose response
Lower in fiber	Higher in fiber
Lighter texture	Denser texture
Lower in nutrient density but enriched	Higher in vitamins, minerals, and antioxidants

WHOLE GRAINS

The *Dietary Guidelines* recommends that we consume at least half of all grains as whole grains. We can increase whole grain intake by replacing highly processed refined grains with whole grains and limiting the consumption of foods that contain refined grains, solid fats, added sugars, and sodium. The *Dietary Guidelines* defines whole grain as the entire grain seed or kernel made of three components: bran, germ, and endosperm (Fig. 4-5). When the term *whole grain* is used on a food package, it also means that the product contains a minimum of 51% whole grain ingredients by weight per serving. Examples of whole grains include amaranth, barley (not pearled), brown rice, buck-wheat, bulgur, millet, oats, popcorn, quinoa, dark rye, whole-grain cornmeal, whole-wheat bread, whole-wheat chapati, whole-grain cereals and crackers, and wild rice. In contrast, refined grains have been milled, a process that removes the bran and germ. This process gives grains a finer texture and improves their shelf life, but it also removes dietary fiber, iron, and many B vitamins (Table 4-2). Some examples of refined grain products are white breads, refined grain cereals and crackers, corn grits, cream of rice, cream of wheat, barley (pearled), masa, pasta, and white rice. Refined-grain choices should be enriched.

Although more fiber is one of the primary advantages of whole grains, many benefits of whole grains are thought to be due to the combined effects of several compounds. These compounds include fiber, minerals, vitamins, and an abundance of phytochemicals. These are mainly contained in the bran and germ parts of the grains. The *Dietary Guidelines* recommends consuming two to four servings of whole grains per day so that half of all the grains eaten are whole grains. Studies have shown that this is enough to impart numerous health benefits, including reducing risks of cardiovascular disease, diabetes, metabolic syndrome, some cancers, and obesity. Scientific evidence also supports the role of fiber in maintaining a healthy gut microbiota.

On average, the total grain intakes of Americans meet the recommendations of the *Dietary Guidelines*. However, intakes of refined grains exceed recommendations, whereas intakes of whole grains are too low. In fact, 98% of Americans ages 1 and older are below whole grain recommendation from total grains[5] (Fig. 4-9). Because so few adults meet the recommendations for fiber, it is highlighted as a nutrient of public health concern (in addition to vitamin D, calcium, iron, and potassium). The reasons Americans are reluctant to consume whole grains include preferences in the taste, texture, cost, and availability of whole grains, compared to products made with refined flour.

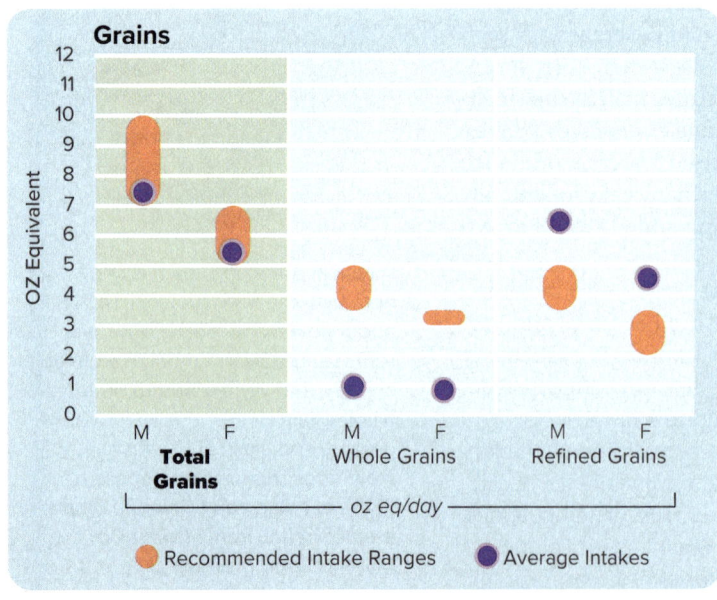

FIGURE 4-9 Average intakes of the grains subgroups compared to recommended intake ranges: ages 31 through 59.

Source: Analysis of *What We Eat in America*, NHANES 2015-2016. Recommended Intake Ranges: Healthy U.S.-Style Dietary Patterns

In addition to our preference for refined grains, many consumers who are trying to choose a whole grain product are very confused by the deceptive marketing messages on the labels of grain products. For example, a label that says a cereal is *made with whole grains* does not guarantee that the cereal contains 100% whole grain. Terms such as *cracked wheat, stoneground wheat, enriched wheat flour, 12-grain,* and *multigrain* can be confusing because these products may contain little to no whole grains. Multigrain cereals may contain several grains, but many of them may be refined with just a small amount of whole grains. Some whole grain breads are actually white bread in disguise after brown coloring is added to enriched white flour.[6]

With all of the confusion, it is crucial to look beyond the front-of-the-package marketing claims and examine the list of ingredients. To confirm that products contain 100% whole grain, look for *whole* as the first word on the ingredient list. Sugary breakfast cereals that claim to be whole grain may list the first ingredient as a whole grain such as corn, rice, oat, or wheat, but then the next several ingredients may be various forms of sugar that together weigh more than the sum of the whole grains.[7]

Although whole grains make up only a small fraction of grains on grocery shelves, it is getting easier to find a variety of whole grain products. To help simplify the process even further, the Whole Grains Council developed the Whole Grain Stamp (Fig. 4-10). This stamp is on more than 13,000 different products in more than 65 countries.[8] Choosing products with the 100% whole grain stamp will help us reach the minimum goal of getting 3 ounce-equivalents of whole grains per day.[9] Schools are also doing their part to increase whole grain consumption. Foods must contain at least 50% whole grains to meet the whole grain–rich criteria for the federal school breakfast and lunch programs.[10] See Table 4-3 for information on some whole grains that are available, including their potential health benefits.

VEGETABLES

Vegetables are a valuable source of carbohydrates in the form of starch and fiber. They are naturally low in fat and calories and come packed with nutrients that are vital for health, including potassium, folate, vitamin A, and vitamin C. Potatoes, as featured in this chapter's *Farm to Fork*, contain many nutrients as well as a healthy dose of fiber. Eating the recommended amount of vegetables has been shown to improve weight and reduce the risk of several chronic diseases.

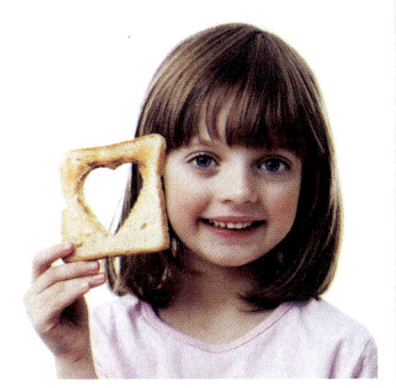

White whole wheat has the nutritional benefits of whole wheat but a milder taste, softer texture, and the lighter color of white bread. Traditional whole wheat is made from red wheat, which has a darker color and strongly flavored phenolic compounds. Switching to white whole wheat may be an acceptable option for those who prefer the taste and texture of white bread. **Based upon this information, is white whole wheat really a whole grain?**
verastuchelova/123RF

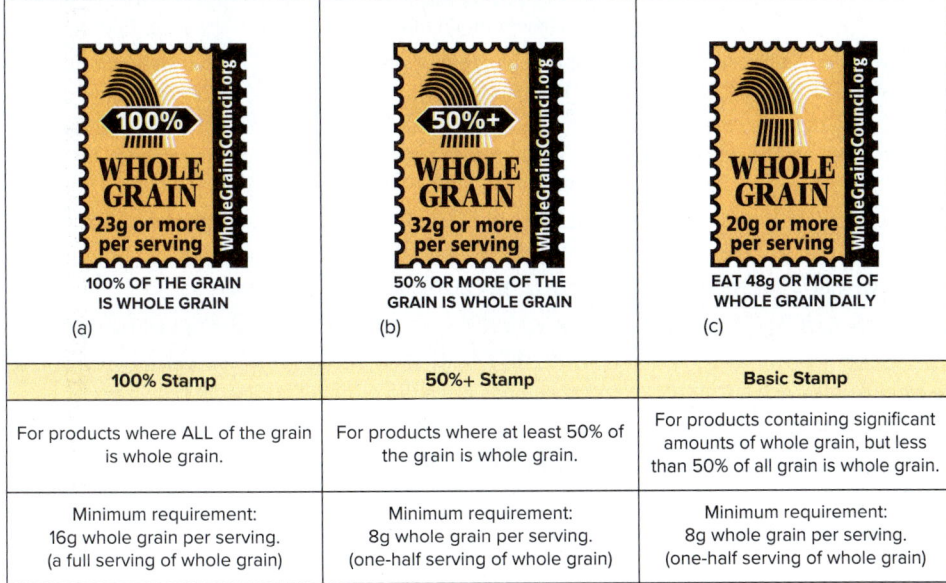

FIGURE 4-10 The whole grain stamp is used on grain products to identify whole grain foods. There are three versions of the stamp: (a) 100% stamp; (b) 50% stamp; (c) basic stamp. Wholegraincouncil.org

100% Stamp	50%+ Stamp	Basic Stamp
For products where ALL of the grain is whole grain.	For products where at least 50% of the grain is whole grain.	For products containing significant amounts of whole grain, but less than 50% of all grain is whole grain.
Minimum requirement: 16g whole grain per serving. (a full serving of whole grain)	Minimum requirement: 8g whole grain per serving. (one-half serving of whole grain)	Minimum requirement: 8g whole grain per serving. (one-half serving of whole grain)

TABLE 4-3 ■ Know Your Whole Grains

Grain	Characteristics	Health Benefits
Amaranth*	High-protein kernels that are tiny and have a peppery taste; gluten-free.	Contains a high level of complete protein, including lysine, an amino acid often missing in grains.
Barley	Highest in fiber; very slow cooking. Note: pearled barley is not technically a whole grain.	Barley may lower cholesterol even more effectively than oat fiber. Look for *whole barley, hulled barley,* or *hull-less barley.*
Buckwheat*	High levels of the antioxidant *rutin* and a high level of protein; gluten-free.	Rutin improves circulation and prevents LDL cholesterol from blocking blood vessels.
Bulgur*	Quick cooking time and mild flavor; often used in tabbouleh.	More fiber than quinoa, oats, millet, buckwheat, or corn.
Corn	Known for its sweet flavor; gluten-free.	Highest level of antioxidants of any grain or vegetable. Avoid labels that say *degerminated* and look for the words *whole corn*.
Einkorn*	An ancient strain of wheat that has a strong hull.	May contain more protein, phosphorus, potassium, and beta-carotene than traditional wheat.
Farro	Also known as *emmer,* an ancient strain of wheat. Has a strong hull and chewy texture, and can be used to make pasta.	May be much higher in antioxidants than traditional wheat. Avoid pearled farro, and look for the words *whole farro* on labels.
Freekeh*	A hard wheat with a smoky flavor that is similar to bulgur.	Harvested while it is young, yielding a higher nutritional value.
Kamut	An heirloom grain with a rich, buttery taste.	Higher in protein and vitamin E than traditional wheat. Look for *whole kamut* in the ingredient list.
Kañiwa*	A cousin of quinoa that is high in protein; gluten-free.	May be higher in certain antioxidants than other whole grains.
Millet*	A versatile family of grains in white, gray, yellow, and red varieties; gluten-free.	Naturally high in protein and antioxidants and can help control blood sugar and cholesterol.
Oats	High in protein, oats are popular for breakfast; although inherently gluten-free, oats are often contaminated with wheat during growing and processing.	Oat fiber is especially effective in lowering cholesterol. *Steel-cut oats* contain the entire oat kernel.
Quinoa*	Rich in high-quality protein, this is a small, light-colored round grain; gluten-free.	Quinoa contains complete protein, with all of the essential amino acids.
Rice	Many whole grain varieties, including brown, black, purple, or red. Brown rice is lower in fiber than other whole grains but rich in nutrients. White rice is refined; gluten-free.	One of the most easily digested grains, ideal for those on a restricted diet or who are gluten intolerant. Brown rice, and most other colored rice, is always whole.
Rye	Unusual among grains for the high level of fiber in its endosperm—not just in its bran.	Rye promotes a feeling of fullness, and it generally has a lower glycemic index than most other grains. Look for *whole rye* or *rye berries* in the ingredient list.
Sorghum*	Easily grown grain that can be eaten like popcorn, made into porridge, ground into flour, or brewed into beer; gluten-free.	Another gluten-free grain, popular among those with celiac disease.
Spelt	Variety of wheat that can be used as an alternative to traditional strains.	Spelt is higher in protein than common wheat. Look for *whole spelt* in the ingredient list.
Teff*	Versatile and easy to grow with a sweet, molasses-like flavor; gluten-free.	Twice the iron and three times the calcium of many other grains.
Triticale*	A hybrid of durum wheat and rye that is easily grown.	Shares many of the same health benefits as rye.
Wheat	Contains large amounts of gluten, a stretchy protein that enables bakers to create risen breads.	Look for *whole wheat* (in Canada, for the term *whole grain whole wheat*).
Wild Rice*	Not technically rice but a type of grass with a strong flavor; gluten-free.	Wild rice has twice the protein and fiber of brown rice.

Source: Adapted from the Whole Grains Council, Whole grains A to Z, at http://wholegrainscouncil.org/whole-grains-101/whole-grains-a-to-z.

*When found on an ingredient list, it almost always indicates a whole grain.

Sustainable Solutions

Whole Grains

Grains are leading sources of energy and dietary fiber in global eating patterns. They also provide protein, B vitamins, and phytochemicals. A dietary pattern that includes whole grains promotes human health, reducing the risk for chronic diseases like cancer and heart disease. Not only are whole grains good for you, but they are also good for the planet! Many varieties are drought-resistant and can withstand high temperatures, which makes grains a reliable food choice amid global climate change. For comparison, it takes 10.19 liters (2.7 gallons) of water to produce 1 kcal of beef, whereas grains require, on average, 0.51 liter (0.1 gallon) of water to produce 1 kcal. In addition, many grain farmers use low-till or no-till methods of tending the land, which means that the stalks are left to decompose in the field after harvest. This helps to return vital nutrients to the soil and prevents erosion. To improve the sustainability of the global food system, experts advocate a shift toward a plant-based dietary pattern. Whole grains are a crucial part of this solution.

Source: Sluyter C. Whole grains: good for the planet and good for you. Oldways. Published April 20, 2017. https://oldwayspt.org/blog/whole-grains-good-planet-and-good-you

According to the *Dietary Guidelines,* any vegetable or 100% vegetable juice counts as a member of the vegetables group. Vegetables are organized into five subgroups based on their nutrient content:

1. Dark-green vegetables
2. Starchy vegetables
3. Red and orange vegetables
4. Beans, peas, and lentils
5. Other vegetables

Vegetable choices should be selected from among the vegetable subgroups but may be raw or cooked; fresh, frozen, canned, or dried/dehydrated; and whole, cut up, or mashed.

Nearly 90% of the U.S. population falls short of the *Dietary Guidelines* recommendations for vegetables.[9] Furthermore, when vegetables are consumed, they are often combined with high-sodium condiments and seasonings. The amount of vegetables you need depends on your age, sex, and level of physical activity. For example, recommended total daily amounts for females ages 19 to 50 years are 2½ cups. In general, 1 cup of raw or cooked vegetables or vegetable juice or 2 cups of raw leafy greens can be considered as a "1 cup equivalent" from the vegetables group. Recommended weekly amounts from each vegetable subgroup are given as amounts to eat weekly. For example, the weekly recommendations for females ages 19 to 50 years are 1½ cups of dark-green vegetables; 5½ cups of red and orange vegetables; 1½ cups of beans, peas, and lentils; 5 cups of starchy vegetables; and 4 cups of other vegetables such as cauliflower or mushrooms.

FARM to FORK: Potatoes

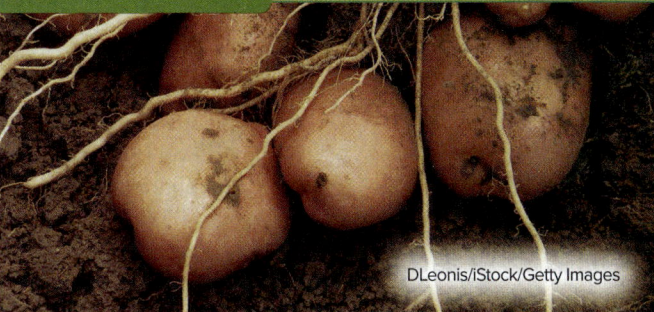
DLeonis/iStock/Getty Images

Potatoes are one of the most productive and consumed crops around the world. This is good news because the average adult eats more than 125 pounds of potatoes each year!

Grow
- Potatoes can be easily grown in most climates with little maintenance.
- Plant one seed potato in the bottom third of a gallon container. As the plant grows, mound more soil/compost mix around the stem until you reach the top of the vessel. Stop watering for 2 weeks after the foliage dies.
- Harvest by hand, allow the harvest to dry for one day, then brush off the soil, wash, and enjoy!

Shop
- New potatoes (harvested early in the season) have thin skins and a waxy flesh. They cause a slower rise in blood glucose than potatoes harvested late in the season, which have thick skins and are typically used for baking.
- Of the most common varieties, russet potatoes contain the most phytochemicals. They are good sources of potassium, vitamin C, and several B vitamins. Sweet potatoes also contain these nutrients in addition to being rich in vitamin A and fiber.
- Try colorful novelty potatoes (red-, blue-, and black-skinned) with deep-colored flesh to get a more varied boost of phytochemicals.
- Consider buying organic potatoes to reduce pesticide residues.

Store
- Store new potatoes in the refrigerator and eat within 1 week of purchase.
- Thicker-skin potatoes can be stored for months in a cool, dark, well-ventilated location but away from onions. The gases from the onions may speed the potato spouting process.
- Green potatoes contain solanine, a toxic compound that should be avoided.

Prep
- Scrub potatoes before cooking, and eat with the skins to increase nutrient consumption by up to 50%.
- Most varieties of potatoes contain rapidly digested starch, which causes a sharp rise in blood glucose.
- For those concerned with blood glucose control, leftovers are better! Cook potatoes, refrigerate overnight, then reheat and eat them the next day. The cooler temperatures, post-cooking, change the structure of the starch, which will delay a sharp rise in blood glucose.
- To add flavor and nutrients without extra fat, opt for toppings such as yogurt, vegetarian chili, salsa, herbs, and spices.
- Try to limit consumption of French fries and potato chips and aim for less highly processed potatoes.

Source: Robinson J. Potatoes: from wild to fries. In *Eating on the Wild Side*. New York: Little, Brown and Company, 2013.

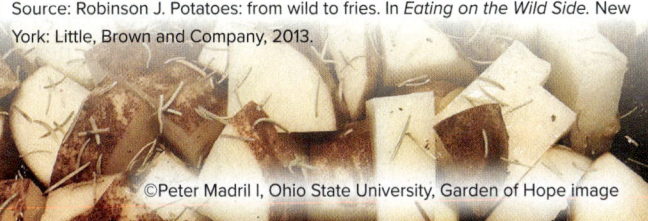
©Peter Madril I, Ohio State University, Garden of Hope image

FRUITS

Fruits provide carbohydrates primarily in the form of natural sugar and fiber. Eating fruits provides health benefits similar to those discussed for vegetables. People who eat more fruits as part of an overall healthy dietary pattern are more likely to have lower body weight and a reduced risk of several chronic diseases. Dietary fiber from fruits helps reduce blood cholesterol levels, lower risk of disease, and promote proper bowel function. The fiber in fruits helps with weight maintenance by providing a feeling of fullness (satiety) with fewer calories. The MyPlate fruit group includes whole fruits and 100% fruit juice. Whole fruits include fresh, canned, frozen, and dried forms. It is recommended that at least half of the recommended amount of fruit should come from whole fruit, rather than 100% juice. Fruit juices should be 100% juice and always pasteurized. Diluting 100% juice with water (without added sugars) is an even healthier choice. When selecting canned fruit, choose options that are canned with 100% juice and without added sugars.

About 80% of the U.S. population does not meet the fruit recommendations. Although fruit is generally consumed in nutrient-dense forms such as bananas, apples, oranges, or grapes, some fruit is consumed in energy-dense forms such as fruit pies or similar desserts.

DAIRY

The dairy group includes fat-free and low-fat (1%) milk, yogurt, and cheese, as well as fortified soy alternatives. Fortified soy products have added calcium, vitamin A, and vitamin D to match the nutritional profile of most dairy products. Other plant-based dairy alternatives (e.g., almond, rice, coconut, oat, and hemp "milks") may or may not be fortified with these nutrients and are typically much lower in protein than cow's milk or fortified soy alternatives, so they are not included as part of the dairy group. Servings of dairy foods are expressed in cup-equivalents. One cup of milk, yogurt, or fortified soy beverage; 1½ ounces of natural cheese; or 1 ounce of processed cheese are considered as "1 cup equivalent" from the dairy group. Foods made from milk that are primarily fat, such as cream cheese, cream, and butter, are not part of the dairy group.

Recommended intakes of dairy or fortified soy alternatives vary across the life span. Older children and most adults need 3 cup equivalents per day. However, approximately 90% of the U.S. population falls short of the recommendations. Indeed, only 20% of adults consume milk at all on any given day. To make matters worse, dairy in the U.S. is often consumed in combination dishes with high amounts of sodium, saturated fat, and added sugars (e.g., pizza, ice cream).

The main carbohydrate in cow's milk is lactose. Individuals with lactose maldigestion or lactose intolerance may experience gastrointestinal distress when they consume foods that contain lactose (Table 4-4). Section 4.4 covers lactose maldigestion in more detail. Individuals with lactose maldigestion can choose low-lactose and lactose-free dairy products or fortified soy alternatives.

NUTRITIVE SWEETENERS

The various substances that impart sweetness to foods fall into two broad classes: nutritive sweeteners, which can provide calories for the body, and artificial sweeteners, which, for the most part, provide no calories.[11] Artificial sweeteners are much sweeter on a per-gram basis than the nutritive sweeteners that provide calories. The taste and sweetness of sucrose (table sugar) make it the benchmark against which all other sweeteners are measured. Sucrose is obtained from sugarcane and sugar beet plants. Both sugars and sugar alcohols provide calories along with sweetness. Sugars are found in many different food products, whereas sugar alcohols have rather limited uses.

Sugars. All of the monosaccharides (glucose, fructose, and galactose) and disaccharides (sucrose, lactose, and maltose) discussed earlier are designated nutritive sweeteners because they provide calories. The *Dietary Guidelines* recommends that we reduce the intake of calories from added sugars. Added sugars are defined as caloric sweeteners added to foods during processing or preparation or before consumption. It is estimated that adults consume almost 270 calories (13%) of added sugars per day, far exceeding the recommendation of no more than 10% of total of calories per day.[5] As you might guess, almost 40% of added sugars come from sugar-sweetened beverages, including soft drinks, fruit drinks, sports and energy drinks, and sweetened coffee and tea (Fig. 4-11). Desserts and sweet snacks are the next biggest source of added sugars.[5] Fortunately, the amount of added sugars must now be present on the Nutrition Facts label.

High-fructose corn syrup (HFCS) is a sweetener used in a wide variety of foods, from soft drinks to barbecue sauce. It is called high-fructose corn syrup because it contains up to 55% fructose, compared to sucrose, which contains only 50% fructose. HFCS is made by an enzymatic process that converts some of the glucose in cornstarch into fructose, which tastes sweeter than glucose. In the United States, corn is abundant and inexpensive compared to sugarcane or sugar beets, much of which is imported. Food manufacturers prefer HFCS because of its low cost and broad range of food-processing applications, and because it is easy to transport, has better shelf stability, and improves food properties. There has been much confusion and controversy surrounding the use and possible health effects of HFCS. After extensive review, the scientific community has concluded that there are no metabolic or endocrine differences between HFCS and sucrose related to obesity or any other adverse health outcome.[12]

Honey is a product of plant nectar that has been altered by bee enzymes. The enzymes break down much of the nectar's sucrose into fructose and glucose. Honey offers essentially the same nutritional value as other simple sugars—a source of energy and little else. However, honey is not safe for infants because it can contain spores of the bacterium *Clostridium botulinum* that causes fatal foodborne illness. Unlike the acidic environment of an adult's stomach, which inhibits the growth of the bacterium, an infant's stomach does not produce much acid, making infants more susceptible to the threat that this bacterium poses.

Agave nectar comes from the same plant used to make tequila. Like high-fructose corn syrup, it's highly processed before it can be added to products. Agave contains about 60 calories per tablespoon compared to 40 calories per tablespoon for table sugar. Agave is sweeter than granular sugar, so you can use less to reduce calories.

In addition to sucrose and HFCS, brown sugar, turbinado sugar, honey, maple syrup, agave nectar, and other sugars are also added to foods. Brown sugar is essentially sucrose containing some molasses that is not completely removed from the sucrose during processing or is added to the sucrose crystals. Turbinado sugar is a partially refined version of raw sucrose that is often marketed as raw sugar. Maple syrup is made by boiling down and concentrating the sap from sugar maple trees. Because pure maple syrup is expensive, most pancake syrup is primarily corn syrup and HFCS with maple flavor added.

Sugar Alcohols. Food manufacturers and consumers have numerous options for obtaining sweetness while using less sugar and calories. Sugar alcohols are carbohydrates with a chemical structure that partially resembles both sugar and alcohol, but they don't contain ethanol. They are incompletely absorbed and metabolized by the body, and consequently contribute fewer calories than most sugars. This allows people with diabetes to enjoy the flavor of sweetness while controlling sugars; they also provide noncaloric or very-low-calorie sugar substitutes for persons trying to lose (or control) body weight.

TABLE 4-4 ■ Lactose in Common Dairy Foods

Food Product	Lactose (grams)
Cheese (1 oz, American)	1.5
Cheese (1 oz, Swiss)	0
Cottage cheese (½ cup)	4
Ice cream (½ cup)	3
Lactaid® milk (1 cup)	0
Milk (1 cup)	11
Sour cream (½ cup)	4
Yogurt (8 oz, Greek)	7
Yogurt (8 oz, 12 g protein)	15

Source: USDA, ARS National Agriculture Library: Nutrient Data Laboratory. Lactose may vary by brand. Read labels carefully.

Drink (12-ounce serving)	Added Sugars (Teaspoons)	Added Sugars (Grams)	Total Calories
Plain Water	0	0	0
Unsweetened Tea	0	0	0
Sports Drinks	5	20	97
Cafe Mocha	5	21	290
Chai Tea Latte	5½	23	180
Sweetened Tea	7	29	115
Regular Soda	9	37	156
Lemonade	10	43	171
Fruit Drinks	14	59	238

FIGURE 4-11 Common sources of added sugars.

Source: U.S. Department of Agriculture, Agricultural Research Service. 2020. USDA Food and Nutrient Database for Dietary Studies and USDA Food Patterns Equivalents Database *2017-2018*. Food Surveys Research Group Home Page, **ars.usda.gov/nea/bhnrc/fsrg**.

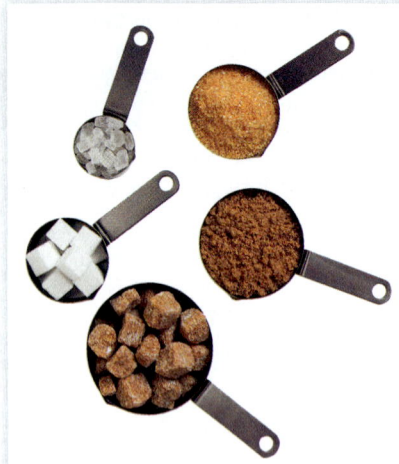

There are many forms of sugar on the market. Together they contribute to our average daily intake of approximately 17 teaspoons of sugar. **How many calories are in 1 gram of sugar?** C Squared Studios/Photodisc/Getty Images

Sugar alcohols, or polyols, such as sorbitol and **xylitol,** are used as nutritive sweeteners but contribute fewer calories (about 2.6 kcal per gram) than sugars. Unlike sucrose, sugar alcohols are not readily metabolized by bacteria to acids in the mouth and thus do not promote tooth decay. They are also absorbed and metabolized to glucose more slowly than are simple sugars. Because of this, they remain in the intestinal tract for a longer time and, in large quantities, can cause diarrhea.

Sugar alcohols are used in sugarless gum, breath mints, and candy. Sugar alcohols must be listed on labels. If only one sugar alcohol is used in a product, its name must be listed; however, if two or more are used in one product, they are grouped together under the heading sugar alcohols. The caloric value of each sugar alcohol used in a food product is calculated so that when one reads the total amount of calories a product provides, it includes the sugar alcohols in the overall amount.

ARTIFICIAL SWEETENERS

 Artificial sweeteners, also called nonnutritive sweeteners or sugar substitutes, yield few or no calories when consumed in amounts typically used in food products. They also are not metabolized by bacteria in the mouth, so they do not promote dental caries. High-intensity sweeteners are regulated as food additives, unless their use as a sweetener is **generally recognized as safe (GRAS).** For use as a food additive, these sweeteners must undergo premarket review and approval by FDA before they can be used in food products.

A growing number of artificial sweeteners are currently available in the United States with an industry value of approximately $2.2 billion.[11] Replacing added sugars with low- and no-calorie sweeteners may reduce overall calorie intake in the short term and support weight management, yet questions still remain about their long-term weight effectiveness as a weight management strategy.[5]

For each sweetener, the FDA determines an Acceptable Daily Intake (ADI) guideline. ADIs are set at a level 100 times less than the level at which no harmful effects were noted in animal studies. Current evidence suggests that artificial sweeteners can be used safely by adults and children, and they are considered safe during pregnancy. Note that large, long-term studies have yet to be conducted in humans. A summary of the most popular artificial sweeteners can be found in Table 4-5, and additional information can be found below.

Acesulfame-K. Acesulfame-K is an organic acid linked to potassium (K). It is sold as Sunette® and can be used in baking. In the United States, it is currently approved for use as a general-purpose sweetener.

Advantame. A general-purpose sweetener and flavor enhancer, **advantame** is stable at higher temperatures and can be used as a tabletop sweetener as well as in cooking. Chemically, advantame is similar to aspartame but is much sweeter. Because only a small amount is

xylitol Alcohol derivative of the five-carbon monosaccharide xylose. Absorbed more slowly than sucrose, xylitol supplies 40% fewer calories than table sugar.

generally recognized as safe (GRAS) A list of food additives that in 1958 were considered safe for human consumption. FDA continues to bear responsibility for proving the additives are not safe and can remove unsafe products from the list.

acesulfame-K Artificial sweetener that yields no energy to the body; 200 times sweeter than sucrose.

advantame A sweetener similar in structure to aspartame; 20,000 times sweeter than sucrose.

TABLE 4-5 ■ Artificial Sweeteners

Sweetener	Brand Names	Sweetness Intensity (Compared to Sucrose)	Acceptable Daily Intake (ADI) (mg/kg/day)	Approximate # Packets to Reach ADI*	Heat Stable
Aspartame	Nutrasweet®, Equal®, Sugar Twin®	200 ×	50	75	No
Saccharin	Sweet and Low®, Sweet Twin®, Sweet'N Low®, Necta Sweet®	200–700 ×	15	45 (400 × sucrose)	Yes
Stevia	Truvia®, PureVia®, Enliten®	200–400 ×	4**	9 (300 × sucrose)	Yes
Sucralose	Splenda®	600 ×	5	23	Yes

Source: Adapted from U.S. Food & Drug Administration at https://www.fda.gov/food/food-additives-petitions/additional-information-about-high-intensity-sweeteners-permitted-use-food-united-states
*Number of Tabletop Sweetener Packets a 60 kg (132 pound) person would need to consume to reach the ADI. Calculations assume 1 packet of high-intensity sweetener is as sweet as 2 teaspoons of sugar.
**ADI established by the Joint FAO/WHO Expert Committee on Food Additives (JECFA).

needed to achieve the same level of sweetness (it is 20,000 times sweeter than sucrose), foods that contain advantame do not need to include alerts for people with **phenylketonuria (PKU)**.

Allulose. Allulose (D-allulose or D-psicose) is a monosaccharide that is nearly identical to fructose in chemical structure and present in small quantities in natural products including wheat, figs, jackfruit, and raisins. Delivering about 0.2 kcal per gram, or about 5% of the calories of sugar, this compound is absorbed in the small intestine but not metabolized, and excreted primarily in the urine. In terms of Nutrition Facts labeling, allulose is unique in that the FDA has exempted it from inclusion in the total and added sugars declaration, but it must be listed in the ingredient list, total carbohydrates, and total calories sections on a food label.

Aspartame. Aspartame is in widespread use throughout the world (typically packaged in blue packets, including Equal®). The components of aspartame are the amino acids phenylalanine and aspartic acid, along with methanol. Recall that amino acids are the building blocks of proteins, so aspartame is more like a protein than a carbohydrate. Like protein, aspartame yields about 4 kcal per gram, but because it is about 200 times sweeter than sucrose, only a small amount is needed to obtain the desired sweetness.

Assessments of the health impacts of aspartame were recently reassessed and cited *limited evidence* for carcinogenicity in humans.[13] There is also limited evidence for cancer in animal trials and limited evidence related to the possible mechanisms for causing cancer. As mentioned in this Chapter's *Fact Check*, safe consumption was reaffirmed that equates to more than 9 to 14 cans of diet soda pop per day to exceed the acceptable daily intake, assuming no other intake from other food sources.

Persons with the rare disease called phenylketonuria (PKU), which interferes with the metabolism of phenylalanine, should avoid aspartame because of its high phenylalanine content. People with PKU will find a mandatory warning label on products containing aspartame.

Luo Han Guo. Luo han guo is an extract of the monk fruit. It was approved by the FDA and is sold as the sweeteners Nectresse™ and Monk Fruit in the Raw™.

Neotame. Neotame was approved by the FDA for use as a general-purpose sweetener but is used in few foods. Neotame is heat stable and can be used as a tabletop sweetener as well as in cooking. Neotame is safe for use by the general population, including children, during pregnancy and lactation, and for people with diabetes. Although similar to aspartame, neotame does not require labeling for people with PKU because it is not broken down in the body to individual amino acid components.

Saccharin. Discovered and used since 1879, **saccharin** represents about half of the artificial sweetener market in the United States (typically packaged in pink packets, including Sweet 'N Low®).

Stevia. Stevia, sold as Truvia® and Sweet Leaf®, is an artificial sweetener derived from a South American plant and provides no energy. It has been used in teas and as a sweetener in Japan since the 1970s, and it is considered generally recognized as safe (GRAS) for use in foods.

Sucralose. Sucralose (Splenda®) is made by adding three chlorine molecules to sucrose. It cannot be broken down or absorbed, so it yields no calories. Sucralose is approved as an additive to foods such as soft drinks, gum, baked goods, syrups, gelatins, frozen dairy desserts such as ice cream, jams, processed fruits, and fruit juices, and for tabletop use.

To Sugar or Not to Sugar . . . That Is the Question! There is much controversy surrounding which is a healthier option—consuming artificially sweetened diet soft drinks or natural sugar–sweetened beverages. Like most of the field of nutrition, the answer is quite complex. In some studies, high consumption of artificial sweeteners has been

phenylketonuria (PKU) Disease caused by a defect in the liver's ability to metabolize the amino acid phenylalanine. If left untreated, toxic by-products of phenylalanine build up in the body and lead to brain damage and severe health issues.

allulose Naturally occurring sugar in some food sources that is about 70% as sweet as sugar.

luo han guo Extract of the monk fruit, this artificial sweetener is 100 to 250 times sweeter than sucrose.

neotame General-purpose, nonnutritive sweetener that is approximately 7000 to 13,000 times sweeter than table sugar. It has a chemical structure similar to aspartame.

saccharin Artificial sweetener that yields no energy to the body; 200 to 700 times sweeter than sucrose.

stevia Artificial sweetener derived from a South American shrub; 200 to 400 times sweeter than sucrose.

sucralose Artificial sweetener that has chlorines in place of 3 hydroxyl (—OH) groups on sucrose; 600 times sweeter than sucrose.

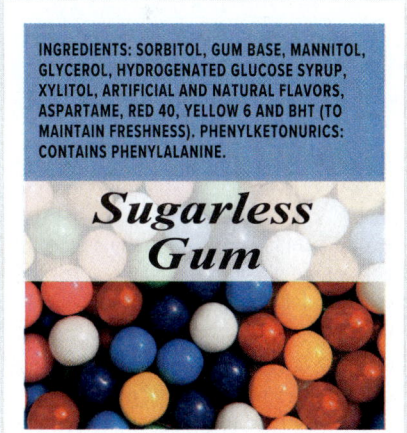

Sugar alcohols and the artificial sweetener aspartame are used to sweeten this product. Note the warning for people with phenylketonuria (PKU) that this product is made with aspartame. **What is the significance behind this health warning?** Nancy R. Cohen/Photodisc/Getty Images

linked with appetite alterations, obesity promotion, and even changes in gut microbes. On the other hand, we have definitive scientific evidence that large quantities of added sugars (such as those found in soda and in sports and energy drinks) are related to dental caries, obesity, risk of obesity-related chronic disease, and even alterations in brain function. Until we know more, reputable scientific organizations recommend that people replace sugar-sweetened and artificially sweetened drinks with carbonated, plain, or unsweetened flavored water.[14]

✓ CONCEPT CHECK 4.3

1. Which food groups are the primary sources of carbohydrate?
2. What specific foods contain the highest percentage of calories from carbohydrates?
3. List three common nutritive sweeteners.
4. Name two artificial sweeteners that are approved for use in food.

4.4 Making Carbohydrates Available for Body Use

As discussed previously, simply consuming a food or beverage does not supply nutrients to body cells. Digestion and absorption must occur first.

STARCH AND SUGAR DIGESTION

Food preparation can be viewed as the start of carbohydrate digestion because cooking softens tough connective structures in the fibrous parts of plants, such as broccoli stalks. When starches are heated, the starch granules swell as they soak up water, making them much easier to digest. All of these effects of cooking generally make carbohydrate-containing foods easier to chew, swallow, and break down during digestion.

The enzymatic digestion of starch begins in the mouth, when the saliva, which contains an enzyme called salivary amylase, mixes with carbohydrate-containing food products during the chewing of food. This amylase immediately breaks down starch into many smaller units, primarily disaccharides, such as maltose (Fig. 4-12). You can taste this conversion while chewing a saltine cracker. Prolonged chewing of the cracker causes it to taste sweeter as some starch breaks down into the sweeter disaccharides, such as maltose. Usually, food is in the mouth for such a short amount of time that this phase of digestion is negligible. In addition, once the food moves down the esophagus and reaches the stomach, the acidic environment inactivates salivary amylase.

When the carbohydrates reach the small intestine, the more alkaline environment of the intestine is better suited for further carbohydrate digestion. The pancreas releases enzymes, such as pancreatic amylase, to aid the last stage of starch digestion. After amylase action, the original carbohydrates in a food are now present in the small intestine as disaccharides (maltose from starch breakdown, lactose mainly from dairy products, and sucrose from food and added at the table) as well as the monosaccharides glucose and fructose initially present as such in food.

The disaccharides are digested to their single monosaccharide units once they reach the wall of the small intestine, where the specialized enzymes on the absorptive cells digest each disaccharide into monosaccharides. The enzyme **maltase** acts on maltose to produce two glucose molecules. **Sucrase** acts on sucrose to produce glucose and fructose. **Lactase** acts on lactose to produce glucose and galactose.

LACTOSE MALDIGESTION AND LACTOSE INTOLERANCE

Deficient production of the enzyme lactase will impair the digestion of lactose. The most common form of this condition is **primary lactose maldigestion,** a normal pattern of physiology that often begins to develop around ages 2 to 5 years.[15] This primary

maltase An enzyme made by absorptive cells of the small intestine; this enzyme digests maltose to two glucose molecules.

sucrase An enzyme made by absorptive cells of the small intestine; this enzyme digests sucrose to glucose and fructose.

lactase An enzyme made by absorptive cells of the small intestine; this enzyme digests lactose to glucose and galactose.

primary lactose maldigestion Develops at about age 2 to 5 years when the production of the enzyme lactase decreases. When significant symptoms develop after lactose intake, it is then called *lactose intolerance.*

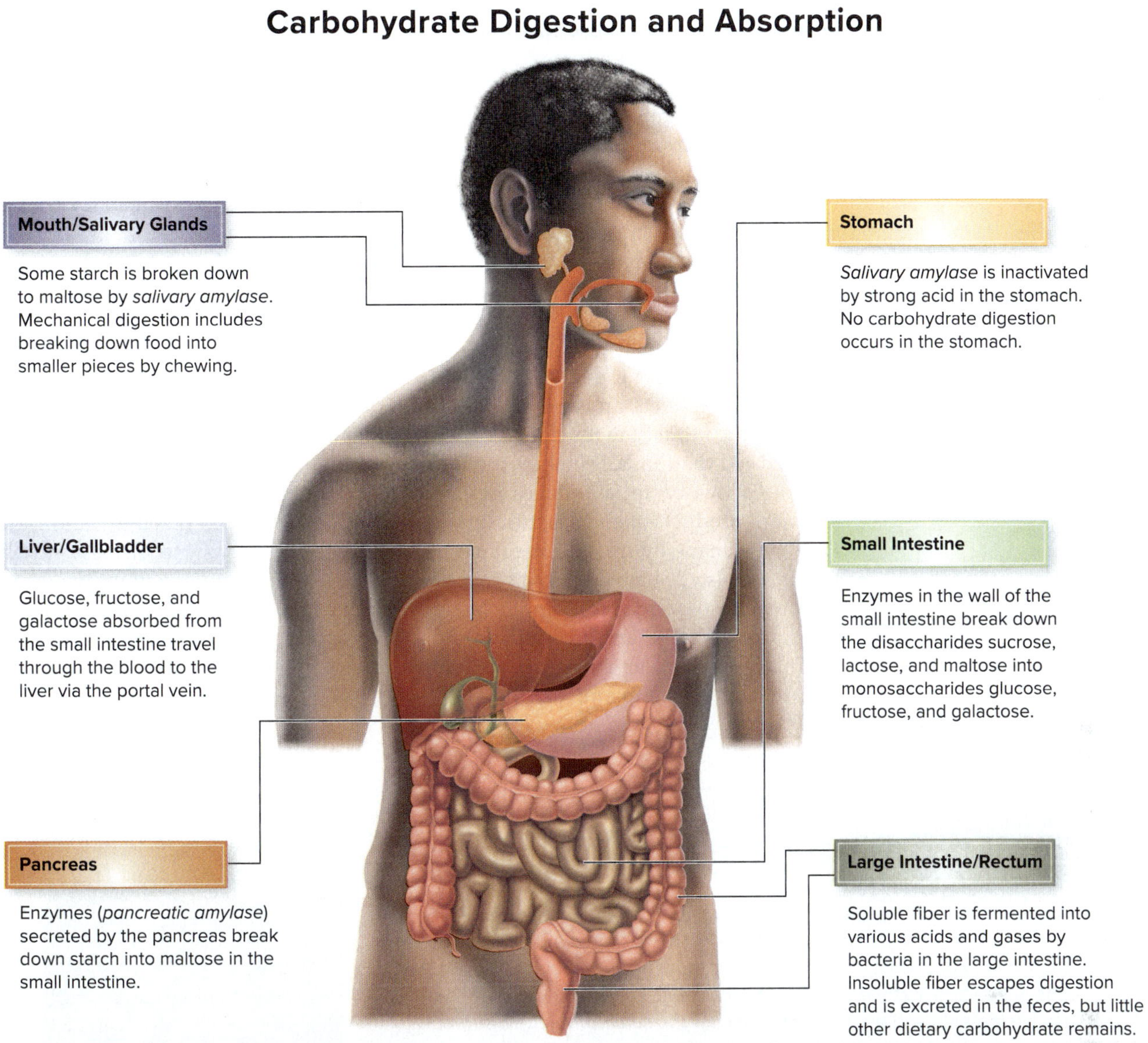

Carbohydrate Digestion and Absorption

Mouth/Salivary Glands
Some starch is broken down to maltose by *salivary amylase*. Mechanical digestion includes breaking down food into smaller pieces by chewing.

Stomach
Salivary amylase is inactivated by strong acid in the stomach. No carbohydrate digestion occurs in the stomach.

Liver/Gallbladder
Glucose, fructose, and galactose absorbed from the small intestine travel through the blood to the liver via the portal vein.

Small Intestine
Enzymes in the wall of the small intestine break down the disaccharides sucrose, lactose, and maltose into monosaccharides glucose, fructose, and galactose.

Pancreas
Enzymes (*pancreatic amylase*) secreted by the pancreas break down starch into maltose in the small intestine.

Large Intestine/Rectum
Soluble fiber is fermented into various acids and gases by bacteria in the large intestine. Insoluble fiber escapes digestion and is excreted in the feces, but little other dietary carbohydrate remains.

FIGURE 4-12 Carbohydrate digestion and absorption. Enzymes made by the mouth, pancreas, and small intestine participate in the process of digestion. Most carbohydrate digestion and absorption take place in the small intestine.

form of lactose maldigestion is estimated to be present in about 68% of the world's population, although not all of these individuals experience symptoms and most continue to produce some lactase.[16]

Secondary lactose maldigestion is a temporary condition in which lactase production is decreased in response to another condition, such as intestinal diarrhea. Rarely, lactase production is absent from birth, a condition known as **congenital lactase deficiency**. Any of these types of lactose maldigestion can lead to symptoms of gas, abdominal bloating, cramps, and diarrhea when lactose is consumed. The bloating and gas are caused by bacterial fermentation of lactose in the large intestine. The diarrhea is caused by undigested lactose in the large intestine as it draws water from the circulatory system into the large intestine. When significant symptoms develop after lactose intake, it is then called **lactose intolerance**. It is important to note that lactose maldigestion and resultant lactose intolerance are not equivalent to a milk allergy.

Lactose intolerance is most prevalent in people of East Asian descent. It is also common in people of West African, Arab, Jewish, Greek, and Italian descent, and the occurrence increases as people age. Individuals with lactose intolerance can handle

secondary lactose maldigestion Temporary condition in which lactase production is decreased in response to illness or surgery.

congenital lactase deficiency A rare birth defect resulting in the inability to produce lactase, such that a lactose-free diet is required from birth.

lactose intolerance A condition in which symptoms such as abdominal gas and bloating appear as a result of severe lactose maldigestion.

varying amounts of lactose. Research suggests that many people can tolerate approximately 12 grams of lactose (the amount in about 1 cup of milk) without symptoms or with only mild symptoms.[16] Thus, it is unnecessary for these people to totally restrict or avoid their intake of lactose-containing foods, such as milk and milk products, which are important for maintaining bone health. Obtaining enough calcium and vitamin D from food and beverages is much easier if milk and milk products are included in a dietary pattern.

Recall that the dairy group includes fat-free and low-fat milk and fortified soy alternatives. Be sure to check the Nutrition Facts label to be sure your soy alternative contains added calcium, vitamin A, and vitamin D. Again, other plant-based dairy alternatives may not be fortified with these key nutrients and, therefore, not included as part of the dairy group.

Individuals with lactose maldigestion usually still produce some lactase. Combining lactose-containing foods with other foods is helpful because certain foods can have positive effects on rates of digestion. For example, fat in a meal slows digestion, leaving more time for lactase action. Hard cheese and yogurt are also more easily tolerated than milk. Much of the lactose is lost during the production of cheese, and the active bacteria cultures in yogurt digest the lactose with their lactase. In addition, products such as lactose-free or lactose-reduced milk (Lactaid® and Dairy Ease®) are made by treating regular milk with the lactase enzyme. Lactase supplements are also available to assist those with lactose maldigestion when they decide to consume products containing lactose. Many plant-based milks, including soy milk, almond milk, and rice milk, are naturally lactose free and can be used as an alternative to regular milk. Just be sure to read labels to see if these products are fortified with calcium and vitamin D.

CASE STUDY   Problems with Milk Intake

Myeshia is a 19-year-old African-American female who recently read about the health benefits of calcium and decided to increase her intake of dairy products. To start, she drank a cup of 1% milk at lunch. Not long afterward, she experienced bloating, cramping, and increased gas production. She suspected that the culprit of this pain was the milk she consumed, especially because her parents and her sister complain of the same problem. She wanted to determine if other milk products were, in fact, the cause of her discomfort, so the next day she substituted a cup of yogurt for the glass of milk at lunch. Consuming the yogurt did not cause any pain.

Answer the following questions about Myeshia:

1. Why did Myeshia believe that she was sensitive to milk?
2. What component of milk is likely causing the problems that Myeshia experiences after drinking milk?
3. Why does this component cause intestinal discomfort in some individuals?
4. What is the name of this condition?
5. What groups of people are most likely to experience this condition?
6. Why did consuming yogurt not cause the same effects for Myeshia?
7. Are there any other products on the market that can replace regular milk or otherwise alleviate symptoms for individuals with this problem?
8. Can people with this condition ever drink regular milk?
9. What other foods should Myeshia include to supply the calcium, potassium, vitamin A, and vitamin D that are typically found in cow's milk?
10. Why do some individuals have trouble tolerating milk products during or immediately after an intestinal viral infection?

Complete the Case Study. Responses to these questions can be provided by your instructor.

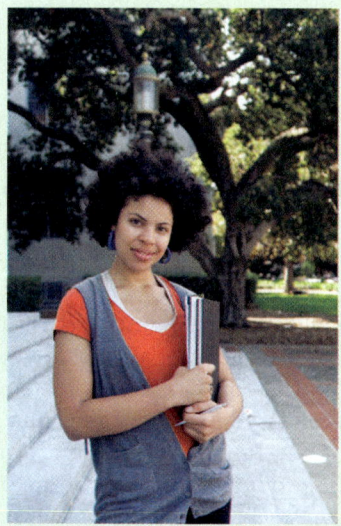

College students, like Myeshia, are wise to listen to their bodies and seek professional assistance when needed. Chuckstock/Shutterstock

CARBOHYDRATE ABSORPTION

Monosaccharides found naturally in foods and those formed as byproducts of starch and disaccharide digestion in the mouth and small intestine generally follow an active absorption process. Recall that this is a process that requires a specific carrier and energy input for the substance to be taken up by the absorptive cells in the small intestine. Glucose and its close relative galactose undergo active absorption. They are pumped into the absorptive cells along with sodium.

Fructose is taken up by the absorptive cells via facilitated diffusion. In this case, a carrier is used, but no energy input is needed. This absorptive process is thus slower than that seen with glucose or galactose. So, large doses of fructose are not readily absorbed and can contribute to diarrhea as the monosaccharide remains in the small intestine and attracts water.

Once glucose, galactose, and fructose enter the absorptive cells, some fructose is metabolized into glucose. The single sugars in the absorptive cells are then transferred to the portal vein that goes directly to the liver. The liver then metabolizes those sugars by transforming the monosaccharides galactose and fructose into glucose and:

- Releases it directly into the bloodstream for transport to organs such as the brain and kidneys and to muscles and adipose tissues;
- Produces glycogen for storage of carbohydrate; and
- Produces fat when carbohydrates are consumed in high amounts and overall calorie needs are exceeded.

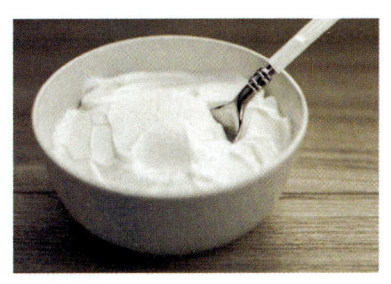

Use of yogurt helps those with lactose maldigestion meet calcium needs. **What other foods might you recommend for individuals affected by lactose maldigestion?**
Anastasios71/Shutterstock

Unless an individual has a condition that causes malabsorption or an intolerance to a carbohydrate such as lactose (or fructose), only a minor amount of some sugars (about 10%) escapes digestion. Any undigested carbohydrate travels to the large intestine. Some of that undigested carbohydrate (i.e., fermentable fiber) can be fermented by bacteria. The acids and gases produced by bacterial metabolism of the undigested carbohydrate are absorbed into the bloodstream. Scientists suspect that some of these products of bacterial metabolism promote the health of the large intestine by providing it with a source of calories.

FIBER AND INTESTINAL HEALTH

Bacteria in the large intestine ferment soluble fibers into such products as acids and gases. The acids, once absorbed, also provide calories for the body. In this way, soluble fibers provide about 1.5 kcal per gram. Although the intestinal gas (flatulence) produced by this bacterial fermentation is not harmful, it can be painful and sometimes embarrassing. Over time, however, the body tends to adapt to a high-fiber dietary pattern, eventually producing less gas. Many gas-forming foods are good sources of soluble fiber.

Because insoluble fiber is an indigestible carbohydrate, it remains in the intestinal tract and supplies bulk to the feces, making elimination much easier. When enough fiber is consumed, the stool is large and soft because many types of plant fibers attract water. The larger size stimulates the intestinal muscles to contract, which aids elimination. Consequently, less pressure is necessary to expel the stool. When too little fiber is eaten, the opposite can occur: very little water is present in the feces, making it small and hard. Constipation may result, which forces one to exert excessive pressure in the large intestine during defecation. Hemorrhoids may also result from excessive straining during defecation.

Increased fluid intake is extremely important with a high-fiber dietary pattern. Inadequate fluid intake can leave the stool very hard and painful to eliminate. In more severe cases, the combination of excess fiber and insufficient fluid may contribute to blockages in the intestine, which may require surgery. Aside from problems with the passage of materials through the GI tract, a high-fiber dietary pattern may also decrease the availability of nutrients. Certain components of fiber may bind to essential minerals, blocking them from being absorbed. For example, when fiber is consumed in large amounts, zinc, calcium, magnesium, and iron absorption may be hindered. Although there is no Upper Intake Level set for fiber, dangerous levels could occur with excessive fiber supplement use.

magnificent microbiome

Microbiota-Accessible Carbohydrates
One function of the gut microbiota is to consume carbohydrates. Microbiota-accessible carbohydrates (MACs) are indigestible complex carbohydrates found in fruits, vegetables, whole grains, and legumes that our microbiota feeds on. By consuming MACs, we can cultivate healthy microorganisms to improve overall health, reduce inflammation, support immunity, and even promote positive mental health.

Many population studies have shown a link between increased fiber intake and a decrease in colon cancer development. Most research on dietary patterns and colon cancer focuses on the potential preventive effects of fruits, vegetables, whole grain breads and cereals, and beans. It is more advisable to increase fiber intake by using fiber-rich foods than by relying on fiber supplements. Overall, the health benefits to the colon that stem from a high-fiber dietary pattern are partially due to the nutrients that are commonly present in most high-fiber foods, such as vitamins, minerals, phytochemicals, and, in some cases, essential fatty acids.

A group of carbohydrates known as FODMAPs (fermentable oligo-, di-, and monosaccharides and polyols) may cause gastrointestinal symptoms such as gas, bloating, and diarrhea in some people. The FODMAPs include fructose, lactose, fructans (in wheat, onions, and garlic), galactans (in legumes), and polyols (sugar alcohols). Some individuals appear to be poor digesters of FODMAPs; thus, these carbohydrates reach the large intestine without being digested, leading to bloating and gas. A low-FODMAP diet may provide relief for some people who experience gastrointestinal distress after meals, but this is not a cure-all. It is important to work with a gastroenterologist and RDN when limiting FODMAPs. Ideally, you should eliminate only those foods that trigger digestive problems; overly restrictive dietary patterns can lead to nutrient inadequacies.[17]

✓ CONCEPT CHECK 4.4

1. In what form are carbohydrates absorbed, and what happens to these compounds after absorption?
2. What are the names of the enzymes that digest carbohydrates?
3. What are the beneficial effects of fiber in the intestinal tract?

4.5 Putting Carbohydrates to Work in the Body

As discussed, all of the digestible carbohydrate that we eat is eventually converted into glucose. Glucose then goes on to function in body metabolism. The other sugars can generally be converted into glucose, and the starches are broken down to yield glucose, so the functions described here apply to most carbohydrates. The functions of glucose in the body start with supplying calories to fuel the body.

PROVIDING ENERGY

The main function of glucose is to supply calories for use by the body. Certain tissues in the body, such as red blood cells, can use only glucose and other simple carbohydrate forms for fuel. Most parts of the brain and central nervous system also derive energy only from glucose, unless the dietary pattern contains almost no available glucose. In that case, the brain can use partial breakdown products of fat—called **ketone bodies**—for energy needs. Other body cells, including muscle cells, can use simple carbohydrates as fuel, but many of these cells can also use fat or protein for energy needs.

A dietary pattern that supplies enough carbohydrates to prevent breakdown of proteins for energy needs is considered protein sparing. Under normal circumstances, digestible carbohydrates end up as blood glucose, and protein is reserved for functions such as building and maintaining muscles and vital organs. However, if you don't eat enough carbohydrates, your body is forced to make glucose from body proteins, draining the pool of amino acids available in cells for other critical functions. During long-term starvation, the continuous withdrawal of proteins from the muscles, heart, liver, kidneys, and other vital organs can result in weakness, poor function, and even failure of body systems.

ketone bodies Partial breakdown products of fat that contain three or four carbons.

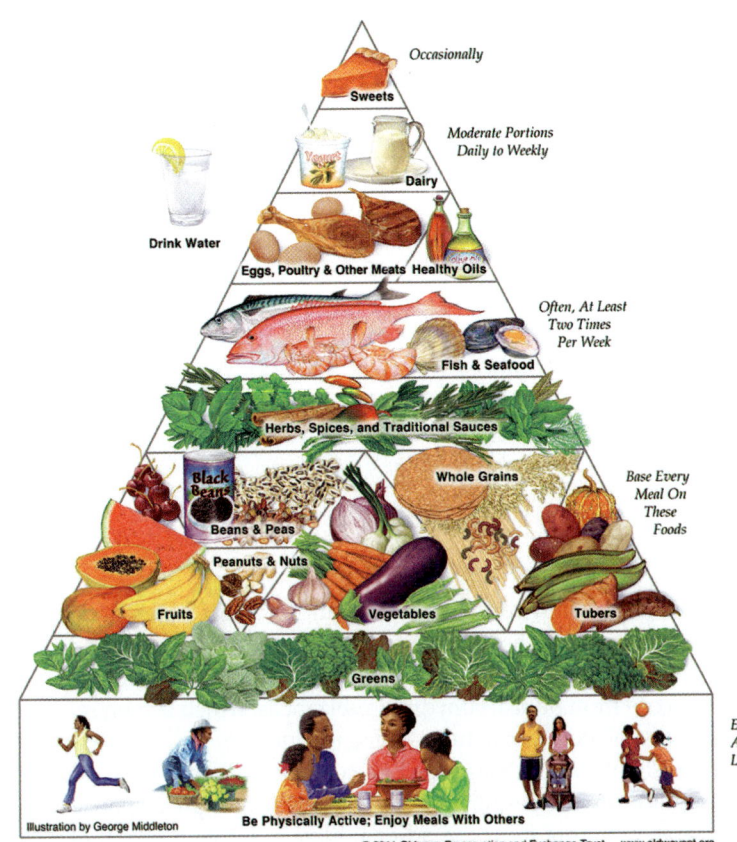

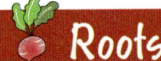

African Heritage Dietary Pattern

We belong to a beautiful and diverse country where one size does not fit all. The African Heritage Diet Pyramid (Fig. 4-13) illustrates a dietary pattern that incorporates traditional foods and flavors from many regions of the world. For instance, did you know that crops like rice, peanuts, okra, and black-eyed peas originated in Africa? Indeed, individuals with African roots enjoy foods steeped in history and tradition while embracing a varied dietary pattern. With more recent influences shared by our southern U.S. states, South America, and the Caribbean, we can appreciate and celebrate the African framework that permeates through all our dietary patterns.

FIGURE 4-13 The African Heritage Diet Pyramid is based on dietary patterns from the African region. Oldways, www.oldwayspt.org

In addition to the loss of protein, when you don't eat enough carbohydrates, the metabolism of fats is inefficient. In the absence of adequate carbohydrates, fats are not broken down completely in metabolism and instead form ketone bodies. This condition, known as **ketosis,** should be avoided because it disturbs the body's normal acid–base balance and leads to other health problems. This is a good reason to question the long-term safety of the low-carbohydrate diets that have been popular. Therapeutic ketogenic diets have proven effective for treating epilepsy for some individuals. Research is underway to evaluate keto diets in cancer therapies, sports nutrition, diabetes, and weight loss.

ketosis The condition of having a high concentration of ketone bodies and related breakdown products in the bloodstream and tissues.

REGULATING BLOOD GLUCOSE

Under normal circumstances, your blood glucose concentration is regulated within a narrow range. When carbohydrates are digested and taken up by the absorptive cells of the small intestine, the resulting monosaccharides are transported directly to the liver. One of the liver's roles, then, is to guard against excess glucose entering the bloodstream after a meal. The liver works together with the pancreas to regulate blood glucose.

When the concentration of glucose in the blood is high, such as during and immediately after a meal, the pancreas releases the hormone insulin into the bloodstream. Insulin delivers two different messages to various body cells to cause the level of glucose in the blood to fall. First, insulin directs muscle, adipose, and other cells to remove glucose from the bloodstream by taking it into those cells. Second, insulin directs the liver to store glucose as glycogen. By triggering both glycogen synthesis in the liver and glucose movement out of the bloodstream into certain cells, insulin keeps the concentration of glucose from rising too high in the blood (Fig. 4-14).

FIGURE 4-14 Regulation of blood glucose. Insulin and glucagon are key factors in controlling blood glucose. When blood glucose rises above the normal range (100 mg/dl or above) and blood glucose becomes elevated: (1) insulin is released from the pancreas (2) to lower it (3) and (4) blood glucose then falls back into the normal range (5). Inversely, when blood glucose falls below the normal range (6), glucagon is released (7), which has the opposite effect of insulin (8) and (9), and this then restores blood glucose to the normal range (10). Other hormones, such as epinephrine, norepinephrine, cortisol, and growth hormone, also affect blood glucose levels.

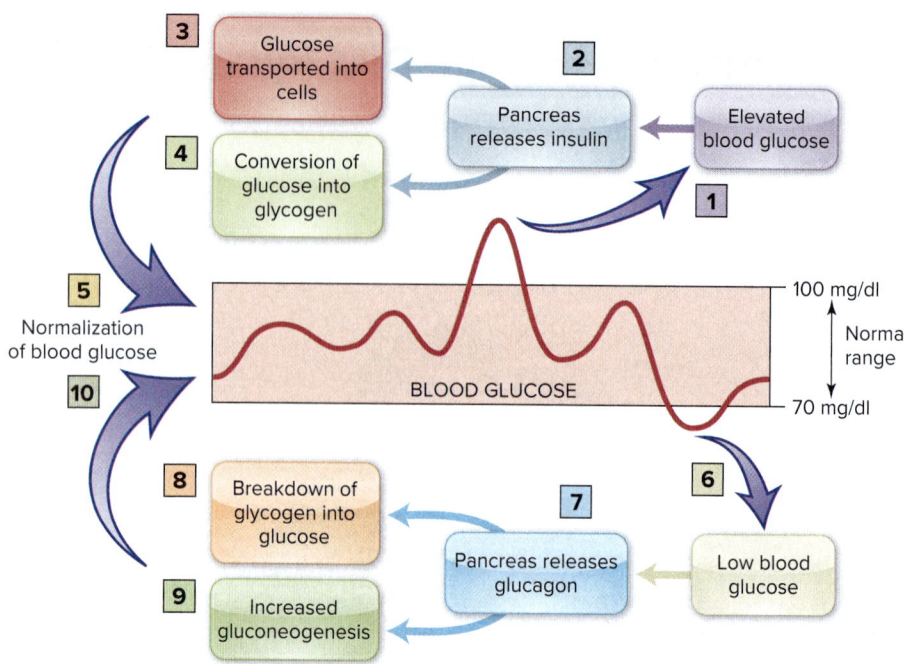

hyperglycemia High blood glucose, typically defined as above 125 mg/dl while in a fasted state.

hypoglycemia A condition caused by low levels of blood sugar that is often related to the treatment of diabetes and often defined by 70 mg/dl or less.

type 1 diabetes A form of diabetes characterized by total insulin deficiency due to destruction of insulin-producing cells of the pancreas. Insulin therapy is required.

prediabetes A serious health condition in which blood sugar levels are higher than normal, but not high enough to be diagnosed as type 2 diabetes.

On the other hand, when you have not eaten for a few hours and blood glucose begins to fall, the pancreas releases the hormone glucagon. This hormone has the opposite effect of insulin. It prompts the breakdown of liver glycogen into glucose and the generation of glucose from noncarbohydrate substances, which is then released into the bloodstream to keep blood glucose from falling too low.

A different mechanism increases blood glucose during times of stress. Epinephrine (adrenaline) is the hormone responsible for the flight-or-fight response. Epinephrine is released in large amounts from the adrenal glands (located on top of each kidney) in response to a perceived threat, such as a car approaching head-on. These hormones cause glycogen in the liver to be quickly broken down into glucose. The resulting rapid flood of glucose from the liver into the bloodstream helps fuel quick mental and physical reactions.

This complex regulatory system is responsible for maintaining blood glucose within an acceptable range. It provides a safeguard against extremely high blood glucose **(hyperglycemia)** or low blood glucose **(hypoglycemia).** In essence, the actions of insulin on blood glucose are balanced by the actions of glucagon, epinephrine, and other hormones. If hormonal balance is not maintained, major changes in blood glucose concentrations occur. The disease **type 1 diabetes** is an example of the underproduction of insulin.

Lifestyle Management and Blood Glucose Control. Continued evidence supports lifestyle management techniques to improve blood glucose control. Directly aligning with the *Dietary Guidelines*, individuals are encouraged to consume a healthy dietary pattern rich in vegetables; fruits; whole grains; seafood; eggs; beans, peas, and lentils; unsalted nuts and seeds; fat-free and low-fat dairy products; and lean meats and poultry. Fat quality (selecting monounsaturated and polyunsaturated fats over saturated fats) has been found to be more important than fat quantity. Recommendations also encourage limiting or avoiding intake of sugar-sweetened beverages, reducing sodium to less than 2300 mg per day, and eating fatty fish at least two times (2 servings) per week. Note that dietary patterns that align to the majority of these guidelines include the Mediterranean, vegan, vegetarian, low-fat, low-carb, and DASH diets. To be safe, individuals with inadequate blood glucose control or those diagnosed with **prediabetes** or diabetes should work closely with an endocrinologist and registered dietitian to obtain individualized lifestyle recommendations. If insulin is prescribed, it may be necessary to count carbohydrates, protein, and fat until insulin dosing and blood glucose levels are controlled.

Glycemic Response and Blood Glucose. Our bodies react uniquely to different sources of carbohydrates. For example, a serving of a high-fiber food, such as black beans, results in lower blood glucose levels compared to the same size serving of mashed white potatoes. The effects of various foods on blood glucose are important to know because foods that result in a higher blood glucose level cause a larger release of insulin from the pancreas. When this higher insulin output occurs frequently, it leads to deleterious effects on the body. Some of these undesirable effects are high blood triglycerides, increased fat deposition in the adipose tissue, increased tendency for blood to clot, and increased fat synthesis in the liver. In addition, as insulin rapidly pulls glucose from the blood and into cells, hunger-regulating hormones are released, thus promoting increased refined carbohydrate intake. Over time, this increase in insulin output may also cause the muscles to become resistant to the action of insulin and eventually lead to **type 2 diabetes** in some people.

The **glycemic index (GI)** is a measurement of how the carbohydrate in a food raises blood glucose and has been used as a measure for planning dietary patterns for those with diabetes. Glycemic index is a ratio of the blood glucose response to a given food compared to the response to a reference such as glucose or white bread. Foods are ranked based on this comparison with a high GI food raising blood glucose more than a medium or low GI food.

The GI of a food is influenced by starch structure, fiber content, and food processing. In an effort to explain why glycemic responses to the same foods differ so greatly between people, scientists are now studying the interactions between individual physiological and genetic characteristics as well as the gut microbiome in regulation of individual glycemic responses.[18] Also keep in mind that the GI value only describes the type, not the amount, of carbohydrate in a food. The **glycemic load (GL)** measures both the quality and quantity of carbohydrates in meals. Knowing how different foods affect blood glucose can be helpful in meal planning. Portion sizes are important to manage in order to control blood glucose and maintain weight. Maintaining a healthy body weight and performing regular physical activity further reduce the effects of a high GI dietary pattern. The International Glycemic Index (GI) Database was developed to provide a public-use database of the glycemic index and glycemic load of foods.[19]

FIBER: REDUCING CHOLESTEROL ABSORPTION AND OBESITY RISK

Aside from its role in maintaining bowel regularity, the consumption of fiber has many additional health benefits. A high intake of soluble fiber also inhibits absorption of cholesterol and cholesterol-rich bile acids from the small intestine, thereby reducing blood cholesterol and possibly reducing the risk of cardiovascular disease and gallstones. Recall good sources of soluble fiber include apples, bananas, oranges, carrots, barley, oats, and kidney beans. The beneficial bacteria in the large intestine degrade soluble fiber and produce certain fatty acids that probably also reduce cholesterol synthesis in the liver. In addition, the slower glucose absorption that occurs with dietary patterns high in soluble fiber is linked to a decrease in insulin release. One of the effects of insulin is to stimulate cholesterol synthesis in the liver, so this reduction in insulin may contribute to the ability of soluble fiber to lower blood cholesterol. Overall, a fiber-rich dietary pattern containing fruits, vegetables, beans, and whole grains is advocated as part of a strategy to reduce risk of cardiovascular disease. Again, this is something that a low-carbohydrate dietary pattern cannot promise.

A dietary pattern high in fiber helps control weight and reduces the risk of developing obesity.[20] Due to their bulky nature, high-fiber foods require more time to chew and move out of the stomach, and thus they fill us up without yielding many calories. Increasing intake of foods rich in fiber is one strategy for feeling satisfied or full after a meal.

type 2 diabetes A form of diabetes characterized by insulin resistance and often associated with obesity. Insulin therapy may be required in advanced stages of the disease.

glycemic index (GI) The blood glucose response of a given food, compared to a standard (typically, glucose or white bread). Glycemic index is influenced by starch structure, fiber content, food processing, physical structure, and macronutrients such as fat in the meal.

glycemic load (GL) A measure of both the quality (GI value) and quantity (grams per serving) of a carbohydrate in a meal.

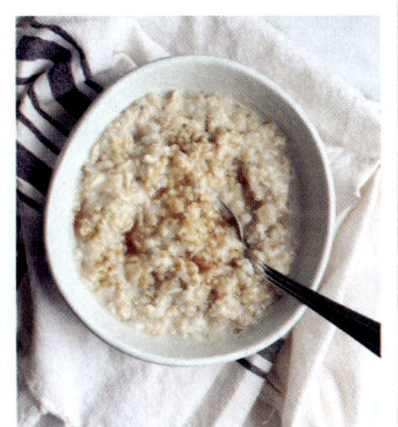

Oatmeal is a rich source of soluble fiber. The FDA allows a health claim for the benefits of oatmeal to lower blood cholesterol because of the effects of this soluble fiber. **How does soluble fiber help to reduce blood cholesterol?** Alexis Joseph/McGraw Hill

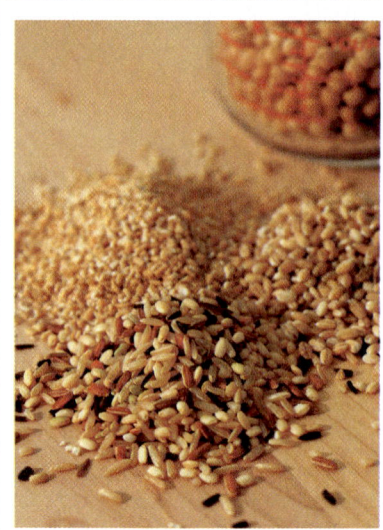

The *Dietary Guidelines* recommends half of all grains come from whole grains in your dietary pattern. Recall that whole grains contain all parts of the kernel. **What are the three components of the kernel?** Nancy R. Cohen/Photodisc /Getty Images

FIGURE 4-15 Carbohydrate-specific recommendations from the *Dietary Guidelines for Americans.*
Source: DietaryGuidelines.gov

✓ **CONCEPT CHECK 4.5**

1. What is the primary role of carbohydrates in the body?
2. How does the body respond when too little carbohydrate is consumed?
3. What are the mechanisms by which blood glucose levels are maintained within a narrow range?
4. What are some of the important functions of fiber?

4.6 Carbohydrate Needs

The RDA for carbohydrates is 130 grams per day for adults. This is based on the amount needed to supply adequate glucose for the brain and nervous system, without having to rely on ketone bodies from incomplete fat breakdown as a calorie source. Somewhat exceeding this amount is fine; the recommended carbohydrate intake ranges from 45% to 65% of total calories. The Nutrition Facts label on foods uses 55% of calorie intake as the standard for recommended carbohydrate intake. This would be 275 grams of carbohydrate when consuming a dietary pattern of 2000 kcal.

Recommendations for carbohydrate consumption, however, emphasize the type of carbohydrates we should consume rather than just the total amount. Experts agree that one's carbohydrate intake should be based primarily on vegetables (dark green; red and orange; beans, peas, and lentils), fruits (especially whole fruit), and grains (at least half of which are whole grain), rather than on refined grains, starchy foods, and added sugars.

The *Dietary Guidelines* recommends that we choose fiber-rich fruits, vegetables, and whole grains often (Fig. 4-15). More specifically, 3 or more ounce equivalents of grains—roughly one-half of one's grains—should be whole. Whole grain is defined as the entire grain

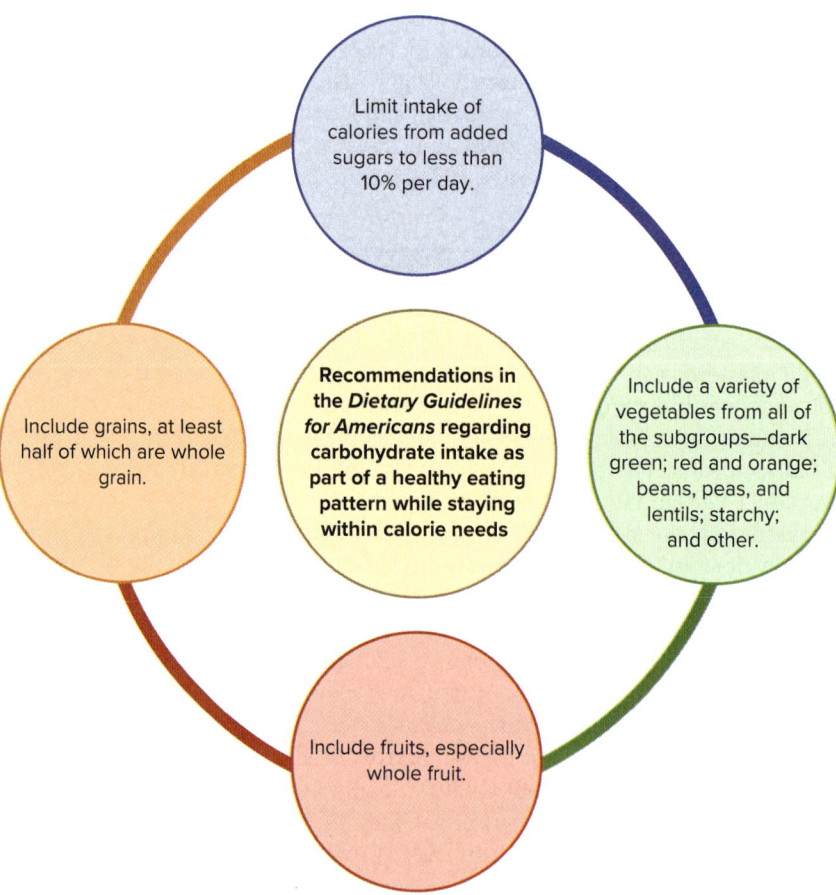

seed or kernel made of three components: the bran, germ, and endosperm, which must be in nearly the same relative proportions as the original grain if cracked, crushed, or flaked.[7]

HOW MUCH FIBER DO WE NEED?

An Adequate Intake for fiber has been set based on the ability of fiber to reduce risk of disease. The Adequate Intake for fiber for adults is 25 grams per day for females and 38 grams per day for males. The goal is to provide at least 14 grams per 1000 kcal in a dietary pattern. After age 50, the Adequate Intake falls to 21 grams per day and 30 grams per day, respectively. The Daily Value used for fiber on food and supplement labels is 28 grams for a 2000 kcal dietary pattern.[21]

In the United States, fiber intake remains well below the recommended values. More than 90% of women and 97% of men do not meet recommended intakes for dietary fiber.[5] This low intake is attributed to the lack of knowledge on the benefits of whole grains and the inability to recognize whole grain products at the time of purchase. Thus, most of us could benefit from increasing our fiber intake. At least 3 ounce equivalents of whole grains per day are recommended. Eating a high-fiber cereal (at least 3 grams of fiber per serving) for breakfast is one easy way to increase fiber intake (Fig. 4-16).[4] Other strategies include increasing dietary intakes of fruits and vegetables, and replacing refined grains with whole grains.

HOW MUCH SUGAR IS TOO MUCH?

The main problems with consuming an excess amount of sugar are that it provides discretionary calories and increases the risk for dental decay, weight gain, and other health issues.

Dietary Quality Declines When Sugar Intake Is Excessive. Overconsumption of sweet treats can leave little room for important, nutrient-dense foods, such as fruits and vegetables. Children and teenagers are at the highest risk for consuming too many discretionary calories in place of nutrients essential for growth. Many children and teenagers are drinking an excess of sugar-sweetened soft drinks and other sugar-containing beverages, including energy and sports drinks, and much less milk than ever before. Replacing sugar-laden drinks for milk can compromise bone health because milk contains calcium and vitamin D, which are both essential for bone health.

Remember that added sugars are sugars added to foods during processing and preparation. The *Dietary Guidelines* continues to strongly recommend that added sugars provide no more than 10% of total daily calorie intake. Dietary patterns that go beyond this upper limit are likely to be deficient in vitamins and minerals. A moderate intake of about 10% of calorie intake corresponds to a maximum of approximately 50 grams (or 12.5 teaspoons) of sugars per day, based on a 2000 kcal dietary pattern. Because of the association between excessive consumption of sugars and several metabolic abnormalities and adverse health conditions, the American Heart Association recommends reductions in the intake of added sugars such that the upper limit of intake for most American females is no more than 100 kcal (25 grams) per day from added sugars and no more than 150 kcal (36 grams) per day for most American males.[22]

Most of the sugars we consume come from foods and beverages to which sugar has been added during processing or manufacturing. Major sources of added sugars include sugar-sweetened beverages, desserts and sweet snacks, and sweetened coffee and tea (Fig. 4-17).

Supersizing sugar-rich beverages has also become common and has led to more sugar consumption. For example, in the 1950s, a typical serving size of a cola soft drink was a 6.5-ounce bottle, and now a 20-ounce plastic bottle is a typical serving. This one change in serving size contributes an extra 164 kcal to the dietary pattern—all from added sugars. Most convenience stores now offer cups that will hold 64 ounces of soft drink. Health messages about the sugary beverages appear to be having some positive effects, resulting in a decrease in soft drink sales over the past decade. Market research

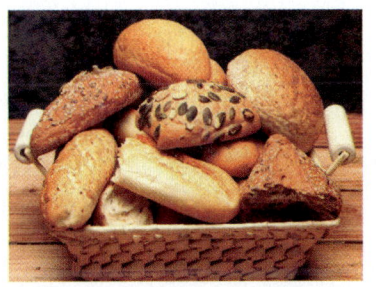

When buying a bread labeled as *wheat bread*, most people think they are buying a whole wheat product. Because the flour is from the wheat plant, manufacturers can correctly list enriched white (refined) flour as wheat flour on food labels; however, if *whole wheat flour* is not listed first on the ingredient list, then the product is not primarily a whole wheat bread. **Look for 100% whole grain or whole wheat flour on the label for breads that are an excellent source of fiber.** ninikas /iStockphoto/Getty Images

FIGURE 4-16 When choosing a breakfast cereal, it is generally wise to focus on those that are rich sources of fiber. Sugar content can also be used for evaluation; strive for no more than 8 grams of added sugars per serving. Reading the Nutrition Facts label helps us choose more nutritious foods. **Based on the information from these nutrition labels, which cereal is the better choice for breakfast?** Which has more fiber?

Cereal 1

Nutrition Facts

10 servings per container
Serving size: 1 cup (55g)

Amount per serving	Cereal	Cereal with ½ Cup Skim Milk
Calories	170	210

	% Daily Value**	
Total Fat 1.0g*	2%	2%
Saturated Fat 0g	0%	0%
Trans Fat 0g		*
Cholesterol 0mg	0%	0%
Sodium 300mg	13%	15%
Potassium 340mg	10%	16%
Total Carbohydrate 43g	14%	16%
Dietary Fiber 7g	25%	25%
Total Sugars 16g		
Includes 10g Added Sugars	20%	20%
Protein 4g		
Vitamin D 1mcg, 2.5mcg	10%	25%
Calcium 20mg, 120mg	2%	12%
Iron 12mg, 12mg	65%	65%
Potassium 225mg, 402mg	6%	11%
Vitamin A 225mcg, 300mcg	15%	20%
Vitamin C 12mg, 13mg	20%	22%
Thiamin 0.3mg, 0.5mg	25%	30%
Riboflavin 0.4mg, 0.6mg	25%	35%
Niacin 5mg, 5mg	25%	25%
Vitamin B$_6$ 0.5mg, 0.5mg	25%	25%
Folic acid 120mcg, 120mcg	30%	30%
Vitamin B$_{12}$ 1.5mcg, 2.1mcg	25%	35%
Phosphorus 200mg, 300mg	20%	30%
Magnesium 80mg, 100mg	20%	25%
Zinc 3.7mg, 3.7mg	25%	25%
Copper 0.2mg, 0.2mg	22%	22%

* Amount in cereal. One half cup skim milk contributes an additional 40 calories, 65mg sodium, 6g total carbohydrate (6g sugars), and 4g protein.

** The % Daily Value (DV) tells you how much a nutrient in a serving of food contributes to a daily diet. 2,000 calories a day is used for general nutrition advice.

Cereal 2

Nutrition Facts

17 servings per container
Serving size: ¾ cup (30g)

Amount per serving	Cereal	Cereal with ½ Cup Skim Milk
Calories	170	210

	% Daily Value**	
Total Fat 0g*	0%	1%
Saturated Fat 0g	0%	1%
Trans Fat 0g		*
Cholesterol 0mg	0%	1%
Sodium 60mg	2%	4%
Potassium 80mg	2%	8%
Total Carbohydrate 35g	9%	11%
Dietary Fiber 1g	4%	4%
Total Sugars 20g		
Includes 15g Added Sugars	30%	30%
Protein 3g		
Vitamin D 1mcg, 2mcg	10%	20%
Calcium 0mg, 150mg	0%	15%
Iron 1.8mg, 1.8mg	10%	10%
Potassium 95mg, 272mg	3%	8%
Vitamin A 375mcg, 450mcg	25%	30%
Vitamin C 0mg, 1.2mg	0%	2%
Thiamin 0.3mg, 0.3mg	25%	25%
Riboflavin 0.4mg, 0.6mg	25%	35%
Niacin 5mg, 5mg	25%	25%
Vitamin B$_6$ 0.5mg, 0.5mg	25%	25%
Folic acid 100mcg, 100mcg	25%	25%
Vitamin B$_{12}$ 1.5mcg, 1.8mcg	25%	30%
Phosphorus 40mg, 150mg	4%	15%
Magnesium 16mg, 32mg	4%	8%
Zinc 1.5mg, 1.5mg	10%	10%
Copper 0.04mg, 0.04mg	4%	4%

* Amount in cereal. One-half cup skim milk contributes an additional 40 calories, 65mg sodium, 6g total carbohydrate (6g sugars), and 4g protein.

** The % Daily Value (DV) tells you how much a nutrient in a serving of food contributes to a daily diet. 2,000 calories a day is used for general nutrition advice.

indicates that youth are choosing more water, energy drinks, and coffee in place of soft drinks. Refer to Table 4-6 for suggestions on how to reduce added sugars in your dietary pattern, and read more about trends in added sugar consumption in *Newsworthy Nutrition* in this section.[23]

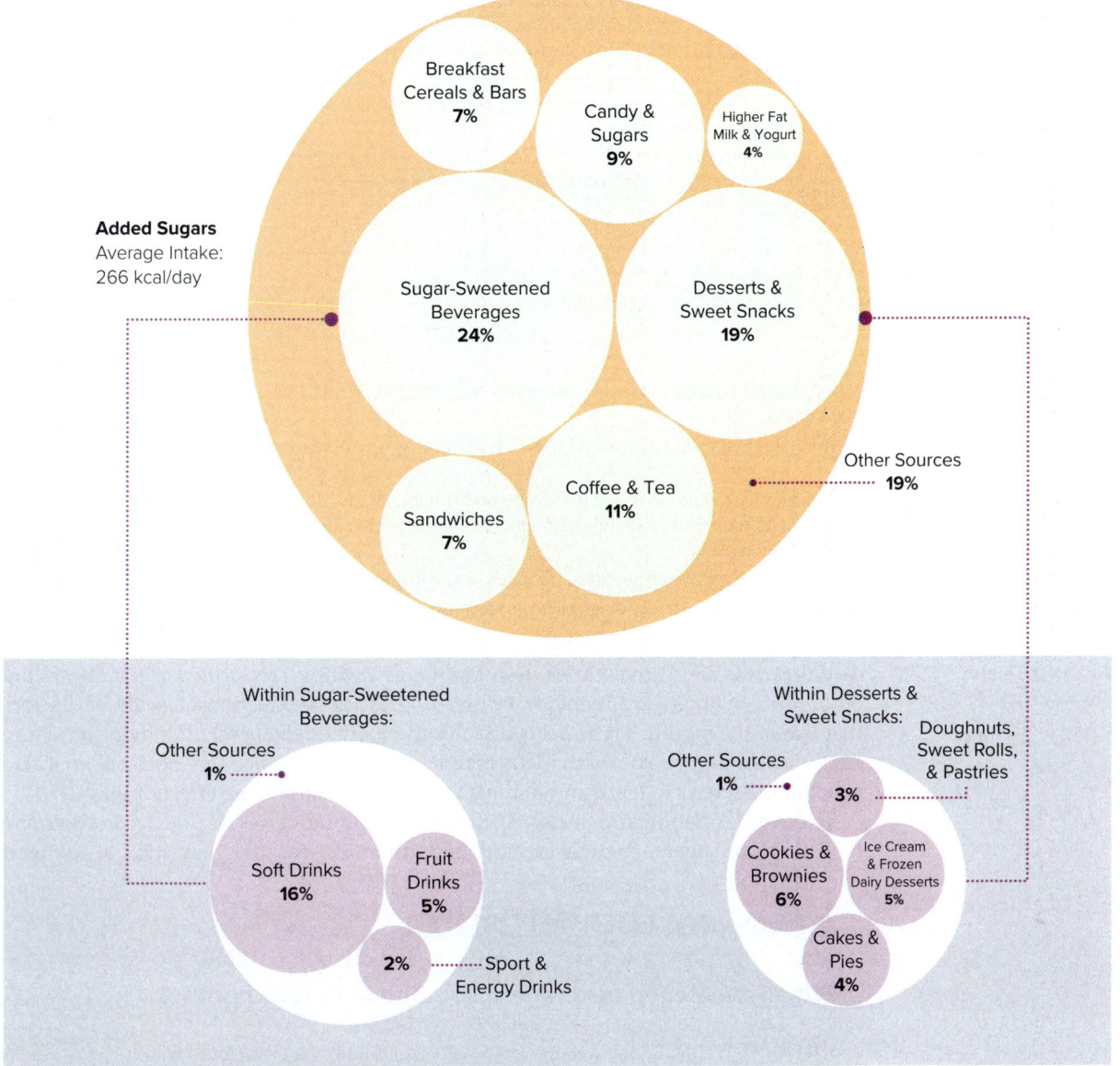

FIGURE 4-17 Sources of added sugars in the dietary patterns of the U.S. population.
Source: Analysis of *What We Eat in America*, NHANES, 2013-2016, USDA *Dietary Guidelines for Americans*, *2020–2025*. https://www.dietaryguidelines.gov/sites/default/files/2020-12/Dietary_Guidelines_for_Americans_2020–2025.pdf

Sugar and Hyperactivity. There is a widespread notion that high sugar intake causes hyperactivity in children, typically part of the syndrome called attention deficit hyperactivity disorder (ADHD). However, several well-controlled studies found that sugar in the dietary patterns did not affect children's behavior.[24] Some researchers suggest that expecting sugar to affect a child can influence parents' interpretation of what they see. A study of parents' perceptions showed that parents who believe a child's behavior is affected by sugar are more likely to perceive their child as hyperactive when they believe the child just had a sugary drink. Experts recommend that other factors associated with hyperactivity, including temperament, emotional disturbances, learning disorders, overstimulation, and sleep problems, be considered.[24]

Sugar and Oral Health. Sugars in the dietary pattern (and starches readily fermented in the mouth, such as crackers and white bread) also increase the risk of developing

TABLE 4-6 ■ Tips for Reducing Added Sugars

At the Grocery Store
- Read the ingredients list on food labels. Look for all forms of added sugars. Added sugars are often hidden in tomato sauce, crackers, condiments, and salad dressings. Added sugars also hide under names such as high-fructose corn syrup, invert sugar, sucrose, dried cane syrup, brown rice syrup, honey, molasses, and maple syrup. These can be listed separately on ingredients lists and add up!
- Buy unsweetened versions of foods typically high in sugar such as cereals, applesauce, yogurt, and canned fruit (in heavy syrup). Look for foods labeled no added sugar or unsweetened.
- Buy nuts and unsweetened dried fruits to replace candy for snacks.

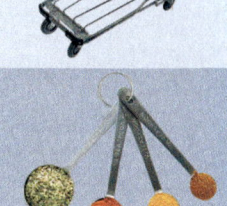

In the Kitchen
- Reduce the sugar in foods prepared at home. Try low-sugar recipes or adjust the sugar on your own. The amount of sugar can be decreased in recipes for foods such as pancakes, waffles, cookies, and cakes that will still taste great. Start by reducing the sugar gradually until you've decreased it by one-third or more.
- Add sweetness to foods with flavors and spices such as vanilla, citrus zest, cinnamon, cardamom, coriander, nutmeg, ginger, and mace.

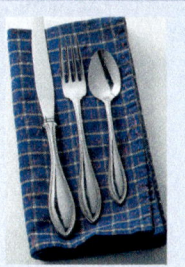

At the Table
- Choose fewer foods high in sugar, such as prepared baked goods and sweet desserts. Reach for fresh fruit instead of cookies or candy for dessert and between-meal snacks.
- Include more protein, such as eggs and turkey, and healthy fats, such as nuts, seeds, and olive oil, to decrease the desire for sugar.
- Add less sugar to foods such as coffee, tea, cereal, and fruit. Reduce the use of white and brown sugars, honey, molasses, syrups, jams, and jellies. Cut back gradually to a quarter or half the amount. Use artificial sweeteners sparingly, as these may actually increase your desire for sweets.
- Substitute water for sugared soft drinks, sweet tea, coffee drinks, energy drinks, punches, and fruit juices.

(top) Stockbyte/Getty Images; (middle) Elenathewise/Stockbrokerxtra Images/Photolibrary/Getty Images; (bottom) Jack Holtel/McGraw Hill

dental caries Erosions in the surface of a tooth caused by acids made by bacteria as they metabolize sugars.

dental caries. Recall that caries, also known as cavities, are formed when sugars and other carbohydrates are metabolized, leading to the production of acids by bacteria that live in the mouth. These acids dissolve the tooth enamel and underlying structure. Bacteria also use the sugars to make plaque, a sticky substance that both adheres acid-producing bacteria to teeth and diminishes the acid-neutralizing effect of saliva.

The worst offenders in terms of promoting dental caries are sticky and gummy foods high in sugars, such as caramel and gummies, because they stick to the teeth

Newsworthy Nutrition

Sugar-sweetened beverage consumption in 185 countries

INTRODUCTION: Sugar-sweetened beverages (SSBs) are associated with cardiometabolic diseases and social inequities, but for most nations, estimates and trends of intake are not available. **OBJECTIVE:** To provide estimates for SSB intake in 185 countries between 1990 to 2018, and to examine if SSB intake trends differ by education or urbanicity. **METHODS:** This *cross-sectional* study utilized SSB data from the Global Dietary Database from 1990 to 2018 in 185 countries. **RESULTS:** In 2018, the mean global SSB intake was 2.7 (8 oz = 248 grams) servings/week (range: 0.7 (0.5–1.1) in South Asia to 7.8 (7.1–8.6) in Latin America/Caribbean). SSB intakes were higher in males vs. females, younger vs. older individuals, higher vs. lower education level, and urban vs. rural adults. Variations by education and location were largest in Sub-Saharan Africa. In addition, between 1990 and 2018, SSB intakes increased by +0.37 (+0.29, +0.47), with the largest increase in Sub-Saharan Africa. **CONCLUSION:** These results on global SSB intakes, trends, and inequities can inform future interventions, surveillance, and global policy actions, highlighting the public policy concerns related to the increasing intake of SSBs consumption in Sub-Saharan Africa.

Source: Lara-Castor L, Micha R, Cudhea F, et al. Sugar-sweetened beverage intakes among adults between 1990 and 2018 in 185 countries. *Nat Commun.* 2023;14:5957. doi: org/10.1038/s41467-023-41269-8

and supply the bacteria with a long-lived carbohydrate source. For this reason, snacking regularly on sugary foods is likely to cause caries because it gives the bacteria on the teeth a steady source of carbohydrates from which to continually make acid. Frequent consumption of liquid sugar sources (e.g., fruit juices, soda, sports beverages, energy drinks, and even many smoothies) can also cause dental caries. Chewing sugar-laden gum between meals is a prime example of a poor dental habit. Still, sugar-containing foods are not the only foods that promote acid production by bacteria in the mouth. As mentioned, if starch-containing foods (e.g., crackers and bread) are stuck to the teeth for a long time, the starch will be broken down to sugars by enzymes in the mouth; bacteria can then produce acid from these sugars. Overall, the sugar and starch contents of a food and its ability to remain in the mouth largely determine its potential to cause caries.

Fluoridated water and toothpaste are major factors in the prevention of dental caries in children due to fluoride's tooth-strengthening effect. Research has also indicated that certain foods—such as cheese, peanuts, and sugar-free chewing gum—can help reduce the amount of acid on teeth. In addition, rinsing the mouth after meals, drinking plenty of water, and eating healthy snacks reduce the acidity in the mouth. Certainly, good nutrition habits that do not present an overwhelming challenge to oral health (e.g., drinking plenty of water, chewing sugar-free gum) and routine visits to the dentist all contribute to improved dental health.

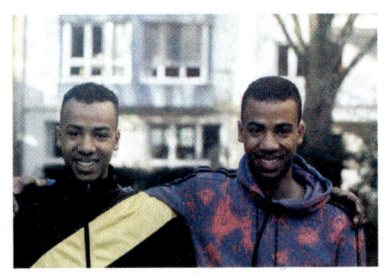

John and Mike are identical twins who like the same games, sports, and foods. However, John likes to chew sugar-free gum and Mike doesn't. At their last dental visit, John had no cavities but Mike had two. Mike wants to know why John, who chews sugar-free gum after eating, doesn't have cavities and he does. **How would you explain this to him?** Image Source Trading Ltd /Shutterstock

✅ CONCEPT CHECK 4.6

1. What is the recommended intake of total carbohydrate per day?
2. How much fiber is recommended per day?
3. How can we reduce our consumption of added sugars?

4.7 Nutrition and Your Health: Diabetes—When Blood Glucose Regulation Fails

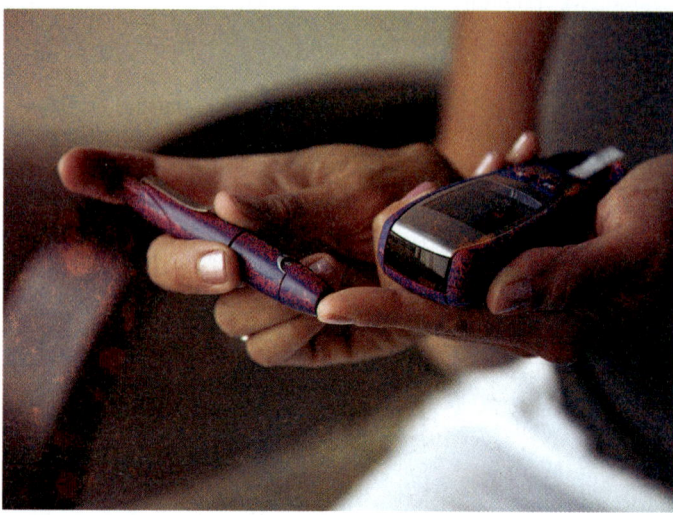
Purestock/Getty Images

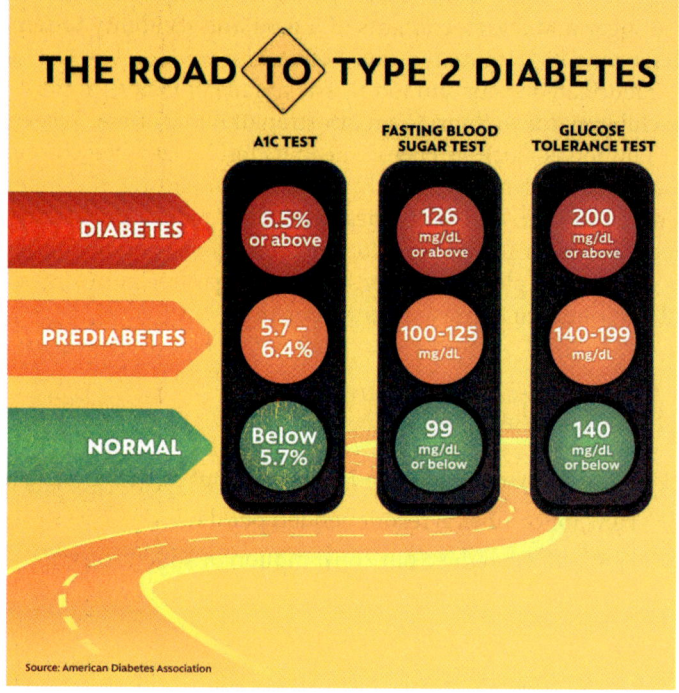

FIGURE 4-18 CDC guide to the criteria for diabetes.
Source: CDC, https://www.cdc.gov/diabetes/library/socialmedia/infographics.html

Improper regulation of blood glucose results in either *hyperglycemia* (high blood glucose) or *hypoglycemia* (low blood glucose). High blood glucose is most commonly associated with diabetes (technically, diabetes mellitus), a disease that affects over 37 million adults, or 11% of the U.S. population 20 years or older.[25] It is estimated that over 23%, or 8.5 million, of these individuals do not know that they have the disease. Diabetes remains the seventh leading cause of death in the U.S. And as with most chronic disease, **health disparities** exist. A Nutrition and Health Disparities *Ask the RDN* in this section covers this extremely important and timely topic.

The American Diabetes Association (ADA) recommends testing fasting blood glucose in adults over age 45 every 3 years to screen for diabetes for asymptomatic individuals and more often for those with symptoms (history of gestational diabetes, prediabetes, or other risk factors like overweight or obese). Your primary care physician may also order a blood glucose test as part of a routine appointment. Figure 4-18 details the diagnostic criteria and categories for normal, prediabetes, and diabetes according to the CDC. Diabetes is often diagnosed using a **hemoglobin** A1c (HbA1c) test to diagnose diabetes with a threshold ≥ 6.5%. The HbA1c is a more sensitive, long-term indicator of poor blood glucose control than the fasting blood glucose level. When blood glucose is too high, the glucose builds up in the blood and combines with hemoglobin (protein in red blood cells), making it glycated. The amount of glycated hemoglobin, or HbA1c, reflects the last several weeks or months of blood glucose levels.[26]

Prediabetes

Prediabetes describes the condition for individuals whose blood glucose levels do not meet the criteria for diabetes but are higher than normal. Often people with type 2 diabetes did not develop the disease suddenly. Prediabetes is a condition in which the concentration of blood glucose drifts up higher than normal. By the time symptoms are noticeable, organs and tissues may already be damaged. Simple tests of your fasting blood glucose level or HbA1c can determine if you are prediabetic. If you have a family history of diabetes or if your behaviors (being physically inactive and overweight, and having a poor dietary pattern) put you at risk, it is important to discover if your blood glucose is still in the prediabetic stage. Prediabetes, also called impaired fasting glucose, is diagnosed if the fasting blood glucose is 100 to 125 milligrams per deciliter or the HbA1c is 5.7% to 6.4%.[24]

The National Diabetes Prevention Program was a large, multisite study designed to improve glucose control and prevent the onset of diabetes. The DPP found that participants who lost even a modest amount of weight via dietary and physical activity changes sharply reduced their chances of developing diabetes. More impressive is

health disparities Preventable differences in the burden of disease, injury, violence, or opportunities to achieve optimal health that are experienced by socially disadvantaged populations.

hemoglobin The iron-containing part of the red blood cell that carries oxygen to the cells and carbon dioxide away from the cells. The heme iron portion is also responsible for the red color of blood.

that the DPP lifestyle intervention had health outcomes that were better than those in the medication-treated cohort.[27]

Diabetes remission is the preferred term to describe the condition in which an individual who was previously diagnosed with diabetes has successfully maintained HbA1c < 6.5% for at least 3 months after stopping glucose-lowering pharmacotherapy. This definition holds true whether it is attained by lifestyle changes, metabolic surgery, or other means.

Diabetes

There are two major forms of diabetes: type 1 (formerly called insulin-dependent or juvenile-onset diabetes) and type 2 (formerly called noninsulin-dependent or adult-onset diabetes) (Table 4-7). The change in names to type 1 and type 2 diabetes stems from the fact that many individuals with type 2 diabetes eventually must also rely on insulin injections as part of their treatment. In addition, many children today have type 2 diabetes. A third form, called gestational diabetes, occurs in some females who are pregnant. It is usually treated with an insulin regimen and dietary changes, and then resolves after delivery of the baby. However, females who have gestational diabetes during pregnancy are at high risk for developing type 2 diabetes later in life.

Type 1 Diabetes

Type 1 diabetes occurs at every age and in people of every race and ethnicity, shape, and body size. Approximately 1.6 million Americans have type 1 diabetes, and an estimated 64,000 people will be diagnosed with the disease each year in the U.S.[25] Children usually are admitted to the hospital with abnormally high blood glucose after eating, as well as evidence of ketosis.

The onset of type 1 diabetes is generally associated with decreased release of insulin from the pancreas. As insulin in the blood declines, blood glucose increases, especially after eating. When blood glucose levels are high, the kidneys let excess glucose spill into the urine, resulting in frequent urination that is high in sugar.

Most cases of type 1 diabetes begin with an immune system disorder that causes destruction of the insulin-producing cells in the pancreas. The disease may stem from genetic, autoimmune, or environmental factors. Eventually, the pancreas loses its ability to synthesize insulin, and the clinical stage of the disease begins. Hyperglycemia and other symptoms develop slowly and only after 90% or more of the insulin-secreting cells have been destroyed. HbA1c, fasting blood glucose, or an oral glucose tolerance test can be used to diagnose diabetes (Fig. 4-18). Remember that HbA1c is the recommended measure, and an HbA1c value of 7% or over indicates poor blood glucose control.[24]

Type 1 diabetes is treated primarily by insulin therapy, either with injections or with an insulin infusion pump. Advantages of using an insulin pump include eliminating individual insulin injections; delivering insulin more accurately than injections; achieving improved stabilization of blood glucose levels; enabling more dietary and physical activity flexibility; reducing severe low blood glucose episodes; and eliminating unpredictable effects of intermediate- or long-acting insulin. Now, an amazing innovation is showing promise for management of type 1 diabetes. The bionic pancreas is a novel device that would fully automate blood glucose tracking and adjust the hormonal response accordingly. Several biotech companies are testing models.[28]

Medical nutrition therapy includes tailoring dietary pattern recommendations to the individual. It includes balancing carbohydrate intake with the insulin regimen and physical activity schedule to manage blood glucose levels. The amount and timing of carbohydrates eaten should be consistent from day to day to maintain blood glucose control. Insulin should be adjusted to match carbohydrate intake in persons who adjust their mealtime insulin doses or who are using an insulin pump. There are several methods available to estimate carbohydrate content of foods, including carbohydrate counting, exchange lists, and the glycemic index and glycemic load of foods (Appendix B).[29,30] If one does not eat often enough, the injected insulin can cause a severe drop in blood glucose or hypoglycemia because it acts on whatever glucose is available. Dietary patterns should be moderate or low in simple carbohydrates, include ample fiber and unsaturated fat, be low in saturated fats, and supply an amount of calories to balance with needs. Providing adequate calories and nutrients to promote growth and development in children is crucial for young individuals with diabetes.[26,30,31]

The hormone imbalances that occur in people with untreated type 1 diabetes—primarily, not enough insulin—lead to mobilization of body fat, taken up by liver cells. Ketosis is the result because the fat is partially broken down to ketone bodies. Ketone bodies can rise excessively in the blood and eventually spill into the urine. These pull sodium and potassium ions as well as water into the urine. This series of events also causes frequent urination and can contribute to dehydration, ion imbalance, coma, and even death. Treatment includes provision of insulin, fluids, and minerals such as sodium and potassium.

Several degenerative complications, including cardiovascular disease, blindness, kidney disease, and nerve damage, result from poor blood glucose regulation, specifically long-term hyperglycemia. The high blood sugar concentration physically deteriorates small blood vessels (capillaries) and nerves. When improper nerve stimulation occurs in the intestinal tract, intermittent diarrhea

TABLE 4-7 ■ Comparison of Type 1 and 2 Diabetes

Type 1 Diabetes	Type 2 Diabetes
Occurrence	
5% to 10%	90% to 95%
Risk Factors	
Moderate genetic predisposition	Strong genetic predisposition, obesity, physical inactivity, ethnicity, metabolic syndrome, prediabetes
Prevention	
No known preventive measures	Most cases can be prevented
Insulin Response	
Insulin dependent Not enough insulin produced	Insulin resistant Dysfunctional insulin response
Symptoms	
Distinct symptoms: frequent thirst and urination, weight loss, fatigue, blurred vision, frequent infections	Mild symptoms: fatigue and nighttime urination, weight loss, fatigue, blurred vision, frequent infections
Treatment	
Insulin Healthy dietary pattern Increased physical activity	Healthy dietary pattern Increased physical activity Oral medications

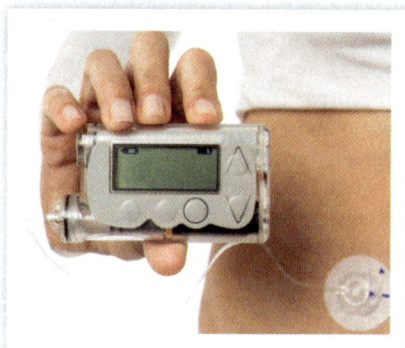

Insulin pumps alleviate the discomfort of injecting insulin under the skin multiple times per day. **How does this device work?** Oscar Gimeno Baldo/Alamy Stock Photo

and constipation result. Because of nerve deterioration in the extremities, many people with diabetes lose the sensation of pain associated with injuries or infections. They do not have as much pain, so they often delay treatment of hand or foot problems. This delay, combined with a rich environment for bacterial growth (bacteria thrive on glucose), sets the stage for damage and death of tissues in the extremities, sometimes leading to the need for amputation of feet and legs.

Current research has shown that aggressive treatment directed at keeping blood glucose within the normal range can slow the development of blood vessel and nerve complications of diabetes. A person with diabetes must work closely with a primary care provider and dietitian to make the correct alterations in the dietary pattern and medications and to perform physical activity safely. Physical activity enhances glucose uptake by muscles independent of insulin action, which in turn can lower blood glucose. This outcome is beneficial, but people with type 1 diabetes need to be aware of their blood glucose response to physical activity and compensate appropriately to avoid hypoglycemia.

Type 2 Diabetes

Type 2 diabetes usually begins after age 45 but increasingly, more children and young adults are developing it. This is the most common type of diabetes, accounting for about 90% to 95% of the cases diagnosed in the U.S.[25] The disease is progressive and is present, in many cases, long before it is diagnosed. Hyperglycemia develops slowly such that the classic symptoms are not noticed in the early stages of the disease. Risk factors for type 2 diabetes are both genetic and environmental and include a family history of diabetes; older age; obesity, especially **upper-body obesity;** physical inactivity; prior history of gestational diabetes; prediabetes; and race or ethnicity. Latino/Hispanic Americans, African Americans, Asian Americans, Native Americans, and Pacific Islanders are at particular risk. The overall number of people affected is also on the rise, primarily because of widespread inactivity and obesity. There has also been a substantial increase in type 2 diabetes in children, due mostly to an increase in body fat in this population (coupled with limited physical activity).

Type 2 diabetes arises when the insulin receptors on the cell surfaces of certain body tissues, especially muscle and fat tissue, become **insulin resistant** (Fig. 4-19). During the onset of the disease, there is an abundance of insulin that is not used properly, and blood glucose is not readily transferred into cells. The person develops high blood glucose as a result of the glucose remaining in the bloodstream. As the pancreas attempts to increase insulin output to compensate, the beta cells in the pancreas lose the ability to produce sufficient quantities of the hormone. As the disease develops, pancreatic function can fail, eventually leading to reduced insulin output. Because of the genetic link for type 2 diabetes, those who have a family history should schedule regular diabetes screening and be careful to avoid risk factors such as obesity and inactivity.

upper-body obesity The type of obesity in which fat is stored primarily in the abdominal area; defined as a waist circumference more than 40 inches (102 centimeters) in males and more than 35 inches (88 centimeters) in females; closely associated with a high risk for cardiovascular disease, hypertension, and type 2 diabetes. Also known as *android, visceral,* or *central obesity.*

insulin resistance Also known as *impaired insulin sensitivity,* insulin resistance refers to an impaired biological response to insulin that makes it less effective.

INSULIN RESISTANCE EXPLAINED

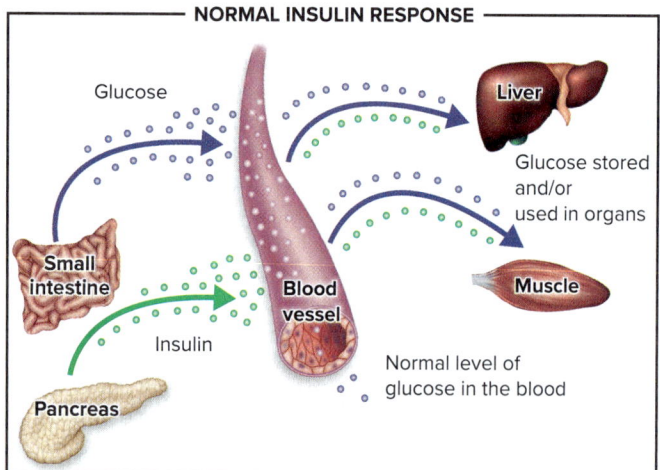

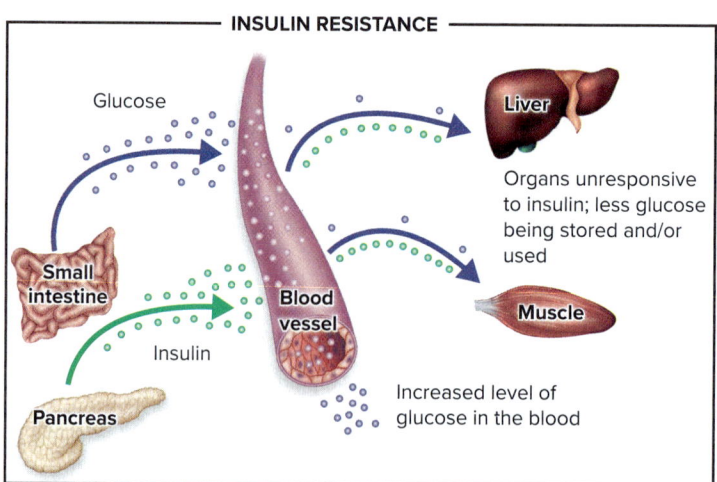

FIGURE 4-19 During a normal insulin response (figure on left), glucose is absorbed from the small intestine after digestion into the bloodstream. As blood glucose levels rise, the pancreas secretes the hormone insulin to signal cells to take up glucose from the bloodstream. Insulin resistance (figure on the right) occurs when the cells do not respond to normal insulin signals to take up glucose from the bloodstream.

Almost 90% of type 2 diabetes cases are associated with overweight and obesity, but high blood glucose is not directly caused by the obesity. Obesity associated with oversized adipose cells increases the risk for insulin resistance by the body as more fat is added to these cells during weight gain. Because type 2 diabetes is linked to obesity, achieving a healthy weight should be a primary goal of treatment, with even limited weight loss leading to better blood glucose regulation. Although many cases of type 2 diabetes can be relieved by reducing excess fat, many people struggle to lose weight. They remain affected with diabetes and may experience the degenerative complications seen in the type 1 form of the disease. Ketosis, however, is not usually seen in type 2 diabetes. Glucose-lowering medications and insulin are used as needed in patients with type 2 diabetes. New classes of drugs that mimic gut hormones are helping individuals with diabetes overcome the chronic problems that conventional treatments alone have been unable to control.

Nutrition, physical activity, and behavioral therapy are recommended to support individuals with type 2 diabetes achieve and maintain a 5% weight loss.[32] Additional weight loss usually results in further improvements in the management of diabetes and cardiovascular risk. Medical nutrition therapy should emphasize overall calorie control, increased intakes of plant-based and fiber-rich foods and fish, and reduced intake of added sugars and unhealthy fats. Physical activity helps the muscles take up more glucose. As in type 1 diabetes, it is critical that discussions include a dietitian and primary care provider to create a tailored lifestyle management plan to meet the needs of each individual.[33] It is also important to consume the recommended 25 to 38 grams of fiber, with emphasis on soluble fiber sources, which will help regulate glucose.[34]

Although sugar does not have to be completely eliminated, persons with diabetes will benefit from adhering to the recommendation to reduce consumption of added sugars. Because persons with diabetes are at increased risk of cardiovascular disease, heart-healthy choices should also be included in their diabetic meal plan. For more information on living healthy with diabetes, visit https://care.diabetesjournals.org/content/44/Supplement_1/S15.

Hypoglycemia

People with diabetes who are taking insulin sometimes have hypoglycemia if they do not eat frequently enough. The first signs of diabetic hypoglycemia include shakiness, sweating, palpitations, anxiety, and hunger. Later symptoms are the result of insufficient glucose reaching the brain and include mental confusion, extreme fatigue, seizures, and unconsciousness. Symptoms should be treated immediately with consumption of glucose or food containing carbohydrate.

Metabolic Syndrome

Metabolic syndrome is characterized by the presence of several risk factors for diabetes and cardiovascular disease. A person with metabolic syndrome must have at least three of the following metabolic risk factors (or be on medication to treat these risk factors) to be diagnosed with metabolic syndrome: a large waistline from abdominal obesity, high blood triglycerides, low HDL (or good cholesterol), hypertension, and high fasting blood glucose (Fig. 4-20). Each aspect of metabolic syndrome is a unique health problem with its own treatment. In metabolic syndrome, however,

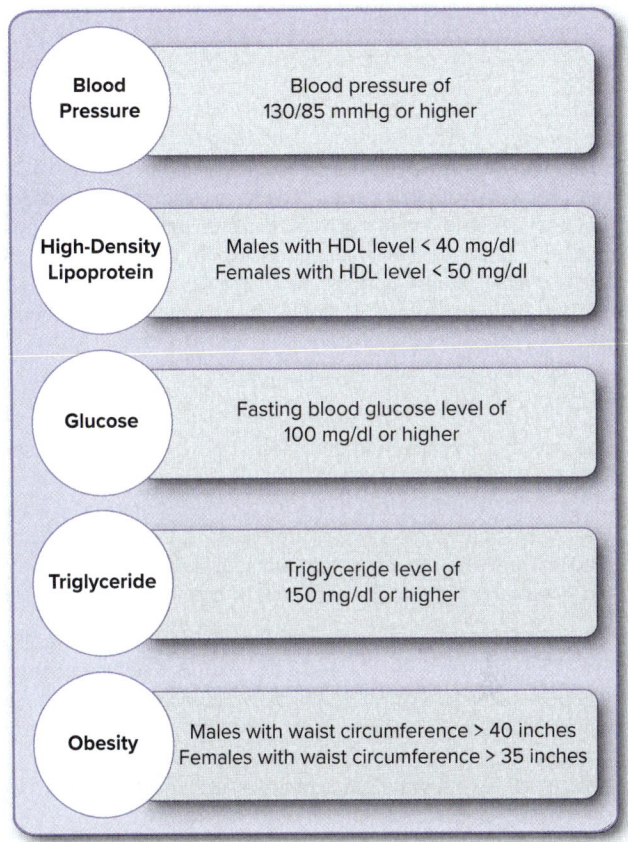

FIGURE 4-20 Metabolic syndrome is characterized by the presence of several risk factors for diabetes and cardiovascular disease.

these risk factors are clustered together, making a person twice as likely to develop cardiovascular disease and five times more likely to develop diabetes.

It is generally accepted that one key element that unifies metabolic syndrome is insulin resistance. As you learned, insulin is a hormone that directs tissues to pull glucose out of the blood and into cells for storage or fuel. With insulin resistance, the pancreas produces plenty of insulin, but the cells of the body do not respond to it effectively. Instead, excess glucose stays in the bloodstream. For a while, the pancreas may be able to compensate for the resistance of cells to insulin by overproducing insulin. Over time, however, the pancreas is unable to keep up the accelerated insulin production, and blood glucose levels remain elevated. With metabolic syndrome, blood glucose is not high enough to be classified as diabetes, but without intervention, it is likely to get worse and eventually lead to diabetes.

Genetics and aging contribute to the development of insulin resistance and the other elements of metabolic syndrome, but environmental factors, such as the dietary pattern and activity,

metabolic syndrome A condition in which a person has poor blood glucose regulation, hypertension, increased blood triglycerides, and other health problems. This condition is usually accompanied by obesity, lack of physical activity, and a dietary pattern high in refined carbohydrates. Also called *Syndrome X*.

ASK THE RDN: Nutrition and Health Disparities

Dear RDN: *What are health disparities and how do they impact nutritional status?*

The CDC broadly defines health disparities as preventable differences in the burden of disease or opportunities to achieve optimal health that are experienced by socially disadvantaged populations. Health disparities in nutrition may specifically impact dietary consumption, behaviors, and patterns and often result in reduced diet quality and adverse health outcomes for groups based upon race and ethnicity, age, income, education, location, disability, sexual orientation, and/or gender identity.

The occurrence of health disparities in the United States has grown as the population has become increasingly diverse in the last century. Recently, the U.S. Census Bureau reported that by the year 2050, minorities (identified as Hispanic, Black, Asian, American Indian, Native Hawaiian, Pacific Islander, or mixed race) will make up 54% of the U.S. population. As these populations grow, it is important to understand diet- and health-related disparities. The goal for all is to acknowledge nutrition and health disparities, educate oneself on the issues, and strive to be a part of the solution!

The following are recommendations that will help decrease health disparities and encourage optimal health in individuals of all races and ethnicities:

- Ask your primary care provider to refer you to a registered dietitian nutritionist (RDN) for all nutrition-related concerns, especially if diagnosed with diabetes or hypertension.
- If hospitalized, request to see an RDN for any diet or nutrition concerns including understanding medical dietary restrictions, addressing food insecurity, supporting behavioral modifications, even requesting healthy and budget-friendly recipes and cooking tips.
- Request an RDN of your own race/ethnicity for more relatable and culturally sensitive care that may reduce health disparities. But do not refuse an RDN simply because there may not be one sharing your specific race/ethnicity, demographics, or beliefs.

Currently in the U.S., there remains a lack of diversity within health care teams. Over 50% of practicing primary care providers are white and male. There is a shift occurring among physicians under 35 years of age with females outnumbering males in most racial and ethnic groups. Specific to nutrition, the makeup of RDNs is approximately 3% Black, 5% Hispanic, 5% Asian, 2% identifying as Other, and 94% identifying as female. Although we have a long way to go, we are making strides nationally in educating the current workforce and improving recruitment strategies to better reflect the world in which we live.

Embracing all,

Carmen Blakely, EdD, MEd, RDN, LD
Associate Professor, Kent State University

Sources: CDC, AAMC

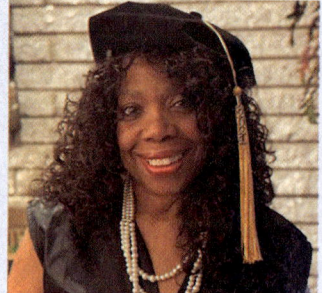

Carmen Blakely/Lucretia Adams

---

play an important role. Body fatness, particularly abdominal obesity, is highly related to insulin resistance. Almost 75% of adults in the U.S. are overweight or obese, and these numbers continue to climb year after year.[35] Increases in body weight among children and adolescents are of great concern because childhood obesity places them at high risk for these health problems. This increase in body weight has precipitated a dramatic surge in cardiovascular disease and diabetes risk.

The insulin resistance that precedes and contributes to type 2 diabetes also leads to several other components of the metabolic syndrome. The chief culprits contributing to the high blood triglycerides of metabolic syndrome are large meals rich in simple sugars and refined starches and low in fiber and whole grains, coupled with little to no physical activity. Nutrition and lifestyle changes are key strategies in addressing all of the unhealthy conditions of metabolic syndrome as a whole. Modifiable behavioral interventions include:

- Decrease body weight. Even small improvements (5% weight loss) for individuals who are overweight or obese can lessen disease risk. The most successful weight-loss and weight-maintenance programs include moderate dietary restriction combined with physical activity.
- Increase physical activity. To alleviate risks for chronic diseases, the *Physical Activity Guidelines* recommend at least 150 minutes of moderate-intensity physical activity each week.
- Limit solid fat consumption, especially saturated fat sources. We will explore the different types and sources of fats and their effects later in the text.

✓ CONCEPT CHECK 4.7

1. List key differences between type 1 and type 2 diabetes.
2. Describe insulin resistance and how it contributes to diabetes.
3. Identify two health consequences of diabetes and three lifestyle behaviors that can reduce these adverse effects.
4. List the risk factors for metabolic syndrome.

Summary (Numbers refer to numbered sections in the chapter)

4.1 Carbohydrates are created in plants through photosynthesis. They are our main fuel source for body cells. Refined and highly processed products lack many of the health benefits provided by the carbohydrates found in whole grains, beans, fruits, and vegetables. The *Dietary Guidelines* suggests making at least half the grains you eat whole grains.

4.2 The common monosaccharides in food are glucose, fructose, and galactose. The major disaccharides are sucrose (glucose + fructose), maltose (glucose + glucose), and lactose (glucose + galactose). When digested, these yield their component monosaccharides. Once these are absorbed from the small intestine and delivered to the liver, much of the fructose and galactose is converted into glucose.

One major group of polysaccharides consists of storage forms of glucose: starches in plants and glycogen in humans. These can be broken down by human digestive enzymes, releasing the glucose units. The main plant starches—straight-chain amylose and branched-chain amylopectin—are digested by enzymes in the mouth and small intestine. In humans, glycogen is synthesized in the liver and muscle tissue from glucose. Under the influence of hormones, liver glycogen is readily broken down to glucose, which can enter the bloodstream to fuel necessary cells.

Fiber is a group of indigestible polysaccharides including cellulose, hemicellulose, pectin, gum, β-glucans, inulin, resistant starch, as well as the noncarbohydrate lignins. These substances are not broken down by human digestive enzymes. Dietary fiber can be categorized by their solubility, viscosity, and fermentation potential. Soluble fiber forms a gel in the intestines, reduces glucose and cholesterol absorption, promotes a sense of satiety, and serves as fuel for the microbiota. Insoluble fiber passes through the GI tract intact, adding bulk to the feces.

4.3 Table sugar, honey, jelly, and fruit are some of the most concentrated sources of carbohydrates. Other high carbohydrate foods, such as pie and fat-free milk, are diluted by either fat or protein. Nutritive (calorie-containing) sweeteners in food include sucrose, high-fructose corn syrup, brown sugar, and maple syrup. Several artificial sweeteners approved for use by the FDA include saccharin, aspartame, sucralose, neotame, stevia, allulose, and acesulfame-K.

4.4 Some starch digestion occurs in the mouth with assistance from the enzyme amylase. Carbohydrate digestion is completed in the small intestine. Some plant fibers are digested by the bacteria present in the large intestine; undigested plant fibers become part of the feces. Monosaccharides in the intestinal contents mostly follow an active absorption process. They are then transported via the portal vein that leads directly to the liver.

The ability to digest lactose often diminishes with age. Undigested lactose travels to the large intestine, resulting in such symptoms as abdominal gas, pain, and diarrhea. The occurrence of severe symptoms after consuming lactose is called lactose intolerance. Most people with lactose maldigestion can tolerate cheese, yogurt, and moderate amounts of milk.

4.5 Carbohydrates provide calories (4 kcal per gram), spare protein from being broken down for fuel, and prevent ketosis. The RDA for carbohydrate is 130 grams per day. If carbohydrate intake is inadequate for the body's needs, protein is metabolized to provide glucose for energy needs. However, the price is loss of body protein, ketosis, and eventually a general body weakening. For this reason, low-carbohydrate diets are not recommended for extended periods.

4.6 A goal of about half of calories as complex carbohydrates is a good one, with about 45% to 65% of total calories coming from carbohydrates in general. The *Dietary Guidelines* encourages fiber-rich fruits, vegetables, and whole grains. Roughly one-half of one's grains should be whole grains. Added sugars should be limited to less than 10% of total calories.

Moderating sugar intake, especially between meals, reduces the risk of dental caries. Artificial sweeteners, such as aspartame, aid in reducing intake of sugars.

4.7 Diabetes is characterized by a persistent high blood glucose concentration. Type 1 diabetes is caused by a lack of insulin, whereas type 2 diabetes is due to insulin resistance. Regular physical activity and a balanced meal plan that emphasizes fiber and limits added sugars and saturated fats are helpful in treating both type 1 and type 2 diabetes. Insulin is the main medication employed: it is required in type 1 diabetes and may be used in type 2 diabetes.

Check Your Knowledge (Answers are available at the end of this question set)

1. Dietary fiber
   a. raises blood cholesterol levels.
   b. speeds up transit time for food through the digestive tract.
   c. causes diverticulosis.
   d. causes constipation.

2. When the pancreas detects excess glucose in the blood, it releases
   a. enzyme amylase.
   b. monosaccharide glucose.
   c. hormone insulin.
   d. hormone glucagon.

3. Cellulose is a(n)
   a. indigestible fiber.
   b. simple carbohydrate.
   c. energy-yielding nutrient.
   d. animal polysaccharide.

4. Digested table sugar is broken into _____ and _____.
   a. glucose, lactose
   b. glucose, fructose
   c. sucrose, maltose
   d. fructose, sucrose

5. Starch is a
   a. complex carbohydrate.
   b. fiber.
   c. simple carbohydrate.
   d. gluten.

6. Fiber content of the dietary pattern can be increased by adding
   a. fresh fruits.
   b. fish and poultry.
   c. eggs.
   d. whole grains and cereals.
   e. both a and d.

7. Which form of diabetes is most common?
   a. Type 1
   b. Type 2
   c. Type 3
   d. Gestational

8. The recommended daily intake for fiber is approximately _____ grams.
   a. 5 to 10
   b. 25 to 38
   c. 45 to 65
   d. 75 to 109

9. Lactose intolerance is the result of
   a. drinking high-fat milk.
   b. eating a large amount of yogurt.
   c. low lactase activity.
   d. a high-fiber dietary pattern.

10. One of the components of metabolic syndrome is
    a. high HDL.
    b. high waist circumference.
    c. low blood sugar.
    d. low blood pressure.

Answer Key: 1. b (LO 4.5), 2. c (LO 4.5), 3. a (LO 4.2), 4. b (LO 4.2), 5. a (LO 4.2), 6. e (LO 4.3), 7. b (LO 4.7), 8. b (LO 4.6), 9. c (LO 4.4), 10. b (LO 4.7)

Study Questions (Numbers refer to Learning Outcomes)

1. Why do we need carbohydrates in our dietary pattern? **(LO 4.1)**
2. What are the three major monosaccharides and the three major disaccharides? Describe how each plays a part in the human dietary pattern. **(LO 4.2)**
3. Why are some foods that are high in carbohydrates, such as cookies and fat-free milk, not considered to be concentrated sources of carbohydrates? **(LO 4.3)**
4. List three alternatives to simple sugars for adding sweetness to the dietary pattern without adding calories. **(LO 4.3)**
5. Describe the digestion of the various types of carbohydrates in the body. **(LO 4.4)**
6. Describe the reason why some people are unable to tolerate high intakes of milk. **(LO 4.4)**
7. Outline the basic steps in blood glucose regulation, including the roles of insulin and glucagon. **(LO 4.5)**
8. What are the important roles that fiber plays in our dietary pattern? **(LO 4.5)**
9. Summarize current carbohydrate intake recommendations. **(LO 4.6)**
10. What, if any, are the proven ill effects of excessive sugar in the dietary pattern? **(LO 4.6)**
11. Type 1 diabetes is caused by a lack of insulin. What leads to type 2 diabetes? **(LO 4.7)**

References

1. AICR Recommendations & Cancer Prevention. 2018. https://healthy10challenge.org/cancer-prevention/. Accessed Sept 24, 2023.
2. Institute of Medicine. *Dietary Reference Intakes for Energy, Carbohydrate, Fiber, Fat, Fatty Acids, Cholesterol, Protein, and Amino Acids.* Washington, DC: The National Academies Press; 2005. https://doi.org/10.17226/10490
3. Prats C, Graham TE, Shearer J. The dynamic life of the glycogen granule. *J Biol Chem.* 2018 May 11;293(19):7089-7098. doi: 10.1074/jbc.R117.802843
4. Veronese N, Solmi M, Caruso MG, et al. Dietary fiber and health outcomes: an umbrella review of systematic reviews and meta-analyses. *Am J Clin Nutr.* 2018 Mar 1;107(3):436-444. doi: 10.1093/ajcn/nqx082
5. U.S. Department of Agriculture; U.S. Department of Health and Human Services. *Dietary Guidelines for Americans, 2020–2025.* 9th ed. December 2020. https://DietaryGuidelines.gov
6. Whole grain statistics. Oldways Whole Grain Council. March 2018. Available at https://wholegrainscouncil.org/newsroom/whole-grain-statistics. Accessed October 5, 2023.
7. Schaeffer J. Consuming more whole grains. *Today's Dietitian.* 2013 Feb;15(2):32.
8. Whole grain stamp. Oldways Whole Grain Council. Available at https://wholegrainscouncil.org/whole-grain-stamp. Accessed October 7, 2023.
9. Ahluwalia N, Herrick KA, Terry AI, Hughes JP. Contribution of whole grains to total grains intake among adults aged 20 and over: United States, 2013–2016. *NCHS Data Brief.* 2019 Jul;(341):1-8. https://www.cdc.gov/nchs/data/databriefs/db341-h.pdf
10. Nutrition standards for school meals. U.S. Department of Agriculture, Food and Nutrition Service. Available at https://www.fns.usda.gov/school-meals/nutrition-standards-school-meals. Accessed October 7, 2023.

11. Fitch C, Keim KS; Academy of Nutrition and Dietetics. Position of the Academy of Nutrition and Dietetics: use of nutritive and nonnutritive sweeteners. *J Acad Nutr Diet.* 2012 May;112(5):739-758. doi: 10.1016/j.jand.2012.03.009

12. Rippe JM, Angelopoulos TJ. Relationship between added sugars consumption and chronic disease risk factors: current understanding. *Nutrients.* 2016 Nov 4;8(11):697. doi: 10.3390/nu8110697

13. World Health Organization. Aspartame hazard and risk assessment results released. July 2023. Available at https://www.who.int/news/item/14-07-2023-aspartame-hazard-and-risk-assessment-results-released

14. How sweet it is: all about sugar substitutes. U.S. Department of Agriculture, Food & Drug Administration. https://www.fda.gov/consumers/consumer-updates/how-sweet-it-all-about-sugar-substitutes. Accessed October 11, 2023.

15. Fassio F, Facioni MS, Guagnini F. Lactose maldigestion, malabsorption, and intolerance: a comprehensive review with a focus on current management and future perspectives. *Nutrients.* 2018 Nov 1;10(11):1599. doi: 10.3390/nu10111599

16. Lactose intolerance. U.S. Department of Health and Human Services, National Institutes of Health, National Institute of Diabetes and Digestive and Kidney Diseases. Accessed December 5, 2023. https://www.niddk.nih.gov/health-information/digestive-diseases/lactose-intolerance

17. Dionne J, Ford AC, Yuan Y, et al. A systematic review and meta-analysis evaluating the efficacy of a gluten-free diet and a low FODMAPs diet in treating symptoms of irritable bowel syndrome. *Am J Gastroenterol.* 2018 Sep;113(9):1290-1300. doi: 10.1038/s41395-018-0195-4

18. Mendes-Soares H, Raveli-Sadka T, Azulay S, et al. Assessment of a personalized approach to predicting postprandial glycemic responses to food among individuals without diabetes. *JAMA Netw Open.* 2019 Feb 1;2(2):e188102. doi: 10.1001/jamanetworkopen.2018.8102

19. Glycemic index research and GI news. University of Sydney: GI Newsletter. Accessed October 11, 2023. http://www.glycemicindex.com

20. Seal CJ, Brownlee IA. Whole-grain foods and chronic disease: evidence from epidemiological and intervention studies. *Proc Nutr Soc.* 2015 Aug;74(3):313-319. doi: 10.1017/S0029665115002104

21. Interactive nutrition facts label: dietary fiber. U.S. Food & Drug Administration. Accessed October 5, 2023. https://www.accessdata.fda.gov/scripts/InteractiveNutritionFactsLabel/assets/InteractiveNFL_DietaryFiber_March2020.pdf

22. How much sugar is too much? American Heart Association, Heart Attack and Stroke Symptoms. Accessed October 5, 2023. https://www.heart.org/en/healthy-living/healthy-eating/eat-smart/sugar/how-much-sugar-is-too-much

23. Bleich SN, Vercammen KA, Koma JW, Li Z. Trends in beverage consumption among children and adults, 2003–2014. *Obesity (Silver Spring).* 2018 Feb;26(2):432-441. doi:10.1002/oby.22622

24. Ansel K. Sugar: does it really cause hyperactivity? Academy of Nutrition and Dietetics. September 21, 2020. Accessed October 5, 2023. https://www.eatright.org/food/nutrition/dietary-guidelines-and-myplate/sugar-does-it-really-cause-hyperactivity

25. Statistics about diabetes. American Diabetes Association. Accessed October 6, 2023. https://www.diabetes.org/resources/statistics/statistics-about-diabetes

26. American Diabetes Association. *Standards of Medical Care in Diabetes—2021* abridged for primary care providers. *Clin Diabetes.* 2021 Jan;39(1):14-43. doi: 10.2337/cd21-as01

27. National Diabetes Prevention Program. U.S. Department of Health and Human Services, Centers for Disease Control and Prevention. January 2018. Accessed October 7, 2023. https://www.cdc.gov/diabetes/prevention/index.html

28. McAdams BH, Rizvi AA. An overview of insulin pumps and glucose sensors for the generalist. *J Clin Med.* 2016 Jan 4;5(1):5. doi: 10.3390/jcm5010005

29. National Diabetes Statistics Report. U.S. Department of Health and Human Services, Centers for Disease Control and Prevention. Accessed October 7, 2023. https://www.cdc.gov/diabetes/data/statistics-report/index.html

30. Young-Hyman D, de Groot M, Hill-Briggs F, Gonzalez JS, Hood K, Peyrot M. Psychosocial care for people with diabetes: a position statement of the American Diabetes Association. *Diabetes Care.* 2016 Dec;39(12): 2126-2140. doi: 10.2337/dc16-2053

31. American Diabetes Association. *Standards of Medical Care in Diabetes—2018* abridged for primary care providers. *Clin Diabetes.* 2018 Jan;36(1):14-37. doi: 10.2337/cd17-0119

32. Nuha AES, Grazia A, Vanita RA, et al.; American Diabetes Association, 5. Facilitating positive health behaviors and well-being to improve health outcomes: standards of care in diabetes—2023. *Diabetes Care* 1 January 2023;46 (Supplement_1):S68-S96. https://doi.org/10.2337/dc23-S005

33. Early KB, Stanley K. Position of the Academy of Nutrition and Dietetics: the role of medical nutrition therapy and registered dietitian nutritionists in the prevention and treatment of prediabetes and type 2 diabetes. *J Acad Nutr Diet.* 2018 Feb;118(2):343-353. doi: 10.1016/j.jand.2017.11.021

34. Evert AB, Dennison M, Garner CD, et al. Nutrition therapy for adults with diabetes or prediabetes: a consensus report. *Diabetes Care.* 2019 May;42(5):731-754. doi: 10.2337/dci19-0014

35. Fryar CD, Carroll MD, Afful J. Prevalence of overweight, obesity, and severe obesity among adults aged 20 and over: United States, 1960–1962 through 2017–2018. National Center for Health Statistics, Health E-Stats. December 2020. Revised January 29, 2021. https://www.cdc.gov/nchs/data/hestat/obesity-adult-17-18/overweight-obesity-adults-H.pdf

Design Element Credits: Fact Check/magnifying glass icon: McGraw Hill; Magnificent Microbiome background image: Alena Ohneva/Shutterstock; Sustainable Solutions icon: McGraw Hill; Roots icon: McGraw Hill; Medicine Cabinet icon: Peter Dazeley/Photographer's Choice/Getty Images

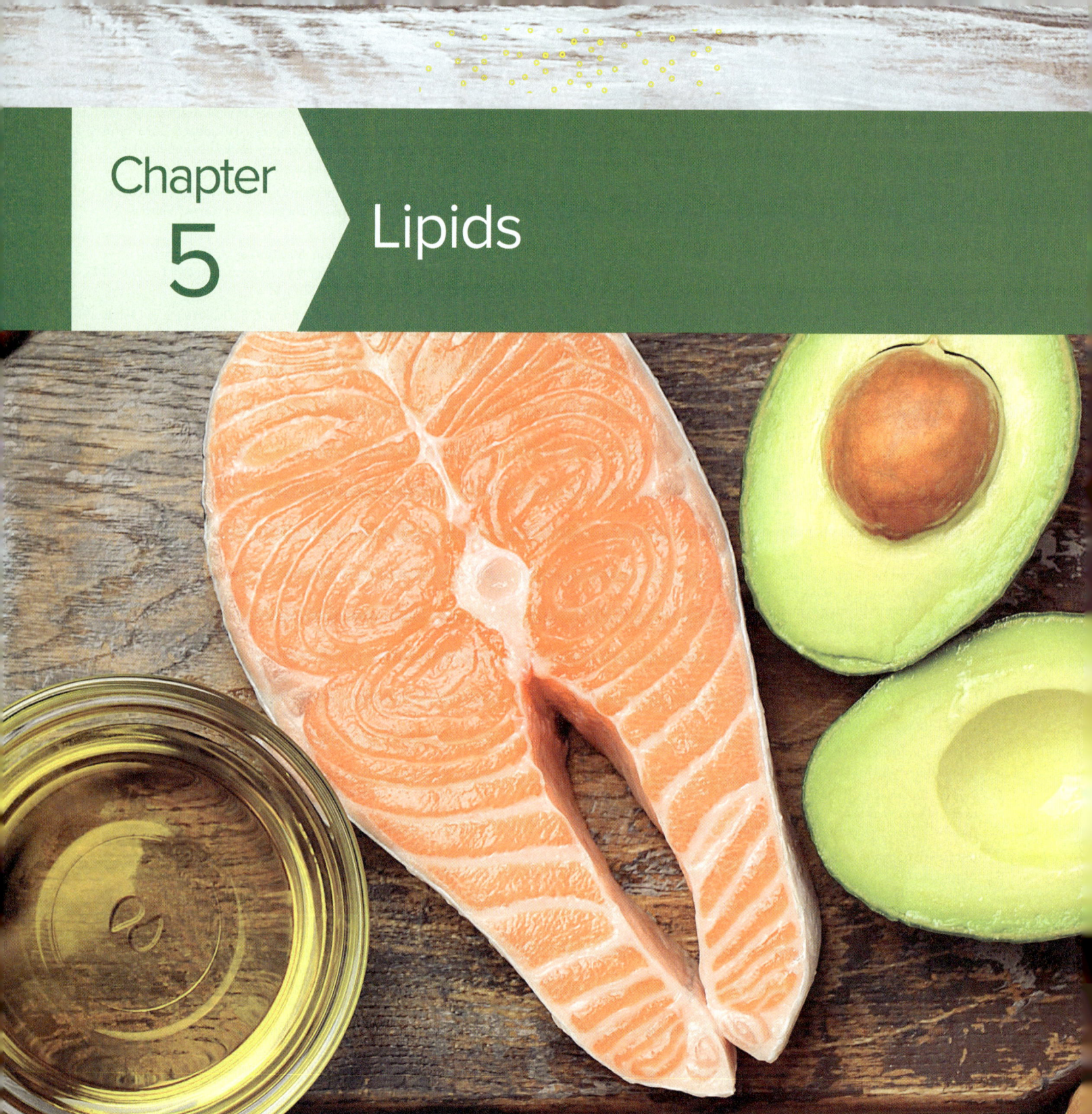

Chapter 5: Lipids

Student Learning Outcomes

Chapter 5 is designed to allow you to:

5.1 Understand the common properties of lipids.

5.2 Describe the structures of the three forms of lipids: triglycerides, phospholipids, and sterols.

5.3 Discuss the importance of the essential fatty acids.

5.4 Identify food sources of saturated, monounsaturated, and polyunsaturated fatty acids; phospholipids; and sterols.

5.5 Explain how lipids are digested and absorbed.

5.6 Name the lipoproteins and classify them according to their functions.

5.7 Describe the functions of the various forms of lipids in the body.

5.8 Summarize current recommendations for fat intake.

5.9 Characterize the relationship between lipids and cardiovascular disease.

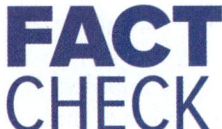

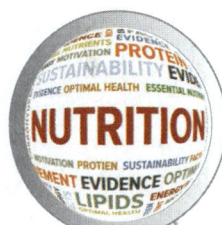

Are eggs bad for your heart?

One large egg (with the yolk) provides about 5 grams of fat, 1.5 grams of saturated fat, and 185 milligrams of cholesterol (and nearly all the lipids in eggs are in the yolks). Consuming too much of any of these nutrients could increase your risk for cardiovascular disease.

While eggs do provide some saturated fat and cholesterol, don't overlook their many nutritional benefits! Eggs are inexpensive sources of protein. The protein in eggs is of high quality, which means that it closely matches the amino acid needs of the human body. Eggs also supply several micronutrients, such as vitamin D and choline, which tend to be low in the dietary patterns of most Americans. Research evidence indicates that eating an average of one whole egg per day (about 7 eggs per week) is reasonable for heart health. See Section 5.6 to learn more about recommendations for fat intake.

Source: Sanlier N, Üstün D. Egg consumption and health effects: a narrative review. *J Food Sci*. 2021 Oct;86(10):4250-4261. doi: 10.1111/1750-3841.15892

5.1 Lipids: What Are They?

triglyceride The major form of lipid in the body and in food. It is composed of three fatty acids attached to glycerol.

sterol A compound containing a multi-ring (steroid) structure and a hydroxyl group (–OH). Cholesterol is a typical example.

Lipid is a general term that includes **triglycerides,** phospholipids, and **sterols.** Food scientists and culinary professionals usually refer to lipids that are solid at room temperature as *fats*, whereas lipids that are liquid at room temperature are called *oils*. To simplify our discussion, this chapter primarily uses the term *fat* to refer to lipids in foods. When necessary for clarity, the name of a specific lipid, such as cholesterol, will be used. This word use is consistent with the way many people use these terms.

As a class of nutrients, lipids share one main characteristic: they do not readily dissolve in water. Think of an oil-and-vinegar salad dressing. The oil is not soluble in the water-based vinegar; on standing, the two separate into distinct layers, with oil on the top and vinegar on the bottom.

Lipids are composed primarily of carbon, hydrogen, and oxygen. Compared to carbohydrates, lipids contain more carbon-hydrogen bonds and fewer carbon-oxygen bonds. Lots of chemical energy is released when those carbon-hydrogen bonds are broken down, so lipids yield more than twice as much energy (9 kcal per gram) as carbohydrates or proteins (4 kcal per gram).

The structures of lipids are diverse. In this section, you will learn about the structures of three categories of lipids: triglycerides, phospholipids, and sterols.

FATTY ACIDS AND TRIGLYCERIDES

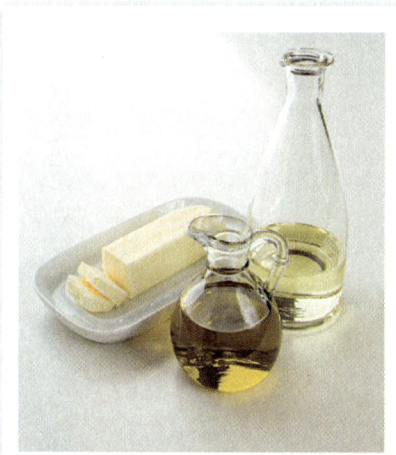

The physical properties of fats and oils depend on their chemical structures. **Why is butter solid at room temperature, while olive oil and corn oil are liquid at room temperature?** Tetra Images/Getty Images

Triglycerides are the primary form of lipids in the body and in foods. Their main purpose is to store energy. A triglyceride is composed of three fatty acids attached to a **glycerol** backbone. Each fatty acid is basically a chain of carbons bonded together and flanked by hydrogens. At one end of a fatty acid (the alpha end) is an **acid group**. At the other end (the omega end) is a **methyl group** (Fig. 5-1).

Here is an important point to remember: triglycerides are not composed of just one type of fatty acid. Rather, triglycerides may contain any combination of three fatty acids, which may vary in size and shape. The complex combination of fatty acids contributes to the unique taste and smell of each food. Food sources of various fatty acids will be discussed in Section 5.2.

glycerol A three-carbon alcohol used to form triglycerides.

acid group In chemistry, a functional group that consists of a carbon atom that shares bonds with two oxygen atoms. This is the site where fatty acids are linked to glycerol to form triglycerides.

methyl group In chemistry, a carbon atom that shares bonds with three hydrogen atoms. The methyl group is the omega end of a fatty acid.

short-chain fatty acid A fatty acid with fewer than 6 carbons.

medium-chain fatty acid A fatty acid that contains 6 to 10 carbons.

long-chain fatty acid A fatty acid that contains 12 or more carbons.

saturated fatty acid A fatty acid containing no carbon-carbon double bonds.

Fatty Acids Vary in Length. A **short-chain fatty acid** has fewer than 6 carbons. A fatty acid that contains 6 to 10 carbons is a **medium-chain fatty acid.** Most of the fatty acids in foods and in the body are **long-chain fatty acids,** which have 12 or more carbons. In foods, the length of a fatty acid affects its melting point. The longer the fatty acid, the higher its melting point. In the body, the length of a fatty acid affects its absorption and metabolism. As you will learn in Section 5.3, short- and medium-chain fatty acids are more easily absorbed and more quickly used by cells as a source of fuel.

Fatty Acids Can Be Saturated or Unsaturated. The terms *saturated* and *unsaturated* refer to the amount of hydrogen atoms that attach to the carbon atoms in a fatty acid. Each carbon atom can form four bonds. Within the carbon chain of a fatty acid, each carbon atom binds to two adjacent carbon atoms and one or two hydrogen atoms. The carbons that make up a **saturated fatty acid** are all connected to each other by single bonds. If only two of the carbon's bonds are used to join with adjacent carbon atoms, this leaves room to bind to two hydrogen atoms—the maximum amount. Just as a sponge can be saturated (full) with water, a saturated fatty acid, such as stearic acid, is saturated with hydrogen [see Fig. 5-1(a)]. The shape of saturated fatty acids is quite linear, so they can pack very close together. This close packing of saturated fatty acids gives them a solid consistency at room temperature.

If the carbon chain of a fatty acid contains at least one double bond, the carbon atoms involved in the double bond have fewer bonds to share with hydrogen, and the

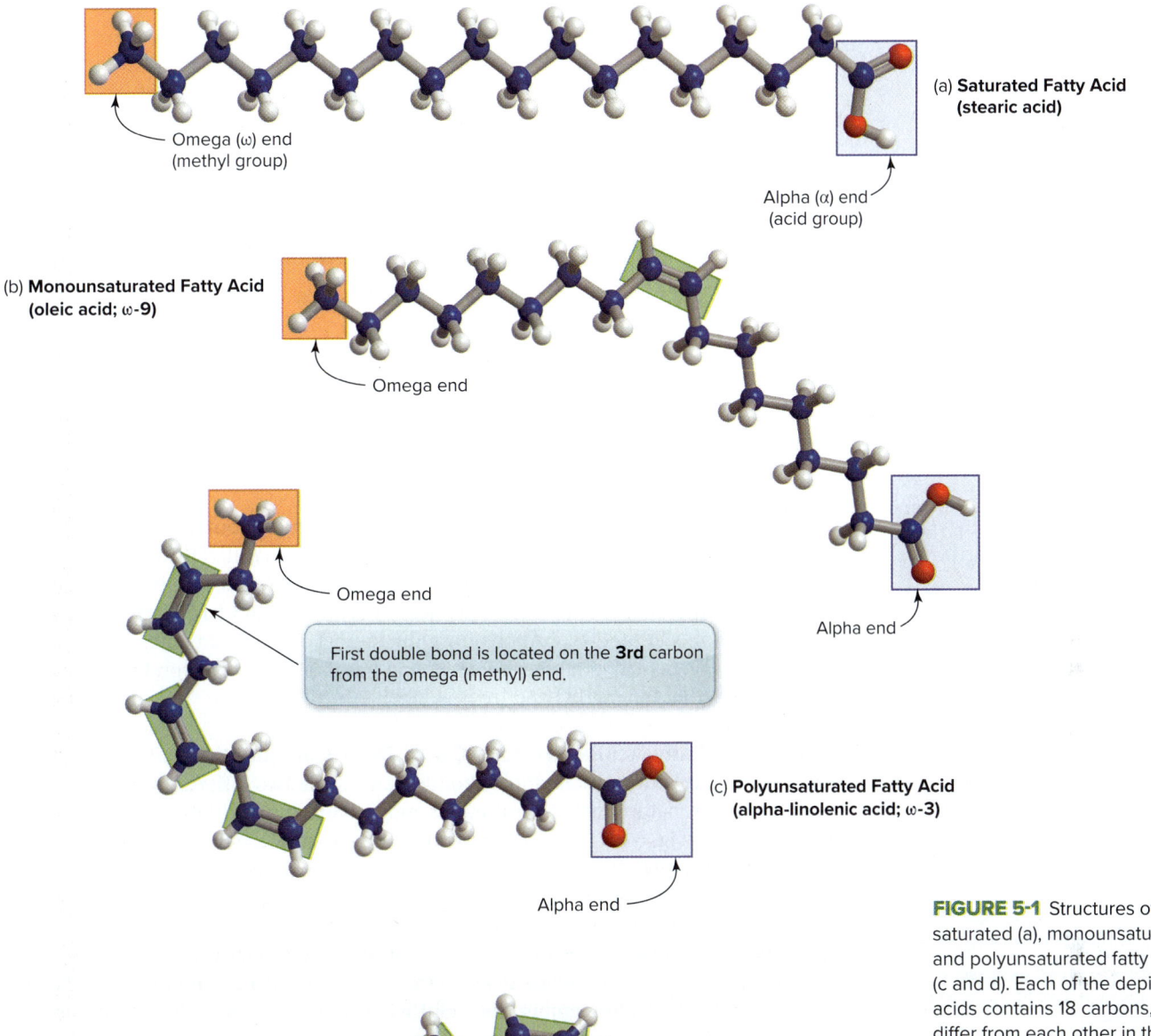

FIGURE 5-1 Structures of saturated (a), monounsaturated (b), and polyunsaturated fatty acids (c and d). Each of the depicted fatty acids contains 18 carbons, but they differ from each other in the number and location of double bonds. The double bonds are shaded green. The linear shape of saturated fatty acids, as shown in (a), allows them to pack tightly together and form a solid at room temperature. In contrast, unsaturated fatty acids (b–d) have "kinks" where double bonds interrupt the carbon chain (Fig. 5-2). Thus, unsaturated fatty acids pack together only loosely and are usually liquid at room temperature.

fatty acid is said to be *unsaturated*. A fatty acid with only one double bond is **monounsaturated** [see Fig. 5-1(b)].

If the carbon chain of a fatty acid contains two or more double bonds, the fatty acid is even less saturated with hydrogens, and so it is **polyunsaturated** [see Fig. 5-1(c), (d)]. The double bonds in unsaturated fatty acids create kinks that keep them from packing closely together, so they are liquid at room temperature.

monounsaturated fatty acid A fatty acid containing one carbon-carbon double bond.

polyunsaturated fatty acid A fatty acid containing two or more carbon-carbon double bonds.

FIGURE 5-2 *Cis* and *trans* fatty acids. In foods, *cis* fatty acids are much more common than *trans* fatty acids.

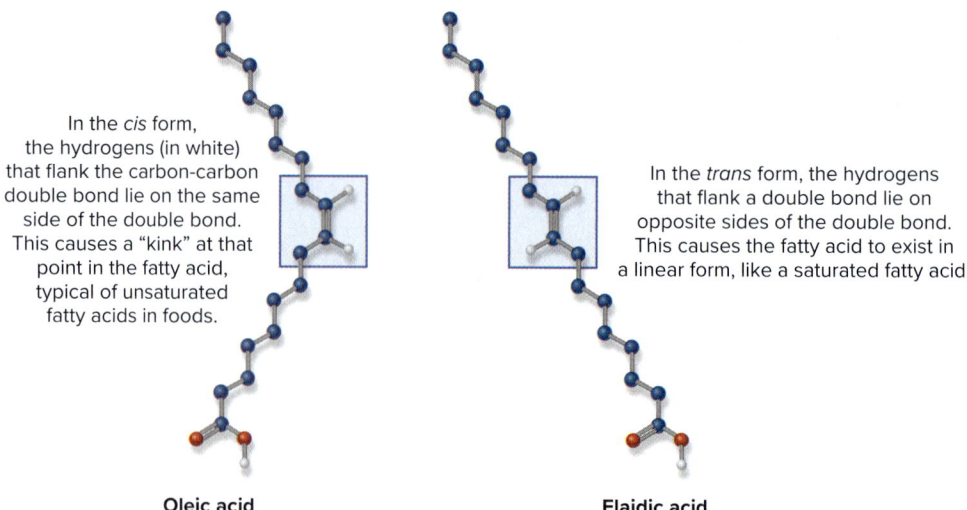

In the *cis* form, the hydrogens (in white) that flank the carbon-carbon double bond lie on the same side of the double bond. This causes a "kink" at that point in the fatty acid, typical of unsaturated fatty acids in foods.

In the *trans* form, the hydrogens that flank a double bond lie on opposite sides of the double bond. This causes the fatty acid to exist in a linear form, like a saturated fatty acid.

Oleic acid Elaidic acid

omega-3 (ω-3) fatty acid An unsaturated fatty acid with the first double bond on the third carbon from the methyl end (—CH₃).

omega-6 (ω-6) fatty acid An unsaturated fatty acid with the first double bond on the sixth carbon from the methyl end (—CH₃).

cis fatty acid A form of an unsaturated fatty acid that has the hydrogens lying on the same side of the carbon-carbon double bond.

trans fatty acid A form of an unsaturated fatty acid, usually a monounsaturated one when found in food, in which the hydrogens lie on opposite sides of the carbon-carbon double bond.

linoleic acid An essential omega-6 fatty acid with 18 carbons and two double bonds.

alpha-linolenic acid An essential omega-3 fatty acid with 18 carbons and three double bonds.

eicosanoids A class of signaling compounds, including the prostaglandins, derived from the essential polyunsaturated fatty acids.

eicosapentaenoic acid (EPA) An omega-3 fatty acid with 20 carbons and 5 carbon-carbon double bonds. It is present in large amounts in fatty fish and is slowly synthesized in the body from alpha-linolenic acid.

docosahexaenoic acid (DHA) An omega-3 fatty acid with 22 carbons and 6 carbon-carbon double bonds. It is present in large amounts in fatty fish and is slowly synthesized in the body from alpha-linolenic acid. In the human body, high levels of DHA are found in the retina and brain.

arachidonic acid (ARA) An omega-6 fatty acid made from linoleic acid with 20 carbon atoms and 4 carbon-carbon double bonds.

Unsaturated Fatty Acids Differ in the Location of Their Double Bonds. The location of the first double bond relative to the methyl end (also called the *omega* end) of an unsaturated fatty acid is another important feature. If the first double bond starts three carbons from the methyl end of the fatty acid, it is an **omega-3 (ω-3) fatty acid** [review Fig. 5-1(c)]. If it is located six carbons from the methyl end, it is an **omega-6 (ω-6) fatty acid** [review Fig. 5-1(d)]. An omega-9 fatty acid has its first double bond starting at the ninth carbon from the methyl end [review Fig. 5-1(b)].

Unsaturated Fatty Acids Can Have *Cis* or *Trans* Configuration. Unsaturated fatty acids, which have one or more double bonds, can exist in two different structural forms: *cis* and *trans*. In nature, monounsaturated and polyunsaturated fatty acids usually are in the *cis* form (Fig. 5-2). In a *cis* **fatty acid,** the hydrogens are on the same side of the carbon-carbon double bond. In a *trans* **fatty acid,** the hydrogens are oriented on opposite sides of the carbon-carbon double bond. As shown in Figure 5-2, the *cis* bond causes the fatty acid's carbon chain to bend, whereas the *trans* bond allows the chain to remain more linear. This change in shape makes a *trans* unsaturated fatty acid look more like a saturated fatty acid. As you might guess, a *trans* fatty acid also acts more like a saturated fatty acid in the body. Remember this point when you learn about the health effects of various fatty acids in Sections 5.6 and 5.7.

Two Fatty Acids Are Essential for Human Health. The various classes of lipids have diverse functions in the body and are necessary for health. Of all the types of lipids found in foods, however, only two polyunsaturated fatty acids are essential. Remember, in nutrition, *essential* means that the substance is necessary for health, but it cannot be made in the body, so it must be consumed as part of the dietary pattern. **Linoleic acid** (an omega-6 fatty acid) and **alpha-linolenic acid** (an omega-3 fatty acid) are the two essential fatty acids for humans. The essential fatty acids form body structures, perform important functions for the immune and nervous systems, and produce regulatory compounds, such as **eicosanoids** and hormones.

Many important *nonessential* fatty acids can be derived from the essential fatty acids (Fig. 5-3). Human enzymes can convert the two essential fatty acids to other long-chain polyunsaturated fatty acids, such as **eicosapentaenoic acid (EPA), docosahexaenoic acid (DHA),** and **arachidonic acid (ARA),** which are particularly important for proper function of the brain and nervous system. Because of its role in brain structure, DHA is especially important during pregnancy for fetal brain and nervous system development. Failing to consume enough of the essential fatty acids will limit the production of many nonessential fatty acids in the body. As you will learn in Section 5.6, a deficiency of essential fatty acids can severely impact the health of all body systems.

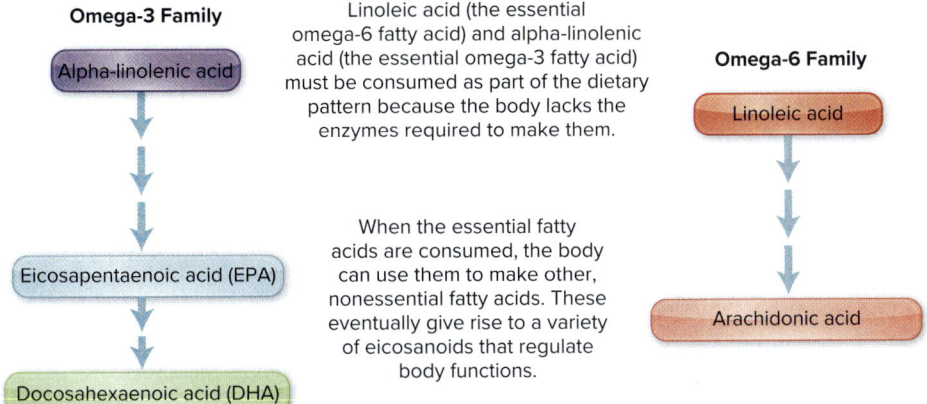

FIGURE 5-3 The essential fatty acid (EFA) family.

Triglycerides Are the Main Form of Lipids in Foods and in the Body. The lipids in foods and in body structures are mostly in the form of triglycerides. Although some free fatty acids are transported in the bloodstream while attached to proteins, most fatty acids in the body are part of triglycerides.

Triglycerides contain a simple three-carbon alcohol, called glycerol, that serves as a backbone for three fatty acids [Fig. 5-4(a)]. Removing one fatty acid from a triglyceride forms a **diglyceride.** Removing two fatty acids from a triglyceride forms a **monoglyceride.** Later in this chapter, you will see that before most dietary fats are absorbed, the two outer fatty acids are typically removed from the triglyceride during digestion in the small intestine. This produces a mixture of fatty acids and monoglycerides that can be absorbed into the intestinal cells. After absorption, the fatty acids and monoglycerides are mostly reformed into triglycerides inside body cells.

diglyceride A breakdown product of a triglyceride consisting of two fatty acids attached to a glycerol backbone.

monoglyceride A breakdown product of a triglyceride consisting of one fatty acid attached to a glycerol backbone.

PHOSPHOLIPIDS

Like triglycerides, phospholipids are made of glycerol and fatty acids. However, at least one fatty acid in the structure is replaced with a compound containing phosphorus (and often other elements, such as nitrogen) [see Fig. 5-4(d)]. This structure gives phospholipids a unique ability: the fatty acid part of a phospholipid is soluble in fat, but the phosphate group at the other end of a phospholipid is soluble in water. Thus, phospholipids are **amphipathic,** which means they are simultaneously soluble in fat and water. The amphipathic property of phospholipids allows them to perform some very important functions in foods and in the body.

Many types of phospholipids exist in the body; they are part of the structure of every cell membrane. Phospholipids participate in fat digestion, absorption, and transport. Even though phospholipids are present in some foods (naturally or as an additive) and are sold as dietary supplements, phospholipids are *not essential* components of the dietary pattern. Rather, the body is able to produce all the phospholipids it needs. **Lecithin** is one example of a phospholipid.

amphipathic Having both hydrophobic (fat-soluble) and hydrophilic (water-soluble) parts. Amphipathic molecules can function as emulsifiers.

lecithin A group of phospholipid compounds that are major components of cell membranes.

STEROLS

Sterols are a class of lipids characterized by a multi-ringed structure that makes them structurally and functionally different from other forms of lipids [see Fig. 5-4(e)]. Although this waxy substance does not look much like the other lipids discussed so far, it is classified as a lipid because it does not readily dissolve in water. The most common example of a sterol is cholesterol, which is synthesized by the liver in animals and humans. Among other functions, cholesterol is a vital part of cell membranes and is used to form hormones and bile acids. It is important to note that the human body can make all the cholesterol it needs, so sterols are *not essential* components of the dietary pattern. Plants produce a different form of sterols called *phytosterols,* which may have benefits for human health (see Section 5.7).

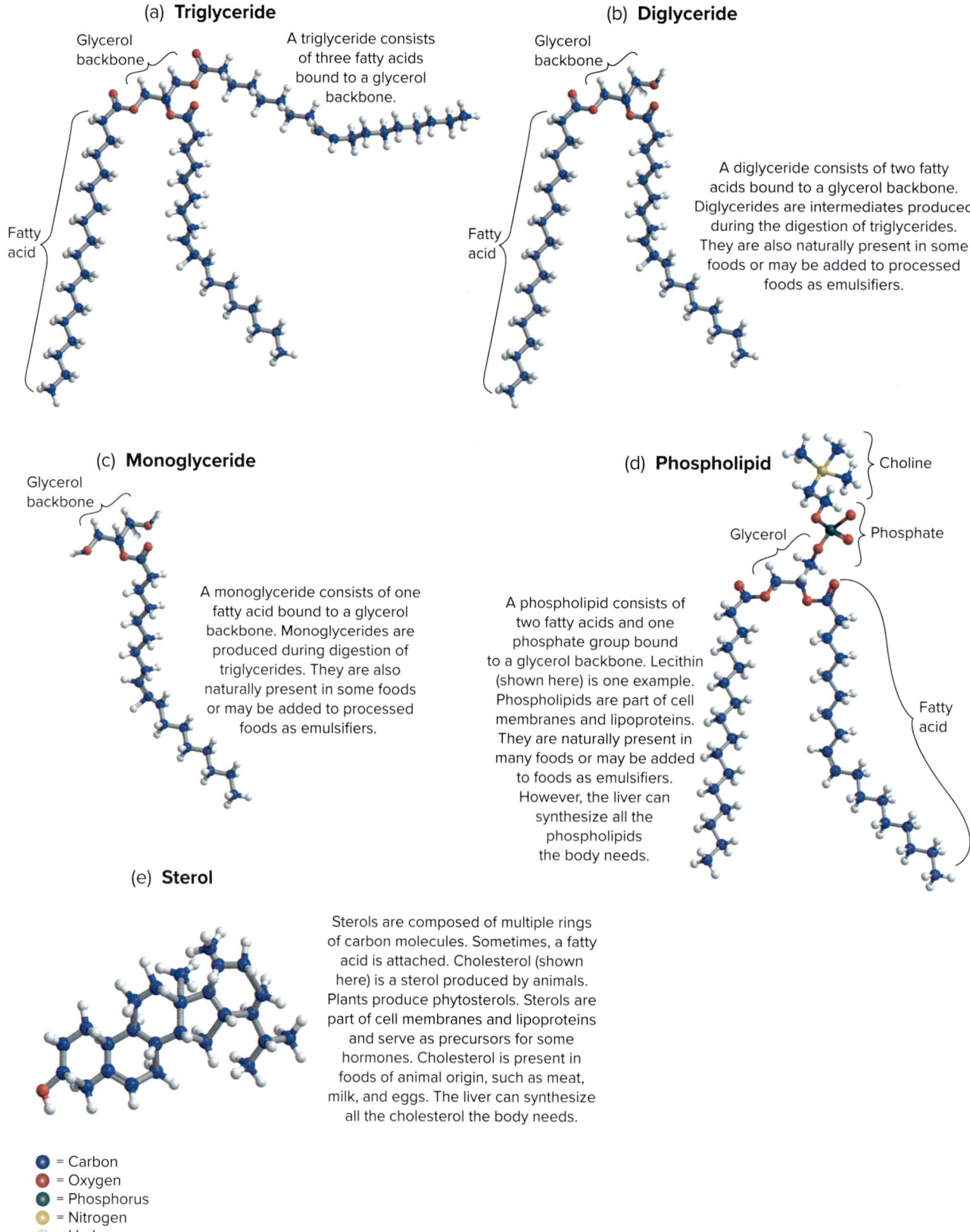

FIGURE 5-4 Chemical forms of common lipids: (a) triglyceride, (b) diglyceride, (c) monoglyceride, (d) phospholipid (in this case, lecithin), and (e) sterol (in this case, cholesterol).

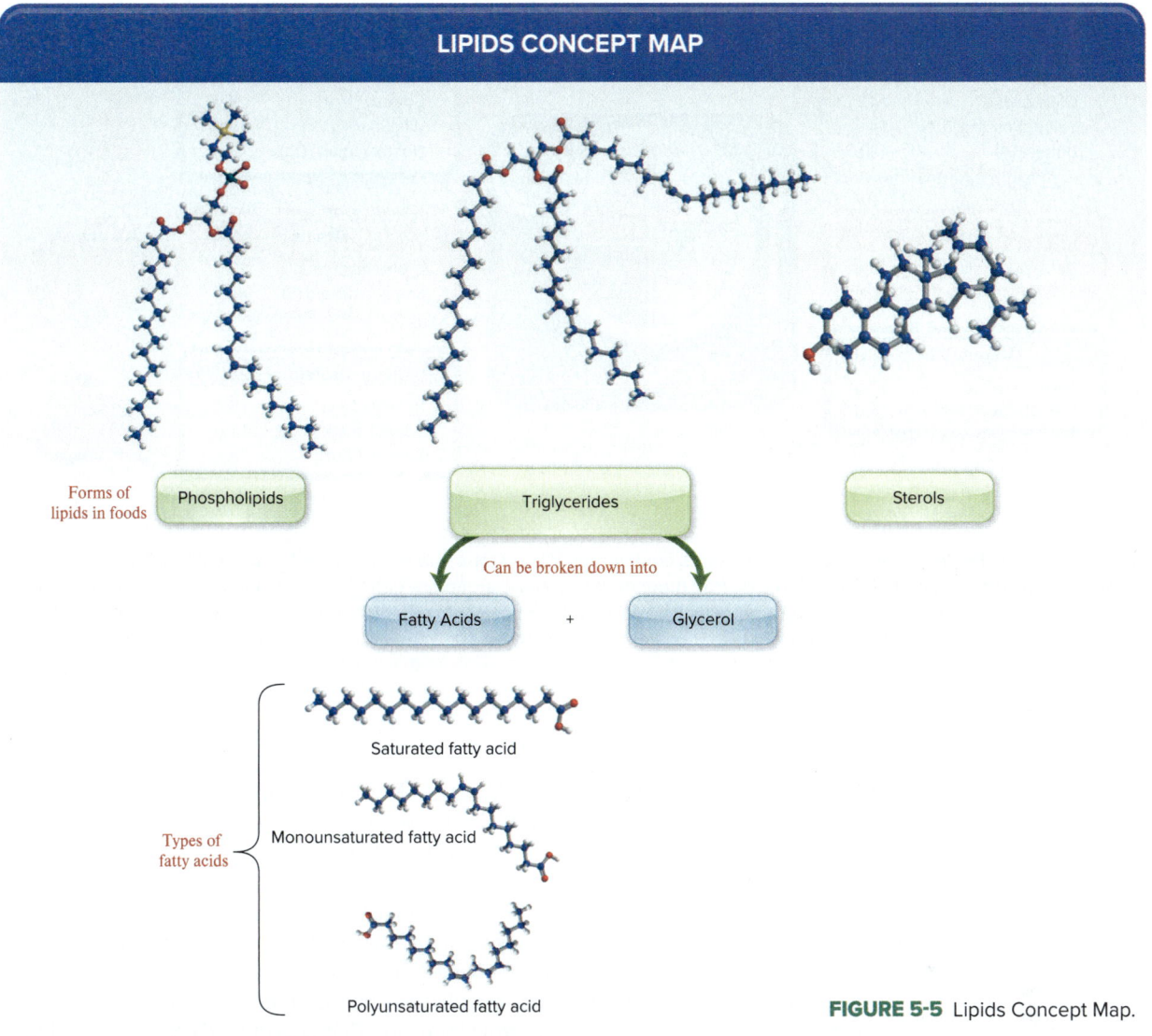

FIGURE 5-5 Lipids Concept Map.

The Lipids Concept Map (Fig. 5-5) summarizes the various forms of lipids.

✓ CONCEPT CHECK 5.1

1. Name the three forms of lipids.
2. What is the structural difference between saturated and unsaturated fatty acids?
3. What is the structural difference between omega-3 and omega-6 fatty acids?
4. Which two fatty acids are essential?
5. How do triglycerides differ from phospholipids?
6. Are phospholipids and sterols essential in the human dietary pattern? Why or why not?

5.2 Fats and Oils in Foods

FOOD SOURCES OF TRIGLYCERIDES

Foods that are high in fat are very energy dense, which means they pack a lot of calories into a small space. While you certainly should monitor the *total amount* of fat, the *type* of fat in foods is another important consideration when it comes to selecting a dietary pattern that promotes optimal health.

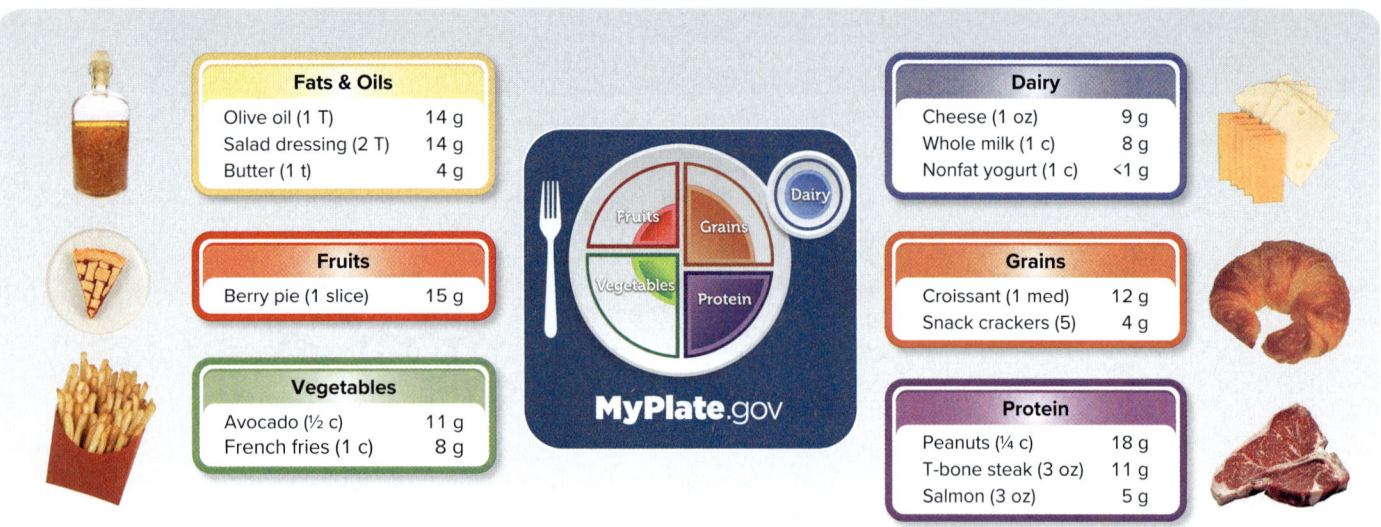

FIGURE 5-6 Sources of fat from MyPlate. The fill of the background color (none, 1/3, 2/3, or completely covered) within each group in the plate indicates the average nutrient density for fat in that group. The fruit group and vegetable group are generally low in fat. In the other groups, both high-fat and low-fat choices are available. In general, any type of frying adds significant amounts of fat to a product, as with French fries and fried chicken. Careful reading of food labels can help you identify the fat content of foods. MyPlate: U.S. Department of Agriculture (USDA); Italian dressing in a flask: Holly Hildreth/McGraw Hill; berry pie: RTsubin/iStock/Getty Images; French fries in container: Comstock/Getty Images; cheeses: Holly Curry/McGraw Hill; croissant: Ingram Publishing/Alamy Stock Photo; frozen steak: Frank Bean/Uppercut/Getty Images

Source: U.S. Department of Agriculture, Agricultural Research Service. FoodData Central, 2019. fdc.nal.usda.gov.

Where Is the Fat on MyPlate? You'll notice there is no food group for fats and oils on MyPlate; it is assumed that fats and oils are incorporated into each food group. The fat content of foods may vary significantly because of fats and oils added during processing or food preparation. Figure 5-6 shows examples of food sources of fat.

In the protein foods group, there is a wide range of fat content. With less than 0.5 gram of fat per ½-cup serving, kidney beans are quite low in fat (4% of total kcal from fat). Lean cuts of meat, such as *loin* and *round* cuts of beef, have about 5 grams of fat per 3-ounce serving (25% of total kcal from fat). Nuts, marbled meats, and some processed meats are quite high in fat. Just 1 ounce of peanuts provides nearly 15 grams of fat (76% of total kcal from fat). A 3-ounce portion of prime rib has 29 grams of fat (76% of total kcal from fat). About 80% of the calories in processed meats, such as pepperoni and bacon, comes from fat.

In the dairy foods group, some items are very low in fat. A serving of 1 cup of skim milk or 1 cup of low-fat yogurt contains less than 1 gram of fat. Whole milk or yogurt made from whole milk contains 8 grams of fat per cup (50% of total kcal). With 9 grams of fat per slice, most types of cheese are fairly high in fat (74% of total kcal). Because it contributes so much to flavor and texture, the butterfat content of ice cream is the factor that determines quality of ice cream: Standard ice cream has about 10 to 12 grams of fat per ½ cup (50% of total kcal), whereas premium ice cream has up to 18 grams of fat per ½ cup (60% of total kcal).

Most grains are quite low in fat. One slice of whole wheat bread, 1 cup of corn flakes cereal, or 1 cup of plain, cooked pasta, for example, provide just 1 gram of fat (about 5% to 10% of total kcal). However, we tend to add fat to grains to make them more palatable. Spreading 1 teaspoon of butter on a slice of bread adds about 4 grams of fat. When we make cookie dough or pie crust, we incorporate fat into flour to give it a delicious flavor and flaky texture. A slice of pie has about 5 grams of fat in the crust alone. Adding ½ cup of creamy alfredo sauce to your pasta will add 20 grams of fat (80% of total kcal from fat).

With less than 1 gram of fat per cup, most fruits and vegetables are low in fat. Avocados, discussed in *Farm to Fork,* are a notable exception. One whole avocado has about 30 grams of fat (82% of total kcal from fat). For most fruits and vegetables, however, what we add to these foods during preparation or processing can increase the fat content. Take the potato, for example. A plain, 3-ounce, baked potato is nearly devoid of fat.

Adding a teaspoon of butter adds about 4 grams of fat. If we take that potato, slice it into fries, and deep-fry it in a vat of sizzling peanut oil, we add about 15 grams of fat (42% of total kcal). Likewise, adding just 2 tablespoons of ranch salad dressing incorporates 13 additional grams of fat into an otherwise fat-free pile of vegetables.

Triglycerides Contain Mixtures of Fatty Acids. Remember that triglycerides contain three fatty acids bound to a glycerol backbone. These three fatty acids could be short, medium, or long. They may be saturated or unsaturated. Furthermore, the unsaturated fatty acids can bend in different directions. Variations in the length, degree of saturation, and shape of fatty acids affect their properties in foods and their functions in the body.

Chain Length of Fatty Acids. Some short-chain fatty acids are naturally present in foods. For example, butterfat contains a 4-carbon fatty acid called butyrate. Short-chain fatty acids are also produced in the colon when certain strains of probiotic bacteria ferment carbohydrates in the colon (Section 3.9).

Foods that provide significant amounts of medium-chain fatty acids include human breast milk, cow's milk, coconut oil, and palm oil. There are also medical products that are formulated to provide triglycerides in which all three fatty acids are medium-chain fatty acids. These are useful for individuals who have conditions that impair fat digestion or absorption because short- and medium-chain fatty acids are absorbed differently than larger fatty acids.

Most of the fatty acids in foods and in the body are long-chain fatty acids. Palmitic acid is a 16-carbon fatty acid found in milk and other dairy products, red meat, and palm oil (commonly used for frying foods). Oleic acid is an 18-carbon fatty acid found in olive oil, nuts, and seeds. Linoleic acid is another 18-carbon fatty acid found in lots of plant oils, including sunflower, safflower, and soybean oils.

Saturation of Fatty Acids. Overall, a fat or an oil is classified as saturated, monounsaturated, or polyunsaturated based on the type of fatty acids present in the greatest concentration (Fig. 5-7). Fats in foods that contain primarily saturated fatty acids are solid at room temperature. In contrast, fats containing primarily monounsaturated or polyunsaturated fatty acids (regardless of the length of the carbon chain) are usually liquid at room temperature.

Animal fats are the chief contributors of saturated fatty acids to the American dietary pattern. About 40% to 60% of total fat in dairy and meat products is in the form of saturated fatty acids. Palm oil and coconut oil are two plant oils that are rich sources of saturated fatty acids. Aside from palm oil and coconut oil, most plant oils are rich in unsaturated fatty acids, ranging from 73% to 94% of total fat. The major sources of monounsaturated fatty acids are canola oil, olive oil, and peanut oil. Corn, cottonseed, sunflower, soybean, and safflower oils contain mostly polyunsaturated fatty acids (54% to 77% of total fat).

FARM to FORK Avocados

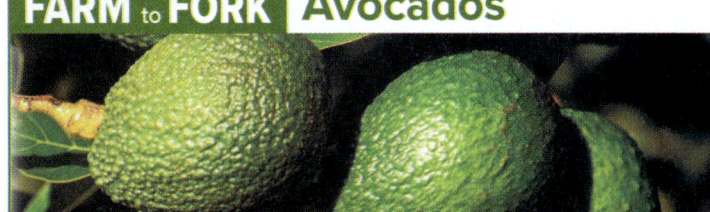

imagebroker/Alamy Stock Photo

Who knew? Although avocados are categorized as vegetables on MyPlate, botanists classify them as berries. Like other berries, they are loaded with antioxidants and fiber.

Grow
- Of the avocados grown in the United States, most are grown in California. Globally, Mexico is the top producer of avocados. The trees grow best in tropical or subtropical climates, but it is possible to grow hardy varieties of the plant in slightly cooler regions or indoors.

Shop
- Most common are the Hass avocados. When ripe, they have dark green, almost black skin. A ripe avocado is soft at the top and yields only slightly when pressed in the middle.
- Another way to check for ripeness is to pluck the stem off the fruit. A vibrant green flesh is best. Light yellow (or if the stem is difficult to pluck) means the fruit is not ripe enough. Dark green or brown is too ripe.
- Don't buy avocados that are dented or mushy, or if you can feel the pit moving inside.

Store
- Unripe avocados will ripen at room temperature. To promote ripening, place the avocado in a paper bag with a banana. Gases produced by the banana will help the avocado to ripen quickly.
- Ripe avocados will remain at peak quality for 2 or 3 days in the refrigerator.
- To prevent cut avocados from browning, sprinkle the cut surface with an acidic juice, such as lemon or lime, and store them in a plastic bag (remove as much air as possible) in the refrigerator.
- Storing cut avocados with sliced onions will prevent browning as well because volatile oils from the onion are very effective antioxidants.
- If you have more ripe avocados than you can use, a good way to reduce food waste is to freeze them. Cut your avocados into slices or chunks, place them on a plate or baking sheet, sprinkle with lemon juice, and place them in the freezer for about 1 hour. After they have partially frozen, transfer the avocados to a plastic bag for long-term storage.

Prep
- Most often, avocados are served raw, chopped in flavorful salsas, or mashed in guacamole. Their mild flavor pairs well with the more defined flavors of onion, citrus, and fresh herbs.
- Avocados are rich in monounsaturated fatty acids, which gives them a creamy, delicate texture. Pureed avocados can substitute 1:1 for butter in recipes for baked goods. The mild flavor of the avocado will be imperceptible, and the final product will be lower in calories but higher in fiber and monounsaturated fats than the original recipe.
- Use half an avocado as a deliciously edible bowl for tuna salad.
- Search online for trendy ways to bake an egg in an avocado or grill it up with lean meats and veggies.
- Frozen avocados are useful for smoothies, guacamole, or baked goods.

Source: Robinson J. Artichoke, asparagus, and avocados: indulge! In: *Eating on the Wild Side: The Missing Link to Optimum Health.* New York: Little, Brown & Co.; 2013.

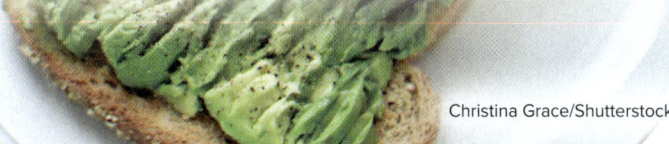

Christina Grace/Shutterstock

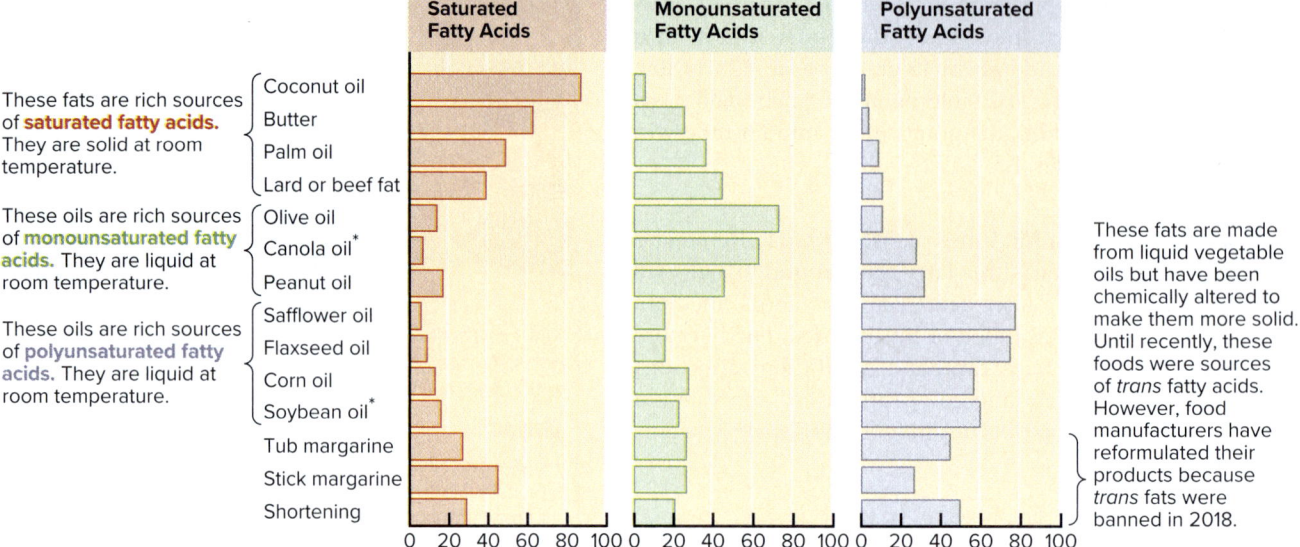

FIGURE 5-7 Saturated, monounsaturated, and polyunsaturated fatty acid composition of common fats and oils (expressed as percent of all fatty acids in the product). Foods contain mixtures of fatty acids.
*Rich source of the essential omega-3 fatty acid alpha-linolenic acid.

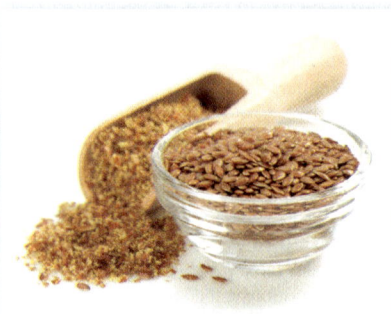

Flaxseeds are rich sources of alpha-linolenic acid, the essential omega-3 fatty acid. Whole flaxseeds must be chewed thoroughly or ground to improve digestibility and nutrient absorption. Flaxseed oil should be refrigerated to prevent it from turning rancid. **Why is flaxseed oil susceptible to rancidity?** Sergii Moskaliuk/123RF

Food Sources of Essential Fatty Acids. Rich food sources of linoleic acid—the essential omega-6 fatty acid—include corn, cottonseed, grapeseed, safflower, soybean, and sunflower oils, as well as nuts and seeds. Linoleic acid is also found in meat, poultry, and eggs.[1]

Two nutrient-dense food sources of alpha-linolenic acid (the essential omega-3 fatty acid) are flaxseeds and walnuts.[2] Compared to other nuts and seeds, walnuts are one of the richest sources of alpha-linolenic acid (2.6 grams per 1-ounce serving, which is 14 walnut halves). In addition, walnuts are a rich source of plant sterols known to inhibit intestinal absorption of cholesterol. Other rich food sources of alpha-linolenic acid include oils from perilla seeds, chia seeds, canola seeds, and soybeans.

Omega-3 Fatty Acids in Fish. Looking at Figure 5-3, you can see that eicosapentaenoic acid (EPA) and docosahexaenoic acid (DHA) can be made in the body, so they are not essential fatty acids. However, by consuming food sources of EPA and DHA, you effectively skip a few rather slow and inefficient steps in the conversion of alpha-linolenic acid to EPA and DHA. These two omega-3 fatty acids are naturally found in fatty fish such as salmon, tuna, sardines, anchovies, striped bass, catfish, herring, mackerel, trout, and halibut (Table 5-1). Recommendations from the

TABLE 5-1 ■ Omega-3 Fatty Acids in Fish

Food Item	Serving Size	Omega-3 Fatty Acids (g)*
Atlantic salmon	3 oz	1.8
Anchovy	3 oz	1.7
Sardines	3 oz	1.4
Rainbow trout	3 oz	1.0
Coho salmon	3 oz	0.9
Bluefish	3 oz	0.8
Striped bass	3 oz	0.8
Tuna, white, canned	3 oz	0.7
Halibut	3 oz	0.4
Catfish	3 oz	0.2

*EPA + DHA

Source: U.S. Department of Agriculture, Agricultural Research Service. FoodData Central, 2019.

Dietary Guidelines for Americans and the American Heart Association (AHA) encourage us to consume two servings of fatty fish per week for optimal cardiovascular health as well as improvements in brain health. An EPA/DHA supplement is useful for people who do not regularly consume fatty fish.

A word of caution: Some types of fish can be a source of mercury, which is toxic in high amounts, especially during pregnancy, infancy, and early childhood (see Section 14.8). Fish species that are highest in mercury include shark, swordfish, king mackerel, tilefish, marlin, orange roughy, and bigeye (ahi) tuna. Salmon, sardines, herring, and albacore or yellowfin tuna are better choices because they are lower in mercury, yet they still provide heart-healthy omega-3 fatty acids. To limit exposure to mercury, vary your choices rather than always eating the same species of fish and limit overall intake to 12 ounces per week (two to three meals of fish or shellfish per week). Overall, research indicates that the benefits of fish intake, especially for heart health and brain health, outweigh the possible risks of mercury contamination.[3]

FOOD SOURCES OF PHOSPHOLIPIDS

Wheat germ, peanuts, egg yolks, soybeans, and organ meats are rich sources of phospholipids. Phospholipids such as lecithin, a component of egg yolks, are often added to salad dressing. Lecithin is used as an **emulsifier** in these and other products because of its ability to keep mixtures of lipids and water from separating (Fig. 5-8). Emulsifiers are added to salad dressings to keep the vegetable oil suspended in water. Likewise, eggs are added to cake batters to emulsify the fat with the milk.

emulsifier A compound that can suspend fat in water by isolating individual fat droplets, using a shell of water molecules or other substances to prevent the fat from coalescing.

FOOD SOURCES OF STEROLS

Your body can make all the cholesterol you need, so cholesterol is not an essential nutrient. However, if you do consume dietary sources of cholesterol, it can be absorbed from your small intestine and perform all the same functions as the cholesterol produced by

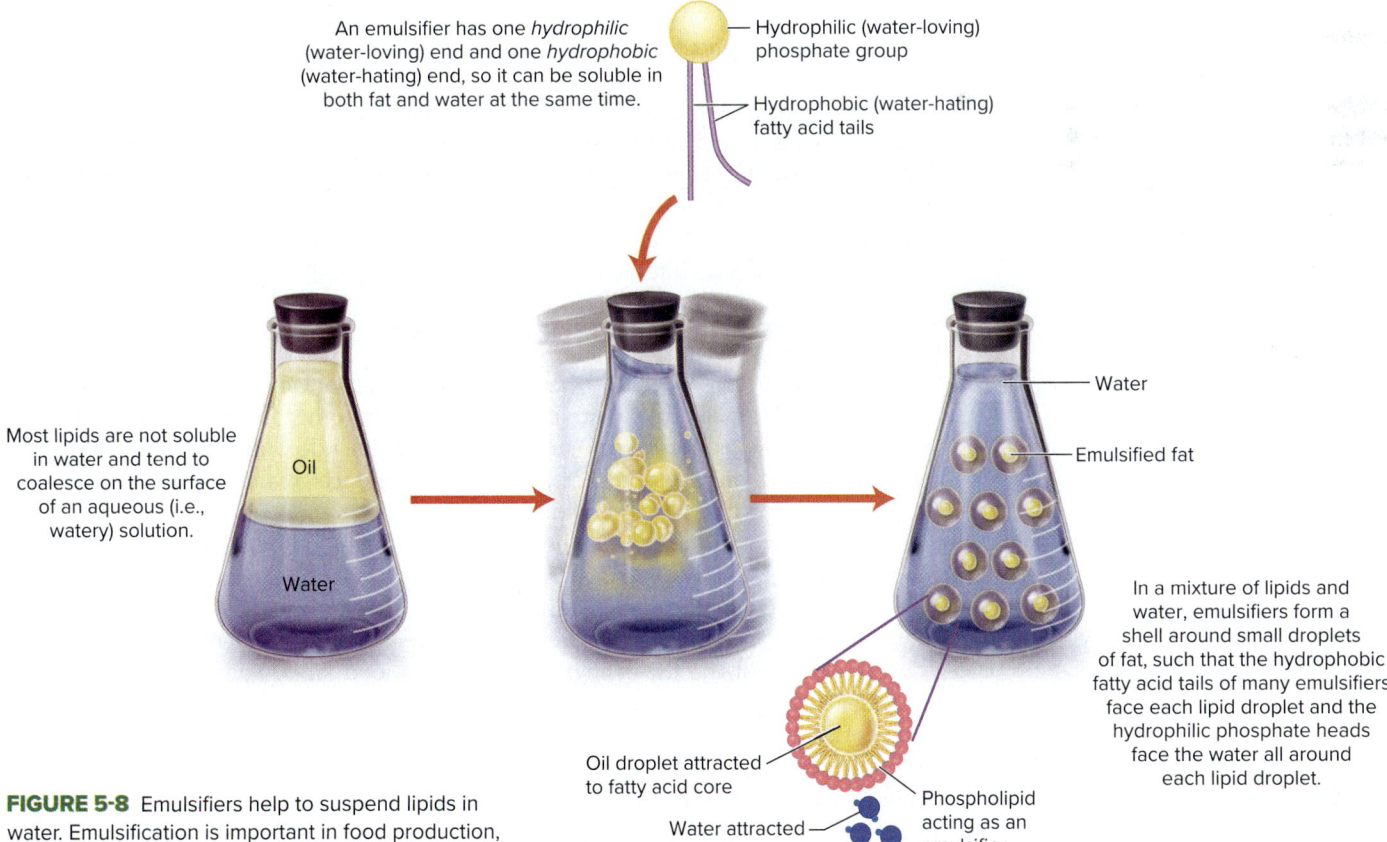

FIGURE 5-8 Emulsifiers help to suspend lipids in water. Emulsification is important in food production, fat digestion, and transport of fats through the blood.

TABLE 5-2 ■ Cholesterol Content of Foods

Food Item	Serving Size	Cholesterol (mg)
Beef brains, cooked	3 oz	2635 mg
Beef liver, braised	3 oz	334 mg
Egg yolk*	1 large	184 mg
Shrimp, cooked	3 oz	123 mg
Beef, pot roast, braised*	3 oz	89 mg
Pork loin, roasted	3 oz	69 mg
Chicken breast, skinless, roasted*	3 oz	85 mg
Trout, broiled	3 oz	63 mg
Ice cream, chocolate, regular	1 cup	50 mg
Tuna, broiled	3 oz	42 mg
Hot dog	1 each	33 mg
Cheddar cheese*	1 oz	28 mg
Whole milk*	1 cup	24 mg
1% milk	1 cup	12 mg
Fat-free milk	1 cup	5 mg
Egg white	1 large	0 mg

*Leading dietary sources of cholesterol in American dietary patterns.
Source: U.S. Department of Agriculture, Agricultural Research Service. FoodData Central, 2019.

your liver. Typically, if cholesterol is part of your dietary pattern, your liver synthesizes less cholesterol.

There are two types of sterols in the food supply: (1) cholesterol and (2) phytosterols. Cholesterol is found only in foods of animal origin. Eggs, meats, and whole milk are our main dietary sources of cholesterol (Table 5-2). One large egg yolk contains about 185 milligrams of cholesterol.

Foods of plant origin are naturally cholesterol free, but they may contain phytosterols (e.g., plant sterols and plant stanols). Some phytosterols can help to lower blood cholesterol because they compete with cholesterol for absorptive sites in the small intestine and thereby limit cholesterol absorption. The highest sources of phytosterols include plant oils, nuts, seeds, beans, peas, lentils, and whole grains (refer to the discussion in Section 5.7 on medical interventions to lower blood lipids).

USING FOOD LABELS TO IDENTIFY FAT

In some foods discussed thus far, the presence of fat is obvious: butter on bread, mayonnaise in potato salad, and marbling in raw meat. In other foods, however, fat is not immediately obvious. Foods that contain hidden fat include whole milk, pastries, cookies, cake, cheese, hot dogs, crackers, French fries, and ice cream. The fat (and calories) in these foods can add up rather quickly!

A good way to find out about the fat content of the foods you eat is by reading the food label (Fig. 5-9). The Nutrition Facts label displays total fat, saturated fat, and *trans* fat. You can use that information to select foods that comply with the recommendations of major health authorities, which urge Americans to limit saturated fat intake.

Also, check out the list of ingredients on the food label. Some examples of food ingredients that you may not immediately recognize as fats include tallow (beef fat), lard (pork fat), egg yolks or egg yolk solids, cream, cocoa butter, modified vegetable oils, or shortening. Conveniently, the label lists ingredients in order by weight in the product. If fat is one of the first ingredients listed, you are probably looking at a high-fat product.

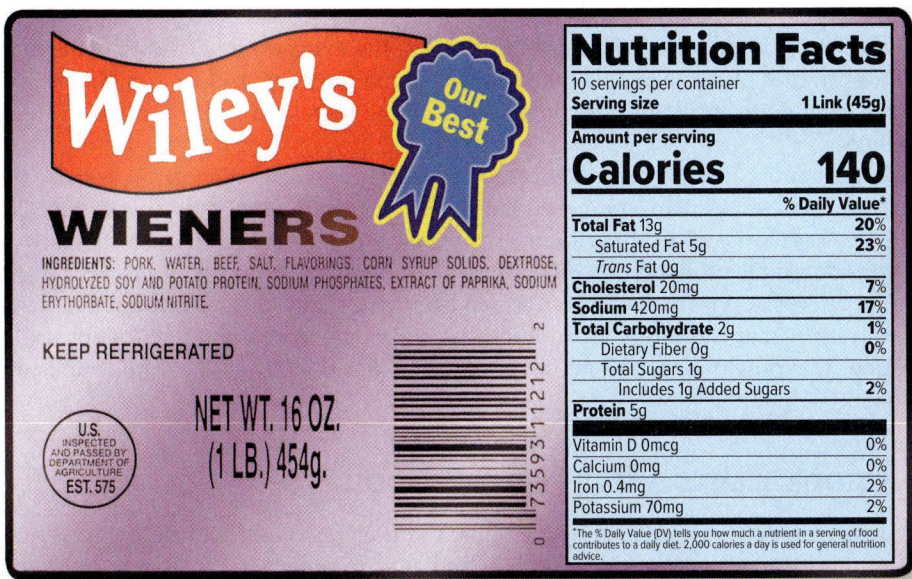

FIGURE 5-9 Food labels can help you identify hidden fat in foods. Who would think that wieners (hot dogs) can contain about 85% of food calories as fat? Looking at the hot dog does not suggest that almost all of its food calories come from fat, but the label shows otherwise. Let us do the math: 13 grams total fat × 9 kcal per gram of fat = 117 kcal from fat; 117 kcal/140 kcal per link = 0.84 or 84% kcal from fat.

FAT IN FOOD PROVIDES SOME SATIETY, FLAVOR, AND TEXTURE

Does fat promote satiety? Fats tend to slow the process of digestion, which could help you to feel full after a meal. However, fats also improve the flavor and texture of foods, so they may stimulate increased food intake. Fat's effect on satiety and eating behaviors may depend on the size and saturation of the fatty acids in foods.[4] What everyone knows for sure is that fats contain more than twice the calories of carbohydrates and proteins. Therefore, a high-fat meal is likely to be a high-calorie meal.

Fat provides texture in foods. If you have ever taken a bite of high-quality milk chocolate, you probably agree that the feel of fat melting on the tongue is good. The fat in milk also provides a richness that fat-free milk lacks. The most tender cuts of meat are high in fat, visible as the marbling of meat. In addition, fat carries flavors in foods. Heating spices in oil intensifies the flavors of an Indian curry or a Mexican dish. You can see why reduced-fat foods may be less appealing than their full-fat counterparts!

FAT-REPLACEMENT STRATEGIES FOR REDUCED-FAT FOODS

Manufacturers have introduced reduced-fat versions of numerous food products. The fat content of these alternatives ranges from 0% in fat-free Fig Newtons to about 75% of the original fat content in other products. However, the total calorie content of most reduced-fat products is not substantially lower than regular products. When fat is removed from a product, what is used in its place? Sugar! It is difficult to reduce both the fat and sugar contents of a product at the same time and maintain flavor and texture. For this reason, many reduced-fat products (e.g., cakes and cookies) are still rich sources of energy. Use the Nutrition Facts label on the food package to choose the portion size that fits into your daily calorie needs.

To lower the fat in foods, manufacturers may replace some of the fat with water, protein (Simplesse®, Dairy-Lo®), or forms of carbohydrates such as starch derivatives (Z-Trim®), fiber (Maltrin®, Stellar™, Oatrim), and gums. In reduced-fat margarines, water replaces some of the fat. While regular margarines are 80% fat by weight

Nutrient Claims You May See on Food Labels

Fat

- **Fat free:** less than 0.5 gram of fat per serving
- **Saturated fat free:** less than 0.5 gram of saturated fat per serving, and the level of *trans* fatty acids does not exceed 0.5 gram per serving
- **Low fat:** 3 grams of fat or less per serving and, if the serving is 30 grams or less or 2 tablespoons or less, per 50 grams of the food; 2% milk cannot be labeled low fat because it exceeds 3 grams per serving. *Reduced fat* is used instead.
- **Low saturated fat:** 1 gram of saturated fat or less per serving and not more than 15% of calories from saturated fatty acids
- **Reduced or less fat:** at least 25% less fat per serving than reference food
- **Reduced or less saturated fat:** at least 25% less saturated fat per serving than reference food

Cholesterol

- **Cholesterol free:** less than 2 milligrams of cholesterol and 2 grams or less of saturated fat per serving
- **Low cholesterol:** 20 milligrams or less of cholesterol and 2 grams or less of saturated fat per serving and, if the serving is 30 grams or less or 2 tablespoons or less, per 50 grams of the food
- **Reduced or less cholesterol:** at least 25% less cholesterol and 2 grams or less of saturated fat per serving than reference food

(11 grams per tablespoon), some reduced-fat margarines are as low as 30% fat by weight (4 grams per tablespoon). When used in recipes, the extra water added to these margarines can cause texture and volume changes in the finished product. Cookbooks can suggest alterations in recipes to compensate for the increased water content of these products.

Manufacturers also may use engineered fats, such as salatrim (Benefat®). Because the triglycerides in salatrim are composed mostly of short-chain fatty acids, this fat replacer yields fewer calories (5 kcal per gram) than typical triglycerides, so it can be used to create reduced-fat products. To date, fat replacements have had little impact on our eating patterns. Consumer acceptance has been poor, and fat replacers are not used extensively by manufacturers. In addition, fat replacements are not practical for use in the foods that provide the most fat in our eating patterns: beef, cheese, whole milk, and pastries.

RANCIDITY LIMITS SHELF LIFE OF FOODS

Decomposing oils emit a disagreeable odor, and they taste sour and stale. Foods with lots of unsaturated fatty acids—especially polyunsaturated fatty acids—are most susceptible to **rancidity** because exposure to ultraviolet light, oxygen, and heat can break down the double bonds in these fatty acids when they are stored or heated to high temperatures. Plant oils, nuts, seeds, whole grains, and fish oils are most susceptible to rancidity because they contain lots of polyunsaturated fatty acids. Saturated fats can more readily resist these effects because they contain fewer carbon-carbon double bonds.

Rancidity is not a major problem for consumers because the odor and taste generally discourage us from eating enough decomposed fats to become sick. However, rancidity is a problem for the food manufacturing and restaurant industries because it can reduce a product's shelf life. How can food manufacturers prevent rancidity in food products?

For nearly a century, food manufacturers used a process called **hydrogenation** to make partially hydrogenated oils, which have an extended shelf life. In hydrogenation, the addition of hydrogen to some of the double bonds in polyunsaturated fatty acids (liquid at room temperature) could make them more saturated (solid at room temperature), and therefore less likely to decompose. Unfortunately, this method of processing liquid plant oils to make them more solid had the unintended effect of producing some *trans* fatty acids. As mentioned, *trans* fatty acids are similar to saturated fatty acids in both shape and function. In fact, over several decades, research emerged to show that these artificial *trans* fats were even worse for cardiovascular health than saturated fats—they negatively impact blood lipids and increase inflammation in the body.

As these harmful effects on health became apparent, major health authorities, such as the World Health Organization, the AHA, and the *Dietary Guidelines* Advisory Committee, recommended minimizing or avoiding *trans* fats. Since 2006, federal regulations have required the disclosure of *trans* fat content on food labels to improve consumer awareness of *trans* fats in foods (review Fig. 5-9). A few city and state governments in the United States made laws to limit the use of *trans* fats by restaurants; some countries banned them altogether. In 2015, the FDA determined that partially hydrogenated oils—the main sources of *trans* fats in typical eating patterns—were no longer "generally recognized as safe" for use in human food products.[5] As of June 2018, partially hydrogenated oils have been banned from use in foods sold in grocery stores and restaurants in the United States.

Now that artificial *trans* fats have been banned, what are food manufacturers using to prevent rancidity in their food products? A different type of engineered fat called *interesterified fat* has been used in some food products to achieve the same shelf stability and food properties as partially hydrogenated oils. Interesterified fats are made by

rancidity Production of decomposed fatty acids that have an unpleasant flavor and odor.

hydrogenation The addition of hydrogen to a carbon-carbon double bond, producing a single carbon-carbon bond with two hydrogens attached to each carbon.

enzymatically removing an unsaturated fatty acid from a triglyceride and replacing it with a saturated fatty acid to make a liquid plant oil into a more stable, solid fat without generating *trans* fatty acids. Other food manufacturers are using **tropical plant oils**, such as coconut oil or palm kernel oil, which are naturally high in saturated fatty acids. Some opt to use the oils from plants that have been genetically modified to produce fatty acids that are more shelf stable. On food labels, these appear as high-oleic soybean oil or high-oleic canola oil.[6]

tropical plant oils Oils derived from tropical plants that are high in saturated fatty acids. Examples: coconut oil, palm oil, and palm kernel oil.

ASK THE RDN: Coconut Oil

Dear RDN: *My friend at the health food store said I should start using coconut oil in my cooking because it has all kinds of health benefits. Is coconut oil a good choice?*

Recently, coconut oil has been promoted for weight loss, heart health, cancer protection, and brain health. Indeed, there is some interesting research on the health effects of the particular fatty acids in coconut oil. At this point, however, there is little evidence to back up the claims that coconut oil is a miracle cure for anything.

Coconut oil is highly saturated. In fact, nearly 90% of the fatty acids in coconut oil are saturated, which is even more than butter or beef fat. This makes for a desirable product: it has that "melt in your mouth" quality and is very shelf stable, which is attractive for food manufacturers and consumers alike. How do saturated fats impact your health? In this chapter, you are seeing the recommendations from all the major health authorities urging Americans to limit their intakes of saturated fat. This is because saturated fatty acids have been shown to increase blood levels of LDL cholesterol, which are linked to atherosclerosis. Proponents of coconut oil point to research showing that the fatty acids in coconut oil, while they do raise LDL, also raise HDL levels. However, the AHA advises against the use of coconut oil (and other sources of saturated fatty acids) because evidence shows replacing saturated fatty acids with sources of unsaturated fatty acids lowers LDLs and positively affects heart health.

When it comes to weight loss, the producers of coconut oil focus on the size of the fatty acids in their product. Most dietary fats are long-chain fatty acids. About 60% of the fatty acids in coconut oil, however, are medium-chain fatty acids, which are more likely to be burned as fuel and less likely to be stored in adipose tissue. Does coconut oil help you lose weight? There are two small human studies that show a decrease in waist circumference with coconut oil, but there is not yet enough evidence to promote coconut oil as a weight-loss aid.

If you like coconut oil, you can use it *in moderation.* Like any dietary fat, coconut oil provides a lot of calories in a small portion. However, adding coconut oil to your dietary pattern is not a wise choice because those extra fat calories can quickly add up. Extra calories from any source inevitably lead to weight gain. You could use it instead of butter or margarine, aiming to keep your total intake of saturated fat less than 10% of total calories. Most of the time, though, choose unsaturated plant oils, which have proven benefits for heart health. Coconut oil is not a cure-all, but it can be included as part of an overall healthy dietary pattern that meets your calorie needs.

Yours in health,

Angela Collene, MS, RDN, LD
Senior Lecturer, The Ohio State University, Author of *Wardlaw's Contemporary Nutrition* and *Wardlaw's Contemporary Nutrition: A Functional Approach*

Tim Klontz

Sources: Jayawardena R, Swarnamali H, Ranasinghe P, Misra A. Health effects of coconut oil: summary of evidence from systematic reviews and meta-analysis of interventional studies. *Diabetes Metab Syndr.* 2021 Mar-Apr;15(2):549-555. doi: 10.1016/j.dsx.2021.02.032

Sacks FM, Lichtenstein AH, Wu JHY, et al.; American Heart Association. Dietary fats and cardiovascular disease: a presidential advisory from the American Heart Association. *Circulation.* 2017 Jul 18;136(3):e1-e23. doi: 10.1161/CIR.0000000000000510

Some *trans* fatty acids occur naturally. Conjugated linoleic acid (CLA) is a family of fatty acids derived from linoleic acid. The bacteria that live in the rumens of some animals (cows, sheep, and goats, for example) produce *trans* fatty acids from the polyunsaturated fats in the grass the animals are fed. These natural *trans* fats eventually appear in foods such as beef, milk, and butter. CLA contains both *cis* and *trans* bonds, and the *trans* bond is in a different location compared to industrial *trans* fats. CLA may improve insulin levels in people with diabetes and decrease the risk of heart disease, cancer, and obesity—the very same diseases that industrial *trans* fats have been shown to increase. Isn't it amazing how a slight difference in the chemical structure of a fatty acid leads to vastly different health effects?

oxidation The process of losing an electron during a chemical reaction.

antioxidant A substance that has the ability to prevent or repair the damage caused by oxidation.

BHA, BHT Butylated hydroxyanisole and butylated hydroxytoluene: two common synthetic antioxidants added to foods.

Another way to prevent rancidity is to carefully package foods to protect them from exposure to light, heat, and oxygen. When you purchase frozen fish, you will notice that it has been vacuum packaged to limit exposure to oxygen. When high-fat snack foods, such as potato chips, are packaged, the bag is filled with an inert gas to prevent **oxidation.** Opaque packaging can limit exposure to light. Dark-colored glass or plastic packages are used for some plant oils and dietary supplements that contain oils. Addition of **antioxidants,** such as vitamin C, vitamin E, **BHA,** or **BHT,** can help to protect foods against rancidity by blocking the oxidation that causes fats to break down. Antioxidants are added to many processed foods that contain fat, such as salad dressings and cake mixes.

✓ CONCEPT CHECK 5.2

1. Name three foods for which at least 50% of total calories come from fat
2. List two dietary sources of cholesterol. List two dietary sources of phytosterols.
3. Which types of fat are used as emulsifiers, and what is their function in food?
4. What are some strategies used to produce reduced-fat foods?
5. What is the benefit of storing plant oils in tinted or opaque containers?

5.3 Making Lipids Available for Body Use

It is no secret that fats and oils make foods more appealing. Their presence in foods adds flavor, moistness, and texture. What happens to lipids once they are eaten? Let us take a closer look at the digestion and absorption of lipids in the body.

DIGESTION

In the first phase of fat digestion, the stomach (and salivary glands to some extent) secretes lipase enzymes. Salivary lipase and gastric lipase act primarily on triglycerides that have fatty acids with short chain lengths, such as those found in butterfat. The actions of salivary lipase and gastric lipase, however, are dwarfed by that of the pancreatic lipase enzyme that is released from the pancreas to digest fats in the small intestine. Most of the triglycerides in a typical dietary pattern contain fatty acids with longer chain lengths; these are generally not digested until they reach the small intestine (Fig. 5-10).

In the small intestine, triglycerides are broken down by pancreatic lipase into smaller products, namely monoglycerides (glycerol backbones with a single fatty acid attached) and fatty acids. Under the right circumstances, digestion is rapid and thorough. The "right" circumstances depend on the presence of bile from the gallbladder. Bile acids (components of bile) act to emulsify fats in the watery digestive juices. This is necessary because the lipid components of food are not soluble in chyme, which is mostly water; lipids tend to coalesce into large globules. Emulsification improves digestion and absorption because it separates large fat globules into smaller ones, thereby increasing the total surface area for pancreatic lipase action (Fig. 5-11).

What happens to the bile acids after their work in fat digestion is complete? They get recycled! After participating in fat digestion, most bile acids are absorbed in the last segment of the small intestine and transported back to the liver. Through this process, approximately 98% of bile acids are recycled. This recycling of bile is called enterohepatic circulation. Only 1% to 2% of bile acids end up in the large intestine to be eliminated in the feces.

Phospholipid digestion is similar to triglyceride digestion. Enzymes from the pancreas and cells in the wall of the small intestine digest phospholipids. The eventual products are glycerol, fatty acids, and the remaining phosphorus-containing parts.

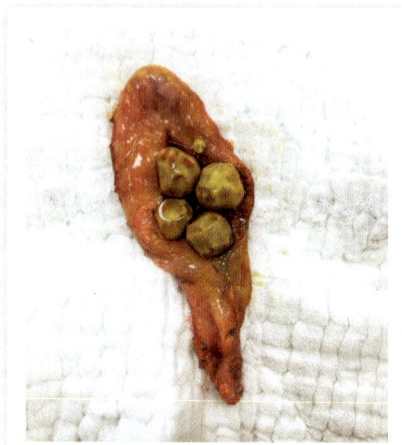

Each year, about 300,000 adults in the United States undergo surgery to remove the gallbladder (usually due to gallstones). For about 1 month after surgery, patients are advised to eat small, frequent meals with low or moderate fat content. **Explain the physiology behind this recommendation.** Pthawatc/Shutterstock

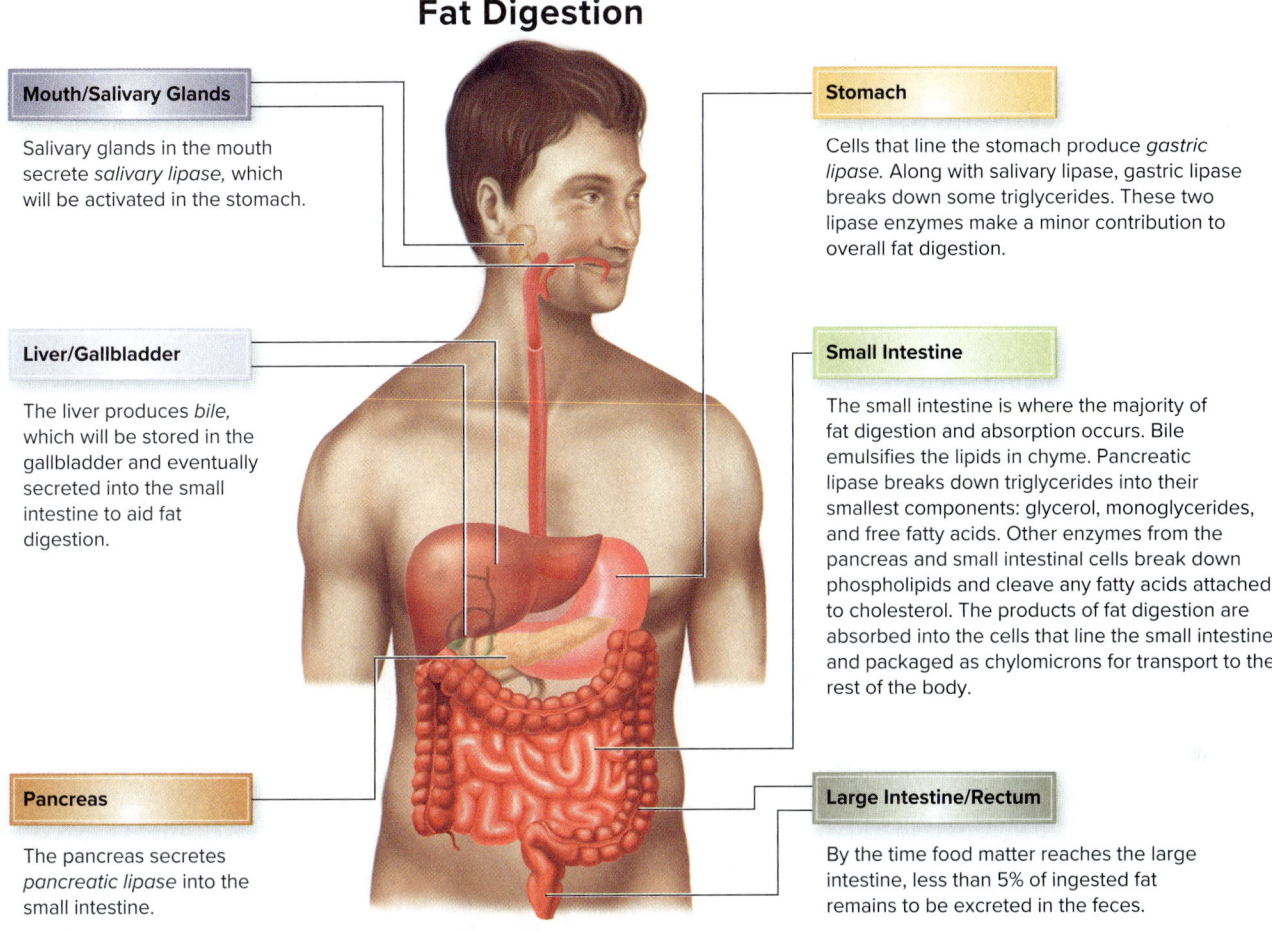

FIGURE 5-10 A summary of fat digestion. Section 3.8 covered general aspects of this process.

With regard to cholesterol digestion, any cholesterol with a fatty acid attached is broken down to free cholesterol and fatty acids by enzymes released from the pancreas. Any fatty acids that are part of these structures could be broken down to yield energy, but their contribution to overall calorie intake is miniscule compared to the energy derived from triglycerides.

ABSORPTION

The free fatty acids, monoglycerides, and glycerol that arise from the digestion of triglycerides diffuse into the absorptive cells that line the small intestine (Fig. 5-11). About 95% of dietary fat is absorbed by the time a meal makes it to the end of the small intestine.

The chain length of fatty acids dictates how they will be distributed to the rest of the body. If the chain length of a fatty acid is less than 12 carbon atoms, it is relatively soluble in water and small enough to be absorbed into the capillaries that surround the small intestine. The capillaries merge into larger blood vessels that eventually connect to the hepatic portal vein, which transports this nutrient-rich blood directly to the liver.

Long-chain fatty acids are too large to be absorbed directly into the capillaries. These larger products of fat digestion are reformed into triglycerides within the absorptive cells of the small intestine, packaged as **chylomicrons,** and absorbed via lacteals into the lymphatic system. The lymphatic system is like a detour for dietary fats on the way to the bloodstream. Chylomicrons eventually get into the blood as lymph vessels empty into the bloodstream through a duct near the heart. Read the next section to find out what happens to lipids as they are transported throughout the body.

chylomicron Lipoprotein made of dietary fats surrounded by a shell of cholesterol, phospholipids, and protein. Chylomicrons are formed in the absorptive cells of the small intestine after fat absorption and travel through the lymphatic system to the bloodstream.

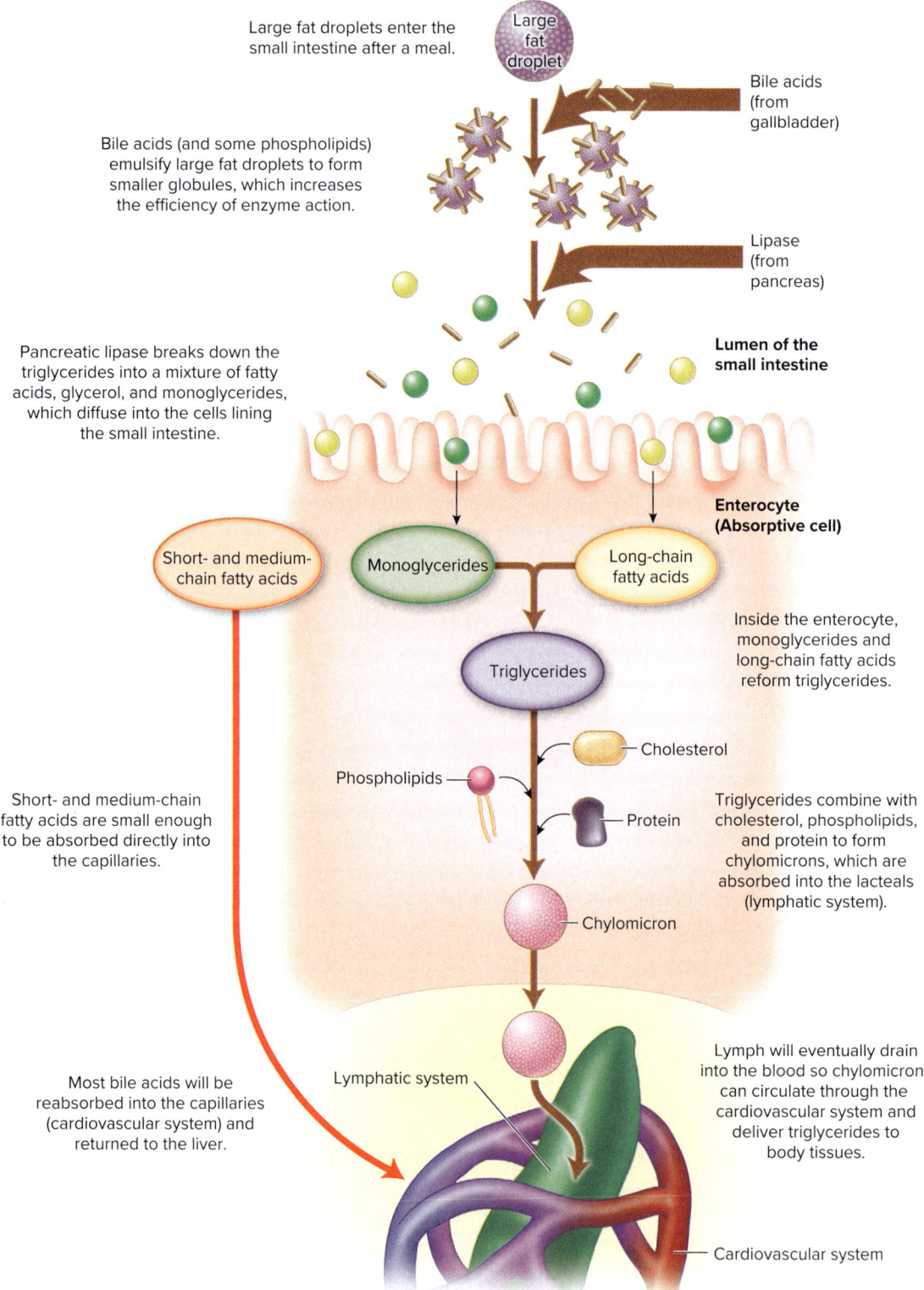

FIGURE 5-11 Summary of fat absorption. Bile acids facilitate the digestion of triglycerides by emulsifying fat droplets in the chyme in the small intestine. This allows for efficient action of pancreatic lipase and subsequent absorption of monoglycerides and fatty acids into the mucosal cells of the small intestine.

✓ CONCEPT CHECK 5.3

1. Describe the role of bile in fat digestion.
2. What enzymes are responsible for digestion of triglycerides?
3. What are the end products of fat digestion?
4. Describe how the absorption of short- or medium-chain fatty acids differs from the absorption of long-chain fatty acids.

5.4 Carrying Lipids in the Bloodstream

As noted earlier, fat and water do not mix easily. This incompatibility presents a challenge for the transport of fats through the blood and lymph, which are mostly water. **Lipoproteins** serve as vehicles for transport of lipids from the small intestine and liver to the body tissues. They consist of a core of triglycerides and cholesterol surrounded by a shell of protein and phospholipids (Fig. 5-12).

Lipoproteins are classified into four groups, as detailed next (Table 5-3). Chylomicrons originate from the cells of the small intestine and are made of dietary fats. **Very-low-density lipoproteins (VLDLs), low-density lipoproteins (LDLs),** and most **high-density lipoproteins (HDLs)** originate from the liver.

CHYLOMICRONS TRANSPORT DIETARY FATS

Digestion of dietary fats results in a mixture of glycerol, monoglycerides, and fatty acids. Once these products are absorbed by the cells of the small intestine, they are reassembled into triglycerides. Then, the intestinal cells package the triglycerides into chylomicrons. Like the other lipoproteins, chylomicrons are composed of large droplets of triglycerides and cholesterol surrounded by a thin, water-soluble shell of phospholipids and protein (Fig. 5-12). The water-soluble shell around a chylomicron allows the lipid to float freely in the lymph and blood, which are both water based. Some of the proteins in the shell may also help other cells identify the lipoprotein as a chylomicron.

Chylomicrons are loaded with dietary fat. They are the largest of the lipoproteins—too large to enter the capillaries that run through each villus. Therefore, they pass from the small intestinal cells into the lacteals, which are the smallest vessels of the lymphatic

lipoprotein A compound found in the bloodstream containing a core of triglycerides and cholesterol surrounded by a shell of protein and phospholipids.

very-low-density lipoprotein (VLDL) The lipoprotein created in the liver that carries cholesterol and lipids that have been taken up or newly synthesized by the liver.

low-density lipoprotein (LDL) The lipoprotein in the blood containing primarily cholesterol; elevated LDL is strongly linked to cardiovascular disease risk, so it is sometimes called *bad cholesterol*.

high-density lipoprotein (HDL) The lipoprotein in the blood that picks up cholesterol from dying cells and other sources and transfers it to the other lipoproteins in the bloodstream or directly to the liver; higher HDL levels are associated with decreased risk for cardiovascular disease, so it is sometimes called *good cholesterol*.

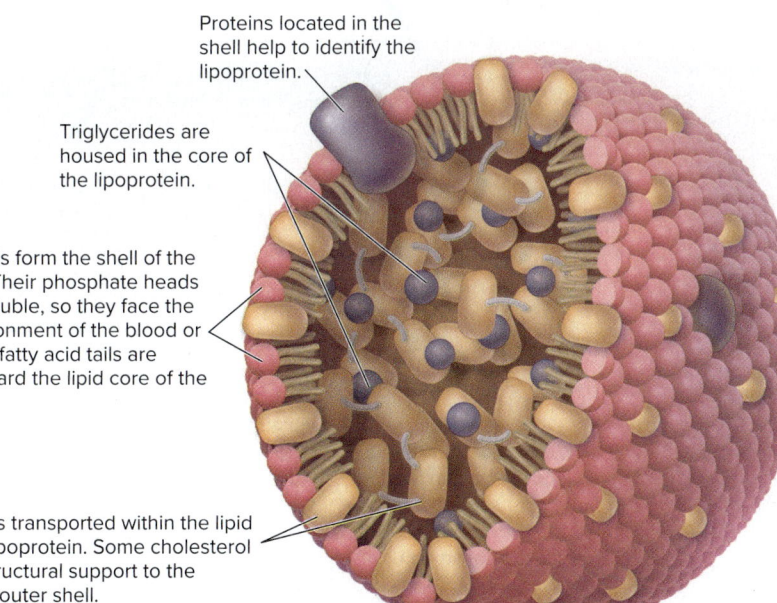

FIGURE 5-12 The general structure of a lipoprotein. All lipoproteins are made of triglycerides, cholesterol, phospholipids, and protein in various proportions. This unique structure allows fats to circulate in the water-based bloodstream.

TABLE 5-3 ■ Composition and Roles of the Major Lipoproteins in the Blood

Lipoprotein	Primary Component	Key Role
Chylomicron	Triglyceride	Carries dietary fat from the small intestine to cells
VLDL	Triglyceride	Carries lipids made and taken up by the liver to cells
LDL	Cholesterol	Carries cholesterol made by the liver and from other sources to cells
HDL	Protein	Contributes to cholesterol removal from cells and, in turn, excretion of it from the body

■ Triglyceride ■ Cholesterol ■ Phospholipid ■ Protein

Torbjorn Lagerwall/Alamy Stock Photo

MedicalRF.com

lipoprotein lipase An enzyme attached to the cells that form the inner lining of blood vessels; it breaks down triglycerides into free fatty acids and glycerol.

system. Chylomicrons travel through the lymph vessels, which eventually empty into the bloodstream through a duct near the heart (Fig. 5-13).

Once a chylomicron enters the bloodstream, the triglycerides in its core are broken down into fatty acids and glycerol by yet another lipase enzyme. This one is called **lipoprotein lipase**, and it is attached to the walls of the blood vessels. As soon as the fatty acids are liberated from triglycerides by lipoprotein lipase, they are absorbed by nearby

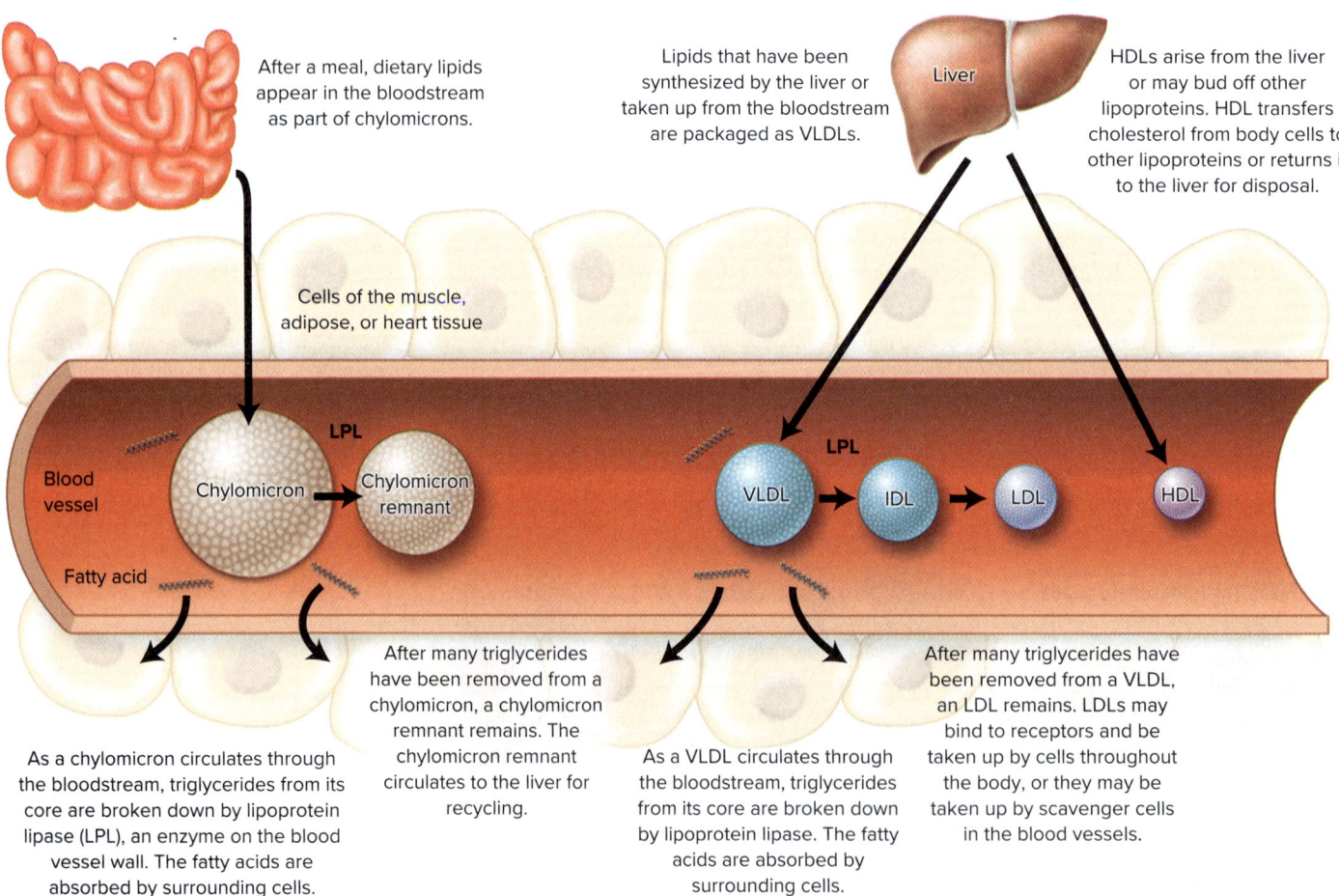

FIGURE 5-13 Transporting lipids through the body.

cells. The remaining glycerol backbone circulates back to the liver. If the cells need energy, they can immediately break down the fatty acids for fuel. Otherwise, cells can reassemble the fatty acids into triglycerides for storage. An **adipose cell** is a type of cell that is specialized for fat storage.

What happens to the rest of the chylomicron after triglycerides have been removed? The leftover materials are called **chylomicron remnants.** Chylomicron remnants are removed from circulation by the liver, and their components are recycled to make other lipoproteins and bile acids.

VLDLs AND LDLs TRANSPORT LIPIDS FROM THE LIVER TO THE BODY CELLS

The liver takes up various lipids from the blood. The liver can also synthesize cholesterol, phospholipids, and some fatty acids. The raw materials for lipid and cholesterol synthesis include free fatty acids taken up from the bloodstream, as well as carbon and hydrogen derived from carbohydrates, protein, and alcohol. The liver then must package the lipids it makes into lipoproteins for transport through the blood to body tissues.

First in our discussion of lipoproteins made by the liver are very-low-density lipoproteins (VLDLs). These particles are composed of cholesterol and triglycerides surrounded by a water-soluble shell of phospholipids and protein. VLDLs are rich in triglycerides and thus are very low in density (Table 5-3). Once in the bloodstream, lipoprotein lipase on the inner surface of the blood vessels breaks down the triglycerides into fatty acids and glycerol. Fatty acids and glycerol are released from the VLDLs into the bloodstream and are taken up by the body cells.

As its triglycerides are released, a VLDL becomes proportionately more dense and is known as a low-density lipoprotein (LDL) (Fig. 5-13). Now, most of what remains in the core of the lipoprotein is cholesterol. The role of LDLs is to transport cholesterol to tissues. LDL particles are taken up from the bloodstream by specific receptors on cells, especially liver cells, and are then broken down. The cholesterol and protein components of LDLs provide some of the building blocks necessary for cell growth and development, such as synthesis of cell membranes and hormones.

HDLs REMOVE CHOLESTEROL FROM THE BLOOD

The final group of lipoproteins, high-density lipoproteins (HDLs), is a critical and beneficial participant in this process of lipid transport. Its high proportion of protein makes it the most dense lipoprotein. The liver synthesizes most of the HDLs in the body (70% to 80%); the intestinal cells make the remainder. It roams the bloodstream, picking up cholesterol from dying cells and other sources. HDLs donate the cholesterol to other lipoproteins for transport back to the liver to be excreted. Some HDLs travel directly back to the liver. This process is called **reverse cholesterol transport.**

A FEW NOTES ABOUT *GOOD* AND *BAD* CHOLESTEROL

HDLs and LDLs are often described as *good* and *bad* cholesterol, respectively. Many studies demonstrate that the amount of HDLs in the bloodstream can closely predict the risk for cardiovascular disease. Risk increases with low HDLs because too little cholesterol is transported back to the liver and excreted. Compared to males, females tend to have higher amounts of HDLs, especially before **menopause.** High amounts of HDLs slow the development of cardiovascular disease, so any cholesterol carried by HDLs can be considered *good* cholesterol.

On the other hand, LDLs are sometimes considered *bad* cholesterol. In our discussion of LDLs, you learned that it is taken up by receptors on various cells. If LDLs are not readily cleared from the bloodstream, **scavenger cells** in the arteries take up the lipoproteins, leading to a buildup of cholesterol on the blood vessel walls. This buildup, known as **atherosclerosis,** greatly increases the risk for cardiovascular disease. Some LDLs are needed as part of routine body functions, but a high level of LDLs is a risk

adipose cell A cell that is specialized for fat storage; also called an *adipocyte*.

chylomicron remnant Lipoprotein that remains after triglycerides have been removed from a chylomicron; composed of protein, phospholipids, and cholesterol.

reverse cholesterol transport Process by which HDL picks up cholesterol from the tissues and blood vessels and takes it to the liver for metabolism or excretion.

menopause The cessation of the menstrual cycle in females, usually beginning at about 50 years of age.

scavenger cells Specific form of white blood cells that can bury themselves in the artery wall and accumulate LDL. As these cells take up LDL, they contribute to the development of atherosclerosis.

atherosclerosis A buildup of fatty material (plaque) in the arteries, including those surrounding the heart.

Newsworthy Nutrition

Effects of almond versus cracker snacks among college students

INTRODUCTION: During the transition to college, changes in dietary patterns, such as breakfast skipping, nutritionally inadequate food choices, and overall energy intake, may negatively impact the cardiometabolic health of young adults. Previous research has demonstrated a positive impact of nut consumption on risks for metabolic syndrome, cardiovascular disease, and type 2 diabetes. However, no intervention has examined the effects of nut consumption on health parameters among young adults, who are forming dietary habits that may persist throughout adulthood. **OBJECTIVES:** To evaluate the effects of snacks of almonds versus snacks of graham crackers on markers of cardiovascular health and blood glucose control among first-year college students. **METHODS:** Using a *randomized, controlled trial design,* 73 first-year college students were randomized to two groups: one group consumed a mid-morning almond snack (2 ounces) and the other group consumed a mid-morning graham cracker snack (5 sheets of crackers) daily for 8 weeks. Anthropometric measurements included body mass, height, waist circumference, and bioelectric impedance analysis of fat mass and fat-free mass. Biochemical analyses included glucose, insulin, and blood lipids, as well as several markers of insulin sensitivity and inflammation. **RESULTS:** Despite an increase in body mass over the 8-week period in both groups, almond snacking resulted in improved blood lipids and insulin sensitivity compared to cracker snacking. The almond snacking group experienced smaller reductions in HDL, 13% lower glucose area under the curve, and 34% lower insulin resistance index compared to the cracker snacking group. Both groups experienced improvements in fasting glucose and LDL. **CONCLUSION:** Snacking on almonds may improve cardiometabolic health among young adults. This is important because dietary behaviors established during young adulthood could influence health outcomes later in life.

Source: Dhillon J, Thorwald M, De La Cruz N, et al. Glucoregulatory and cardiometabolic profiles of almond vs. cracker snacking for 8 weeks in young adults: a randomized controlled trial. *Nutrients.* 2018 Jul 25;10(8):960. doi: 10.3390/nu10080960

factor for cardiovascular disease. Read more about the development of atherosclerosis in Section 5.7.

Here is an important point: The cholesterol in *foods* is not designated as *good* or *bad.* It is only after cholesterol has been made or processed by the *liver* that it shows up in the bloodstream as part of LDLs or HDLs. Nevertheless, dietary patterns can certainly affect the lipoproteins in your blood. The cholesterol in your dietary pattern actually does not have a very big impact on the levels of LDLs and HDLs in your blood. If your body's regulatory mechanisms are working properly, when your dietary intake of cholesterol increases, your liver's synthesis of cholesterol should decrease. Research shows that *saturated fat* is the dietary lipid that has the biggest impact on blood lipid levels. Higher intakes of saturated fat tend to increase blood levels of LDLs. This is why you hear so much dietary advice to limit saturated fat intake!

✓ CONCEPT CHECK 5.4

1. Describe how the structure of lipoproteins allows fats to be transported through the watery environment of the lymph and blood.
2. How are dietary fats packaged in the small intestine and transported?
3. Where are VLDLs made, and what do they contain?
4. Where do LDLs originate, and what is their role in the body?
5. Why are HDLs considered *good* cholesterol?

5.5 Roles of Lipids in the Body

Many vital body functions rely on lipids. They provide energy, serve as structural components of every cell, and regulate cellular processes.

PROVIDING ENERGY

Fatty acids (part of triglycerides) are an important source of fuel for the body. Within cells, the breakdown of the chemical bonds between the carbon, hydrogen, and oxygen atoms in fatty acids releases energy that can be used to synthesize adenosine triphosphate (ATP), the source of energy for all cellular processes. Overall, about half of the energy used by the entire body at rest and during light activity comes from fatty acids; the remainder is derived mostly from carbohydrates.

STORING ENERGY FOR LATER USE

We store energy mainly in the form of triglycerides. The body's ability to store fat is essentially limitless. Our fat storage sites, adipose cells (Fig. 5-14), can increase about 50 times in weight. If the amount of fat to be stored exceeds the ability of the existing cells to expand, the body can form new adipose cells.

An important advantage of using triglycerides to store energy in the body is that they can pack a lot of energy into a small space. Recall that fats yield, on average, 9 kcal per gram, whereas proteins and carbohydrates yield only about 4 kcal per gram. Adipose tissue contains about 80% lipid and only 20% water and protein. In contrast, muscle tissue is about 73% water. What if we had to store energy as muscle tissue? In addition, triglycerides are chemically stable, so they are not likely to react with other cell constituents. Fat is certainly a safe and efficient way to store energy.

FORMING CELL MEMBRANES

Lipids are structural components of all cells. Phospholipids—with their water-soluble phosphate heads and fat-soluble fatty acid tails—have the unique ability to be simultaneously soluble in water and fat. In cell membranes, this amphipathic property allows phospholipids to form a bilayer (Fig. 5-15). The phospholipids line up so that all the fatty acid tails point toward the interior of the membrane and all the phosphate heads face the watery environments on the inside (cytosol) or outside of the cell. The fatty acids, many of which are unsaturated, in the interior of the cell membrane lend fluidity to the cell membrane. Cholesterol, which is also present within the phospholipid bilayer, adds stability to the structure of cell membranes. Because it is made mostly of lipids, the cell membrane is impermeable to most water-soluble substances (e.g., ions, glucose, amino acids, waste products). Thus, the movement of substances across the cell membrane often requires the help of proteins, which serve as gates, pumps, or channels.

Lipids are especially important for the structure of the cells of the nervous system. Although the exact composition changes throughout the life cycle, lipids make up about 60% of the weight of the human brain. Phospholipids and cholesterol are major components of the myelin sheath that surrounds and protects nerve cells. Myelin participates in rapid cell-to-cell communication within the nervous system.

INSULATING AND PROTECTING THE BODY

The layer of fat that lies just below the skin serves as insulation to keep the body warm. Due to its low water content, adipose tissue does not conduct heat very well, so it slows the loss of heat from the body in a cold environment. In addition to insulating the body, fat tissue also surrounds and protects some organs (e.g., kidneys) from injury.

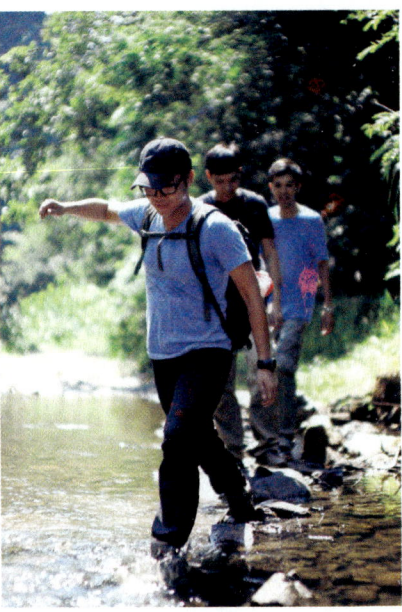

At rest or during light activity, the muscles use mostly fatty acids for fuel. mr.jerry/Flickr RF/Moment/Getty Images

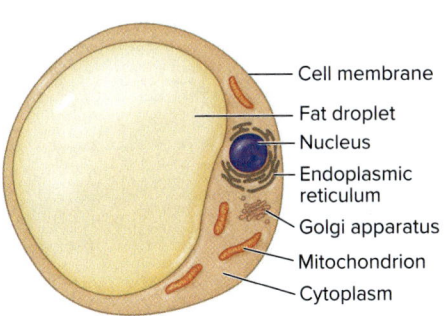

FIGURE 5-14 An adipose cell.

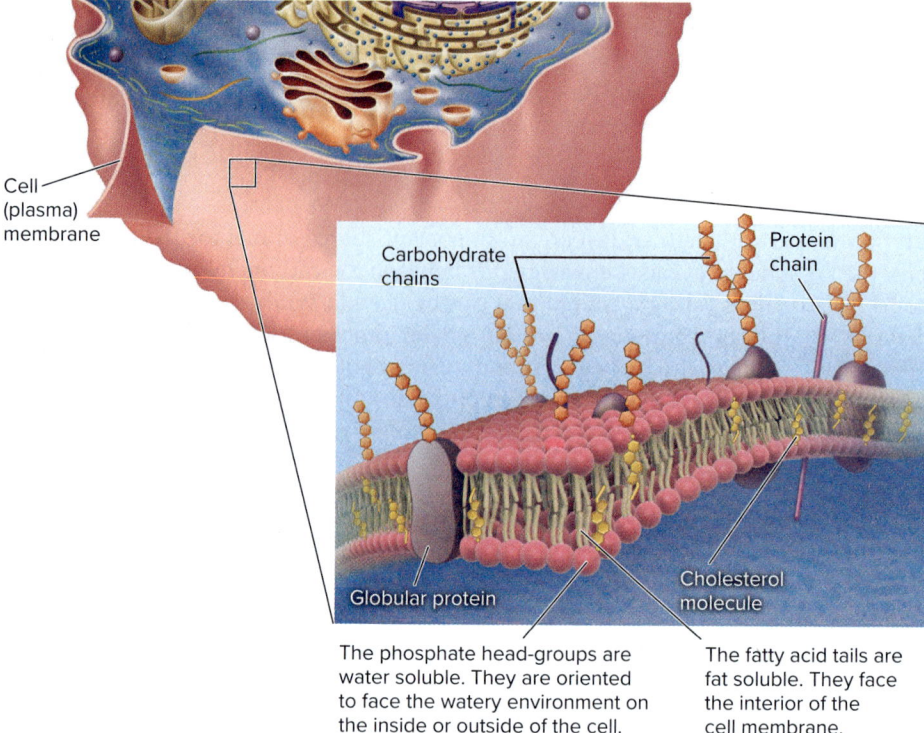

FIGURE 5-15 The phospholipid bilayer. This cross-section of the cell membrane shows that phospholipids are the main components of cell membranes, forming a double layer (bilayer) of lipids.

DIGESTION, ABSORPTION, AND NUTRIENT TRANSPORT

Phospholipids and cholesterol participate in digestion and absorption. Cholesterol is the building block for bile acids, which you learned about in Section 3.8. Bile acids and phospholipids function as emulsifiers, which enable lipids to be suspended in water. During digestion, these emulsifiers help to break apart large droplets of fat into smaller droplets so that digestive enzymes can perform the work of breaking down the fats in a meal.

Lipids in food also carry fat-soluble vitamins to the small intestine and aid their absorption. People who absorb fat poorly (e.g., due to medical conditions or gastrointestinal surgery) are at risk for deficiencies of fat-soluble vitamins, especially vitamin K. A similar problem could result from frequent use of mineral oil as a laxative. The body cannot digest or absorb mineral oil; if taken with a meal, the undigested mineral oil carries fat-soluble vitamins from the meal through the GI tract and out of the body as part of feces. Fat malabsorption can impair mineral status as well. Within the GI tract, unabsorbed fatty acids can bind to some minerals, such as calcium and magnesium, and prevent them from being absorbed. As the fat is eliminated from the body, minerals will be lost, too.

Once absorbed, phospholipids are necessary for the transport of lipid-soluble materials through the lymph and blood. Recall that phospholipids form the outer shell of the lipoproteins: chylomicrons, VLDLs, LDLs, and HDLs.

REGULATION AND COMMUNICATION

Lipids are potent regulators of chemical processes within the body. Sterols are needed for the synthesis of hormones, including estrogen, testosterone, and the active form of vitamin D. Individual fatty acids also orchestrate many aspects of human metabolism.

As you learned in Section 5.1, cells can convert the essential omega-3 and omega-6 fatty acids into other fatty acids, which give rise to eicosanoids. Eicosanoids act as chemical messengers that direct growth and development, immune function, and the work of the central nervous system.

> **CONCEPT CHECK 5.5**
>
> 1. What are the functions of triglycerides in the body?
> 2. Where are phospholipids found in the body?
> 3. What important regulatory compounds are made from cholesterol?

5.6 Recommendations for Fat Intake

TOTAL FAT

There is no Recommended Dietary Allowance (RDA) for total fat for adults. Rather, the Food and Nutrition Board has set an Acceptable Macronutrient Distribution Range (AMDR) of 20% to 35% of total calories. This equates to 44 to 78 grams of fat per day for a person who consumes 2000 kcal daily. Staying within the AMDR for total fat intake helps to ensure that you get enough fat to meet your needs for essential fatty acids, yet not so much fat that you increase your risks for chronic diseases. Typically, the fat intake of Americans is slightly above the recommended amount.[7]

Please note that fat recommendations for infants and children are different from those of adults (see Section 15.2). Youngsters are forming new tissue that requires fat, especially in the brain, so their intake of fat and cholesterol should not be greatly restricted.

TABLE 5-4 ■ **Food and Nutrition Board Recommendations for Essential Fatty Acids**

	Males (g/d)	Females (g/d)
Linoleic acid (omega-6)	17	12
Alpha-linolenic acid (omega-3)	1.6	1.1

ESSENTIAL FATTY ACIDS

As introduced in Section 5.1, there are two fatty acids that are essential in the human diet: linoleic acid and alpha-linolenic acid. If humans fail to consume enough linoleic acid and alpha-linolenic acid, signs of essential fatty acid deficiency may appear. The first signs of essential fatty acid deficiency usually involve epithelial tissues because these cells are rapidly turned over; the skin becomes flaky and itchy, wound healing may be slow, and the individual may experience diarrhea. Over time, hair may fall out or lose its pigment. Due to the role of fatty acids in regulating the immune response, patients with essential fatty acid deficiency are more vulnerable to infections. Among children, growth may be restricted.[8]

The Food and Nutrition Board has set Adequate Intakes (AIs) for linoleic acid and alpha-linolenic acid. Table 5-4 lists the AIs for essential fatty acids for adults. These amounts equate to roughly 5% of our total calorie intake. We can easily get enough essential fatty acids by including moderate amounts of cooking oils, salad dressings, nuts and seeds, and whole grain breads. Even a low-fat eating pattern will provide enough essential fatty acids if it follows a balanced plan such as MyPlate. Except in cases of GI tract diseases, eating disorders, or inadequate intravenous feeding, essential fatty acid deficiencies are quite rare in developed regions of the world.

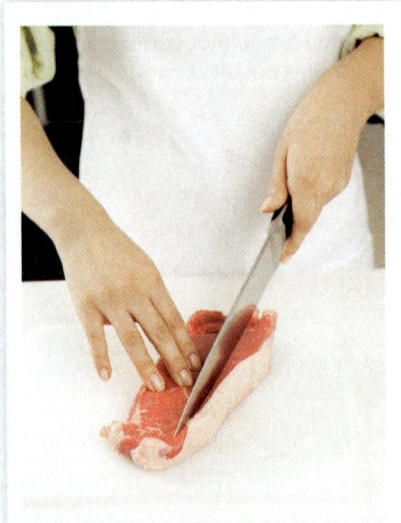

Trimming the visible fat from meats can help reduce saturated fat intake, but you cannot remove the marbling (streaks of fat running through the meat). **Is it possible to incorporate red meats into a heart-healthy dietary pattern?** Chris Stein/DigitalVision/Getty Images

SATURATED FAT

The *Dietary Guidelines* urges all Americans, starting at age 2, to limit saturated fat intake to less than 10% of total calories. The latest dietary guidance from the American Heart Association does not set a numerical limit for saturated fat intake for the general

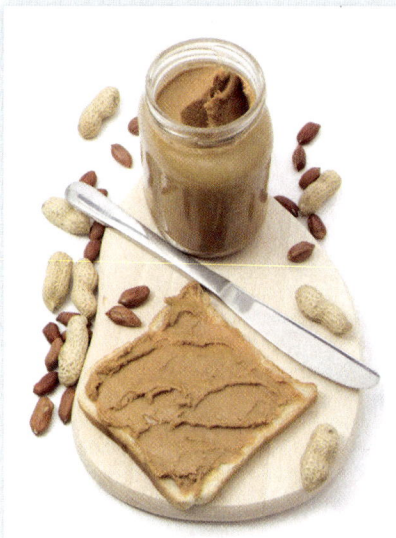

Nut butters are plant products, so they are naturally cholesterol free and provide 2 or 3 grams of fiber per serving, which can lower blood cholesterol. Nuts are also a good source of unsaturated fats, which tend to promote heart health. Be on the lookout for products with high sugar content. Nut butters naturally contain 1 or 2 grams of sugar, but processed varieties (e.g., cinnamon swirl) may contain up to 9 grams of sugar. **How can you determine which nut butters provide heart-healthy fats without added sugars?**
Igor Dutina/iStock/Getty Images

nontropical plant oils Oils derived from plants other than coconut, palm, and palm kernel. Nontropical plant oils are rich in unsaturated fatty acids. Examples: canola oil, grapeseed oil, and olive oil.

ischemic stroke Damage to part of the brain resulting from lack of blood flow to the brain.

hemorrhagic stroke Damage to part of the brain resulting from rupture of a blood vessel and subsequent bleeding within or over the internal surface of the brain.

population but, like the *Dietary Guidelines,* recommends replacing saturated fats with unsaturated fats by choosing a dietary pattern that emphasizes fruits, vegetables, whole grains, plant sources of protein (e.g., beans, peas, lentils, nuts, and seeds), fish, and lean animal proteins.[9] However, for individuals who need to lower their blood cholesterol, the American Heart Association recommends limiting saturated fat intake to 5% to 6% of total calories. These recommendations are based on evidence linking saturated fat intake with increased LDL levels in the blood, which tend to promote atherosclerosis.[10] Typical saturated fat intake among Americans is about 12% of total calories, so there is room for improvement in this area.[7] Remember: Fats that are solid at room temperature tend to be high in saturated fatty acids. Most of the time, choose **nontropical plant oils,** nuts, seeds, and fish (sources of unsaturated fatty acids) in place of tropical oils, fatty cuts of meat, full-fat dairy products, and deep-fried foods to reduce your saturated fat intake.[11]

CHOLESTEROL

About two-thirds of the cholesterol circulating through your body is made by body cells; only one-third comes from a typical dietary pattern. Each day, your body's cells produce approximately 875 milligrams of cholesterol. In addition to the cholesterol that cells make, Americans typically consume about 180 to 325 milligrams of cholesterol per day from animal-derived food products. Most of the time, cholesterol synthesis by the body is well regulated: If you eat more dietary cholesterol, the liver synthesizes less cholesterol.

Notice that the latest guidelines from the AHA set no specific limits on dietary cholesterol. This is because dietary cholesterol intake has little impact on blood cholesterol levels. Instead, evidence shows that saturated fat and *trans* fat have the greatest impact on blood lipids. That doesn't mean you should eat limitless quantities of cholesterol-rich foods. In fact, the *Dietary Guidelines* advises Americans to keep dietary cholesterol intake as low as possible while still meeting your needs for essential nutrients. As it turns out, rich food sources of cholesterol are usually sources of saturated fat as well. Thus, as you reduce the saturated fat in your eating pattern, you will likely reduce your cholesterol intake, too. The relationship between dietary lipids and cardiovascular disease risk will be discussed further in Section 5.7.

OMEGA-3 FATTY ACIDS

Have you heard advice to include seafood in your dietary pattern two times per week? The omega-3 fatty acids in seafood—namely EPA and DHA—help to regulate body processes that may improve heart health, protect brain health, and reduce the inflammation associated with rheumatoid arthritis.

How do these fatty acids influence health? After you eat foods containing fat, the fatty acids are taken up by your cells, where they can be incorporated into cell membranes or used to synthesize signaling molecules that influence blood clotting, inflammation, and heart rhythm. Indeed, many human studies show that people who eat fish once or twice a week (total weekly intake of 8 ounces) have lower risks for sudden cardiac death, coronary heart disease, and **ischemic stroke** compared to people who rarely eat fish. One to two servings per week of seafood that is not breaded or fried seems to be just the right amount for health benefits; higher intakes of seafood do not provide additional benefits.[12]

Although many people would benefit from consuming more omega-3 fatty acids, excessive intakes can be unhealthy, too. Certain groups of people, such as the Greenlandic Inuit, eat so much seafood that their normal blood-clotting ability can be impaired. This increases the risk for uncontrolled bleeding and may cause **hemorrhagic stroke.** An excessive intake of long-chain fatty acids from seafood can also depress immune function.

The *Dietary Guidelines* and the latest dietary guidance from the AHA encourage Americans to eat two or more servings of fatty fish each week. Fish is not only a rich source of omega-3 fatty acids but also a valuable source of protein and trace elements that may protect the cardiovascular system. Broiled or baked fish is recommended rather than fried fish because frying may increase the ratio of omega-6 to omega-3 fatty acids and may produce *trans* fatty acids and **oxidized** lipid products that may be harmful for heart health.

Although consuming fish is thought to have greater benefits, fish oil capsules can be safely substituted for fish if a person does not like fish. Generally, about 1 gram of omega-3 fatty acids (about three capsules) from fish oil per day is recommended, especially for people with evidence of cardiovascular disease. The AHA also recently suggested that fish oil supplements (providing 2 to 4 grams of omega-3 fatty acids per day) could be employed to treat elevated blood triglycerides. However, a recent science advisory from the AHA noted there is insufficient evidence to recommend fish oil supplementation for prevention of cardiovascular diseases among the general population (i.e., individuals without existing cardiovascular disease).[13] Fish oil capsules should be limited for individuals who have bleeding disorders, take anticoagulant medications, or anticipate surgery because the extra omega-3 fatty acids may increase risk of uncontrollable bleeding and hemorrhagic stroke. Thus, for fish oil capsules, as well as other dietary supplements, it is important to follow the recommendations of your primary health care provider. Remember that fish oil supplements are not closely regulated by the FDA; the quality of these supplements is not standardized, and contaminants naturally present in the fish oil may not have been removed.

EATING WELL FOR HEART HEALTH

Despite the potential to control many risk factors through dietary and lifestyle changes, cardiovascular disease remains the leading cause of death and disability worldwide. The latest dietary guidance from the AHA (summarized in Table 5-5) aims to help Americans achieve and maintain a healthy body weight, blood lipid profile, blood pressure, as well as blood glucose levels. Dietary patterns impact cardiovascular health throughout the lifespan.

In recent years, the Mediterranean diet has attracted a lot of attention because of the lower rates of chronic diseases seen among people following such a dietary plan. Reduction of cardiovascular disease has been one of the most consistent results of the

oxidize In the most basic sense, the loss of an electron or gain of an oxygen by a chemical substance. This change typically alters the shape and/or function of the substance.

Sustainable Solutions

Aquaculture

Public health authorities tell us to consume seafood twice per week. However, some species of fish and shellfish are near extinction due to overfishing and damage to their habitats. How can we comply with these recommendations without jeopardizing the global supply of seafood for generations to come? Wild-capture fisheries in the U.S. must adhere to laws that limit overfishing and prevent damage to aquatic habitats. In addition, when managed responsibly, aquaculture (i.e., fish farming) can help to meet the global demand for seafood without harming the environment. Download a consumer guide about sustainable seafood at www.seafoodwatch.org. Also, look for the Aquaculture Stewardship Council (ASC)–certified and Marine Stewardship Council (MSC)–certified labels on packages of seafood sold in stores.

TABLE 5-5 ■ A Summary of Dietary Advice from the American Heart Association

Balance your food and beverage intake with your physical activity to maintain a healthy body weight.
Include a variety of fruits and vegetables.
Select whole grains more often than refined grains.
Choose heart-healthy sources of protein, such as legumes; nuts and seeds; fish and seafood; low-fat or fat-free dairy products; and lean, minimally processed meats.
Prepare foods with liquid oils (e.g., nontropical plant oils) instead of solid fats (e.g., tropical plant oils, butter, and lard).
Select minimally processed foods instead of highly processed foods.*
Limit your intake of sugar-sweetened beverages and foods with added sugars.
Reduce your intake of sodium by choosing unsalted or low-sodium foods and limiting use of salt in food preparation.
If you choose to consume alcohol, do so in moderation.

Source: Lichtenstein AH, Appel LJ, Vadiveloo M, et al. 2021 dietary guidance to improve cardiovascular health: a scientific statement from the American Heart Association. *Circulation.* 2021 Dec 7;144(23):e472-e487. doi: 10.1161/CIR.0000000000001031

* There is no commonly accepted definition for ultraprocessed foods, and some healthy foods may exist within the ultraprocessed food category.

> 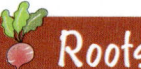 **Roots**
>
> ### Nordic Diet
>
> The Nordic diet (sometimes called the *Viking diet*) refers to a collection of foodways observed in the countries of Denmark, Finland, Norway, Iceland, Sweden, and Greenland. Historically, the short growing season and lack of arable farmland in this area of the world demanded a reliance on wild plants from the forests, wild game, seafood, dairy products, and foods that could be easily preserved. Recently, nutrition, culinary, and environmental experts have joined forces to popularize the *New Nordic diet,* which combines these traditional foods with modern culinary techniques to promote healthier dietary patterns in a region where, like the rest of the world, obesity and chronic diseases are on the rise.
>
> The Nordic diet builds its foundation on a variety of regional fruits (e.g., apples, pears, and wild berries), lots of cruciferous vegetables (e.g., cabbage and broccoli), and root vegetables (e.g., kohlrabi, turnips, parsnips, and beetroot). The grains are mostly whole grains, especially rye, oats, and barley. Locally sourced fish, low-fat dairy products (including fermented dairy products, such as *skyr*), and legumes are the primary sources of protein. Fats are mostly unsaturated, including those from fish and vegetable oils (e.g., rapeseed oil). Sweets, solid fats, and alcohol are consumed in small quantities. Importantly, with its focus on eating locally sourced, seasonal foods, the Nordic diet is a sustainable dietary pattern.
>
> Although not as thoroughly studied as the Mediterranean diet, research shows that adherence to the Nordic diet is linked to reduced risk for cardiovascular disease. Researchers are currently investigating links between the Nordic diet and abdominal obesity, type 2 diabetes, and cancer.

Mediterranean diet.[14] The major sources of fat in the Mediterranean diet include liberal amounts of olive oil (a rich source of monounsaturated fatty acids) and regular intake of fish (rich sources of omega-3 fatty acids). Meats, eggs, and dairy foods (rich sources of saturated fatty acids) are consumed sparingly.

While dietary fat sources definitely play a role in prevention of chronic disease, it is important to remember that other aspects of one's lifestyle also contribute to disease risk. People who follow a Mediterranean diet also tend to consume moderate alcohol (usually in the form of red wine, which contains many antioxidants), eat plenty of whole grains and few highly processed carbohydrates, and also be more physically active than typical Americans.[15]

An alternative plan for reduction of cardiovascular disease is Dr. Dean Ornish's purely vegetarian (**vegan**) dietary plan.[16] This dietary pattern is very low in fat, including only a scant quantity of vegetable oil used in cooking and the small amount of oils present in plant foods. Individuals restricting fat intake below the AMDR (i.e., less than 20% of total calories) should be monitored by a physician, as the resulting increase in carbohydrate intake can increase blood triglycerides in some people, which is not a healthful change. Over time, however, the initial problem of high blood triglycerides on a low-fat dietary pattern may self-correct. Among people following the Ornish plan, blood triglycerides initially increased but, within a year, fell to normal values as long as the individuals emphasized high-fiber carbohydrate sources, controlled (or improved) body weight, and followed a regular exercise program.

vegan Referring to a dietary pattern that only includes foods of plant origin.

FAT *QUALITY* VERSUS FAT *QUANTITY*

Weight control is a vitally important way to minimize risk for a variety of chronic diseases. Because it is a dense source of calories, many people seek to limit fat intake as a way to manage body weight. However, it is important to recognize that excess calories from any source—fat, carbohydrate, protein, or alcohol—contribute to weight gain. If weight loss is needed, understand that your overall calorie intake is more important than the specific macronutrient composition of your eating pattern.

As you have learned, the general consensus among nutrition experts is that fat should comprise 20% to 35% of total calories. When it comes to improving your dietary pattern, it is usually not necessary to drastically lower the *quantity* of fat in your dietary pattern. However, you should aim to choose more foods that provide unsaturated fats, including more omega-3 fatty acids, while choosing fewer sources of saturated and *trans* fats.[17] In short, most Americans need to improve their fat *quality*.

Simply selecting the reduced-fat versions of pastries, cookies, and cakes will not improve the quality of your dietary pattern. Often, extra sugar or salt has been added to these foods to compensate for losses of taste and texture. Instead, focus your efforts on choosing plant sources of fat more often than animal sources (Table 5-6). Fruits, vegetables, and whole grains are usually low in total fat and saturated fat; the (mostly unsaturated) fats they do provide are accompanied by vitamin E, vitamin K, and a variety of health-promoting phytochemicals.[11]

TABLE 5-6 ■ Tips for Cutting Back on Saturated Fats

	Eat Less of These Foods	Eat More of These Foods
Grains	Pasta dishes with cheese or cream sauces Croissants Pastries Doughnuts Pie crust	Whole grain breads Whole grain pasta Brown rice Air-popped popcorn
Vegetables	French fries Potato chips Vegetables cooked in butter, cheese, or cream sauces	Fresh, frozen, baked, or steamed vegetables
Fruit	Fruit pies	Fresh, frozen, or canned fruits
Dairy	Whole milk Ice cream High-fat cheese Cheesecake	Fat-free and reduced-fat milk Low-fat frozen desserts (e.g., yogurt, sherbet, and ice milk) Reduced-fat/part-skim cheese
Protein	Bacon Sausage Organ meats (e.g., liver) Egg yolks	Fish Skinless poultry Lean cuts of meat (with fat trimmed away) Beans, peas, and lentils Egg whites/egg substitutes Nuts and nut butters
Fat and Oils	Butter Lard	Plant oils

CASE STUDY: Planning a Heart-Healthy Dietary Pattern

Avani is a 21-year-old, health-conscious individual majoring in business. She recently learned that an eating pattern high in saturated fat can contribute to high blood cholesterol and that exercise is beneficial for the heart. Avani now takes a brisk 30-minute walk each morning before going to class, and she has started to cut as much fat out of her dietary pattern as she can, replacing it mostly with carbohydrates. A typical day for Avani now begins with a big bowl (approximately 2 cups) of Fruity Pebbles™ with 1 cup of skim milk and ½ cup of apple juice. For lunch, she might pack a turkey sandwich on white bread with lettuce, tomato, and mustard; a 1-ounce package of fat-free pretzels; and five reduced-fat vanilla wafers. Dinner could be 1 cup of dal (lentil stew) served over 1 cup of rice. Her snacks are usually baked chips, low-fat cookies, fat-free frozen yogurt, or fat-free pretzels. She drinks masala chai tea (unsweetened) throughout the day as her main beverage.

1. Avani's recent dietary changes have drastically reduced her overall fat intake. What are the recommendations of the American Heart Association related to fat intake?
2. Avani has replaced most of the fat in her eating pattern with carbohydrates. What concerns, if any, do you have about her carbohydrate choices?
3. Fat *quality* is just as important as fat *quantity*. What types of fat should Avani try to consume? Suggest three examples of foods Avani could incorporate into her eating pattern to obtain high-quality fats.
4. How does Avani's new exercise plan compare to the recommendations for adults in the *Physical Activity Guidelines for Americans*?

Complete the Case Study. Responses to these questions can be provided by your instructor.

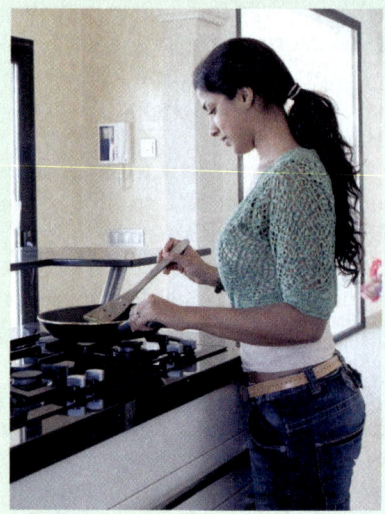

What cooking oils should Avani use to prepare foods? Stuart Pearce/Pixtal/age fotostock

ASK THE RDN: Ketogenic Diet

Dear RDN: *I am thinking about trying a ketogenic diet. Can you share the pros and cons, so I can make an informed decision?*

The ketogenic diet was first used in the 1920s to help reduce seizures in individuals with epilepsy. The diet is still used today in those with drug-resistant epilepsy. In the 1970s, Dr. Robert Atkins began advocating the use of ketogenic diets for weight loss and blood glucose control. Clinical ketogenic diets, such as those used for epilepsy, are moderate in protein, given that some amino acids can be converted to glucose in the body, potentially reducing the formation of ketones. However, the Atkins-style ketogenic diet mainly restricted carbohydrates, with no limitations on protein or fat consumption. In recent years, ketogenic diets have been touted as a potential nutritional therapy for everything from obesity to type 2 diabetes, cancer, neurologic diseases, and even for improving athletic performance.

Today's popular ketogenic diets are very low in carbohydrates (typically less than 50 grams per day), very high in fat (at least 75% of total calories), and variable in protein content. When carbohydrates are largely unavailable as a fuel source, the body must rely on fat as a source of energy. Such dominant use of fat as an energy source results in the incomplete breakdown of fatty acids and the accumulation of small molecules, called ketone bodies, in the blood (hence, the terms *ketosis* or *ketogenic*). In extreme situations (e.g., poorly controlled type 1 diabetes), ketosis can alter the pH of the blood. This condition—*ketoacidosis*—can be life-threatening. However, the mild ketosis induced by popular keto diets (sometimes called *nutritional ketosis*) is not harmful in the short term.

The ketogenic diet has stirred up a lot of controversy, stemming largely from how much it varies from established dietary recommendations like the *Dietary Guidelines*. The total fat and saturated fat content are typically much higher than what is recommended for overall health. In addition, the near elimination of carbohydrates renders these diets low in nutrient-dense foods, such as whole grains, fruits, starchy vegetables, and most dairy products (except cheese). Common concerns from the scientific community regarding ketogenic diets include (1) potential increases in blood cholesterol, especially LDL cholesterol, which could increase heart disease risk; (2) low fiber intakes, which may adversely affect the gut microbiota; and (3) suboptimal intakes of certain vitamins, minerals, and phytochemicals that are beneficial to health. Advocates for these diets, though, counter that ketogenic diets greatly reduce intake of added sugars, refined carbohydrates, and overall energy, leading to rapid weight loss, which may improve other markers of cardiovascular disease risk and help with blood glucose control.

So, who should you believe? It can be quite difficult to sort out these conflicting messages. For example, short-term studies (< 6 months in duration) in individuals with overweight or obesity show that ketogenic diets are associated with greater weight loss and reductions in blood triglycerides compared with commonly recommended low-fat diets. However, in studies lasting 1 year or longer, differences in weight loss between these two types of diets are generally no longer statistically significant, favoring the ketogenic diet by 1 kg (2.2 lbs.) or less. Part of the explanation is likely due to decreased adherence to the diet over time, given its highly restrictive nature. Preliminary evidence also suggests the potential for the ketogenic diet to positively impact markers of blood glucose control in people with diabetes. However, studies of the ketogenic diet for diabetes management often have serious limitations, such as small sample size, inappropriate experimental design, and short duration. As such, there remains no scientific consensus on the value of the ketogenic diet for individuals with diabetes. There is also no high-quality evidence in humans for positive effects of the ketogenic diet in cancer or Parkinson's disease, or for improving athletic performance. And, finally, little is known regarding the long-term safety or sustainability of the ketogenic diet.

In summary, despite a lot of media attention and bold claims for the health and performance effects of the ketogenic diet, the scientific evidence to date is insufficient to support most applications of the ketogenic diet outside of epilepsy management. Even so, some people may be interested in trying the ketogenic diet, and those who do should consult with their health care team (e.g., RDN, primary care provider) for assistance with proper diet planning and medical monitoring.

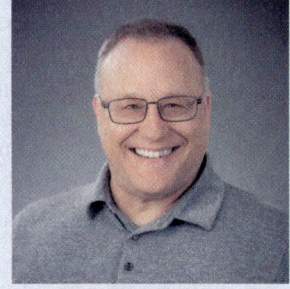

Kathy Bernat Photography

Seeking out the evidence,

Steven Hertzler, PhD, RD, LD
Senior Scientist, Clinical Research, Abbott Nutrition

✓ CONCEPT CHECK 5.6

1. How does the percent of calories from fat in the typical American dietary pattern compare to recommendations?
2. Describe the rationale for the current public health recommendations regarding saturated fat intake.
3. What are the key features of the Mediterranean diet? Why is the Mediterranean diet promoted as a healthy dietary pattern?

5.7 Nutrition and Your Health: Lipids and Cardiovascular Disease

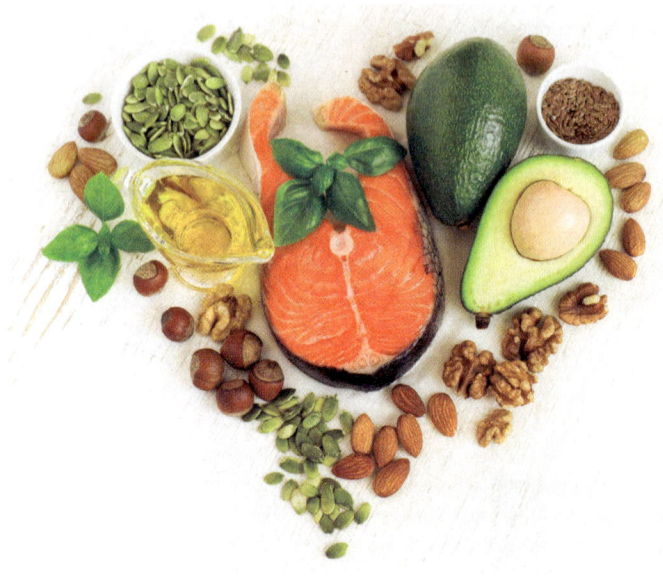

Elena Nazarova/123RF

Cardiovascular disease is the major killer of North Americans. It includes a variety of diseases of the heart and blood vessels. The terms *coronary artery disease, coronary heart disease,* or simply *heart disease* refer to cardiovascular disease that affects the heart. *Cerebrovascular disease* affects the brain and could lead to a stroke. *Peripheral artery disease* impacts the blood vessels that supply other areas of the body, such as the legs. It is estimated that one person dies of a heart attack every 33 seconds in the United States.[18] Females generally lag about 10 years of age behind males in developing cardiovascular disease. Still, it eventually kills more females than any other disease.

Development of Cardiovascular Disease

The symptoms of cardiovascular disease develop over many years and often do not become obvious until older adulthood. Nonetheless, autopsies of young adults under 20 years of age have shown that many of them had atherosclerotic **plaque** in their arteries. This finding indicates that plaque buildup can begin in childhood and continue throughout life, although it usually goes undetected for some time.[19]

The typical forms of cardiovascular disease—coronary heart disease and strokes—are associated with inadequate blood circulation in the heart and brain related to buildup of atherosclerotic plaque. Blood supplies the heart muscle, brain, and other body organs with oxygen and nutrients. When blood flow via the coronary arteries surrounding the heart is interrupted, the heart muscle can be damaged. A heart attack (also called *myocardial infarction*) may result. This may cause the heart to beat irregularly or to stop. Similarly, if blood flow to part of the brain is interrupted long enough, part of the brain suffers damage, causing a stroke (also called *cerebrovascular accident*).

Sometimes, a heart attack can strike with the sudden force of a sledgehammer, with pain radiating up the neck or down the arm. Other times, it can sneak up at night, masquerading as indigestion, with slight pain or pressure in the chest. Crushing chest pain is a more common symptom in males.[20] Many times, the symptoms are so subtle in a female that death occurs before the patient or the health professional realizes that a heart attack is taking place (Fig. 5-16). If there is any suspicion that a heart attack is taking place, the person should first call 911 and then chew an aspirin (325 milligrams) thoroughly. Aspirin helps to reduce the blood clotting that leads to a heart attack.

Atherosclerosis probably first develops as part of an immune response to repair damage in a blood vessel (Fig. 5-17). A healthy blood vessel is smooth and flexible so that blood can easily move through it. What happens to cause damage to a blood vessel? Likely culprits include smoking, diabetes, high blood pressure, high blood cholesterol, infection—basically any process that causes inflammation in the body. (A laboratory test for C-reactive protein in the blood is used to detect inflammation.) Atherosclerosis can be seen in arteries throughout the body. The damage develops especially at points where an artery branches into two smaller vessels. A great deal of stress is placed on the vessel walls at these points due to changes in blood flow.

Over time, plaque continues to build up at the site of initial damage. The rate of plaque buildup is directly related to the amount of LDL in the blood. Specifically, oxidized LDL appears to be responsible for plaque formation. Oxidized LDL has undergone changes that make it more likely to be taken up by scavenger cells in the arterial wall. The body also sends white blood cells called **macrophages** to the location of the cholesterol accumulation on the blood vessel wall. In an attempt to destroy it, the macrophage surrounds the fatty deposit and produces lipid-loaded **foam cells.** Laden with plaque, the blood vessels stiffen, so they cannot dilate or constrict to accommodate normal changes in blood pressure throughout the day. Over years, the buildup of plaque can restrict or block blood flow. Some plaques can become unstable and tear away from the artery. If they rupture, a blood clot will form inside the artery, and within minutes blood flow is cut off, resulting in a heart attack or stroke.

plaque A cholesterol-rich substance deposited in the blood vessels; it contains various white blood cells, smooth muscle cells, various proteins, cholesterol and other lipids, and eventually calcium.

macrophages Large white blood cells that arise from monocytes; one of several types of white blood cells that phagocytize pathogens and signal other white blood cells to mount an immune response.

foam cells Lipid-loaded white blood cells that have surrounded large amounts of a fatty substance, usually cholesterol, on the blood vessel walls.

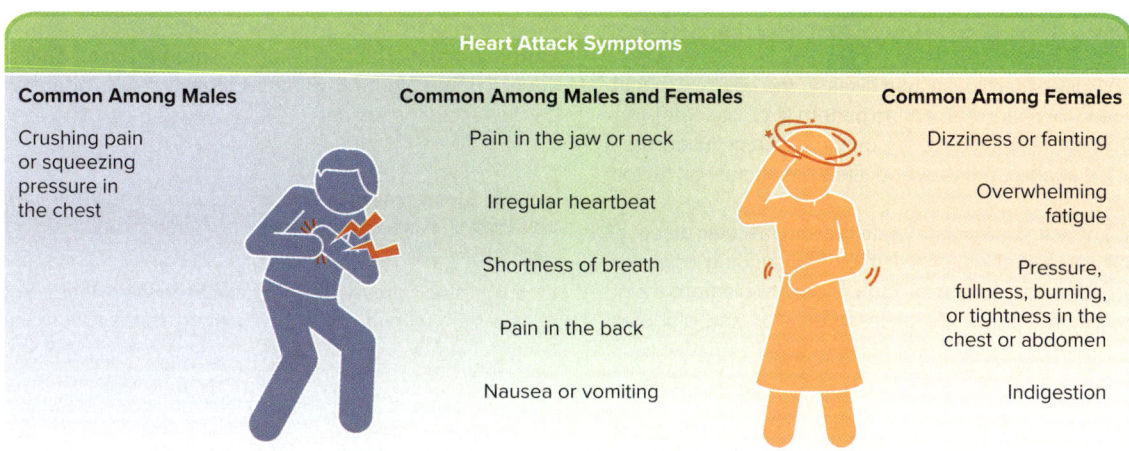

FIGURE 5-16 Be aware of common warning signs of a heart attack. The signs may differ for males and females.

Blood clotting is a normal and necessary process that prevents blood loss in case of injury. Some people, however, develop disorders in which their blood forms clots too frequently. In areas of the blood vessels that are already partially blocked by plaque, a blood clot can cut off blood flow, leading to tissue damage or death.

Some common triggers for a heart attack include dehydration; acute emotional stress (e.g., getting fired from a job); strenuous physical activity when not otherwise physically fit (e.g., shoveling snow); waking during the night or getting up in the morning (linked to an abrupt increase in stress); and consuming large, high-fat meals (increases blood clotting).

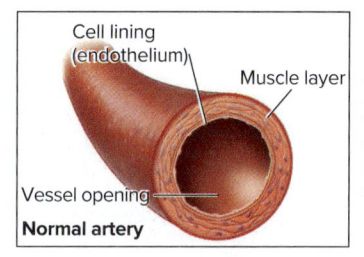

A healthy blood vessel is smooth and flexible. Blood can easily move through the vessel, and it is able to stretch to accommodate changes in blood pressure throughout the course of a day.

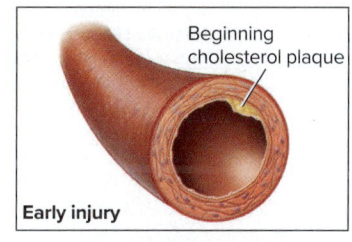

Injury to an artery wall begins the process of plaque formation. Possible causes for injury include smoking, diabetes, high blood pressure, high blood cholesterol, or infection.

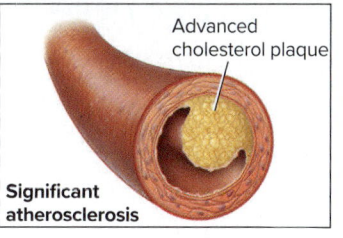

The initial injury is followed by a progressive buildup of plaque in the artery walls. The plaque consists of fatty materials (e.g., oxidized LDL), platelets, and minerals. Over time, the blood vessel narrows.

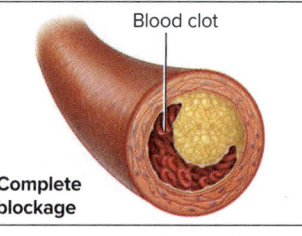

A blood clot becomes lodged in the narrow blood vessel, blocking or greatly restricting blood flow to tissues. Nutrients and oxygen cannot reach the tissue, so it is damaged and may die. A heart attack results when this occurs in a blood vessel that supplies the heart muscle.

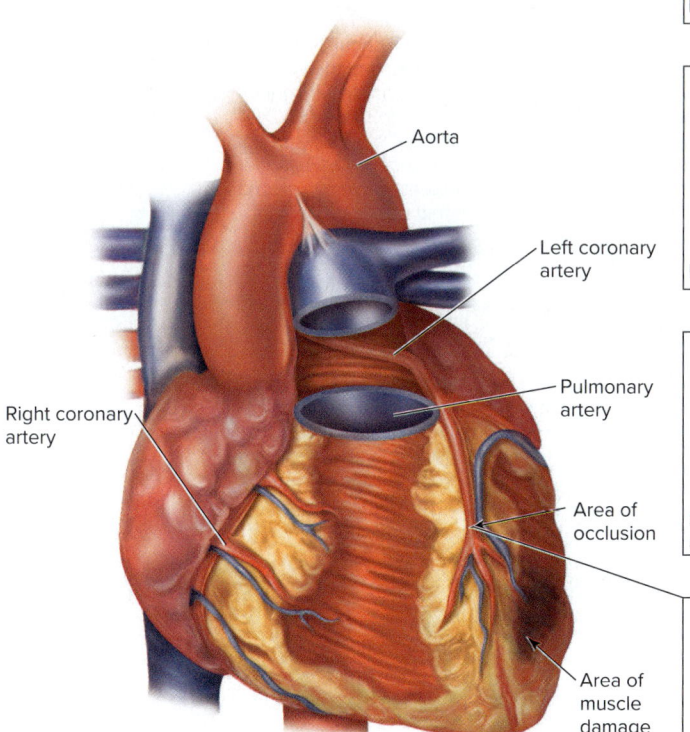

FIGURE 5-17 How atherosclerosis leads to heart attack.

Risk Factors for Cardiovascular Disease

For a person at low risk of cardiovascular disease, the advice of health experts is to adhere to a balanced eating pattern (e.g., MyPlate), perform regular physical activity, have a complete fasting lipoprotein analysis performed at age 20 or beyond, and reevaluate risk factors every 4 to 6 years.

How do you know if you are at risk for cardiovascular disease? The AHA identifies several major risk factors, including age, sex, heredity, use of tobacco products, high blood cholesterol, high blood pressure, physical inactivity, excess body fat, and diabetes. Additional contributing factors include stress, alcohol, and dietary patterns that are high in calories, saturated fat, sodium, and added sugars.[21] See Figure 5-18 for additional details about risk factors for cardiovascular disease.

systolic blood pressure The pressure in blood vessels when the heart beats, squeezing and pushing blood through the arteries to the rest of the body.

diastolic blood pressure The pressure in the arteries when the heart rests between beats and fills with blood and receives oxygen.

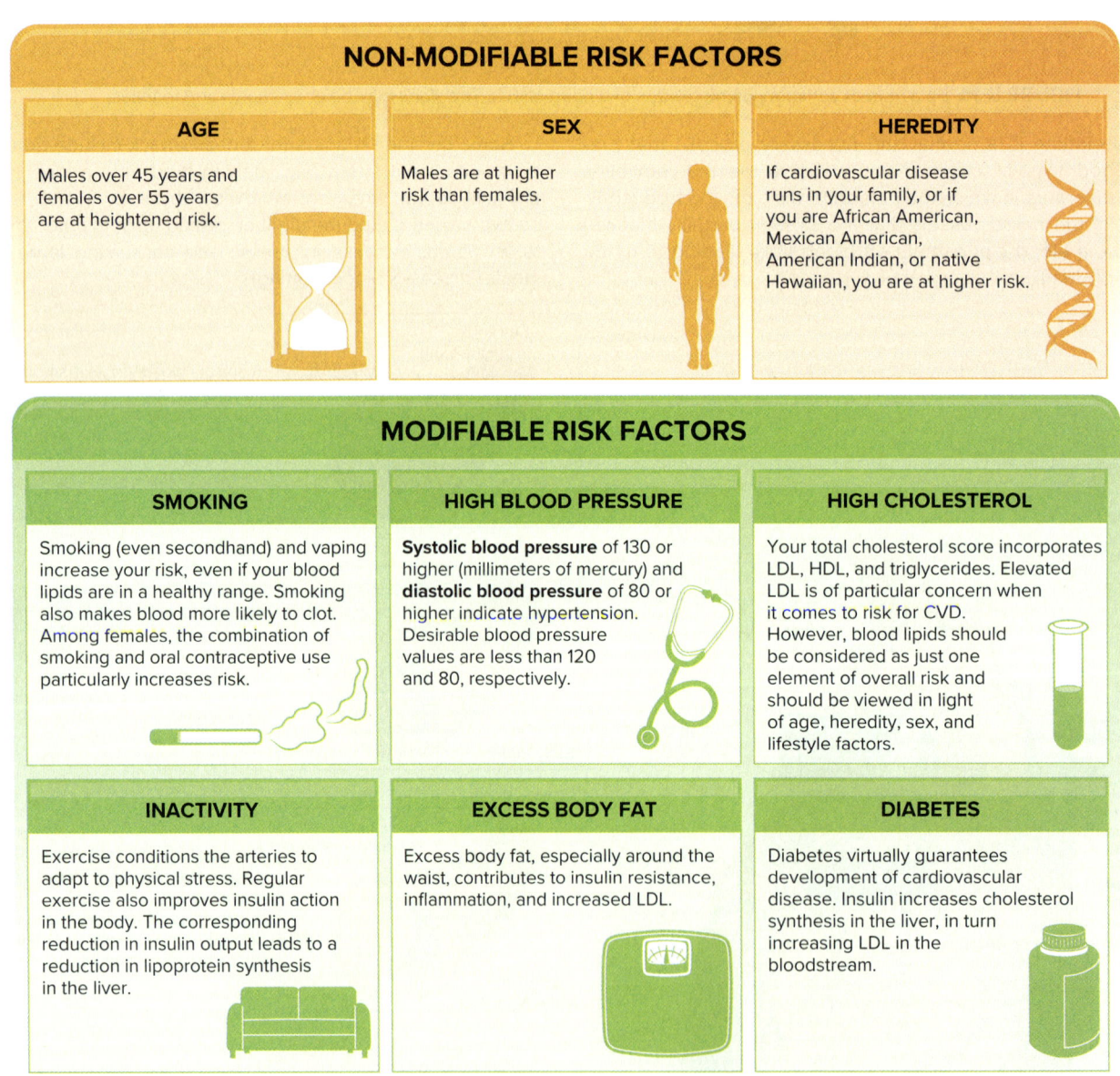

FIGURE 5-18 Risk factors for cardiovascular disease.
Sources: American Diabetes Association Professional Practice Committee. 10. Cardiovascular disease and risk management: standards of care in diabetes—2024. *Diabetes Care*. 2024;47(Suppl 1):S179-S218. doi:10.2337/dc24-S010
Grundy SM and others. AHA/ACC/AACVPR/AAPA/ABC/ACPM/ADA/AGS/APhA/ASPC/NLA/PCNA guideline on the management of blood cholesterol: A report of the American College of Cardiology/American Heart Association Task Force on Clinical Practice Guidelines. *Circulation* 2018. DOI:10.1161/CIR.0000000000000625.

Does this list of risk factors sound familiar? Many of these were introduced in Section 4.7 as part of the discussion of the metabolic syndrome, a cluster of risk factors that increases risk for heart disease, stroke, and type 2 diabetes. Recognize that a *risk factor* is not equivalent to a *cause* for disease. Nevertheless, the more of these risk factors you have, the greater your chances of ultimately developing cardiovascular disease. The good news: By aligning your dietary pattern with the guidance of the AHA and staying physically active, you can control many of these risk factors.

Lifestyle Modifications to Prevent Cardiovascular Disease

In Section 5.6, you read about recommendations to modify fat intake to promote heart health. For the general population, starting at age 2, the *Dietary Guidelines* recommends limiting saturated fat intake to 10% of total calories and avoiding *trans* fats. For people with elevated LDL, the AHA recommends restricting saturated fat intake even further to 5% to 6% of total calories. These recommendations are based on scientific evidence that links saturated and *trans* fat intake to higher levels of LDLs, which promote plaque formation in blood vessels.[22]

Even while cutting back on saturated and *trans* fats, overall fat intake should generally fall within the range of 20% to 35% of total calories. This means you shouldn't simply cut fat out of your eating pattern. Rather, you should choose monounsaturated and polyunsaturated sources of fat, such as fatty fish, plant oils, nuts, and seeds, instead of foods rich in saturated fats. The omega-3 polyunsaturated fatty acids in fish are particularly helpful for promoting heart health.

Remember that eating for heart health extends beyond a focus on dietary fat! Over the past few decades, evidence has accumulated that excessive intakes of added sugars have contributed to the high rate of cardiovascular disease. This is why it is important to replace saturated fat with unsaturated fat, rather than with simple carbohydrates. Excessive intakes of refined carbohydrates and added sugars promote high levels of insulin, inflammation, and increased blood cholesterol. Uncontrolled blood sugar among people with diabetes is a significant risk factor for cardiovascular disease. Review recommendations for healthy carbohydrate choices in Section 4.3.

You also read about the dangers of oxidized LDL—the form of LDL that contributes to plaque formation. Nutrients and phytochemicals that have antioxidant properties may reduce LDL oxidation. Fruits and vegetables are particularly rich in these compounds. Eating fruits and vegetables regularly is one positive step we can make to reduce plaque accumulation and slow the progression of cardiovascular disease. Some plant foods particularly helpful in this regard include beans, peas, lentils, nuts, dried plums (prunes), raisins, berries, plums, apples, cherries, oranges, grapes, spinach, broccoli, red bell peppers, and onions. Tea, coffee, and dark chocolate are also sources of antioxidants. Please note that *foods* are the best choices for antioxidants. The AHA does not support use of antioxidant supplements (such as vitamin E) to reduce cardiovascular disease risk. This is because large-scale studies have shown *no* decrease in cardiovascular disease risk with use of antioxidant supplements.[23]

Some plants contain natural cholesterol-lowering compounds called plant stanols or plant sterols. Rich food sources of plant sterols include wheat germ, sesame seeds, pistachios, and sunflower seeds. These compounds have been clinically shown to reduce LDL (bad) cholesterol, and products that contain these natural cholesterol reducers are backed by the following FDA-approved health claim: *Foods containing at least 0.4 gram per serving of plant sterols, eaten twice a day with meals for a daily total intake of at least 0.8 gram, as part of a diet low in saturated fat and cholesterol, may reduce the risk of heart disease.* CoroWise® is a leading brand of plant sterols. Products such as Smart Balance® margarines and Minute Maid Heart Wise® orange juice contain these plant sterols. The plant sterols work by reducing cholesterol absorption in the small intestine and lowering its return to the liver. The liver responds by taking up more cholesterol from the blood so it can continue to make bile acids. Studies show that 2 to 5 grams of plant sterols per day can reduce total blood cholesterol by 8% to 10% and LDL cholesterol by 9% to 14% (similar to what is seen with some cholesterol-lowering drugs).[24]

The dietary recommendations described above are illustrated in Figure 5-19.

Naturally, in a course about nutrition, we focus primarily on *dietary* changes to prevent or treat cardiovascular disease. However, there are multiple elements of a healthy lifestyle to promote optimal heart health. The AHA educates consumers about *Life's Essential 8*,[25] a list of eight key components of cardiovascular health:

- **Eat better.** Eat plenty of fruits and vegetables; choose lean meats, seafood, and plant sources of protein.
- **Be more active.** Engage in 150 minutes per week of moderate-intensity physical activity or 75 minutes per week of vigorous-intensity physical activity.
- **Quit tobacco.** This includes traditional cigarettes, e-cigarettes, and vaping. Avoid exposure to secondhand smoke.
- **Get healthy sleep.** Adults need about 7 to 9 hours of quality sleep each night.
- **Manage weight.** As described in Chapter 7, lifestyle changes and some medical interventions can help keep body weight within a healthy range.
- **Control cholesterol.** Lifestyle changes or medications can help to keep LDL, HDL, and triglycerides within a healthy range.
- **Manage blood sugar.** As described in Section 4.7, lifestyle changes or medications can help keep blood sugar within a healthy range.
- **Manage blood pressure.** As described in Section 9.17, lifestyle changes and medications can help keep blood pressure under 120/80 millimeters of mercury.

According to the *Physical Activity Guidelines,* heart health benefits begin with about 90 minutes of moderate-intensity physical activity per week. In general, adults should strive to achieve 150 to 300 minutes of moderate-intensity physical activity per week to reduce risks for chronic diseases. Both regular aerobic exercise and resistance exercise are recommended. Older adults and anyone with existing cardiovascular disease should seek physician approval before starting such a program.[26]

FARM to FORK | Olive Oil

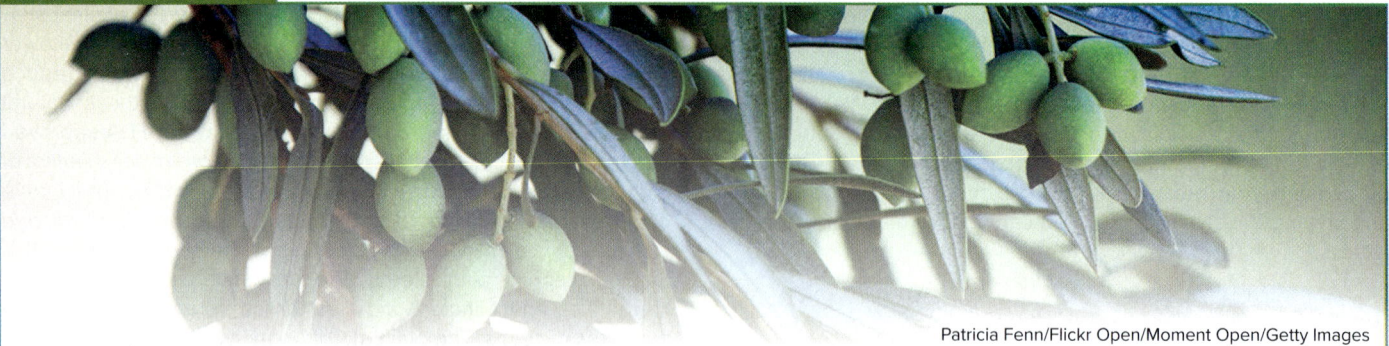

Patricia Fenn/Flickr Open/Moment Open/Getty Images

Olives are members of the drupe family, which includes fruits with soft flesh and hard pits, such as cherries, peaches, and plums. This hero of the heart-healthy Mediterranean diet is a rich source of monounsaturated fatty acids, which can improve blood lipids when used as a replacement for saturated fatty acids.

Grow

- Some olives are grown in California and Florida, but most of the world's supply of olives comes from the Mediterranean nations of Spain, Italy, and Greece. The hot, dry summers and mild winters favor the growth of olive trees.
- With at least 6 to 8 hours of full sun per day, you can grow olive trees in cooler climates, but you may need to bring them indoors in the winter.
- The color of olives depends on their ripeness and curing. Most olives start out green and ripen to a purple or black color. Some curing processes may also change a green olive to a dark hue. Curing is a process that helps to remove the naturally bitter flavor of olives, which is due to the presence of a phytochemical called *oleuropein*.

Shop

- Recognize the different types of olive oil. *Virgin olive oil* is the oil that is mechanically extracted (i.e., crushed) from olives during the first, cold press. No heat or chemicals have been used in this process, so virgin olive oil has the deepest color, most robust flavor, and highest phytochemical content. *Extra virgin olive oil* is the product with the highest quality, measured as the proportion of free acids in the oil. After the oil from the first, cold press has been extracted, the olives undergo further processing with heat and chemicals to extract more oil. This refined product still contains heart-healthy monounsaturated fats, but it is lower in phytochemicals and has a milder flavor. Refined olive oil is sometimes labeled *light* or *extra light*.
- If you can find it, choose *unfiltered* olive oil. Filtering olive oil produces a clear product, but it removes some phytochemicals. Unfiltered olive oil lasts longer than filtered products because it retains more of its natural antioxidants.

Store

- The unsaturated fatty acids in olive oil are susceptible to rancidity, so only buy as much as you can use by the date indicated on the bottle. Once opened, use olive oil within 3 months for the best quality.
- Store olive oil in a tightly sealed container in a cool, dark location to protect it from damage caused by heat, light, and oxygen. An opaque or tinted container provides the best protection from UV light. Use a vacuum stopper to seal your oil if you have one. This is a device that removes the air from inside a container before sealing it.

Prep

- Refined olive oil has a very mild flavor and is suitable for cooking or baking.
- Use higher-quality, extra virgin olive oil for salad dressings and finishing sauces, where the aroma and flavor will shine through. Adding fat to your fresh vegetables will enhance the bioavailability of fat-soluble vitamins and many phytochemicals.
- Olive oil can be used for stir-frying, sautéing, or roasting, but it is not ideal for deep-frying due to its low smoke-point.

Sources: Everything you need to know about olive oil: how to shop for, cook with, and store olive oil. America's Test Kitchen. 2017. https://www.americastestkitchen.com/articles/499-everything-you-need-to-know-about-olive-oil

Levinson JF. Healthful fats: olives in the spotlight—a small fruit with big flavor and hefty health benefits. *Today's Dietitian.* 2020 Jan;22(1):12.

Palmer S. Healthful fats: the skinny on unrefined plant oils. *Today's Dietitian.* 2019 Jun;21(6):12.

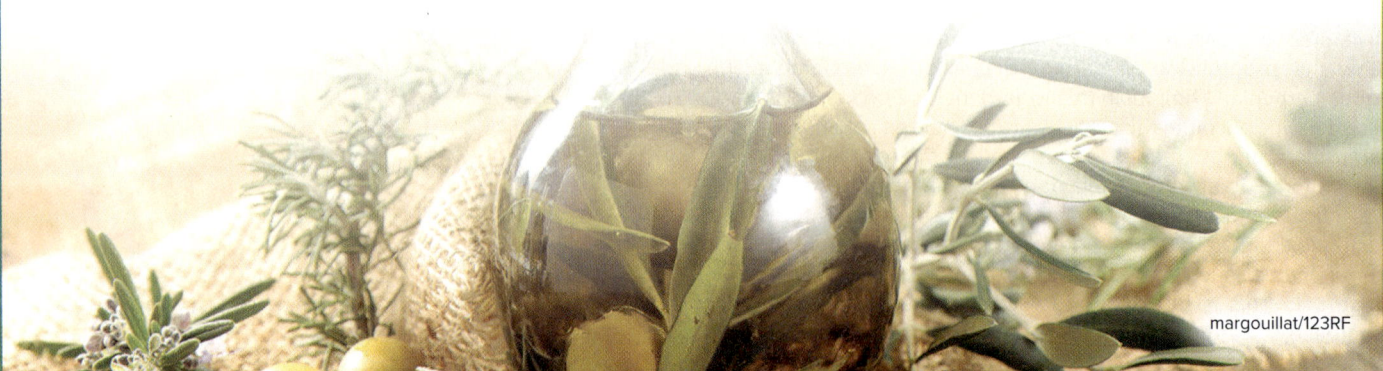

margouillat/123RF

Be sure to choose whole grains. Whole grains have more fiber, potassium, and magnesium but less added sugars than refined grains.

Choose low-fat or fat-free dairy products as you aim to keep saturated fat intake under 10% of total calories (or 5% to 6% of total calories for individuals at risk of cardiovascular disease). Low-fat and fat-free dairy products provide just as much calcium and vitamin D as their full-fat counterparts.

As you fill half your plate with fruits and vegetables, choose a variety of brightly colored produce. Fruits and vegetables provide fiber, potassium, magnesium, vitamin C, and vitamin E. Brightly colored selections, such as spinach and berries, are packed with disease-fighting phytochemicals. Cook vegetables with heart-healthy plant oils, such as olive oil, which are rich in unsaturated fatty acids. Use fresh or frozen fruits and vegetables to limit the amount of sodium in your dietary pattern.

For protein, choose mostly lean options. Substitute plant proteins for animal sources of protein several days per week. This meal illustrates a portion of grilled salmon. Fatty fish, like salmon, provide omega-3 fatty acids, which tend to decrease inflammation and promote healthy blood cholesterol levels.

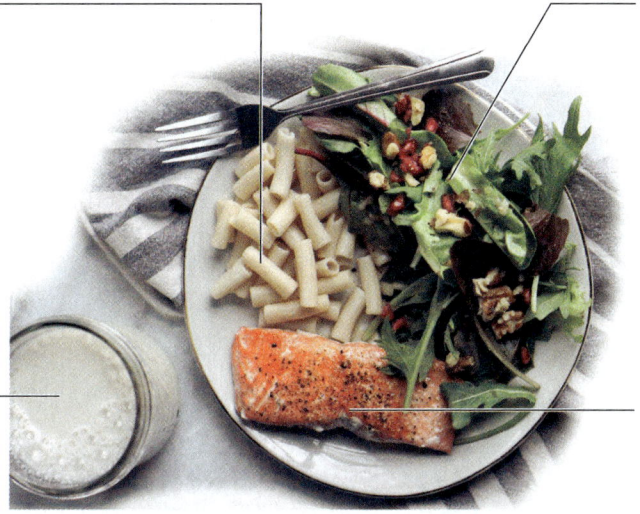

FIGURE 5-19 Use MyPlate with the AHA *2021 Dietary Guidance to Improve Cardiovascular Health* to build a heart-healthy meal. Complement your plan for heart-healthy eating with an active lifestyle. Alexis Joseph/McGraw Hill

Medications to Lower Blood Lipids

For some people, eating and lifestyle changes are simply not enough to lower blood cholesterol. Fortunately, medications offer a more aggressive approach to treating high cholesterol.

Cholesterol-lowering medications may be appropriate for individuals who are at heightened risk for cardiovascular disease. Some factors to take into consideration include clinical evidence of atherosclerosis (see Fig. 5-17), very high LDL levels (e.g., $\geq$ 190 mg/dL), or preexisting diabetes or hypertension.

Medications work to lower blood cholesterol in several ways. Examples are listed in the *Medicine Cabinet* feature in this section. Keep in mind that medications may lead to adverse effects, especially on liver function, so physician monitoring is required. In addition, the cost of treatment with these drugs can vary widely, from as little as $5 per month to nearly $5000.[27]

Medicine Cabinet

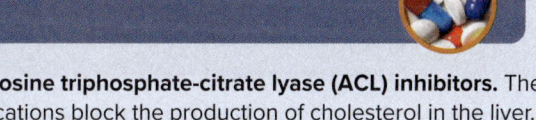

Lipid-Lowering Medications

Statins. Most frequently prescribed cholesterol-lowering drugs block a liver enzyme involved in cholesterol synthesis and thus reduce the amount of cholesterol in the blood. Examples: simvastatin (Zocor®), atorvastatin (Lipitor®), and rosuvastatin (Crestor®).

Selective cholesterol absorption inhibitors. Just as the name would suggest, these drugs keep cholesterol from being absorbed from the small intestine. Cholesterol will still be produced by the liver, but the contribution from dietary cholesterol is minimized. Example: ezetimibe (Zetia®).

Bile acid sequestrants (resins). These medications bind to bile acids in the intestine and are excreted in the feces, reducing their supply. This stimulates the liver to produce more bile acids, which uses more cholesterol and causes a decrease in blood cholesterol levels. Examples: cholestyramine (Questran®) and colesevelam (Welchol®).

PCSK9 inhibitors. These biologic drugs bind to and inactivate an enzyme that blocks LDL cholesterol uptake by the liver. When the enzyme is inhibited, the liver takes up more LDL from the blood. Examples: alirocumab (Praluent®) and evolocumab (Repatha®).

Adenosine triphosphate-citrate lyase (ACL) inhibitors. These medications block the production of cholesterol in the liver. They are intended for use by individuals who are genetically prone to high cholesterol and those who are unable to control cholesterol with other medications. Example: bempedoic acid (Nexletol®)

Fibrates. These drugs lower blood triglycerides by decreasing the production of triglycerides by the liver. Example: gemfibrozil (Lopid®).

Marine oils and derivatives. Dietary supplementation with 2 to 4 grams per day of marine-derived polyunsaturated fatty acids, used under the supervision of a health care provider, can help to lower triglycerides. Chemically altered preparations of these fatty acids may also be prescribed. Example: Lovaza®.

Combination drugs. Some pharmaceutical companies combine medications with different mechanisms of action. For example, a statin drug (simvastatin) has been combined with another drug (ezetimibe) and is marketed as Vytorin®. While the statin reduces the cholesterol made by the liver, the ezetimibe helps to block the absorption of cholesterol from food.

Cholesterol medications. American Heart Association. 2018. https://www.heart.org/en/health-topics/cholesterol/prevention-and-treatment-of-high-cholesterol-hyperlipidemia/cholesterol-medications

magnificent microbiome

Heart Health

There are several mechanisms by which the gut microbiota may influence your risk for developing cardiovascular disease. One way is by reducing the absorption of cholesterol from your GI tract. Cholesterol enters the GI tract from dietary sources and also as a component of the bile acids secreted by the gallbladder during digestion. Certain strains of bacteria in the GI tract are capable of converting cholesterol into a nonabsorbable compound called *coprostanol*. Reduced absorption of cholesterol from the GI tract can lower blood cholesterol levels, and thereby lower the risk for cardiovascular disease.

Source: Kazemian N, Mahmoudi M, Halperin F, Wu JC, Pakpour S. Gut microbiota and cardiovascular disease: opportunities and challenges. *Microbiome*. 2020 Mar 14;8(1):36. doi: 10.1186/s40168-020-00821-0

Surgical Treatment for Cardiovascular Disease

The two most common surgical treatments for coronary artery blockage are percutaneous transluminal coronary angioplasty (PTCA) and coronary artery bypass graft (CABG). PTCA involves the insertion of a balloon catheter into an artery. Once it is advanced to the area of the blockage, the balloon is expanded to crush the buildup of plaque. Afterward, the blood vessel may be held open with metal mesh, called a stent. CABG involves the relocation of a large vein—from the leg, for example—to bypass the blocked blood vessel.

For more information on cardiovascular disease, see the websites of the American Heart Association at www.heart.org or the National Heart, Lung, and Blood Institute at www.nhlbi.nih.gov.

✓ CONCEPT CHECK 5.7

1. List five risk factors for cardiovascular disease. Which of these are modifiable?
2. Define atherosclerosis. How does atherosclerosis cause a heart attack?
3. Identify three specific dietary strategies to lower your risk for cardiovascular disease.

Summary (Numbers refer to numbered sections in the chapter)

5.1 Lipids are a group of compounds that do not dissolve in water. The three main forms of lipids are triglycerides, phospholipids, and sterols. Fatty acids are components of the chemical structure of lipids.

Saturated fatty acids contain no carbon-carbon double bonds, monounsaturated fatty acids contain one carbon-carbon double bond, and polyunsaturated fatty acids contain two or more carbon-carbon double bonds. In omega-3 polyunsaturated fatty acids, the first of the carbon-carbon double bonds is located three carbons from the methyl end of the carbon chain. In omega-6 polyunsaturated fatty acids, the first carbon-carbon double bond counting from the methyl end occurs at the sixth carbon.

The essential fatty acids are linoleic acid (an omega-6 fatty acid) and alpha-linolenic acid (an omega-3 fatty acid). These must be included in the dietary pattern to maintain health.

Triglycerides are formed from a glycerol backbone with three fatty acids. Triglycerides rich in long-chain saturated fatty acids tend to be solid at room temperature, whereas those rich in monounsaturated and polyunsaturated fatty acids are liquid at room temperature. Triglycerides are the major form of fat in both food and the body. They allow for efficient energy storage, protect certain organs, transport fat-soluble vitamins, and help insulate the body.

Phospholipids are derivatives of triglycerides in which one or two of the fatty acids are replaced by phosphorus-containing compounds. Sterols are lipids made of multiple carbon rings.

5.2 Lipids have several functions as components of foods. Triglycerides (i.e., fats and oils) add flavor and texture to foods and provide some satiety after meals. Some phospholipids are used in foods as emulsifiers, which suspend fat in water.

Foods that are almost entirely fat include vegetable oils, butter, margarine, and mayonnaise. In the dairy group, whole milk and cheese are highest in fat. In the protein foods group, marbled meats, poultry with skin, cold water fish, and nuts are highest in fat. In the grains group, baked goods often have lots of fat added. In the fruits and vegetables groups, most foods are naturally low in fat, but fat may be added during food preparation (e.g., vegetable dip, butter).

Linoleic acid, the essential omega-6 fatty acid, is found in many plant oils, nuts, seeds, and poultry. Two rich sources of alpha-linolenic acid, the essential omega-3 fatty acid, are walnuts and flaxseed oil. Fatty fish are good sources of some nonessential omega-3 fatty acids, including eicosapentaenoic acid (EPA) and docosahexaenoic acid (DHA).

Food sources of phospholipids include organ meats, legumes (i.e., beans, peas, and lentils), eggs, and wheat germ. Cholesterol is only found in foods of animal origin, especially organ meats, egg yolks, and shellfish. Phytosterols are found in plant oils, nuts, seeds, and legumes.

5.3 Salivary lipase and gastric lipase make a small contribution to fat digestion in the stomach, but fat digestion takes place primarily in the small intestine. Bile is released into the small intestine to emulsify the lipids in the chyme. Pancreatic lipase breaks down triglycerides into diglycerides, then into monoglycerides (glycerol backbone with a single fatty acid attached) and fatty acids. The products of fat digestion are taken up by the absorptive cells of the small intestine, packaged as chylomicrons, and enter the lymphatic system before they eventually pass into the bloodstream.

5.4 Lipids are carried in the bloodstream as part of lipoproteins, which consist of a lipid core encased in a shell of protein, cholesterol, and phospholipids. There are four main types of lipoproteins. Chylomicrons are released from intestinal cells and carry lipids arising from dietary intake. Very-low-density lipoproteins (VLDLs) and low-density lipoproteins (LDLs) carry lipids both taken up by and synthesized in the liver. High-density lipoproteins (HDLs) pick up cholesterol from cells and facilitate its transport back to the liver.

5.5 Triglycerides are used for energy storage, insulation, and transportation of fat-soluble vitamins. Phospholipids are important parts of cell membranes, and some act as emulsifiers.

Cholesterol forms vital biological compounds, such as hormones, cell membranes, and bile acids. Cells in the body make cholesterol whether we eat it or not. It is not an essential part of an adult's dietary pattern.

5.6 The AMDR for fat is 20% to 35% of total calories. There is currently no RDA for total fat for adults, although Adequate Intakes (AIs) have been set for the essential fatty acids. Fatty fish are a rich source of omega-3 fatty acids and should be consumed at least twice per week.

The *Dietary Guidelines* advises Americans, starting at 2 years of age, to limit saturated fat intake to less than 10% of total calories. For those who need to lower their blood cholesterol levels, the AHA recommends further restriction of saturated fat to 5% to 6% of total calories. *Trans* fat intake should be avoided; as of 2018, the use of partially hydrogenated oils (the leading dietary source of *trans* fatty acids) has been banned in the United States. Although there are no strict, numerical limits on dietary cholesterol intake for the general population, the *Dietary Guidelines* recommends keeping dietary cholesterol intake as low as possible while still meeting daily needs for essential nutrients.

5.7 In the blood, elevated amounts of LDL and low amounts of HDL are strong predictors of risk for cardiovascular disease. Additional risk factors for the disease are smoking, hypertension, diabetes, obesity, and inactivity. Lifestyle modifications to improve heart health include choosing fish and plant oils instead of food sources of saturated fats; limiting added sugar intake; consuming plenty of fruits, vegetables, and whole grains to obtain antioxidants; incorporating phytosterols; and exercising regularly.

Check Your Knowledge (Answers are available at the end of this question set)

1. The main form of lipid found in the food we eat is
   a. cholesterol.
   b. phospholipids.
   c. triglycerides.
   d. diglycerides.

2. Which of the following is an essential fatty acid?
   a. Linoleic acid
   b. Oleic acid
   c. Docosahexaenoic acid
   d. Eicosapentaenoic acid

3. Which of the following foods are rich sources of saturated fatty acids?
   a. Olive oil, peanut oil, canola oil
   b. Palm oil, palm kernel oil, coconut oil
   c. Safflower oil, corn oil, soybean oil
   d. All of the above

4. Which of the following foods is the best source of omega-3 fatty acids?
   a. Fatty fish
   b. Peanut butter
   c. Lard and shortening
   d. Beef and other red meats

5. Lipoproteins are important for
   a. transport of fats in the blood and lymphatic system.
   b. synthesis of triglycerides.
   c. synthesis of adipose tissue.
   d. enzyme production.

6. Immediately after a meal, newly digested and absorbed dietary fats appear in the lymph and then the blood as part of which of the following?
   a. LDL
   b. HDL
   c. Chylomicrons
   d. Cholesterol

7. High blood concentrations of _____ decrease the risk for cardiovascular disease.
   a. low-density lipoproteins
   b. chylomicrons
   c. high-density lipoproteins
   d. cholesterol

8. _____ are unique among the lipids because they have one end that is soluble in water and one end that is soluble in fat.
   a. Saturated fatty acids
   b. Unsaturated fatty acids
   c. Sterols
   d. Phospholipids

9. Cholesterol is
   a. an essential nutrient.
   b. found in foods of plant origin.
   c. an important part of human cell membranes.
   d. all of the above.

10. The *Dietary Guidelines* recommends that Americans age 2 and older limit their intake of saturated fat to less than _____ of total calories.
    a. 5%
    b. 10%
    c. 35%
    d. 50%

Answer Key: 1. c (LO 5.2), 2. a (LO 5.3), 3. b (LO 5.4), 4. a (LO 5.4), 5. a (LO 5.6), 6. c (LO 5.6), 7. c (LO 5.9), 8. d (LO 5.7), 9. c (LO 5.7), 10. b (LO 5.8)

Study Questions (Numbers refer to Learning Outcomes)

1. Name a common property of all lipids. **(LO 5.1)**
2. Describe the chemical structures of saturated and unsaturated fatty acids and their different effects in both food and the human body. **(LO 5.2)**
3. Suggest three strategies to lower your saturated fat intake. **(LO 5.4)**
4. Describe the structures, origins, and roles of the four major blood lipoproteins. **(LO 5.6)**
5. What are two important functions of lipids in the human body? **(LO 5.7)**
6. List two possible health benefits of consuming fatty fish at least twice a week. **(LO 5.8)**
7. What are the recommendations from various health care organizations regarding total fat intake? Saturated fat intake? **(LO 5.8)**
8. Does the total cholesterol concentration in the bloodstream tell the whole story with respect to cardiovascular disease risk? **(LO 5.9)**
9. List three risk factors for the development of cardiovascular disease. **(LO 5.9)**
10. Describe three lifestyle changes to decrease the risk of cardiovascular disease. **(LO 5.9)**

References

1. Whelan J, Fritsche K. Linoleic acid. *Adv Nutr.* 2013 May 1;4(3):311-312. doi: 10.3945/an.113.003772
2. Kris-Etherton PM, Fleming JA. Emerging nutrition science on fatty acids and cardiovascular disease: nutritionists' perspectives. *Adv Nutr.* 2015 May 15;6(3):326S-337S. doi: 10.3945/an.114.006981
3. Gil A, Gil F. Fish, a Mediterranean source of n-3 PUFA: benefits do not justify limiting consumption. *Br J Nutr.* 2015 Apr;113 Suppl 2:S58-S67. doi: 10.1017/S0007114514003742
4. Maher T, Clegg ME. Dietary lipids with potential to affect satiety: mechanisms and evidence. *Crit Rev Food Sci Nutr.* 2019;59(10):1619-1644. doi: 10.1080/10408398.2017.1423277
5. *Trans* fat. U.S. Food & Drug Administration. May 18, 2018. https://www.fda.gov/food/food-additives-petitions/trans-fat
6. Atchley C. Replacing phos with customizable alternatives. *Food Business News.* October 3, 2018. https://www.foodbusinessnews.net/articles/12034-replacing-phos-with-customizable-alternatives
7. USDA, Agricultural Research Service. Usual nutrient intake from food and beverages, by gender and age. *What We Eat in America.* NHANES 2017-March 2020 Prepandemic. Available http://www.ars.usda.gov/nea/bhnrc/fsrg
8. Mogensen KM. Essential fatty acid deficiency. *Practical Gastro.* 2017 Jun;41(6):37. https://practicalgastro.com/2017/06/01/essential-fatty-acid-deficiency
9. Lichtenstein AH, Appel LJ, Vadiveloo M, et al. 2021 dietary guidance to improve cardiovascular health: a scientific statement from the American Heart Association. *Circulation.* 2021 Dec 7;144(23):e472-e487. doi: 10.1161/CIR.0000000000001031
10. Eckel RH, Jakicic JM, Ard JD, et al.; American College of Cardiology/American Heart Association Task Force on Practice Guidelines. 2013 AHA/ACC guideline on lifestyle management to reduce cardiovascular risk: a report of the American College of Cardiology/American Heart Association Task Force on Practice Guidelines. *Circulation.* 2014 Jun 24;129(25 Suppl 2):S76-S99. doi: 10.1161/01.cir.0000437740.48606.d1
11. Sacks FM, Lichtenstein AH, Wu JHY, et al.; American Heart Association. Dietary fats and cardiovascular disease: a presidential advisory from the American Heart Association. *Circulation.* 2017 Jul 18;136(3):e1-e23. doi: 10.1161/CIR.0000000000000510
12. Rimm EB, Appel LJ, Chiuve SE; American Heart Association Nutrition Committee of Council on Lifestyle and Cardiometabolic Health; Council on Epidemiology and Prevention; Council on Cardiovascular Disease in Young; Council on Cardiovascular and Stroke Nursing; Council on Clinical Cardiology. Seafood long-chain n-3 polyunsaturated fatty acids and cardiovascular disease: a science advisory from the American Heart Association. *Circulation.* 2018 Jul 3;138(1):e35-e47. doi: 10.1161/CIR.0000000000000574
13. Siscovick DS, Barringer TA, Fretts AM, et al.; American Heart Association Nutrition Committee of Council on Lifestyle and Cardiometabolic

Health; Council on Epidemiology and Prevention; Council on Cardiovascular Disease in Young; Council on Cardiovascular and Stroke Nursing; Council on Clinical Cardiology. Omega-3 polyunsaturated fatty acid (fish oil) supplementation and the prevention of clinical cardiovascular disease: a science advisory from the American Heart Association. *Circulation.* 2017 Apr 11;135(15):e867-e884. doi: 10.1161/CIR.0000000000000482

14. Shen J, Wilmot KA, Ghasemzadeh N, et al. Mediterranean dietary patterns and cardiovascular health. *Annu Rev Nutr.* 2015;35:425-449. doi: 10.1146/annurev-nutr-011215-025104

15. Dennett C. Key ingredients of the Mediterranean diet—the nutritious sum of delicious parts. *Today's Dietitian.* 2016 May;18(5):28.

16. Palmer S. Low-fat vegan diets. *Today's Dietitian.* 2016 Oct;18(10):20.

17. Vannice G, Rasmussen H. Position of the Academy of Nutrition and Dietetics: dietary fatty acids for healthy adults. *J Acad Nutr Diet.* 2014 Jan;114(1):136-153. doi: 10.1016/j.jand.2013.11.001

18. Heart disease facts. Centers for Disease Control and Prevention. 2023. Accessed October 27, 2023. https://www.cdc.gov/heartdisease/facts.htm

19. Expert Panel on Integrated Guidelines for Cardiovascular Health and Risk Reduction in Children and Adolescents; National Heart, Lung, and Blood Institute. Expert Panel on Integrated Guidelines for Cardiovascular Health and Risk Reduction in Children and Adolescents: summary report. *Pediatrics.* 2011 Dec;128(Suppl 5):S213-S256. doi: 10.1542/peds.2009-2107C

20. What are the warning signs of heart attack? American Heart Association. 2015. https://www.heart.org/-/media/Files/Health-Topics/Answers-by-Heart/What-Are-the-Warning-Signs-of-Heart-Attack.pdf

21. Understand your risks to prevent a heart attack. American Heart Association. June 30, 2016. Accessed October 29, 2023. https://www.heart.org/en/health-topics/heart-attack/understand-your-risks-to-prevent-a-heart-attack

22. Arnett DK, Khera A, Blumenthal RS. 2019 ACC/AHA guideline on the primary prevention of cardiovascular disease: part 1, lifestyle and behavioral factors. *JAMA Cardiol.* 2019 Oct 1;4(10):1043-1044. doi: 10.1001/jamacardio.2019.2604

23. Moyer VA; U.S. Preventive Services Task Force. Vitamin, mineral, and multivitamin supplements for the primary prevention of cardiovascular disease and cancer: U.S. Preventive Services Task Force recommendation statement. *Ann Intern Med.* 2014 Apr 15;160(8):558-564. doi: 10.7326/M14-0198

24. Cofán M, Ros E. Use of plant sterol and stanol fortified foods in clinical practice. *Curr Med Chem.* 2019;26(37):6691-6703. doi: 10.2174/0929867325666180709114524

25. Lloyd-Jones DM, Allen NB, Anderson CAM, et al. Life's Essential 8: updating and enhancing the American Heart Association's construct of cardiovascular health: a presidential advisory from the American Heart Association. *Circulation.* 2022;146(5):e18–e43. doi:10.1161/CIR.0000000000001078

26. U.S. Department of Health and Human Services. *Physical Activity Guidelines for Americans.* 2nd ed. Washington, DC: U.S. Department of Health and Human Services; 2018.

27. High cholesterol medications. GoodRx. 2023. Accessed October 27, 2023. https://www.goodrx.com/high-cholesterol/drugs

Design Element Credits: Fact Check/magnifying glass icon: McGraw Hill; Magnificent Microbiome background image: Alena Ohneva/Shutterstock; Sustainable Solutions icon: McGraw Hill; Roots icon: McGraw Hill; Medicine Cabinet icon: Peter Dazeley/Photographer's Choice/Getty Images

Chapter 6: Proteins

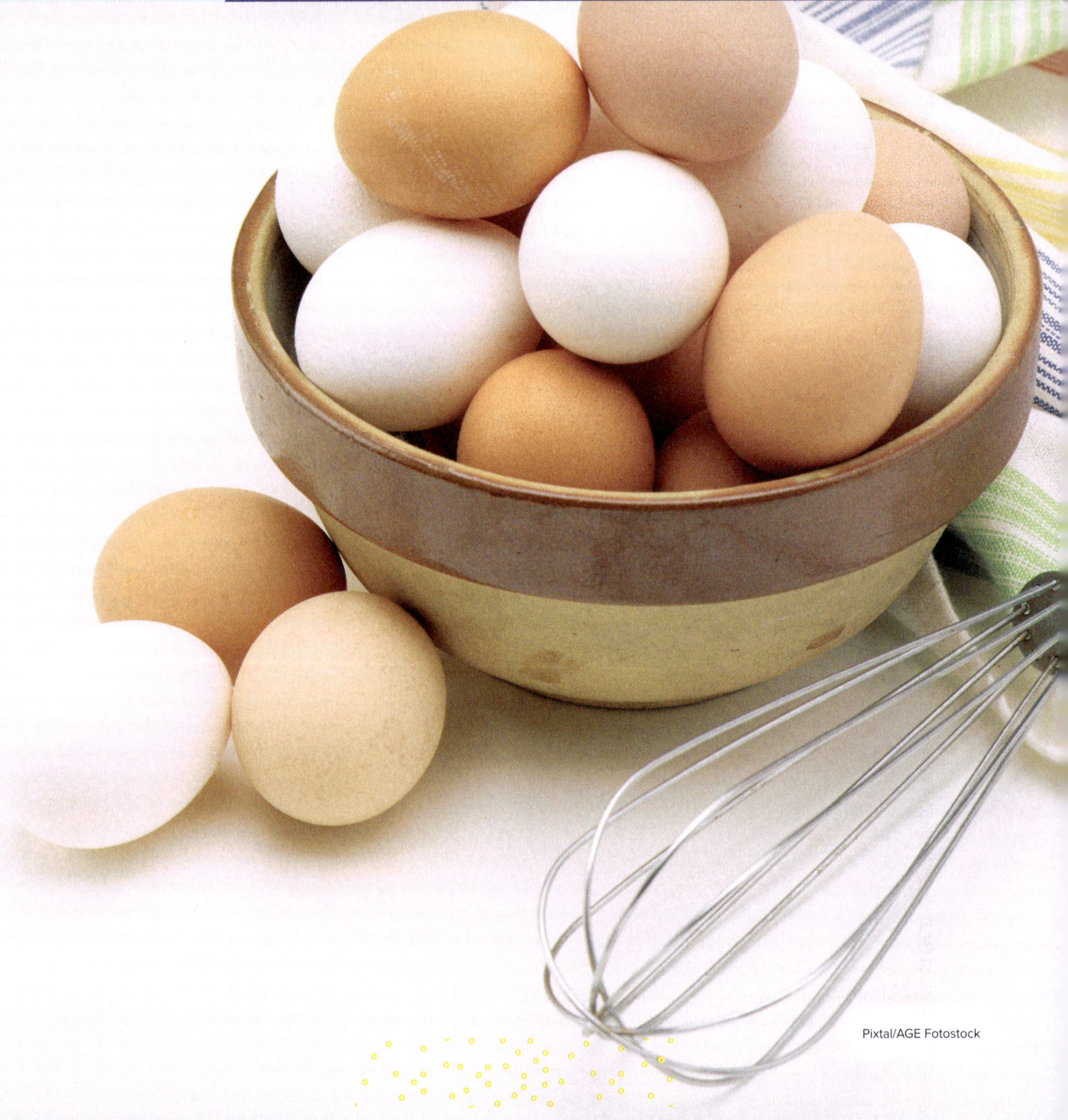

Pixtal/AGE Fotostock

Student Learning Outcomes

Chapter 6 is designed to allow you to:

6.1 Describe the structure and role of amino acids, distinguish essential from nonessential amino acids, and explain why adequate amounts of each of the essential amino acids are required for protein synthesis.

6.2 Describe how amino acids are organized and used to form proteins.

6.3 Identify food sources of protein, distinguish between high-quality and low-quality proteins, and describe the concept of complementary proteins.

6.4 Plan a healthy plant-based eating pattern that meets the body's nutritional needs.

6.5 Describe how protein is digested, absorbed, and metabolized in the body.

6.6 List the primary functions of protein in the body.

6.7 Apply current recommendations for protein intake to determine protein needs for healthy adults, and describe what is meant by positive protein balance, negative protein balance, and protein equilibrium.

6.8 Describe several health concerns related to protein intake, including protein-calorie malnutrition, food allergies, kidney disease, and inborn errors of metabolism.

6.9 Define nutritional genomics.

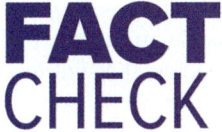

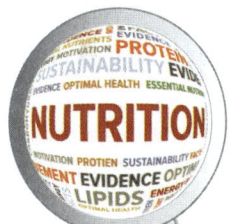

Should I take collagen for healthy skin?

Collagen accounts for approximately one-third of all the proteins in your body. It has a structural role in bones, joints, muscles, blood vessels, and skin. Many people are interested in the potential for collagen supplements to improve the elasticity, hydration, and firmness of skin to reduce the signs of skin aging. Collagen proteins in food are not absorbed intact but are broken down into small peptides and individual amino acids during digestion. The collagen found in dietary supplements comes from cows, pigs, chickens, and fish and has been hydrolyzed (broken down into small peptides) to promote absorption. Once absorbed, these raw materials can be used to synthesize collagen in cells if it is needed. Other nutrients, such as vitamin C and zinc (sometimes added to collagen supplements), are also required for collagen synthesis. Besides providing the building blocks for protein synthesis, collagen peptides may play a role in regulating the breakdown and synthesis of proteins within the cell. Results of clinical trials show that collagen supplements are well tolerated and can increase skin hydration and elasticity, which decreases the appearance of skin aging. However, further research is underway to determine the best dose and combination of ingredients to support skin health. Should you take a collagen supplement? There is no evidence of adverse effects, and studies do show a benefit for skin outcomes. However, the cost of supplements is a consideration. A varied dietary pattern can provide the building blocks necessary for collagen synthesis at a reasonable cost. In Section 6.6 you will learn more about the structural role of collagen in the body.

Source: de Miranda RB, Weimer P, Rossi RC. Effects of hydrolyzed collagen supplementation on skin aging: a systematic review and meta-analysis. *Int J Dermatol.* 2021;60(12):1449-1461. doi:10.1111/ijd.15518

6.1 Amino Acids—Building Blocks of Proteins

Thousands of substances in your body are made of protein. Aside from water, protein is the major component of lean body tissue, totaling about 17% of body weight. Proteins are crucial for the *regulation* and *maintenance* of the body. Functions such as blood clotting, fluid balance, hormone and enzyme production, vision, transport of many substances in the bloodstream, and cell repair require specific proteins. Proteins can also be broken down to *supply energy* for the body—on average, 4 kcal per gram.

Proteins are an essential part of a healthy eating pattern because, in addition to carbon, oxygen, and hydrogen, they supply *nitrogen* in a form we can readily use. Plants combine nitrogen from the soil with carbon and other elements to form **amino acids,** which are the building blocks of protein. Plants then link these amino acids together to make proteins. Figure 6-1 shows the general structure of an amino acid and two examples of specific amino acids. The various amino acids used to make proteins are slight variations of the generic amino acid shown below (see Appendix D). Each amino acid has an "acid" group, an "amino" group, and a "side" group (sometimes called an "R" group). The acid group and amino group look the same in every amino acid, but the side group is what distinguishes one amino acid from another.

ESSENTIAL AND NONESSENTIAL AMINO ACIDS

Your body uses 20 different amino acids to function (Table 6-1). Although all of these commonly found amino acids are important, only nine of them are considered **essential amino acids.** Remember, when a nutrient is *essential,* that means your body needs it, but your cells cannot make it in sufficient quantities to meet your body's requirements, so you must consume that nutrient as part of your dietary pattern. The nine essential amino acids are histidine, isoleucine, leucine, lysine, methionine, phenylalanine, threonine, tryptophan, and valine. If you do not eat enough essential amino acids, the synthesis of body proteins will slow down until, at some point, your cells will break protein down faster than they can make it. When that happens, health deteriorates (Section 6.8). Fortunately, about half of the amino acids in dietary proteins are essential amino acids, which is more than enough to meet human requirements.

The other 11 amino acids (alanine, arginine, asparagine, aspartic acid, cysteine, glutamic acid, glutamine, glycine, proline, serine, and tyrosine) are considered **nonessential amino acids.** Your tissues have the ability to make the nonessential amino acids as long as the essential amino acids are present.

Both nonessential and essential amino acids are present in foods. Animal sources of protein, such as meat and dairy products, and plant sources of protein, such as beans, nuts, and seeds, can supply us with both the essential and nonessential amino acid building blocks needed to maintain good health.

TABLE 6-1 ■ Amino Acids

Essential Amino Acids	Nonessential Amino Acids
Histidine	Alanine
Isoleucine*	Arginine
Leucine*	Asparagine
Lysine	Aspartic acid
Methionine	Cysteine
Phenylalanine	Glutamic acid
Threonine	Glutamine
Tryptophan	Glycine
Valine*	Proline
	Serine
	Tyrosine

*A branched-chain amino acid.

amino acid The building block for proteins containing a central carbon atom with nitrogen and other atoms attached.

essential amino acids The amino acids that cannot be synthesized by humans in sufficient amounts or at all and therefore must be included in the dietary pattern; there are nine essential amino acids. These are also called *indispensable amino acids.*

nonessential amino acids Amino acids that can be synthesized by a healthy body in sufficient amounts; there are 11 nonessential amino acids. These are also called *dispensable amino acids.*

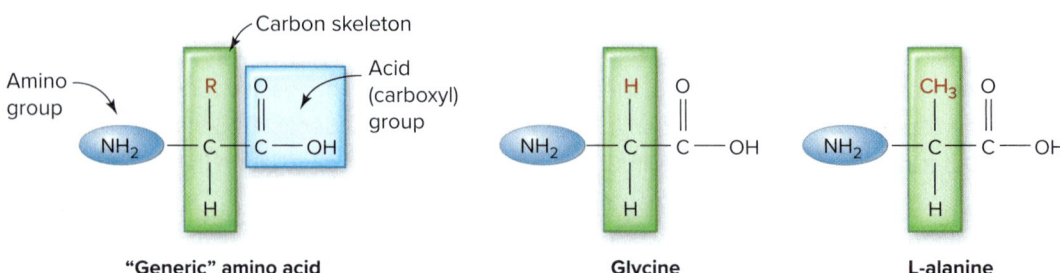

FIGURE 6-1 Amino acid structure. The side group (R) differentiates glycine (H) and alanine (CH_3).

CONDITIONALLY ESSENTIAL AMINO ACIDS

Some of the nonessential amino acids, which are usually synthesized in the body, can become **conditionally essential amino acids** during times of rapid growth, disease, or metabolic stress. For example, the need for amino acids to promote healing during recovery from surgery or burns is so high that synthesis of nonessential amino acids, especially arginine and glutamine, cannot keep up with demands. Studies have shown that supplementation with these nonessential amino acids is effective in improving the healing of surgical and burn wounds.[1]

BRANCHED-CHAIN AMINO ACIDS

The R group of some amino acids has a branched shape, like a tree. There are three so-called **branched-chain amino acids:** leucine, isoleucine, and valine (marked with asterisks in Table 6-1). The branched-chain amino acids get a lot of attention, especially in sports nutrition, because they are the primary amino acids that promote and signal protein synthesis and turnover in muscles. Whey protein (from milk) is popular among strength-training athletes because it is particularly rich in branched-chain amino acids.

> ✓ **CONCEPT CHECK 6.1**
>
> 1. Describe the basic structure of an amino acid.
> 2. What is the difference between the essential and nonessential amino acids?
> 3. What are some examples of conditions in which a nonessential amino acid becomes essential?

conditionally essential amino acids Nonessential amino acids that cannot be made in adequate amounts to support the body's increased requirements during conditions of rapid growth, disease, or metabolic stress, and therefore become essential (i.e., must be obtained from food).

branched-chain amino acids Amino acids with a branching carbon backbone; these are leucine, isoleucine, and valine. All are essential amino acids.

peptide bond A chemical bond formed between amino acids in a protein.

polypeptide A group of 10 to 2000 or more amino acids bonded together to form proteins.

6.2 Protein Synthesis and Organization

Some of the amino acids in your cells come from the foods you eat, some can be synthesized within your cells, and others arise from the breakdown of old and worn-out proteins in your body. Within your cells, those individual amino acids can be linked together by **peptide bonds** to form proteins of many different sizes and configurations (Fig. 6-2). Peptide bonds form between the amino group of one amino acid and the acid (carboxyl) group of another. Once formed, peptide bonds are difficult to break, but heat, acids, enzymes, and other agents are able to break apart peptide bonds during cooking and chemical digestion.

Through peptide bonding of amino acids, cells can synthesize dipeptides (two amino acids bound together), tripeptides (three amino acids bound together), oligopeptides (four to nine amino acids bound together), and **polypeptides** (10 or more amino acids bound together). Most of the proteins in your body are polypeptides, ranging from about 50 to 2000 amino acids.

PROTEIN SYNTHESIS

As we describe protein synthesis, let's use an analogy of preparing a meal from an online database of recipes. Before you prepare a meal, you search the recipe database and download a recipe or two, which tells you all the ingredients you will need and the sequence of steps to prepare each food in the meal. You must gather all the ingredients for the meal on your kitchen counter, then set to work to prepare the recipe. For your meal to turn out perfectly, the recipes must download successfully, you must have all the ingredients, and you must follow the sequence of steps described in each recipe.

In protein synthesis, the recipe database is the deoxyribonucleic acid (DNA), which is housed in the nucleus of the cell (online). Recall from Chapter 3, DNA is a double strand of nucleic acids that stores the information to direct synthesis of proteins. Your cells must make thousands of different proteins (foods), and DNA includes the genes (recipes) to make each and every protein your cells need. Protein synthesis, however, does not take

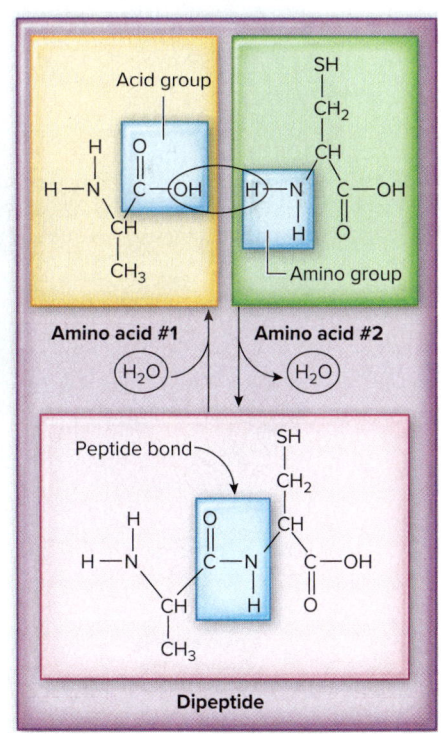

FIGURE 6-2 Peptide bonds link amino acids together. During synthesis of a peptide bond, a molecule of water is removed (dehydration). When peptide bonds are broken (as in digestion), a molecule of water is added (hydrolysis).

messenger RNA (mRNA) A strand of ribonucleic acid that corresponds to a gene to encode a specific protein. In the process of gene expression, mRNA is involved in transcription.

transcription The process by which the code or gene for a protein on a DNA sequence is copied into a single-stranded mRNA molecule that is ready to leave the nucleus.

translation The process of adding amino acids one at a time to a growing polypeptide chain, according to the instructions on the mRNA.

transfer RNA (tRNA) A type of ribonucleic acid that delivers amino acids to the ribosomes for protein synthesis; tRNA is involved in translation.

place in the nucleus; it takes place in the cytoplasm of the cell (your kitchen), on a ribosome (your kitchen counter—the specific site in your kitchen where you prepare foods). Thus, before a protein can be synthesized, the information from a gene must be transferred from the nucleus to the cytoplasm. Because the DNA cannot leave the nucleus to get to the cytoplasm, the information coded on a gene must be transcribed into a form that can leave the nucleus. This is the job of **messenger RNA (mRNA).** During a step called **transcription** (downloading the recipe), a gene that codes for a specific protein is transcribed into a single-stranded mRNA molecule that is ready to leave the nucleus.

Once in the cytoplasm, mRNA travels to a ribosome. During the process of **translation,** the ribosome interprets the information from the mRNA to produce a specific protein. In this process, **transfer RNA (tRNA)** delivers amino acids to the ribosome so they can be combined according to the specific instructions encoded by the mRNA. In our analogy, amino acids are the ingredients required for the recipe and you are the tRNA, bringing ingredients to the kitchen counter to assemble the recipe. Figure 6-3 illustrates the process of protein synthesis.

PROTEIN ORGANIZATION

After the synthesis of a polypeptide is complete, it twists and folds into the specific three-dimensional shape of the intended protein. These structural changes occur based

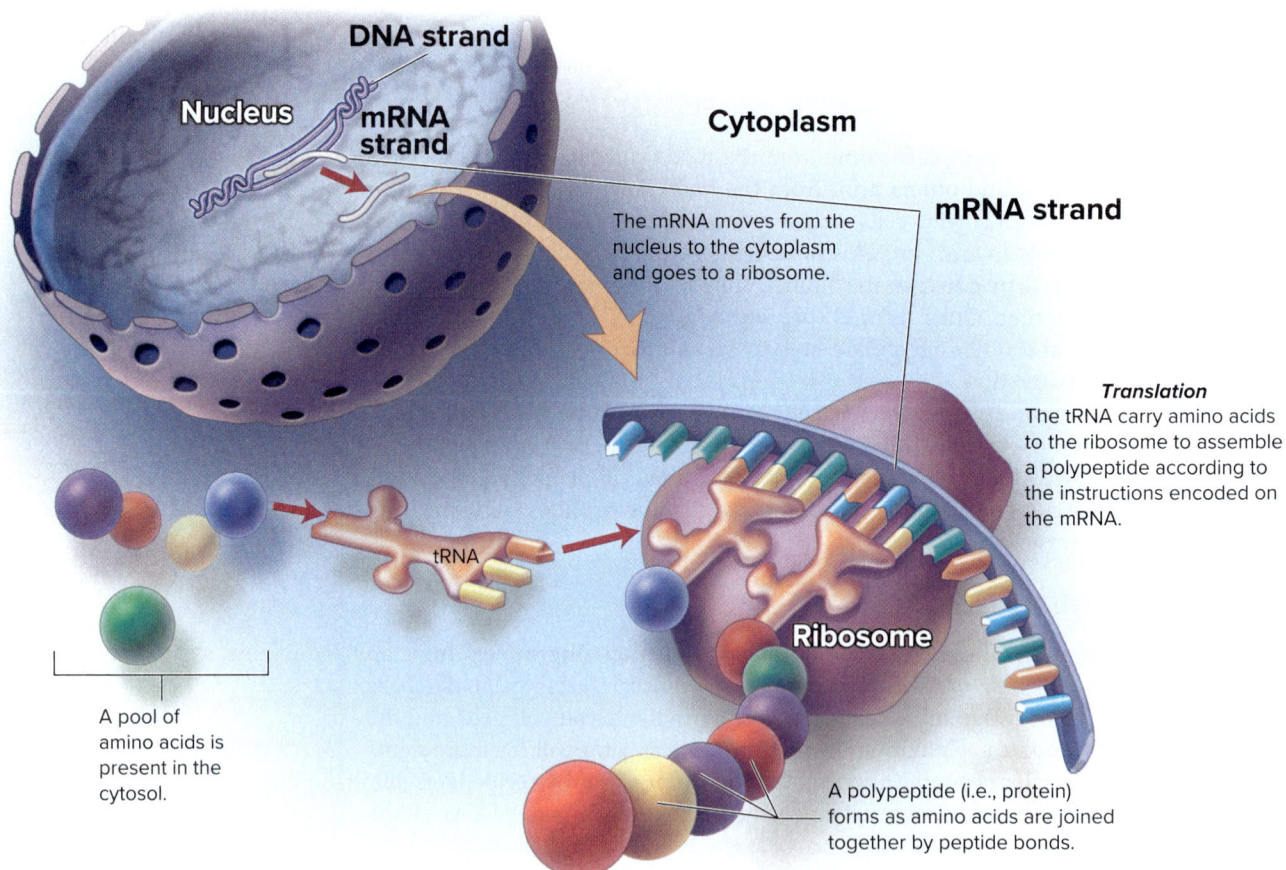

FIGURE 6-3 Protein synthesis is also called *gene expression*. During transcription, the information from a segment of DNA (a gene) is copied to mRNA, which moves through nuclear pores to the cytosol. During translation, tRNA bring amino acids to the ribosomes, where they are joined together according to the information coded on mRNA to form a polypeptide. The polypeptide may then undergo further processing to become a functioning protein.

on interactions among the amino acids in the polypeptide chain. Only correctly positioned amino acids can interact and fold properly to form the intended shape for the protein. The resulting unique, three-dimensional form, such as that shown for the protein hemoglobin in Figure 6-4, dictates the function of each particular protein.

Do you recognize the direct relationship between DNA and the characteristics of the proteins produced by a cell? If the DNA code contains errors, one or more incorrect amino acids will be added, resulting in the synthesis of an incorrect polypeptide chain that may fold into an incorrect shape. If it lacks the proper structure, a protein cannot function. Many health problems, including inherited diseases and certain cancers, stem from errors in the DNA code.

Sickle cell disease (also called *sickle cell anemia*) is one example of an inherited genetic disease in which amino acids are out of order on a protein. Individuals of African descent are especially prone to this genetic disease. Sickle cell disease is not a nutritional disease; rather, it is caused by a mutation in the genetic code for hemoglobin, the protein depicted in Figure 6-4 that carries oxygen in red blood cells. The mutation causes the amino acid glutamic acid to be replaced with the amino acid valine. This error produces a profound change in hemoglobin's structure. It can no longer form the concave disk shape needed to carry oxygen efficiently inside the red blood cell. Instead, the red blood cells collapse into crescent (or sickle) shapes (Fig. 6-5). Sickle-shaped red blood cells become hard and sticky, causing them to clog blood flow and break apart. This can cause severe bone and joint pain, abdominal pain, headache, convulsions, paralysis, and even death due to the lack of oxygen.

DENATURATION OF PROTEINS

Changing the shape of a protein often destroys its biological activity and thus its ability to function normally. Exposure to acid or alkaline substances, heat, or agitation (e.g., whipping egg whites) can alter a protein's structure, leaving it uncoiled or otherwise deformed. This process of altering the three-dimensional structure of a protein is called **denaturation** (Fig. 6-6).

Denaturation of dietary proteins does not alter their nutritional value and is a necessary part of digestion and other body processes. The heat produced during cooking starts the denaturation of some proteins. After food is ingested, the secretion of stomach acid denatures many forms of proteins in foods, making them safer to eat. These include bacterial proteins, plant hormones, and many active enzymes. Denaturation also enhances digestion because the unraveling of the polypeptide chain increases its exposure to digestive enzymes. Denaturing proteins in some foods can also reduce their ability to cause allergic reactions.

CAN WE CHANGE THE GENETIC CODE?

The growth, development, and maintenance of cells, and ultimately of the entire organism, are directed by the DNA present in the cells. If we could somehow alter the DNA, we could control what proteins are produced. By placing a new or modified segment into the DNA code in the nucleus, scientists could alter gene expression in such a way to change the proteins that are made by the ribosomes. This type of manipulation of DNA is called **genetic engineering.** It is used extensively in agriculture to introduce beneficial traits (e.g., pest resistance or drought resistance) into plants grown for food. It is also used to induce microorganisms to produce proteins such as insulin or clotting factors that can be used to treat human diseases. In humans, it is possible to use a type of genetic engineering called **gene therapy** to correct some gene defects or alter the risk for heritable diseases. However, gene therapy in humans remains controversial and is currently only being investigated in clinical trials.[2]

You may be surprised to learn that many nutrients and other dietary components taken up by cells can interact with our genes and affect gene expression and protein synthesis. While our human genome contains the code for all the proteins

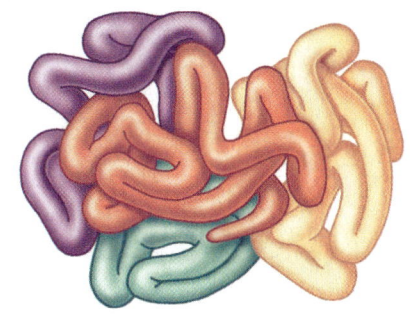

FIGURE 6-4 The polypeptides that make up hemoglobin coil into a specific shape. Four polypeptides join together to make the functional hemoglobin protein. To get an idea of its size, consider that each teaspoon (5 milliliters) of blood contains about 10^{18} hemoglobin molecules. (One billion is 10^9.)

sickle cell disease An illness that results from a malformation of the red blood cell because of an incorrect structure in part of its hemoglobin protein chains; also called *sickle cell anemia*.

denaturation Alteration of a protein's three-dimensional structure, usually because of treatment by heat, enzymes, acid or alkaline solutions, or agitation.

genetic engineering Manipulation of the genetic makeup of any organism with recombinant DNA technology. This includes DNA insertion, deletion, modification, or replacement. Also referred to as *gene editing* or *genetic editing*.

gene therapy Altering, replacing, or regulating the expression of genes to prevent or treat disease.

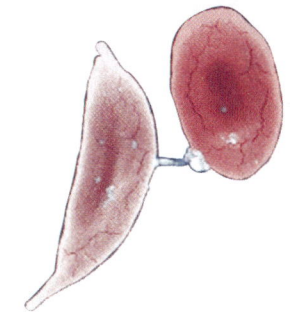

FIGURE 6-5 Sickle cell disease is one example of the consequences of errors in DNA coding of proteins. A normal disk-shaped red blood cell is shown on the right. An abnormal sickle-shaped red blood cell is shown on the left.
Janice Haney Carr/CDC

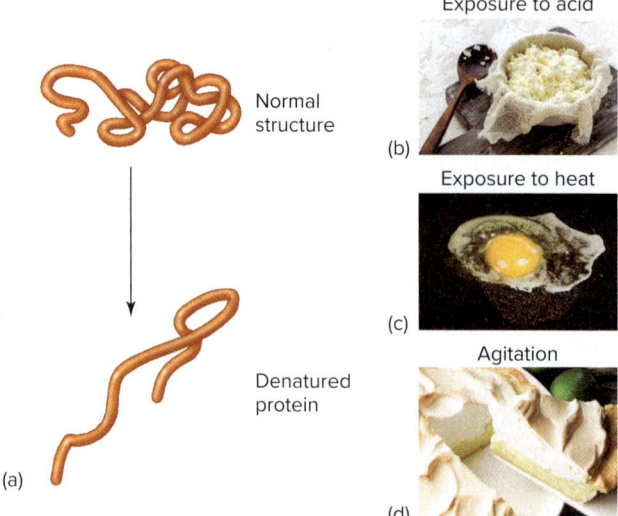

FIGURE 6-6 Denaturation alters the functions and properties of proteins. (a) The amino acid chain of a functioning protein is folded into a specific shape as a result of weak chemical interactions between the amino acids. Agitation or exposure to acids, bases, or heat can disrupt (i.e., denature) those chemical interactions. This unfolds the protein, leaving a chain of amino acids that no longer functions. (b) During cheese production, exposure to acid causes milk proteins to coagulate (curdle). (c) During cooking, exposure to heat causes the proteins in egg whites to solidify. (d) Agitation breaks the bonds between amino acids in egg whites, which allows them to form the stiff matrix of the meringue on top of this key lime pie.
Source (b): Marina Saprunova/123RF; (c) Sven Kahns/McGraw Hill; (d) Michael Lamotte/Cole Group/Photodisc/Getty Images

epigenome A network of chemical compounds surrounding DNA that modify the genome without altering the DNA sequences and have a role in determining which genes are active (expressed) or inactive (silenced) in a particular cell.

epigenetics The study of heritable changes in gene function that are independent of DNA sequence. For example, malnutrition during pregnancy may modify gene expression in the fetus and affect long-term body weight regulation in the offspring.

nutritional genomics Study of interactions between nutrition and genetics; includes nutrigenetics and nutrigenomics.

that can be made by our bodies, our **epigenome** is an extra layer of instructions that can be altered by environmental and dietary factors and influence gene activity. **Epigenetics** refers to changes in gene expression caused by mechanisms other than changes in the underlying DNA sequence.

Through research, our understanding of the links between nutrition and genetics is becoming clearer. To some extent, health professionals can now personalize nutrition recommendations based on their client's genetic information. Collectively, the interactions between genetics and nutrition are known as **nutritional genomics,** which is discussed in more detail in Section 6.9.

✓ CONCEPT CHECK 6.2

1. With reference to protein synthesis, explain what happens during transcription and translation.
2. Why is the order of the amino acids in a protein important?
3. What are some of the ways a protein can become denatured?
4. What is the difference between the genome and the epigenome?

6.3 Protein in Foods

Protein is found in all of the MyPlate food groups, but about two-thirds of the protein in the typical American dietary pattern comes from animal sources in the dairy and protein sections of MyPlate (Fig. 6-7).[3] Animal sources of protein, such as meat, poultry, and fish, provide about 7 grams of protein per ounce, or around 24 grams in a typical serving. One cup of cow's milk or yogurt has about 8 grams of protein. (Soy milk is similar to cow's milk in protein content, but most other plant-based dairy alternatives have very little protein.) Cooked beans, peas, and lentils provide about 5 grams of protein per 1/4 cup. A handful of nuts has about 5 grams of protein. Most grains provide 1 to 3 grams of protein per serving.

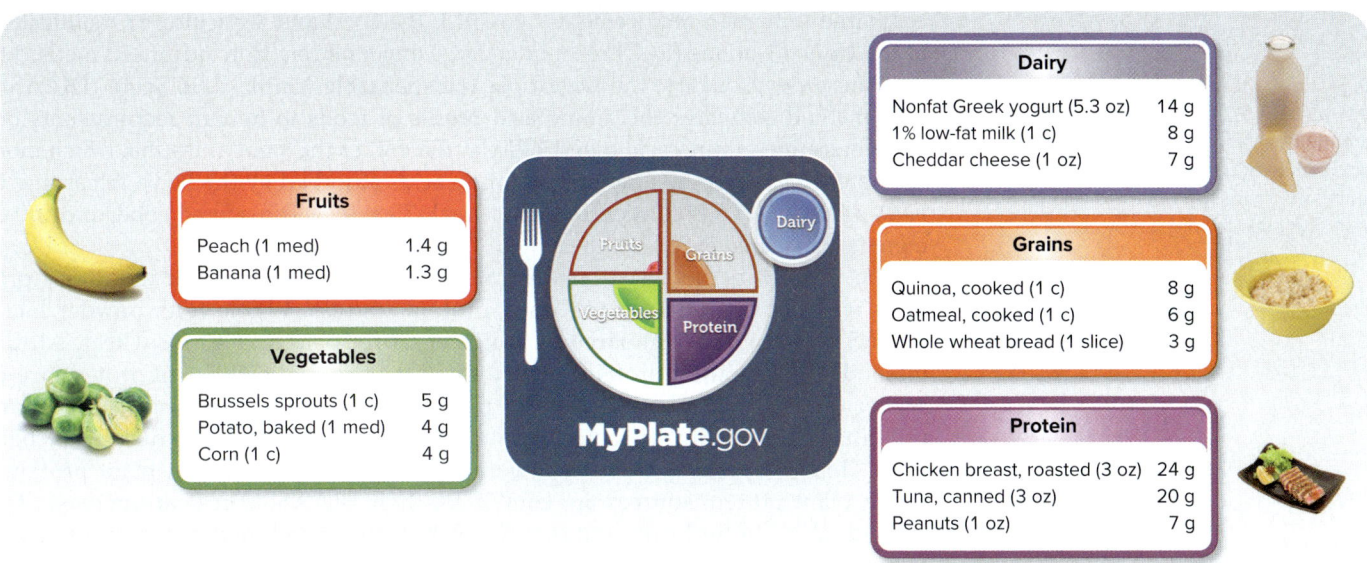

FIGURE 6-7 Food sources of protein. The fill of the background color (none, 1/3, 2/3, or completely covered) within each food group on MyPlate indicates the average nutrient density for protein in that group. Overall, the dairy group (7 to 14 grams of protein per serving) and the protein foods group (7 to 24 grams of protein per serving) are the most nutrient-dense sources of protein. The fruits group provides little or no protein (about 1 gram per serving). Food choices from the vegetables group and grains group provide moderate amounts of protein (3 to 8 grams per serving). banana: David Cook/blueshiftstudios/Alamy Stock Photo; Brussels Sprouts: Pixtal/age fotostock; MyPlate: U.S. Department of Agriculture (USDA); milk: Photodisc/Photodisc/Getty Images; oatmeal: Holly Hildreth/McGraw Hill; tuna: Vladislav Ostancov/123RF
Source: U.S. Department of Agriculture, Agricultural Research Service. FoodData Central, 2019.

PROTEIN QUALITY OF FOODS

Besides accounting for the total amount of protein in foods, we must also consider the quality of food proteins. Basically, *protein quality* refers to how effectively a food source of protein meets the amino acid requirements of humans. As you know by now, some amino acids are essential, meaning our cells cannot synthesize them, so we need to consume them as part of our dietary pattern. Food sources of protein vary in their amino acid composition and bioavailability.

High-quality proteins (sometimes called *complete proteins*) are those that are readily digestible and contain all the essential amino acids in quantities that humans require. To support growth and maintenance, humans generally are able to use proteins from any single animal source more efficiently than from any single plant source. Animal proteins (except for gelatin, which is made from collagen) contain ample amounts of all nine essential amino acids, so they are considered high-quality proteins.

There are a few plant proteins that are considered high-quality proteins. For example, soy and quinoa provide ample quantities of all nine essential amino acids to match human protein requirements. A few others (e.g., buckwheat and the seeds of amaranth, chia, hemp, and pumpkin) have all nine essential amino acids, albeit in smaller amounts than soy and quinoa. Many plant proteins, however, do not match our needs for essential amino acids as precisely as animal proteins because they are low in one or more of the nine essential amino acids. Because their amino acid patterns can be quite different from human requirements, the majority of individual plant sources of proteins are considered **lower-quality proteins** (also called *incomplete proteins*). Typically, a single plant protein source, such as corn, cannot easily support human growth and maintenance. Nevertheless, if you consume a *variety* of plant proteins throughout the day, you can easily obtain sufficient quantities of all nine essential amino acids.

How do food scientists measure protein quality? Historically, several methods of assessing protein quality have been used, including Protein Digestibility Corrected Amino Acid Score (PDCAAS), Biological Value (BV), and Protein Efficiency Ratio (PER). In various ways, these methods attempt to rate the amino acid profile or bioavailability

high-quality proteins Dietary proteins that contain ample amounts of all nine essential amino acids; also called *complete proteins*.

lower-quality proteins Dietary proteins that are low in or lack one or more essential amino acids; also called *incomplete proteins*.

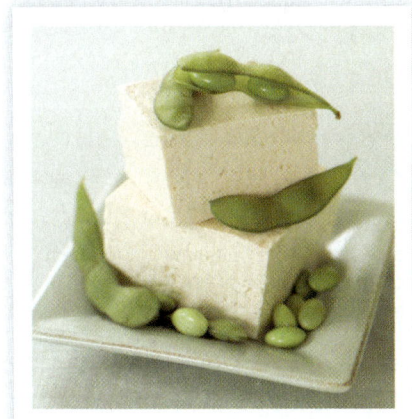

Soy provides a sufficient quantity of all nine essential amino acids, so it is considered a high-quality protein. Make a stir-fry with tofu (pressed soybean curds) or top your salad with mukimame (shelled soybeans). **How could you incorporate more plant proteins into your dietary pattern?** D. Hurst/Alamy Stock Photo

Digestible Indispensable Amino Acid Score (DIAAS) A method of assessing protein quality that compares the amino acid profile of a food protein to human amino acid requirements and also factors in the digestibility of food proteins.

compared to human requirements.[4] In 2013, the Food and Agriculture Organization of the United Nations (FAO) recommended using a newer, more advanced method to evaluate protein quality: the **Digestible Indispensable Amino Acid Score (DIAAS)**.[5] This method compares the amino acid profile of foods to human requirements but also determines amino acid digestibility at the end of the small intestine, which more accurately measures the amounts of amino acids absorbed by the body. According to FAO, a DIAAS < 75 is considered suboptimal, 75 to 99 is considered good, and 100 or more is considered excellent.

The DIAAS method has demonstrated the higher bioavailability of dairy proteins when compared to plant-based protein sources. Whole milk powder has a DIAAS score of 122, compared to scores of 64 for peas and 40 for wheat. All the methods of evaluating protein quality show that animal sources of protein are of higher quality than plant sources of protein, but that does not mean that plant proteins are unhealthy. In fact, plant sources of protein offer many nutritional benefits! This is especially true if you consume a variety of different plant proteins. When plant protein sources are combined, their DIAAS scores can increase. The individual scores for beans and rice are 60, but when combined, the score increases to nearly 80.

LIMITING AMINO ACIDS

An inadequate supply of just one of the essential amino acids prevents protein synthesis. This is known as the *all-or-none* principle: unless all the essential amino acids are available for protein synthesis, none can be used. The essential amino acid in smallest supply in a food or meal in relation to body needs becomes the limiting factor or **limiting amino acid** because it limits the amount of protein the body can synthesize. Once the limiting amino acid is used up, protein synthesis comes to a halt. The remaining amino acids may be used for energy needs or converted into carbohydrate or fat, but they will not be used for protein synthesis.

limiting amino acid The essential amino acid in lowest concentration in a food or dietary pattern relative to body needs.

Adults need only about 11% of their total protein requirement to be supplied by essential amino acids. Typically, 50% of the amino acids in the foods we eat are essential amino acids. However, when only lower-quality protein foods are consumed, the amount of the essential amino acids needed for protein synthesis may not be obtained. In this case, a greater amount of lower-quality protein is needed to meet the demands of protein synthesis, compared to high-quality proteins.

COMPLEMENTARY PROTEINS

When two or more lower-quality protein sources are combined, one lower-quality protein can compensate for the lack of an essential amino acid in another lower-quality protein. Two lower-quality proteins that, when combined, supply an ample quantity of all nine essential amino acids are called **complementary proteins.**

complementary proteins Two food protein sources that make up for each other's inadequate supply of specific essential amino acids; together, they yield a sufficient amount of all nine essential amino acids and so provide high-quality (complete) protein for the diet.

Meals with a variety of protein sources generally result in a complementary protein pattern. Figure 6-8 provides examples of food combinations in which the proteins complement each other based on their limiting amino acids. Many legumes, for example, are deficient in the essential amino acid methionine, whereas grains are limited in lysine. Eating a combination of legumes and grains, such as beans and rice, will supply the body with adequate amounts of all essential amino acids. Likewise, vegetables, which are limited in methionine, can be combined with nuts, which are limited in lysine.

pool The amount of a nutrient stored within the body that can be mobilized when needed.

Please note that complementary proteins need not be consumed at the same meal. Each cell contains a **pool** of amino acids that is available for protein synthesis. The amino acids in that pool come from recent dietary intake as well as endogenous sources (e.g., breakdown of old and worn-out cell components). Thus, healthy adults who consume an adequate quantity of a variety of plant sources of protein over the course of a day should have little concern about obtaining sufficient amino acids to support protein synthesis and maintenance.

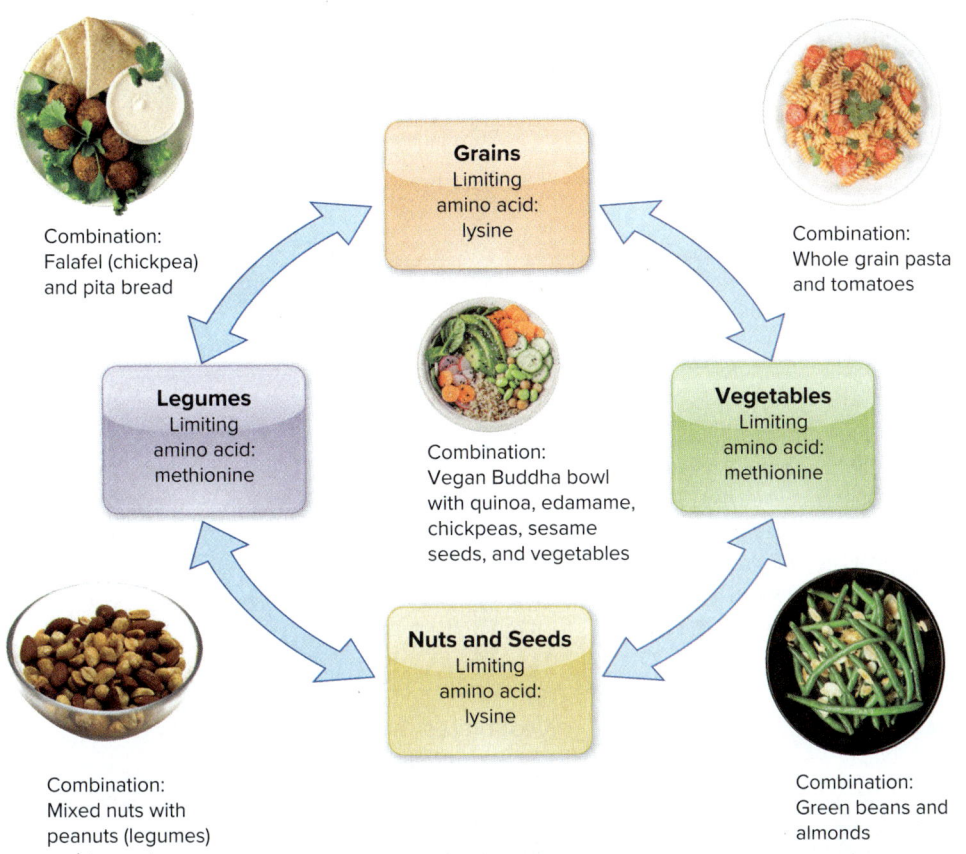

FIGURE 6-8 Plant group combinations in which the proteins complement each other based on their limiting amino acids. falafel: jenifoto/123RF; mixed nuts; L A Heusinkveld/Alamy Stock Photo; pasta: olegdudko/123RF; green beans with toasted almonds: robynmac/123RF; vegan Buddha bowl salad: Ekaterina Kondratova/nblxer/123RF

CHOOSING HEALTHY SOURCES OF PROTEIN

Plant Proteins. Plant-based protein sources include dairy alternatives, whole grains, legumes (beans, peas, and lentils), nuts, seeds, and vegetables (Fig. 6-9). Per serving, these plant foods provide more magnesium, fiber, folate, and vitamin E than animal sources of protein. Despite lower bioavailability, plant sources also provide iron, zinc, and calcium. Also, foods rich in phytochemicals help reduce the risk of a wide variety of chronic diseases.

Legumes are a plant family with pods that contain a single row of seeds. Examples include garden and black-eyed peas, chickpeas, black beans, pinto beans, kidney beans, great northern beans, lentils, soybeans, and peanuts. Mature legume seeds—what we know as *beans*—make an impressive contribution to the protein, vitamin, mineral, and fiber content of a meal.[6] A ½-cup serving of legumes provides 100 to 150 kcal, 5 to 10 grams of protein, less than 1 gram of fat, and about 5 grams of fiber.

Legumes are also naturally high in **lectins,** a class of proteins that bind carbohydrates and play a protective role in plants. Lectins have recently been wrongly blamed for causing a variety of health problems, including obesity, cancers, and inflammatory diseases. Although lectins are "natural pesticides" in plants, they are not toxic to humans because we cook legumes before consuming them. Eating raw or undercooked legumes would allow unbound lectins to attach to intestinal cells, resulting in vomiting, diarrhea, and abdominal pain. However, when legumes are cooked, fermented, sprouted, or processed for canning, the lectins bind to carbohydrates, which deactivates them and causes them to pass through the digestive tract and be eliminated. To prevent gastrointestinal distress, only consume beans that have been adequately cooked. Keep in mind that canned beans are already cooked. Read more about legumes in the *Farm to Fork* feature in this chapter.

Nuts and seeds are also excellent sources of plant protein. Commonly consumed nuts include almonds, cashews, pistachios, walnuts, and pecans. The defining characteristic of a nut is that it grows on a tree. Remember that peanuts, because they grow

lectins Proteins that serve as part of a plant's natural defense system. When ingested intact and in large amounts, they may cause gastrointestinal distress or inflammation or decrease the bioavailability of nutrients.

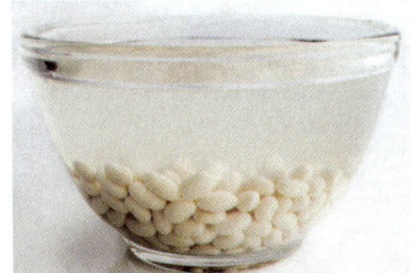

Consumption of beans can lead to intestinal gas because our bodies lack the enzymes to break down certain carbohydrates in beans. Gas production can be decreased by soaking dry beans in water before cooking. Some of the indigestible carbohydrates leach into the water, which then can be discarded. Ksenia Shachmester/123RF

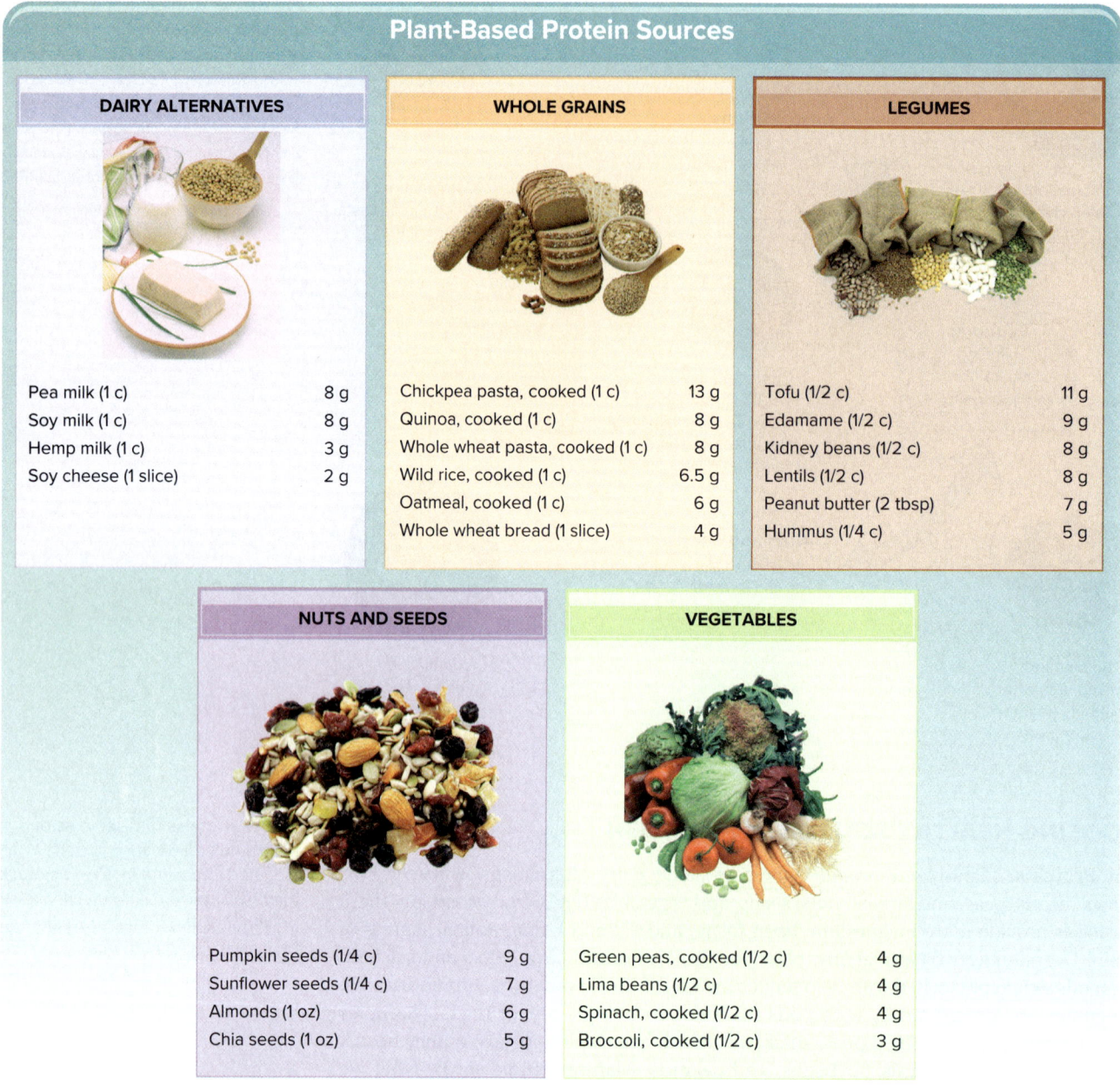

FIGURE 6-9 Plant-based proteins are found in a variety of food sources. dairy alternatives: Pixtal/age fotostock; whole grains: Tetra Images/Getty Images.; nuts and seeds: Thomas Northcut/Photodisc/Getty Images; vegetables: Pixtal/age fotostock; legumes: viperagp/123RF

underground, are legumes. Seeds, including pumpkin, sesame, and sunflower seeds, are similar to nuts in nutrient composition. A 1-ounce serving of nuts or seeds generally supplies 160 to 190 kcal, 6 to 10 grams of protein, and 14 to 19 grams of fat. Although they are a dense source of calories, nuts and seeds make a powerful contribution to health when consumed in moderation. Chia and pumpkin seeds have the added advantage of being sources of high-quality protein with all of the essential amino acids.

In summary, plant proteins are a nutritious alternative to animal proteins. They are inexpensive, versatile, tasty, a colorful addition to your plate, and beneficial to health beyond their contribution of protein to the dietary pattern. Learning to use plant proteins in place of or alongside animal sources of protein may help to reduce your risk for many diseases. The impact of plant proteins on health is discussed in Section 6.4.

Animal Proteins. As mentioned, in developed regions of the world, most of the protein we eat comes from animal sources (Fig. 6-7). For example, milk and eggs both contain very-high-quality protein and are often used as standards against which other food proteins are compared. Milks with various fat contents, ranging from whole milk to fat-free milk, are rich sources of protein (8 grams per cup) and several other nutrients, including calcium and vitamin D. One egg has only 75 calories but 7 grams of high-quality protein.

Although these animal products are rich sources of high-quality protein, eating patterns that rely heavily on animal products—especially red and processed meats—are associated with an increased risk for several chronic diseases.[7,8] Animal products are leading sources of saturated fat, cholesterol, and several compounds that may promote cancer. Furthermore, an overemphasis on animal products may crowd out plant sources, leaving the dietary pattern short on food components (e.g., fiber, folate, magnesium, and phytochemicals) known to decrease risk for chronic diseases.

The link between high intake of animal products and cardiovascular disease is most likely mediated by excessive intakes of saturated fat (review Chapter 5). Saturated fat intake is associated with increased blood levels of LDL, which promote the formation of atherosclerotic plaque in blood vessels. Atherosclerosis narrows the blood vessels, which limits blood flow to vital organs and may lead to a heart attack or stroke. Other compounds in animal products that have been associated with an increased risk for cardiovascular disease include dietary cholesterol, choline, heme iron, and specific types of amino acids.[7,8] For processed meats, added sodium and other preservatives may also contribute to risk.

Consumption of high levels of red and processed meat has been associated with an increased risk of cancer, particularly colorectal cancer.[8] This connection could be due to the curing agents used to process meat such as ham and salami, as well as substances that form during cooking of meat at high temperatures. Any type of meat should be trimmed of all visible fat before cooking, especially grilling. The excessive fat or low fiber contents of dietary patterns high in red meat may also be a contributing factor. These concerns could be avoided by focusing more on poultry, fish, nuts, legumes, and seeds to meet protein needs.

Red and processed meats have also been shown to be associated with increased risk of kidney disease.[9] Some researchers have expressed concern that a high-protein intake in general may overburden the kidneys by forcing them to excrete the extra nitrogen as urea. Also, animal proteins may contribute to kidney stone formation in certain individuals. A high-protein dietary pattern is not recommended for persons with limited kidney function such as those who have diabetes, early signs of kidney disease, or only one functioning kidney. There is evidence that low-protein dietary patterns (i.e., meeting but not exceeding the RDA for protein) are somewhat helpful in slowing the decline in kidney function. High-protein dietary patterns increase urine output, which can lead to dehydration, especially in athletes.

FARM to FORK Legumes

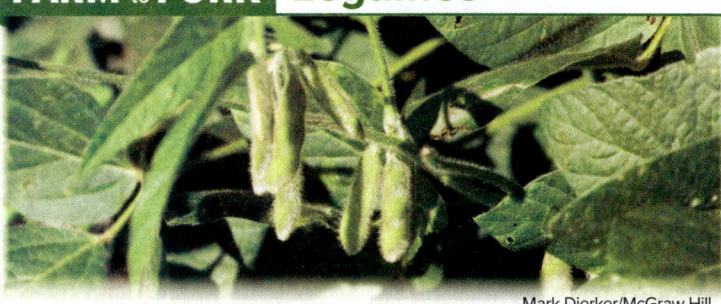

Mark Dierker/McGraw Hill

Legumes are seeds that grow in pods, such as beans, peas, lentils, and peanuts. Beans have an oval or kidney shape, while peas are round, and lentils are flat disks.

Grow
- Legumes have a beneficial relationship with bacteria in the soil. The bacteria take nitrogen from the soil and feed this nitrogen to the legumes. Legumes provide carbohydrates to the bacteria and nitrogen to support plants growing nearby.
- Pole beans can grow tall on trellises or in containers, making the most of limited garden spaces.
- Stagger the planting of beans to enjoy beans throughout the growing season. Some legumes (e.g., fava beans, chickpeas, and lentils) grow best in the cooler weather of spring or autumn, while others (e.g., soybeans and cowpeas) prefer a warmer growing season.

Shop
- Look for multicolored legumes—kidney beans, black beans, yellow peas, black-eyed peas, and lentils—to obtain abundant and varied phytochemicals.
- Buy canned beans. The heating that takes place during the canning process increases their nutritional value.
- Choose fresh or frozen pod peas to get the most fiber and antioxidants. Canned peas have lost up to 50% of their antioxidant content.

Store
- Store fresh beans in a moisture-proof, airtight container to maintain freshness. Beans tend to get tough quickly after harvest.
- Canned beans remain highly nutritious over a long shelf life.
- To prevent dried beans from drying out further, keep them in a food-safe storage container with a tight lid and place in a cool, dry place away from sunlight.

Prep
- Soak dry beans in water overnight prior to cooking. Discarding the water will help to reduce the flatulence that often occurs after eating legumes.
- During cooking, more than half of the antioxidants in dried beans will be leached into cooking water. Consume this water or allow the cooked beans to soak for 1 hour after cooking to help retain much of the nutrient content.
- Cook beans in a multifunction cooker or instant pot to save time, produce a tender product, and retain the most nutrients. If you prepare dried beans in a crockpot or slow cooker, make sure they are cooked adequately to deactivate the lectins.
- For the greatest convenience, use canned beans in cooking because they are higher in antioxidant content than fresh beans. Because canned beans are typically high in sodium, drain and rinse them under cold water to remove nearly half of the sodium.
- Most legumes are low in the essential amino acid methionine. Complement legumes with whole grains, which are a good source of methionine, to achieve an eating pattern that provides all the essential amino acids.

Source: Robinson J. Legumes: beans, peas and lentils. In: *Eating on the Wild Side: The Missing Link to Optimum Health.* New York: Little, Brown & Co.; 2013.

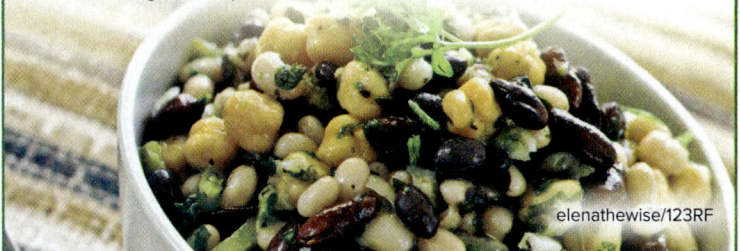

elenathewise/123RF

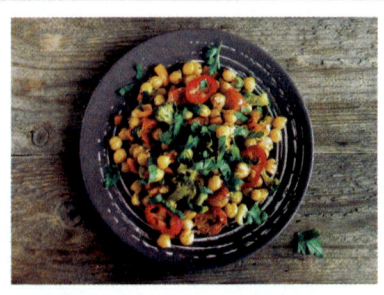

Meatless Monday is a nonprofit initiative that began in the United States in 2003 to reduce dietary saturated fat and is now active in more than 40 countries. The Meatless Monday campaign recommends that we cut meat from our meals on Monday and thus encourages us to increase our consumption of fruits, vegetables, whole grains, and legumes. **Visit www.mondaycampaigns.org /meatless-monday and pick out one new meatless recipe to try this week.** Mizina/iStock/Getty Images

Beyond these negative effects on personal health, our heavy reliance on animal sources of protein impacts the environment, as well. Overall, the increases in demand and consumption of animal products have had a substantial impact on agriculture over the past three decades.[10] Raising livestock for food has a significant environmental impact globally because of the large amount of land and water used and the high level of waste produced, including agricultural greenhouse gas emissions.[11]

PROTEIN POWDERS AND AMINO ACID SUPPLEMENTS

Protein powders and amino acid supplements are used primarily by those trying to lose weight and by athletes hoping to build muscle. Do you need a supplemental source of protein? Are there any risks associated with these products?

Most protein powders are made from cow's milk or soy protein, which are both high-quality proteins. Whey protein is one of the proteins in cow's milk that is especially popular with athletes because it is a source of branched-chain amino acids, which support muscle protein synthesis. In response to consumer demand, a wide variety of plant-based protein powders are available. Besides soy-based formulas, there are other plant-based products, which are made from grains, beans, peas, seeds, or blends of various plant proteins.[12]

Protein powders can be convenient—quickly mix a scoop of protein powder with water and breakfast is ready. They are also lean sources of protein, which can be beneficial for individuals who are trying to lose weight or gain muscle mass. However, depending on the brand, protein powders can be quite expensive. Most people can obtain adequate protein (along with other essential nutrients) from a dietary pattern that includes a variety of foods from each food group and meets energy needs. Populations who may benefit most from these protein supplements are those with calorie-restricted diets (whether for weight loss or due to limited appetite) and individuals with acutely increased protein needs (e.g., during recovery from illness or injury).

If you choose to use a protein powder, carefully examine the Supplement Facts label. Many of these supplements are highly fortified with vitamins and minerals. Avoid products that exceed 100% of the Daily Value for nutrients, especially if you consume multiple servings per day. Also, look for products that are lower in added sugars.

Sustainable Solutions

The Role of Livestock in Planetary Health

Many advocates for sustainability promote plant-based dietary patterns as the most environmentally friendly way to produce food to feed people. Compared to raising crops, raising animals for food uses more land and water and generates more greenhouse gases. However, sustainability is not only about preserving the planet; it is also about protecting the quality of life, health, education, and economic growth of the people who live on the planet! Foods of animal origin have many desirable nutritional benefits to support human health. Animal-sourced proteins are more digestible and absorbable than plant proteins. In addition, foods of animal origin provide micronutrients, such as iron, zinc, calcium, and vitamin B-12, which are less abundant and/or less bioavailable from plant sources. These nutrients have critical roles in preventing global nutrition problems such as stunting (decreased growth), suboptimal intellectual development, and impaired immune function that result from protein-energy malnutrition and micronutrient deficiencies. Furthermore, livestock production is a vital means of economic growth, particularly for families in developing nations. Improvements in the efficiency of livestock production are needed, but eliminating animal products as a source of nutrition would be short-sighted. As discussed throughout this chapter, plant-based dietary patterns have many health benefits, but foods of animal origin also perform important functions in sustaining human health.

Source: The Dublin Declaration of Scientists on the Societal Role of Livestock. *Anim Front.* 2023;13(2):10. Published 2023 Apr 15. doi:10.1093/af/vfad013

Although they may not be necessary, protein powders are generally safe to use. This is not the case, however, for dietary supplements of individual amino acids. In Canada, the sale of individual amino acids to consumers is banned. Because your gastrointestinal system is adapted to handle whole proteins as a dietary source of amino acids, individual amino acid supplements can overwhelm the absorptive mechanisms in the small intestine. When amino acids are ingested as supplements, amino acid imbalances occur in the intestinal tract because chemically similar amino acids compete for absorption sites in the absorptive cells. For example, an excess of lysine can impair absorption of arginine because these two amino acids are absorbed by the same transporter. The amino acids methionine, cysteine, and histidine are most likely to cause toxicity when consumed in large amounts. Due to this potential for imbalances and toxicities, the best advice is to stick to whole foods as sources of amino acids rather than supplements. Amino acid supplements also have a disagreeable odor and flavor and are much more expensive than food protein.

✓ CONCEPT CHECK 6.3

1. List three food sources of high-quality proteins.
2. What are complementary proteins? Give an example of a meal containing complementary proteins.
3. Describe two nutrition benefits of consuming animal sources of protein. Describe two nutrition benefits of consuming plant sources of protein.

6.4 Plant-Based Dietary Patterns

Vegetarianism has evolved over the centuries from a necessity into an option. A 2023 Gallup poll found approximately 4% of U.S. adults follow a vegetarian dietary pattern, and about 1% are strictly vegan.[13] The popularity of vegetarian dietary patterns has prompted changes in the marketplace. Many restaurants offer vegetarian meals in response to the growing number of customers who want a vegetarian option when they eat out. Campus dining services offer vegetarian options at every meal.

It is the position of the Academy of Nutrition and Dietetics that appropriately planned vegetarian diets are healthful and nutritionally adequate and may provide health benefits for the prevention and treatment of certain diseases. These diets are appropriate for all stages of the life cycle.[14]

There are many documented health benefits of plant-based eating patterns. Plant-based dietary patterns are linked to lower rates of obesity, which may translate into lower risk for several chronic diseases.[15] Indeed, studies show that death rates from certain forms of cardiovascular disease, many cancers, and type 2 diabetes are lower for vegetarians than for nonvegetarians. In general, vegetarians live longer than omnivores, as shown in religious groups that practice vegetarianism. It is important to note that other healthful lifestyle factors (e.g., not smoking, abstaining from alcohol and drugs, and engaging in regular physical activity) may partially account for the increased quantity and quality of life observed among populations that adhere to plant-based eating patterns.

Advances in nutrition science help to ensure the nutritional adequacy of vegetarian dietary patterns. This information is important for vegetarians because an eating pattern of only plant-based foods has the potential to leave gaps between nutrient intake and nutrient needs. Nutrient deficiencies can diminish health at any life stage, but infants and children are at particular risk for stunting of growth and developmental delays. However, with some nutrition knowledge and a bit of creativity, a plant-based dietary pattern can supply high-quality protein and other key nutrients without animal products.

fruitarian Referring to a dietary pattern that primarily includes fruits, nuts, honey, and vegetable oils.

lactovegetarian Referring to a dietary pattern that is primarily plant-based but also includes dairy products.

ovovegetarian Referring to a dietary pattern that is primarily plant-based but also includes egg products.

lactoovovegetarian Referring to a dietary pattern that is primarily plant-based but also includes dairy products and eggs.

pescovegetarian Referring to a dietary pattern that is primarily plant-based but also includes fish and other aquatic animal protein. Also called *pescatarian*.

pollovegetarian Referring to a dietary pattern that is primarily plant-based but also includes chicken, turkey, and other poultry.

The *Dietary Guidelines for Americans* and MyPlate emphasize that a healthy vegetarian dietary pattern can be achieved by incorporating protein foods from plants. In addition, the American Institute for Cancer Research promotes "The New American Plate," which includes plant-based foods covering two-thirds (or more) of the plate, leaving meat, fish, poultry, or low-fat dairy covering only one-third (or less) of the plate (aicr.org/cancer-prevention/healthy-eating/new-american-plate/).

TYPES OF PLANT-BASED EATING PATTERNS

There are several different types or degrees of plant-based eating (Fig. 6-10). Of the estimated 4% of American adults who call themselves vegetarians, about half are total vegetarians, or vegans, who eat only plant foods. **Fruitarians** primarily eat fruits, nuts, honey, and vegetable oils. This plan is not recommended because it can lead to nutrient deficiencies in people of all ages. **Lactovegetarians** and **ovovegetarians** allow dairy and egg products, respectively, in their plant-based eating pattern. **Lactoovovegetarians** include both dairy products and eggs in their plant-based eating pattern. These inclusions make food planning easier because the dairy and eggs are rich in some nutrients, such as vitamin B-12 and calcium, that are missing or minimal in plants.

The more variety in the dietary pattern, the easier it is to meet nutritional needs. A **pescovegetarian** dietary pattern, one that includes fish and other aquatic animal protein, has been associated with a lower risk of colon cancer.[16] A **pollovegetarian** eating plan includes chicken, turkey, and other poultry. Anyone who goes meatless most of the time can call themselves a semivegetarian or a flexitarian.

FIGURE 6-10 The different types of vegetarians and the protein sources they consume.

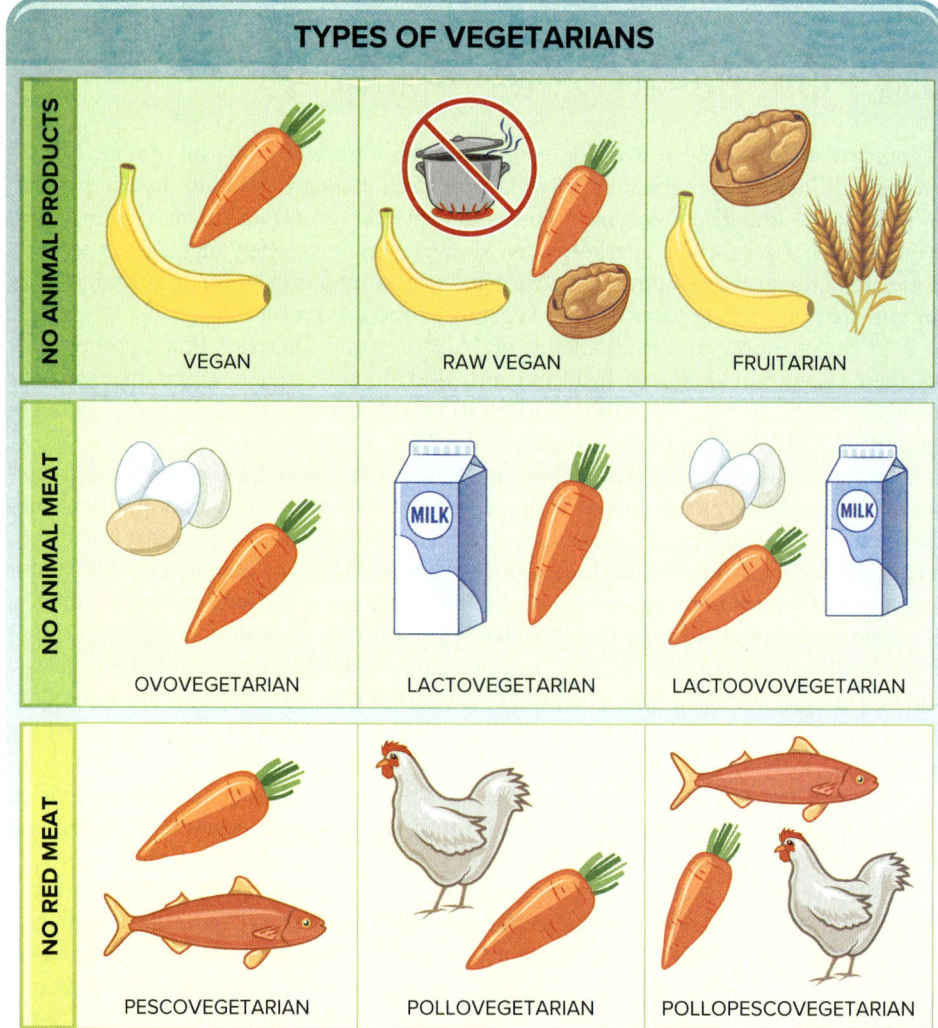

WHY DO PEOPLE BECOME VEGETARIANS?

People choose plant-based dietary patterns for a variety of reasons.

Personal Health Concerns. Health concerns are the most common reason why people choose plant-based dietary patterns.[17] Compared to omnivorous eating patterns in the United States, plant-based dietary patterns are lower in energy, total fat, saturated fat, cholesterol, and sodium and higher in fiber.[18] As detailed in the next subsection, these dietary changes may impact the risk of developing several chronic diseases.

Religion or Ethical Concerns. Some believe that killing animals for food is unethical. Hindus and Trappist monks eat vegetarian meals as a practice of their religion. Many Seventh-day Adventists base their practice of vegetarianism on biblical texts and believe it is a more healthful way to live.

Environmental Concerns. Some individuals may choose plant-based dietary patterns due to concerns about the environmental impact of raising animals for food. Per kilocalorie of food energy produced, raising livestock uses more land and water than raising crops. Runoff from farms that raise livestock may pollute nearby land and water. Livestock also contribute to greenhouse gas emissions, which may affect global climate change.[19]

Economic Concerns. Plant proteins are more affordable than animal sources of protein, so switching from an omnivorous to a vegan or vegetarian dietary pattern could directly decrease household food costs. In developed nations, where people typically rely heavily on plant sources of protein, switching to a vegetarian or vegan dietary pattern could cut household food costs by 22% to 34%.[20] Beyond direct food costs, shifting to a plant-based dietary pattern may result in additional savings in health care costs.

GOOD FOR DISEASE PREVENTION

Heart Health. Plant sources of proteins can positively impact heart health in several ways (see *Newsworthy Nutrition*). First, the plant foods we eat contain no cholesterol or *trans* fat and little saturated fat. The major types of fat in plant foods are monounsaturated and polyunsaturated fats. A vegan dietary pattern coupled with regular exercise and other lifestyle changes can lead to a reversal of atherosclerotic plaque in various arteries in the body.[15]

Beans and nuts contain soluble fiber, which binds to cholesterol in the small intestine and prevents it from being absorbed by the intestinal cells. Also, due to the activity of some phytochemicals, foods made from soybeans can lower the production of cholesterol by the liver. The Food and Drug Administration (FDA) allows health claims for the cholesterol-lowering properties of soy foods, and the American Heart Association has recommended the inclusion of some soy protein in the dietary patterns of people with high blood cholesterol. To list a health claim for soy on the label, a food product must have at least 6.25 grams of soy protein and less than 3 grams of total fat, less than 1 gram of saturated fat, and less than 20 milligrams of cholesterol per serving. Based on inconsistent findings from recent studies of the ability of soy protein to lower LDL cholesterol, the FDA is proposing to downgrade the soy health claim from "authorized" to "qualified." The FDA is not questioning whether soy protein lowers cholesterol but, rather, by how much.[21] Today soy products are readily available to consumers and can certainly play a role in reducing heart disease risk when combined with other cholesterol-reducing changes in the eating pattern.

There are several other heart-protective compounds in plant foods. Some of the phytochemicals may help to prevent blood clots and relax the blood vessels. Nuts are an especially good source of nutrients implicated in heart health, including vitamin E, folate, magnesium, and copper. Frequent consumption of nuts (about 1 ounce of nuts five times per week) is associated with a decreased risk of cardiovascular disease.

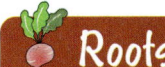

Roots

Vegetarian Dietary Patterns Among Seventh-Day Adventists

Seventh-day Adventists are a religious group in which physical health is closely intertwined with spirituality. Members of the church believe that the body is a temple and that wholesome living—eating well and avoiding harmful substances—is an important way to care for the temple and honor God. Of the church's 21 million adherents worldwide, about 5% are vegan, 14% are vegetarian, 11% are pescatarian, and another 32% report eating meat only once per week or less. In the United States and Canada, more than half of Seventh-day Adventists follow a vegan or vegetarian lifestyle. Furthermore, more than 90% of Seventh-day Adventists abstain from drinking alcohol. Members of this religious group have been the focus of many longitudinal studies of lifestyle and health outcomes. Indeed, the Adventist Health Studies have demonstrated that vegetarian lifestyles are associated with lower risk for obesity, hypertension, type 2 diabetes, and cancer. Their adherence to the Health Message of the Church certainly contributes to the fact that Seventh-day Adventists live, on average, 10 years longer than the general population. Read more about the dietary patterns of the Seventh-day Adventists and other long-lived population groups in Section 16.5.

Sources: McBride DC, Bailey KGD, Landless PN, et al. Health beliefs, behavior, spiritual growth, and salvation in a global population of Seventh-day Adventists. *Rev Relig Res*. 2021 Mar 6;63:535-557. doi: 10.1007/s13644-021-00451-4

Orlich MJ, Fraser GE. Vegetarian diets in the Adventist Health Study 2: a review of initial published findings. *Am J Clin Nutr*. 2014 Jul;100 Suppl 1(1):353S-358S. doi: 10.3945/ajcn.113.071233

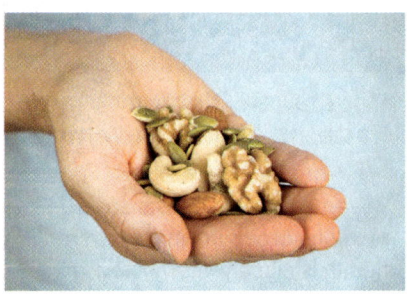

A small handful of nuts is a heart-healthy snack. The FDA allows a qualified health claim on food labels to link nuts with a reduced risk of developing cardiovascular disease. Johan Larson/123RF

Newsworthy Nutrition

Plant-based dietary patterns linked to lower risk for cardiovascular disease

INTRODUCTION: Cardiovascular disease (CVD) is the leading cause of death worldwide. Adherence to a healthy, plant-based dietary pattern—low in energy density, saturated fat, and cholesterol and high in dietary fiber, vitamins, minerals, and phytochemicals—may reduce the risk for CVD (which includes both coronary heart disease and stroke). **OBJECTIVE:** In this *systematic review and meta-analysis* of cohort studies, the researchers wanted to examine correlations between plant-based dietary patterns and incidence of total CVD, coronary heart disease, and stroke. In addition, they wanted to determine if there is a dose-response relationship between the degree of adherence to a healthy, plant-based dietary pattern and the risk for CVD. **METHODS:** The researchers identified 923 published articles related to plant-based dietary patterns and CVD risk. Of those, they reviewed 122 articles that met their inclusion criteria (longitudinal cohort studies investigating the relationship between plant-based dietary patterns and CVD incidence among adults who were free of CVD at enrollment). Finally, 10 different articles describing 9 different cohort studies were included in the systematic review and meta-analysis. The researchers extracted data from these studies that scored the participants' adherence to plant-based dietary patterns (the provegetarian diet index, the overall plant-based index, the healthful plant-based index, and the unhealthful plant-based index) and estimated risk for incidence of cardiovascular disease. **RESULTS:** The meta-analysis included 698,707 study participants with 137,968 cases of CVD. The mean age of study subjects ranged from 36 to 64 years and the duration of follow-up ranged from 5 to 36 years. Data from six publications that examined the association between plant-based dietary patterns and incidence of CVD showed that the plant-based dietary pattern was associated with a lower risk of total CVD. Data from five publications that specifically reported the incidence of coronary heart disease showed a plant-based dietary pattern was associated with a lower risk for CHD. Data from five publications that specifically reported the incidence of stroke showed there was a trend for lower risk for stroke with higher adherence to a plant-based dietary pattern. **CONCLUSION:** This systematic review and meta-analysis of prospective cohort studies demonstrated a statistically significantly lower risk for total cardiovascular disease and coronary heart disease with adherence to a healthy, plant-based dietary pattern. Higher adherence to a healthy, plant-based dietary pattern was associated with the greatest reductions in CVD risk. Furthermore, subgroup analyses demonstrated the most significant effects for younger adults. There seems to be a trend for a protective effect of a plant-based dietary pattern on risk for stroke as well, but additional research is needed to clearly assess the impact of plant-based dietary patterns on stroke risk.

Source: Gan ZH, Cheong HC, Tu Y-K, Kuo P-H. Association between plant-based dietary patterns and risk of cardiovascular disease: a systematic review and meta-analysis of prospective cohort studies. *Nutrients.* 2021 Nov 5;13(11):3952. doi: 10.3390/nu13113952

Cancer Prevention. Excess body fat is a risk factor for 13 types of cancer, including cancers of the digestive, reproductive, and endocrine organs.[22] Because an eating pattern rich in plant foods can assist with achieving and maintaining a healthy weight, this may be one mechanism whereby plant-based dietary patterns are linked to lower risk for cancer. Also, dietary fiber, specific micronutrients, and numerous phytochemicals in plant foods may aid in the prevention of some types of cancers. The American Institute for Cancer Research maintains a website that summarizes the current and emerging evidence on various foods and cancer risk. The site provides information on the potential benefits of several fruits, vegetables, legumes, nuts, seeds, spices, coffee, and tea.[23] Visit AICR's Foods that Fight Cancer™ site at https://www.aicr.org/cancer-prevention/food-facts/. Chapter 8 provides additional information about the connections between nutrition and cancer.

Diabetes Prevention and Control. Plant-based dietary patterns are associated with lower risk for developing type 2 diabetes. Among individuals with existing type 2

diabetes, shifting to a plant-based dietary pattern tends to improve blood glucose control. Some studies indicate long-term adherence to a plant-based dietary pattern may even reverse type 2 diabetes.[15]

There are several features of a plant-based dietary pattern that may explain these metabolic outcomes. Improvements in blood glucose control may be partly due to reductions in body weight. Plant-based dietary patterns, especially those that focus on whole foods (as opposed to highly processed plant-based products) tend to be lower in energy density, which leads to an overall reduction in calorie intake and loss of body fat. Reductions in body fat (especially from the abdominal region) are associated with better glycemic control. In addition, plants also may be particularly good sources of protein for people with diabetes or impaired glucose tolerance because the high fiber content of plant foods leads to a slower increase in blood glucose after meals. Higher intakes of whole grains, legumes, and nuts have all been linked to reduced risk for type 2 diabetes.[24]

We must also consider what is *left out* of a plant-based eating pattern. Several studies have linked high intakes of red and/or processed meats with increased risk for type 2 diabetes. In fact, replacing at least 35% of animal protein with plant protein is associated with improvements in markers of glucose control, including HbA1c, fasting glucose, and fasting insulin levels.[25]

ENSURING NUTRIENT ADEQUACY

While many people assume that plant-based dietary patterns are deficient in protein, this is not usually the case. As you learned in Section 6.3, there are many good plant sources of protein. Although some plant proteins are considered lower-quality proteins, consuming a variety of plant proteins throughout the day can provide ample amounts of all nine essential amino acids to support growth and maintenance (review Fig. 6-8). As with any meal plan, variety is an especially important characteristic of a nutritious plant-based dietary pattern (Fig. 6-9). Table 6-2 outlines various types of vegetarian food plans, which emphasize grains, legumes, nuts, and seeds to help meet protein needs.

Aside from amino acids, low intakes of certain micronutrients and fatty acids can be a problem for those who avoid animal products, especially for those who adhere to a vegan dietary pattern. At the forefront of nutritional concerns are riboflavin, vitamin B-12, iron, zinc, iodine, calcium, and vitamin D. Although use of a balanced multivitamin and mineral supplement can help, the following dietary advice should be implemented.

TABLE 6-2 ■ Food Plan for Vegetarians Based on MyPlate

Food Group	MyPlate Servings Lactovegetarian*	Vegan†	Key Nutrients Supplied‡
Grains	6–11	8–11	Protein, thiamin, niacin, folate, vitamin E, zinc, magnesium, iron, and fiber
Beans and other legumes	2–3	3	Protein, vitamin B-6, zinc, magnesium, and fiber
Nuts, seeds	2–3	3	Protein, vitamin E, and magnesium
Vegetables	3–5 (include 1 dark-green or leafy variety daily)	4–6 (include 1 dark-green or leafy variety daily)	Vitamin A, vitamin C, folate, vitamin K, potassium, and magnesium
Fruits	2–4	4	Vitamin A, vitamin C, and folate
Dairy	3	—	Protein, riboflavin, vitamin D, vitamin B-12, and calcium
Fortified soy milk	—	3	

*This plan contains about 75 grams of protein in 1650 kcal.

†This plan contains about 79 grams of protein in 1800 kcal.

‡One serving of vitamin- and mineral-enriched ready-to-eat breakfast cereal is recommended to meet possible nutrient gaps. Alternatively, a balanced multivitamin and mineral supplement can be used. Vegans also may benefit from the use of fortified soy milk to provide calcium, vitamin D, and vitamin B-12.

B Vitamins. A few B vitamins may be more difficult to obtain from a strict vegetarian dietary pattern. In the typical American dietary pattern, dairy foods are a major source of riboflavin (vitamin B-2). For those who exclude dairy foods, riboflavin can be obtained from green leafy vegetables, whole grains, yeast, and legumes—components of most vegan plans.

Vitamin B-12 only occurs naturally in animal foods. Vegans can prevent a vitamin B-12 deficiency by finding a reliable source of this vitamin, such as fortified soy milk, ready-to-eat breakfast cereals fortified with vitamin B-12, and special nutritional yeast grown on media rich in vitamin B-12. Plants can contain soil or microbial contaminants that provide trace amounts of vitamin B-12, but these are negligible sources of the vitamin. Because the liver can store vitamin B-12 for about 4 years, it may take a long time for a vitamin B-12 deficiency to surface after removal of animal foods from the dietary pattern. If dietary vitamin B-12 inadequacy persists, deficiency can lead to anemia, nerve damage, and mental dysfunction. These deficiency consequences have been noted in the infants of vegetarian mothers whose breast milk was low in vitamin B-12.

Iron. Iron is a mineral that is found in both plant and animal food sources, but the form of iron in plant sources is not absorbed as efficiently as iron in animal sources. However, consuming plant sources of iron along with a good source of vitamin C can enhance iron absorption. For those who exclude animal products, whole grains and ready-to-eat breakfast cereals, dried fruits, nuts, and legumes are good sources of iron. Cooking in iron pots and skillets can also add iron to food.

Zinc. Zinc is another mineral that is more bioavailable from animal sources. Phytic acid and other substances in foods of plant origin can limit zinc absorption. Plant sources of zinc include whole grains (especially ready-to-eat breakfast cereals), nuts, and legumes. Breads are a good source of zinc because the leavening process (rising of the bread dough) reduces the influence of phytic acid.

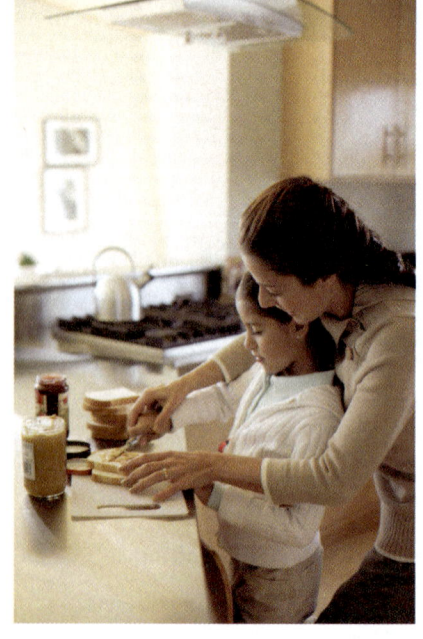

A plant-based dietary pattern is naturally low in energy density. Dietary planning for children should specifically incorporate energy-dense foods, such as plant oils, avocados, and nut butters, to make sure children have adequate energy to support growth and development. Digital Vision/Alamy Stock Photo

Iodine. During certain stages of the life cycle, iodine can be a nutrient of concern for those who follow a plant-based dietary pattern.[24] Iodine is required for synthesis of thyroid hormones, which regulate growth, development, and metabolic rate. Thus, infants, children, and women who are pregnant may be at risk for health problems related to iodine deficiency. Common sources of iodine in the typical American dietary pattern include iodized salt, seafood, and dairy products. Although sea vegetables (i.e., seaweed) supply iodine, the amount is highly variable. For those who follow a strict vegetarian dietary pattern, iodized salt is a reliable source of iodine. It should be used instead of plain salt. Check the label to find out if your salt is iodized.

Calcium and Vitamin D. Dietary requirements for calcium and vitamin D are difficult to meet for individuals who avoid dairy foods. Green leafy vegetables, legumes, and nuts do contain calcium, but the mineral is either not well absorbed or not very plentiful from these sources. As for vitamin D, this prohormone can be synthesized in the skin with regular sun exposure, but most people do not receive adequate sun exposure to meet the body's requirements during all times of the year. Furthermore, only a few varieties of mushrooms are natural plant sources of vitamin D. Thus, fortified foods including fortified soy milk, fortified orange juice, calcium-rich tofu, and certain ready-to-eat breakfast cereals and snacks are the vegan's best options for obtaining these nutrients. Dietary supplements are a viable option, but even a multivitamin and mineral supplement will not supply enough calcium to completely meet daily needs for bone health.

Omega-3 Fatty Acids. Consuming adequate quantities of omega-3 fatty acids is yet another nutritional concern for those who adhere to a vegetarian dietary pattern. Fish and fish oils, abundant sources of these heart-healthy fats, are omitted from many types of vegetarian plans. Alternative plant sources of omega-3 fatty acids include canola oil, soybean oil, seaweed, microalgae, flax seeds, chia seeds, and walnuts.

ASK THE RDN | Plant-Based Eating

Dear RDN: I am hearing more and more about the health benefits of a plant-based eating pattern. Can you give me some tips on replacing meat and dairy with high-quality plant proteins?

Regularly consuming foods high in plant proteins such as legumes (including tofu and other soybean products), whole grains, nuts, and seeds can help prevent and reverse a slew of chronic conditions, including cancers, diabetes, and heart disease. Plant foods are packed with fiber and phytochemicals that support immunity, combat inflammation, and promote healthy bacteria in our gut. As an added bonus, plant proteins are far more affordable, sustainable, and lower in terms of environmental impact than animal proteins.

The good news is that you don't have to swear off meat forever to reap these benefits. Research suggests that following a flexitarian diet (increasing plant-based foods and reducing, but not eliminating, animal foods) yields similar health benefits, like reduced risk of heart disease and diabetes. Eating less meat doesn't mean you're going to suffer from protein deficiency any time soon, either. It is important to note that protein is found in *almost all* foods, and it is nearly impossible not to get enough protein if you're eating enough calories.

In order to transition to a more plant-centric dietary pattern, start small. Overturning your entire eating pattern in a day can be a bit overwhelming initially. Instead of jumping to extremes, pick two small changes to implement each week. First, it may be swapping cow's milk with unsweetened almond or coconut milk. The great thing about nondairy beverages is that they're lower in calories, and some pack more calcium and vitamin D than dairy milk. Make your morning oatmeal with almond milk and stir in a tablespoon of peanut butter and chia seeds for a protein boost. Chia seeds are a hydrating powerhouse, made up of 20% protein and 25% fiber while absorbing up to 30 times their weight in water.

Did you know ¼ cup of pumpkin seeds has 7 grams of protein? Or that hemp seeds are the highest-protein seed, with 3 grams of protein per tablespoon? Peanuts boast the most protein in the nut category, with 7 grams per serving. For a tasty chocolate-banana shake, blend together 1 large frozen overripe banana, 1 tablespoon peanut butter, 1 tablespoon hemp seeds, 1 tablespoon cocoa powder, a handful of spinach, and 1 cup unsweetened vanilla almond milk. Breakfast is served!

For lunches, try power bowls made with a base of wild rice or quinoa, which yield 6 and 8 grams of protein per 1-cup serving, respectively. Top with ½ cup beans, chickpeas, or baked tempeh; a handful of arugula; avocado slices; a drizzle of tahini and lemon juice; and a sprinkle of hemp seeds for a calcium boost. If you're craving a sandwich, stuff a sprouted wheat wrap with ½ cup of black beans, a sprinkle of corn, salsa, avocado, crunchy romaine, and hot sauce.

Consider pasta night. Instead of refined white pasta, try one of the many bean- or lentil-based noodles on the market. You can find spaghetti, fusilli, and penne made from black beans, lentils, or chickpeas that all boast 13 grams of protein or more per 1-cup serving. Stick with 100% whole grain pasta, and you've still got 8 grams of protein and 25% of the Daily Value of fiber per 1-cup serving. On top of pasta, instead of parmesan, sprinkle nutritional yeast, a cheesy-tasting inactive yeast that's packed with protein and vitamin B-12. Drizzle a tablespoon of tahini and a tablespoon of hemp seeds on your green salad for another 6 grams of protein.

For stir-fry night, swap the chicken for high-protein edamame, which you can usually find in the freezer section of your grocery store. Soy not only is a complete plant protein, but it also has a high concentration of branched-chain amino acids, which are beneficial to athletic performance. Many stores sell marinated tofu (or try tempeh) that's delicious in stir-fry as well. For a tasty peanut sauce, whisk together ¼ cup natural peanut butter, ¼ cup almond milk, 4 teaspoons honey, and 4 teaspoons reduced-sodium soy sauce.

When you're craving chili, swap the meat for a couple cans of kidney beans. Adding sautéed mushrooms to the mix will up the umami factor and add meatiness. Boost spices like oregano and chili powder for extra flavor. High-plant-protein dinner is served!

When it comes to baking, experiment with nut- and seed-based flours. Peruse your favorite food blogs for chocolate chip cookies or banana bread made with almond flour or coconut flour for a protein boost. These versions are lower in carbohydrates and super moist thanks to the healthy fat content.

There's no doubt about it—plant proteins are trending *for good.* Do your health and wallet a favor and hop on the bandwagon!

Enjoy your plant proteins,

Alexis Joseph, MS, RD, LD

Dietitian, Nutrition Consultant, Founder of Hummusapien; Co-Owner of Alchemy Brands

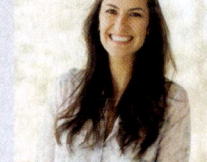
Raul Velasco

SPECIAL CONCERNS FOR INFANTS AND CHILDREN

Infants and children, notoriously picky eaters in the first place, are at the highest risk for nutrient deficiencies as a result of improperly planned vegetarian and vegan dietary patterns. However, with the use of complementary proteins and good sources of the nutrients just discussed, the calorie and nutrient needs of vegetarian and vegan infants and children can be met.[26] The most common nutritional concerns for vegetarian and vegan infants and children are deficiencies of iron, vitamin B-12, vitamin D, and calcium.

Vegetarian and vegan plans tend to be high in bulky, high-fiber, low-calorie foods that cause a feeling of fullness. While this is a welcome advantage for most adults, children have a small stomach capacity and relatively high nutrient needs and thus may feel full before their calorie needs are met. The fiber content of a child's dietary pattern may need to be decreased by replacing high-fiber sources with some refined grain products, fruit juices, and peeled fruit. Other concentrated sources of calories for children who are vegetarian and vegan include fortified soy milk, nuts, dried fruits, and avocados.

✓ CONCEPT CHECK 6.4

1. What are some of the major health benefits of following a vegetarian eating pattern?
2. Describe the major types of plant-based eating patterns.
3. What are some nutritional concerns of following a vegan eating pattern?

6.5 Protein Digestion and Absorption

The digestion of most proteins begins with the cooking of food. Cooking unfolds (denatures) proteins (Fig. 6-6) and softens tough connective tissue in meat. The cooking process makes many protein-rich foods easier to chew and swallow, and facilitates their breakdown during later digestion and absorption. Cooking also makes many protein-rich foods, such as meats, eggs, fish, and poultry, much safer to eat.

DIGESTION

The enzymatic digestion of protein begins in the stomach (Fig. 6-11). Thinking about food or chewing food stimulates the release of the hormone gastrin in the stomach. Gastrin then stimulates the stomach to produce acid and release pepsin. Proteins are first denatured by stomach acid. **Pepsin,** a major stomach enzyme for digesting proteins, then goes to work on the unraveled polypeptide chains. Pepsin can break only a few of the many peptide bonds found in these large polypeptide molecules, resulting in shorter chains of amino acids.

The partially digested proteins move from the stomach into the small intestine along with the rest of the nutrients and other substances in a meal (chyme). Once in the small intestine, the partially digested proteins (and any fats accompanying them) trigger the release of the hormone cholecystokinin (CCK) from the walls of the small intestine. CCK, in turn, travels through the bloodstream to the pancreas, where it causes the pancreas to release protein-splitting enzymes, such as **trypsin** and **chymotrypsin.** These digestive enzymes work in the small intestine to further divide the chains of amino acids into segments of two to three amino acids and some individual amino acids. Eventually, this mixture is digested into amino acids, using other enzymes from the lining of the small intestine and enzymes present in the absorptive cells themselves.

pepsin A protein-digesting enzyme produced by the stomach.

trypsin A protein-digesting enzyme secreted by the pancreas to act in the small intestine.

chymotrypsin A protein-digesting enzyme secreted by the pancreas to act in the small intestine.

ABSORPTION

The short chains of amino acids and any individual amino acids in the small intestine are taken up by active transport into the absorptive cells lining the small intestine. Any remaining peptide bonds are broken inside intestinal cells to yield individual amino acids. Because amino acids are water soluble, they travel to the liver via the hepatic portal vein, which transports absorbed nutrients from the intestinal tract directly to the liver (Fig. 6-11). In the liver, individual amino acids can undergo several modifications, depending on the needs of various body tissues. Individual amino acids may be (1) combined to form the proteins needed by specific cells, (2) broken down to meet energy needs, (3) released into the bloodstream, or (4) converted into nonessential amino acids, glucose, or fat. With excess protein intake, amino acids are converted into fat as a last resort.

magnificent microbiome

Protein Feeds Microbes
Different sources of protein can impact the gut microbiota in both positive and negative ways. The high BCAA content of dairy proteins has a positive effect on gut microbiota and the prevention of obesity. Protein sources such as red meats and eggs, however, contain compounds that the gut microbiota may convert into trimethylamine and trimethylamine oxide (TMAO), which have been associated with increased risks for atherosclerosis and obesity.

Source: Madsen L, Myrmel LS, Fjære E, Liaset B, Kristiansen K. Links between dietary protein sources, the gut microbiota, and obesity. *Front Physiol.* 2017 Dec 19;8:1047. doi: 10.3389/fphys.2017.01047

Protein Digestion and Absorption

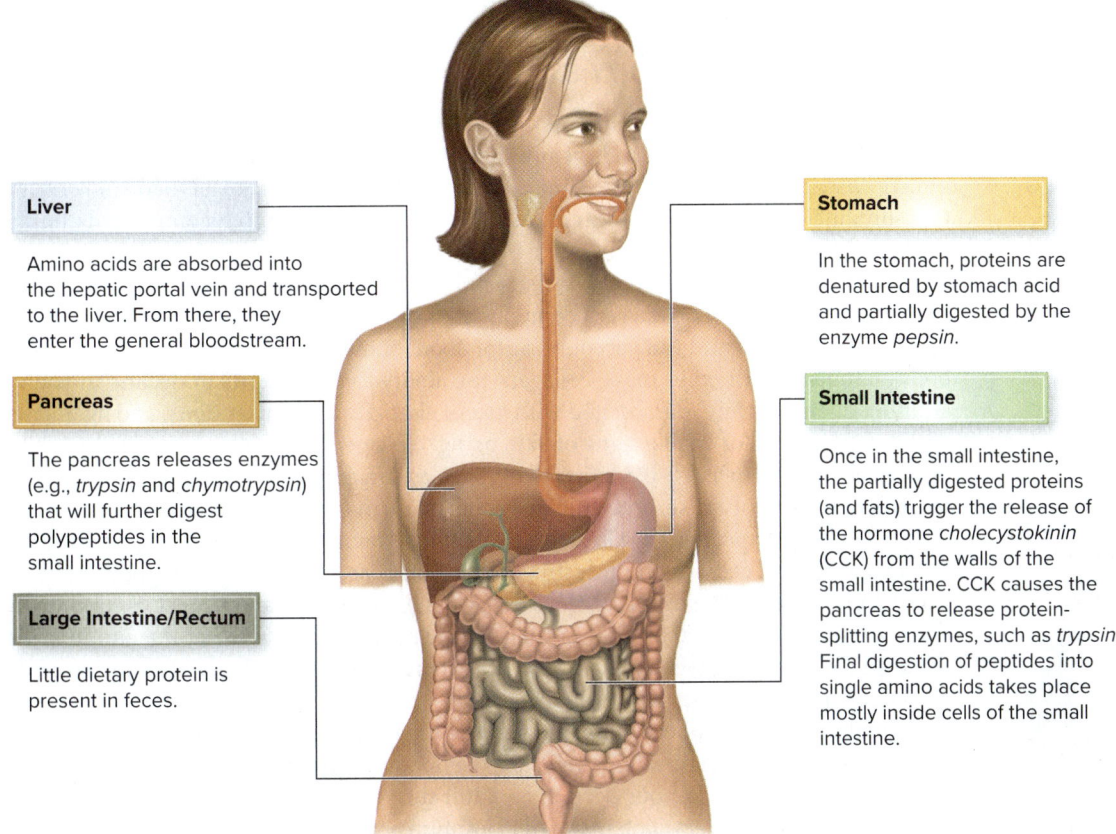

Liver

Amino acids are absorbed into the hepatic portal vein and transported to the liver. From there, they enter the general bloodstream.

Pancreas

The pancreas releases enzymes (e.g., *trypsin* and *chymotrypsin*) that will further digest polypeptides in the small intestine.

Large Intestine/Rectum

Little dietary protein is present in feces.

Stomach

In the stomach, proteins are denatured by stomach acid and partially digested by the enzyme *pepsin*.

Small Intestine

Once in the small intestine, the partially digested proteins (and fats) trigger the release of the hormone *cholecystokinin* (CCK) from the walls of the small intestine. CCK causes the pancreas to release protein-splitting enzymes, such as *trypsin*. Final digestion of peptides into single amino acids takes place mostly inside cells of the small intestine.

FIGURE 6-11 A summary of protein digestion and absorption. Enzymatic protein digestion begins in the stomach and ends in the absorptive cells of the small intestine, where any remaining short groupings of amino acids are broken down into single amino acids. Stomach acid and enzymes contribute to protein digestion. Absorption from the intestinal lumen into the absorptive cells requires energy input.

Throughout most of the life span, it is uncommon for intact proteins to be absorbed from the digestive tract. However, in infants up to 4 to 5 months of age, the gastrointestinal tract is somewhat permeable to small proteins, so some whole proteins can be absorbed. Because proteins from some foods (e.g., cow's milk and egg whites) may predispose an infant to food allergies, experts recommend waiting until an infant reaches 4 to 6 months of age to introduce solid foods.[27]

✓ CONCEPT CHECK 6.5

1. Where and how does the chemical digestion of protein begin?
2. What digestion steps take place in the stomach and small intestine?
3. What are the final products of protein digestion, and where do they go after absorption?

6.6 Putting Proteins to Work in the Body

Proteins perform various roles in human metabolism and in the formation of body structures. Dietary sources of protein can supply sufficient amino acids to meet our physiological requirements, but to ensure that amino acids are used efficiently, we must also consume adequate amounts of carbohydrates and fat. If there are not enough carbohydrates and fat to meet the body's energy demands, amino acids will be broken down to supply energy to cells. This renders the amino acids unavailable for growth and repair of body tissues.

PRODUCING VITAL BODY STRUCTURES

Every cell contains protein. Muscles, connective tissue, mucus, blood-clotting factors, transport proteins in the bloodstream, lipoproteins, enzymes, antibodies, some hormones, visual pigments, and the support structure inside bones are all made of protein. Consuming excess protein does not enhance the synthesis of these body components, but eating too little protein can prevent it.

Collagen is one example of a structural protein that has gotten lots of attention in recent years. Collagen is a component of connective tissues, such as bones, cartilage, tendons, and skin, accounting for about one-third of the protein in the human body. Although our bodies make collagen, the ability to do so starts to decline in young adulthood. This decline is associated with loss of elasticity in skin, tendons, and ligaments and is responsible for visible signs of skin aging. Collagen production can also be inhibited by factors that increase **oxidative stress** such as sun exposure, smoking, environmental pollution, alcohol abuse, and a dietary pattern low in fruits and vegetables.

Most vital body proteins are in a constant state of breakdown, rebuilding, and repair. For example, the cells of the intestinal tract lining are constantly sloughed off (i.e., shed) and replaced. The digestive tract treats sloughed intestinal cells just like food particles, digesting them and absorbing their amino acids. In fact, most of the amino acids released throughout the body can be recycled to become part of the pool of amino acids available for the synthesis of future proteins.

Overall, **protein turnover** is a process by which a cell can respond to its changing environment by making proteins that are needed and disassembling proteins that are not needed. During a 24-hour period, an adult turns over (makes and degrades) about 250 grams of protein, recycling many of the amino acids. When you compare this to the 70 to 100 grams of protein per day typically consumed by American adults, you can see that recycled amino acids make an important contribution to total protein metabolism. If a person's dietary pattern is low in protein for a long period, the processes of rebuilding and repairing body proteins will slow down. Over time, skeletal muscles, blood proteins, and vital organs such as the heart and liver will lose protein and decrease in size or volume. Only the brain resists protein breakdown.

REGULATORY FUNCTIONS

Maintaining Fluid Balance. Blood proteins help maintain body fluid balance. Recall from Section 3.3 that blood flows from the heart to the rest of the body via arteries, which branch into smaller vessels called capillaries. The walls of the capillaries are very thin. With every heartbeat, the pressure of blood rushing through blood vessels forces some fluid out of the capillaries into the spaces between nearby cells **(extracellular spaces)**. This is normal and necessary to allow for the exchange of oxygen, nutrients, and wastes with the surrounding tissues (Fig. 6-12). Proteins in the bloodstream are too large, however, to move out of the capillaries into the tissues. In fact, the presence of these proteins within the capillaries attracts the proper amount of fluid back to the bloodstream, partially counteracting the force of blood pressure. (The lymphatic system also helps maintain fluid balance by collecting excess fluid and returning it to the bloodstream.)

When protein intake is too low, the concentration of proteins in the bloodstream drops below normal. Excessive fluid then builds up in the surrounding tissues because the osmotic pressure from the smaller amount of blood proteins is too weak to pull enough of the fluid back from the tissues into the bloodstream. As fluids accumulate in the tissues, the tissues swell, causing **edema**. Because edema can also be a symptom of other medical problems, an important step in diagnosing its cause is to measure the concentration of blood proteins.

---

oxidative stress Imbalance between the production of reactive compounds and the body's ability to protect against their adverse effects.

protein turnover The process by which cells break down old proteins and resynthesize new proteins. In this way, the cell will have the proteins it needs to function at that time.

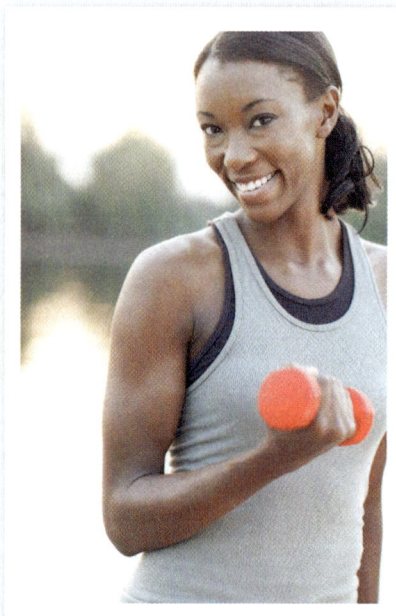

Protein contributes to the structure and function of muscle. **Will eating protein in excess of requirements help this athlete build muscle mass?**
Laura Doss/Fancy Collection/SuperStock

extracellular space The space outside cells; represents one-third of body fluid.

edema The buildup of excess fluid in extracellular spaces.

(a) Normal blood protein levels

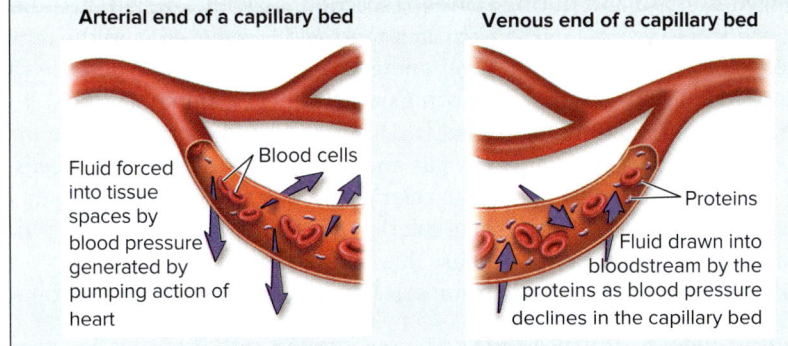
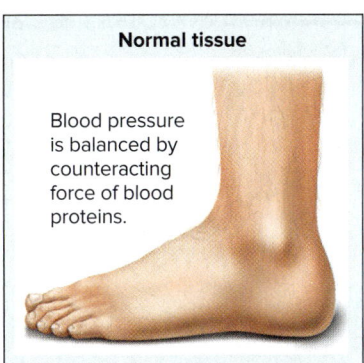

(b) Low blood protein levels

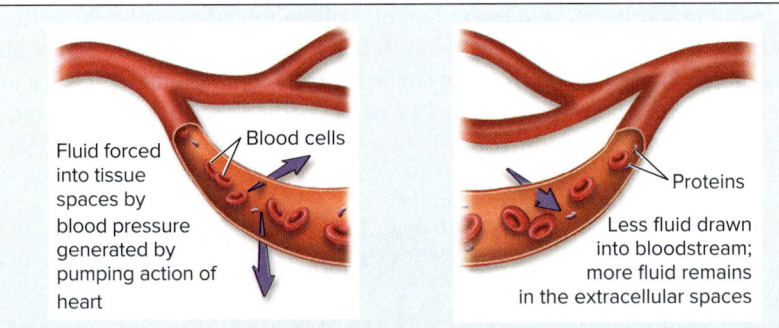
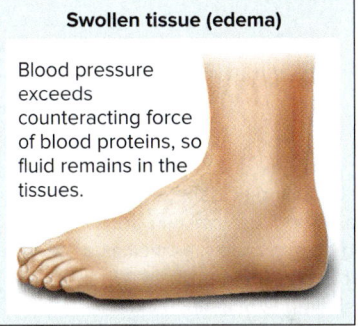

FIGURE 6-12 Proteins help to maintain fluid balance. (a) As blood is pumped through the cardiovascular system, some fluid leaks out of the vessels. When blood protein levels are normal, proteins in the blood draw water back into the blood vessels. (b) When blood protein levels are low, fluid remains in the tissues and edema develops.

Contributing to Acid–Base Balance. Proteins located in cell membranes help to regulate acid–base balance in the blood by pumping chemical ions in and out of cells. This pumping of ions, among other factors, occurs in an effort to keep the blood slightly alkaline. In addition, some amino acids are especially good **buffers** in the bloodstream. Buffers are compounds that maintain acid–base conditions within a narrow range.

Forming Hormones and Enzymes. Many hormones, our internal body messengers, are proteins and therefore require amino acids for synthesis. The thyroid hormones are made from two molecules of only one type of amino acid: tyrosine. Insulin, on the other hand, is a hormone composed of 51 amino acids. Almost all enzymes are proteins or have a protein component.

Contributing to Immune Function. Without sufficient dietary protein, the immune system lacks the materials needed to function properly. The body's first layer of immune defense is the healthy, intact epithelial tissue that forms the skin and the gastrointestinal tract. These barriers keep pathogens out of the body. Because the cells of the epithelial tissues are exposed to lots of stressors from the external environment, they are rapidly turned over. Maintenance of healthy epithelial tissue requires plenty of protein.

If pathogens make it past the body's barrier defenses and enter the blood, the cells of the immune system mount an immune response. An immune response involves the release of chemical messengers that trigger inflammation and recruit white blood cells to the site of infection or injury. Some immune cells synthesize antibodies, which are like protein tags that mark a pathogen for destruction. Other immune cells can destroy pathogens. Proteins serve as the building blocks to produce and maintain the immune cells, make antibodies, and synthesize those chemical messengers.

SOURCE OF ENERGY

Providing Energy. Typically, proteins are not a major source of energy. However, two situations in which a person does use protein to meet energy needs are during

> Some neurotransmitters are derivatives of amino acids. For example, dopamine and norepinephrine are both synthesized from the amino acid tyrosine, and serotonin is synthesized from the amino acid tryptophan.

buffer Compounds that cause a solution to resist changes in acid–base conditions.

prolonged exercise and during calorie restriction, as with a weight-loss diet. In these cases, the amino group ($-NH_2$) from an amino acid is removed, and the remaining carbon skeleton is metabolized to meet energy needs (Fig. 6-13). When the carbon skeletons of amino acids are broken down to supply energy, ammonia (NH_3) is a resulting waste product. The ammonia is converted into urea and excreted in the urine. Under most conditions, cells primarily use fats and carbohydrates for energy needs. Although proteins contain the same amount of calories (on average, 4 kcal per gram) as carbohydrates, proteins are a costly source of calories, considering the amount of processing the liver and kidneys must perform to use this calorie source.

The functions of proteins are summarized in Figure 6-14, the Protein Concept Map.

Forming Glucose. If you do not consume enough carbohydrates to supply glucose, your liver (and kidneys, to a lesser extent) will be forced to make glucose from amino acids present in body tissues (Fig. 6-13). A fairly constant concentration of glucose must be maintained in the blood to supply energy for the brain, red blood cells, and nervous tissue. At rest, the brain uses about 19% of the body's energy requirements, and it gets most of that energy from glucose.[28]

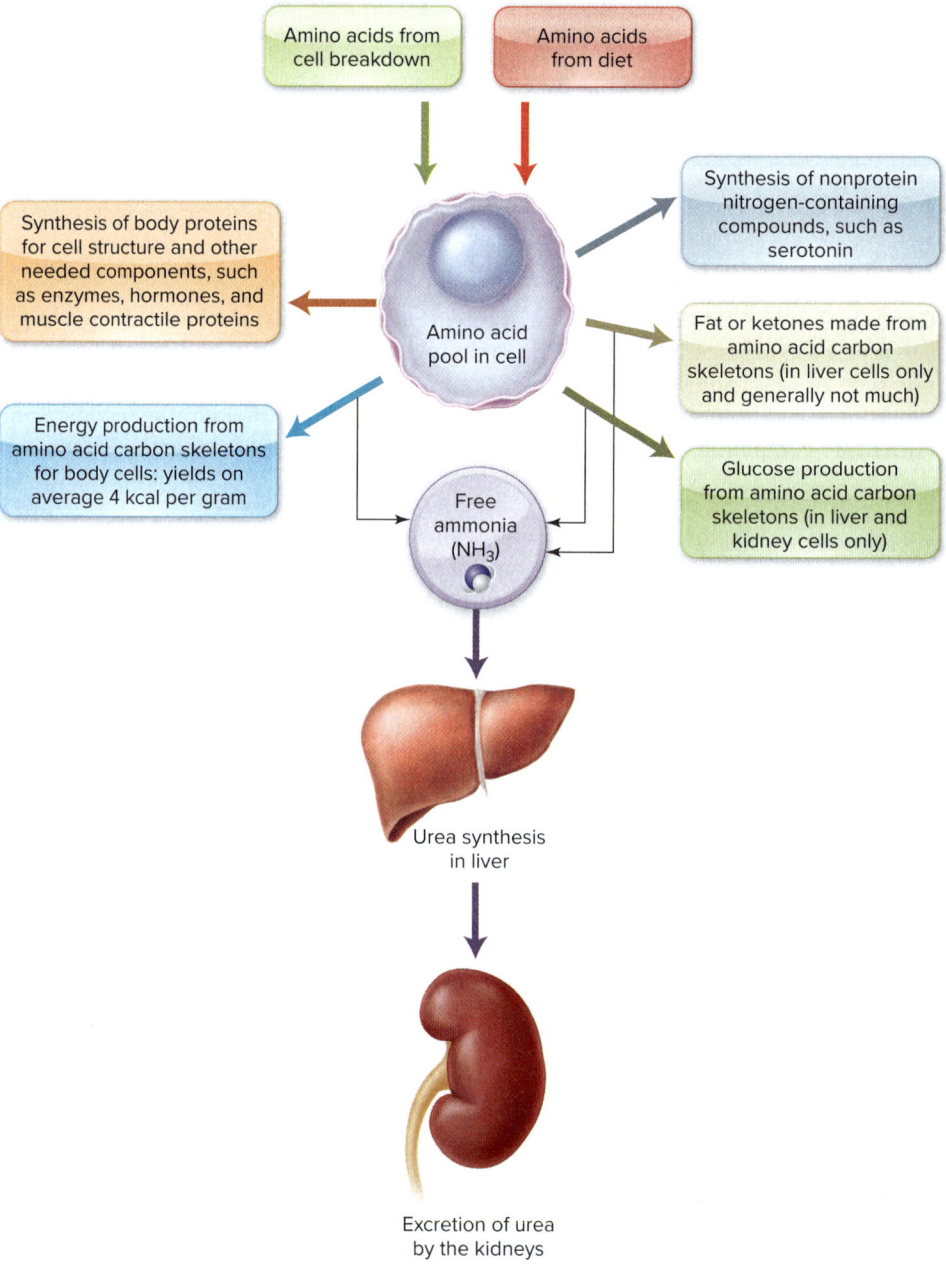

FIGURE 6-13 Amino acid metabolism. The amino acid pool in a cell can be used to form body proteins, as well as a variety of other possible products. When the carbon skeletons of amino acids are metabolized to produce glucose or fat, ammonia (NH_3) is a resulting waste product. The ammonia is converted into urea and excreted in the urine.

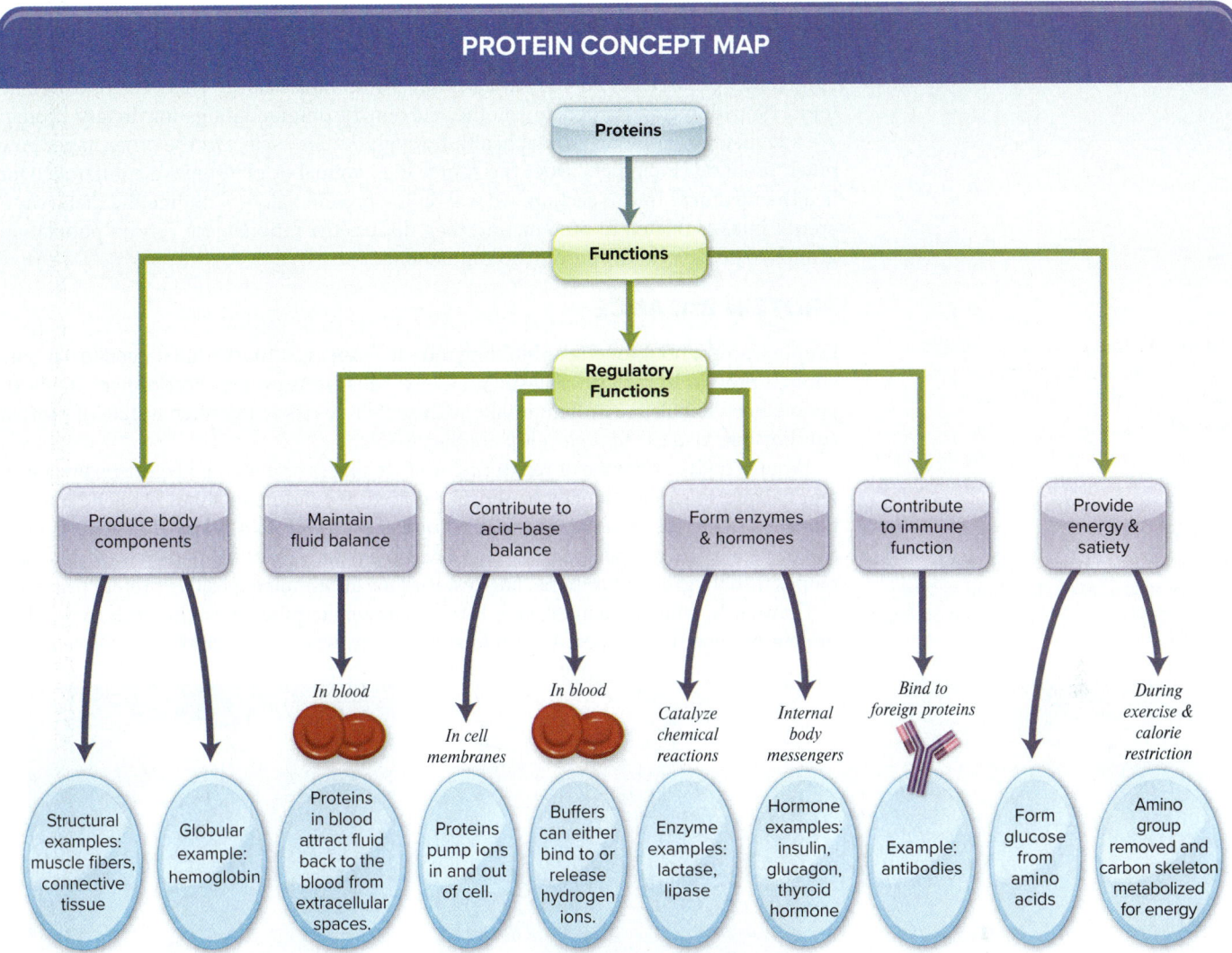

FIGURE 6-14 Protein Concept Map illustrating the functions of protein throughout the body.

Making some glucose from amino acids is normal. For example, when you skip breakfast and have not eaten since early the previous evening, glucose must be manufactured. In extreme situations, however, such as starvation, the use of amino acids to synthesize glucose and yield energy will lead to the breakdown of skeletal muscles and organs.

Contributing to Satiety. Of all the macronutrients, protein appears to have the greatest impact on feelings of satiety.[29] Indeed, many popular weight management programs recommend an increased amount of protein to enhance feelings of fullness to facilitate reduced calorie intake. Several effective weight-loss programs include a percentage of calories from protein at the upper end of the Acceptable Macronutrient Distribution Range of 10% to 35% for protein. In general, these diets are appropriate if otherwise nutritionally sound, especially if they include a variety of foods from each food group.

> The vitamin niacin can be made from the amino acid tryptophan, illustrating another role of proteins.

✓ CONCEPT CHECK 6.6

1. Name three body structures that are made of protein.
2. Define *protein turnover*. How many grams of protein does the body typically turn over each day?
3. What is *edema*? Explain why low blood protein levels can lead to edema.
4. If amino acids can be broken down to yield energy for cells, why do we need to convert some amino acids into glucose?

6.7 Protein Needs

How much protein should you eat each day for optimal health? This is a controversial topic. Nutrition experts debate whether current recommendations for dietary protein are adequate to promote optimal health through the life cycle. On the other hand, how much protein is too much? Does the source (i.e., animal or plant) make a difference for health outcomes? In this section, we will define protein balance, outline the dietary reference intakes related to protein, and then discuss the rationale for certain population groups to go beyond the current recommendations.

PROTEIN BALANCE

People who are not growing or building muscle tissue (i.e., most adults) need to eat only enough protein to match whatever they lose daily from protein breakdown. In short, people need to balance protein intake with protein losses to maintain a state of **protein equilibrium,** also called *protein balance* (Fig. 6-15).

When a body is growing or recovering from an illness or injury, it needs a **positive protein balance** to supply the raw materials required to build new tissues. Athletic training that aims to increase muscle mass also requires positive protein balance. To achieve positive protein balance, a person must eat more protein daily than that person loses. The hormones insulin, growth hormone, and testosterone all stimulate positive protein balance.

Conversely, when protein intake is less than protein requirements, this leads to **negative protein balance.** This can occur with food insecurity, when a person does not have access

protein equilibrium A state in which protein intake is equal to related protein losses; the person is said to be in *protein balance.*

positive protein balance A state in which protein intake exceeds related protein losses, as is needed during times of growth.

negative protein balance A state in which protein intake is less than related protein losses, such as often seen during acute illness.

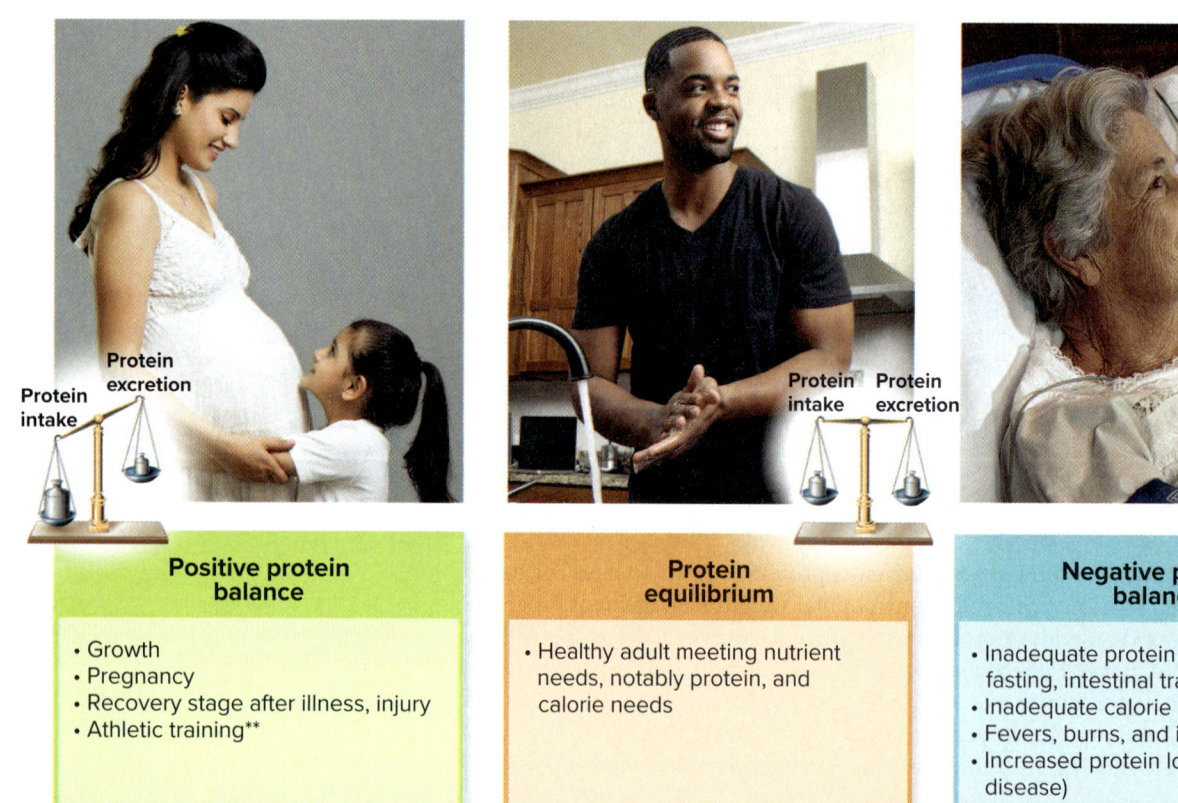

*Based on losses of urea and other nitrogen-containing compounds in the urine, as well as protein lost from feces, skin, hair, nails, and other minor routes.
**Only when additional lean body mass is being gained. Nevertheless, the athlete is probably already eating enough protein to support this extra protein synthesis; protein supplements are not needed.

FIGURE 6-15 Protein balance in practical terms: (a) positive protein balance, (b) protein equilibrium, and (c) negative protein balance.
(left): Sudipta Halder/IndiaPicture/Getty Images; (middle) Nina Shannon/Getty Images; (right): Dynamic Graphics Group/Getty Images

to enough food. Acute illness may reduce the appetite, such that a person fails to consume enough protein to compensate for daily protein losses. Some mental health conditions, such as eating disorders, may also lead to inadequate intakes of protein and other nutrients.

ACCEPTABLE MACRONUTRIENT DISTRIBUTION RANGE FOR PROTEIN

The Food and Nutrition Board of the National Academies of Sciences, Engineering, and Medicine has set an Acceptable Macronutrient Distribution Range (AMDR) for protein. This is a range of protein intake (given as a proportion of total calories) that is sufficient to meet nutrient requirements and is associated with low risk for chronic diseases. The AMDR for protein for adults is 10% to 35% of total calories.[30] This wide range of protein intake ensures protein adequacy, but also allows for flexibility in dietary planning. The example below shows how to calculate the AMDR for protein for a healthy adult who consumes 2000 kilocalories per day.

Calculating the AMDR for Protein for a Healthy Adult

The AMDR for protein for adults is 10% to 35% of total calories.

First, calculate the minimum end of the range. What is 10% of 2000 kcal?

2000 kcal × 0.10 = 200 kcal from protein

How many grams of protein would provide 200 kcal? Protein yields approximately 4 kcal/gram, so divide kcal from protein by 4 kcal/gram:

200 kcal from protein ÷ 4 kcal/gram = 50 grams of protein

Next, calculate the maximum end of the range. What is 35% of 2000 kcal?

2000 kcal × 0.35 = 700 kcal from protein

How many grams of protein would provide 700 kcal?

700 kcal from protein ÷ 4 kcal/gram = 175 grams of protein

The AMDR for protein for an adult who consumes 2000 kcal is 50 to 175 grams of protein per day.

RECOMMENDED DIETARY ALLOWANCE FOR PROTEIN

The Food and Nutrition Board also sets the Recommended Dietary Allowance (RDA) for protein. The RDA for the amount of protein required for nearly all adults to maintain protein equilibrium is 0.8 gram of protein per kilogram of healthy body weight.[30] Requirements are higher during periods of growth, such as infancy, childhood, and pregnancy. Healthy weight (see Section 7.3) is used in the calculation of protein needs because excess body fat does not contribute significantly to protein needs. The calculations below demonstrate how to calculate the protein RDA for a healthy female who weighs 125 pounds (57 kilograms).

Calculating the Protein RDA for a Healthy Adult Female

The units given for the RDA are grams per kilogram. If weight is measured in pounds, start by converting weight from pounds to kilograms:

$$\frac{125 \text{ pounds}}{2.2 \text{ pounds/kilogram}} = 57 \text{ kilograms}$$

Multiply weight in kilograms by 0.8 gram per kilogram to calculate protein RDA:

$$57 \text{ kilograms} \times \frac{0.8 \text{ gram of protein}}{\text{kilogram body weight}} = 46 \text{ grams of protein}$$

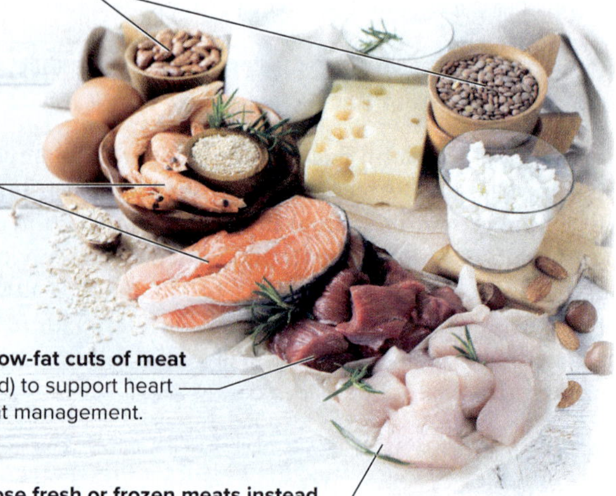

FIGURE 6-16 Protein-specific recommendations from the *Dietary Guidelines.* Antonina Vlasova/123RF

Select beans, peas, and lentils more often. These foods provide protein along with fiber, potassium, and magnesium.

Include seafood twice per week. These foods provide protein along with omega-3 fatty acids to support heart health and brain health.

Choose lean or low-fat cuts of meat (e.g., loin or round) to support heart health and weight management.

Choose fresh or frozen meats instead of highly processed meats to limit sodium intake. If you do consume some processed meats, **choose lower-sodium options.**

The RDA for protein equates to about 10% of total calories—the lower end of the AMDR. When it comes to making healthy protein choices, the *Dietary Guidelines* encourages the consumption of a variety of nutrient-dense protein foods from several subgroups including meats, poultry, and eggs; seafood; and nuts, seeds, and soy products (Fig 6-16).

Many Americans consume more protein than the RDA because they enjoy a variety of high-protein foods and can afford to buy them. Moderately exceeding the RDA for protein is fine for healthy individuals (i.e., with normal liver and kidney function). However, do not be fooled into believing that simply consuming extra protein will result in increased muscle mass. Our bodies do not store excess protein as muscle tissue. Gains in lean mass require the stimulus of resistance training. Without this stimulus, excess amino acids that are not used for protein synthesis will be stripped of their nitrogen-containing amino group and metabolized for fuel or stored as fat (Fig. 6-13).

Most nutrition experts agree that the RDA for protein should be viewed as a *minimum* to prevent the breakdown of lean tissues. For many individuals, an *optimal* protein intake is probably higher than the RDA.[4] For example, sports nutrition research shows that protein intakes within the range of 1.2 to 2.0 grams per kilogram of body weight are needed to support the increased use of amino acids for fuel and muscle protein synthesis among athletes (see Section 10.4). Also, a protein intake of more than 1.0 gram per kilogram of body weight per day has been recommended for older adults to prevent age-related declines in bone and muscle mass (see Section 16.2).[31] Still, protein supplements are rarely necessary. Many Americans already consume more than the RDA for protein. Table 6-3 illustrates how easy it is to plan a realistic dietary pattern with adequate protein.

Protein Requirements per Meal. Many adults have an unbalanced meal distribution of protein with more than 60% of daily protein consumed during a single evening meal and less than 15 grams at breakfast. Recent research, however, shows that distributing protein more evenly throughout the day is optimal for body functions.[32] Many protein functions, such as maintaining body composition and regulating

TABLE 6-3 ■ Protein Content of Sample Menus Containing 1600 and 2000 kcal

Menu	1600 kcal Serving Size	1600 kcal Protein (g)	2000 kcal Serving Size	2000 kcal Protein (g)
Breakfast				
Low-fat granola	⅔ cup	6	⅔ cup	6
Blueberries	1 cup	1	1 cup	1
Greek yogurt, low-fat	8 ounces	23	8 ounces	23
Coffee	1 cup	0	1 cup	0
Lunch				
Broiled chicken breast	3 ounces	26	4 ounces	35
Salad greens	3 cups	2	3 cups	2
Croutons	½ cup	2	½ cup	2
Low-fat salad dressing	2 tbsp	0	2 tbsp	0
Snack				
Apple			1 medium	1
Peanut butter			2 tbsp	7
Dinner				
Fat-free (skim) milk	1 cup	8	1 cup	8
Rice	1 cup	5	1.25 cups	6
Shrimp	4 large	5	4 large	5
Red kidney beans	½ cup	8	¾ cup	12
Sweet red pepper	½ cup	1	½ cup	1
Snack				
Woven wheat crackers	6 crackers	3	6 crackers	3
Cheddar cheese	1 ounce	7	1 ounce	7
Banana	1 medium	1	1 medium	1
Total		98		120

breakfast: Floortje/E+/Getty Images; lunch: Olga Nayashkova/Shutterstock; snack: William Berry/123RF; dinner: John A. Rizzo /Pixtal/age fotostock; snack: CWLawrence/E+/Getty Images

glucose, are sensitive to the concentration of amino acids in blood and cells after meals. Certain amino acids (e.g., leucine) function as a signal to stimulate the synthesis of skeletal muscle.

Studies have found that consuming at least 20 to 30 grams of protein at a given meal has positive effects on muscle protein synthesis, compared with spreading the same total amount of protein across multiple small meals. Researchers now recommend that adults consume at least 30 grams of protein at more than one meal in order to maintain healthy muscles and bones. Protein at breakfast is especially critical to regulate appetite and daily food intake and to replenish body proteins after an overnight fast.

CASE STUDY: Planning a Vegetarian Dietary Pattern

Jordan is a freshman in college. He lives in a campus residence hall and teaches martial arts in the afternoon. He eats two or three meals a day at the residence hall cafeteria and snacks between meals. Jordan and his roommate both decided to become vegetarians because they recently read an article on a fitness website describing the health benefits of a vegetarian dietary pattern. Yesterday, Jordan's vegetarian plan consisted of a Danish pastry for breakfast and a tomato-rice dish (no meat) with pretzels and a diet soft drink for lunch. In the afternoon, after his martial arts class, he had a milkshake and two cookies. At dinnertime, he had a vegetarian sub sandwich consisting of lettuce, sprouts, tomatoes, cucumbers, and cheese, with two glasses of fruit punch. In the evening, he had a bowl of popcorn.

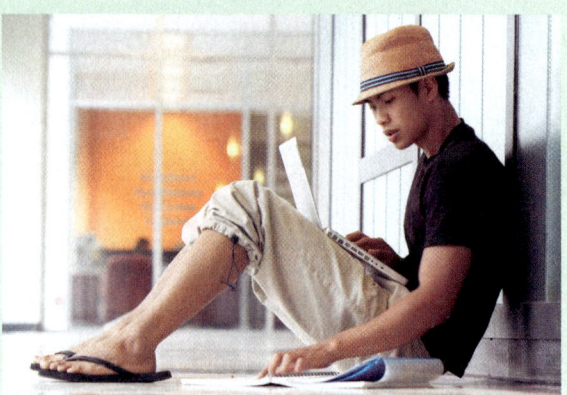

Has Jordan planned a healthy and nutritious vegetarian dietary pattern? Purestock/SuperStock

1. What type of plant-based eating pattern is Jordan following?
2. What health benefits can Jordan expect from following a well-planned vegetarian dietary pattern?
3. Evaluate Jordan's current dietary plan. Are there any food groups he seems to be over- or underconsuming?
4. Based on what you have learned so far in this course, which macronutrient(s) is(are) missing in Jordan's current dietary plan?
5. Are there any food components in the current eating pattern that should be minimized or avoided?
6. How could Jordan improve his new dietary pattern at each meal and snack to meet his nutritional needs and avoid undesirable food components?
7. Would you consider adopting a vegetarian dietary pattern? If so, which type of plant-based dietary pattern would you choose? What would be some potential barriers to shifting your dietary pattern? List some possible health benefits of shifting your dietary pattern.

Complete the Case Study. Responses to these questions can be provided by your instructor.

✓ CONCEPT CHECK 6.7

1. During what situations is the body in positive protein balance?
2. What is the RDA for protein for a person weighing 70 kilograms?
3. What is your favorite way to get 20 to 30 grams of protein at breakfast?

6.8 Special Health Concerns Related to Protein Intake

PROTEIN-CALORIE MALNUTRITION

Protein deficiency is rarely an isolated condition; it is usually accompanied by a deficiency of calories and other nutrients resulting from insufficient food intake. This form of undernutrition is called **protein-calorie malnutrition (PCM)**. In developing areas of the world, where famine or civil unrest lead to widespread disruptions in the food supply, PCM stunts the growth of children and makes them more susceptible to infectious diseases throughout life. In developed nations, extreme poverty can lead to PCM, but it more commonly arises secondary to other diseases, such as alcohol use disorders, eating disorders, or conditions that impair nutrient intake or absorption. PCM is a significant problem among hospitalized patients of all ages and can negatively impact recovery from illness or injury.[33]

protein-calorie malnutrition (PCM) A condition resulting from regularly consuming insufficient amounts of calories and protein. The deficiency eventually results in body wasting, primarily of lean tissue, and an increased susceptibility to infections. Also known as *protein-energy malnutrition (PEM)*.

The consequences of PCM are severe, especially among infants and children. Physical growth is stunted and cognitive development may be impaired. The immune system cannot function normally. For example, a condition such as measles, a disease that normally makes a well-nourished child ill for only a week or so, can become severely debilitating and even fatal when combined with PCM.

Let's examine two severe forms of PCM: **kwashiorkor** and **marasmus.** Both conditions are seen primarily in children but also may develop in adults. These two conditions form the tip of the iceberg with respect to states of undernutrition. Symptoms of both conditions may be present in the same person.

Kwashiorkor. *Kwashiorkor* is a word from Ghana that means "the disease that the first child gets when the new child comes." Infants in developing areas of the world are usually breastfed from birth. Human breast milk is well suited to support infant growth and development. However, by the time the child reaches 1 to 1.5 years of age, the mother is pregnant or has already given birth again, and the newborn infant gets preference for breastfeeding. The older child's diet then abruptly changes from nutritious human milk to starchy roots and **gruels,** which provide marginally adequate calories but are low in protein. Bulky plant fibers fill the child's stomach before nutrient and energy needs are fully met. Infections (e.g., diarrheal disease from unsafe water) may simultaneously increase the demand for nutrients and impair nutrient absorption. These conditions make it challenging to meet calorie, protein, and micronutrient requirements.

The major symptoms of kwashiorkor are apathy, diarrhea, listlessness, failure to grow and gain weight, and withdrawal from the environment. Advanced symptoms include changes in hair color, potassium deficiency, flaky skin, fatty liver, reduced muscle mass, and massive edema in the abdomen and legs. The presence of edema in a child who has some subcutaneous fat (i.e., fat directly under the skin) is the hallmark of kwashiorkor (Fig. 6-17).

How do these symptoms of kwashiorkor relate to what you know about the roles of protein in the body? Proteins play important roles in fluid balance, lipoprotein transport, immune function, and production of tissues such as skin, cells lining the GI tract, and hair.

Marasmus. The word *marasmus* means "to waste away" in Greek. Marasmus results from a severe deficit of both protein and energy. Victims have a "skin-and-bones" appearance, with little or no subcutaneous fat (Fig. 6-17). Marasmus in infants

kwashiorkor A form of protein-calorie malnutrition occurring primarily in young children who have an existing disease and consume a marginal amount of calories and insufficient protein in relation to needs. The child generally suffers from infections and exhibits edema, poor growth, weakness, and an increased susceptibility to further illness.

marasmus A form of protein-calorie malnutrition resulting from consuming a grossly insufficient amount of protein and calories. Victims have little or no fat stores, little muscle mass, and poor strength. Death from infections is common.

gruel A thin mixture of grains or legumes in milk or water.

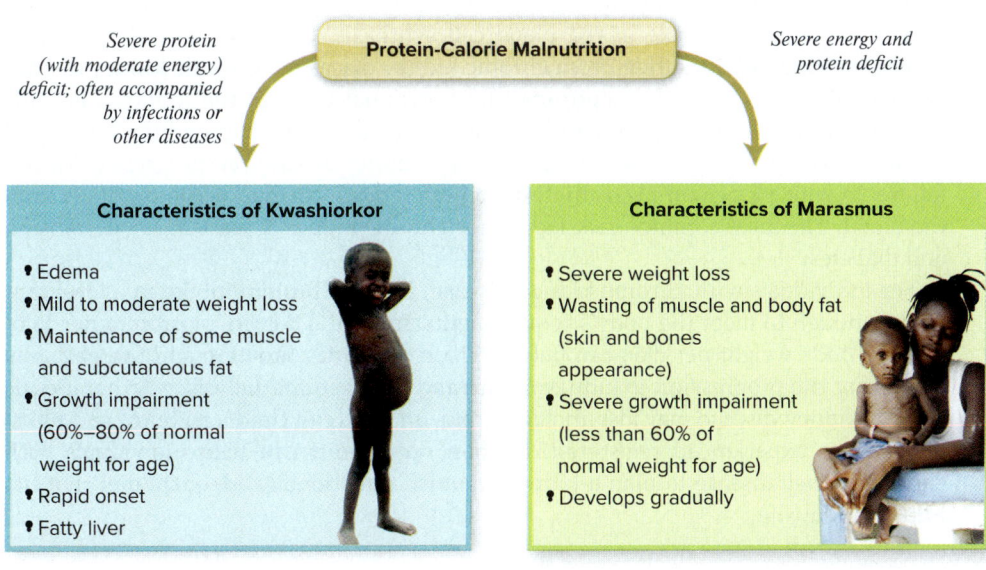

FIGURE 6-17 Classification of protein-calorie malnutrition occurring primarily in children (kwashiorkor and marasmus). (left): Christine Osborne Pictures/Alamy Stock Photo; (right): Phanie/Alamy Stock Photo

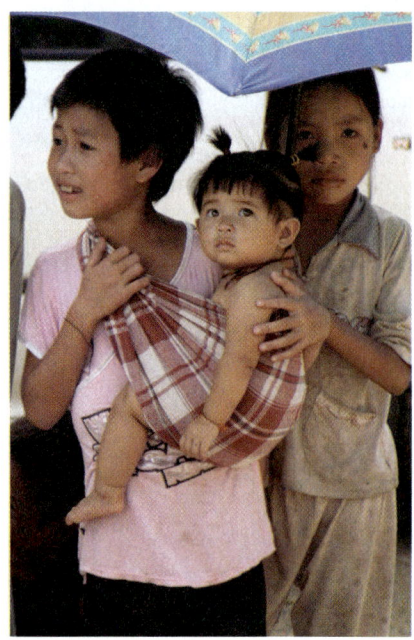

Aims of the United Nations Sustainable Development Goals include drastically decreasing global poverty and hunger, including protein-calorie malnutrition, by 2030. Lissa Harrison

food allergy An adverse reaction to food that involves an immune response; also called *food hypersensitivity*.

chronic kidney disease A condition characterized by the gradual loss of kidney function over time, which can lead to the buildup of waste products in the blood.

nephrons The functional units of kidney cells that filter wastes from the bloodstream and deposit them into the urine.

dialysis A medical procedure that removes excess fluid and wastes from the blood when the kidneys are not functioning properly.

commonly occurs in the large cities of poverty-stricken countries. In these settings, bottle-feeding (rather than breastfeeding) is often necessary because mothers must go off to work and leave the infant with a caregiver. Although infant formula certainly can be a nutritious alternative to human milk, it must be prepared properly: powdered or concentrated liquid formula must be mixed with an appropriate amount of clean water. When families lack education, economic resources, and sanitation, infant formula may be prepared with unsafe water (leading to diarrheal disease) or diluted with too much water (leading to undernutrition). Marasmus results in growth restriction, impaired cognitive development, increased susceptibility to disease, and high rates of infant mortality.

If children with PCM are helped in time—if infections are treated and appropriate calories and nutrients are supplied—then the disease process reverses. They begin to grow again and may even show no signs of their previous condition, except perhaps shortness of stature. Unfortunately, by the time many of these children reach a hospital or care center, they already have severe infections. Despite the best care, they may become ill again or die.

FOOD ALLERGIES

A healthy immune system recognizes and mounts an immune response to foreign proteins. Allergies occur when the immune system mistakenly reacts to a harmless protein. In the case of **food allergies,** specific food proteins trigger an inappropriate immune response. Overall, food allergies occur in about 8% of children and about 11% of adults.[34,35] Most allergic reactions are mild (e.g., itchy skin, runny nose, gastrointestinal distress), but some can be fatal, involving the cardiovascular and respiratory systems. Nine foods account for about 90% of all food-related allergies. In order of prevalence (among all ages), these include shellfish, milk, peanuts, tree nuts, eggs, fin fish, wheat, soy, and sesame (Fig. 6-18). Section 15.7 provides additional information about food allergies.

KIDNEY DISEASE

As described in Section 6.6, protein metabolism generates some waste products that must be processed by the liver and excreted via the kidneys. Individuals with healthy kidney function have no problem processing and excreting these waste products, even when protein intake is double or triple the RDA. However, for individuals with impaired kidney function, consuming too much protein can be harmful.

Your kidneys are busy organs. They filter wastes out of your blood, maintain a steady level of hundreds of solutes in your blood, and help to regulate your blood pressure. They also play a role in red blood cell synthesis. Unfortunately, about one in seven American adults suffers from chronic kidney disease.[36] **Chronic kidney disease** is a condition in which the **nephrons** (the functional units of the kidneys) become less efficient at filtering blood, which can lead to fluid imbalances and the buildup of harmful wastes in the blood. Over time, chronic kidney disease can progress to kidney failure, in which a person needs **dialysis** to help remove harmful waste products from the blood. The most common risk factors for chronic kidney disease are hypertension and diabetes.

For individuals with chronic kidney disease, limiting protein intake to a level that is just enough to meet the body's requirements (around 0.8 gram of protein per kilogram of body weight per day) can help to preserve kidney function and thereby slow or prevent the progression to kidney failure and the need for dialysis.[37] A therapeutic diet for kidney disease may also include limits on intake of fluids, sodium, and phosphorus. An experienced registered dietitian nutritionist can help individuals with chronic kidney disease to plan a kidney-friendly, nutritionally adequate diet that fits into everyday life.

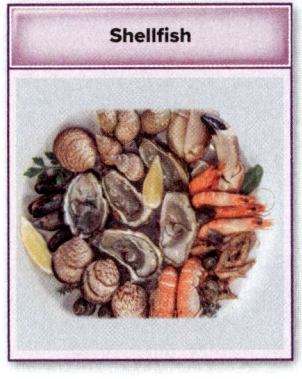
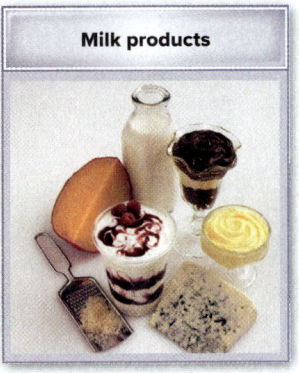
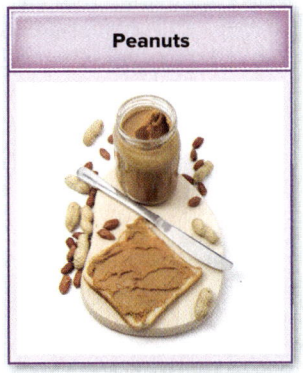
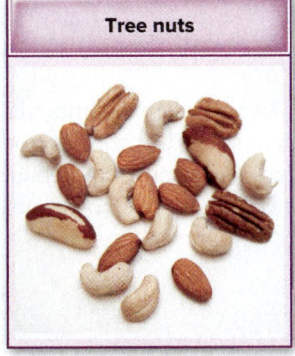
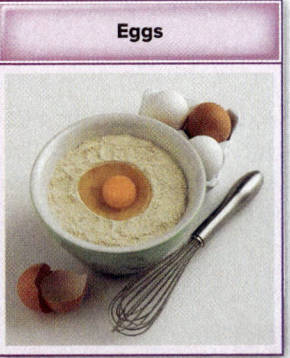
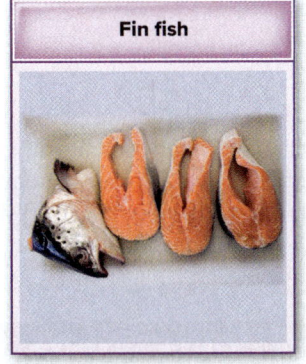
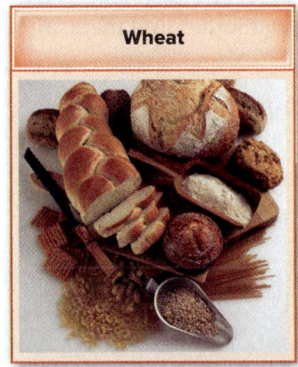
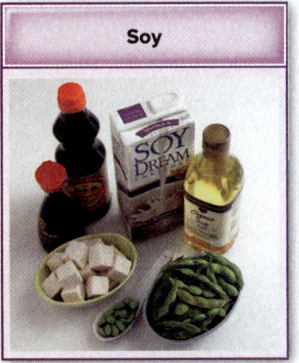
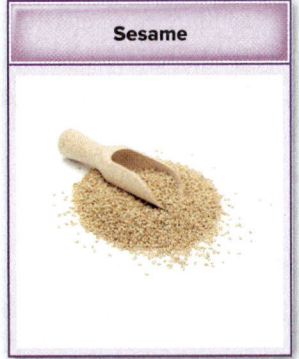

FIGURE 6-18 Most common food allergens. peanut butter: Igor Dutina/iStock/Getty Images; tree nuts: Lucy Stein/Image Source/Glow Images; milk products, soy, wheat, eggs: Dennis Gottlieb; fish: Javier Larrea/Pixtal/age fotostock; shellfish: Jean-Bernard Nadeau/freeprod/123RF; sesame: imstock/123RF

> **Celiac Disease or Wheat Allergy?**
>
> Gluten is one type of protein found in wheat, rye, and barley. Some individuals have an allergic response to gluten or other proteins in wheat. However, a food allergy to wheat is not the same as celiac disease (see Section 3.11). Celiac disease is an autoimmune disorder, in which the immune system attacks the body's own cells. Small peptides that arise from partial gluten digestion can be absorbed into the cells lining the small intestine and cause an autoimmune reaction in people with a genetic predisposition for celiac disease. Strict dietary avoidance of food products containing wheat, rye, and barley is the only proven way to manage celiac disease.
>
> Source: Aljada B, Zohni A, El-Matary W. The gluten-free diet for celiac disease and beyond. *Nutrients*. 2021 Nov 9;13(11):3993. doi: 10.3390/nu13113993

inborn error of metabolism A genetic condition that affects how specific compounds (e.g., amino acids, fatty acids) are used or broken down in the body.

INBORN ERRORS OF METABOLISM

The chemical reactions that take place in the human body are regulated by enzymes, which are proteins. As you learned in Section 6.2, protein synthesis is directed by DNA, and if there is an error in the information encoded by DNA, a faulty protein may result. Errors in the genetic code that cause problems with enzyme function are called **inborn errors of metabolism**. Although these genetic disorders are rare, the consequences can be devastating, so newborns are routinely screened for a variety of inborn errors of metabolism shortly after birth.[38]

Many inborn errors of metabolism affect how nutrients are handled in the body, and nutrition therapy is part of treatment for some conditions. One example of an inborn error of metabolism that is related to our discussion of protein is phenylketonuria (PKU). For an individual with PKU, the ability to convert phenylalanine (an essential amino acid) into tyrosine (a nonessential amino acid) is either partially or fully impaired due to a faulty enzyme (Fig. 6-19). The consequences of PKU are that (1) tyrosine becomes essential (i.e., it must be consumed as part of the dietary pattern), whereas

PKU: Metabolism of Phenylalanine to Tyrosine Is Blocked

Phenylalanine (Phe) (essential) — Phenylalanine hydroxylase ✗ → Tyrosine (Tyr) (becomes conditionally essential)

FIGURE 6-19 In the genetic disorder phenylketonuria, tyrosine, a nonessential amino acid, becomes a conditionally essential amino acid because its production from phenylalanine is blocked.

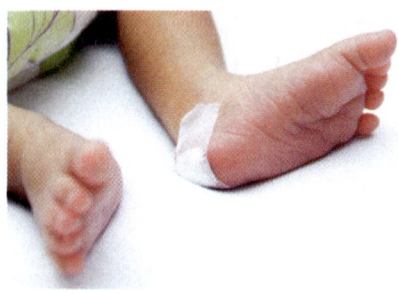

All newborns are tested for phenylketonuria and some other amino acid disorders within the first few days of life using blood collected by a heel prick. If PKU is diagnosed, a special diet should begin as soon as possible after birth to ensure normal brain development. Noor Haswan Noor Azman/Shutterstock

(2) phenylalanine can build up to toxic levels in the blood. Elevated phenylalanine disrupts brain function, leading to intellectual disability. Treatment for PKU involves a special diet that provides adequate protein but limits phenylalanine. Recall from Section 4.3 that individuals with PKU should avoid the artificial sweetener aspartame because it contains phenylalanine.

✓ CONCEPT CHECK 6.8

1. Identify two similarities and two differences between kwashiorkor and marasmus.
2. List the nine most common food allergens.
3. Why do some individuals with kidney disease need to restrict dietary protein intake?
4. Why must individuals with PKU avoid the artificial sweetener aspartame? (HINT: Review Section 4.3)

6.9 Nutrition and Your Health: Nutritional Genomics

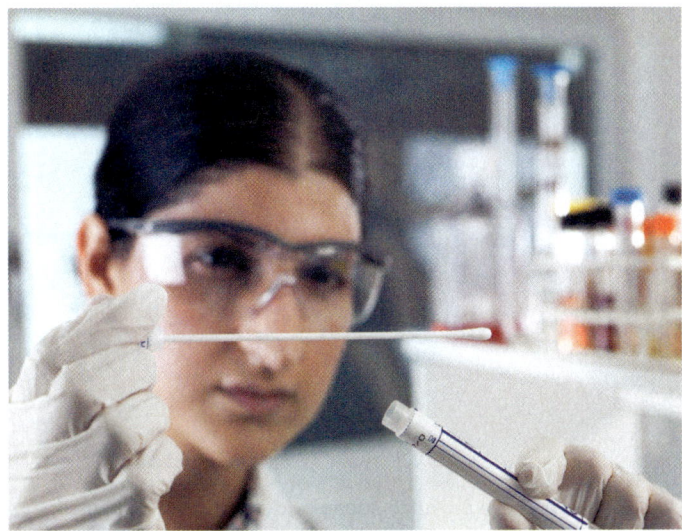

Andrew Brookes/Cultura/Getty Images

We discuss nutrition and genetics in the protein chapter because the primary function of our genes is to produce proteins. The availability of genetic information is now enabling health professionals to personalize nutrition recommendations that can optimize nutritional status and improve the outcomes of nutrition-related diseases. It is evident that nutritional status can both *affect* and *be affected by* an individual's genetic makeup.

The Emerging Field of Nutritional Genomics

The study of interactions between nutrition and genetics is known as nutritional genomics (Fig. 6-20). **Nutrigenetics** is the branch of nutritional genomics that examines how variations in genes can affect nutritional health. For example, the efficiency of absorption, metabolism, and excretion of a particular nutrient is controlled by genes. On the other hand, **nutrigenomics** refers to the many ways dietary components affect gene expression—particularly as it relates to development and treatment of nutrition-related diseases. In this section, we will examine each of these branches of nutritional genomics more closely.

NUTRIGENETICS

Recall that nutrient recommendations, such as RDAs, are not absolute but are actually estimates of a level of intake that is likely to meet the needs of most (97% to 98%) of the population. For

nutrigenetics A branch of nutritional genomics that studies how genes affect nutritional health, such as variations in nutrient requirements and responsiveness to dietary modifications.

nutrigenomics A branch of nutritional genomics that studies how food impacts health through its interaction with our genes and its subsequent effect on gene expression.

example, the RDA for folic acid (a B vitamin) is 400 micrograms per day. For most of the population, consuming this much folic acid from foods or supplemental sources will supply enough of the vitamin to optimize its functions in the body. There are certain subgroups of the population, however, that have dietary requirements for folic acid that are as much as 10 times higher than the RDA because of a genetic variation that alters the function of an enzyme necessary for amino acid metabolism. *Nutrigenetics* may help to explain why some individuals respond to a dietary intervention and others do not. Nutrigenetics researchers are actively examining how genetic variations like this can affect individual nutrient requirements, how we can identify individuals at risk for adverse outcomes of such genetic variations, and how we can personalize nutrition advice based on this knowledge.[39]

NUTRIGENOMICS

With *nutrigenomics*, researchers are interested in finding out how nutrients or other dietary components can influence gene expression, particularly as it relates to development of chronic diseases. Nutrigenomics research is now making it clear that generalized nutrition recommendations may not apply to all individuals within a population group.

The nutrients or other compounds we consume can turn certain genes on (gene expression) or off (gene suppression), just like a light switch. Thus, certain dietary components can manipulate the production of proteins that can affect—positively or negatively—the development or progression of diseases. Current areas of

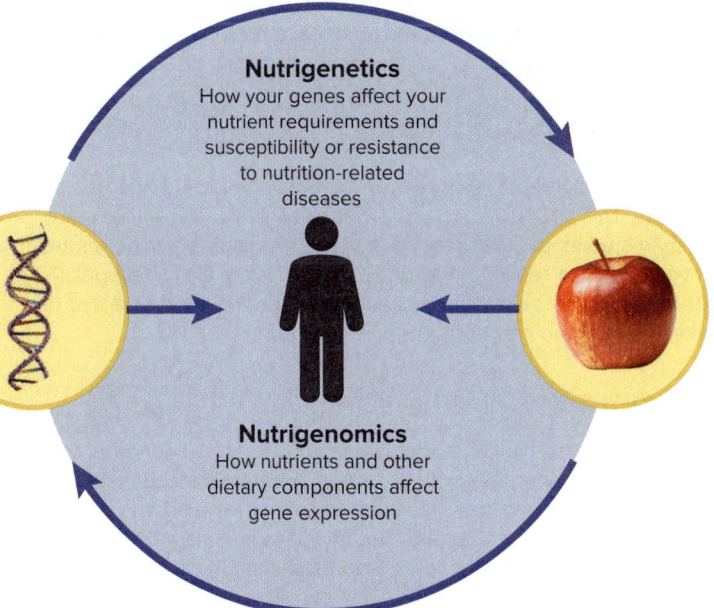

FIGURE 6-20 Nutrigenetics and nutrigenomics are two branches of nutritional genomics. DNA helix: Comstock/Stockbyte/Getty Images; red apple: Turnervisual/iStock/Getty Images

nutrigenomics research include obesity, diabetes, cardiovascular disease, celiac disease, cancer, osteoporosis, and Alzheimer's disease. Beyond the human genome, researchers are also interested in the impact of dietary components on the microbiome and how those changes can affect human health.[40] With a better understanding of the interactions between genes and our eating patterns, it will not be long before dietary recommendations can be tailored to help those with genetically linked diseases.

Nutritional Diseases with a Genetic Link

Studies of families, including those with identical twins and adopted children, provide strong support for the effects of genetics in various disorders. In fact, a family history of disease is considered to be an important risk factor in the development of many nutrition-related diseases.

However, as we study nutrition, we must recognize that a genetic *predisposition* is not a *predestination;* environmental factors (which include dietary and physical activity behaviors) do influence the way each person's genetic potential is expressed. Although not every person with a genetic tendency toward obesity becomes obese, those genetically predisposed to weight gain have a higher lifetime risk than individuals without a genetic predisposition for obesity.

CARDIOVASCULAR DISEASE

There is strong evidence that cardiovascular disease is the result of gene–environment interactions. An estimated 1 of every 311 people in the general population worldwide has a defective gene that greatly delays cholesterol removal from the bloodstream.[41] Elevated blood cholesterol is one of the risk factors for development of cardiovascular disease. Discoveries of interactions between genes and our eating patterns will allow for personalized treatment plans to manage blood lipids using medications and nutrition therapy that will help reduce disease risk and improve health outcomes. Although dietary modifications are important and can make a difference, medications and even surgery are often needed to fully address these problems.

OBESITY

Most individuals with obesity have at least one parent affected by obesity. This strongly suggests a genetic link. Findings from many human studies suggest that a variety of genes (500 or more) are involved in the regulation of body weight.[42] For example, specific gene variations have been linked to the propensity to overeat or alterations in the way nutrients are metabolized.

DIABETES

Both type 1 and type 2 diabetes are influenced by genetics. Evidence for these genetic links comes from studies of families, including twins, and from the high incidence of diabetes among certain population groups (e.g., South Asians or Pima Indians). Type 2 diabetes, in fact, is a complex disease with more than 200 genes identified as possible causes.[43] Only sensitive and expensive testing can identify who is at greatest risk. Type 2 diabetes, the most common form of diabetes (90% of all cases), is typically diagnosed after a person becomes obese, not before. In this case, a lifestyle leading to obesity affects genetic expression.

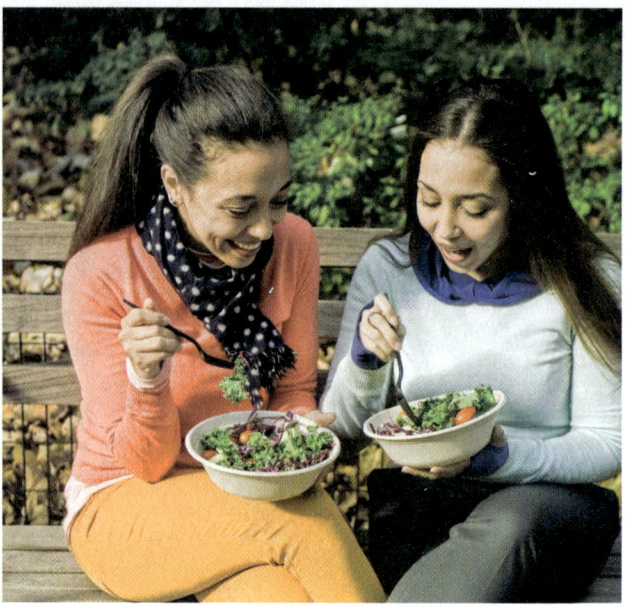

Studies of twins have provided strong evidence for the interaction between genes and dietary patterns and their combined effects on disease risk. Leland Bobbe/Image Source/Getty Images

CANCER

It is estimated that about 10% of cancers have a genetic link.[44] A much higher percentage (about 90%) of cancers are related to environmental and lifestyle factors. Body weight and eating patterns have been estimated to account for approximately 60% of all cancers.[45] Other environmental influences on cancer risk include tobacco, sedentary lifestyles, family history, viruses, radiation, and toxic exposures.

Your Genetic Profile

From this discussion, you can see that your genes certainly influence your risk of developing certain diseases. By recognizing your potential for developing a particular disease, you can avoid behaviors and exposures that further raise your risk. Genetic testing can be valuable if it confirms that you carry a genetic mutation associated with a disease, and the results of testing might alter the course of treatment. Testing is also of interest when you do not know your family medical history or there are gaps in your family tree. Depending on the gene of interest, it typically costs under $1000 to have your DNA sequenced to reveal susceptibility for diseases or disorders. Many genetic tests are covered by health insurance plans, and the Genetic Information Nondiscrimination Act prohibits health insurers from raising premiums or denying coverage based on genetic information. DNA testing requires providing a DNA sample (blood, saliva, hair). Areas of interest in the genome are sequenced and read in a process known as genotyping. If you are considering genetic testing, it is best to consult a Certified Genetic Counselor. You can find one at www.nsgc.org.

Many of the genes involved in common diseases, such as diabetes, are still unknown. Although there are genetic tests available for some diseases, your family history of certain diseases is still a much better indicator of your genetic profile and risk of disease.

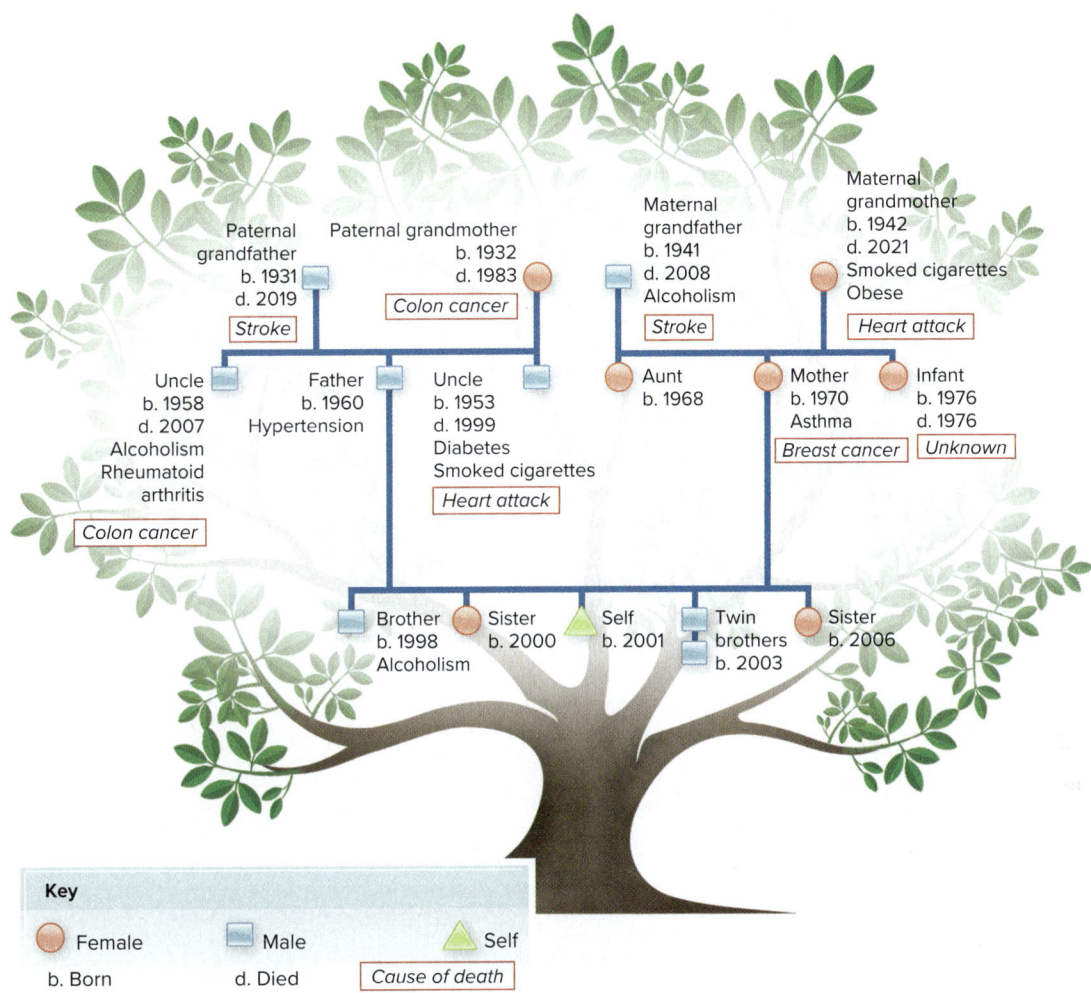

FIGURE 6-21 Example of a family tree for Justin, designated as "Self" at the trunk of the tree. The sex of each family member is identified by color (blue squares for males and red circles for females). Dates of birth (b) and death (d) are listed below each family member. If deceased, the cause of death is highlighted with a red box. Other medical conditions the family members experienced are noted beneath each name. Create your own family tree of frequent diseases using the interactive tool available at https://cbiit.github.io/FHH/html/index.html. Then show your family tree to your health care provider to discuss a more complete picture of what the information means for your health.

Put together a family tree of illnesses and deaths by compiling a few key facts about your primary relatives: siblings, parents, aunts and uncles, and grandparents. In general, the greater the number of your relatives who had a genetically transmitted disease and the closer they are related to you, the greater your risk. If there is a significant family history of a certain disease, lifestyle changes may help decrease your risk of developing this disease.

Figure 6-21 shows an example of a medical family tree (also called a *genogram*). Risk is high when two or more first-degree relatives in a family have a specific disease (first-degree relatives include one's biological parents, siblings, and offspring) or when a first-degree relative develops a disease before age 50 to 60 years. In the family depicted in Figure 6-21, prostate cancer killed the man's father. Knowing this, the man should be tested regularly for prostate cancer. His sisters should have frequent mammograms and breast exams because their mother was diagnosed with breast cancer. Because heart attack and stroke are also common in the family, all the children should adopt a lifestyle that minimizes

The following websites will help you gather more information about genetic conditions and testing:

https://geneticalliance.org/

The Genetic Alliance is a nonprofit health advocacy group that provides a variety of publications for families about genetic conditions.

http://learn.genetics.utah.edu

The Genetic Science Learning Center maintained by the University of Utah provides an online tour of basic genetics.

http://www.cancer.gov/publications/pdq/information-summaries/genetics

The National Cancer Institute of the National Institutes of Health provides fact sheets pertaining to genetics and cancer for health professionals.

https://www.genome.gov/26524162/bringing-the-genomic-revolution-to-the-public

The National Human Genome Research Institute website, from the National Institutes of Health, describes the latest research findings, discusses some ethical issues, and provides a talking glossary.

the risk of developing these conditions, such as avoiding excessive saturated fat and salt intake. Colon cancer is also evident, so careful screening throughout life is important.

Information about our genetic makeup should inform our eating patterns and lifestyle choices. Throughout this text, we discuss modifiable (i.e., controllable) risk factors that could contribute to the development of genetically linked diseases present in your family. This information will help you personalize nutrition advice based on your genetic background and identify and avoid or minimize exposure to the risk factors that could lead to the diseases present in your family.

Personalizing Nutrition Advice

Nutrition professionals already recognize that dietary advice must be tailored to personal and cultural preferences.[46] Research is now paving the way for even more personalized nutrition (sometimes called *precision nutrition*) that incorporates the results of genetic testing when designing the most effective eating pattern for each person. There are genetic tests available for at least 1500 diseases and conditions. Many companies—most of them online—are already offering dietary advice and supplements based on direct-to-consumer genetic tests.

Remember that caution is always needed when evaluating nutrition information and claims. Some DNA-testing companies are responsible organizations, but many are not. Marketing schemes may belittle the science of genetics to consumers. Even though there have been some great advancements in nutritional genomics in recent years, there is still much to learn. Not only is the science of nutritional genomics in its infancy, but application of this technology will require advanced training for health practitioners. Most health professionals agree that genetic testing complements carefully planned nutrient recommendations and dietary guidelines.

✓ CONCEPT CHECK 6.9

1. What is the difference between nutrigenetics and nutrigenomics?
2. List two nutrition-related diseases that are strongly affected by genetics.
3. Predict how nutritional genomics will affect nutrition recommendations in the future.

Summary (Numbers refer to numbered sections in the chapter)

6.1 Amino acids, the building blocks of proteins, contain a very usable form of nitrogen for humans. Of the 20 common types of amino acids found in food, nine must be consumed in food (essential) and the rest can be synthesized by the body (nonessential).

6.2 Individual amino acids are bonded together to form proteins. The sequential order of amino acids determines the protein's ultimate shape and function. This order is directed by DNA in the cell nucleus. Diseases such as sickle cell anemia can occur when the amino acids are assembled incorrectly in a polypeptide chain. When the three-dimensional shape of a protein is denatured by treatment with heat, acid or alkaline solutions, agitation, or other processes, the protein loses its biological activity but not its nutritional value.

6.3 Protein is available from both animal and plant sources. High-quality (complete) protein foods contain ample amounts of all nine essential amino acids and closely match the amino acid requirements of humans. Except for gelatin, all animal sources of protein are high-quality proteins. Lower-quality (incomplete) protein foods lack sufficient amounts of one or more essential amino acids. However, consuming different sources of plant proteins (complementary proteins) throughout the day will help to ensure that all essential amino acids are available for protein synthesis. Excellent plant sources of protein include legumes, nuts, and seeds.

Excessive intake of red meat, especially processed forms, has been linked to colon cancer and deaths caused by cardiovascular disease and cancers.

6.4 Vegetarian and other plant-based dietary patterns provide many health benefits, including lower risks for chronic diseases such as cardiovascular disease, diabetes, and certain cancers. The benefits associated with plant-based dietary patterns appear to stem from the lower content of saturated fat and cholesterol and the higher amount of fiber, vitamins, minerals, and phytochemicals.

6.5 Protein digestion begins in the stomach, where stomach acid and pepsin break down proteins into shorter polypeptide chains. In the small intestine, these polypeptide chains are further digested to yield small peptides and amino acids, which can be absorbed by the cells that line the small intestine. Absorbed amino acids travel via the hepatic portal vein to the liver, where they can be metabolized or exported to other tissues via the bloodstream.

6.6 Important body components—such as muscles, connective tissue, transport proteins in the bloodstream, visual pigments, enzymes, some hormones, and immune cells—are made of proteins. These proteins are in a state of constant turnover. The carbon chains of proteins may be used to produce glucose (or fat) when necessary.

6.7 The protein RDA for adults is 0.8 gram per kilogram of healthy body weight. The typical American dietary pattern generally supplies plenty of protein, with males consuming about 100 grams of protein daily and females consuming about 70 grams. These protein intakes are typically sufficient to support body functions. To maintain a state of protein balance, an individual needs to consume enough protein to compensate for protein losses. A positive protein balance is needed to supply the raw materials required to build new tissues during growth or recovery from an illness or injury. To achieve this, a person must eat more protein daily than that person loses. Consuming less protein than needed leads to negative protein balance, such as when acute illness reduces the desire to eat. Researchers now recommend that adults consume 20 to 30 grams of protein at each of three meals daily in order to maintain healthy muscles and bones. Due to the potential for imbalances and toxicities, the best practice to ensure adequacy is to rely on whole foods as sources of amino acids rather than supplements.

6.8 Kwashiorkor and marasmus are two severe forms of protein-calorie malnutrition, which is most common among children in developing regions of the world. Food allergies occur when the immune system mistakes a food protein for a harmful invader. Nine foods account for 90% of food-related allergies (shellfish, milk, peanuts, tree nuts, eggs, fin fish, wheat, soy, and sesame). Individuals with kidney disease may need to restrict protein intake to a level that is just enough to meet daily requirements to preserve kidney function. Inborn errors of metabolism are inherited conditions that arise from the dysfunction of enzymes that regulate the use or breakdown of nutrients in the body.

6.9 Nutritional genomics includes the study of how genes influence nutritional status (nutrigenetics) and how nutrients and other dietary components influence gene expression (nutrigenomics). Genograms and gene testing can be useful tools for identifying the prevalence of disease. Personalized nutritional prescriptions can then be applied to promote optimal health.

Check Your Knowledge (Answers are available at the end of this question set)

1. Which of the following groups accounts for the differences among amino acids?
   a. Amino group
   b. Side chain
   c. Acid group
   d. Keto group

2. The "instructions" for making proteins are located in the
   a. cell membrane.
   b. cell nucleus.
   c. cytoplasm.
   d. lysosome.

3. If an essential amino acid is unavailable for protein synthesis,
   a. the cell will make the amino acid.
   b. protein synthesis will stop.
   c. the cell will continue to attach amino acids to the protein.
   d. the partially completed protein will be stored for later completion.

4. An example of complementary proteins used in vegan dietary planning would be the combination of
   a. cereal and milk.
   b. bacon and eggs.
   c. rice and beans.
   d. macaroni and cheese.

5. A nutrient that could easily be deficient in the dietary pattern of a vegan would be
   a. vitamin C.
   b. folic acid.
   c. calcium.
   d. carbohydrate.

6. Absorption of amino acids primarily takes place in the
   a. stomach.
   b. liver.
   c. small intestine.
   d. large intestine.

7. Which of the following is an example of a protein with a structural role in the body?
   a. Hydroxyapatite
   b. Insulin
   c. Collagen
   d. Dopamine

8. Jack is not an athlete and weighs 176 pounds (80 kilograms). His daily protein requirement is _____ grams.
   a. 32
   b. 40
   c. 64
   d. 80

9. Maple syrup urine disease is a rare genetic condition in which an individual lacks the enzymes to break down branched-chain amino acids. The accumulation of branched-chain amino acids and their toxic byproducts in body fluids can cause neurological damage. The disorder can be detected by the sweet smell of the urine. Maple syrup urine disease is an example of
   a. protein-calorie malnutrition.
   b. a food allergy.
   c. a kidney disorder.
   d. an inborn error of metabolism.

10. The study of how food impacts health through interaction with genes is
    a. epidemiology.
    b. nutrigenomics.
    c. nutrigenetics.
    d. genealogy.

Answer Key: 1. b (LO 6.1), 2. b (LO 6.2), 3. b (LO 6.3), 4. c (LO 6.3), 5. c (LO 6.4), 6. c (LO 6.5), 7. c (LO 6.6), 8. c (LO 6.7), 9. d (LO 6.8), 10. b (LO 6.9)

Study Questions (Numbers refer to Learning Outcomes)

1. What makes an amino acid *essential*? **(LO 6.1)**
2. Briefly describe the organization of proteins. How can this organization be altered or damaged? What might be a result of damaged protein organization? **(LO 6.2)**
3. What is a limiting amino acid? Explain why this concept is a concern in a vegetarian dietary pattern. How can an individual following a vegetarian dietary pattern compensate for limiting amino acids in specific foods? **(LO 6.3)**
4. Describe three different types of plant-based eating patterns. Plan one balanced meal that would be acceptable for each of the three dietary patterns you described. **(LO 6.4)**
5. What is the role of cholecystokinin (CCK) in protein digestion? **(LO 6.5)**
6. Describe four functions of proteins. Provide an example of how the structure of a protein relates to its function. **(LO 6.6)**
7. Describe how protein intake should be distributed throughout the day for more optimal function of protein. **(LO 6.7)**
8. Outline the major differences between kwashiorkor and marasmus. **(LO 6.8)**
9. Which nine foods are the major sources of proteins that cause food allergies? **(LO 6.8)**
10. Describe the nutrition-related diseases for which genetics or family history is considered to be an important risk factor. **(LO 6.9)**

References

1. Ellinger S. Micronutrients, arginine, and glutamine: does supplementation provide an efficient tool for prevention and treatment of different kinds of wounds? *Adv Wound Care (New Rochelle).* 2014 Nov 1;3(11):691-707. doi: 10.1089/wound.2013.0482
2. What is gene therapy? National Library of Medicine (US), MedlinePlus. Updated February 28, 2022. Accessed November 3, 2023. https://medlineplus.gov/genetics/understanding/therapy/genetherapy/
3. Hoy MK, Murayi T, Moshfegh AJ. Diet quality and food intakes among US adults by level of animal protein intake, *What We Eat in America,* NHANES 2015–2018. *Curr Dev Nutr.* 2022;6(5):nzac035. Published 2022 Mar 17. doi:10.1093/cdn/nzac035
4. Paddon-Jones D, Coss-Bu JA, Morris CR, Phillips SM, Wernerman J. Variation in protein origin and utilization: research and clinical application. *Nutr Clin Pract.* 2017 Apr;32(1_suppl):48S-57S. doi: 10.1177/0884533617691244
5. Food and Agriculture Organization of the United Nations. Dietary protein quality evaluation in human nutrition: report of an FAO expert consultation. *FAO Food Nutr Pap.* 2013;92:1-66. PMID: 26369006
6. Messina V. Nutritional and health benefits of dried beans. *Am J Clin Nutr.* 2014 Jul;100 Suppl 1:437S-442S. doi: 10.3945/ajcn.113.071472
7. Pan A, Sun Q, Bernstein AM, et al. Red meat consumption and mortality: results from 2 prospective cohort studies. *Arch Intern Med.* 2012 Apr 9;172(7):555-563. doi: 10.1001/archinternmed.2011.2287
8. Sun Y, Liu B, Snetselaar LG, et al. Association of major dietary protein sources with all-cause and cause-specific mortality: prospective cohort study. *J Am Heart Assoc.* 2021 Feb;10(5):e015553. doi: 10.1161/JAHA.119.015553
9. Haring B, Selvin E, Liang M, et al. Dietary protein sources and risk for incident chronic kidney disease: results from the Atherosclerosis Risk in Communities (ARIC) Study. *J Ren Nutr.* 2017 Jul;27(4):233-242. doi: 10.1053/j.jrn.2016.11.004
10. Tilman D, Clark M. Global diets link environmental sustainability and human health. *Nature.* 2014 Nov 27;515(7528):518-522. doi: 10.1038/nature13959
11. Hilborn R, Banobi J, Hall SJ, Pucylowski T, Walsworth TE. The environmental cost of animal source foods. *Front Ecol Environ.* 2018 Aug;16(6):329-335. doi: 10.1002/fee.1822
12. Hultin G. Plant protein powders. *Today's Dietitian.* 2020 Mar;22(3):16.
13. Jones J. In U.S., 4% identify as vegetarian, 1% as vegan. Updated August 24, 2023. Accessed November 4, 2023. https://news.gallup.com/poll/510038/identify-vegetarian-vegan.aspx
14. Melina V, Craig W, Levin S. Position of the Academy of Nutrition and Dietetics: vegetarian diets. *J Acad Nutr Diet.* 2016 Dec;116(12):1970-1980. doi: 10.1016/j.jand.2016.09.025
15. Remde A, DeTurk SN, Almardini A, Steiner L, Wojda T. Plant-predominant eating patterns—how effective are they for treating obesity and related cardiometabolic health outcomes?—a systematic review. *Nutr Rev.* 2022 Apr 8;80(5):1094-1104. doi: 10.1093/nutrit/nuab060
16. Orlich MJ, Singh PN, Sabaté J, et al. Vegetarian dietary patterns and the risk of colorectal cancers. *JAMA Intern Med.* 2015 May;175(5):767-776. doi: 10.1001/jamainternmed.2015.59
17. Hopwood CJ, Bleidorn W, Schwaba T, Chen S. Health, environmental, and animal rights motives for vegetarian eating. *PLoS One.* 2020;15(4):e0230609. Published 2020 Apr 2. doi:10.1371/journal.pone.0230609
18. Bowman SA. A vegetarian-style dietary pattern is associated with lower energy, saturated fat, and sodium intakes; and higher whole grains, legumes, nuts, and soy intakes by adults: National Health and Nutrition Examination Surveys 2013–2016. *Nutrients.* 2020;12(9):2668. Published 2020 Sep 1. doi:10.3390/nu12092668
19. Alexandropoulou I, Goulis DG, Merou T, Vassilakou T, Bogdanos DP, Grammatikopoulou MG. Basics of sustainable diets and tools for assessing dietary sustainability: a primer for researchers and policy actors. *Healthcare (Basel).* 2022;10(9):1668. Published 2022 Aug 31. doi:10.3390/healthcare10091668
20. Springmann M, Clark MA, Rayner M, Scarborough P, Webb P. The global and regional costs of healthy and sustainable dietary patterns: a modelling study [published correction appears in *Lancet Planet Health.* 2021 Dec;5(12):e861]. *Lancet Planet Health.* 2021;5(11):e797-e807. doi:10.1016/S2542-5196(21)00251-5
21. Petersen KS. The dilemma with the soy protein health claim. *J Am Heart Assoc.* 2019 Jul 2;8(13):e013202. doi: 10.1161/JAHA.119.013202
22. Obesity and cancer. Centers for Disease Control and Prevention. Reviewed August 9, 2023. Accessed November 9, 2023. https://www.cdc.gov/cancer/obesity/index.htm

23. AICR'S Foods that Fight Cancer™. American Institute for Cancer Research. Accessed November 9, 2023. https://www.aicr.org/cancer-prevention/food-facts/

24. Craig WJ, Mangels AR, Fresán U, et al. The safe and effective use of plant-based diets with guidelines for health professionals. *Nutrients.* 2021 Nov 19;13(11):4144. doi: 10.3390/nu13114144

25. Viguiliouk E, Stewart SE, Jayalath VH, et al. Effect of replacing animal protein with plant protein on glycemic control in diabetes: a systematic review and meta-analysis of randomized controlled trials. *Nutrients.* 2015 Dec 1;7(12):9804-9824. doi: 10.3390/nu7125509

26. Academy of Nutrition and Dietetics. Position of the Academy of Nutrition and Dietetics: vegetarian diets. *J Acad Nutr Diet.* 116:1970, 2016. doi:10.1016/j.jand.2016.09.025.

27. Fleischer DM, Spergel, JM, Ass'ad AH, Pongracic JA. Primary prevention of allergic disease through nutritional interventions. *J Allergy Clin Immunol Prac.* 2013 Jan;1(1):29-36. doi: 10.1016/j.jaip.2012.09.003

28. Raichle ME, Gusnard DA. Appraising the brain's energy budget. *Proc Natl Acad Sci U S A.* 2002 Aug 6;99(16):10237-10239. doi: 10.1073/pnas.172399499

29. James Stubbs R, Horgan G, Robinson E, Hopkins M, Dakin C, Finlayson G. Diet composition and energy intake in humans. *Philos Trans R Soc Lond B Biol Sci.* 2023;378(1888):20220449. doi:10.1098/rstb.2022.0449

30. Institute of Medicine. *Dietary Reference Intakes for Energy, Carbohydrate, Fiber, Fat, Fatty Acids, Cholesterol, Protein, and Amino Acids.* The National Academies Press; 2005. doi: 10.17226/10490

31. Bauer J, Biolo G, Cederholm T, et al. Evidence-based recommendations for optimal dietary protein intake in older people: a position paper from the PROT-AGE Study Group. *J Am Med Dir Assoc.* 2013 Aug:14(8): 542-559. doi: 10.1016/j.jamda.2013.05.021

32. Layman DK, Anthony TG, Rasmussen BB, et al. Defining meal requirements for protein to optimize metabolic roles of amino acids. *Am J Clin Nutr.* 2015 Jun;101(6):1330S-1338S. doi: 10.3945/ajcn.114.084053

33. Correia MITD, Hegazi RA, Higashiguchi T, et al. Evidence-based recommendations for addressing malnutrition in health care: an updated strategy from the feedM.E. Global Study Group. *J Am Med Dir Assoc.* 2014 Aug;15(8):544-550. doi: 10.1016/j.jamda.2014.05.011

34. Gupta RS, Warren CM, Smith BM, et al. The public health impact of parent-reported childhood food allergies in the United States [published correction appears in *Pediatrics.* 2019 Mar;143(3):e20183835]. *Pediatrics.* 2018:142(6):e20181235. doi: 10.1542/peds.2018-3835

35. Gupta RS, Warren CM, Smith BM, et al. Prevalence and severity of food allergies among US adults. *JAMA Netw Open.* 2019 Jan 4;2(1):e185630. doi: 10.1001/jamanetworkopen.2018.5630

36. Chronic kidney disease basics. Centers for Disease Control and Prevention. Reviewed February 28, 2022. Accessed November 9, 2023. https://www.cdc.gov/kidneydisease/basics.html

37. Ko GJ, Obi Y, Tortorici AR, Kalantar-Zadeh K. Dietary protein intake and chronic kidney disease. *Curr Opin Clin Nutr Metab Care.* 2017 Jan;20(1):77-85. doi: 10.1097/MCO.0000000000000342

38. Kruszka P, Regier D. Inborn errors of metabolism: from preconception to adulthood. *Am Fam Physician.* 2019 Jan 1;99(1):25-32. PMID: 30600976

39. Singh V. Current challenges and future implications of exploiting the omics data into nutrigenetics and nutrigenomics for personalized diagnosis and nutrition-based care. *Nutrition.* 2023;110:112002. doi:10.1016/j.nut.2023.112002

40. Riscuta G, Xi D, Pierre-Victor D, Starke-Reed P, Khalsa J, Duffy L. Diet, microbiome, and epigenetics in the era of precision medicine. *Methods Mol Biol.* 2018;1856:141-156. doi: 10.1007/978-1-4939-8751-1_8

41. Hu P, Dharmayat KI, Stevens CAT, et al. Prevalence of familial hypercholesterolemia among the general population and patients with atherosclerotic cardiovascular disease: a systematic review and meta-analysis. *Circulation.* 2020 Jun 2;141(22):1742-1759. doi: 10.1161/CIRCULATIONAHA.119.044795

42. Loos RJ. The genetics of adiposity. *Curr Opin Genet Dev.* 2018 Jun;50: 86-95. doi: 10.1016/j.gde.2018.02.009

43. Witka BZ, Oktaviani DJ, Marcellino M, Barliana MI, Abdulah R. Type 2 diabetes-associated genetic polymorphisms as potential disease predictors. *Diabetes Metab Syndr Obes.* 2019 Dec 18;12:2689-2706. doi: 10.2147/DMSO.S230061

44. The genetics of cancer. National Institutes of Health, National Cancer Institute. Updated August 17, 2022. Accessed November 9, 2023. https://www.cancer.gov/about-cancer/causes-prevention/genetics

45. Anand P, Kunnumakkara AB, Sundaram C, et al. Cancer is a preventable disease that requires major lifestyle changes [published correction appears in *Pharm Res.* 2008 Sep;25(9):2200. Kunnumakara, Ajaikumar B [corrected to Kunnumakkara, Ajaikumar B]]. *Pharm Res.* 2008 Sep;25(9):2097-2116. doi: 10.1007/s11095-008-9661-9

46. Dennett C. The future of nutrigenomics. *Today's Dietitian.* 2017 Oct;19(10):30.

Design Element Credits: Fact Check/magnifying glass icon: McGraw Hill; Magnificent Microbiome background image: Alena Ohneva/Shutterstock; Sustainable Solutions icon: McGraw Hill; Roots icon: McGraw Hill; Medicine Cabinet icon: Peter Dazeley/Photographer's Choice/Getty Images

Chapter 7: Energy Balance

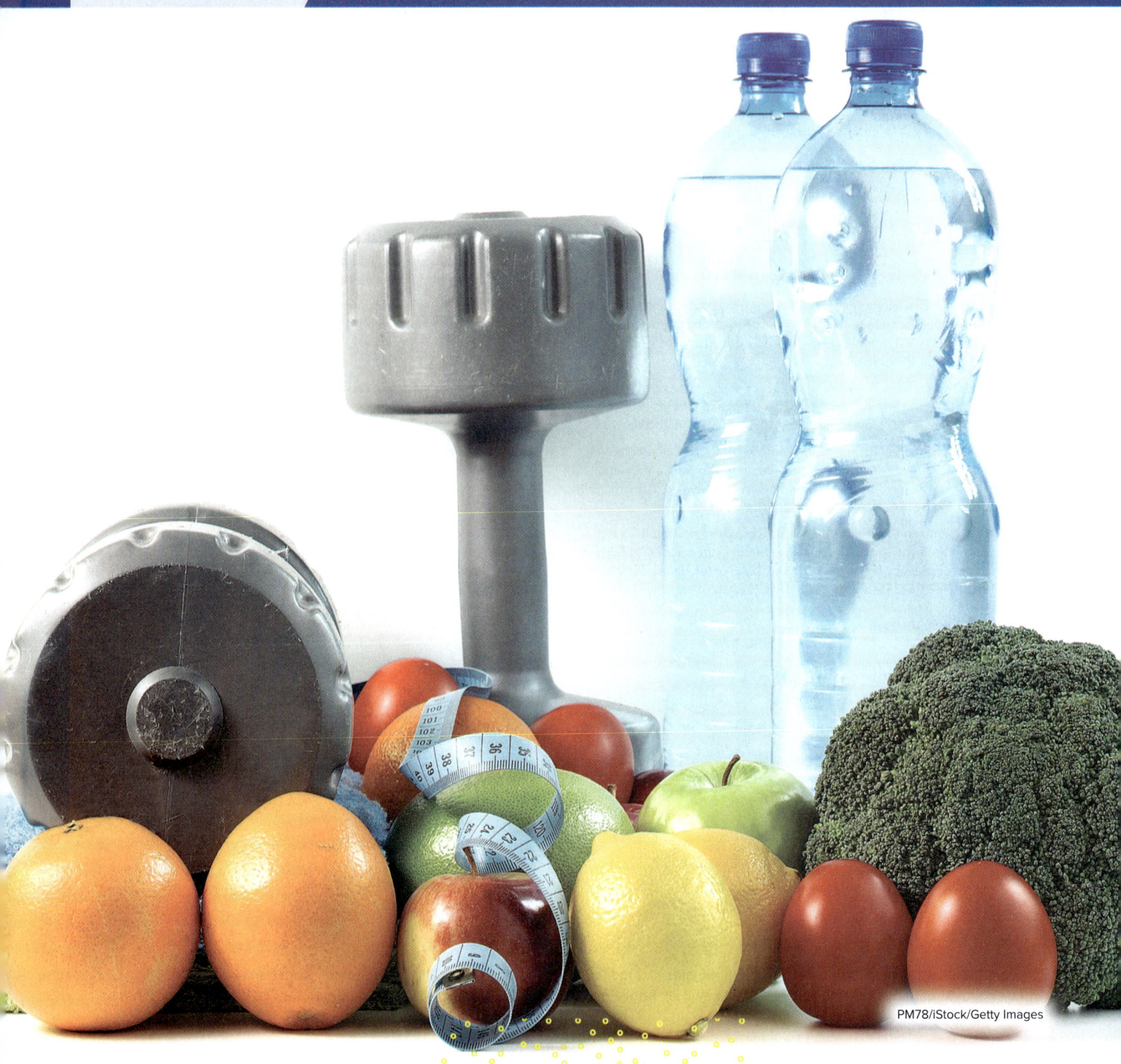

PM78/iStock/Getty Images

Student Learning Outcomes

Chapter 7 is designed to allow you to:

7.1 Describe energy balance and its use by the body.

7.2 Compare methods to determine energy use by the body.

7.3 Discuss methods for assessing and classifying body composition.

7.4 Explain risk factors associated with overweight and obesity and related health consequences.

7.5 Describe how energy balance is fundamental to weight management.

7.6 Discuss how physical activity is a key component of health and weight management.

7.7 Describe how modifying lifestyle behaviors fits into a sound and sustainable energy balance program.

7.8 List and discuss characteristics of a sound weight management program.

7.9 Outline the pros and cons of weight-loss methods for severe obesity.

7.10 Discuss the causes and treatment of underweight.

7.11 Evaluate popular weight-reduction methods, and determine which are safest and most successful.

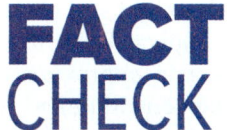

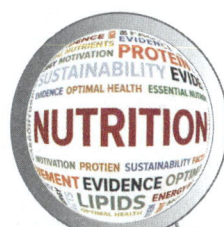

Does weight bias impact health outcomes?

Weight bias, also known as weight stigma or weight discrimination, refers to negative attitudes and stereotypes directed toward individuals based on their body weight or size. This bias is both a social determinant of health and a human rights issue that can have significant and far-reaching impacts on the physical and mental health of those who experience it.

It is essential to address weight bias at both the individual and societal levels. The World Obesity Federation (WOF) recently convened a global working group of practitioners, researchers, policymakers, youth advocates, and individuals with lived experience of obesity to consider the ways that global obesity narratives may contribute to weight stigma.[1]

Promoting acceptance, inclusivity, and respect for individuals of all body sizes can help decrease the negative health impacts of weight bias. Health care providers also can play a key role. Practitioners should strive to provide compassionate and unbiased care to all patients, regardless of their weight, to ensure equitable health outcomes. Learn how weight bias can specifically impact health outcomes in Section 7.1.

Source: https://www.cdc.gov/healthyweight/healthy_eating/energy_density.html

weight bias Negative attitudes toward, and beliefs about, others because of their weight that are often manifested by stereotypes or prejudice toward people with overweight and obesity.

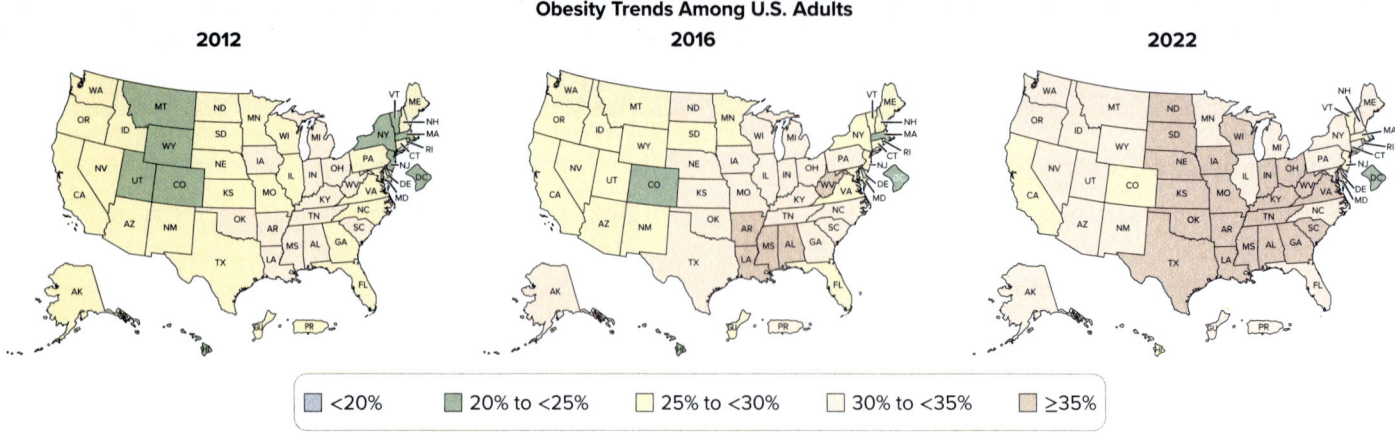

FIGURE 7-1 Self-reported obesity prevalence by U.S. state and territory; 2012, 2016, 2022.
Source: Behavioral Risk Factor Surveillance System, CDC.

7.1 Energy Balance and Health Promotion

energy balance The state in which energy intake, in the form of food and beverages, matches the energy expended, primarily through basal metabolism and physical activity.

This chapter sets the stage for presenting the science related to **energy balance** and health promotion. Energy is required to sustain the body's various functions, including respiration, circulation, physical activity, and protein synthesis. As you have learned, this energy is derived from dietary carbohydrates, proteins, fats, and to a lesser extent, alcohol.[2]

Obtaining and maintaining a healthy body weight can lead to positive lifelong physical and mental health outcomes. Yet the prevalence of overweight and obesity continues to increase with almost 75% of all U.S. adults now impacted (Fig. 7-1).[3] From early to middle adulthood, the majority of U.S. adults gain approximately 1.1 to 2.2 pounds per year. This modest weight gain over time contributes to the fact that 60% of adults are affected by obesity-related health issues and chronic diseases.[4]

As introduced in this chapter's *Fact Check*, there are many ways in which weight bias can affect a person's health and well-being. For instance, weight bias can contribute to an increased risk of developing depression, anxiety, disordered eating, and other harmful behaviors. The chronic stress of weight discrimination can increase the production of stress hormones that are associated with various health problems.

Those experiencing weight bias may have a history of substandard health care or feeling medically discriminated against. In turn, individuals may avoid seeking medical care to avoid feeling mistreated or feeling judged by health care providers. Paradoxically, experiencing weight bias may contribute to weight gain due to emotional eating, reduced physical activity, and avoidance of health care. Taken together, chronic weight bias can result in social isolation and discrimination, resulting in a lack of social support, which is important for overall health and well-being.

There is no quick cure for overweight or obesity, despite what many weight-loss marketing advertisements and fad diets claim. The most reliable and successful weight management approaches come from long-term behavior change and adoption of lifestyle behaviors that improve dietary and physical activity patterns. A combination of improved energy balance, increased physical activity, and behavior modification is considered the most reliable treatment for overweight and obesity. And without a doubt, prevention of overweight and obesity in the first place is the most successful approach.

POSITIVE AND NEGATIVE ENERGY BALANCE

A healthy weight can result from understanding the important concept of energy balance (Fig. 7-2). Think of energy balance as an equation consisting of energy input (calories in) and energy output (calories out):

> **Energy Balance**
> **Energy input = Energy output**
> (calories in from dietary intake) (calories out from metabolism; digestion, absorption, and transport of nutrients; physical activity)

The balance of energy (or calories, measured in kilocalories) on the two sides of this equation can influence energy stores, especially the amount of fat stored in adipose

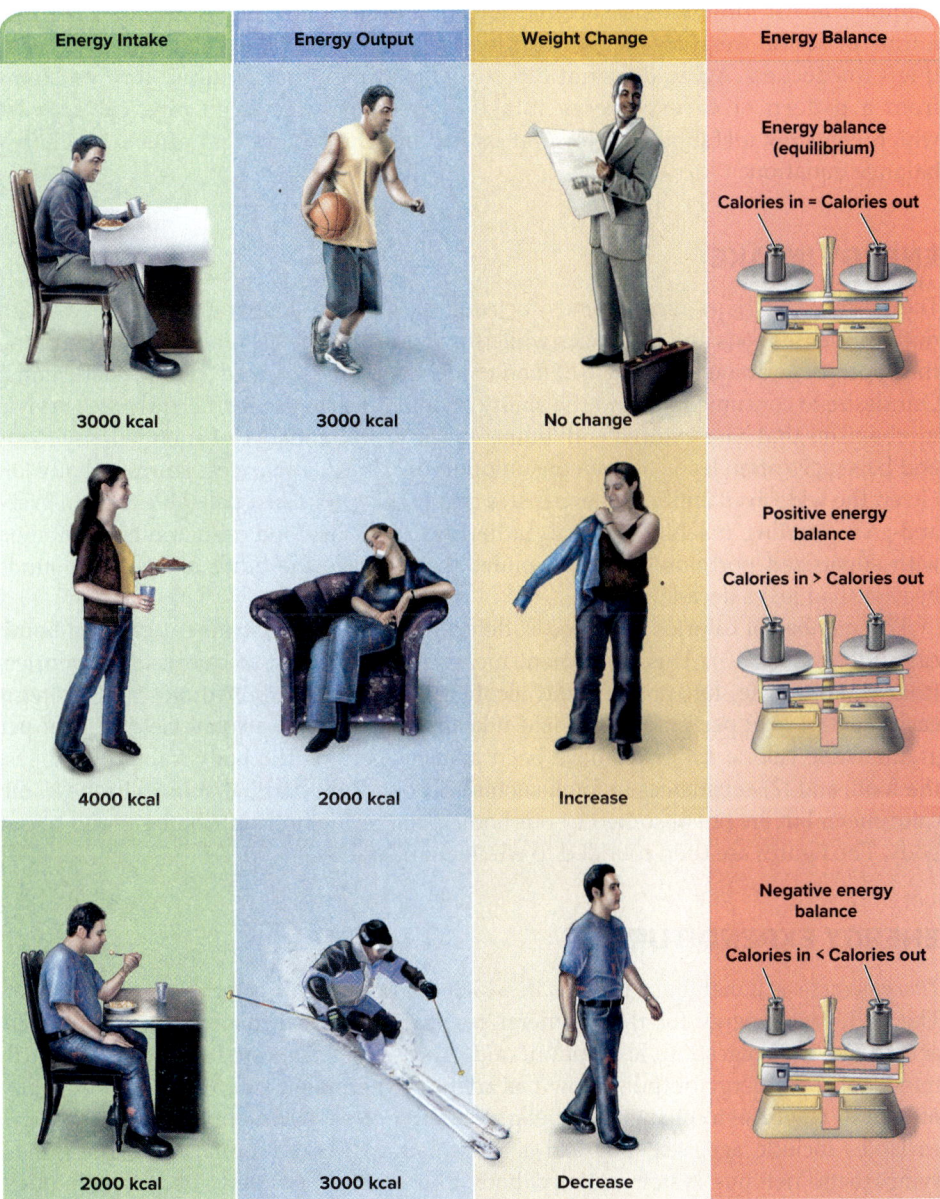

FIGURE 7-2 A model for energy balance: intake versus output. This figure depicts energy balance in practical terms. Energy balance helps maintain weight. Positive energy balance promotes weight gain, and negative energy balance promotes weight loss.

positive energy balance The state in which energy intake is greater than energy expended, generally resulting in weight gain.

tissue. When energy input (calories in) is greater than energy output (calories out), the result is **positive energy balance.** The excess calories consumed are stored in the body, which results in weight gain.

There are some situations in which positive energy balance is normal and healthy. During pregnancy and lactation (breastfeeding), a surplus of calories supports the developing fetus and infants, respectively. Infants and children also require a positive energy balance for normal growth and development during youth and puberty. In adults, however, even a small positive energy balance can result in fat storage, and, over time, this can contribute to increased body fatness.

negative energy balance The state in which energy intake is less than energy expended, resulting in weight loss.

On the other hand, if energy input (calories in) is less than energy output (calories out), there is a calorie deficit, and **negative energy balance** results. A negative energy balance is necessary for weight loss. It is important to realize that when we lose weight, we typically lose some lean tissue in addition to adipose tissue.

The maintenance of energy balance while at an optimal weight substantially contributes to health and well-being by minimizing the risk of developing many common health problems associated with increased body fat. Adulthood is often a time of subtle weight gain that can lead to obesity and a greater risk of disease if left unchecked. Aging does not directly cause weight gain; rather, it often stems from a pattern of excess energy intake coupled with reduced physical activity, which can slow metabolism. Now, let us explore the factors that affect the energy balance equation.

ENERGY INTAKE

bomb calorimeter An instrument used to determine the calorie content of a food.

adaptive thermogenesis The ability of humans to regulate body temperature within narrow limits (thermoregulation) in response to changes in dietary patterns or environmental temperatures.

The *Dietary Guidelines* recommends focusing on meeting your nutritional needs with nutrient-dense foods and beverages while staying within calorie limits. Yet determining the appropriate amount and type of food to meet your energy needs can be challenging. Our desire to consume food and the ability of our bodies to use it efficiently are survival mechanisms that have evolved with humans. The overabundance of energy-dense foods and beverages often leads to overconsumption of calories and excess stores of body fat. Given the wide availability of inexpensive and highly processed palatable food in grab-and-go's, vending machines, social gatherings, and fast-food restaurants—combined with supersized portions—it is no wonder that the average adult is over 10 pounds heavier than just a decade ago!

The number of calories in a food is determined with an instrument called a **bomb calorimeter** (Fig. 7-3). This instrument measures the amount of calories (kilocalories) from carbohydrate, fat, protein, and alcohol. Recall that carbohydrates and proteins each yields 4 kcal per gram, fats yield 9 kcal per gram, and alcohol yields 7 kcal per gram. These calorie estimates have been adjusted for: (1) the body's ability to digest the food; and (2) substances in food, such as fibrous plant parts, that burn in the bomb calorimeter but are not absorbed by our bodies, so they do not contribute calories to our body. The figures are then rounded to whole numbers.

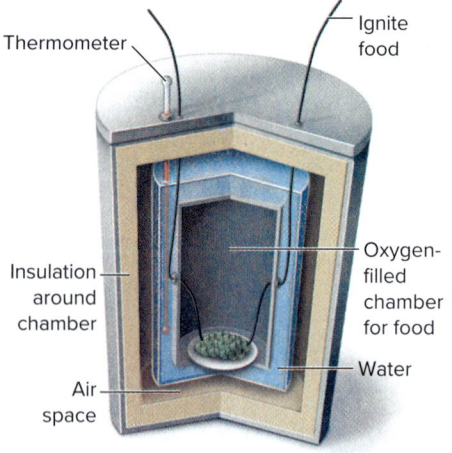

FIGURE 7-3 Bomb calorimeters measure calorie content by igniting and burning a dried portion of food. The burning food raises the temperature of the water surrounding the chamber holding the food. The increase in water temperature indicates the number of calories in the food because 1 kcal equals the amount of heat needed to raise the temperature of 1 kilogram of water by 1 degree Celsius.

ENERGY EXPENDITURE

Thermogenesis is a metabolic process in which the body burns calories to produce heat. The body uses energy for three general purposes: (1) basal metabolism; (2) physical activity; and (3) digestion, absorption, and processing of ingested nutrients. A fourth minor form of energy output, known as **adaptive thermogenesis,** refers to production of heat in response to changes in dietary patterns or environmental exposures. These variables include age, sex, physical activity patterns, body composition, hormones, sympathetic nervous system activity, body and ambient temperature, comorbidities, and medications (Fig. 7-4).

Adaptive thermogenesis (AT) is complex and refers to the change in the BMR in response to environmental stresses. Although weight loss can lead to AT, systematic

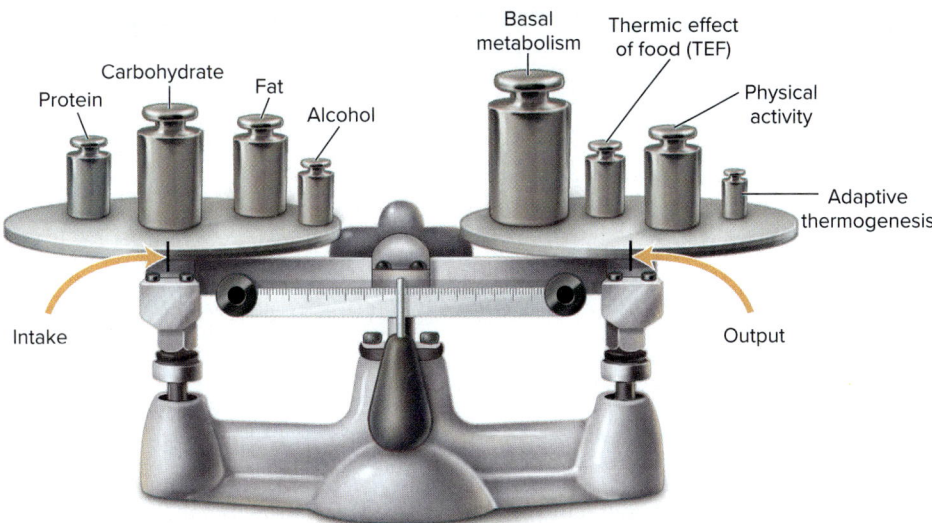

FIGURE 7-4 The components of energy intake and expenditure. This figure incorporates the major variables that influence energy balance. Remember that alcohol is an additional source of energy. The size of each weight on the scale represents the relative contribution of that component to energy balance.

reviews have documented these values are small or nonsignificant in high-quality trials. Furthermore, AT seems to be attenuated, or nonexistent, after periods of weight stabilization or neutral energy balance. More high-quality studies are warranted to understand the impact of AT and its clinical implications on weight management outcomes.[5]

Many students are surprised to learn that a very low calorie intake decreases basal metabolism by about 10% to 20% (about 150 to 300 kcal per day) as the body shifts into a conservation or starvation mode. In addition, the effects of aging also can make weight maintenance a challenge. Metabolism peaks at one year of age and declines until age 20. It remains stable from ages 20 to 60, and declines again in older adulthood.[6]

AT also represents the increase in nonvoluntary physical activity triggered by reflex responses (versus intentional physical activity). For instance, body temperature is tightly regulated by the hypothalamus. When your temperature begins to drop when exposed to cold temperatures, the hypothalamus signals your muscles to contract. These involuntary muscle contractions, known as *shivering thermogenesis,* serve as a defense mechanism to warm your body. Thus, exposure to colder climates can temporarily boost your metabolism. It is interesting to think that some activities, such as eating, include both voluntary and involuntary movement. Chewing is a voluntary movement, while the muscular contractions of the esophagus and intestine are under subconscious control.

Brown adipose tissue is a specialized form of adipose tissue that is brown in color and participates in thermogenesis. The brown appearance results from its greater number of mitochondria. Brown fat contributes to thermogenesis by releasing some of the energy from energy-yielding nutrients into the environment as heat instead of producing ATP. Hibernating animals use brown adipose tissue to generate heat to withstand long winters. In humans, brown adipose tissue contributes as much as 5% of body weight. It is metabolically active and regulates heat to protect our internal organs. Unlike the muscle-contracting shivering thermogenesis, *nonshivering thermogenesis* occurs in the brown adipose tissue. Compared to infants, adults have very little brown adipose tissue, and its role in adulthood remains poorly understood.

brown adipose tissue A specialized form of adipose (fat) tissue that produces large amounts of heat by metabolizing energy-yielding nutrients without synthesizing much useful energy for the body. The unused energy is released as heat.

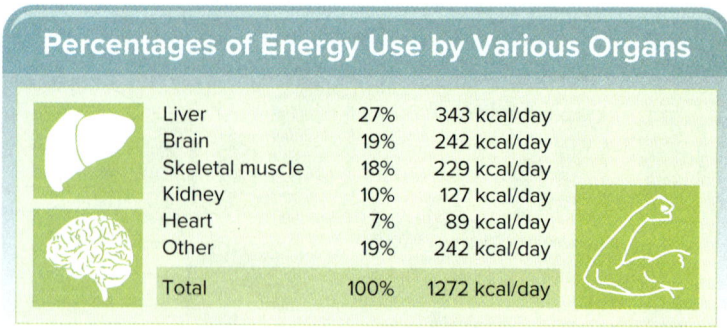

FIGURE 7-5 Percentages of energy use by various organs.
Source: Passmore R, Draper M. The chemical anatomy of the human body. In: Thompson RHS, Wootton IDP, eds. *Biochemical Disorders in Human Disease*. 3rd ed. J. & A. Churchill; 1970:1-14.

basal metabolism The minimal amount of calories the body uses to support itself in a fasting state when resting and awake in a warm, quiet environment. It amounts to roughly 1 kcal per kilogram per hour for males and 0.9 kcal per kilogram per hour for females; these values are often referred to as *basal metabolic rate (BMR)*.

resting metabolism The amount of calories the body uses when the person has not eaten in 4 hours and is resting (e.g., 15 to 30 minutes) and awake in a warm, quiet environment. It is usually slightly higher (~10%) than basal metabolism due to the more flexible testing criteria; often referred to as *resting metabolic rate (RMR)*.

Basal Metabolism. Basal metabolism is expressed as basal metabolic rate (BMR) and represents the minimal amount of calories expended in a fasting state to keep a resting, awake body alive in a warm, quiet environment. For a sedentary person, basal metabolism accounts for about 60% to 80% of total energy use by the body. Some of the processes that utilize energy include the beating of your heart, respiration by the lungs, and the activity required by other organs, such as the liver, brain, and kidneys (Fig. 7-5). It does not include energy used for physical activity or digestion, absorption, and processing of recently consumed nutrients. If you are not fasting or are completely rested, the term **resting metabolism** is used and expressed as resting metabolic rate (RMR). An individual's RMR is slightly higher than their BMR.

How to Estimate Your Basal Metabolic Rate (BMR)

To see how basal metabolism contributes to energy needs, we will consider a 130-pound female (named Maria), as our example.

First, knowing that there are 2.2 pounds (lbs) for every kilogram (kg), convert Maria's weight in pounds into kilograms:

$$130 \text{ lb} \div 2.2 \text{ lb/kg} = 59 \text{ kg}$$

Then, using a rough estimate of BMR of 0.9 kcal per kilogram per hour for an average female (note 1 kcal per kilogram per hour is used for an average male), calculate Maria's BMR:

$$59 \text{ kg} \times 0.9 \text{ kcal/kg/hr} = 53 \text{ kcal/hr}$$

Finally, use this hourly BMR to find Maria's BMR for an entire day (24 hours):

$$53 \text{ kcal/hr} \times 24 \text{ hr/day} = 1272 \text{ kcal/day}$$

These calculations provide an estimate of basal metabolism, as it can vary as much as 25% to 30% among individuals.

In this example, Maria's estimated BMR is 1292 kcal/day

lean body mass Body weight minus fat storage weight equals lean body mass. This includes organs such as the brain, muscles, and liver, as well as bone and blood and other body fluids.

Many factors influence BMR (Fig. 7-6). Of these, **lean body mass** (LBM) is the most important. Persons with higher amounts of LBM have a higher BMR because lean tissue is more metabolically active than adipose tissue (fat mass). The lean tissue, therefore, requires more energy to support its metabolic activity. Although persons who are overweight or obese have an increased amount of body fat, they also typically have a high amount of LBM to support their body weight and therefore a higher BMR to go along with it (Fig. 7-7).

Energy for Physical Activity. Your daily energy needs include your basal metabolic rate, plus the thermic effect of the foods you eat, plus factors called *non-exercise activity thermogenesis (NEAT)* or *non-exercise physical activity (NEPA)*. These terms refer to the energy burned through movement outside of planned physical activity. This includes singing, dancing, getting dressed, fidgeting, and similar movements. While these movements may seem insignificant, it turns out that NEAT can have quite a substantial impact on our metabolic rates and calorie expenditures. For instance, studies have found that fidgeting may reduce the risk of death associated with excessive sedentary time.[7]

During intentional physical activity, your muscles burn calories to provide ample energy to fuel muscle contractions. The calorie expenditure from physical activity varies widely among individuals and is categorized as *exercise-activity thermogenesis (EAT)*.[8] EAT and NEAT may account for 15% to 30% of your total energy expenditure. Although we can't do much to alter our BMR, we can incorporate more NEAT into our regular routines. For instance, climbing stairs rather than riding the elevator, walking to class rather than riding an electric scooter, and standing at a workstation rather than sitting for long periods of time all increase physical activity throughout the day and, hence, energy output. Over time, this energy expenditure adds up and can help with long-term weight management.

Thermic Effect of Food. In addition to basal metabolism and physical activity, the body uses energy to digest food and to absorb and metabolize the nutrients recently consumed. Energy used for these tasks is referred to as the **thermic effect of food (TEF)** or *diet-induced thermogenesis*. TEF is similar to a sales tax; it is like being charged about 8% to 15% for the total amount of calories you eat to cover the cost of processing that food. This metabolic tax equates to between 8 and 15 extra kcal for every 100 kcal needed for basal metabolism and physical activity. For instance, if your daily calorie intake is 2000 kcal per day, TEF would account for 160 to 300 kcal of those calories.[9] As with other components of energy output, note the total amount can vary somewhat among individuals.

Energy Output

Basal Metabolic Rate (BMR) 60% to 80% of Total Energy Expenditure (TEE)
Factors That Increase BMR
Acute illness or injury
Certain medical conditions
Excess thyroid hormones
Greater body surface area (e.g., tall height)
Increased body temperature
Lactation
Lean body mass
Periods of growth (pregnancy, infancy, adolescence)
Post-exercise recovery
Stimulant drugs (e.g., caffeine)
Stress
Factors That Decrease BMR
Aging
Insufficient thyroid hormone production
Less body surface area (e.g., short stature)
Starvation or very-low-calorie diets

Physical Activity (PA) 15% to 30% of TEE	Thermic Effect of Food (TEF) 8% to 15% of TEE

FIGURE 7-6 Contributions of basal metabolic rate, physical activity, and thermic effect of food to energy output.

thermic effect of food (TEF) The increase in metabolism that occurs during the digestion, absorption, and metabolism of energy-yielding nutrients. This typically represents 8% to 15% of calories consumed. Also called *diet-induced thermogenesis*.

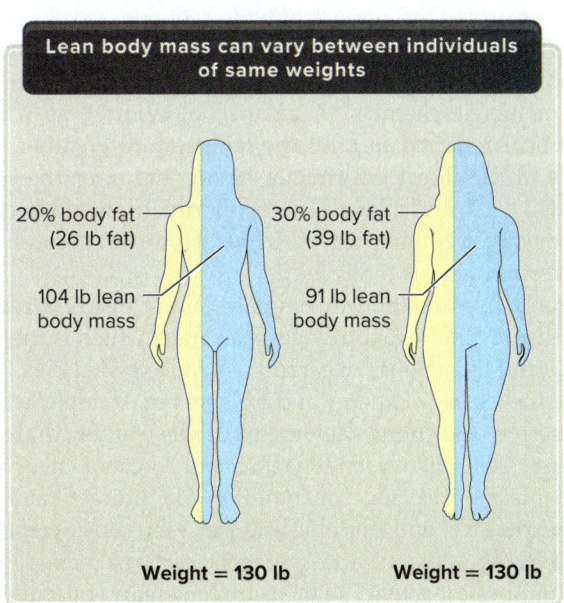

FIGURE 7-7 Lean body mass (LBM), the most significant contributor to basal metabolic rate, varies greatly between individuals. Persons of the same body weight can have different amounts of LBM and body fat and, therefore, have varying energy needs and body types.

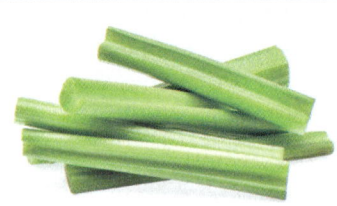

A few foods, such as celery, have been hypothesized to use more calories for TEF than they contain, making them a *negative calorie* food. Despite its recurring popularity in fad diets, there is no scientific evidence supporting the idea that any food, including celery, is calorically negative. Although celery still yields some calories, it remains an excellent choice to include in a healthy dietary pattern. **Are celery and other vegetables considered a low or high energy-dense food option?** Wealthylady/Shutterstock

Food composition also influences TEF. For example, the TEF value for a protein-rich meal is 20% to 30% of the calories consumed, which is higher than that of a carbohydrate-rich (5% to 10%) or a fat-rich (0% to 3%) meal. The TEF value for alcohol is 10% to 30%.[10]

Protein foods have the highest TEF at 20% to 30% of the macronutrients. This means that if you eat 100 kcal of lean chicken breast, almost 30 of those calories (or 30%) are burned off (energy out) during the process of digestion. This is because it takes more energy to metabolize amino acids (from protein sources) into fat than to convert glucose (from carbohydrate sources) into glycogen or transfer absorbed fat into adipose stores. In sum, consuming a nutritious dietary pattern and engaging in regular physical activity are still the best way to increase your metabolism and burn extra calories.

✅ CONCEPT CHECK 7.1

1. What are the main components of energy balance?
2. How is the energy content of food determined and expressed?
3. What are the main purposes for which the body uses energy?
4. List three factors that increase and three factors that decrease basal metabolic rate.

7.2 Determination of Energy Use by the Body

Energy is required to sustain the body's various functions, including respiration, circulation, physical work, and protein synthesis. This energy is derived from dietary carbohydrates, proteins, fats, and to a lesser extent, alcohol. The amount of energy our body uses can be measured by both direct and indirect calorimetry or can be estimated based on height, weight, degree of physical activity, and age.

DIRECT AND INDIRECT CALORIMETRY

Direct calorimetry measures the amount of body heat released. To assess, an individual enters an insulated metabolic chamber (often the size of a small bedroom), and over the course of 24 hours, any body heat released raises the temperature of a layer of water surrounding the metabolic chamber. A calorie (kilocalorie), as you recall, is related to the amount of heat required to raise the temperature of water. By measuring the water temperature in the direct calorimeter before and after the body releases heat, the energy expended can be calculated. Direct calorimetry works because almost all the energy used by the body eventually leaves as heat. However, because of its expense and complexity, direct calorimetry is rarely used.

A more commonly used method to estimate calorie needs is **indirect calorimetry**. This technique measures the respiratory gas exchange, which is the amount of oxygen a person consumes and the amount of carbon dioxide expelled (Fig. 7-8). A relationship exists between the body's use of energy and oxygen. For example, when metabolizing a mixed dietary pattern of the energy-yielding nutrients (carbohydrate, fat, and protein), the human body uses 1 liter of oxygen to yield about 5 kcal of energy.

Instruments to measure oxygen consumption for indirect calorimetry are widely used, relatively inexpensive, and portable and can vary considerably in terms of their accuracy. They can be mounted on carts (metabolic carts) or carried in a backpack while a person engages in physical activity to measure how many calories are burned during these activities. Tables presenting energy costs of various forms of physical activity rely on information gained from indirect calorimetry studies. You will also see an estimation of calories burned during a workout on most exercise equipment and wearable fitness tracking devices.

direct calorimetry A method of determining a body's energy use by measuring heat released from the body. An insulated metabolic chamber is typically used.

indirect calorimetry A method to measure energy use by the body by measuring oxygen uptake and carbon dioxide output. Formulas are then used to convert this gas exchange value into energy use, estimating the proportion of energy nutrients that are being oxidized for energy in the fuel mix.

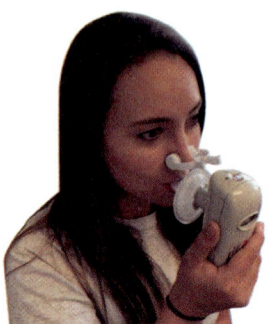

FIGURE 7-8 Indirect calorimetry measures oxygen intake and carbon dioxide output from respirations to predict energy expended during activities. Sarah Rusnak

ESTIMATES OF ENERGY NEEDS

Energy has no Recommended Dietary Allowance (RDA) nor a Tolerable Upper Intake Level (UL). Instead, the EER equation is used to predict appropriate energy intakes for individuals and groups. The Dietary Reference Intake (DRI) value for energy is the Estimated Energy Requirement (EER),[2] defined as the average dietary energy intake that is predicted to maintain energy balance in an adult. The EER calculation considers age, sex, weight, height, physical activity level, and life stage, consistent with maintaining health. And although this is a comprehensive tool, it remains just a prediction. We have limited data on how certain variables, such as dietary macronutrient composition, the gut microbiome, dietary fiber, and genetic factors, affect energy requirements throughout various life stages. See Appendix F for a complete set of EER equations for individuals at various stages of the life cycle.

> **Estimating Energy Requirements**
>
> The following is a sample calculation for a male who is 25 years old, 5 feet 9 inches (175 centimeters), and 154 pounds (70 kilograms) and has an active physical activity level. His EER is calculated as follows:
>
> EER = 1004.82 − (10.83 × age) + (6.52 × height) + (15.91 × weight)
>
> EER = 1004.82 − (10.83 × 25 years) + (6.52 × 175 cm) + (15.91 × 70 kg)
>
> EER = 1004.82 − 270.75 + 1141 + 113.70 = 2988.77 kcal

> **Track Your Energy Needs**
>
> Have you ever wondered how many calories you burn each day? Use *NutritionCalc Plus* (available in Connect) to estimate your usual energy expenditure. On the Activities tab in *NutritionCalc Plus*, enter all your activities (everything from sleeping to studying to eating to working out) for a 24-hour period. Be sure your activities for each day total 1440 minutes (i.e., 24 hours). Doing this for one or more days will help you get a personalized estimate of your usual energy expenditure.

The National Institutes of Health has a Body Weight Planner to help adults balance food and activities. This is a four-step online calculator that can be accessed at https://www.niddk.nih.gov/bwp.

The *Dietary Guidelines* also provides estimated calorie needs (Fig. 7-9) using activity levels and calorie recommendations for various age and sex groups. Visit https://www.myplate.gov/myplate-plan to get your own MyPlate Plan!

✓ CONCEPT CHECK 7.2

1. What methods can be used to measure energy use by the body?
2. Estimated Energy Requirement (EER) can be calculated based on what six factors?

7.3 Assessing Body Weight

Numerous methods are used to establish a person's healthy weight. Several tables exist, generally based on weight-for-height criteria. When applied to a population, they provide adequate estimates of weight associated with health and longevity; however, they do not indicate the healthiest body weight for an individual.

Healthy body weight is based upon many factors. Body weight must be considered in terms of overall health, not merely a mathematical calculation. Under the guidance of a registered dietitian nutritionist (RDN) or primary care provider, you can obtain estimates of your personal healthy weight based on weight and medical history, body fat distribution patterns, physical activity, dietary patterns, family history, and current health status.

Red flags that your body weight may be contributing to poor health or increasing your risk of disease include:

- Hypertension (high blood pressure)
- Hypercholesterolemia (high cholesterol)
- Family history of obesity or obesity-related diseases
- Upper-body (apple-shaped) android fat distribution
- Hyperglycemia (high blood sugar)

MyPlate Calorie Guidelines		
Children	**Sedentary** →	**Active**
2–3 years	1000 →	1400
Females	**Sedentary** →	**Active**
4–8 years	1200 →	1800
9–13	1400 →	2200
14–18	1800 →	2400
19–30	1800 →	2400
31–50	1800 →	2200
51+	1600 →	2200
Males	**Sedentary** →	**Active**
4–8 years	1200 →	2000
9–13	1600 →	2600
14–18	2000 →	3200
19–30	2400 →	3000
31–50	2200 →	3000
51+	2000 →	2800

FIGURE 7-9 *Dietary Guidelines for Americans* recommendations for estimated calorie needs per day by age, sex, and physical activity level.

Again, these criteria and current height/weight standards serve only as a rough estimate of health status. A healthy lifestyle may make a more important contribution to your overall health status than the number on your scale. Being fit and overweight are not necessarily mutually exclusive, and neither is *thin* synonymous with *healthy* if the person is not physically active.

BODY MASS INDEX

body mass index (BMI) Weight (in kilograms) divided by height (in meters) squared; a value of 25 and above indicates overweight, and a value of 30 and above indicates obesity.

The **body mass index (BMI)** considers body weight and height to calculate health risk. The concept of BMI is convenient to use because it is inexpensive, noninvasive, and easy to obtain, and the values apply to both sexes. However, any weight-for-height standard remains a very crude measure and does not consider body composition or fatness. For instance, a BMI of 25 to 29.9 is a marker of overweight (compared to a standard population) and not necessarily a marker of excessive body fatness.

TABLE 7-1 ■ Body Mass Index Categories

Category	BMI
Underweight	< 18.50
Severe thinness	< 16.00
Moderate thinness	16.00–16.99
Mild thinness	17.00–18.49
Normal	18.50–24.99
Overweight	≥ 25.00
Pre-obese	25.00–29.99
Obese	≥ 30.00
Obese class I	30.00–34.99
Obese class II	35.00–39.99
Obese class III	≥ 40.00

BMI categories should only be used as a screening tool and not for diagnostic purposes given individual and cultural variations exist.
Source: Adapted from World Health Organization 1995, 2000, 2004, and 2018.

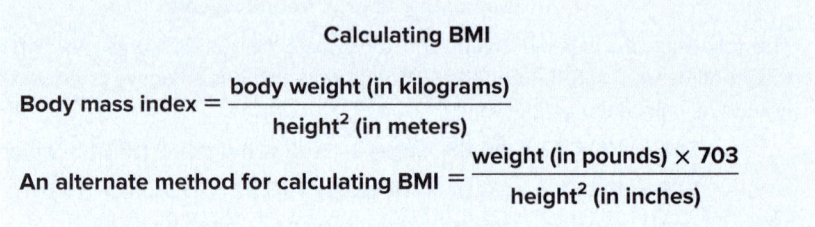

$$\text{Body mass index} = \frac{\text{body weight (in kilograms)}}{\text{height}^2 \text{ (in meters)}}$$

$$\text{An alternate method for calculating BMI} = \frac{\text{weight (in pounds)} \times 703}{\text{height}^2 \text{ (in inches)}}$$

The BMI weight classifications are shown in Table 7-1. A healthy weight for height is defined by a BMI between 18.5 and 24.9. Overweight- and obesity-related health risks increase when BMI is 25 or more (Fig. 7-10). Note these are general cutoff values for overweight and obesity respectively and, therefore, only provides estimated risk of nutrition-related disease. BMI is not a diagnostic tool.

Historically, body mass index (BMI) has been the most widely used weight-for-height standard because it is a noninvasive clinical measurement related to risk of disease for most individuals. Medical experts recommend that an individual's diagnosis of obesity should not be based solely on body weight or BMI but, rather, on the total amount of fat within the body, its location and distribution, and the presence or absence of weight-related medical conditions.

The American Medical Association acknowledged that BMI is primarily based on data from white people, even though body shape and composition vary among racial and ethnic groups, sexes, and age groups. There are subgroups where BMI is not useful. For instance, many athletic individuals have a BMI greater than 25 because lean body mass is more dense than fat mass. Also, adults under 5 feet tall may have a high BMI

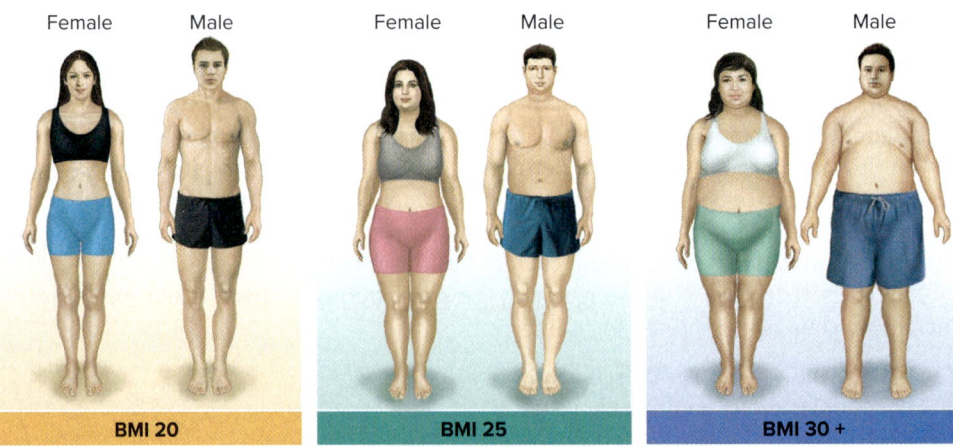

FIGURE 7-10 Estimates of body shapes at different BMI classifications.

that may not necessarily reflect overweight or fatness. Some ethnic groups, such as Asians, have higher health risks at lower BMIs.[11] Adult BMIs should not be applied to children, growing adolescents, older individuals who are frail, females during pregnancy or lactation, some ethnic groups, and individuals with higher lean body mass. BMI is interpreted differently in these cohorts and will be discussed throughout the relevant chapters.

Thankfully, views on proper weight and causes of obesity are changing along with new approaches to weight management. On the other end of the spectrum, medical experts also caution against an overemphasis of bodily thinness. Primary care providers are encouraged to avoid promoting dieting and instead focus on individualized approaches to determining the most appropriate body weight for patients.

ESTIMATING BODY COMPOSITION

Body composition varies widely among individuals. According to the American Council on Exercise, average amounts of body fat are about 18% to 24% for males and 25% to 31% for females. A higher range of body fat percentage for females is physiologically acceptable to maintain reproductive functions, including estrogen production. Males with over 25% body fat and females with over 32% body fat are typically categorized as obese. Now, let's examine some tools used to measure body composition in clinical settings.

Densitometry. To measure body fat content accurately, both body weight and body volume of the person are used to calculate body density. Body weight is easy to measure on a conventional scale. Of the typical methods used to estimate body volume, **underwater (hydrostatic) weighing** remains quite accurate (Fig. 7-11).

Air displacement (Bod Pod®) is another method of determining body volume. Body volume is quantified by measuring the space a person takes up inside a measurement chamber (Fig. 7-12).

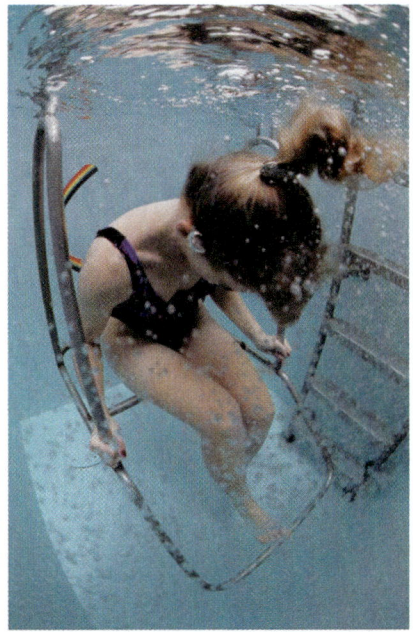

FIGURE 7-11 Underwater (hydrostatic) weighing. This procedure requires that an individual be totally submerged in a tank of water, with a trained technician directing the procedure. This technique determines body volume using the difference between conventional body weight and body weight measured while submerged under water and the relative densities of fat tissue and lean tissue. David Madison/Getty Images

underwater (hydrostatic) weighing This is a method of estimating total body fat by weighing the individual on a standard scale, then weighing the individual again submerged in water. The difference between the two weights is used to estimate total body volume. Also known as *hydrodensitometry*.

air displacement A method for estimating body composition that makes use of the volume of space taken up by a body inside a small chamber (Bod Pod®). This tool is also known as *air displacement plethysmography*.

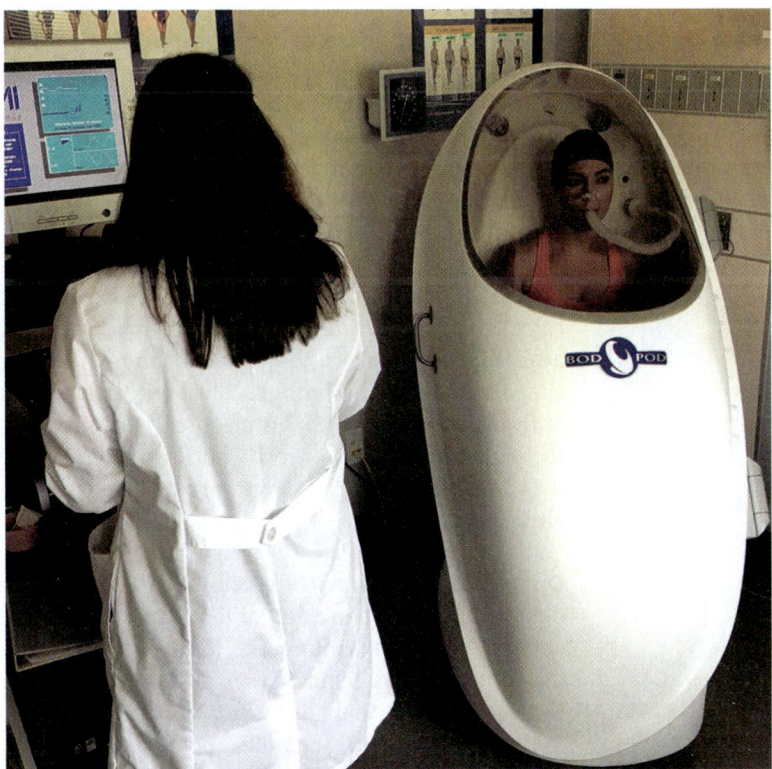

FIGURE 7-12 Bod Pod®. This device determines body volume based on the volume of displaced air, measured as a person sits in a sealed chamber. Sarah Rusnak

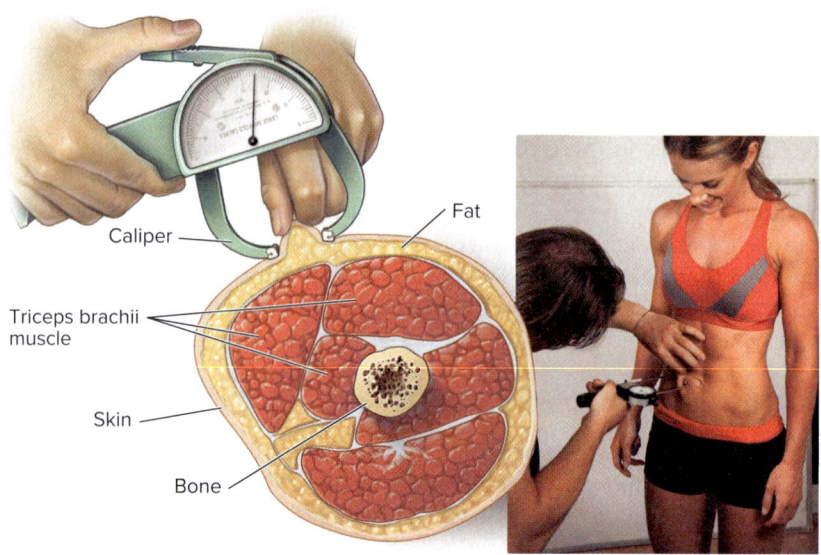

FIGURE 7-13 Skinfold measurements. With proper technique and calibrated equipment, skinfold measurements taken at various body sites can be used to predict body fat content in about 10 minutes. Ian Thraves/Alamy Stock Photo

skinfold measurements Skinfold or caliper testing is a common method to determine body fat percentage. This utilizes prediction equations that are population-specific to estimate fat.

Skinfold Measures. **Skinfold measurements** are also a common anthropometric method to estimate total body fat content, although there are some limits to its accuracy. Clinicians use skinfold calipers to measure the fat layer directly under the skin at multiple sites and then plug these values into a mathematical formula (Fig. 7-13). The most common measurements are made at the triceps, biceps, abdomen, and thigh, then compared to standards for adult males and females across different stages of the life cycle.

bioelectrical impedance analysis (BIA) The method to estimate total body fat that uses a low-energy electrical current. The more fat storage a person has, the more impedance (resistance) to electrical flow will be exhibited.

dual energy X-ray absorptiometry (DXA) A scientific tool used to measure bone mineral density and body composition.

Bioelectrical Impedance Analysis. The measurement of **bioelectrical impedance analysis (BIA)** is also used to estimate body fat. This procedure sends a painless, low-energy, and safe electrical current through the body to estimate body fat (Fig. 7-14). This estimation is based on the assumption that adipose (fat) tissue has proportionately greater electrical resistance than lean tissue. Within a few seconds, bioelectrical impedance analyzers convert body electrical resistance into an approximate estimate of total body fat, as long as hydration is adequate in the person being measured.

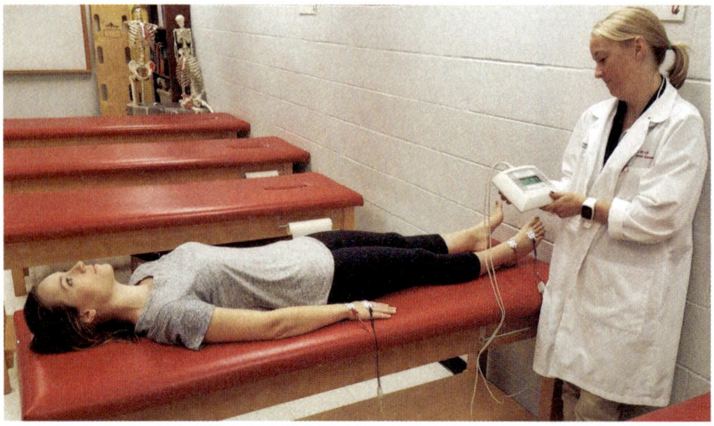

Body composition monitors, better known as body fat calculators, which use bioelectric impedance, are now available for home use. These machines are similar in shape and use to bathroom scales, but their main purpose is to measure body fat. An electrical current passes easily through conductive foot pads and/or handheld electrodes. It is important to know that varying hydration levels can alter the results.

FIGURE 7-14 Bioelectrical impedance. This estimates total body fat in less than 5 minutes. This device sends an electrical current through the body and gives a percentage of body fat when it has completed its process. Sarah Rusnak

Dual Energy X-ray Absorptiometry. A more advanced determination of body fat content can be made using **dual energy X-ray absorptiometry (DXA)**. DXA is considered one of the most accurate ways to determine body fat, but the equipment is expensive and not widely available. This X-ray-based system separates body weight into distinct components: fat, fat-free soft tissue, and bone mineral. Additional software can determine segmental body fat distribution. An assessment of bone mineral density and the risk of osteoporosis can also be made using DXA (Fig. 7-15). The typical whole-body scan requires about 10 to 25 minutes, and the dose of radiation is less than a chest X-ray.

There are other methods of assessing body composition, but those detailed here are the most commonly used in health clinics, fitness centers, and research. In the hands of a trained clinician, these assessments provide valuable information about body fat beyond simple measures of height and weight.

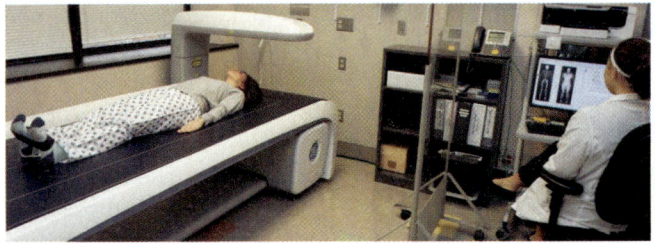

FIGURE 7-15 Dual energy X-ray absorptiometry (DXA). The scanner arm moves from head to toe and, in doing so, can determine body fat and bone density. Sarah Rusnak

BODY FAT DISTRIBUTION

In addition to the amount of fat we store, the location of that body fat is an important predictor of health risks. Some people store fat in upper-body areas, whereas others store fat lower on the body. Recall that upper-body obesity, characterized by a large abdomen or waist, is more often called *abdominal, visceral,* or *central* obesity and is related to insulin resistance and a fatty liver leading to chronic diseases. Because males typically develop upper-body obesity, it is also known as *android* obesity. While other adipose cells empty fat into general blood circulation, the fat released from abdominal adipose cells goes directly to the liver, by way of the portal vein. This influx of fat interferes with the liver's ability to use insulin and negatively affects lipoprotein metabolism by the liver. These upper-body adipose cells are not just storage depots; they are metabolically active cells that release many hormones and other cellular signals involved in long-term energy regulation. When they fill with excess fat, the cells become dysfunctional, resulting in inflammation, insulin resistance, and other adverse health conditions leading to chronic disease. High testosterone levels, excessive alcohol intake, and smoking all promote upper-body obesity. This pattern of fat storage is commonly known as the *apple shape* given individuals are characterized by a large abdomen and small buttocks and thighs (Fig. 7-16).

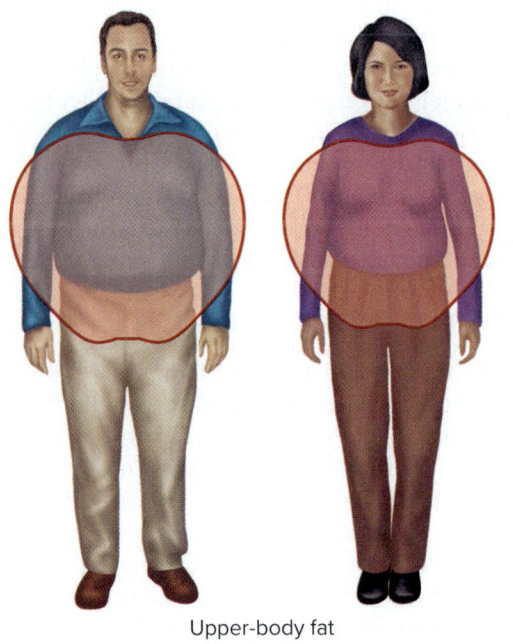

Upper-body fat distribution
(android: apple shape)

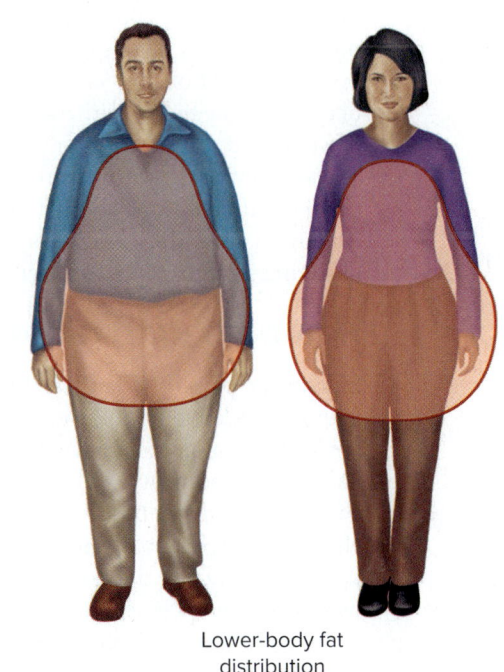

Lower-body fat distribution
(gynoid: pear shape)

FIGURE 7-16 Body fat stored primarily in the upper body (android) brings higher risks of obesity-related diseases than lower-body (gynoid) obesity. A waist circumference > 40 for males and > 35 for females indicates increased risk of disease.

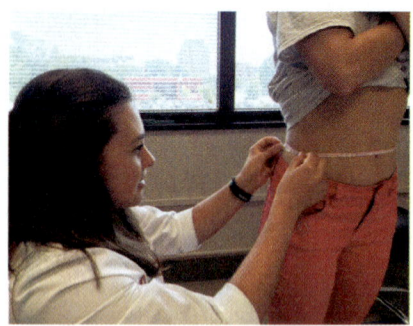

FIGURE 7-17 Waist circumference. This is a measure of weight-related health risk. Note there are multiple protocols to measure waist circumference. Sarah Rusnak

lower-body obesity The type of obesity in which fat storage is primarily located in the buttocks and thigh area. Also known as *gynoid* or *gynecoid obesity*.

identical twins Two offspring that develop from a single ovum and sperm and, consequently, are born with the same genetic makeup.

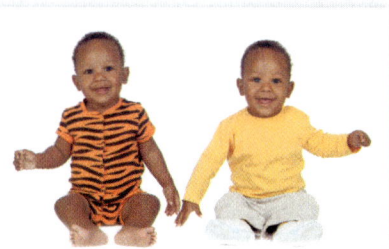

Studies in identical twins give us insight into the genetic contribution to obesity. **Does nature or nurture play a larger role in adult body weight?** José Manuel Gelpi Díaz/Melba Photo Agency/Alamy Stock Photo

Upper-body obesity is assessed by measuring the circumference of the abdomen at the waist. A waist circumference more than 40 inches (102 centimeters) in males and more than 35 inches (88 centimeters) in females indicates risk for upper-body obesity (Fig. 7-17). The combination of a large waist circumference and a BMI of 25 or more significantly increases health risks.

The other classification is **lower-body obesity**—the typical female pattern correlated with estrogen and progesterone hormone levels. The small abdomen and much larger buttocks and thighs give a *pear shape* appearance. Fat deposited in the lower body is not mobilized as easily as android fat cells and often resists being released. After menopause, blood estrogen levels fall, encouraging greater upper-body fat distribution and raising the risk of chronic disease for postmenopausal females.

✓ CONCEPT CHECK 7.3

1. How is body mass index (BMI) determined? What are the limitations of BMI?
2. What are the BMI, body fat percentage, and waist circumference values for males and females that are associated with increased risk of health problems related to being overweight or obese?
3. List three methods by which body composition can be estimated.

7.4 Nature Versus Nurture

The energy imbalance that promotes weight gain (positive energy balance) stems from many factors, including individual characteristics and behaviors in addition to one's environment, culture, and social and economic status.[4] Many studies of obesity attribute increasing trends to the growth of the global food system, including advancements in energy-dense food processing, persuasive marketing, and the widespread availability of more affordable and accessible energy-dense foods.

Both genetic (nature) and environmental (nurture) factors increase the risk for obesity (Table 7-2). Both nature and nurture may help explain why offspring born to mothers affected by obesity are at heightened risk of obesity later in life. Consider the possibility that obesity is nurture allowing nature to express itself. Some people with obesity may begin life with a slower basal metabolism (genetic) but maintain a sedentary lifestyle and consume highly refined, calorie-dense dietary patterns (environment). These individuals are nurtured into gaining weight, promoting their natural genetic predisposition toward obesity. Even with a genetic tendency toward obesity, individuals can attain a healthier body weight by engaging in positive lifestyle behaviors including engaging in regular physical activity and adopting nutrient-dense dietary patterns.

HOW DOES NATURE CONTRIBUTE TO WEIGHT MANAGEMENT?

Studies in pairs of **identical twins** provide insight into the contribution of nature (genetics) relative to obesity. Even when identical twins are raised apart with different environmental and behavioral influences, they tend to show similar weight gain patterns, in both overall weight and body fat distribution. A child with no biologic parent affected by obesity has approximately a 10% chance of becoming obese. When a child has one parent affected by obesity, that risk increases to 40%, and with two parents having obesity, the risk soars to 80%.[12] Our genes play a role in our metabolic rate, fuel use, and differences in brain chemistry—all of which ultimately affect body weight.

In early human history, our genes adapted to an environment where food was sometimes scarce; thus, a metabolism that efficiently stored fat would have been a safeguard against starvation in times of famine. Now, with a constant overabundance of accessible food, we require wise food choices and regular physical activity to maintain energy balance. This so-called *thrifty* metabolism enables us to store fat more readily.[13] So depending on genetic traits we inherit from our parents, some of us are more prone to weight gain in the modern food environment than others.

TABLE 7-2 ■ Factors That Encourage Excess Body Fat Stores and Obesity

Factor	How Fat Storage Is Affected
Age	Excess body fat is more common in adults over 60 years of age due to loss of lean body mass and often a reduction in physical activity.
Basal metabolism	A low BMR due to factors such as genetics, thyroid problems, or energy restriction is linked to weight gain.
Childbearing years	A pattern of excessive weight gain during the childbearing years can occur to support a fetus. Fat stored during pregnancy to support lactation may not be fully lost in females who do not breastfeed.
Energy balance	Over time, dietary patterns consistent with positive energy balance promote storage of excess body fat.
Ethnicity	In some groups, higher body weight is socially acceptable.
Fat uptake	Fat storage efficiency is higher in some individuals and may even increase with weight loss.
Genetics	Genetic factors may affect metabolism, energy expenditure, deposition of adipose tissue or lean tissue, satiety, and the relative proportion of fuels used by the body.
Hunger sensations	Blunted satiety mechanisms may alter brain signals involved in food reward pathways.
Medications	Changes in hunger and appetite can be a side effect of many medications.
Menopause	Hormonal changes result in increased abdominal fat deposition.
Physical activity	Sedentary behavior promotes positive energy balance and body fat storage.
Ratio of fat to lean tissue	A high ratio of fat mass to lean body mass is correlated with weight gain.
Residence	Regional environmental and lifestyle differences, such as calorie-laden diets and sedentary lifestyles, especially in the South and Midwest, are associated with higher rates of obesity.
Sex	Females have more fat mass than males due to less lean body mass and reduced surface area (height).
Social and behavioral factors	Obesity is associated with socioeconomic status, environment, social networks, obesogenic dietary patterns, sedentary lifestyles, smoking cessation, excessive alcohol intake, and frequency dining out.
Thermic effect of food	Some individuals are efficient metabolizers and thus expend fewer calories for digestion and absorption.

We also inherit specific body types. Tall, thin people typically have an inherently easier time maintaining healthy body weight. This is likely due to the fact that BMR increases as body surface increases; therefore, people who are taller utilize more calories than people who are shorter, even at rest. Although we cannot overlook the impact of nurture, it appears that nature is a strong influencer of body weight and body composition.

Influences on Weight. The **set-point theory** of weight maintenance proposes that humans have a genetically predetermined body weight or body fat content, which the body closely regulates.[14] Several physiological changes that occur during calorie reduction and weight loss support this theory. For example, research suggests that the hypothalamus monitors the amount of body fat in humans and tries to keep that amount constant over time. The release and circulation of the hormone leptin, from adipose cells, promotes satiety and a sense of fullness, thus reducing appetite. As adipose cells increase in size and number, overall production of leptin increases, which should suppress appetite. If fat mass is reduced, leptin levels are reduced, so appetite should be increased. This system, however, is not foolproof. Research has shown that persons who are overweight can have large amounts of leptin coming from the excess body fat, but their brains seem to be leptin resistant and are not receiving a functional signal to stop eating.

Thyroid hormone levels change in relation to body composition, too. When calorie intake is reduced, the blood concentration of thyroid hormones falls, which slows BMR. Also, the calorie cost of weight-bearing activity decreases, so an activity that burned 100 kcal before weight loss may only burn 90 kcal after weight loss. Furthermore, as

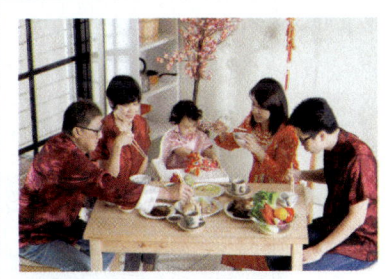

Body weight is influenced by many factors related to both nature and nurture. **Thinking back to your childhood, what influences do you think impacted your current weight?** szefei/123RF

set-point theory Theory of weight status that refers to the close regulation of body weight. Although the details remain unclear, there is evidence that complex mechanisms exist that help regulate weight.

magnificent microbiome

Appetite

Think of the possibilities.... What if you could regulate your appetite by simply flipping a switch! Now, researchers are doing just that with engineered mice. For some time, we have known that our brains influence hunger and appetite. Now we have growing evidence that our gut microbes are also involved. The gut-brain axis refers to the bidirectional communication between the GI tract and the brain that affects appetite and metabolism. Understanding the key mechanisms by which the gut microbiota can influence appetite and metabolism can provide clues to implement effective treatments for obesity, eating disorders, and other metabolic conditions.

Source: Han H, Yi B, Zhong R, et al. From gut microbiota to host appetite: gut microbiota-derived metabolites as key regulators. *Microbiome*. 2021 Jul 20;9(1):162. doi: 10.1186/s40168-021-01093-y

weight loss occurs, the body becomes more efficient at storing fat by increasing the activity of the enzyme lipoprotein lipase, which permits fat entry into cells. All of these changes protect the body from losing weight.

If a person overeats, in the short term the BMR tends to increase. This causes some resistance to weight gain. In the long run, however, resistance to weight gain is much less than resistance to weight loss. When a person gains weight and stays at a stable weight for some time, the body tends to establish energy balance at a new set point.

Opponents of the set-point theory argue that weight does not remain constant throughout adulthood: the average person gains weight slowly through old age. Also, if an individual is placed in a different social, emotional, or physical environment, weight can be altered and maintained at a markedly higher or lower point. These arguments suggest that humans, rather than having a set point determined by genetics or the number of adipose cells, settle into a particular stable weight based on their circumstances, often regarded as a settling point.

DOES NURTURE PLAY A ROLE?

Environmental factors, such as consuming an energy-dense dietary pattern and failing to meet physical activity guidelines, literally shape us. This seems reasonable when we consider that our gene pool has not significantly changed in the past century, yet the ranks of people having obesity have grown to epidemic proportions.

Some would argue that body weight similarities between family members stem more from learned behaviors than genetic similarities. Even couples, who have no genetic link, may behave similarly toward food and eventually assume similar degrees of leanness or fatness. Adult obesity is correlated with childhood obesity.

Is poverty associated with obesity? Ironically, in developed nations the answer is yes. North Americans of lower socioeconomic status, especially mothers who are single, are more likely to be affected by obesity than those of higher socioeconomic status. Several social and behavioral factors promote fat storage and support the link between socioeconomic status and obesity. These factors may include social networks afflicted by overweight, a cultural or ethnic group that prefers higher body weight, a lifestyle that discourages healthy meals and adequate physical activity, easy availability of inexpensive energy-dense foods, limited access to fresh fruits and vegetables, excessive screen time, lack of adequate sleep, emotional stress, meals frequently eaten away from home, and inadequate access to health care.

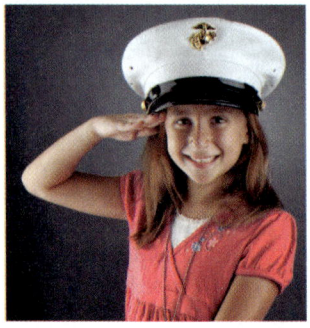

The U.S. military acknowledges overweight and obesity as serious threats to our nation. Over 70% of potential recruits between the ages of 17 and 24 currently do not qualify for military service, and obesity accounts for over 30% of those disqualified. Promoting healthy dietary and physical activity patterns is paramount to ensuring that all children grow up healthy, and that military enlistees are prepared to meet the strict eligibility requirements. Straight 8 Photography/Shutterstock

Source: Maxey H, Bishop-Josef S, Goodman B; Council for a Strong America; Mission: Readiness. Unhealthy and unprepared: national security depends on promoting healthy lifestyles from an early age. October 2018. Accessed October 21, 2023. https://www.strongnation.org/articles/737-unhealthy-and-unprepared

✓ CONCEPT CHECK 7.4

1. List three factors that promote energy imbalance.
2. Explain how body weight is influenced by nature (genetics).
3. What role does nurture (environment) play in determining body weight?

7.5 Energy Balance Throughout the Life Course

Following a healthy dietary pattern, engaging in regular physical activity, and managing body weight are critical during all life stages. As you learned earlier, the average female (ages 19 through 30) requires about 1800 to 2400 kcal/day. Males in this age group need about 2400 to 3000 kcal/day. Calorie needs for adults ages 31 through 59 are generally lower, with females requiring about 1600 to 2200 kcal/day and males requiring about 2200 to 3000 kcal/day.[15] A goal of losing 1 pound of stored fat per week may require reducing energy intake by 500 kcal per day (or increasing energy output) initially.

The primary determinant of weight loss is the number of calories you consume, exerting a more substantial influence than the proportions of macronutrients (carbohydrates, fat, or protein) in your dietary pattern.[16] Weight loss occurs with an energy deficit over time. Of course, various *experts* offer recommendations, such as reducing saturated fat, minimizing added sugars, or elevating protein intake. Currently, the prevailing evidence supports the idea that a nutritious dietary pattern, predominantly plant-based and high in fiber, combined with regular physical activity, offers the most effective strategy for sustained body fat reduction and weight maintenance.

Portion control is another challenge that influences our calorie intake and requires a change in our approach to eating. As you learned in Chapter 2, the concept of energy density can help you choose more nutrient-rich foods with fewer calories per gram. With this technique, you can fill your plate with larger portions of foods with high nutrient density and low energy density. Fruits and vegetables are great examples of low energy-dense foods (low in calories but high in water, fiber, and key nutrients) that promote satiety. Stone fruits are featured in the *Farm to Fork* and are a great example of a low energy-dense fruit.

One way to monitor calorie intake at the start of a weight-reduction program is by reading Nutrition Facts labels. Label reading is critical because many foods are more energy dense than people realize (Fig. 7-18). With knowledge of current calorie intake, future food choices can be adjusted as needed. The *Newsworthy Nutrition* in this chapter also documents that adopting a healthy plant-based dietary pattern may reduce weight gain over time. In addition, the *Roots* feature highlights the Asian Diet Pyramid. This dietary pattern is rich in plants and tradition!

CONTROLLING HUNGER

A challenge to most weight-loss programs is to regulate appetite while eating less and engaging in more physical

FARM to FORK — Stone Fruits

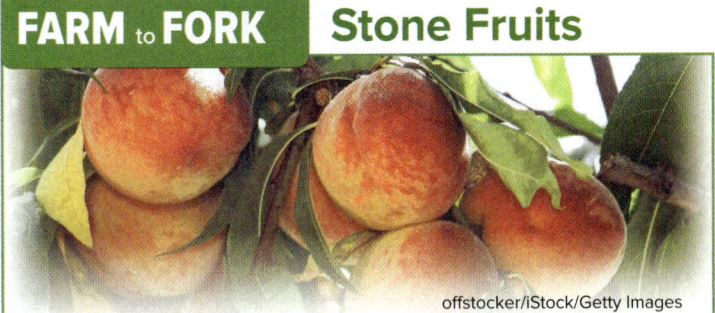
offstocker/iStock/Getty Images

Stone fruits, such as peaches, nectarines, apricots, cherries, and plums, are soft-fleshed fruits with a hard (*stone*) seed. These fruits can contribute to a sound weight management plan while providing key nutrients.

Grow
- The best time to plant stone fruit trees is in winter, when they are dormant. They prefer cold winters and warm, dry summers to produce flowers and fruit.
- Dwarf or semi-dwarf fruit trees allow those with small yards to grow stone fruits. Most trees produce their first viable crops after 3 to 4 years.
- Harvest stone fruits, such as peaches, at a U-pick orchard for fruit picked at the height of ripeness.

Shop
- While the most flavorful stone fruits are locally grown and harvested when ripe, shipped fruits are often harvested prior to ripening and exposed to cold temperatures, resulting in mealy, leathery, and dry fruit.
- Choose stone fruit that is dent-free and without bruises. Ripe stone fruit has a slight give when gently pressed between your palms.
- Select peaches and nectarines by their background color, not their blush. White-fleshed peaches and nectarines are higher in antioxidants than the yellow varieties, and the less common red-flesh, or blood, peaches are the most nutritious.
- When selecting cherries, look for bright green and flexible stems. Darker cherries contain higher levels of anthocyanins and can reduce inflammation.
- Apricots are one of the most nutritious stone fruits; deep orange and red dried apricots pack the most nutrients.
- Dark skins and flesh of plums have more anthocyanins. Dried plums (also known as prunes) are highly nutritious and rich in both soluble and insoluble fibers and have a reputation for relieving constipation.

Store
- Store cherries in a microperforated plastic bag (with pin-size holes to allow moisture to escape) in the crisper drawer to allow gas exchange and decrease oxidation.
- For long-term storage of stone fruits, freezing preserves more antioxidants than canning. Before freezing, slice the fruit and sprinkle with lemon juice and sugar to retain the highest levels of nutrients and prevent browning.

Prep
- Dried plums (prunes) are an excellent source of antioxidants and have been linked to everything from reduced inflammation to bone health. To stew prunes, cover with water in a saucepan, bring to a boil, then reduce heat to simmer for 20 minutes. Add a sprinkle of sugar or slice of lemon for flavor.
- Eating the skin will provide the most fiber and nutrients. To de-fuzz stone fruits, wipe gently with a clean cloth.
- If frozen, thaw stone fruits in the microwave to retain the most antioxidants.

Source: Robinson J. Stone fruits: time for a flavor revival. In: *Eating on the Wild Side: The Missing Link to Optimum Health*. New York: Little, Brown & Co.; 2013.

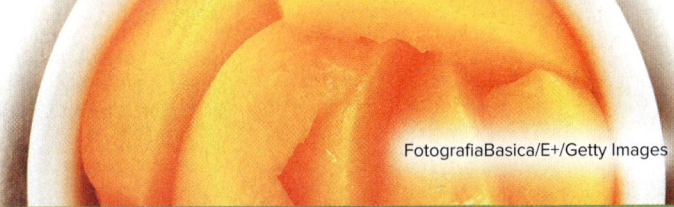
FotografiaBasica/E+/Getty Images

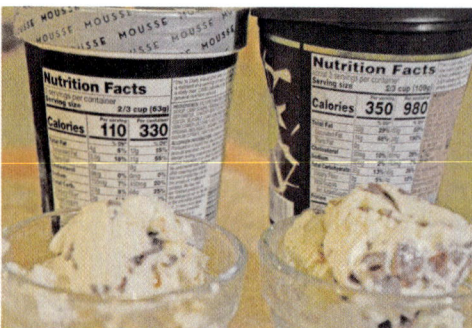

FIGURE 7-18 Reading labels helps you choose more nutrient-dense foods and beverages. Which of these frozen desserts is the better choice, per 2/3-cup serving? The percent Daily Values are based on a 2000 kcal diet. Mary-Jon Ludy/McGraw Hill

Newsworthy Nutrition

Plant-based dietary patterns are associated with improved weight management

INTRODUCTION: Beneficial health effects, including weight loss, have been documented with the adoption of healthy plant-focused dietary patterns.
OBJECTIVE: The purpose of this *cohort study* was to examine the associations between three plant-based dietary patterns (overall, healthful, and unhealthful) with weight change over 4-year intervals spanning more than 20 years. The hypothesis of this study was that healthful plant-based dietary patterns would promote healthier body weight. **METHODS:** Self-reported data from over 126,000 adults from the Nurses' Health Study (NHS & NHS2) and the Health Professionals Follow-Up Study (HPFS) were collected every 4 years to assess the effect of diet quality over time on body weight. **RESULTS:** Study participants gained an average of 0.90 kg (1.98 lbs.) to 1.98 kg (4.36 lbs.) over 4-year intervals. Those following a healthful version of a plant-based dietary pattern (emphasizing whole grains, fruits/vegetables, nuts/legumes, vegetable oils, tea/coffee) were associated with significantly less weight gain over 4-year periods ($p < 0.001$). Conversely, those following an unhealthful version of a plant-based dietary pattern (emphasizing refined grains, potatoes/fries, sweets, sweetened drinks/juices) were associated with significantly more weight gain over 4-year periods (0.36 kg/0.79 lb., $p < 0.001$). **CONCLUSION:** Plant-based dietary patterns that are rich in healthier plant foods are associated with less weight gain over 4-year intervals than overall or unhealthful plant based patterns.

Source: Satija A, Malik V, Rimm EB, Sacks F, Willett W, Hu FB. Changes in intake of plant-based diets and weight change: results from 3 prospective cohort studies. *Am J Clin Nutr.* 2019 Sep 1;110(3):574-582. doi: 10.1093/ajcn/nqz049

Roots

Asian Diet Pyramid

The Asian Diet Pyramid covers a large geographic and culinary base with Bangladesh, Cambodia, China, India, Indonesia, Japan, Laos, Malaysia, Mongolia, Myanmar, Nepal, North Korea, Philippines, Singapore, South Korea, Taiwan, Thailand, and Vietnam included. Asian countries enjoy dietary patterns rich in vegetables, spices, seafood, rice and noodles, and tofu and soy-based products. Yet despite the regional variations, rice remains a staple of many dishes in Asian countries—often found fermented in alcoholic drinks and in confections like candy and cakes. Compare the Asian Diet Pyramid in Figure 7-19 with the *Dietary Guidelines*. What similarities and differences are most notable?

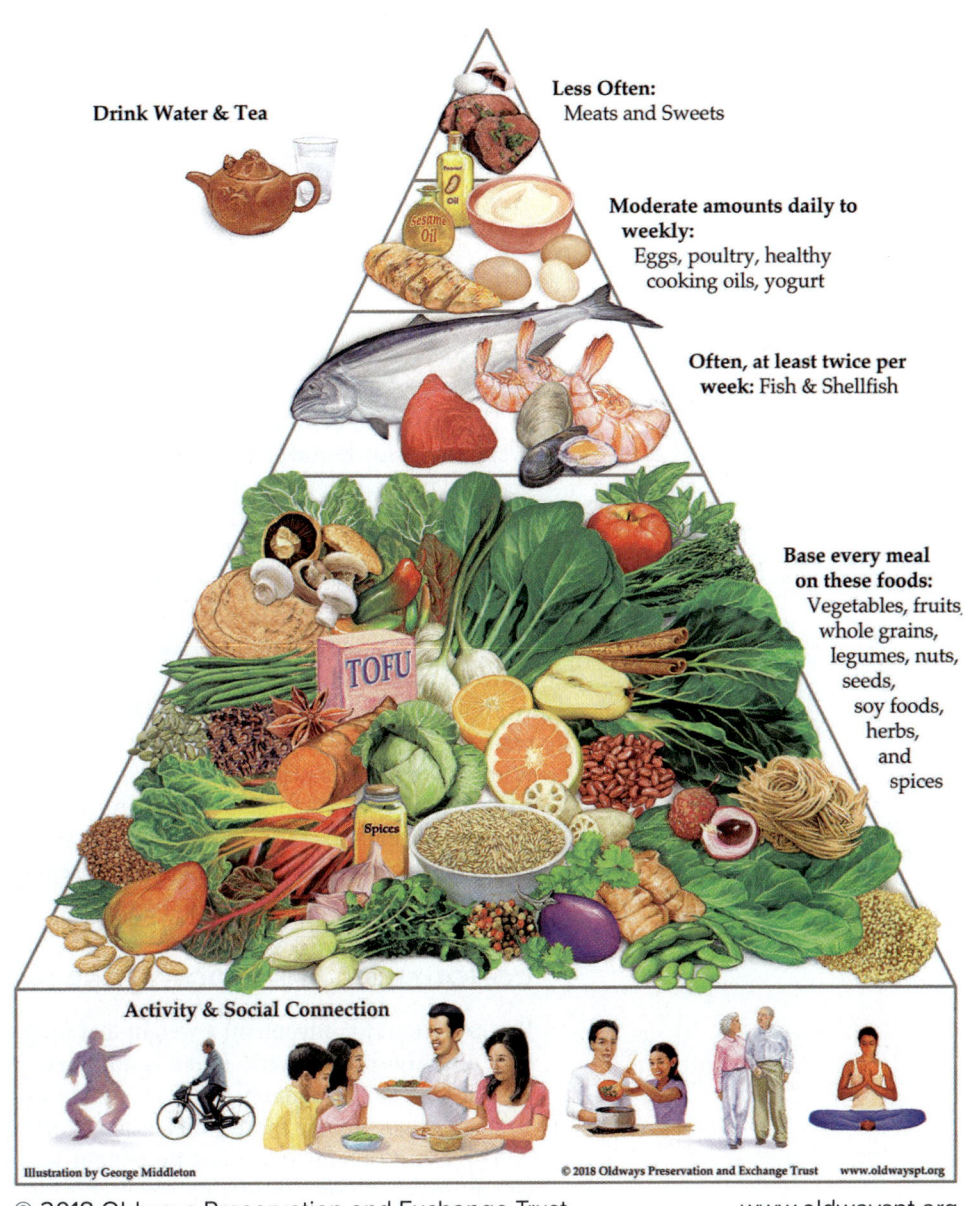

© 2018 Oldways Preservation and Exchange Trust   www.oldwayspt.org

FIGURE 7-19 The Asian Diet Pyramid is based on dietary patterns from the Asian region.
Source: Oldways

activity. Separating true hunger from habit or emotional eating is the first step toward controlling the drive to eat that can sabotage eating patterns. Hormones and your nervous system tell you when you are hungry. The blood hormones, along with an empty stomach, signal the brain that you are hungry. Likewise, nerves in the stomach signal the brain when you are full, but it can take up to 20 minutes for these satiety signals to reach the brain.

TABLE 7-3 ■ Saving Calories: Ideas for Getting Started

Kcal Saving	By Choosing This . . .	Instead of This . . .
45 kcal	1 cup 1% milk	1 cup whole milk
80 kcal	2 slices whole wheat toast	1 whole wheat bagel
120 kcal	1 cup broth-based vegetable soup	1 cup cream-based vegetable soup
120 kcal	3 oz lean beef	3 oz marbled beef
120 kcal	1 cup plain popcorn	1 oz potato chips
155 kcal	12 oz water	12 oz regular soft drink
260 kcal	1 apple	1 slice apple pie
290 kcal	1 English muffin	1 Danish pastry
380 kcal	1 roasted chicken breast	1 batter-fried chicken breast

The goal is to be hungry at mealtime but not so ravenous that you are tempted to overeat. Eat slowly and stop eating when you are comfortably full. If you are craving food between meals, determine if you are feeling true hunger; if you are, then choose a small, high-fiber snack (like a handful of nuts) to satisfy you until the next meal. Including lean protein (low-fat dairy, soy protein, or lean meat, fish, or chicken) in meals and snacks will also keep hunger at bay. Eating high-volume foods that are rich in water and fiber (like fresh fruit) will provide bulk with fewer calories, fill your stomach, and send satiety signals to the brain. Drinking a glass of water can also help decrease hunger sensations between meals.

Table 7-3 shows some simple strategies to reduce energy intake. As you should realize, it is best to consider healthy eating as a lifestyle pattern, rather than a fad diet or rapid weight-loss plan. Also, liquids deserve attention because liquid calories do not appear to stimulate satiety mechanisms to the same extent as solid foods. In terms of artificial sweeteners, the World Health Organization (WHO) has advised against the use of non-sugar sweeteners to control weight, citing a lack of evidence that these products have any long-term weight loss benefits.[17]

CONQUERING THE WEIGHT-LOSS PLATEAU

It is important for anyone on a weight-loss program to know that healthy weight loss is slow and sometimes erratic, and it is normal to reach a weight-loss plateau. After losing weight for weeks, suddenly weight loss may stop abruptly. Fortunately, there are some strategies to overcome these plateaus and start obtaining results again.

There are several reasons why weight loss may stall. During the first part of a weight-loss program, individuals are typically losing fluid in addition to fat, causing a weight loss larger than the expected 1 to 2 pounds per week. Because a healthy weight-loss program is designed to reduce fat rather than muscle or fluid loss, your weight loss will begin to slow after the first week or so. The level of calorie deprivation needed to lose weight is hard to maintain, and you may begin to eat a few more calories. This calorie creep can contribute to the weight-loss plateau and eventually lead to weight gain. When this happens, it is important to go back to tracking your calories by recording what you eat and drink and weighing yourself frequently.

Another possible reason for the weight-loss plateau is that your metabolism is adjusting to your lower calorie intake. In this case, it may be time to reduce your calories somewhat and drink plenty of water. Your metabolism may also be adapting to your physical activity routine. Varying the intensity of your workout routine, therefore, will help your muscles burn more calories and can help get you past the weight plateau. Strength training, along with the calorie-burning physical activities, is important to build muscle mass, which ultimately uses more calories for metabolism. Try not to get discouraged during this time. Simply stay the course while your body adjusts and continue your healthy behaviors!

✅ CONCEPT CHECK 7.5

1. What MyPlate food groups are the best examples of low-energy-dense foods that promote satiety?
2. What mechanisms are involved in hunger control?
3. Why can weight-loss plateaus occur, and what strategies can be used to overcome these plateaus?

7.6 Physical Activity Promotes Weight Management

Adults who engage in regular physical activity are healthier, feel better, and are less likely to develop chronic disease than adults who are inactive.[15] Regular physical activity can provide both immediate and long-term benefits ranging from improving sleep to reducing stress to improving bone health. All adults should move more and sit less, and ANY physical activity is better than none. The greatest health benefits are realized with at least 150 to 300 minutes of moderate-intensity aerobic activity each week. Muscle-strengthening activities, like lifting weights or doing push-ups, should be included at least 2 days each week (Fig. 7-20).

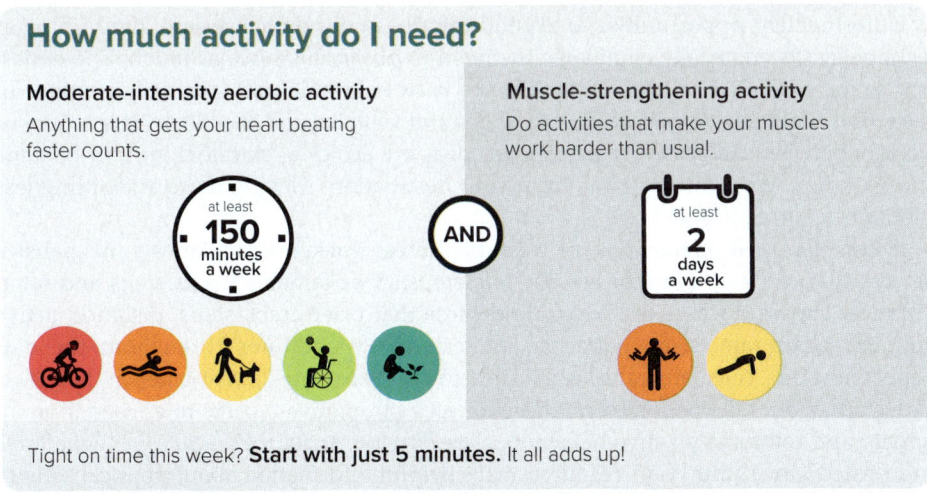

FIGURE 7-20 CDC physical activity recommendations: amount of activity recommended for healthy adults.
Source: CDC

TABLE 7-4 ■ Approximate Calorie Costs of Various Activities and Specific Calorie Costs Projected for a 150-Pound (68 kg) Person

Activity	Kcal per kg per Hour	Total kcal per Hour
Basketball	6.0	408
Cycling (12–13 mph)	8.0	544
Dancing	3.0	204
Housework	3.0	204
Jumping rope	8.0	544
Rowing machine	7.0	476
Running (10-minute mile)	10.0	680
Sitting	1.0	68
Swimming	7.0	476
Walking (3.5 mph, brisk pace)	3.8	258
Weight training	3.0	204

The values above refer to total energy expenditure, including that needed to perform the physical activity, plus that needed for basal metabolism, the thermic effect of food, and thermogenesis.

Source: Physical Activity Calorie Counter at https://www.acefitness.org/education-and-resources/lifestyle/tools-calculators/physical-activity-calorie-counter/

Physical activity should be enjoyable so that it becomes part of a healthy pattern of living. Moving your body expends calories and will promote health and result in weight loss and maintenance over time (Table 7-4). If you can't squeeze in 30 minutes a day, try shorter bouts of activity in 5- to 10-minute intervals. Muscle-strengthening activities will increase and retain lean body mass. As lean muscle mass increases, so will your BMR. Remember, all movement counts!

Unfortunately, opportunities to expend calories in our daily lives are diminishing as technology systematically eliminates the need to physically move as much. The easiest way to increase physical activity is to make it an enjoyable part of a daily routine. To start, one might pack a pair of athletic shoes and walk around the block after school or work or between classes every day. Other ideas are avoiding elevators in favor of stairs and parking the car farther away from your destination. Moving more and sitting less should be your daily goal!

Pedometers, cell phone apps, or wearable fitness trackers are relatively inexpensive devices that can help monitor activity and steps. A pedometer tracks steps and often distance. Fitness trackers are wearable devices that often track steps, distance, active minutes, heart rate, sleep patterns, and calorie expenditures throughout the day. Fitness trackers calculate calories by measuring heart rate, sweat rate, or heat loss and production. Like pedometers, these devices can motivate users to engage in more activity and reinforce positive behaviors. The *Physical Activity Guidelines for Americans* and related Move Your Way® resources have helpful information about physical activity and tips on how to get started at health.gov/paguidelines.

Calorie Estimation on Fitness Machines

The control panel of fitness machines will typically display time, speed, distance covered, and calories burned. Time, speed, and distance are generally accurate values, but calories burned is a rough estimate based on the weight you enter before you start your workout. The calories burned are estimates that are not completely accurate because they do not consider factors other than weight, such as body fat percentage, fitness level, form, and fitness efficiency.

The accuracy of wearable and optically based heart rate monitors is variable and depends on the type of physical activity. It appears most reliable on some treadmills and less reliable on elliptical trainers. Chest monitors with electrodes worn to obtain accurate heart rate measurements are imperative.[18]

✓ CONCEPT CHECK 7.6

1. What should individuals remember about physical activity as part of a healthy lifestyle?
2. What are some simple ways one can incorporate more physical activity into a busy schedule?

7.7 Behavioral Strategies for Weight Management

A healthy weight is not about dieting. Instead, it involves adopting a lifestyle of healthy dietary patterns, regular physical activity, and stress management.[19] The most effective behavioral interventions for weight loss and maintenance include self-monitoring, regular physical activity, and group support.[20] Individuals can benefit from working closely with registered dietitian nutritionists to set individualized and realistic weight-loss goals. Such goals will keep you focused and motivated and help to guarantee success. For instance, if reducing cardiovascular risk is a goal or risk factors are already present, a long-term goal of losing 5% to 10% of your baseline body weight has been shown to produce clinically meaningful health outcomes, including improving blood glucose and blood lipids and reducing the risk of developing type 2 diabetes.[21] Larger weight loss reduces additional risk factors of CVD (e.g., low-density and high-density lipoprotein cholesterol and blood pressure) and decreases the need for medication to control CVD and type 2 diabetes. Thus, a weight-loss goal of 5% to 10% within 6 months is recommended.

***Dietary Guidelines* Promote Weight Management.** Recall the *Dietary Guidelines* provide guidance that can empower you to make healthy shifts in your dietary pattern to encourage healthy weight management.[22] This includes focusing on nutrient-dense foods and beverages within calorie limits. A healthy dietary pattern has little room for extra added sugars, saturated fat, sodium, or alcoholic beverages. Certainly, limited amounts of these discretionary items are permissible once your key nutrient needs are met. These recommendations can give you a start:

- Limit added sugars to less than 10% of calories per day (starting at age 2).
- Limit saturated fat intake to less than 10% of calories per day (starting at age 2).
- Limit sodium intake to less than 2300 milligrams per day (and even less for children younger than 14).
- Limit alcoholic beverages; if consumed at all, should be limited to two drinks or less in a day for males and one drink or less in a day for females.

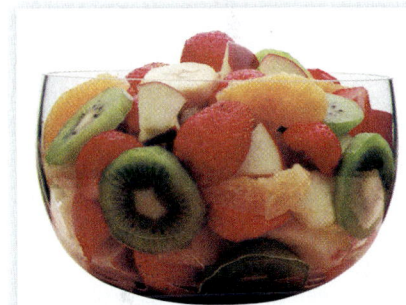

Fruit is a great snack—high in nutrients and low in calories. **Do you recall what type of natural sugar is in fruit?** Dennis Gray/Cole Group/Photodisc/Getty Images

TOOLS FOR SUCCESSFUL WEIGHT MANAGEMENT

Self-Monitoring. For most individuals, adopting positive lifestyle behaviors begins with making simple substitutions that are manageable and fit within your personal budget, traditions, and cultural framework. Over time, these new behaviors will become sustainable and allow for additional changes to promote an even healthier lifestyle over each stage of life!

There is not a cookie-cutter, or one-size-fits-all, approach to weight loss. Therefore, it is important to incorporate proven tools for success into your program. Self-monitoring is effective in helping individuals keep track of specific foods and beverages consumed, the amount of physical activity performed, and other factors that impact your behaviors. The goal of closely monitoring your lifestyle behaviors is to increase self-awareness, at least initially, of your choices and make modifications where necessary.

Many convenient and free self-monitoring tools are now widely available—dietary intake and activity trackers and apps, wearable fitness trackers, digital scales, and food journals. These tools can track your daily patterns and lifestyle choices. You can then assess your own patterns to determine which ones may be promoting weight gain and which ones promote weight loss. Experiment with different trackers to find one that works well for your lifestyle. It is less about the specific tool and more about the importance of self-monitoring to identify patterns of behavior to promote success!

TABLE 7-5 ■ SMART Goals Worksheet

Goal	Question	Physical Activity Example
S = Specific	What do you want to accomplish?	I will walk with my neighbor after dinner.
M = Measurable	How can you measure your progress?	I will walk 3 to 5 days per week for at least 30 minutes each time.
A = Achievable	Do you have the necessary skills?	I enjoy walking and know it can work into my schedule most days.
R = Relevant	Why are you setting this goal?	I want to move more and sit less!
T = Time-bound	What is your deadline?	I will try this for the full semester.

SMART Goals. Setting short-term SMART goals are recommended to help individuals determine small behavior changes that fit into their lifestyles. SMART goals provide a framework for setting specific, measurable, achievable, relevant, and time-bound goals that can help you focus on small and specific behavior changes rather than solely focusing broadly on weight or calories. Table 7-5 provides a sample worksheet to help you draft your own SMART goals for success.

Physical Activity. As you learned in Section 7.6, regular physical activity is essential for optimal mental and physical health. If weight loss is your goal, physical activity, combined with a nutrient-dense dietary pattern, creates a caloric deficit (calories out) that will promote weight loss over time. As a starting point, strive to meet the *Physical Activity Guidelines* of 150 minutes of moderate-intensity aerobic activity, 75 minutes of vigorous-intensity aerobic activity, or an equivalent mix of the two each week. Although strong scientific evidence supports these general recommendations, the exact amount of physical activity needed varies from person to person.

Social Networking and Support Groups. Support groups are an effective component of successful weight management interventions. These groups offer a wonderful platform for individuals to share their experiences, goals, successes, and even setbacks with others in a supportive and nonjudgmental community. Family and friends can also provide praise and encouragement. Unfortunately, social networks may also sabotage your efforts, so be aware of whom you can trust for support.

Today, there are numerous opportunities for social networking surrounding weight management, physical activity, and behavior change. As with self-monitoring, you should experiment with different types and platforms to find what works best for you. Some individuals thrive in organized exercise groups or clubs, others enjoy online forums with teams or competitions, and others may prefer in-person support groups recommended by their health care team. Supportive environments remind you that you are not alone on your journey. Use today's technology and resources to find your people!

BEHAVIORAL TRIGGERS

The average person makes hundreds of food-related decisions every day. Many of us overeat in response to a constant barrage of triggers in our environment—social networks, sights, sounds, smells, schedules, and other prompts throughout our day. Becoming aware of your eating patterns and behavior triggers will ultimately help you achieve and maintain a healthy weight (Fig. 7-21).

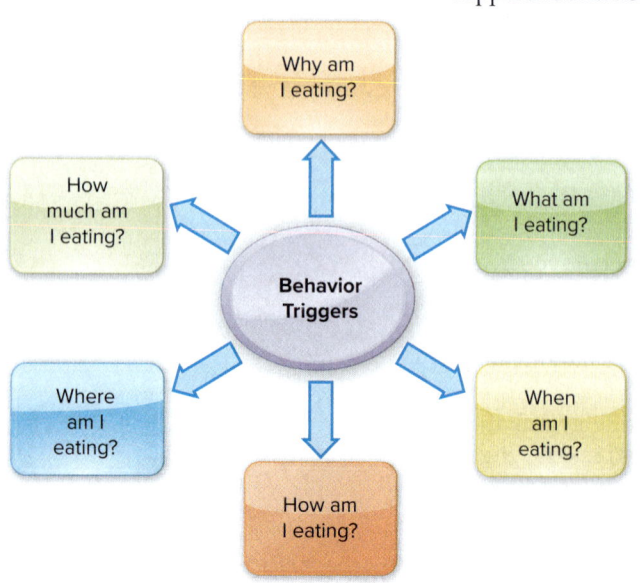

FIGURE 7-21 This figure captures the questions you can ask yourself to help you identify and define your behavior triggers.

When changing behaviors, experiment with different approaches and find what works for you! Modifying behaviors and changing thinking patterns are critical components of weight management and maintenance (Table 7-6). For instance, some

TABLE 7-6 ■ Behavioral Tactics for Weight Management

Shopping
1. Shop for food after eating, so you are not hungry.
2. Shop from a list or use a shopping app.
3. Limit purchases of irresistible "problem" foods.
4. Shop for fresh foods around the perimeter of the store.
5. Read food labels to make educated purchases.

Meal Planning
1. Plan meals in advance.
2. Keep healthy foods washed and prepared.
3. Substitute periods of physical activity for snacking.
4. Eat meals and snacks at scheduled times; don't skip meals.
5. Drink plenty of water throughout the day.

Reduce Triggers
1. Store food out of sight to discourage impulsive eating.
2. Eat all food in a designated dining area.
3. Avoid buffet-type meals.
4. Keep serving dishes off the table.

Holidays and Parties
1. Drink fewer alcoholic beverages; alternate water with alcohol.
2. Eat a low-calorie, high-fiber snack before parties.
3. Plan eating behavior before parties.
4. Practice polite ways to decline food.
5. Don't get discouraged by an occasional setback.

Eating Behavior
1. Eat slowly to avoid overeating.
2. Leave some food on your plate.
3. Take small bites and chew your food thoroughly.
4. Avoid distractions when eating.

Rewards
1. Plan specific rewards for positive behavior; allow for a small treat on physical activity days.
2. Solicit help from family and friends; engage in physical activity and healthy cooking together.
3. Use self-monitoring records (diet, physical activity, body weight) as basis for rewards. Many tracking apps are available.

Self-Monitoring
1. Note the time and place of eating.
2. List the type and amount of food and beverages consumed.
3. Record who is present and how you feel.
4. Use a dietary intake diary to identify problem areas.
5. Use online or mobile apps to track your progress, including your new nutrition and health goals and habits.

Portion Control
1. Make healthy substitutions, such as small fries instead of large fries or add nuts or seeds instead of croutons to salads.
2. Think small. Order the entrée and share it with another person. Order a cup of soup instead of a bowl or an appetizer in place of an entrée.
3. Use a take-home box. Ask your server to pack half the entrée in a take-home box before bringing it to the table.

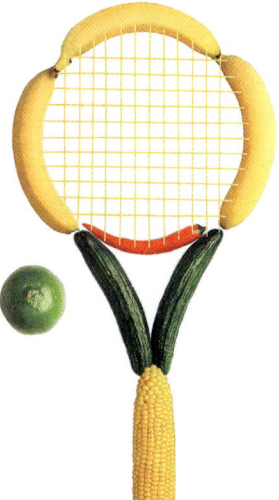
Fisher Photostudio/Shutterstock

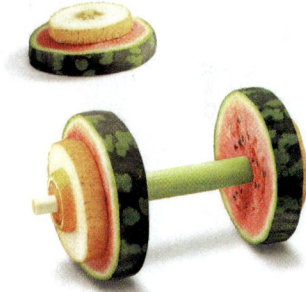
Fisher Photostudio/Shutterstock

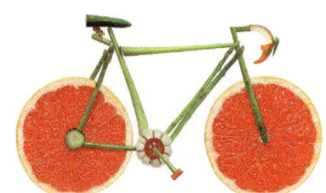
Fisher Photostudio/Shutterstock

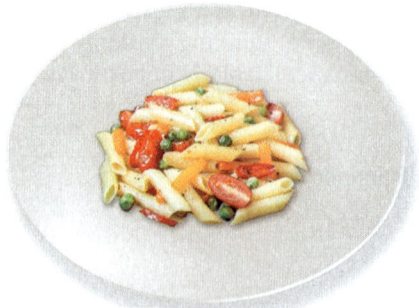
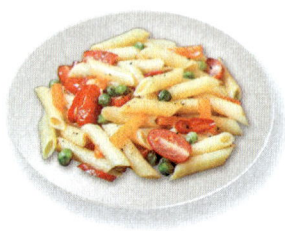

Large dinner plate **Small dinner plate**

FIGURE 7-22 The dinner plate on the left is larger and makes the serving size of the food appear smaller. This optical illusion was first documented in 1865 and termed the Delboeuf Illusion. Nesavinov/Shutterstock

individuals may eat less when using smaller plates (Fig 7-22). Although not proven to work for everyone, it may be worth a try.[23] Without identifying behavioral tactics that work for you, it may be difficult to adopt lifelong lifestyle changes needed to achieve your weight-control goals.

NON-DIET APPROACHES

Non-diet strategies have been proposed as methods to improve health and well-being without specifically targeting weight loss. Yet the science is clear, obesity is a serious medical condition, and those seeking management deserve compassionate, evidence-based, and efficacious care. The Academy of Nutrition and Dietetics conducted a recent systematic review stating that approaches that did not include dietary restriction may be associated with body satisfaction and psychological outcomes but do not result in improved cardiovascular risk factors or biomarkers of physical health.[24]

Strategies such as promoting mindful eating or intuitive eating may be used to help the client in lieu of prescribing caloric restriction; however, little evidence is available that supports the premise that these strategies reduce energy intake or enhance dietary quality. Clinicians should be transparent with clients regarding the strength of the evidence for non-diet approaches as a treatment for overweight and obesity compared with the evidence supporting other interventions for adult overweight and obesity management.

Current evidence does not support that supervised weight management interventions result in eating disorders. In fact, research examining the psychological effects of a year long weight-loss intervention showed improvements in depression, quality of life, and self-efficacy. There was no effect on anxiety, binge eating, body image, emotional eating, life satisfaction, self-esteem, or stress.[24]

RELAPSE PREVENTION

Preventing *relapse* is thought to be the hardest part of weight control—often harder than losing weight. Successful weight managers plan for lapses, do not panic, and take charge immediately. Modifying your language can include changing your internal language from "I ate that cookie; I'm a failure" to "I ate that cookie, but I did well to stop after only one!"

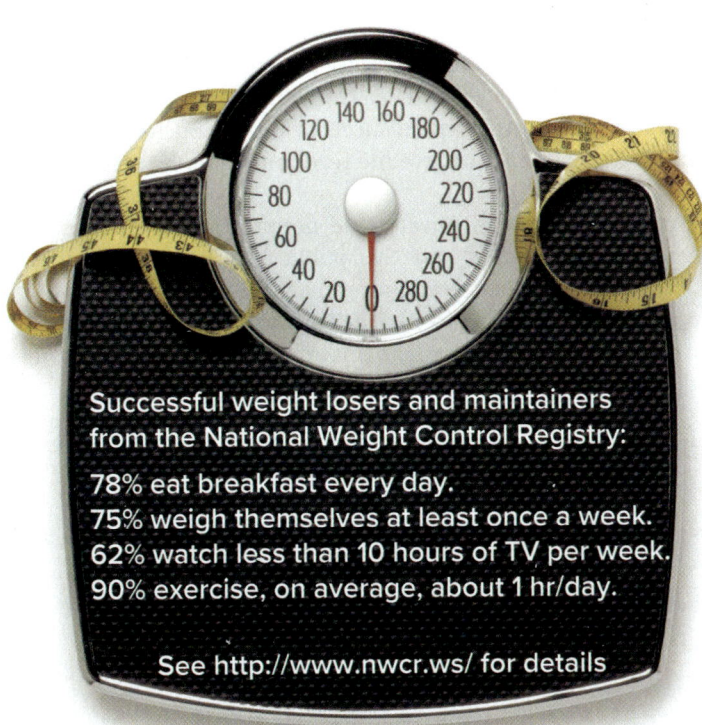

FIGURE 7-23 The National Weight Control Registry (NWCR) was developed to identify the characteristics of individuals who have succeeded at long-term weight loss and kept it off for long periods of time. DNY59/E+/Getty Images

relapse prevention A series of strategies used to help prevent and cope with weight-control lapses, such as recognizing high-risk situations and deciding beforehand on appropriate responses.

Weight Bias

Understand Weight Bias

Weight bias refers to the negative stereotypes, judgments, and discrimination often associated with individuals affected by overweight and obesity.

Understand the Impact

Weight bias often directly or indirectly results in inappropriate or inadequate treatment from members of society.

Understand How You Can Help

Using and promoting People-First Language helps to reframe the conversation to avoid weight bias.

Understand People-First Language

NO: "The obese man..."
YES: "The male affected by obesity..."

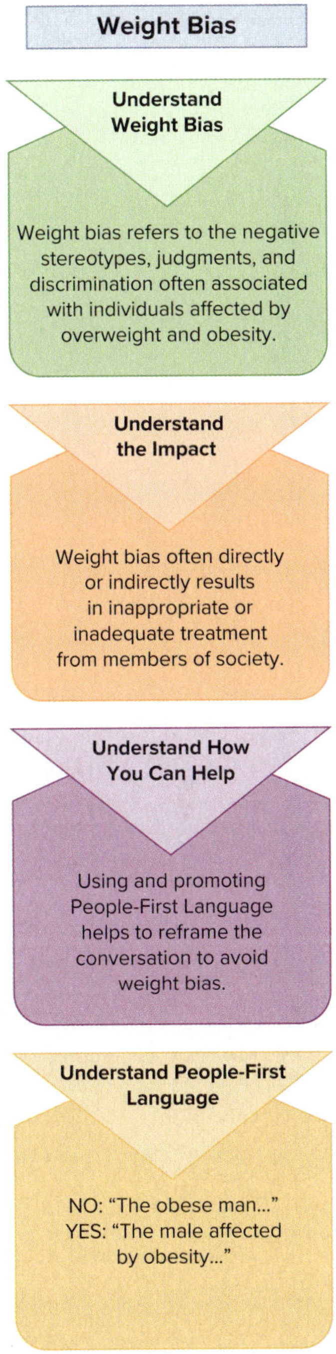

FIGURE 7-24 Weight bias. The term *weight bias* refers to negative attitudes, judgments, stereotypes, beliefs, and discrimination targeting individuals because of their weight.

When you lapse from your plan, newly learned behaviors will steer you back on track. Without a strong behavioral program for **relapse prevention** in place, a lapse frequently turns into a relapse and a potential collapse. Once a pattern of poor food choices begins, individuals may feel failure and stray farther from the plan. As the relapse lengthens, the entire plan collapses and falls short of the weight-loss goal. Losing weight is difficult. Overall, maintenance of weight loss is fostered by the 3 Ms: motivation, movement, and monitoring. The most successful weight loss and maintenance strategies reported are having healthy foods available at home, consuming breakfast, increasing vegetable consumption, decreasing sugary and fatty foods, limiting certain foods, and reducing fat in meals. Increased physical activity is the most consistent positive correlate of weight-loss maintenance.[25] Other successful strategies are listed in Fig. 7-23.

SOCIETAL EFFORTS TO ADDRESS OBESITY

The incidence of obesity in the United States is now considered an *epidemic*. An epidemic is a public health problem, and such problems call for collective action. In fact, improvement in the health of our nation requires an approach that includes many sectors. Partnerships, programs, and policies that support healthy eating and active living must be coordinated. In an effort to eradicate weight bias and stigma associated with obesity, the Obesity Action Coalition (OAC) has joined forces with other obesity-focused organizations to raise awareness of the **People-First Language** initiative. People-First Language is not new. For many years, others with a chronic disease, including the mental health and disabilities communities, have embraced People-First Language (Fig. 7-24).

People-First Language Linguistic prescription that aims to avoid perceived and subconscious dehumanization when discussing people with disabilities. It can also be applied to any group that is defined by a condition rather than as a people: for example, "those with obesity" rather than "the obese."

We all play an important role in promoting health within our communities. To make healthy eating a societal norm, changes must occur on multiple levels. For instance, providing access to safe, affordable, and healthy foods and beverages for all is a goal that will require collaborative efforts across all facets of society. Such changes are paramount in ensuring that Americans can achieve the recommendations set forth by the *Dietary Guidelines*.

The good news is that public, private, and nonprofit organizations have begun to work together to address and reverse this public health crisis. Food manufacturers are reformulating many products resulting in healthier options. Restaurants are now offering more plant-focused options with smaller portion sizes to align with the *Dietary Guidelines*. All of these small steps have an additive effect in nudging Americans in the right direction, so they can benefit from positive lifestyle behaviors.

✓ CONCEPT CHECK 7.7

1. What behavioral techniques are helpful in changing problem eating behaviors to improve weight-loss success?
2. List five behavioral tactics for weight loss.
3. What is weight bias? How can you help to reduce weight bias?

7.8 Management of Overweight and Obesity

The decision to lose weight is an individual one. No person should be shamed or judged for the decisions they make about their own health. If someone elects to attempt weight loss, so they can improve their health, that decision is also valid and should be supported. Treatment of overweight and obesity should be long term and similar to that for any chronic disease.

Effective weight loss maintenance requires sustainable lifestyle changes rather than quick fixes promoted by many popular fad diets. We often view a diet as something one attempts temporarily, only to resume prior behaviors once satisfactory results have been achieved. This is a primary reason so many people regain lost weight. Instead, an emphasis on healthy, active living will promote safe weight loss and sustained weight maintenance.

BODY FAT

Losing weight involves a complex interplay of various bodily components. For example, losing one pound of body weight includes adipose tissue plus supporting lean tissues and fluids. Because there are approximately 3500 kcal in one pound of fat, the past 50 years of weight-loss advice has centered on the notion that a deficit of approximately 500 kcal per day is required to lose 1 pound of fat tissue per week. This fairly simple 3500 kcal rule, however, may be an inaccurate predictor of weight change over time, resulting in unrealistic expectations. When individuals lose weight, compensatory mechanisms kick in to prevent further weight loss and may promote weight regain. To account for these variations, experts have developed new weight-loss prediction formulas that estimate a slower and more realistic pattern of weight loss that is not linear. In reality, weight loss often occurs most rapidly during the first 6 months after a period of negative energy balance and tapers off over time.

A web-based body weight simulator can help you predict your expected weight loss over time. The Body Weight Planner, which can be found at https://www.niddk.nih.gov/bwp, projects weight loss over time based on an individual's height, weight, sex,

According to the *Dietary Guidelines*, Americans should focus on meeting food group needs with nutrient-dense foods and beverages and **stay within calorie limits.**

age, current calorie intake, calorie reduction, and activity level. As always, guidelines emphasize that the daily calorie deficit can come from decreased calorie intake, increased physical activity, or, ideally, a combination of both.

WEIGHT-LOSS PLANS

Overall, a sound weight-loss program should include the components listed in Figure 7-25. Conversely, a one-sided approach that focuses only on restricting calories is a difficult plan of action. Instead, adding physical activity and an appropriate behavioral component will contribute to success in weight loss and eventual weight maintenance (Fig. 7-26).

RATE OF WEIGHT LOSS

- ☐ Encourages slow and steady weight loss, rather than rapid weight loss
- ☐ Sets goal of no more than 1 to 2 pounds of weight loss per week
- ☐ Includes a period of weight maintenance for a few months after about 10% of body weight is lost
- ☐ Evaluates need for further weight loss before more weight loss begins

FLEXIBILITY

- ☐ Supports participation in normal social activities (e.g., dining out, attending parties)
- ☐ Adapts the plan to individual habits and tastes

DIETARY PATTERN

- ☐ Meets nutrient needs and focuses on nutrient-dense options
- ☐ Includes common foods, with no foods being promoted as magical or special
- ☐ Uses MyPlate or a comparable food guide as a pattern for food choices

BEHAVIOR CHANGE

- ☐ Promotes reasonable changes that can be adopted
- ☐ Encourages social support
- ☐ Includes plans for relapse for those suffering setbacks
- ☐ Empowers individuals to manage behaviors
- ☐ Promotes self-monitoring practices such as keeping food diaries and setting goals

OVERALL HEALTH

- ☐ Requires screening by a primary care provider for people with existing health problems, those over 45 (males) to 55 (females) years of age who plan to increase physical activity substantially, and those who plan to lose weight rapidly
- ☐ Encourages regular physical activity, sufficient sleep, stress reduction, and other healthy changes in lifestyle
- ☐ Addresses underlying psychological weight issues, such as depression or stress

FIGURE 7-25 Characteristics of a sound weight-loss plan. Use this checklist to evaluate any weight-loss plan before putting it into practice.

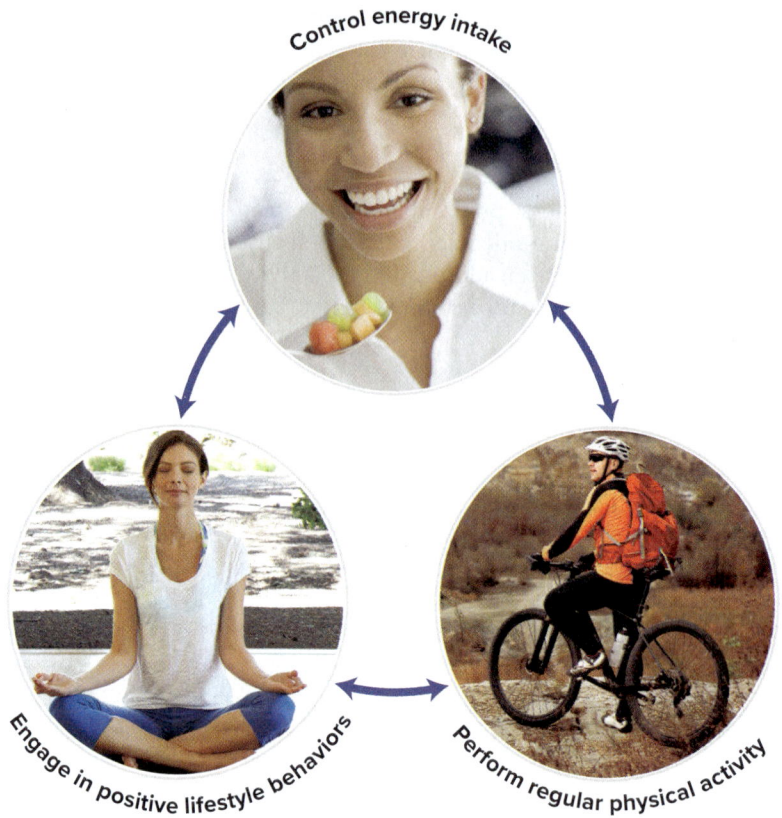

FIGURE 7-26 A successful weight-loss and maintenance strategy incorporates three interrelated components: (1) controlling energy intake, (2) performing regular physical activity, and (3) engaging in positive lifestyle behaviors. Without one component of the triad, weight loss and later maintenance become less likely. (top) Sam Edwards/OJO Images/age fotostock; (left) Chrisgramly/E+/Getty Images; (right) Oleksiy Rezin/Shutterstock

WEIGHT MANAGEMENT IN PERSPECTIVE

Three principles point to the importance of preventing obesity. Public health strategies to address the current obesity problem must speak to all age groups. There is a particular need to focus on children and adolescents because patterns of excess weight and sedentary lifestyles developed during youth may form the basis for a lifetime of weight-related conditions and ill health. In the adult population, attention should be directed toward weight management and maintenance by encouraging:

1. **Improved diet quality** by emphasizing a dietary pattern rich in nutrient-dense plant-focused foods and low-calorie beverages.
2. **Increased physical activity** to the equivalent of 150 to 300 minutes or more of moderate-intensity aerobic activity each week.
3. **Making positive behavior changes** to sustain lifestyle modifications promoting health.

✓ CONCEPT CHECK 7.8

1. What are the characteristics of an appropriate weight-control program?
2. What advice from the *Dietary Guidelines* will help Americans manage body weight over time?

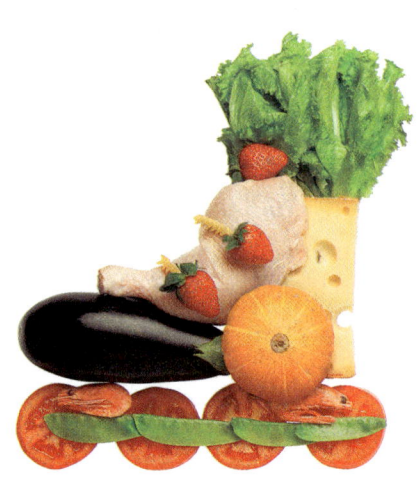

Fisher Photostudio/Shutterstock

7.9 Professional Help for Weight Loss

Your primary care provider can assist with setting up a weight-loss program. This professional is equipped to assess overall health and current weight status by examining health parameters such as blood pressure, blood lipids, and blood glucose that are affected by excess weight. In addition, they may refer you to a dietitian given they are uniquely qualified professionals trained to design personalized weight-loss plans and understand food composition, physiology, and the psychological aspects of behavior change. The expense for such professional interventions is tax deductible in the United States and, in some cases, is covered by health insurance if prescribed by a primary care provider. Some schools offer free services on a student wellness plan.

MEDICATIONS FOR WEIGHT LOSS

Candidates for medications to treat obesity, also called anti-obesity drugs or diet pills, include those with a BMI ≥ 30 or BMI ≥ 27 with at least one obesity-associated comorbid condition (e.g., type 2 diabetes, cardiovascular disease, hypertension) and who are motivated to lose weight.[26] For specific populations, medication, also known as pharmacotherapy, may be considered to supplement lifestyle interventions to help achieve targeted weight loss and health goals. For a drug to be considered effective in treating obesity, it must meet FDA guidelines and prove to be relatively safe (Table 7-7). To date, drug therapy alone has not been found to be successful for long-term weight management. Success with medications has been shown only in those who also modify their behavior, decrease calorie intake, and increase physical activity.

TABLE 7-7 ■ Medications Approved for Obesity Treatment

Medication	Approval	Action	Possible Side Effects
Orlistat (Xenical® or Alli® over-the-counter)	Over age 12	Blocks fat absorption	Stomach pain, gas, diarrhea, leaky and oily stools Rare cases of severe liver injury; avoid taking with cyclosporine Take daily multivitamin to replace nutrients lost
Phentermine-topiramate (Qsymia®)	Adults	Combination of appetite suppressor and migraine/seizure medication	Constipation, dizziness, dry mouth, taste changes, tingling of hands and feet, trouble sleeping Do not use if pregnant, planning to become pregnant, or breastfeeding
Liraglutide (Saxenda®)	Over age 12	Slows gastric emptying and enhances satiety	Nausea, diarrhea, constipation, headache, stomach pain, increased heart rate Increased risk of pancreatitis
Naltrexone-bupropion (Contrave®)	Adults	Mimics hormone that targets areas of the brain that regulate appetite and food intake	Nausea, diarrhea, constipation, headache, stomach pain, headache, fatigue, vomiting, liver damage, insomnia, hypertension, dry mouth, dizziness Do not use if history of disordered eating, hypertension, seizures, drug abuse, taking bupropion May increase suicidal thoughts or actions
Semaglutide (Wegovy®)	Adults	Mimics hormone that targets areas of the brain that regulate appetite and food intake	Nausea, diarrhea, constipation, headache, stomach pain, fatigue Increased risk of pancreatitis
Others: Diethylpropion, Benzphetamine, Phendimetrazine, Phentermine	Adults	Alter brain chemicals to promote appetite suppression. Approved by FDA for use up to 12 weeks only	Dry mouth, difficulty sleeping, dizziness, headache, feeling nervous, upset stomach, diarrhea, constipation, restlessness, hypertension, increased heart rate

Sources: Food and Drug Administration (FDA) and https://www.niddk.nih.gov/health-information/weight-management/prescription-medications-treat-overweight-obesity

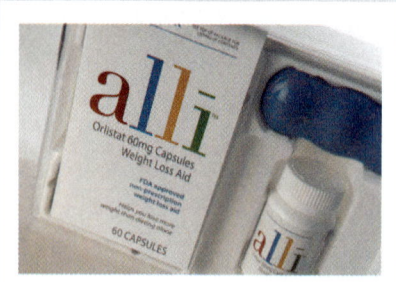

Alli® (orlistat) is an over-the-counter weight-loss drug that blocks fat absorption. **Why should people who take orlistat also take a dietary supplement of vitamins A, D, E, and K?** Jill Braaten/McGraw Hill

The fastest growing class of weight-loss medications are injectable GLP-1 agonists. Initially used to manage type 2 diabetes, these meds trigger insulin release, block glucagon secretion, slow stomach emptying, and increase satiety. Two types of GLP-1 agonists are approved for chronic weight management: Wegovy and Saxenda. Ozempic is approved for the treatment of type 2 diabetes but is often prescribed off-label for weight loss.

Other approved weight-loss medications work in various ways to curb appetite. The FDA has approved a novel weight-loss device called Plenity® for individuals with a BMI of 25 to 40. This is a hydrogel capsule made with cellulose (fiber) and citric acid. Plenity is designed to be taken with water before meals to absorb the water and increase satiety. The FDA cautions that Plenity should be used alongside diet and exercise. It may also be used with other weight-loss medications.

Sometimes, primary care providers may prescribe medications that are not approved for weight loss but have weight loss as a side effect. Such an application is termed off-label. Over-the-counter medications and supplements are widely marketed as miracle cures for obesity, but in some cases they do more harm than good. Today more than ever, let the buyer beware concerning any purported weight-loss aid not prescribed by a primary care provider.

In sum, although prescription medications can aid weight loss in some instances, they do not replace the need for reducing calorie intake, modifying behaviors, and increasing physical activity, both during and after therapy. Often, any weight loss during drug treatment can be attributed mostly to the individual's hard work at balancing calorie intake with calorie output.

TREATMENT OF SEVERE OBESITY

Having severe obesity (BMI ≥ 40), weighing at least 100 pounds over ideal body weight, or having BMI ≥ 35 plus at least one serious obesity-related condition often requires professional treatment. Because of the serious health implications of severe obesity, drastic measures may be necessary. Such treatments are recommended only when traditional diets and medications fail. Drastic weight-loss procedures are not without side effects, both physical and psychological, making careful monitoring by a primary care provider a necessity.

Very-Low-Calorie Diets. If more traditional diets have failed, treating severe obesity with a **very-low-calorie diet (VLCD)** is possible, especially if the person has obesity-related diseases that are not well controlled (e.g., hypertension, type 2 diabetes). A VLCD can be dangerous because of its rapid weight loss and potential for severe health complications, including heart problems and gallstones. Often providing fewer than 800 kcal per day, they require close monitoring during periods of rapid weight loss and should be administered under strict medical supervision by trained medical professionals.

Optifast® and other VLCD meal replacements are only available through medically supervised clinics. In general, these diets allow a person to consume only 400 to 800 kcal per day, often in liquid form. These diets were previously known as protein-sparing modified fasts. Of this amount, approximately 30 to 120 grams (120 to 480 kcal) are carbohydrates. The rest are typically from high-quality protein in the amount of 70 to 100 grams per day (280 to 400 kcal).

Recall that ketosis is an accumulation of ketone bodies in the blood that occurs when fatty acids are broken down for fuel in the absence of carbohydrates. The main reasons for weight loss, however, are the minimal energy consumption and restricted food choices. About 2 to 4 pounds can be lost per week, primarily water and lean body mass losses. When physical activity and resistance training augment this diet, a greater loss of adipose tissue occurs.

Weight regain remains a common reality, especially without a behavioral and physical activity component. If behavioral therapy and physical activity supplement a long-term support program, maintenance of the weight loss is more likely but still difficult. Any program under consideration should include a detailed maintenance plan. Today, anti-obesity medications may also be included in this phase of the program.

very-low-calorie diet (VLCD) This diet allows a person fewer than 800 calories per day, often in liquid form. Of this, 120 to 480 calories are typically from carbohydrate, and the rest are mostly from high-quality protein.

Intermittent Fasting. The dietary practice known as *intermittent fasting,* where one cycles days of so-called normal eating with a day or days of eating little to nothing, is gaining popularity. Research shows that intermittent fasting regimens yield weight-loss results that are similar to traditional weight-loss plans (i.e., moderate calorie restriction). Some individuals may experience improved blood sugar control and blood lipids. More specific information on intermittent fasting, binge eating, and other weight-loss methods can be found in the *Ask the RDN* feature.

ASK THE RDN: Intermittent Fasting

Dear RDN: I have had bad luck with traditional diets, but I've heard rave reviews of "The Fast Diet." Is an intermittent fasting program a good way to lose weight and keep it off?

There are three basic methods of intermittent fasting: whole-day fasting, alternate-day fasting, and time-restricted feeding. The definition of *fasting* can vary from one plan to the next; some plans allow only calorie-free beverages and sugar-free gum during fasts, whereas other plans recommend reducing energy intake to 20% to 25% of your usual intake (i.e., a modified fast) on fast days. Plans also differ in recommendations for food choices during feeding phases; some prescribe specific calorie and nutrient goals, while others allow unrestricted food intake during feeding phases. Proponents of intermittent fasting recommend that individuals experiment to find the method that best fits their lifestyle.

With whole-day fasting, like *The Fast Diet,* you would eat normally on most days of the week but undertake a complete or modified fast 1 or 2 days each week. With alternate-day fasting, days of normal eating alternate with complete or modified fasts. For time-restricted feeding protocols, you would delay the first meal of the day to achieve a fast of 14 to 20 hours (including overnight), but an unrestricted feeding period would be allowed for the remaining hours of the day.

Besides weight loss, purported benefits of intermittent fasting include improved insulin sensitivity, enhanced ability to use fat for energy, decreased triglyceride levels, and reduced inflammation—changes that may potentially decrease risks for chronic diseases and lead to a longer life. Much of the research to date, however, has been conducted in animals, with few controlled studies in humans.

Reviews of current (although sparse) studies of the effects of intermittent fasting suggest that it may be a reasonable alternative to the traditional weight-loss method of moderate daily calorie restriction for some people. Weight loss and improvements in metabolic effects are similar with these two weight-loss methods. However, intermittent fasting is not a good fit for everyone. If you struggle with blood sugar control (e.g., hypoglycemia or diabetes) or are pregnant, you should not attempt intermittent fasting. Quite predictably, some side effects of any fasting regimen include hunger, headaches, fatigue, and irritability. Some critics of intermittent fasting point out that underfeeding in this way could lead to nutrient deficiencies.

Dietitians can help you choose nutrient-dense foods during the feeding phases of any of these dietary patterns. Also, there is some concern that prolonged fasting may decrease your metabolic rate, which would make long-term weight maintenance very difficult. Because we have limited data on the long-term safety of intermittent fasting, it is not clear how much fasting is too much. Fasting too frequently may result in malnutrition, reduced immune function, organ damage, or eating disorders.

Wait—eating disorders?

Take a step back and look at the basic dietary patterns advocated here. Much like the dietary patterns of individuals with anorexia nervosa, intermittent-fasting programs involve calorie counting and extended periods of hunger. For some plans, foods are classified as *safe* or *off limits*, which promotes an unhealthy view of foods and ties eating into emotions such as guilt, shame, and fear. Intermittent fasting programs that advise fasting (deprivation) followed by several hours or days of unrestricted eating (indulgence) may foster binge eating. Participants may feel as if they've failed themselves and others when they have trouble adhering to a strict regimen. For a person who already exhibits anxiety, depression, or obsessive traits, intermittent fasting may be a gateway to pathological dieting and eating disorders.

Although intermittent fasting may be a reasonable alternative to daily moderate calorie restriction for some people, more research is needed to determine which protocol is best and if mental and physical health are affected over the long term. If you are determined to try intermittent fasting, continue to seek the advice of an RDN to ensure that your dietary pattern still meets your nutritional needs. If you tend to obsess about food and body weight or you already have problems with depression or anxiety, it is important to steer clear of this dietary pattern. As you will learn later, eating disorders often begin with a simple diet. If efforts to control weight begin to interfere with daily activities and are linked to physiological and emotional changes, professional help will be needed to treat an eating disorder.

Fueling, not fasting,

Angela Collene, MS, RDN, LD

Senior Lecturer, The Ohio State University, Author of *Wardlaw's Contemporary Nutrition* and *Wardlaw's Contemporary Nutrition: A Functional Approach*

Sources: Patterson RE, Laughlin GA, LaCroix AZ, et al. Intermittent fasting and human metabolic health. *J Acad Nutr Diet.* 2015 Aug:115(8):120312-12. doi: 10.1016/j.jand.2015.02.018

Webb D. Fasting regimens for weight loss. *Today's Dietitian.* 2018;20(2):34.

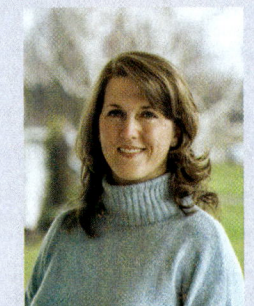
Tim Klontz

bariatrics The medical specialty focusing on the treatment of obesity.

Bariatric Surgery. **Bariatrics** is the medical specialty focusing on the treatment of obesity. Bariatric (or metabolic) surgery is considered for people with a BMI ≥ 30 and includes surgery aimed at promoting weight loss.[27] In addition to BMI for screening, the health care team also considers a person's nutrition and weight history, medical condition, motivation, age, and psychological status. Figure 7-27 provides details about the most common bariatric procedures. Gastric sleeves are the most common bariatric procedure.

The risks of bariatric surgery are serious and include both early and late postoperative complications, such as bleeding, blood clots, hernias, electrolyte imbalances, and severe infections. These risks depend on many factors related to the surgeon and facility, the patient, and the procedure. The procedures that are simply restrictive (e.g., adjustable gastric banding and sleeve gastrectomy) do not cause malabsorption and rarely affect bowel function. However, for those procedures

Select Types of Bariatric Surgery

GASTRIC BYPASS
This procedure, also called Roux-en-Y gastric bypass, creates a small pouch that significantly limits the stomach volume. The stomach continues to make digestive juices, so this permits the digestive juices to flow to the small intestine. Because food now bypasses a portion of the small intestine, fewer calories and nutrients are absorbed.

Benefits: Greater weight loss than gastric band with no foreign objects used in the procedure.

Limitations: Increased risk of surgery-related issues with longer recovery. This procedure is difficult to reverse and nutrient deficiencies may occur.

LAPAROSCOPIC ADJUSTABLE GASTRIC BANDING
This procedure involves placing an inflatable band around the top portion of the stomach. This limits the space available for food and increases satiety. LAGB is often recommended for people who have tried other weight-loss plans without long-term success.

Benefits: The surgical procedure is rapid (30–60 minutes) and can be reversed. This surgery has the lowest risk of vitamin and mineral deficits.

Limitations: Results in less weight loss than other surgeries. The surgical procedure is challenging and requires multiple steps. In addition, the band may slip, so frequent follow-up is required.

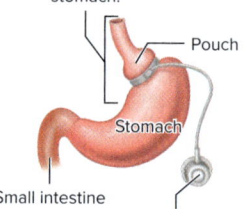

This procedure divides stomach into two sections. This creates a small pouch with a narrow opening that goes into the larger section of the stomach.

Port is used to adjust the gastric band after surgery.

GASTRIC PLICATION
This is a restrictive procedure that shrinks the size of the stomach by suturing large folds in the stomach's lining. This reduces the stomach volume by approximately 80% and increases satiety. The procedure typically takes between 40 minutes and 2 hours to complete.

Benefits: Increased weight loss over gastric band with no change in the intestines. This procedure has a relatively rapid recovery period.

Limitations: This procedure cannot be reversed, and there is an increased risk of acid reflux. As with most bariatric procedures, vitamin and mineral deficiencies are a serious concern.

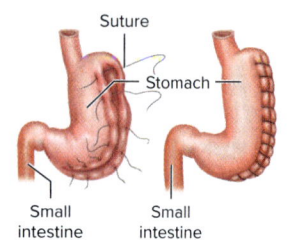

VERTICAL SLEEVE GASTRECTOMY
In this bariatric procedure, 80% to 85% of the stomach is removed to create a smaller stomach pouch. This limits the amount of food consumed and increases satiety. Vertical sleeve gastrectomy has most often been done on people who are too heavy to safely have other types of weight-loss surgery.

Benefits: This is a rapid surgical procedure, taking 30–60 minutes, that is safer than other procedures.

Limitations: This procedure cannot be reversed. Weight loss is typically slower than with other bariatric procedures.

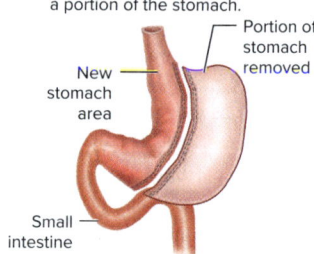

1. Using a video monitor to guide the instruments, surgeon removes a portion of the stomach.
2. The remaining portion of the stomach is closed using staples.

ILEAL TRANSPOSITION
This metabolic procedure is often used for individuals who are overweight with type 2 diabetes. The technique relocates the distal part of the small intestine to the proximal part of the small intestine. This is a longer operation than other procedures (3–3.5 hours) and requires more advanced equipment, longer hospital stays, and higher costs than other commonly used, simpler procedures.

Benefits: Results in greater glycemic control than other procedures; considered key to managing the twin epidemics of obesity and diabetes.

Limitations: As with all invasive procedures, surgical complications are possible.

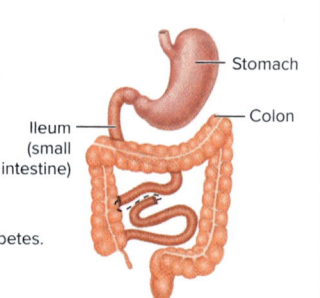

FIGURE 7-27 Bariatric surgery promotes weight loss by altering the digestive tract anatomy or limiting the volume of food that can be consumed and digested. These surgical procedures are not appropriate for everyone, and candidates must be screened carefully. In addition, many of the procedures are relatively new (e.g., intragastric balloon) and long-term effects remain unknown.

TABLE 7-8 ■ Select Bariatric Surgeries Performed on Youth

	Adjustable Gastric Banding	Gastric Bypass	Sleeve Gastrectomy
Strengths	Low rate of complications and quicker recovery Vitamin deficiencies are rare	Most frequent bariatric procedure High success rate	Rapid surgical procedure Considered safer than alternatives
Limitations	Weight loss not as rapid May require replacement surgery	Longer recovery Irreversible procedure	Weight loss not as rapid Irreversible procedure
Possible Side Effects	Infection, bleeding, band slippage or erosion, stomach pouch enlargement, stoma blockage	Infection, bleeding, blood clots, bowel obstruction, *leaky* abdomen	Gastritis, heartburn, stomach ulcers, leaking from the surgical stitches on the stomach, intestinal blockage

Source: American Society for Metabolic and Bariatric Surgery, available at www.asmbs.org/patients/adolescent-obesity

that induce malabsorption (e.g., Roux-en-Y gastric bypass), nutrient deficiencies are of greater concern if the person is not adequately treated in the years following the surgery. Anemia and bone loss might then be the result.

Bariatric surgery is costly and may not be covered by medical insurance. The average cost for bariatric procedures is typically between $15,000 and $35,000. In addition, follow-up surgery is often needed after weight loss to correct stretched skin, previously filled with fat. Furthermore, the surgery necessitates major lifestyle changes, such as the need to plan frequent, small meals. Therefore, the individual who is dieting and has chosen this drastic approach to weight loss faces months of difficult adjustments.

Despite potential adverse effects, the benefits of bariatric surgery for those who are eligible usually outweigh the risks. Interestingly, research has uncovered that bariatric surgery may lead to long-term changes in gut bacteria (increased diversity and quantity) that contribute to weight loss. An increasing number of youth are turning to bariatric surgery to treat obesity. Table 7-8 details the pros and cons of the most common bariatric procedures for children. Weight-loss statistics vary by surgical method, but on average about 95% of people will keep off 50% or more of excess body weight.[28] By no means is bariatric surgery a quick and easy fix for obesity, but with a serious commitment to permanent lifestyle changes and long-term follow-up with a health professional, these procedures can positively impact both quality and quantity of life.

Youth and Adolescent Bariatric Surgery. The American Academy of Pediatrics (AAP) recommends greater access to surgical treatments for severe obesity, defined as a BMI of ≥ 120% of the 95th percentile for age and sex in youth.[29] In the policy statement, the AAP details the health consequences of severe obesity leading to a dramatically shortened life expectancy for today's youth as compared to their parents. Research of adolescents and young adults who have undergone bariatric surgery have better long-term outcomes, including reductions in weight and chronic diseases. The AAP recommends pediatricians refer eligible youth to reputable multidisciplinary centers that have extensive pediatric bariatric surgical experience. The AAP also notes that access to bariatric surgery is often limited by a lack of insurance coverage, especially for youth from lower socioeconomic groups and racial and ethnic minorities. The AAP calls for primary care providers, governments, medical centers, and insurers to collaborate on strategies to improve access to bariatric surgery for those children and adolescents in need.[28]

✓ CONCEPT CHECK 7.9

1. How restrictive is a very-low-calorie diet plan? Why is monitoring by a qualified health professional important?
2. What are the surgical options for people with severe obesity who have failed to lose weight with other weight-loss strategies?

7.10 Treatment of Underweight

underweight Ratio of weight to height that is lower than what is associated with optimal health. For adults, this is defined as BMI less than 18.5. For children, this is defined as BMI-for-age below the 5th percentile.

Underweight is defined by a BMI < 18.5 and can be caused by a variety of factors, such as cancer, infectious disease (e.g., tuberculosis), malabsorption or digestive tract disorders (e.g., inflammatory bowel disease), and excessive dieting or physical activity. Genetic factors may also lead to a higher resting metabolic rate, a slight body frame, or both. Health problems associated with underweight include the loss of menstrual function (amenorrhea), low bone mass, complications with pregnancy and surgery, and slow recovery after illness. Significant underweight is also associated with increased death rates, especially when combined with smoking. We frequently hear about the risks of obesity but seldom of underweight. In our culture, being underweight is much more socially acceptable than being overweight or obese.

Sometimes being underweight requires medical intervention. A thorough physical exam should be obtained first to rule out hormonal imbalances, depression, cancer, infectious disease, digestive tract disorders, excessive physical activity, and other hidden diseases such as a serious eating disorder.

Yet the causes of underweight are not altogether different from the causes of obesity. Internal and external satiety-signal irregularities, the rate of metabolism, genetic factors, and psychological traits can all contribute to underweight.

In children who are growing, the high demand for calories to support physical activity and growth can also cause underweight. During growth spurts, active children and adolescents may not take the time to consume enough calories to support their needs. Moreover, gaining weight can be a formidable task for a person who is underweight. An extra 500 kcal per day or more may be required to gain weight, and this can prove challenging, especially for children who are active. Individuals attempting to gain weight may need to increase portion sizes and include frequent snacks.

When weight gain is necessary, one approach for treating adults is to gradually increase their consumption of energy-dense foods, especially those high in vegetable fats (Fig. 7-28). Nuts, seeds, and granola can be good calorie sources with low saturated fat content. Dried fruits and bananas are good fruit choices. Individuals who are underweight should replace sugar-free drinks with good calorie sources, such as 100% fruit juices and nutrient-rich smoothies.

Encouraging a regular meal and snack schedule also can aid in weight gain and maintenance. Sometimes individuals affected by underweight have experienced stress at work or school or have been too busy to eat. Making regular meals a priority may not only help them attain an appropriate weight but also may help with digestive disorders, such as constipation, sometimes associated with irregular eating patterns.

HEALTHY WEIGHT GAIN

A combination of high-quality nutrition and strength training is needed to gain weight as muscle. Strength training slows muscle loss that comes with dieting and aging, increases the strength of your muscles and connective tissues, and increases bone density. When weight is lost, up to a quarter of the loss may come from muscle mass, which can slow basal metabolism. Strength training helps protect against lean body mass losses and rebuilds any muscle lost by dieting—or prevents it from being lost in the first place. The best bet when starting a strength-training program is to seek individualized counseling from a qualified sports dietitian or certified athletic trainer who can address personal goals and limitations and can help with alignment and execution of each exercise.

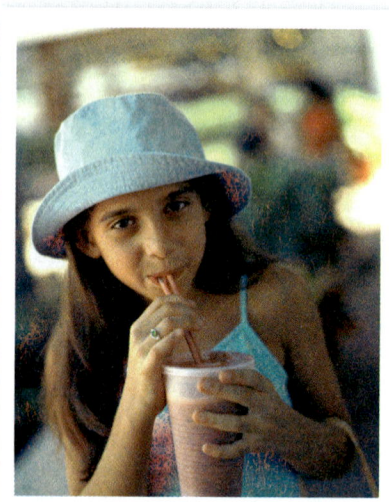

Individuals who are underweight should increase their consumption of calorie-dense foods, such as smoothies, that are also loaded with nutrients. **What are other good sources of nutritious foods that are energy dense?** Dynamic Graphics Group/Creatas/IT Stock/Alamy Stock Photo

Weight Gain Checklist

FRUITS
- ☐ Dried fruit
- ☐ Bananas
- ☐ Mangos
- ☐ Mixed fruit

VEGETABLES
- ☐ Avocados
- ☐ Potatoes and root vegetables

GRAINS
- ☐ Bran muffins
- ☐ Granola, oats, and cereal
- ☐ Brown rice, pasta
- ☐ Quinoa
- ☐ Whole grains

PROTEIN
- ☐ Eggs
- ☐ Peanut or nut butters
- ☐ Beans, nuts, legumes and seeds
- ☐ Salmon (fatty fish)
- ☐ Lean meats

DAIRY
- ☐ Greek yogurt
- ☐ Cheese

OTHER
- ☐ Trail mix
- ☐ Granola bars
- ☐ Smoothies

FIGURE 7-28 Energy-dense foods can be added to any dietary patterns to promote healthy weight gain.

There are several things to consider when designing dietary patterns to accompany training. During a workout, it is normal for the body to break down some muscles due to the stress placed on them. Once you're finished strength training, you want to repair and build muscle again. It is very important to get proper nutrients into the body after a workout to promote recovery and muscle building. Immediately before and again after strength training, a serving of high-quality protein should be consumed to optimize performance and build lean muscle mass. It is also important to have some carbohydrate along with protein to increase the protein absorption, replenish glycogen stores, and provide future fuel for workouts. Low-fat chocolate milk has been shown to be a great source of protein, carbohydrate, and fluid immediately post-activity.

Although a quick protein bar or shake is great when you're at the gym, it should not be the only source of protein. During meals, high-quality lean protein sources such as tuna, chicken, soy, and beans are recommended. Those who work out but eat nothing but food high in saturated fat and calories will gain fat in addition to any muscle gains.

To gain lean muscle mass, one needs a balanced dietary pattern rich in protein and carbohydrates, including plenty of fruits, vegetables, and whole grains. The number of calories you require each day varies greatly and will depend on your weight, activity level, age, and muscle mass. If you are working out 3 days a week, you can eat about 15 kcal per pound of body weight. If you work out 5 days a week, you can increase that calorie count to 20 kcal per pound.

✓ CONCEPT CHECK 7.10

1. How is underweight defined, and what are some of its primary causes?
2. What are the components necessary to gain weight as muscle and not as fat?

7.11 Nutrition and Your Health: Popular Fad Diets—Cause for Concern

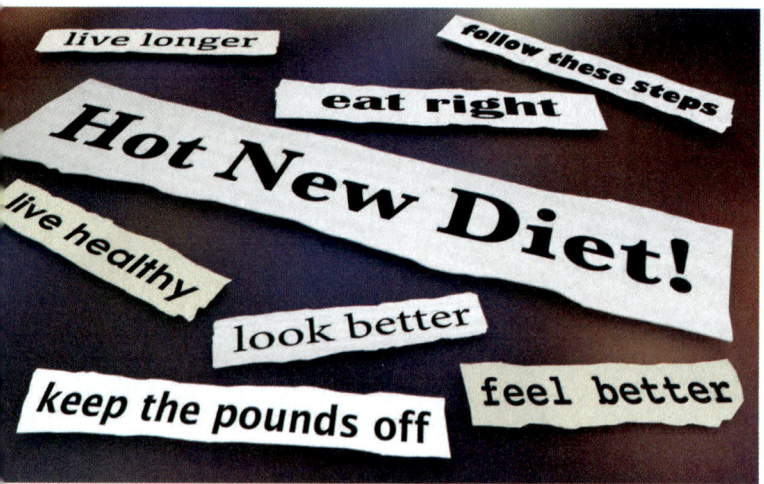
iqoncept/123RF

Many individuals who are overweight try to help themselves by using the latest popular (also called fad) diets. But, as you will see, most of these fad diets do not help, and some can actually harm those who follow them. Research has shown that early dieting and unhealthful weight-control practices in adolescents can lead to an increased risk of weight gain, overweight, and eating disorders.

To achieve weight loss and maintain it over time, experts agree that individuals should strive for reducing overall caloric intake in addition to increasing physical activity. People need a plan they can live with in the long run so that a healthy weight becomes permanent. The goal should be weight management over a lifetime, not immediate weight loss. Every popular diet leads to some immediate weight loss simply because daily intake is monitored and monotonous food choices are typically part of the plan.

People following diets often fall within a healthy weight range. Rather than worrying about weight loss, these individuals should focus on a healthy lifestyle that allows for weight maintenance. Incorporating necessary lifestyle changes, especially regular physical activity, and learning to accept one's individual body characteristics should be the overriding goals.

How to Recognize a Fad Diet

The criteria for evaluating weight-loss programs with regard to their safety and effectiveness were discussed earlier. In contrast, unreliable fad diets typically share some common characteristics:

1. They promote rapid weight loss. As mentioned, this initial weight loss primarily results from water loss and lean muscle mass depletion, not adipose tissue depletion.
2. They often limit food selections and dictate specific rituals, such as eating only fruit for breakfast or cabbage soup every day.
3. They use testimonials from famous people and tie the diet to well-known cities, such as Beverly Hills or South Beach.
4. They present themselves as cure-alls. These diets claim to work for everyone, whatever the type of obesity or the person's genetic or environmental makeup.
5. They often recommend expensive supplements or meal replacements.
6. They typically do not encourage permanent changes to eating behaviors. Individuals follow the diet until their desired weight is reached and then revert to old behaviors.
7. They are generally critical of and skeptical about the scientific community. The lack of a quick fix from medical and dietetic professionals has led some of the public to seek advice from those who appear to have the answer.
8. They claim that there is no need to exercise or engage in regular physical activity.

Probably the cruelest characteristic of these diets is that they essentially guarantee failure. Fad diets are not designed for permanent weight loss. Behaviors are not changed, and the food selection is so limited that the person cannot follow the diet over time. Although individuals assume that they have lost fat when dieting, they often have lost mainly muscle mass and body fluids. As soon as they begin eating normally again, much of the lost tissue is replaced as fat mass. In a matter of weeks or months, most of the lost weight is back. The individual did not fail; the diet failed.

Repetitive weight cycling or yo-yo dieting can add more blame and guilt, challenging the self-worth of the individual. It can also come with some health costs, such as increased upper-body fat deposition. If someone needs help losing weight, consult a nutrition expert, such as a dietitian. It is unfortunate that people spend more time and money on quick fixes rather than on professional help.

Popular Diet Approaches

A list of the best diet plans is presented in Table 7-9. Note that these plans promote the key recommendations of the *Dietary Guidelines* and include an abundance of plant-based foods rich in fiber, key nutrients, and phytochemicals. Dietary patterns that exclude entire food groups are not associated with long-term health benefits.

Top Rated Weight-Loss Plans

The top-rated diet plans specific to weight loss are WW (Weight Watchers), the Flexitarian Diet, and the Vegan Diet.

WW (WEIGHT WATCHERS)

Focused on weight loss, WW has expanded over the years to embrace a more holistic approach to eating healthier, moving more, and improving overall well-being. The myWW program was launched in 2019 and provides an even more flexible and

TABLE 7-9 ■ Best Diet Plans

Diet Plan	#1 Diet Rankings
Mediterranean Diet	Best overall diet Best plant-based diet Best heart-healthy diet (tie) Best diet for bone and joint health (tie) Best diet for healthy eating (tie) Best family-friendly (tie)
DASH Diet (tie)	Best heart-healthy diet (tie) Best diet for diabetes Best diet for bone and joint health (tie)
Flexitarian Diet (tie)	Best weight-loss diet (tie) Best family-friendly (tie) Easiest to follow (tie)
WW (Weight Watchers)	Best weight-loss diet Best diet program
Ornish Diet	Best heart-healthy diet (tie) Best family-friendly (tie) Easiest to follow (tie)

Source: U.S. News & World Report Best Diet Rankings 2019, available here: https://health.usnews.com/best-diet

customized behavioral approach to weight management. Using a point-based system for self-monitoring, this plan is easy to navigate and follow for most. Expert-led workshops and Digital 360 plans provide additional tools and behavior-change techniques to support subscribers. The main drawback to this program is the cost.

FLEXITARIAN DIET

Tied with WW in the rankings, this plan combines two concepts, as inferred in the name: flexible and vegetarian. Although you do not have to eliminate meat completely to follow this plan, it does promote a plant-based dietary pattern that is balanced in nutrient content. Although this plan is flexible and includes many recipes, it may prove challenging for those who do not cook at home or those who do not like fruits and vegetables.

VEGAN DIET

Vegans exclude all animal products from their dietary patterns: meat, fish, poultry, dairy, and eggs. Staple products of vegan dietary patterns include fruits, vegetables, leafy greens, nuts, seeds, legumes, and whole grains. Daily, this pattern aims for six servings of grains; five servings of legumes, nuts, or other plant-based proteins; four servings of vegetables; two servings of fruit; and two servings of healthy fats. The pros of this pattern are that it is rich in high-fiber foods and environmentally friendly. The cons are that it can be challenging to meet all nutrient needs, so it is important to be well-versed and educated in appropriate substitutions.

Other Popular Diet Plans

HIGH-PROTEIN DIETS

High-protein, low-carbohydrate diets continue to be a popular approach to losing weight. These diets typically recommend at least 30% to 50% of their total calories from protein and drastically restrict carbohydrate intake. Low carbohydrate intake leads to less glycogen synthesis and therefore less water in the body (about 3 grams of water are stored per gram of glycogen). As discussed, a very-low-carbohydrate intake also forces the liver to produce some glucose. The source of carbons for this glucose is mostly proteins from tissues such as muscle, resulting in loss of protein tissue, which is about 72% water. Essential ions, such as potassium, are also lost in the urine. In the initial stages of a low-carbohydrate diet, losses of glycogen stores, lean tissue, and water cause rapid weight loss. When a normal dietary pattern is resumed, the protein tissue is rebuilt and the weight is regained.

In addition, restricting carbohydrate causes your body to burn fat instead of carbohydrate for fuel. In theory, this burning of excess fat stores makes sense for weight loss. Remember, however, that when we burn fat without carbohydrate, it causes the body to go into the metabolic state called ketosis. For a person who is trying to lose weight, one benefit of ketone accumulation in body fluids is mild suppression of appetite. Increased excretion of electrolytes can cause nausea and headaches with some of the most restrictive plans. Taken to the extreme over time, ketosis can disrupt the body's acid–base balance and become quite dangerous.

For most individuals dieting, a low-carb plan is such a major change from normal habits that it is very difficult to maintain. However, research indicates that low-carbohydrate diets may be an effective alternative to low-fat diets for some people.[30] Popular low-carb diets include the Ketogenic (Keto) Diet, Atkins, and Paleo. If you elect to follow a high-protein diet, experts agree it's important to choose your protein wisely. Protein sources like beans, nuts, fish, and poultry are healthier options than red and processed meat and full-fat dairy, which have been linked to increased risks of heart disease.

LOW-CALORIE DIETS

Low-calorie diet plans promote rapid weight loss, often by limiting daily caloric intake to less than 1200 calories. In the short term, low-calorie diets can be effective, but they are not sustainable for the long term. Some use a low-calorie diet to jumpstart their weight loss, but experts recommend quickly transitioning to a balanced diet with a modest calorie deficit for long-term behavior change. Because low-calorie diets often deprive your body of key nutrients, it is critical to work with your primary care physician or registered dietitian before initiating this plan on your own.

LOW-CARB DIETS

Low-carbohydrate diet plans limit the amount of carbohydrates in your diet. Diabetes-friendly diet plans have shown that low-carb diets can stabilize blood sugar levels and improve insulin sensitivity given this plan limits consumption of starchy, refined, and sugary foods. The plan calls for avoidance of foods such as breads, pastas, rice, beans, and potatoes, and often includes more meat, fish, eggs, and vegetables. The key to a healthy low-carb diet is consuming rich sources of fiber (leafy greens) because most obtain dietary fiber from grains. Also keep in mind that the *Dietary Guidelines* recommend that carbs provide 45% to 65% percent of your daily calorie intake.

LOW-FAT DIETS

Low-fat diets historically were designed to reduce the risk of heart disease and obesity. As you recall, fat provides 9 calories per gram as compared to 4 calories per gram for both carbohydrates and protein. A typical low-fat diet plan is defined as less than 30% of your daily calories from fat, while a very-low-fat diet plan may contain just 10% to 15% of daily calories from fat. Low-saturated-fat diet plans have proven to lower blood cholesterol and reduce the risk of cardiovascular disease. Yet a low-fat diet does not mean you should avoid all fats. Recommended and healthy sources of fats include mono- and polyunsaturated fats.

WEIGHT-LOSS APPS

Although not ranked as a top weight-loss diet plan, Noom is an example of an app for tech-savvy individuals focusing on self-awareness, accountability, and behaviors that promote weight loss or weight gain. As mentioned in Section 7.7, self-monitoring is a successful behavioral strategy. Noom encourages subscribers to log dietary intake, daily weight, and physical activity. The app uses consistent feedback and messaging along with support from a group coach. In terms of dietary patterns, Noom encourages foods with low caloric density (higher in water, lower in calories by volume).

ELIMINATION DIETS

Individuals use elimination diets to help identify food allergies and intolerances. These plans involve eliminating foods and reintroducing them one at a time to determine which foods or ingredients may be the culprit for specific health issues. The Whole30 diet, gluten-free diet, and low FODMAP diets are considered elimination diets. Although there is some scientific justification for these diets, close supervision by your primary care provider is necessary to ensure safety and monitor symptoms.

DIET QUACKERY

Many popular diets fall under the category of quackery—people taking advantage of others. They usually involve a product or service that costs a considerable amount of money. Often, those offering the product or service don't realize that they are promoting quackery because they themselves were victims. For example, they tried the product and, by pure coincidence, felt it worked for them, so they promote it to all their friends and relatives.

Numerous other gimmicks for weight loss have come and gone and are likely to resurface. If in the future an important aid for weight loss is discovered, you can feel confident that reputable organizations such as the National Academy of Medicine, Academy of Nutrition and Dietetics, or the Centers for Disease Control and Prevention (CDC) will report it. Quackwatch.com is an online resource for consumers to help identify quackery.

✓ CONCEPT CHECK 7.11

1. What are the common characteristics of a fad diet?
2. Why do popular diets often fail?
3. What is the primary mechanism by which all diets lead to weight loss?

CASE STUDY: Choosing a Weight-Management Program

Joe has a hectic schedule. During the day, he works full time at a warehouse distribution center filling orders. At night, three times a week, he attends class at the local community college in pursuit of computer certification. On weekends, he likes to watch sports on television, spend time with family and friends, and study. Joe has little time to exercise or think about what he eats—that is, convenience rules. He stops for coffee and a pastry on his way to work, has a burger or pizza for lunch at a fast-food restaurant, and for dinner picks up fried chicken or fish at the drive-through on his way to class. Unfortunately, over the past few years, Joe's weight has been climbing. He is 5 feet, 10 inches tall and weighs 200 pounds. Lately, he has frequently been short of breath during his shift at work. Watching a game on television a few nights ago, he saw an infomercial for a weight-loss supplement that promises to increase his energy level and allow him to continue to eat large portions of tasty foods but not gain weight. A famous actor supports the claim that this product allows one to eat at will and not gain weight. This claim is tempting to Joe.

1. Has Joe been experiencing positive or negative energy balance over the past few years? What is his current BMI?
2. What aspects of Joe's lifestyle (other than diet) are causing this effect on his energy balance?
3. What changes could Joe make to his dietary and physical activity patterns that would promote weight loss or maintenance?
4. Why should Joe be skeptical of the claims he heard about the weight-loss product in the infomercial?
5. Referring back to the characteristics of fad diets, what advice can you offer Joe for evaluating weight-loss programs?

Complete the Case Study. Responses to these questions can be provided by your instructor.

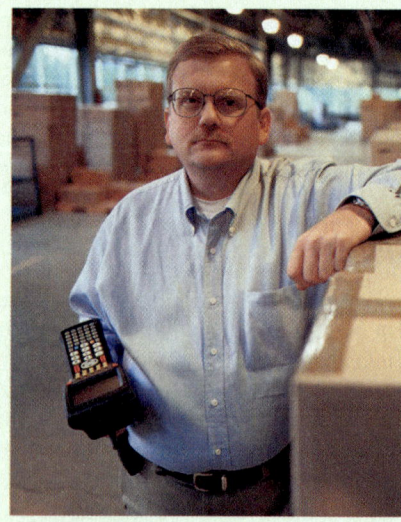

What changes can Joe make in his daily routine and diet to prevent weight gain?
Ryan McVay/Photodisc/Getty Images

Summary (Numbers refer to numbered sections in the chapter)

7.1 Energy balance considers energy intake and energy output. Negative energy balance occurs when energy output surpasses energy intake, resulting in weight loss. Positive energy balance occurs when calorie intake is greater than output, resulting in weight gain.

Basal metabolism, the thermic effect of food, physical activity, and adaptive thermogenesis account for total energy use by the body. Basal metabolism, which represents the minimum amount of calories required to keep the resting, awake body alive, is primarily affected by lean body mass. Physical activity is energy use above that expended at rest. The thermic effect of food describes the increase in metabolism that facilitates digestion, absorption, and processing of the nutrients recently consumed. Adaptive thermogenesis includes nonvoluntary activities, such as shivering and fidgeting, that increase energy use and may counter extra calories from overeating. In a sedentary person, about 60% to 80% of energy use is accounted for by basal metabolism.

7.2 Energy use by the body can be measured as heat given off by direct calorimetry or as oxygen used by indirect calorimetry. A person's Estimated Energy Requirement (EER) can be calculated based on age, sex, weight, height, physical activity level, and life stage, consistent with maintaining health.

7.3 A body mass index (weight in kilograms ÷ height^2 in meters) of 18.5 to 24.9 is one measure of normal (healthy) weight. A body mass index of 25 to 29.9 represents overweight. Obesity is defined as a body mass index of 30 or more or a total body fat percentage over 25% (males) or 32% (females). A healthy weight is best determined in conjunction with a thorough health evaluation by a clinician.

Fat distribution greatly determines health risks associated with obesity. Upper-body fat storage (android), as measured by a waist circumference greater than 40 inches (102 centimeters) for males or 35 inches (88 centimeters) for females, typically results in higher risks of hypertension, cardiovascular disease, and type 2 diabetes than lower-body fat storage (gynoid).

7.4 Both genetic (nature) and environmental (nurture) factors can increase the risk of obesity. The set-point theory proposes that we have a genetically predetermined body weight or body fat content, which the body strives to regulate.

7.5 For those attempting to lose weight, the evidence-based recommendations encourage an initial calorie deficit of approximately 500 kcal per day, increased physical activity, or a combination of both. This should result in approximately 1 pound of weight loss per week initially. Note that weight change is not linear; it occurs most rapidly during the first year after a change in energy balance but tapers off over the next 2 years if changes in energy intake and physical activity are strictly maintained over time.

7.6 Physical activity as part of a weight-management program should be focused on duration rather than just intensity. The recommendations promote 150 to 300 minutes of physical activity per week. Ideally, about 60 minutes of moderate-intensity physical activity should be part of each day to prevent adult weight gain.

7.7 Behavior changes are a vital part of weight-loss and management programs because individuals may have many behaviors that promote obesity. Specific behavior modification techniques, such as self-monitoring, goal setting, and enlisting the aid of social support, can be used to help change lifestyle behaviors.

7.8 A sound weight-loss and maintenance program should meet the individual's nutritional needs by emphasizing a wide variety of nutrient-dense, high-fiber foods; adapting to one's diet with readily obtainable foods; emphasizing regular physical activity; and stipulating the supervision by a clinician if weight is to be lost rapidly, if the person is severely obese (body mass index over 40), or if the individual is over the age of 45 (males) or 55 (females) and plans to perform substantially greater physical activity than recommended.

7.9 Medications to blunt appetite can aid weight loss. Orlistat (Xenical) reduces fat absorption from a meal when taken with the meal. The fastest growing class of weight-loss medications are injectable GLP-1 agonists. Initially used to manage type 2 diabetes, these meds trigger insulin release, block glucagon secretion, slow stomach emptying, and increase satiety. Although prescription medications can aid weight loss in some instances, they do not replace the need for reducing calorie intake, modifying behaviors, and increasing physical activity, both during and after therapy.

The treatment of severe obesity may include very-low-calorie diets containing 400 to 800 kcal per day or bariatric surgery, often to reduce stomach volume to approximately 30 milliliters (1 ounce). Both of these measures should be reserved for people who have failed at more conservative approaches to weight loss. They also require close medical supervision.

7.10 Underweight can be caused by a variety of factors, such as excessive physical activity and genetics. Sometimes being underweight requires medical attention. A primary care provider should be consulted first to rule out underlying health issues. The underweight person may need to increase portion sizes, learn to incorporate calorie-dense foods frequently, and drink fluids between meals. In addition, encouraging a regular meal and snack schedule aids in both weight gain and weight maintenance.

7.11 Many people who are overweight try popular fad diets that most often are not helpful and may actually be harmful. Fad diets typically share some common characteristics, including promoting quick weight loss, limiting food selections, using personal testimonials as proof, and requiring no physical activity.

Check Your Knowledge (Answers are available at the end of this question set)

1. For most adults, the greatest portion of their energy expenditure is for
   a. physical activity.
   b. sleeping.
   c. basal metabolism.
   d. the thermic effect of food.

2. When energy input is greater than energy output, the result is
   a. negative energy balance.
   b. energy balance.
   c. positive energy balance.
   d. thermic effect of food.

3. Which factor is associated with a lower basal metabolic rate
   a. stress.
   b. low calorie intake.
   c. fever.
   d. pregnancy.

4. Thermic effect of food represents the energy cost of
   a. chewing food.
   b. peristalsis.
   c. basal metabolism.
   d. digesting, absorbing, and packaging nutrients.

5. An energy deficit of 500 kcal per day would result in a total weight loss of about 1 pound over a _____ period.
   a. 1-week
   b. 1-month
   c. 1-year
   d. 3-year

6. The major goal for weight reduction in the treatment of obesity is the loss of
   a. weight.
   b. body fat.
   c. body water.
   d. body protein.

7. A well-designed weight-loss and management program should
   a. increase physical activity.
   b. alter problem behaviors.
   c. reduce energy intake.
   d. include all of the above.

8. For weight loss and to achieve and maintain a healthy body weight, adults should complete the equivalent of _____ minutes of moderate-intensity aerobic activity each week.
   a. 30 to 60
   b. 90 to 120
   c. 150 to 300
   d. 400 to 600

9. Probably the most important contributing factor for obesity rates today in the United States is
   a. food advertising.
   b. snacking practices.
   c. physical inactivity.
   d. eating processed food.

10. The mechanism of bariatric surgery is to
    a. reduce stomach volume.
    b. slow transit time.
    c. surgically remove adipose tissue.
    d. prevent snacking.

Answer Key: 1. c (LO 7.1), 2. c (LO 7.1), 3. b (LO 7.1), 4. d (LO 7.2), 5. a (LO 7.5), 6. b (LO 7.5), 7. d (LO 7.5), 8. c (LO 7.7), 9. c (LO 7.8), 10. a (LO 7.10)

Study Questions (Numbers refer to Learning Outcomes)

1. How does energy imbalance lead to weight gain and obesity over time? **(LO 7.1)**

2. What are the five components that are included in calculating estimated energy requirements? **(LO 7.2)**

3. Define how a healthy weight may be determined. **(LO 7.3)**

4. List three health issues that are related to obesity and the mechanism or reason that each condition occurs. **(LO 7.3)**

5. Explain how nurture and nature can contribute to the development of obesity. What are the two most convincing pieces of evidence that both genetic and environmental factors play significant roles in the development of obesity? **(LO 7.4)**

6. List examples of positive behaviors that can lead to weight management. **(LO 7.7)**

7. List three key characteristics of a sound weight-loss program. **(LO 7.8)**

8. Why is the claim for quick, effortless weight loss by any method always misleading? **(LO 7.8)**

9. Why should obesity treatment be viewed as a lifelong commitment rather than a short-term diet? **(LO 7.8)**

10. What steps are important to remember when a person who is underweight wants to gain muscle mass? **(LO 7.10)**

References

1. Nutter S, Eggerichs LA, Nagpal TS, et al. Changing the global obesity narrative to recognize and reduce weight stigma: a position statement from the World Obesity Federation. *Obesity Reviews.* 2023;e13642. doi:10.1111/obr.13642

2. National Academies of Sciences, Engineering, and Medicine. *Dietary Reference Intakes for Energy.* Washington, DC: The National Academies Press; 2023. https://doi.org/10.17226/26818.

3. Centers for Disease Control. Division of Nutrition, Physical Activity, and Obesity, National Center for Chronic Disease Prevention and Health Promotion. Last, updated May 17, 2022. Available at https://www.cdc.gov/obesity/data/adult.html. Accessed October 29, 2023.

4. Zheng Y, Manson JE, Yuan C, et al. Associations of weight gain from early to middle adulthood with major health outcomes later in life. *JAMA.* 2017 Jul 18;318(3):255-269. doi: 10.1001/jama.2017.7092

5. Nunes C, Casanova N, Francisco R, et al. Does adaptive thermogenesis occur after weight loss in adults? A systematic review. *Br J Nutr.* 2022 Feb 14;127(3):451-469. doi: 10.1017/S0007114521001094

6. Pontzer H, Yamada Y, Sagayama H, et al.; IAEA DLW Database Consortium. Daily energy expenditure through the human life course. *Science.* 2021 Aug 13;373(6556):808-812. doi: 10.1126/science.abe5017

7. Levine JA. The Fidget Factor and the obesity paradox. How small movements have big impact. *Front Sports Act Living.* 2023 Apr 3;5:1122938. doi: 10.3389/fspor.2023.1122938. PMID: 37077429; PMCID: PMC10106700.

8. Chung N, Park M-Y, Kim J, et al. Non-exercise activity thermogenesis (NEAT): a component of total daily energy expenditure. *J Exerc Nutrition Biochem.* 2018 Jun 30;22(2):23-30. doi: 10.20463/jenb.2018.0013

9. Calcagno M, Kahleova H, Alwarith J, et al. The thermic effect of food: a review. *J Am Coll Nutr.* 2019 Aug;38(6):547-551. doi: 10.1080/07315724.2018.1552544

10. Westerterp KR. Diet induced thermogenesis. *Nutr Metab (Lond).* 2004 Aug 18;1(1):5. doi: 10.1186/1743-7075-1-5

11. Shai I, Jiang R, Manson JE, et al. Ethnicity, obesity, and risk of type 2 diabetes in women: a 20-year follow-up study. *Diabetes Care.* 2006 Jul;29(7):1585-90. doi: 10.2337/dc06-0057

12. Lifshitz F. Obesity in children. *J Clin Res Pediatr Endocrinol.* 2008;1(2): 53-60. doi: 10.4008/jcrpe.v1i2.35

13. Behavior, environment, and genetic factors all have a role in causing people to be overweight and obese. Centers for Disease Control and Prevention, Genomics and Precision Health. Updated January 19, 2018. Accessed October 15, 2023. https://www.cdc.gov/genomics/resources/diseases/obesity/index.htm

14. Woods SC. Body weight "set point"—what we know and what we don't know. Obesity Action Coalition. Available at https://www.obesityaction.org/community/article-library/body-weight-set-point-what-we-know-and-what-we-dont-know

15. Eat more, weigh less? Centers for Disease Control and Prevention. Updated August 17, 2020. Accessed October 20, 2023. https://www.cdc.gov/healthyweight/healthy_eating/energy_density.html

16. Centers for Disease Control and Prevention. Division of Nutrition, Physical Activity, and Obesity, National Center for Chronic Disease Prevention and Health Promotion. *Cutting Calories.* Jul 26, 2023. Available at https://www.cdc.gov/healthyweight/healthy_eating/cutting_calories.html?CDC_AA_refVal=https%3A%2F%2Fwww.cdc.gov%2Fhealthyweight%2Fhealthy_eating%2Fenergy_density.html. Accessed Nov 5 2023.

17. WHO advises not to use non-sugar sweeteners for weight control in newly released guideline. World Health Organization. May 2023. Available at https://www.who.int/news/item/15-05-2023-who-advises-not-to-use-non-sugar-sweeteners-for-weight-control-in-newly-released-guideline. Accessed Nov 3, 2023.

18. Glave AP, Didier JJ, Oden GL, Wagner MC. Caloric expenditure estimation differences between an elliptical machine and indirect calorimetry. *Exercise Medicine.* 2018;2:8. doi: 10.26644/em.2018.008

19. Wharton S, Lau DCW, Vallis M, et al. Obesity in adults: a clinical practice guideline. *CMAJ.* 2020 Aug 4;192(31):E875-E891. doi: 10.1503/cmaj.191707. PMID: 32753461; PMCID: PMC7828878.

20. LeBlanc EL, Patnode CD, Webber EM, Redmond N, Rushkin M, O'Connor EA. *Behavioral and Pharmacotherapy Weight Loss Interventions to Prevent Obesity-Related Morbidity and Mortality in Adults: An Updated Systematic Review for the U.S. Preventive Services Task Force.* Rockville (MD): Agency for Healthcare Research and Quality (US); September 2018.

21. Raynor HA, Champagne CM. Position of the Academy of Nutrition and Dietetics: interventions for the treatment of overweight and obesity in adults. *J Acad Nutr Diet.* 2016 Jan;116(1):129-147. doi: 10.1016/j.jand.2015.10.031

22. U.S. Department of Agriculture; U.S. Department of Health & Human Services. *Dietary Guidelines for Americans, 2020–2025.* 9th ed. December 2020. https://DietaryGuidelines.gov

23. Peng M. How does plate size affect estimated satiation and intake for individuals in normal-weight and overweight groups? *Obes Sci Pract.* 2017 Jun 27;3(3):282-288. doi: 10.1002/osp4.119

24. Morgan-Bathke M, Raynor HA, Baxter SD, Halliday TM, Lynch A, Malik N, Garay JL, Rozga M. Medical nutrition therapy interventions provided by dietitians for adult overweight and obesity management: an Academy of Nutrition and Dietetics evidence-based practice guideline. *J Acad Nutr Diet.* 2023 Mar;123(3):520-545.e10. doi: 10.1016/j.jand.2022.11.014. Epub 2022 Dec 1. PMID: 36462613.

25. Paixão C, Dias CM, Jorge R, et al. Successful weight loss maintenance: a systematic review of weight control registries. *Obes Rev.* 2020 May;21(5):e13003. doi: 10.1111/obr.13003

26. Prescription medications to treat overweight & obesity. National Institutes of Health, National Institute of Diabetes and Digestive and Kidney Diseases. Updated June 2021. Accessed October 21, 2023. https://www.niddk.nih.gov/health-information/weight-management/prescription-medications-treat-overweight-obesity#who

27. Aminian A, Chang J, Brethauer SA, Kim JJ; American Society for Metabolic and Bariatric Surgery Clinical Issues Committee. ASMBS updated position statement on bariatric surgery in class I obesity. *Surg Obes Relat Dis.* 2018 Aug;14(8):1071-1087. doi: 10.1016/j.soard.2018.05.025

28. FAQs of bariatric surgery. American Society for Metabolic and Bariatric Surgery, Public Education Committee. Updated September 2020. Accessed December 21, 2021. https://asmbs.org/patients/faqs-of-bariatric-surgery#

29. Armstrong SC, Bolling CF, Michalsky MP, Reichard KW; Section on Obesity; Section on Surgery. Pediatric metabolic and bariatric surgery: evidence, barriers, and best practices. *Pediatrics.* 2019 Dec;144(6):e20193223. doi: 10.1542/peds.2019-3223

30. Gardner CD, Trepanowski JF, Del Gobbo LC, et al. Effect of low-fat vs low-carbohydrate diet on 12-month weight loss in overweight adults and the association with genotype pattern or insulin secretion: The DIETFITS randomized clinical trial. *JAMA.* 2018 Feb 20;319(7):667-679. doi: 10.1001/jama.2018.0245

Design Element Credits: Fact Check/magnifying glass icon: McGraw Hill; Magnificent Microbiome background image: Alena Ohneva/Shutterstock; Sustainable Solutions icon: McGraw Hill; Roots icon: McGraw Hill; Medicine Cabinet icon: Peter Dazeley/Photographer's Choice/Getty Images

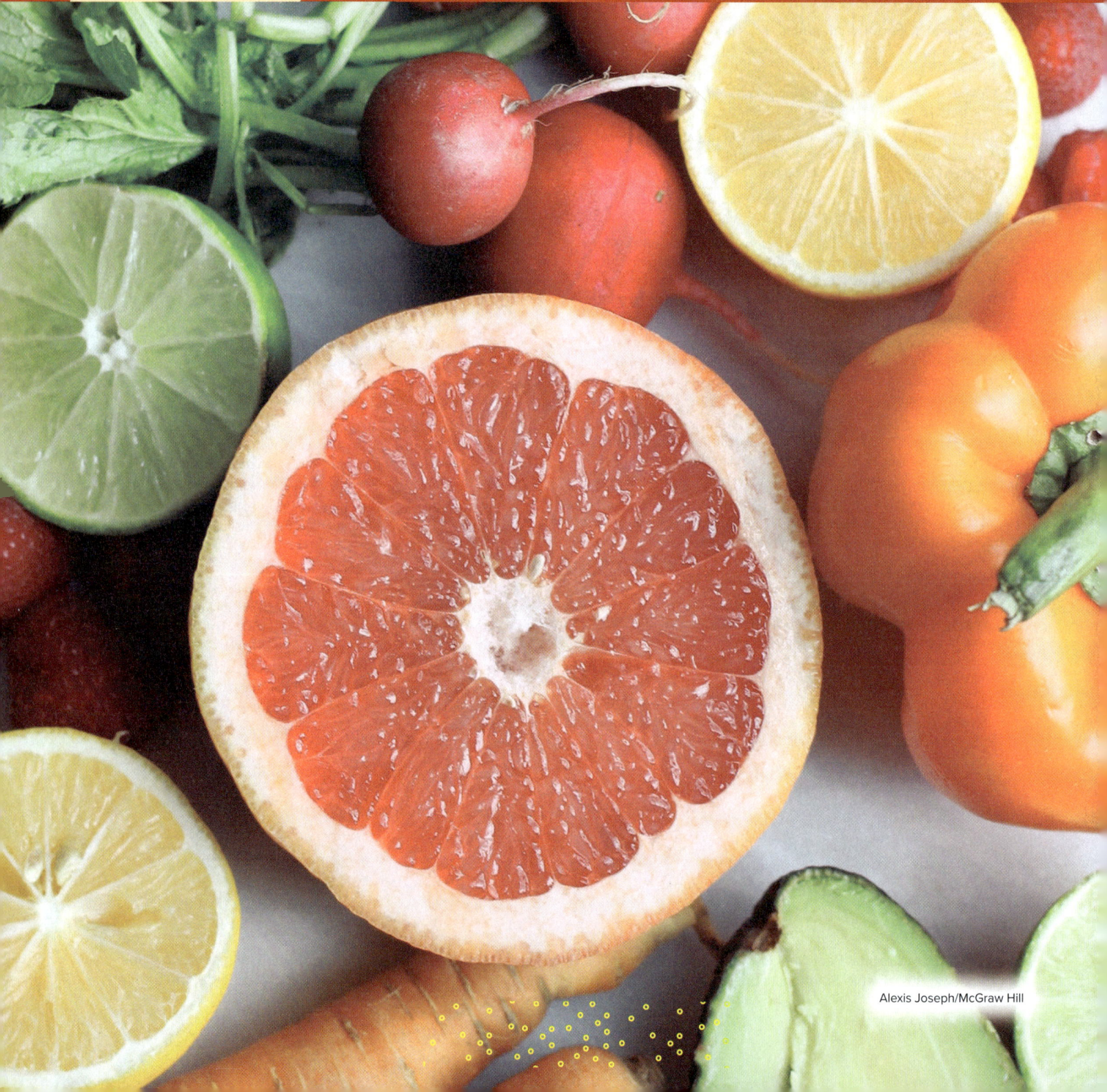

Chapter 8
Vitamins and Phytochemicals

Alexis Joseph/McGraw Hill

Student Learning Outcomes

Chapter 8 is designed to allow you to:

8.1 Describe the general characteristics of the fat- and water-soluble vitamins, absorption, and storage.

8.2 List ways to preserve vitamins in foods and explain the sources and benefits of phytochemicals.

8.3 Describe the roles of the fat-soluble vitamins (A, D, E, and K) in body defenses and bone health.

8.4 Describe the roles of the B vitamins (thiamin, riboflavin, niacin, pantothenic acid, biotin, vitamin B-6, folate, and vitamin B-12) in energy metabolism and in blood and brain health; vitamin C in immune function; and choline in cell structures and metabolism.

8.5 List the dietary sources and requirements for each fat- and water-soluble vitamin and choline as well as the dangers of exceeding the recommendations.

8.6 Describe the signs and symptoms of vitamin deficiencies and risk factors leading to vitamin deficiencies.

8.7 Evaluate dietary supplements, current recommendations, and potential benefits and hazards of use.

8.8 Describe modifiable risk factors that contribute to cancer risk and understand the role of food constituents in cancer prevention, treatment, and survivorship.

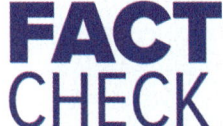

FACT CHECK

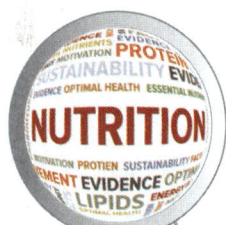

What type of milk is the best source of vitamin D?

Many people associate vitamin D with *whole* milk—and whole milk *is* a rich source of this nutrient. However, if you compare the Nutrition Facts labels from the various types of cow's milk in the grocery store, you will see they all provide about 250 milligrams of calcium and 2.5 micrograms of vitamin D. Fortification of milk with vitamin D is not mandatory in the United States, but most dairy producers voluntarily fortify their milk. If fortified, milk must contain at least 400 IU (10 micrograms) of vitamin D per quart. This regulation applies to all types of cow's milk—whole, reduced fat, or skim milk. It also applies to plant-based milk alternatives, such as soy milk, almond milk, and cashew milk, which are often voluntarily fortified to match the bone-building nutrients present in cow's milk. See Section 8.4 to learn more about the vitamin D content of foods.

Source: Food additives permitted for direct addition to food for human consumption; vitamin D_2 and vitamin D_3. *Fed. Regist.* 2016;81(137):46578-46582.

8.1 Vitamins: Vital Dietary Components

By definition, vitamins are essential organic (carbon-containing) substances needed in small amounts in the dietary pattern for normal function, growth, and maintenance of the body. All humans require the same essential vitamins, but the amount required can vary depending on age, sex, and presence of illness. Although vitamin requirements are very small, each vitamin is essential for one or more functions in the body (Fig. 8-1). Vitamins can be divided into two broad classes based on solubility: vitamins A, D, E, and K are **fat-soluble vitamins,** whereas the B vitamins and vitamin C are **water-soluble vitamins.** The B vitamins include thiamin, riboflavin, niacin, pantothenic acid, biotin, vitamin B-6, folate, and vitamin B-12. Choline is a vitamin-like nutrient but is not technically classified as a vitamin.

Vitamins are essential in human dietary patterns because they cannot be synthesized in the human body or produced in sufficient amounts. Notable exceptions to having a strict dietary need for a vitamin are vitamin A, which we can synthesize from

fat-soluble vitamins Vitamins that dissolve in fat and some chemical compounds but not readily in water. These vitamins are A, D, E, and K.

water-soluble vitamins Vitamins that dissolve in water. These vitamins are the B vitamins and vitamin C.

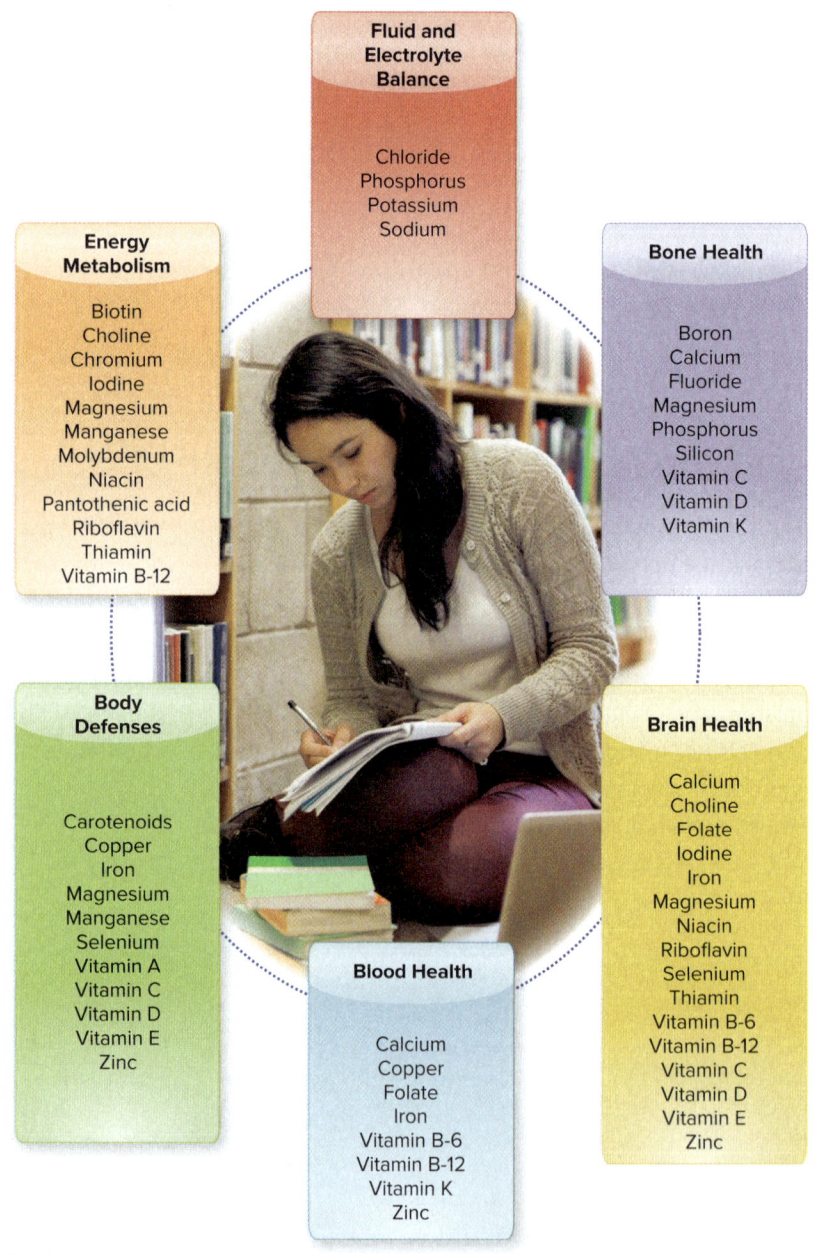

FIGURE 8-1 Micronutrients contribute to many functions in the body. wavebreakmedia/Shutterstock

certain pigments in plants; vitamin D, synthesized in the body if the skin is exposed to adequate sunlight; niacin, synthesized from the amino acid tryptophan; and vitamin K, biotin, and others that are synthesized by the bacteria in the intestinal tract.

To be classified as a vitamin, a compound must meet the following criteria: (1) the body is unable to synthesize enough of the compound to maintain health; and (2) absence of the compound from the dietary pattern for a defined period produces deficiency symptoms. If caught in time, these symptoms can be quickly reversed when the compound is reintroduced. A compound does not qualify as a vitamin merely because the body cannot make it. Evidence must suggest that health eventually declines when the substance is not consumed.

As scientists began to identify various vitamins, related deficiency diseases such as scurvy (vitamin C) and rickets (vitamin D) were dramatically cured. For the most part, as the vitamins were discovered, they were named alphabetically: A, B, C, D, E, and so on. Later, many substances originally classified as vitamins were found not to be essential for humans and were removed from the list. Other vitamins, thought at first to be only one chemical, turned out to be several chemicals, so the alphabetical names had to be broken down by numbers (B-6, B-12, and so on).

In addition to their use in correcting deficiency diseases, a few vitamins have also proved useful in treating several nondeficiency diseases. These medical applications require administration of megadoses, amounts well above typical human needs for the vitamins. Understand that claimed benefits from use of vitamin supplements, especially intakes in excess of the Tolerable Upper Intake Level (UL) (if established), should be viewed critically because unproved claims are common. Remember, whenever you take a supplement at high doses, you are taking it at a pharmacological dose—that of a drug. Expect side effects as you would from any drug.

Vitamins isolated from foods (*natural*) or manufactured in the laboratory (*synthetic*) are the same chemical compounds and work equally well in the body. Contrary to claims on social media and in health food stores, natural vitamins isolated from foods are, with few exceptions, no different than those labeled synthetic. Of note, however, the natural form of vitamin E is much more potent than the synthetic form. In contrast, synthetic folic acid, the form of the vitamin added to ready-to-eat breakfast cereals and flour, is almost twice as potent as the natural vitamin form.[1]

ABSORPTION AND STORAGE OF VITAMINS IN THE BODY

The fat-soluble vitamins (A, D, E, and K) are absorbed in the presence of dietary fat. These vitamins then travel with dietary fats as part of chylomicrons through the bloodstream to reach body cells. Special carriers in the bloodstream help distribute some of these vitamins. Fat-soluble vitamins are stored mostly in the liver and fatty tissues.

When fat absorption is efficient, about 40% to 90% of the fat-soluble vitamins are absorbed. Anything that interferes with normal digestion and absorption of fats, however, also interferes with fat-soluble vitamin absorption. For example, people with cystic fibrosis, a disease that often hampers fat absorption, may develop deficiencies of fat-soluble vitamins. Some medications, such as certain weight-loss drugs, also interfere with fat absorption. Unabsorbed fat carries these vitamins to the large intestine, and they are excreted in the feces. People with fat-malabsorption conditions are especially susceptible to vitamin K deficiency because body stores of vitamin K are lower than those of the other fat-soluble vitamins. Vitamin supplements, taken under a primary care provider's guidance, are part of the treatment for preventing a vitamin deficiency associated with fat malabsorption. Finally, people who use mineral oil as a laxative risk fat-soluble vitamin deficiencies. Fat-soluble vitamins dissolve in the mineral oil, but the intestine does not absorb mineral oil. Hence, the fat-soluble vitamins are eliminated with the mineral oil in the feces.

Vitamin Production
You have learned that the beneficial bacteria in the gut microbiome help us to digest our food, regulate our immune system, offer protection against diseases, and confer other health benefits. Did you also know that your microbiome is responsible for producing vitamins, including vitamin B-12, thiamin, riboflavin, biotin, and vitamin K?

magnificent microbiome

Water-soluble vitamins are handled much differently than fat-soluble vitamins. After being ingested, the B vitamins from food are first broken down from their active coenzyme forms into free vitamins in the stomach and small intestine. The vitamins are then absorbed, primarily in the small intestine. Typically, about 50% to 90% of the water-soluble vitamins in the diet are absorbed, which means they have relatively high bioavailability. Water-soluble vitamins are transported to the liver via the hepatic portal vein and are distributed to body tissues. Once inside cells, the active coenzyme forms are resynthesized. Although some supplement manufacturers sell vitamins in their coenzyme forms, there is no benefit in consuming the coenzyme forms as these are broken down during digestion and activated inside cells as needed.

Excretion of vitamins varies primarily on their solubility. Except for vitamin K, fat-soluble vitamins are not readily excreted from the body. Hence, toxicity can be an issue. Water-soluble vitamins are excreted based on **tissue saturation,** the degree to which the tissue vitamin stores are full. Tissue storage capacity is limited. As the tissues become saturated, the rate of excretion via the kidney increases sharply, preventing potential toxicity. Unlike other water-soluble vitamins, B-6 and B-12 are stored in the liver and not easily excreted in the urine.

tissue saturation The limited storage capacity of water-soluble vitamins in the tissues.

In light of the limits of tissue saturation for many water-soluble vitamins, these vitamins should be consumed in your daily dietary pattern. However, an occasional lapse in the intake of water-soluble vitamins causes no harm. Symptoms of a vitamin deficiency occur only when that vitamin is lacking in one's dietary pattern, and the body stores are essentially exhausted. For example, for an average person, the dietary pattern must be devoid of thiamin for 2 to 3 weeks or lacking in vitamin C for a month before the first symptoms of deficiencies of these vitamins appear.

VITAMIN TOXICITY

For most water-soluble vitamins, when you consume more than the RDA or AI, the kidneys efficiently filter the excess from the blood and excrete these compounds in urine. Notable exceptions are vitamin B-6 and vitamin B-12, which are stored in the liver. Although they are water-soluble, these two B vitamins may accumulate to toxic levels.

In contrast to the water-soluble vitamins, fat-soluble vitamins are not readily excreted, so some can easily accumulate in the body and cause toxic effects (Fig. 8-2). Although a toxic effect from an excessive intake of any vitamin is theoretically possible, toxicity of the fat-soluble vitamin A is the most frequently observed. Vitamin A causes toxicity at intakes as little as two times the RDA.[2] Vitamin E and the water-soluble vitamins niacin, vitamin B-6, and vitamin C can also cause toxic effects but only when consumed in large amounts. Overall, vitamins are unlikely to cause toxic effects unless taken in supplement (pill) form.

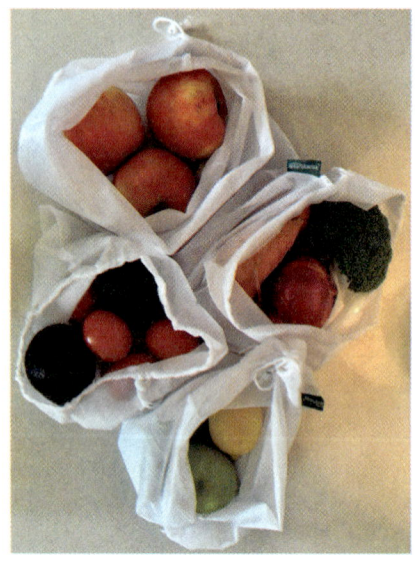

Looking for a way to purchase fruits and vegetables at the grocery or farmers' market without wasting so many plastic bags? Consider reusable produce bags. These environmentally friendly bags are durable, breathable, and washable, and come in a variety of sizes. Anne Smith

Some people believe that consuming vitamins far in excess of their needs provides them with extra energy, protection from disease, and prolonged youth. They seem to think that if a little is good, then more must be better. A *one-a-day* type of multivitamin and mineral supplement (MVM) usually contains less than two times the Daily Values of its components, so daily use of these products is unlikely to cause toxic effects. However, consuming multiple pills, especially single-dose supplements such as vitamin A, can lead to toxicity.

PRESERVATION OF VITAMINS IN FOODS

community-supported agriculture (CSA) Farms that are supported by a community of growers and consumers who provide mutual support and share the risks and benefits of food production, usually including a system of weekly delivery or pickup of vegetables and fruit, and sometimes dairy products and meat.

Good sources of vitamins can be found in all food groups, especially fruits and vegetables (Fig. 8-3). However, storage time and environmental factors can impact the vitamin content of foods. Fully ripe food contains more vitamins, but substantial amounts of vitamins can be lost from the time produce is harvested until it is eaten. Therefore, it is best to eat fresh produce as soon as possible after harvest. Food cooperatives, **community-supported agriculture (CSA),** and farmers' markets are great sources of freshly harvested fruits and vegetables.[3] The water-soluble vitamins, particularly thiamin, vitamin C, and folate, are particularly vulnerable to destruction by environmental exposures.

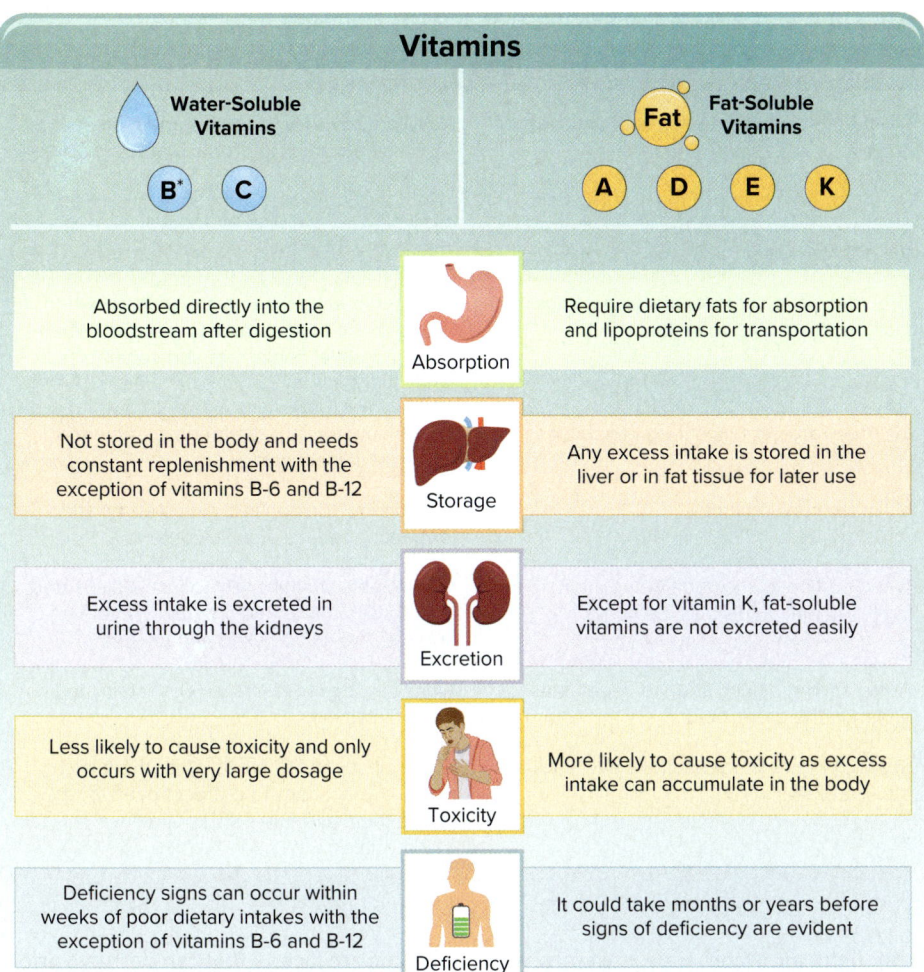

FIGURE 8-2 Comparison of water-soluble and fat-soluble vitamins.

*B vitamins include: thiamin, riboflavin, niacin, pantothenic acid, vitamin B-6, biotin, folic acid, and vitamin B-12. Choline is a vitamin-like substance that is often grouped with B vitamins due its similarities.

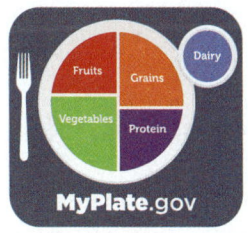

**MyPlate:
Sources of Vitamins and Choline**

FIGURE 8-3 Certain food groups on MyPlate are especially rich sources of various vitamins and choline. Each may also be found in other MyPlate groups but in lower amounts. In addition to those vitamins listed here, pantothenic acid is present in moderate amounts in many groups, and vitamin E is abundant in plant oils. U.S. Department of Agriculture

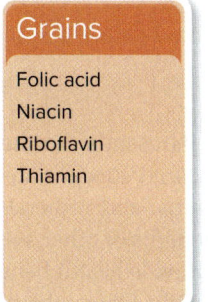

Grains

Folic acid
Niacin
Riboflavin
Thiamin

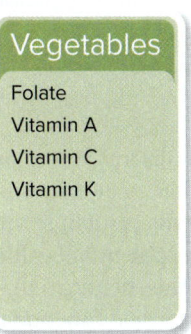

Vegetables

Folate
Vitamin A
Vitamin C
Vitamin K

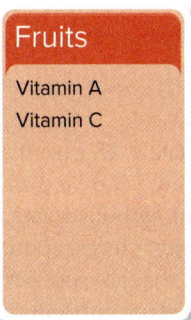

Fruits

Vitamin A
Vitamin C

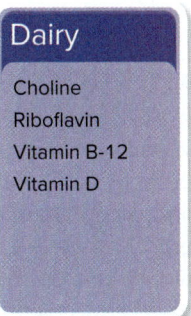

Dairy

Choline
Riboflavin
Vitamin B-12
Vitamin D

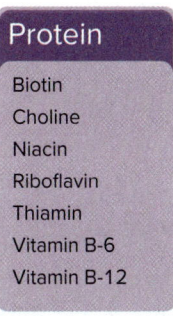

Protein

Biotin
Choline
Niacin
Riboflavin
Thiamin
Vitamin B-6
Vitamin B-12

TABLE 8-1 ■ Tips for Preserving Vitamins in Fruits and Vegetables

Preservation Methods	Mechanism
Keep fruits and vegetables cool until eaten.	Chilling slows down the degradation of vitamins by enzymes in produce once harvested.
Refrigerate fruits and vegetables (except bananas, onions, potatoes, and tomatoes) in the crisper drawer.	Nutrients keep best at temperatures near freezing, at high humidity, and away from air.
Trim, peel, and cut fruits and vegetables minimally and just prior to eating.	Oxygen breaks down vitamins faster when more of the food surface is exposed. Whenever possible, cook fruits and vegetables in their skins.
Microwave, steam, or stir-fry vegetables.	More nutrients are retained when there is minimal contact with water.
Minimize cooking time.	Prolonged cooking (slow simmering) and reheating reduce vitamin content.
Avoid adding fats to vegetables during cooking if you plan to discard the liquid.	Fat-soluble vitamins will be lost in discarded fat. If you want to add fats, do so after vegetables are fully cooked and drained.
Avoid adding baking soda to vegetables to enhance the green color.	Alkalinity destroys vitamin D, thiamin, and other vitamins.
Store canned and frozen fruits and vegetables carefully.	To protect canned foods, store them in a cool, dry location. To protect frozen foods, store them at 0°F (−18°C) or colder. Eat within 12 months.

Heat, light, air, water, time, enzymes, acid, and alkali are factors that can destroy various vitamins. Some foods, like tomatoes, have improved bioavailability once cooked.

There are several steps you can take to preserve nutrients when you are purchasing, storing, and preparing fruits and vegetables (Table 8-1). Frozen vegetables and fruits are often as nutrient-rich as freshly harvested ones because fruits and vegetables are typically frozen immediately after harvesting. As part of the freezing process, vegetables are quickly blanched in boiling water. Blanching destroys the enzymes that would otherwise degrade the vitamins over time. If produce will not be eaten within a few days of harvest, freezing is the best preservation method to retain nutrients.

✓ CONCEPT CHECK 8.1

1. What is a megadose? Are there any negative consequences of consuming megadoses of vitamins?
2. List at least three differences between fat-soluble and water-soluble vitamins.
3. List three ways to preserve vitamin content when storing, preparing, or cooking foods.

8.2 Phytochemicals

In addition to the approximately 45 essential nutrients, there are thousands of other compounds in food. For many years, a great deal of nutrition research concentrated on gaining knowledge about carbohydrates, lipids, proteins, vitamins, and minerals. More recently, there is growing interest about the potential health benefits of other substances found in food. Foods that are sources of the chemicals that provide health benefits beyond being essential dietary nutrients are termed **functional foods.** Oatmeal is an

functional foods Foods that are sources of the chemicals that provide health benefits beyond being essential dietary nutrients.

PHYTOCHEMICALS FOUND IN PLANT PIGMENT COLORS	FOUND IN	GOOD FOR
CAROTENOIDS & HESPERETIN	Carrots, sweet potatoes, oranges, lemons	Eye health, immune function, heart health
ANTHOCYANOSIDES & RESVERATROL	Blueberries, blackberries, grapes, beets, eggplants	Antioxidants, anti-inflammatory, heart health, cognition
SULFORAPHANE & LUTEIN	Leafy greens, broccoli, cabbages, green tea	Anti-carcinogenic, anti-inflammatory, liver function, eye health
ALLYL SULFIDES & FLAVONOIDS	Garlic, onions, leeks, apples, buckwheat	Cholesterol lowering, immune function, anti-allergy, estrogen metabolism
LYCOPENE & ELLAGIC ACID	Tomatoes, cherries, radishes, strawberries	Antioxidants, heart health, immune function

FIGURE 8-4 Plant foods are packed with colorful phytochemicals that support health. Eating plant foods from a variety of color families is associated with a variety of health benefits. oranges: Lluis Real/Pixtal/age fotostock; berries: Noppadon sakulsom/Janecocoa/123RF; broccoli: spafra/iStock/Getty Images; garlic: Maks Narodenko/Shutterstock; tomatoes: Tim UR/Shutterstock

Source: AICR at https://mt-1.aicr.org/reduce-your-cancer-risk/diet/elements_phytochemicals.html

example of a functional food as it contains soluble fiber that can lower cholesterol levels. Other foods are fortified or modified to improve health benefits. For example, some orange juice is fortified with calcium for bone health. Functional foods can be placed into two categories: (1) **zoochemicals,** health-promoting compounds found in animal food; and (2) phytochemicals, health-promoting compounds found in plant foods (*phyto* means "plant" in Greek). Examples of zoochemicals include omega-3 fatty acids in fish and prebiotics and probiotics in the GI tract of animals (including humans).

Phytochemicals are responsible for the unique colors, flavors, and odors observed in plants (Fig 8-4). For plants, phytochemicals serve as an environmental protective mechanism to help plants survive the elements (UV exposure, insects, and other predators). Interestingly, these chemicals improve human health when dietary patterns high in plant foods are consumed. In addition to the **carotenoids,** some of the phytochemicals being studied include allicin, phytosterols, isothiocyanates, lignans, stanols, ellagic acid, **flavonoids,** saponins, glucosinolates, polyphenols, phytoestrogens, sulfides, lectins, and many more. Select examples of phytochemicals include **isoflavones** in soy, sulforaphane in cruciferous vegetables, and resveratrol in grapes and wine. Other examples of foods that are rich sources of phytochemicals include fruits, vegetables, whole grains, beans, peas, lentils, herbs, spices, nuts, and seeds.

Over 4400 molecular features have been identified in a single black raspberry,[4] and over 750 carotenoid pigments found in plants.[5] The full extent of these health benefits are just beginning to be elucidated. What we do know is that phytochemicals cannot be synthesized in the body, so we must obtain them from food; however, they are not considered essential nutrients because a deficiency disease is not observed when they are removed from the dietary pattern. Thus, even though you may see the word *phytonutrient* in some sources, *phytochemical* remains the most accurate term.

PHYTOCHEMICAL FUNCTIONS

Although the study of the metabolic actions of phytochemicals is relatively new, numerous mechanistic protective health benefits of these plant-based foods have been noted, beyond those conferred by their vitamin and mineral contents:

- Stimulate the immune system.
- Reduce inflammation.

zoochemicals Chemicals found in animal products that have health-protective actions.

carotenoids Phytochemicals with red, orange, and yellow colors found in squash, tomatoes, and stone fruits; some can be converted to vitamin A in the body.

flavonoids Phytochemicals with yellow, red, or blue colors found in citrus fruits, berries, red onion, tea, red wine, and dark chocolate.

isoflavones Phytochemicals produced in legumes; some have hormone-like activities in the body.

antioxidant A substance that has the ability to prevent or repair the damage caused by oxidation.

- Prevent DNA damage and aid in DNA repair.
- Reduce oxidative damage to cells.
- Promote cardiovascular, neurocognitive, eye, and bone health.
- Regulate intracellular signaling of hormones and gene expression.
- Activate insulin receptors.
- Inhibit the initiation and proliferation of cancer, and stimulate spontaneous cell death.
- Alter the absorption, production, and metabolism of cholesterol.
- Mimic or inhibit hormones and enzymes.
- Decrease the formation of blood clots.

PHYTOCHEMICAL RECOMMENDATIONS

There are no specific dietary recommendations for the amount of phytochemicals that should be consumed, except that they should be consumed as food. At present, we know that phytochemicals have protective functions with minimal side effects when consumed naturally in a variety of foods. Therefore, it is wise to eat a wide variety of whole plant foods to obtain the optimum amount of macronutrients, vitamins, minerals, fiber, and phytochemicals. A combination of different plant foods will also increase the **antioxidant** capacity of the total dietary pattern, and there is no doubt that we need to consume a greater variety and quantity of antioxidant-rich foods (Table 8-2).

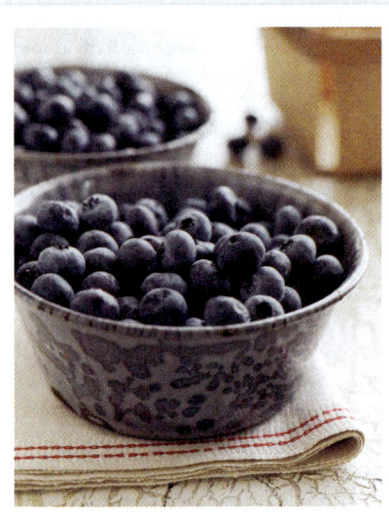

Blueberries are rich in health-promoting phytochemicals. They have been shown to have anti-cancer effects and therefore could be an important part of dietary cancer-prevention strategies. **What is your favorite way to incorporate phytochemicals into your daily menu?** Alexandra Grablewski/Lifesize/Getty Images

TABLE 8-2 ■ Tips for Boosting the Phytochemical Content of Your Eating Pattern

Include vegetables in main and side dishes. Add vegetables to rice, omelets, potato salad, and pastas. Try broccoli or cauliflower florets, mushrooms, peas, carrots, corn, or peppers.
Look for quick-to-fix whole grain side dishes in the supermarket. Pilafs, couscous, rice mixes, and tabbouleh are just a few options.
Choose fruit-filled cookies, such as fig bars, instead of sugar-rich cookies.
Use fresh or canned fruit as a topping for pudding, hot or cold cereal, pancakes, and frozen desserts.
Put raisins, grapes, apple chunks, pineapple, grated carrots, zucchini, or cucumber into coleslaw, chicken salad, or tuna salad.
Be creative at the salad bar: add fresh spinach, leaf lettuce, red cabbage, zucchini, squash, cauliflower, peas, mushrooms, or peppers to your salad.
Pack fresh or dried fruit for snacks away from home instead of grabbing a candy bar or another energy-dense option.
Add slices of cucumber, zucchini, spinach, or carrot slivers to the lettuce and tomato on your sandwiches.
Each week try one or two vegetarian meals such as beans and rice, vegetable stir-fry, or whole-grain pasta with tomato sauce.
If your daily protein intake exceeds the recommended amounts, reduce the meat, fish, or poultry in casseroles, stews, and soups by one-third to one-half and replace with more vegetables and legumes.
Choose a snack from a container of fresh vegetables in the refrigerator or from a bowl of fresh fruit.
Substitute unsweetened tea for sugar-sweetened soft drinks on a regular basis.
Switch from crisp head (iceburg) lettuce to looseleaf lettuce, preferably red or dark green.
Use salsa as a dip for chips in place of creamy dips.
Choose whole grain breakfast cereals, breads, and crackers.
In place of salt, add flavor to your food with onions or herbs such as ginger, rosemary, basil, thyme, garlic, parsley, and chives.
Incorporate soy products, such as tofu, soy milk, soy protein isolate, and roasted soybeans, into your meals.

Roots

Supertasters

Our tongues are covered with small bumps called *papillae* that each contains multiple taste buds. When stimulated, taste receptors send nerve signals to our brains. Normal human taste sensations include sweet, sour, salty, umami, and bitter. In 1931, chemist Arthur Fox inadvertently discovered that individuals had different *bitter* taste perceptions, referring to them as *tasters* and *non-tasters*. Genetic mutations and taste bud density have since contributed to additional stratifications that include supertasters (25% of the population), medium tasters (50%), and non-tasters (25%). Researchers speculate that the ability to taste bitter flavors may have offered an advantage for survival: bitter flavors commonly indicate the presence of toxins!

As you learned in Chapter 1, our food choices and preferences are influenced by many factors. Chapter 15 explores how early and repeated exposures to foods contribute to a child's acceptance of specific foods throughout life. Supertasters have a heightened sensitivity to bitter taste. This could certainly influence both acceptance and rejection of specific foods and beverages, particularity those thought to confer a bitter taste, such as cruciferous vegetables, coffee and tea, alcohol, and tobacco. It is also plausible that supertasters could display more picky eating behaviors.

The good news is that *any* type of taster can adopt the simple tips below to increase their intakes of phytochemical- and antioxidant-rich vegetables!

- Roasting vegetables caramelizes the starches and makes them taste sweeter. Enjoy roasted vegetables in curries, casseroles, lasagna, stir fry, soups, or low-fat creamy soups, or tossed in salads.
- Add steamed and pureed pumpkin or squash to chili, spaghetti sauce, macaroni and cheese, baked goods, and stews.
- Top sliced veggies with low-fat cheese sauce, reduced-fat salad dressing, Greek yogurt, or peanut butter to mask bitter taste.
- Enjoy whole wheat pasta salad with an abundance of sliced raw vegetables and topped with low-fat salad dressing to help mask flavor.
- For bitter greens like broccoli or collard greens, blanch them in boiling water before serving. Blanching reduces their bitter flavor.
- Add leafy greens to fruit smoothies so the sweetness of the fruit can mask the bitter flavors of the vegetables.
- Add shredded zucchini to muffins.
- Make a pesto spaghetti sauce with spinach leaves.

Sources: https://www.psychologytoday.com/us/blog/comfort-cravings/201006/are-you-supertaster-mindless-eating-your-taste-buds; https://thenourishedchild.com/what-supertaster/

FARM to FORK: Crucifers

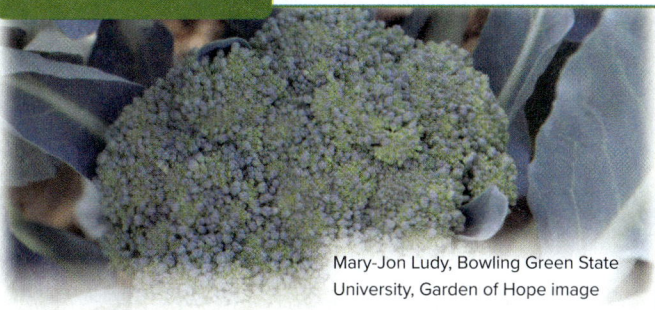

Mary-Jon Ludy, Bowling Green State University, Garden of Hope image

Cruciferous vegetables are cool-weather vegetables with flowers that have four petals that resemble a cross. The most common crucifers include broccoli, cauliflower, cabbage, bok choy, Brussels sprouts, and green leafy vegetables such as kale and arugula. Ounce for ounce, crucifers have it all—vitamins, minerals, fiber, and an abundance of disease-fighting phytochemicals.

Grow

- The freshest and most nutrient-dense crucifers always come straight from the garden. Sadly, up to 80% of nutrients are lost in the transport from farm to fork.
- For crucifer container gardening, estimate 1 broccoli plant per 5 gallons of soil (see https://ofbf.org/2008/06/05/vegetable-container-gardens).
- Most crucifers require full sun and moist, fertile soil that's slightly acidic. Broccoli can germinate in soil with temperatures as low as 40°F, but check online for growing recommendations in your region.

Shop

- Buy broccoli with dark green crowns, tight bud heads, and moist and firm stems. Avoid yellowing and dry produce that is not kept chilled.
- Intact heads of broccoli are not only more nutritious but less expensive than precut florets.

Store

- To preserve the nutrients, antioxidants, and phytochemicals in crucifers, keep them cool and eat within days of harvest.
- If storing for any period, place in a plastic bag with about 20 pinprick holes (*micro-perforated* bag) in the crisper drawer.
- Prior to freezing broccoli, it is essential to *blanch* the produce to deactivate its enzymes (see https://ohioline.osu.edu/factsheet/HYG-5333).

Prep

- In most cases, the leaves or flower buds of crucifers are eaten, but there are a few where either the roots or seeds are also eaten.
- Compounds known as glucosinolates are responsible for much of the bitterness and the health benefits offered by these amazing plants.
- Cooking and preservation expose crucifers to heat, oxygen, and light—all significantly decreasing nutrient and phytochemical content. Lower temperatures as well as drier and shorter cooking times reduce losses.
- Steaming for less than 5 minutes or sautéing with a small amount of extra virgin olive oil is recommended.

Source: Robinson J. The incredible crucifers: tame their bitterness and reap the rewards. In: *Eating on the Wild Side: The Missing Link to Optimum Health*. New York: Little, Brown & Co.; 2013.

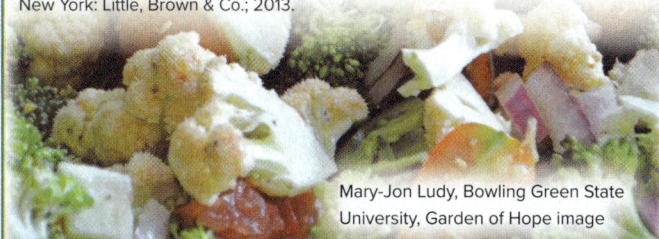

Mary-Jon Ludy, Bowling Green State University, Garden of Hope image

> ✓ **CONCEPT CHECK 8.2**
>
> 1. Give one example of a functional food.
> 2. Which food groups have the richest supply of phytochemicals?
> 3. Dietary patterns rich in phytochemicals are associated with a decreased risk of which diseases?

8.3 Vitamin A (Retinoids) and Carotenoids

Vitamin A was the first fat-soluble vitamin to be recognized as an important component of food essential for human health.[2] Almost all (90%) of vitamin A is stored in the liver; the remaining 10% is in adipose tissue, kidneys, and the lungs. Either a deficiency or toxicity can cause severe problems, and there is a narrow range of optimal intakes between these two states.

Vitamin A is in a group of compounds known as **retinoids.** There are three active forms of vitamin A: (1) **retinol,** (2) **retinal,** and (3) **retinoic acid.** Collectively, these three are often called *preformed* vitamin A. They are only naturally present in animal products. When retinol is stored, it is *esterified* (joined to a fatty acid) and becomes **retinyl.** In supplements, you will often find vitamin A listed as *retinyl acetate* or *retinyl palmitate*.

Besides the retinoids, which come from animal sources, many foods of plant origin contain carotenoids, some of which can be converted into vitamin A in the body. Note that carotenoids are not essential nutrients; they are categorized as phytochemicals. Although hundreds of carotenoids have been identified, just three can be converted to retinol in the body: alpha carotene, **beta-carotene,** and beta-cryptoxanthin. Because these carotenoids can be turned into vitamin A, they are termed **provitamin A.** Of these three, only beta-carotene serves as a significant source of vitamin A. Neither the absorption of carotenoids nor the conversion of the provitamin A carotenoids into vitamin A is an efficient process. Other carotenoids that may play a role in human health but are not vitamin A precursors include lycopene, zeaxanthin, and lutein.

retinoids Chemical forms of preformed vitamin A found in animal foods.

retinol Alcohol form of vitamin A.

retinal Aldehyde form of vitamin A.

retinoic acid Acid form of vitamin A.

retinyl Storage form of vitamin A.

beta-carotene The orange-yellow pigment in carrots; beta-carotene is the only carotenoid that can be sufficiently absorbed and converted into retinol in the body.

provitamin A A substance that can be converted into vitamin A.

FUNCTIONS OF VITAMIN A AND CAROTENOIDS

Epithelial Cell Health and Immune Function. For many years, vitamin A has been dubbed the *anti-infection* vitamin. Vitamin A maintains the health of epithelial cells, which line the surfaces of the lungs, intestines, stomach, vagina, urinary tract, and bladder, as well as those of the eyes and skin. Retinoic acid is required for immature epithelial cells to develop into mature, functional epithelial cells. Epithelial tissues, such as those that form the skin and GI tract, serve as important barriers to infection. Vitamin A also supports the activity of certain immune system cells, specifically the T-lymphocytes, or T-cells.

Eye Health and Vision. The link between vitamin A and night vision has been known since ancient Egyptians used juice extracted from liver to cure **night blindness.** Vitamin A performs important functions in light–dark vision and, to a lesser extent, color vision. Light entering the eye reaches a lining called the **retina.** The retina consists of various cells, such as rods, cones, and nerve cells. Rods detect black and white, and they are responsible for night vision. Cones are responsible for color vision. Rods and cones require vitamin A for normal function. One form of vitamin A (retinal) allows certain cells in the eye to adjust to dim light (such as after seeing the headlights of an oncoming car; Fig. 8-5).

night blindness Vitamin A deficiency disorder that results in loss of the ability to see under low-light conditions.

retina A light-sensitive lining in the back of the eye. It contains retinal.

Some carotenoids are also important for vision. The macula (also known as the *macula lutea,* meaning "yellow spot") is in the central area of the retina and is responsible for the most detailed central vision. It contains the carotenoids lutein and zeaxanthin in high enough concentrations to impart a yellow color. *Age-related macular degeneration* (Fig. 8-6), the leading cause of blindness among older adults in the United States, occurs because of changes in this macular area of the retina. Research studies indicate that higher intakes of these carotenoids may help to prevent or slow the progression of age-related macular degeneration. Carotenoids may also decrease the risk of cataracts in the eyes. Although

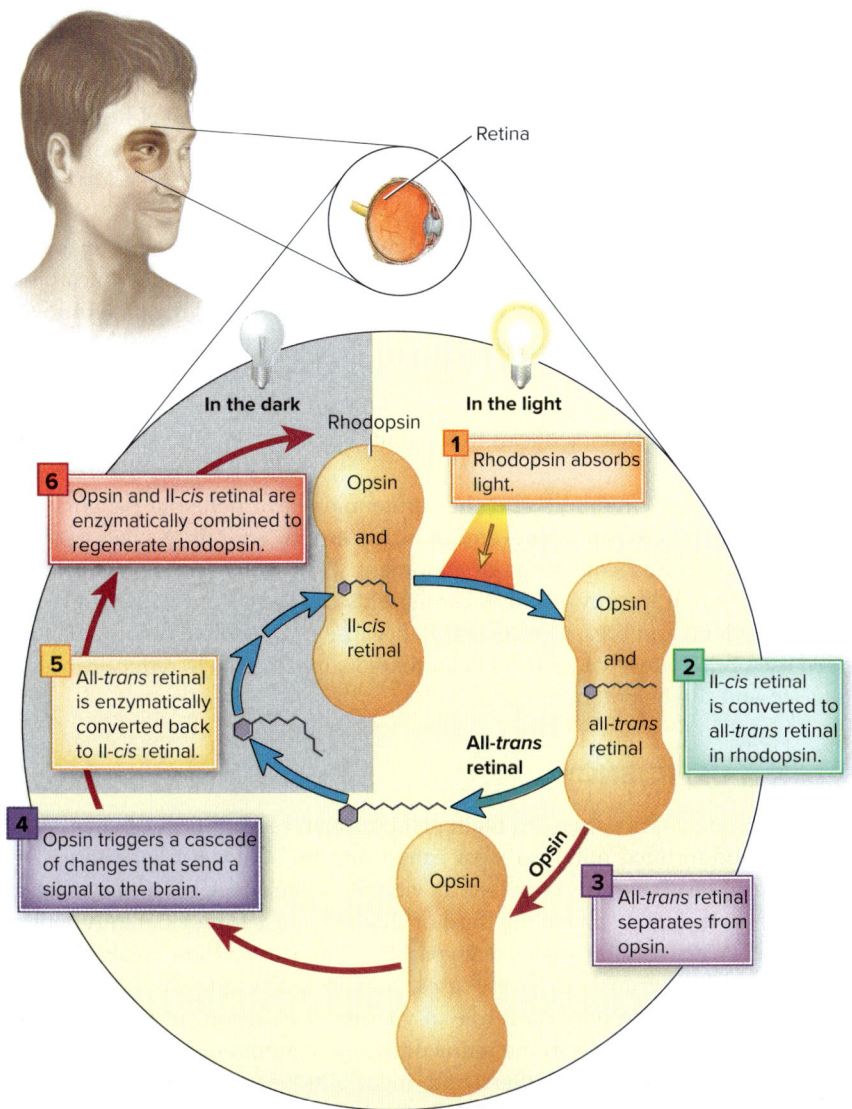

FIGURE 8-5 Vitamin A functions to maintain vision. Light enters the eye through the cornea and lens, and then hits the retina. The light reacts with vitamin A–containing rhodopsin, which is stored in the rod cells of the retina. Rod cells allow us to see black-and-white images. When light reacts with rhodopsin, retinal is cleaved from rhodopsin (bleaching), a process that stimulates an electrical impulse to the brain. A new molecule of vitamin A then combines with opsin to regenerate rhodopsin. The yellow background indicates the bleaching events that occur in the light; the gray background indicates the regenerative events that can occur in either light or dark conditions.

supplements containing carotenoids are marketed to older adults as a way to protect eye health, current research points to the safety and benefits of *dietary* sources of carotenoids. Overall, the richest sources of lutein and zeaxanthin are green leafy vegetables (Table 8-3).

Growth, Development, and Reproduction. Vitamin A participates in the processes of growth, development, and reproduction in several ways. At the genetic level, vitamin A binds to receptors on DNA to increase synthesis of a variety of proteins. Some of these

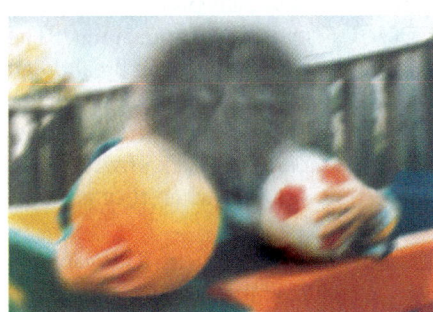

FIGURE 8-6 The blurry center of the image simulates the vision of a person with macular degeneration. National Eye Institute/National Institutes of Health

TABLE 8-3 ■ **Vegetables Rich in Lutein and Zeaxanthin**

Vegetables (serving size)	Lutein and Zeaxanthin (mg)
Broccoli (½ cup cooked)	0.8
Brussels sprouts (½ cup cooked)	1.0
Kale (½ cup cooked)	11.9
Peas (½ cup cooked)	1.9
Romaine lettuce (1 cup raw)	1.5
Spinach (½ cup cooked)	10.2
Spinach (1 cup raw)	3.1
Zucchini (½ cup cooked)	2.0

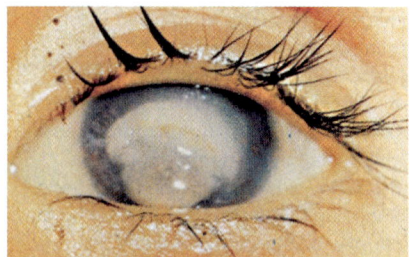

FIGURE 8-7 Vitamin A deficiency eventually leads to blindness. The buildup of scar tissue on the surface of the eye leads to Bitot's spots. This problem is commonly seen today in Southeast Asia. Dr. Alfred Sommer

xerophthalmia Hardening of the cornea and drying of the surface of the eye, which can result in blindness as a result of vitamin A deficiency.

Bitot's spots Dry, foamy spots made from an accumulation of keratin (a protein) on the surface of the eye; caused by vitamin A deficiency.

hyperkeratosis A condition in which patches of skin become thicker, rougher, or drier than usual; a possible consequence of vitamin A deficiency.

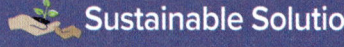

Biofortification

Biofortification increases the nutrient density of food crops through conventional plant breeding, enhanced agronomic practices, or biotechnology without sacrificing consumer and farmer preferences. So far, its application has been applied to iron-biofortification of beans, cowpea, and pearl millet; zinc-biofortification of maize, rice, and wheat; and provitamin A carotenoid-biofortification of cassava, maize, rice, and sweet potato.

Source: WHO Biofortification of Crops with Minerals and Vitamins.

proteins are required for growth. During early fetal growth, vitamin A functions in the differentiation and maturation of cells that will ultimately form tissues and organs. For bones to grow and elongate, old bone must be remodeled (broken down) so that new bone can be formed. Vitamin A assists with the breakdown and formation of healthy bone tissue. Adequate intake of vitamin A is needed for reproduction; it aids in sperm production (associated with its epithelial role) and in a normal reproductive cycle for adult females.

Cardiovascular Disease Prevention. Carotenoids may play a role in preventing cardiovascular disease in individuals at high risk. This role may be linked to carotenoids' ability to inhibit the oxidation of low-density lipoproteins (LDLs). Until definitive studies are complete, many scientists recommend that we consume a total of at least five servings of a combination of fruits and vegetables per day as part of an overall effort to reduce the risk of cardiovascular disease. Until we have more answers, focus on an eating pattern rich in phytochemicals from whole foods.

Cancer Prevention. Vitamin A and the carotenoids have potential benefits but also potential dangers where cancer prevention is concerned. Vitamin A plays a role in cellular differentiation and embryonic development. Numerous studies have found that dietary patterns rich in provitamin A carotenoids are associated with a lower risk of skin, lung, bladder, and breast cancers. Still, because of the potential for toxicity, unsupervised use of megadose vitamin A or carotenoid supplements to reduce cancer risk is not advised and can be potentially dangerous.

VITAMIN A DEFICIENCY

Typical American dietary patterns contain plentiful sources of preformed vitamin A (e.g., meats, eggs, and fortified milk), so most Americans are at low risk for vitamin A deficiency. However, in other parts of the world, vitamin A deficiency is a major public health concern. Across the globe, about one-third of children suffer from vitamin A deficiency.[6] Vitamin A deficiency results in three main problems: impaired vision, weakened immune function, and stunted growth. In severe cases, vitamin A deficiency contributes to death.

You learned about the important role of vitamin A in vision. In the early stages of vitamin A deficiency, the cells in the retina of the eye cannot quickly adjust from bright to dim light and the individual suffers from night blindness. Vitamin A deficiency can also lead to an eye disease called **xerophthalmia**. As vitamin A deficiency progresses, the cells that line the cornea of the eye (the clear window of the eye) lose the ability to produce mucus. The eye then becomes very dry. Eventually, dirt particles scratch and scar the dry surface of the eye. This can lead to accumulations of dead cells and secretions on the surface of the eye, which are called **Bitot's spots** (Fig. 8-7). Over time, impairments in the visual cycle and damage to the cornea lead to blindness. In fact, vitamin A deficiency is the leading cause of preventable blindness among children worldwide.

So, for the eye, unhealthy epithelial tissue contributes to blindness. Lack of vitamin A also affects the integrity of other epithelial tissues, such as the skin, respiratory tract, and GI tract. **Hyperkeratosis** is a condition in which skin cells produce too much keratin, blocking the hair follicles and causing *gooseflesh* or *toadskin* appearance. The excessive keratin in these skin cells causes the skin to be hard and dry. The breakdown of epithelial tissues of the skin, respiratory tract, and GI tract also makes it easier for pathogens to enter the blood and cause infections. To further complicate immune function, the ability of white blood cells to fight infection is impaired by lack of vitamin A. Vitamin A–deficient humans have an increased infection rate, but when they are supplemented with vitamin A, the immune response improves.

Vitamin A deficiency can also affect normal growth and development. This can lead to problems with fetal development during pregnancy. During infancy and childhood, vitamin A deficiency may lead to stunted growth.

Globally, attempts to address vitamin A deficiency include promoting breastfeeding, providing dietary supplements, and fortifying commonly consumed foods (e.g., sugar, margarine, and monosodium glutamate) with vitamin A. Most recently, **biofortification** of crops has become a viable technique to provide vitamin A to populations who need it most.[7]

biofortification Use of selective breeding or other biotechnology to enhance the nutrient content of crops.

fetus The developing organism from about the beginning of the ninth week after conception until birth.

GETTING ENOUGH VITAMIN A AND CAROTENOIDS

Preformed vitamin A (e.g., retinol, retinal, and retinoic acid) is found in liver, fish, fish oils, fortified milk, butter, yogurt, and eggs (Fig. 8-8). Margarine and other plant oil spreads are also fortified with vitamin A. For individuals who choose dairy alternatives, fortified soy beverages (commonly known as *soy milk*) and soy yogurt also contain vitamin A.

About 70% of the vitamin A in the typical dietary pattern comes from preformed vitamin A sources, whereas provitamin A carotenoids dominate the eating patterns among people in less developed areas of the world. The provitamin A carotenoids are mainly found in dark-green and yellow-orange vegetables and some fruits. Carrots, spinach and other leafy greens, winter squash, sweet potatoes, broccoli, mangoes, cantaloupe, peaches, and apricots are examples of such sources. Beta-carotene accounts for some of the orange color of carrots. The yellow-orange beta-carotene is masked by dark-green chlorophyll pigments. Green, leafy vegetables, such as spinach and kale, have high concentrations of lutein and zeaxanthin. Tomato products contain significant amounts of lycopene. Cooking food and consuming food with small amounts of healthy fat improve the bioavailability of carotenoids. In raw fruits and vegetables, carotenoids are bound to proteins. Cooking disrupts this protein bond and frees the carotenoid for better absorption, and fat increases bioavailability.

The RDA for vitamin A is expressed in retinol activity equivalents (RAE). These RAE units consider the activity of both preformed vitamin A and the carotenoids that are converted into vitamin A in humans. The total RAE value for a food is calculated by adding the concentration of preformed vitamin A to the amount of provitamin A carotenoids in the food that will be converted into vitamin A. There is no separate DRI for beta-carotene or any of the other phytochemicals.

The dietary patterns of adults typically contain adequate vitamin A. Most adults have liver reserves of vitamin A three to five times higher than needed to provide good health. Thus, the use of vitamin A supplements by most people is unnecessary. Populations in the United States that may be at risk for vitamin A deficiency include those with low fruit and vegetable intakes (e.g., some children, older adults, and food-insecure individuals); people with alcoholism or liver disease; or people with severe fat malabsorption.

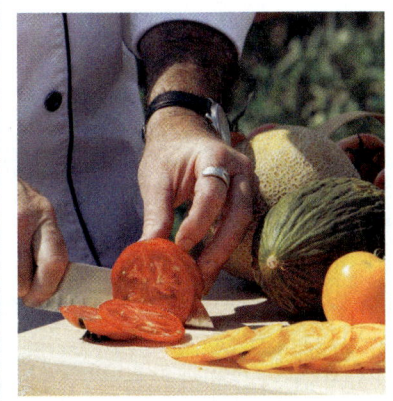

Lycopene is the carotenoid that gives foods such as tomatoes, watermelon, guava, and pink grapefruit their reddish color. **If you want to absorb the most lycopene from tomatoes, is it better to eat them raw or cooked?** Sarah Rusnak

AVOIDING TOO MUCH VITAMIN A AND CAROTENOIDS

Intakes in excess of the UL for vitamin A are linked to birth defects and liver toxicity. Other possible side effects include an increased risk of hip fracture and poor pregnancy outcomes.

During the early months of pregnancy, a high intake of preformed vitamin A is especially dangerous because it may cause fetal malformations and spontaneous abortions. This is because vitamin A binds to DNA and influences cell development. The Food and Drug Administration (FDA) recommends that females of childbearing age limit their overall intake of preformed vitamin A from food and dietary supplements to no more than about 100% of the Daily Value. It is also important to limit consumption of rich food sources of preformed vitamin A, such as liver. In addition, medications that contain derivatives of vitamin A should be avoided during pregnancy. These precautions apply to females who are pregnant and also those who may possibly become pregnant; vitamin A is stored in the body for long periods, so females who ingest large amounts during the months before pregnancy place their **fetus** at risk.

In contrast, ingesting large amounts of vitamin A–yielding carotenoids does not appear to cause toxic effects. A high carotenoid concentration in the blood, *hypercarotenemia*, can occur if someone routinely consumes large amounts of carrots or takes pills containing beta-carotene ($\geq$ 30 milligrams daily) or if infants eat an excessive amount of squash. The skin turns yellow-orange, particularly the palms of the hands and soles of the feet. It differs from jaundice, an accumulation of bilirubin caused by underlying disease, usually involving the liver. In jaundice, the yellow discoloration extends to the sclera (whites) of the eye, whereas in hypercarotenemia it does not. Hypercarotenemia

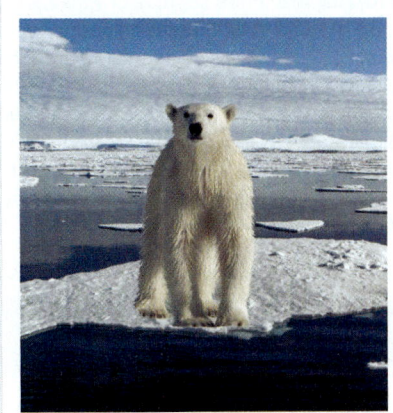

Inuits long knew and explorers soon learned to avoid eating the liver of polar bears. Just 4 ounces of polar bear liver will deliver a toxic dose of 675,000 RAE of vitamin A. **How does this dose compare to the RDA?** M G Therin Weise/Photographer's Choice/Getty Images

does not appear to cause harm and disappears when carotenoid intake decreases. Dietary carotenoids do not produce toxic effects because: (1) their rate of conversion into vitamin A is relatively slow and regulated; and (2) the efficiency of carotenoid absorption from the small intestine decreases markedly as oral intake increases.

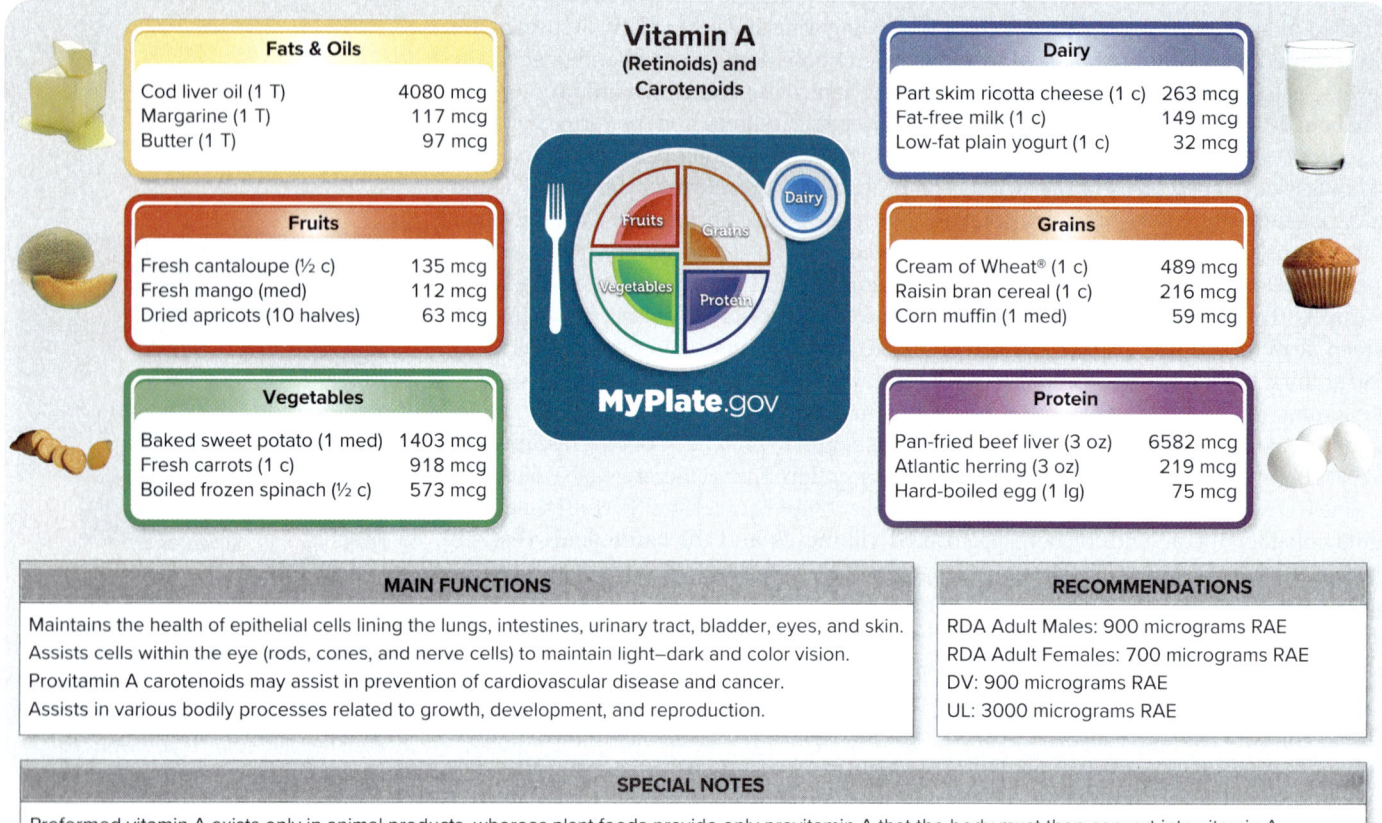

FIGURE 8-8 Food sources of vitamin A and carotenoids. The fill of the background color (none, 1/3, 2/3, or completely covered) within each food group on MyPlate indicates the average nutrient density for vitamin A and provitamin A carotenoids in that group. The figure shows the vitamin A content of several foods from each food group. Overall, the fruits and vegetables groups provide many rich sources of carotenoids, whereas fortified dairy products and certain choices in the protein group are good sources of preformed vitamin A. The grains group also contains some foods that are nutrient dense because they are fortified with vitamin A. butter: 2/James Worrell/Ocean/CORBIS; milk: Nipaporn Panyacharoen/Shutterstock; cantaloupe: Renne Comet/National Cancer Institute; muffin: Anton Prado PHOTO/Shutterstock; sweet potato: lynx/iconotec.com/Glow Images; eggs: Vivian Thode/dancestrokes/123RF; MyPlate: U.S. Department of Agriculture

Sources: Office of Dietary Supplements, Dietary Supplements Fact Sheets, available from https://ods.od.nih.gov/factsheets/list-all; USDA FoodData Central, available from https://fdc.nal.usda.gov

Medicine Cabinet

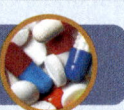

Vitamin A Derivatives

Two derivatives of vitamin A are used to treat moderate to severe acne. Tretinoin (Retin-A®) is used topically (applied to the skin), and isotretinoin (Accutane®) is taken orally. These drugs appear to work by altering genes expressed by the skin cells. However, taking vitamin A supplements or making a paste from supplements and applying it to your skin will have no effect on acne. In fact, high doses of vitamin A can induce toxic symptoms, including birth defects. Accutane's label clearly advises against the use of the medication during pregnancy, and its use is strictly monitored by the Food and Drug Administration (FDA). In order for females to receive this medication, they must have two negative pregnancy tests; sign a patient information/consent form; agree to use two effective forms of birth control; register, along with their primary care providers and pharmacists, with iPLEDGE (https://www.ipledgeprogram.com/iPledgeUI/home.u); and agree to follow all instructions of the program.

Peter Dazeley/Photographer's Choice/Getty Images

> ✓ **CONCEPT CHECK 8.3**
>
> 1. What are the consequences of vitamin A deficiency?
> 2. How are the carotenoids related to vitamin A?
> 3. Name two carotenoids and identify a good food source of each.
> 4. List two rich food sources of retinoids.

8.4 Vitamin D (Calciferol or Calcitriol)

Vitamin D is a fat-soluble vitamin with two unique qualities. First, vitamin D is the only nutrient that is also a hormone. A hormone is a compound manufactured by one organ of the body that then enters the bloodstream and has a physiological effect on another organ or tissue. The cells that participate in the synthesis of vitamin D (skin, liver, and kidneys) are different from the cells that respond to vitamin D, namely bone and intestinal cells; therefore, vitamin D is considered a hormone.[8]

Second, vitamin D is the only nutrient that can be produced in the skin upon exposure to ultraviolet light. The human production of vitamin D begins when the ultraviolet B (UVB) rays of the sun convert a cholesterol precursor of vitamin D (**7-dehydrocholesterol**) in the skin into an inactive, *previtamin* form of **vitamin D_3** (cholecalciferol). As illustrated in Figure 8-9, this compound must be activated to **25-hydroxyvitamin D_3** (calcidiol or calcifediol) in the liver and to **1,25-dihydroxyvitamin D_3** (calcitriol) in the kidney before it can function as the vitamin D hormone. Vitamin D_2 (ergocalciferol) is a synthetic form of vitamin D, which will be discussed later.

Our ability to absorb UVB rays and make vitamin D in the skin is affected by many factors. Dark skin pigmentation, geographic latitude, time of day, season of the year, weather conditions, genetics, and amount of body surface covered with clothing or sunscreen affect the skin's exposure to UVB rays and therefore influence vitamin D synthesis. Something as simple as complete cloud cover or severe pollution can reduce UVB rays by 50%. In addition, UVB rays will not penetrate glass. Aging reduces our ability to synthesize vitamin D—as much as 70% by age 70! Exposure of hands, face, and arms to midday sun for about 10 minutes daily will support adequate vitamin D synthesis for most healthy children and adults during the summer months.[9] However, older adults and individuals with dark skin pigmentation require about three to five times this amount of sun exposure to synthesize an equivalent amount of vitamin D.[10]

7-dehydrocholesterol Precursor of vitamin D found in the skin.

vitamin D_3 Previtamin form synthesized in the skin and found naturally in some animal sources, including fish and egg yolks; also called *cholecalciferol*.

25-hydroxyvitamin D_3 Intermediate form of vitamin D found in blood; also called *calcidiol* or *calcifediol*; sometimes shortened to *25(OH)D_3*.

1,25-dihydroxyvitamin D_3 Biologically active form of vitamin D; also called *calcitriol*; sometimes shortened to *1,25(OH)D_3*.

FUNCTIONS OF VITAMIN D

Did you know the biological effects of vitamin D extend far beyond its role in bone health? The active vitamin D hormone binds to receptors in the nucleus of many cells throughout the body and regulates gene expression. In other words, vitamin D can turn certain genes on and off to control cellular processes. In this way, vitamin D affects many glands and organs, including the parathyroid gland, pancreas, bones, kidneys, intestines, nervous system, skin, muscles, and reproductive organs.[11]

Blood Calcium and Phosphorus Regulation. The most well-known function of the active vitamin D hormone (calcitriol) is to maintain the normal range of calcium and phosphorus in the blood. Together with two other hormones—parathyroid hormone (PTH) and calcitonin—vitamin D maintains blood calcium and phosphorus levels within a narrow range. This tight regulation ensures that an appropriate amount of these minerals is available to all cells. Vitamin D regulates blood mineral levels in three ways: (1) it influences the absorption of calcium and

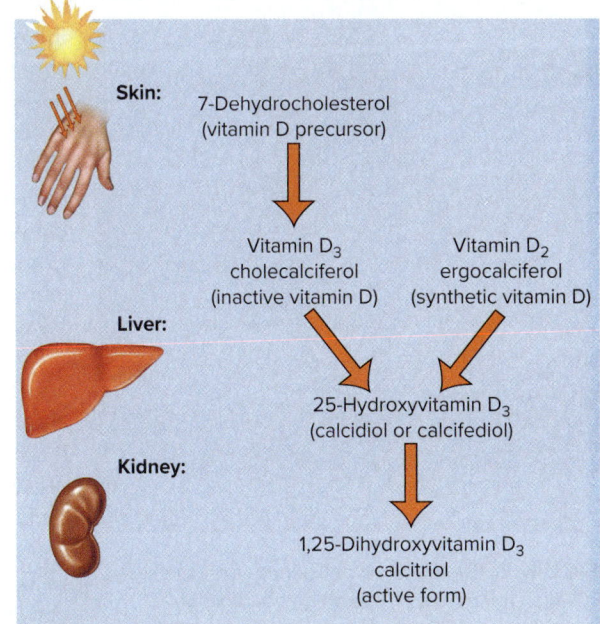

FIGURE 8-9 A precursor to vitamin D is synthesized when skin is exposed to sunlight. Previtamin D must be further modified by the liver and kidney for maximal activity.

phosphorus from the small intestine; (2) in combination with PTH and calcitonin, it regulates calcium excretion via the kidney; and (3) it affects the withdrawal of minerals from the bones.

Cellular Differentiation. Vitamin D is considered one of the most potent regulators of cellular differentiation, the process by which stem cells become specialized for certain roles in the body. Because of its role in normal cell development, vitamin D may prevent mutations and thereby help to reduce cancer risk (e.g., in the skin, colon, prostate, and breast).[12]

Immune Function. Vitamin D helps to regulate the development of immune system cells. Research points to an important role of vitamin D in supporting the innate immune response and in preventing autoimmune diseases, such as type 1 diabetes, multiple sclerosis, and rheumatoid arthritis.

VITAMIN D DEFICIENCY

When vitamin D levels are adequate, about 30% to 40% of dietary calcium is absorbed by the small intestine. If blood levels of vitamin D are low, the small intestine is able to absorb only about 10% to 15% of calcium consumed, which is not enough to maintain the calcium requirements for bone health and other functions. Subsequently, calcium and phosphorus deposition during bone synthesis is reduced, resulting in weaker bones that do not develop properly. Vitamin D deficiency can be traced to inadequate dietary intake, poor absorption (e.g., fat malabsorption in children with cystic fibrosis), specific genetic variants, altered metabolism (e.g., liver or kidney disease), or inadequate sun exposure. Vitamin D deficiency has been known to be a problem in individuals with dark skin and older adults. More recent research found that U.S. adults who were Black, less educated, poor, obese, current smokers, physically inactive, and infrequent milk consumers had a higher prevalence of vitamin D deficiency.[13] Overall, the dietary patterns of more than 90% of all U.S. adults fall short of the RDA for vitamin D.[14] According to the *Dietary Guidelines,* vitamin D is considered a dietary component of public health concern for the general U.S. population.

Vitamin D deficiency can occur at any time, but when it occurs during infancy and early childhood, the resulting disease is known as **rickets.** The skeletal abnormalities of rickets include bowed legs, thick wrists and ankles, curvature of the spine, a pigeon chest (chest protrudes above the sternum), skull malformations, and pelvic deformities (Fig. 8-10). Vitamin D deficiency is a concern among young infants who are not receiving (1) vitamin D supplementation, (2) sufficient exposure to sunlight, or (3) food fortified with vitamin D (e.g., cereal and dairy products). In addition, consumption of non–cow's milk beverages with low vitamin D content has been associated with a decrease in blood vitamin D levels in early childhood compared to levels in children consuming cow's milk fortified with higher levels of vitamin D.[15] Because melanin acts as a natural sunscreen, individuals with darker skin pigmentation are at increased risk for vitamin D deficiency. Compared to non-Hispanic whites, risk for vitamin D deficiency is increased among non-Hispanic Asian and non-Hispanic Black populations. Overall, about 5% of the U.S. population is at risk for vitamin D deficiency.[16]

Osteomalacia, which means "soft bone," is an adult disease comparable to rickets. It can result from inadequate vitamin D or calcium intake, inefficient calcium absorption from the small intestine, or poor conservation of calcium by the kidneys. It occurs most commonly in people with kidney, stomach, gallbladder, or intestinal disease (especially when most of the intestine has been removed) and in people with cirrhosis of the liver. These diseases affect both vitamin D activation and calcium absorption, leading to a decrease in bone mineral density. Bones become porous and weak and break easily. Research shows that treatment with 10 to 20 micrograms per day of vitamin D, in conjunction with adequate dietary calcium, can reduce fracture risk in older adults. Thus, vitamin D is just as important as calcium when it comes to bone health. Table 8-4 summarizes factors that influence vitamin D status.

rickets A disease characterized by poor mineralization of newly synthesized bones because of low calcium content. Arising in infants and children, this deficiency is caused by insufficient amounts of vitamin D in the body.

osteomalacia Adult form of rickets. The bones have low mineral density and consequently are at risk for fracture.

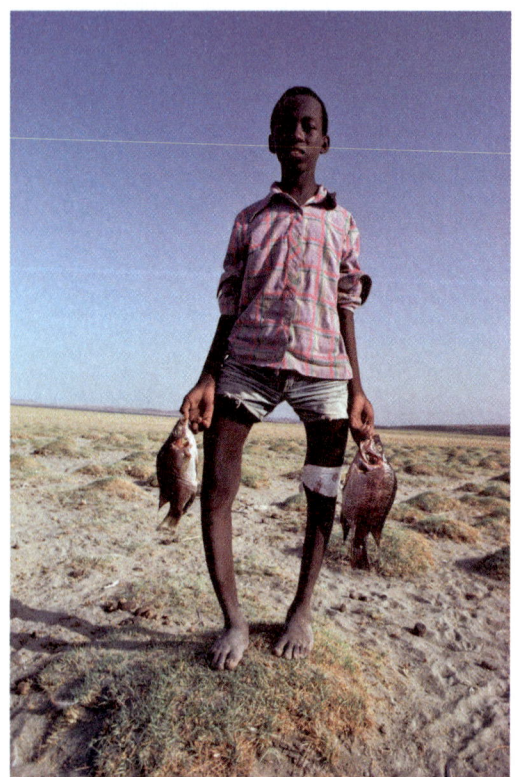

FIGURE 8-10 Vitamin D deficiency causes rickets, in which the bones and teeth do not develop normally. This individual has bowed legs and other skeletal deformities of rickets. Jeff Rotman/Alamy Stock Photo

TABLE 8-4 ■ Factors That Impair Vitamin D Status

Factor	Effect
Inadequate sun exposure • Northern latitudes • Concealing clothing (e.g., robes/veils) • Air pollution (i.e., smog) • Sunscreen with SPF > 8 • Excessive time spent indoors (e.g., due to health, work, or environmental conditions)	Limited exposure to UVB reduces the skin's ability to synthesize vitamin D.
Age	Vitamin D synthesis by the skin decreases. Vitamin D activation by the kidneys decreases.
Dark skin pigmentation	Melanin reduces the skin's ability to produce vitamin D, particularly for older adults and especially among females.
Inadequate dietary intake	Dietary intake of vitamin D is unable to compensate for inadequate skin synthesis of vitamin D.
Exclusive breastfeeding or low consumption of infant formula	Infants typically have limited sun exposure. Breast milk is a poor source of vitamin D. Infant formula contains vitamin D, but young infants may not consume adequate quantities to meet needs.
Fat malabsorption • Liver disease • Cystic fibrosis • Weight-loss medications	Poor absorption of dietary fat limits absorption of vitamin D from the small intestine.
Obesity	Release of vitamin D stored in subcutaneous fat is inefficient.
Liver diseases	Vitamin D activation by the liver decreases.
Kidney diseases	Vitamin D activation by the kidneys decreases.

GETTING ENOUGH VITAMIN D

Although vitamin D can be synthesized in the skin upon exposure to sunlight, there are many factors that can affect vitamin D synthesis (review Table 8-4). Plus, it is difficult to balance the benefits of vitamin D synthesis with the risks of skin damage from excessive exposure to UV light. Therefore, it is important to find dietary sources of vitamin D, especially during the winter months.

There are two forms of vitamin D in foods: vitamin D_2 and vitamin D_3. **Vitamin D_2** (ergocalciferol) is a synthetic product derived from the irradiation of plant sterols (ergosterol) and is used in some supplements. Vitamin D_3 (cholecalciferol)—the form synthesized in the human body and found naturally in a few foods—is more commonly used in supplements and fortified foods. Both forms of vitamin D must be modified by chemical reactions that occur in the kidney and liver (Fig. 8-9) before they can be active in the body.

The RDA for vitamin D is 15 micrograms per day throughout most of adulthood. This is based on a daily intake that is sufficient to maintain bone health and normal calcium metabolism, assuming minimal sun exposure. It is challenging to meet the RDA because dietary sources of vitamin D are limited. Besides fatty fish, organ meats (e.g., beef liver), egg yolks, and select varieties of mushrooms that are grown in the sunlight, very few foods are natural sources of vitamin D (Fig. 8-11 and *Farm to Fork* on mushrooms). However, fortified foods are an effective way to add vitamin D to your dietary pattern. Most cow's milk and many plant-based dairy alternatives you buy in the store are fortified with vitamin D. Use of vitamin D–fortified milk began in the 1930s and effectively wiped out rickets in the United States. Because vitamin D is a fat-soluble vitamin, there is slightly more vitamin D in a cup of whole milk (3.2 micrograms)

vitamin D_2 Form found in nonanimal sources, such as in some mushrooms. Also synthetically produced and included in many supplements; also called *ergocalciferol*.

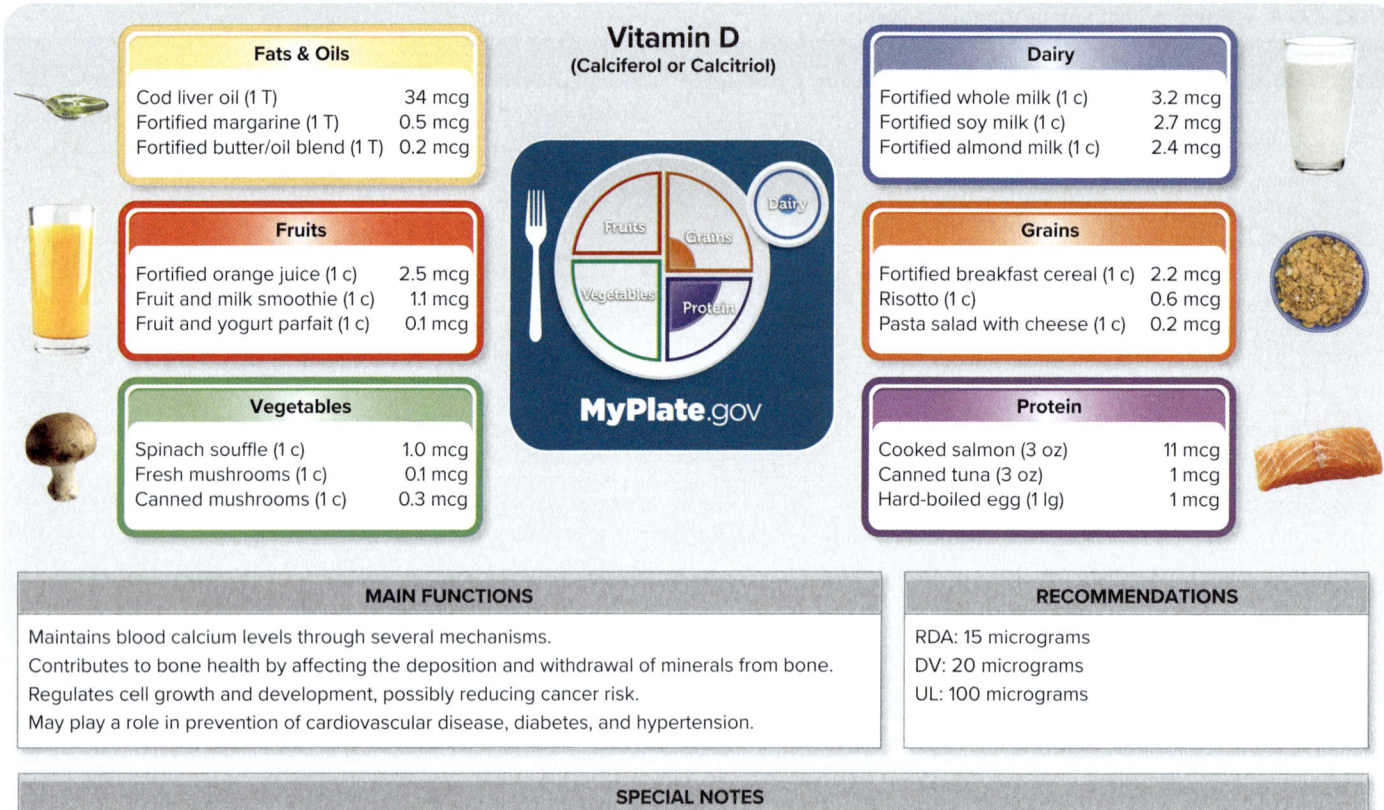

FIGURE 8-11 Food sources of vitamin D. The fill of the background color (none, 1/3, 2/3, or completely covered) within each food group on MyPlate indicates the average nutrient density for vitamin D in that group. The figure shows the vitamin D content of several foods in each food group. Overall, the richest sources of vitamin D are fish, fortified dairy products, and fortified breakfast cereals. Foods from the vegetables group are not a source of vitamin D, except for a select variety of mushrooms. oil: lumusphotography/iStock/Getty Images; milk: NIPAPORN PANYACHAROEN/Shutterstock; juice: Sergei Vinogradov/seralexvi/123RF; cereal: Joe Belanger/iStock/Getty Images; mushrooms: lynx/iconotec.com/Glow Images; salmon: Foodcollection; MyPlate: U.S. Department of Agriculture

Sources: Office of Dietary Supplements, Dietary Supplements Fact Sheets, available from https://ods.od.nih.gov/factsheets/list-all; USDA FoodData Central, available from https://fdc.nal.usda.gov.

compared to 1% milk (3 micrograms) or fat-free milk (2.9 micrograms). Some ready-to-eat breakfast cereals are also fortified with vitamin D (along with many other vitamins and minerals). Fortified breakfast cereals provide as much as 2.2 micrograms per 1-cup serving, but most offer closer to 1 microgram per serving. In addition, some brands of orange juice are fortified with about 2.5 micrograms of vitamin D per 1-cup serving.

The food sources described contain inactive forms of vitamin D that must be converted into the active hormone form in the body. Some foods, such as meat, dairy products, and eggs, contain small amounts of 25-hydroxyvitamin D_3. This is an intermediate form of vitamin D that has gone through one of the two steps required to convert vitamin D to its active form in animal tissues. Although the amount of this form of vitamin D is quite low in the typical American dietary pattern, it is thought to be more bioavailable than other food forms of vitamin D.[17]

It takes some planning to meet your daily vitamin D requirements from food sources. If you work indoors, live in a northern location, habitually use sunscreen, or are not eating fish every day, you may need a supplement. Supplements and fortified foods with vitamin D_3 are most effective at raising blood levels of vitamin D and reducing fracture risk.

During the time of growth from infancy through adolescence, consuming adequate vitamin D supports optimal bone mineralization. The American Academy of Pediatrics recommends that all infants, children, and adolescents should consume a minimum of

FARM to FORK: Mushrooms

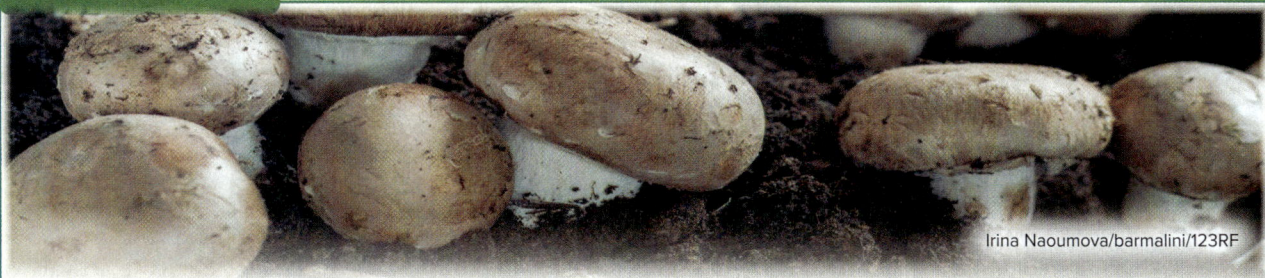

Irina Naoumova/barmalini/123RF

More than 2000 varieties of edible mushrooms are available in all shapes and sizes. They are low in calories (about 20 calories in 1 cup of raw sliced mushrooms) and a good source of fiber. Most varieties are rich in the vitamins riboflavin, niacin, and pantothenic acid and the minerals potassium, selenium, and copper. Mushrooms also contain a vitamin D precursor, ergosterol, which can be converted into vitamin D by exposing mushrooms to the sun's ultraviolet radiation. Mushrooms are a popular meat substitute because of their savory taste called umami.

Grow
- Mushrooms can be cultivated at home or found in the wild (some wild mushrooms are poisonous, so never eat them unless you know they are safe). Mushrooms grow from very tiny spores in a growth mixture of sawdust, composted manure, or straw. This mixture, called spawn, supports growth of the threadlike roots, called mycelium. Mushroom kits are available, packed with mushroom mycelium growing on mushroom spawn.
- Mushrooms grow best in a dark, cool, moist, and humid environment, ideally in a basement or under the sink at home.
- White button mushrooms are the easiest types to grow at home. They should appear within 3 to 4 weeks and can be harvested every day for about 6 months. They are harvested when the caps open and the stalk can be cut from the stem with a sharp knife.

Shop
- White button mushrooms are also the most common and least expensive mushrooms found in grocery stores. When purchasing mushrooms, choose those with a firm texture, even color, and tightly closed caps.
- Crimini mushrooms are young portabellos that look similar to the white button but are darker in color. The large portabellos and shiitakes have a meaty taste and texture.
- Morels have a honeycomb-like shape and are available fresh in spring and summer, whereas dried morels are available year-round and are much less expensive.
- Chanterelles are trumpet-shaped mushrooms and a good substitute for the more expensive morels.
- Porcinis are popular wild mushrooms with a distinct earthy, nutty flavor. Dried porcini mushrooms are less expensive and can be reconstituted and added to recipes.
- Some brands of mushrooms are now exposed to ultraviolet light to stimulate vitamin D production. Vitamin D–enhanced mushrooms providing 10 micrograms of vitamin D per 3-ounce serving (about 1 cup of diced mushrooms) are available in stores. They are usually labeled "UV treated" or "high in vitamin D" and cost more than regular mushrooms. In contrast, wild mushrooms such as chanterelles, maitake, and morels are naturally rich in vitamin D because they get natural sun exposure.

Store
- Mushrooms are best when used within a few days of purchase. They should be stored in the refrigerator in their original package, a paper bag, or a damp cloth bag and used within 1 week. Storing mushrooms in a plastic bag will cause them to deteriorate quickly. Before preparing mushrooms, wipe them off with a clean, damp cloth or paper towel. Soaking fresh mushrooms in water will make them soggy. If they must be rinsed, do it lightly and dry gently.
- You can increase the vitamin D in your mushrooms by slicing them and placing the gills to face the sun for just 15 minutes. This will produce 5 to 20 micrograms of vitamin D (RDA is 15 micrograms) in 3 ounces of mushrooms and at least 90% of the vitamin is retained after storage and cooking.

Prep
- Although mushrooms can be eaten raw, cooking mushrooms releases more of their nutrients and intensifies their color and flavor.
- Most mushrooms can be sautéed, grilled, or stir-fried. Searing mushrooms first in a dry pan browns the mushrooms and quickly drives off excess moisture. Adding a bit of butter and white wine or vinegar gives the mushrooms a nice sauce.
- Mushrooms can also be baked and filled with your favorite stuffing.

Source: Moore M. Mushrooms: taste of the earth. *Food & Nutrition Mag.* 2013 June 26. https://foodandnutrition.org/july-august-2013/mushrooms-taste-earth/

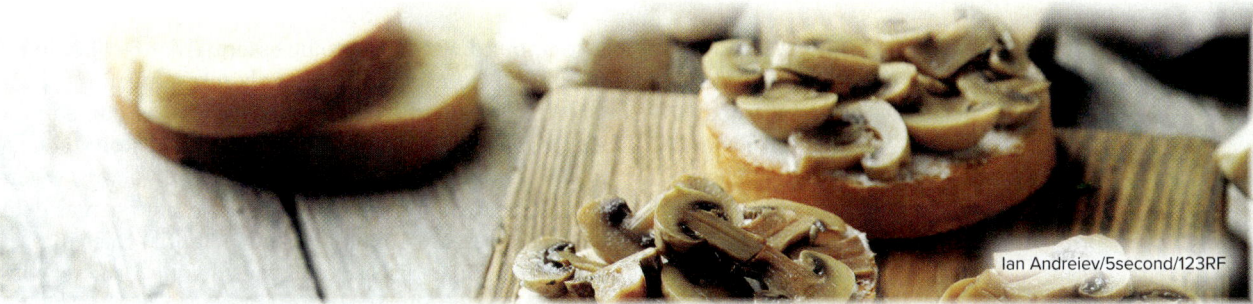

Ian Andreiev/5second/123RF

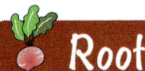

Roots

Religious Customs Affect Vitamin D Status

In this chapter, you have learned that vitamin D can be synthesized by the skin upon exposure to sunlight. How do religious customs, such as the Quran dress code for Muslim females, affect vitamin D status? The Quran dress code requires Muslim females to cover their bodies except for their hands and face. Some conservative branches of Islam require females to cover the hands and face, as well. Clinical research shows that vitamin D status is significantly lower among Muslim females who wear concealing clothing compared to females who do not follow religious dress codes. Recognizing that vitamin D deficiency may affect not only bone health but also immune function and risk for some chronic diseases, females who are not able to expose skin to natural sunlight must emphasize dietary or supplemental sources of vitamin D to prevent vitamin D deficiency.

Source: Chouraqui J-P, Turck D, Briend A, Darmaun D; Committee on Nutrition of the French Society of Pediatrics. Religious dietary rules and their potential nutritional and health consequences. *Int J Epidemiol.* 2021 Mar 3;50(1):12-26. doi: 10.1093/ije/dyaa182

---

10 micrograms of vitamin D daily. Vitamin D supplementation is recommended for all infants (exclusively breastfed, partially breastfed, or formula fed) until adequate vitamin D can be obtained from foods.[18] Breast milk is a poor source of vitamin D, and even though infant formula has vitamin D, the total intake of formula among young infants may not provide adequate vitamin D to meet the RDA. Keep in mind, however, that supplements must be used carefully, and under a primary care provider's guidance, to avoid vitamin D toxicity in the infant.

For adults over the age of 70, the RDA increases to 20 micrograms per day.[19] Older adults have high rates of bone turnover and are at increased risk for fractures. There are many factors that may compromise vitamin D status among older adults, such as decreased synthesis of vitamin D in the skin and a decreased ability to activate vitamin D in the liver and kidneys. Although not all experts agree on the value of vitamin D supplementation for prevention of osteoporosis, the International Osteoporosis Foundation suggests older adults over age 60 take dietary supplements that provide 20 to 25 micrograms of vitamin D per day.[20]

Other population groups that have difficulty meeting vitamin D needs include individuals who follow a vegan dietary pattern or who have milk allergies or lactose malabsorption. Vitamin D supplements or vitamin D–fortified foods are options for people who do not consume dairy products.

AVOIDING TOO MUCH VITAMIN D

Too much vitamin D taken regularly can create serious health consequences in infants and children. Due to the role of vitamin D in calcium absorption, excretion, and release of calcium from bone, supplementation with high doses of vitamin D can cause calcium levels in the blood to increase above the normal range. The UL of 100 micrograms is based on the risk of overabsorption of calcium and eventual calcium deposits in the kidneys and other organs. Calcium deposits in organs can cause metabolic disturbances and cell death. Toxicity symptoms also include weakness, loss of appetite, diarrhea, vomiting, mental confusion, and increased urine output. Please note that vitamin D toxicity does not result from excessive exposure to the sun because the body regulates the amount made in the skin (i.e., as exposure to sunlight increases, the efficiency of vitamin D synthesis decreases).

✓ CONCEPT CHECK 8.4

1. Why is vitamin D sometimes not considered an *essential* nutrient?
2. What is the association between vitamin D and sun exposure?
3. Which two organs are involved in the activation of vitamin D in the body?
4. How does vitamin D work to maintain blood calcium levels?
5. What are some rich food sources of vitamin D?
6. Can vitamin D be toxic?

8.5 Vitamin E (Tocopherols)

In the 1920s, a fat-soluble compound was found to be essential for fertility in rats. This compound was named **tocopherol** from the Greek words *tokos*, meaning "birth," and *phero*, meaning "to bring forth." Later, this essential nutrient was named vitamin E. Vitamin E is a family of four tocopherols and four tocotrienols called alpha, beta, gamma, and delta. They differ in that tocopherols have a saturated side chain, whereas the tocotrienols have an unsaturated side chain. Tocotrienols have not been as extensively studied as tocopherols, but recent research explores their potential roles in prevention of cancers, diabetes, and cardiovascular diseases. Of these eight forms of vitamin E, alpha (α)-tocopherol is the most biologically active and the most potent.

---

tocopherols The chemical name for some forms of vitamin E. The alpha form is the most potent.

FUNCTIONS OF VITAMIN E

Antioxidant. The principal function of vitamin E in humans is as an antioxidant.[21] Vitamin E is a fat-soluble vitamin found primarily in adipose tissue and in the lipid bilayers of cell membranes (Fig. 8-12). Many of the lipids within these membranes are polyunsaturated fatty acids (PUFA), which are particularly susceptible to oxidative attack by free radicals. The formation of **free radicals** may destabilize the cell membrane, which may ultimately alter the ability of the cell to function properly. Vitamin E can donate electrons or hydrogen to free radicals found in membranes, thereby making them more stable. The antioxidant function of vitamin E appears to be critical in cells continually exposed to high levels of oxygen, particularly red blood cells and the cells lining the lungs.

Increasing vitamin E intake has been suggested as a way to prevent several chronic diseases that are linked to oxidative damage. For example, oxidized LDL cholesterol is a major component of the plaque that develops in arteries, which leads to atherosclerosis. Vitamin E is thought to attenuate the development of atherogenic plaque due to its ability to prevent or reduce the formation of oxidized LDL cholesterol. In addition, oxidative damage to proteins in the eye leads to the development of cataracts. Oxidized proteins combine and precipitate in the lens, causing cloudiness and decreasing visual acuity. Insufficient consumption of antioxidants from foods increases one's risk of these diseases.

Experts do not know whether supplementation with megadoses of vitamin E can confer any significant protection against diseases linked to oxidative damage. The consensus among the scientific community is that the established benefits of lifestyle choices have a far greater effect than any proposed benefits of antioxidant supplementation. The consensus of scientific research organizations is that it is premature to recommend vitamin E supplements to the general population, based on current knowledge and the failure of large clinical trials to show any consistent benefit. In addition, the FDA has denied the request of the dietary supplement industry to make a health claim that vitamin E supplements reduce the risk of cardiovascular disease or cancer.

Other Roles of Vitamin E. Although vitamin E is essential for fertility in many animal species, it does not appear to serve this role in humans. It is, however, important for the formation of muscles and the central nervous system in early human development. Vitamin E has been shown to improve vitamin A absorption if the dietary intake of vitamin A is low. It also functions in the metabolism of iron within cells, and it helps maintain nervous tissue and immune function. Current research on vitamin E is focused on its ability to influence the expression of some genes involved in the development of chronic diseases.[22]

VITAMIN E DEFICIENCY

Specific population groups are especially susceptible to developing marginal vitamin E status. Infants who are born preterm tend to have low vitamin E stores because this vitamin is transferred from mother to baby during the late stages of pregnancy. Hence, the potential for oxidative damage, which could cause the cell membranes of red blood cells to break **(hemolysis)**, is of particular concern for infants who are born preterm. The rapid growth of infants who are born preterm, coupled with the high oxygen needs of their immature lungs, greatly increases the stress on red blood cells. Special vitamin E–fortified formulas and supplements designed for infants who are born preterm compensate for this lack of vitamin E. Individuals who use tobacco products are another group at high risk for vitamin E deficiency, as smoking readily destroys vitamin E in the lungs.

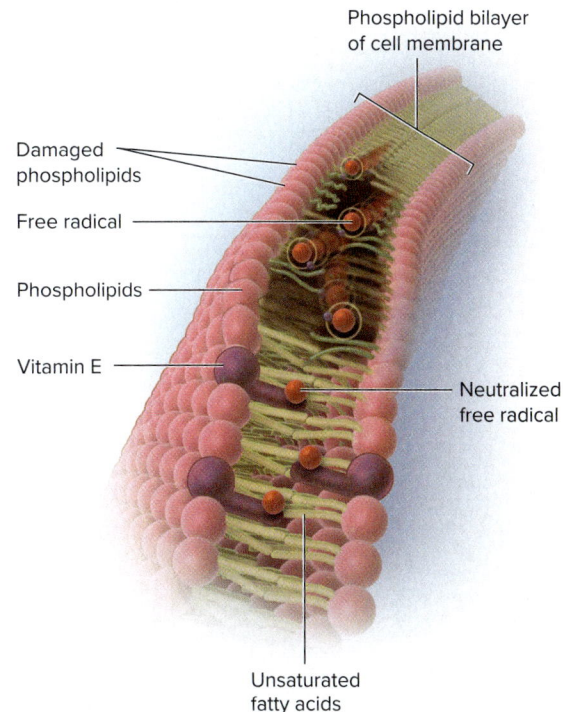

FIGURE 8-12 Because it is fat soluble, vitamin E can insert itself into cell membranes, where it helps stop free-radical chain reactions. If not interrupted, these reactions cause extensive oxidative damage to cells and, ultimately, cell death.

free radical An unstable atom with an unpaired electron in its outermost shell; also called *reactive oxygen species.*

hemolysis Destruction of red blood cells.

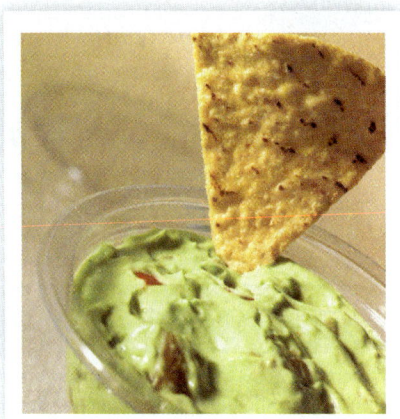

The avocado in guacamole and the sunflower oil in the tortilla chip in this image are good sources of vitamin E. **How can you tell what type of oil is in your tortilla chips?** Andrew Bret Wallis/BananaStock/Getty Images

Others at risk of vitamin E deficiency include adults on very low-fat diets (<15% total fat) or those with fat-malabsorption disorders.

GETTING ENOUGH VITAMIN E

Because vitamin E is only synthesized by plants, plant products (especially the oils) are the best sources. In the U.S. dietary pattern, nearly two-thirds of vitamin E is supplied by salad oils, margarines, spreads (low-fat margarine), and shortening (Fig. 8-13). Breakfast cereals fortified with vitamin E are good sources, but other than wheat germ, few other grain products provide much vitamin E. Milling of grains removes the germ, which contains the oils (mostly polyunsaturated fatty acids or PUFAs) and vitamin E. By removing the germ, the resulting grain product has less chance of spoiling (i.e., rancidity of the PUFAs) and thus a longer shelf life. Other good sources of vitamin E are nuts and seeds.

Because plant oils contain mostly unsaturated fatty acids, the relatively high amount of vitamin E in plant oils naturally protects these unsaturated lipids from oxidation. Animal products (meat, dairy, and eggs) and fish oils, on the other hand, contain almost no vitamin E. Vitamin E is susceptible to destruction by oxygen, metals, light, and heat, especially when oil is repeatedly reused in deep-fat frying; thus, the vitamin E content of a food depends on how it is harvested, processed, stored, and cooked.

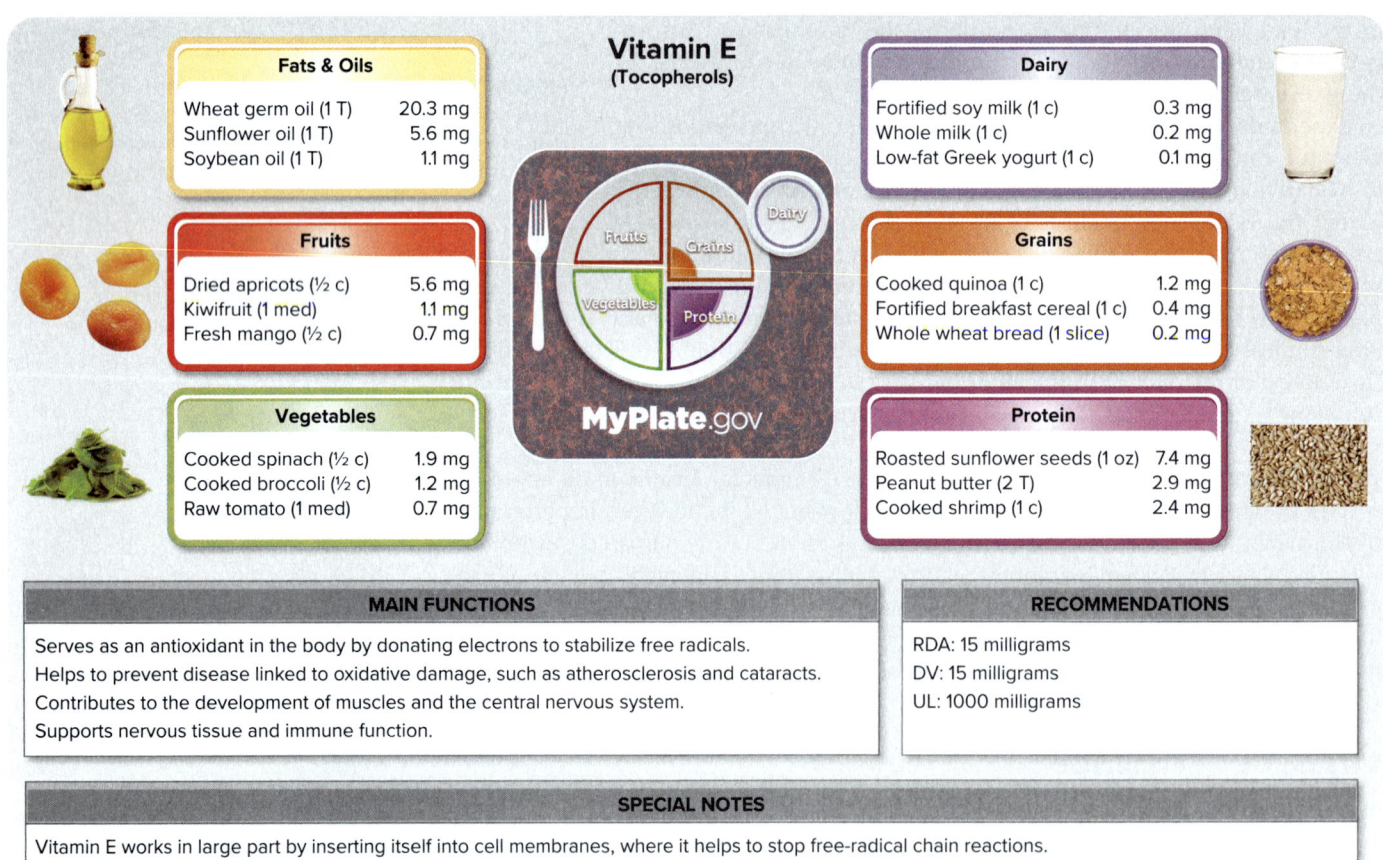

FIGURE 8-13 Food sources of vitamin E. The fill of the background color (none, 1/3, 2/3, or completely covered) within each food group on MyPlate indicates the average nutrient density for vitamin E in that group. The figure shows the vitamin E content of several foods in each food group. Overall, the richest sources of vitamin E are nuts, seeds, plant oils, and quinoa. oil: Iconotec/Glow Images; milk: Nipaporn Panyacharoen/Shutterstock; apricots: lynx/iconotec/Glowimages; cereal: Joe Belanger/iStock/Getty Images; spinach: Elena Elisseeva/Shutterstock; seeds: Glow Images; MyPlate: U.S. Department of Agriculture

Sources: Office of Dietary Supplements, Dietary Supplements Fact Sheets, available from https://ods.od.nih.gov/factsheets/list-all; USDA FoodData Central, available from https://fdc.nal.usda.gov.

Newsworthy Nutrition

Selenium and vitamin E supplements offer no benefit for cancer prevention

INTRODUCTION: In the late 1990s and early 2000s, secondary analysis of a landmark *randomized controlled trial* of nutrient supplementation in cancer prevention hinted at possible roles for micronutrients in the prevention of prostate cancer. **OBJECTIVE:** The 12-year SELECT (Selenium and Vitamin E Cancer Prevention Trial) was designed to further explore the roles of selenium and vitamin E for the prevention of prostate cancer. **METHODS:** Enrollment for the trial included more than 400 sites in the United States, Puerto Rico, and Canada. Over 35,000 males age 50 and older, participated in SELECT. Data were then collected on patients 18 months after the trial ended. **RESULTS:** After 7 years, the trial was stopped due to a lack of any beneficial effects of the supplements on cancer-related endpoints. The trial found that neither selenium (200 mcg/d) nor vitamin E (400 IU/d), either alone or in combination, reduced the risk for prostate cancer. Results from the 18-month follow-up showed that the males who took vitamin E alone had a 17% relative increase in numbers of prostate cancers compared to males on placebo. **CONCLUSION:** These studies emphasize the importance of longitudinal studies and secondary data analyses to fully assess cancer risk over time. The observation that the risk of prostate cancer continued to increase suggests that vitamin E, even after cessation of supplements, may have long-term effects on prostate cancer risk. There remain no clinical trials that show a benefit from taking vitamin E or selenium to reduce the risk of prostate cancer or any other cancer or heart disease.

Source: Klein EA, Thompson IM Jr, Tangen CM, et al. Vitamin E and the risk of prostate cancer: the Selenium and Vitamin E Cancer Prevention Trial (SELECT). *JAMA*. 2011 Oct 12;306(14):1549-1556. doi: 10.1001/jama.2011.1437; https://www.ncbi.nlm.nih.gov/pmc/articles/PMC4169010/

The RDA of vitamin E for adults is 15 milligrams per day of alpha-tocopherol, the most active, natural form of vitamin E. This amount equals 30 milligrams of the less active, synthetic source. Typically, adults consume only about two-thirds of the RDA for vitamin E from food sources. On revised food and supplement labels, the Daily Value for vitamin E is 15 milligrams of alpha-tocopherol.

AVOIDING TOO MUCH VITAMIN E

Unlike other fat-soluble vitamins, vitamin E is not as readily stored in the liver. It is stored in adipose tissue throughout the body. The UL for vitamin E is 1000 milligrams per day of supplemental alpha-tocopherol. Excessive intake of vitamin E can interfere with vitamin K's role in the clotting mechanism, leading to **hemorrhage**. The risk of insufficient blood clotting is especially high if vitamin E is taken in conjunction with anticoagulant medications (e.g., Coumadin® or high-dose aspirin). Always be cautious about using dietary supplements. See the *Newsworthy Nutrition* on the SELECT Trial. In addition to the significant risk of drug interference and prolonged bleeding, vitamin E supplements can produce nausea, gastrointestinal distress, and diarrhea.

hemorrhage An escape of blood from blood vessels.

✓ CONCEPT CHECK 8.5

1. How does vitamin E work to prevent oxidative damage?
2. What are some rich food sources of vitamin E?
3. Why are infants who are born preterm, individuals who smoke, and people with fat-malabsorption disorders particularly susceptible to oxidative damage to cell membranes?
4. What are the possible results of vitamin E toxicity?

8.6 Vitamin K (Quinone)

A family of compounds known collectively as vitamin K is found in plants, plant oils, fish oils, and some animal products.[23] Vitamin K is also synthesized by bacteria in the human colon, which normally fulfills approximately 10% of human requirements. Vitamin K has three forms: (1) phylloquinone, the most abundant form of vitamin K, is synthesized by green plants; (2) menaquinone is synthesized by gut bacteria; and (3) menadione is the synthetic form found in supplements. Interestingly, the synthetic menadione form of vitamin K is twice as biologically available as the other two.

FUNCTIONS OF VITAMIN K

Vitamin K serves as a **cofactor** in chemical reactions that add carbon dioxide (CO_2) molecules to various proteins, thus enabling these proteins to bind to calcium. This is the biochemical basis for vitamin K's role in the life-and-death process of blood clotting. In the clotting cascade, vitamin K imparts calcium-binding ability to seven different proteins, eventually leading to the conversion of soluble fibrinogen into insoluble **fibrin** (i.e., the clot). The "K" stands for *koagulation* in the language spoken by the Danish researchers who first noted the relationship between vitamin K and blood clotting.

Besides its role in blood clotting, vitamin K is also important for bone health. The calcium-binding protein in the bone, **osteocalcin,** depends upon vitamin K for its function in bone mineralization. Other vitamin K–dependent proteins are involved in cardiovascular health, energy metabolism, and glucose regulation.

VITAMIN K DEFICIENCY

Vitamin K deficiency is rare, but its consequences can be life-threatening. Even though it is a fat-soluble vitamin, the body does not store vitamin K to a great extent. Because of its important role in blood clotting, a deficiency of vitamin K can lead to excessive bleeding. In milder forms, this may cause easy bruising. In severe forms, vitamin K deficiency leads to hemorrhage, which can be fatal.

Newborn infants are at highest risk for **vitamin K deficiency bleeding** because they are born with low stores of vitamin K. Furthermore, breast milk is quite low in vitamin K, and at birth a newborn's intestinal tract has not yet been populated with the bacteria that can synthesize vitamin K. Low vitamin K status in an infant sets the stage for serious bleeding problems if the infant is injured or needs surgery. Therefore, vitamin K is routinely administered by injection shortly after birth.[24] It is becoming more common, however, for parents to refuse vitamin K supplementation for their infants. In some cases, this has led to hemorrhagic complications, such as severe gastrointestinal or intracranial bleeding.[25]

Beyond blood clotting, low vitamin K status has been linked to poor bone development in children and osteoporosis in older adults. Furthermore, inadequate vitamin K could play a role in the development of cardiovascular disease.[23]

Among adults, deficiencies of vitamin K can occur when a person takes antibiotics for an extended time. This destroys the bacteria that normally synthesize vitamin K. If vitamin K intake and/or absorption is low (e.g., among individuals with celiac disease) and the vitamin K–producing bacteria are knocked out by antibiotics, vitamin K deficiency may occur.

GETTING ENOUGH VITAMIN K

Major food sources of the phylloquinone form of vitamin K are green leafy vegetables, broccoli, asparagus, and peas (Fig. 8-14). Pomegranates are a source of Vitamin K highlighted in the *Farm to Fork*. The menaquinone form of vitamin K is found in some meats, eggs, and dairy products, and it is the form synthesized by bacteria. Compared to that of plant sources, the nutrient density of vitamin K in foods of animal origin is rather low. Vitamin K is resistant to cooking losses.

---

cofactor An inorganic compound (e.g., mineral) that combines with an inactive enzyme to form a catalytically active form.

fibrin An insoluble blood protein that forms a blood clot.

osteocalcin Small protein in the organic matrix of bone.

vitamin K deficiency bleeding Hemorrhage caused by a lack of vitamin K, especially among infants from birth to 6 months of age; also called *hemorrhagic disease of the newborn*.

aril Clear, ruby-colored fruit or seed pod that surrounds a tiny, crisp seed inside a pomegranate.

FARM to FORK: Pomegranates

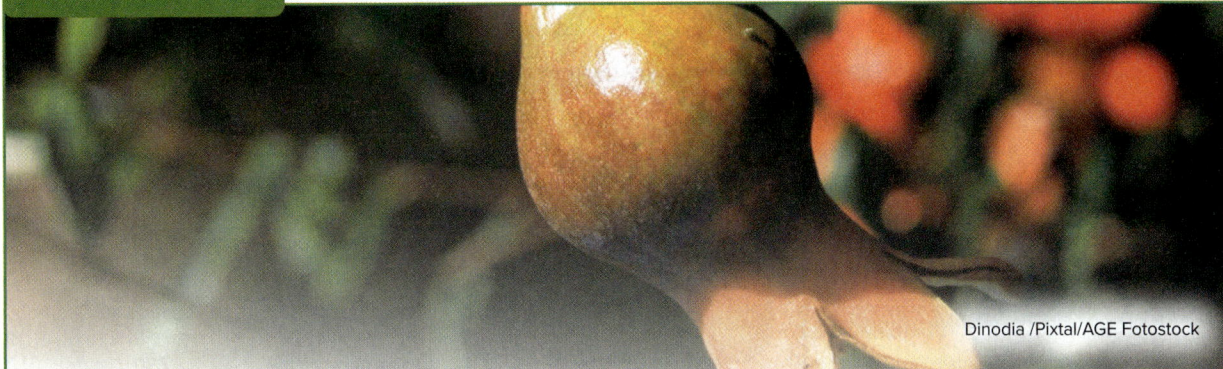
Dinodia /Pixtal/AGE Fotostock

Originally cultivated in the Mediterranean region, most pomegranates now consumed in the U.S. are grown in California and Arizona. Not only are pomegranates rich in polyphenols, antioxidants, and folate, but a single pomegranate delivers about 40% of an adult's daily vitamin K needs. Several clinical trials have linked pomegranate consumption to improved blood pressure.

Grow
- Pomegranates thrive in a semi-arid subtropical climate but can adapt to environments with cool winters and hot summers.
- To successfully grow pomegranate trees or dwarf shrubs outside arid and tropical regions, one must consider container cultures or greenhouse growing.

Shop
- When selecting ripe pomegranate fruits, look for skin that is glossy, unbroken, and bright or dark red. The deeper and richer the color, the sweeter the fruit. The skin of a ripe pomegranate is soft, and when tapped you should hear a metallic sound.
- As ripening continues, the sides of the fruit become slightly squared. This occurs when the seeds (or **arils**) reach their maximum juice content and push against the outer walls.
- Opt for fruits that are heavy for their size.

Store
- Pomegranates have an extended storage life, similar to an apple. They are best stored in a cool, dry, well-ventilated area, free of direct sunlight. When refrigerated, whole fruits should last up to 2 months, and fresh seeds (arils) or juice will last up to 5 days.
- Pomegranate arils can be frozen for up to 1 year. Spread a single layer of arils on a wax paper–lined baking sheet, freeze for no more than 2 hours, then transfer to a moisture-free freezer bag or freezer-safe container for storage.
- Pomegranate juice can be canned or frozen in freezer-safe containers, leaving ½-inch headspace for expansion.

Prep
- To remove the arils, start by cutting a shallow cone shape out of the blossom end. Next, vertically score the husk of the fruit between each lobe. You can peel back the husk to reveal the arils and gently release them from the white pith inside the fruit.
- Fill a large bowl with water and submerge the pomegranate as you loosen the arils. This keeps the bright red juice from splattering your clothing and kitchen! After all the arils have been released, discard the pith and membranes, which naturally float to the surface of the water, then use a strainer to drain off the water.
- Pomegranate arils make a beautiful garnish for fruit cups, salads, desserts, or drinks.
- To juice a pomegranate, remove the arils and run them through a basket press or ordinary orange juicer. This colorful juice can be used to make jellies, sorbets, or sauces. The juice also serves as a natural flavoring and coloring agent for baked goods, chilled desserts, and smoothies.

Sources: Robinson J. Tropical fruits: make the most of eating globally. In: *Eating on the Wild Side: The Missing Link to Optimum Health.* New York: Little, Brown & Co.; 2013.

Sahebkar A, Ferri C, Giorgini P, Bo S, Nachtigal P, Grassi D. Effects of pomegranate juice on blood pressure: a systematic review and meta-analysis of randomized controlled trials. *Pharmacol Res.* 2017;115:149-161. doi: 10.1016/j.phrs.2016.11.018

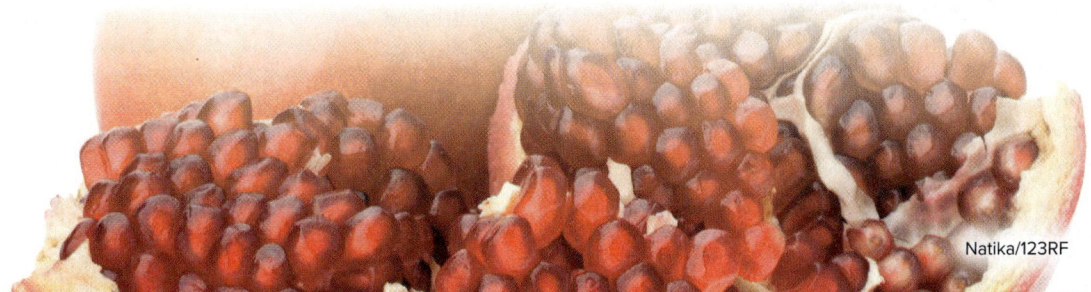
Natika/123RF

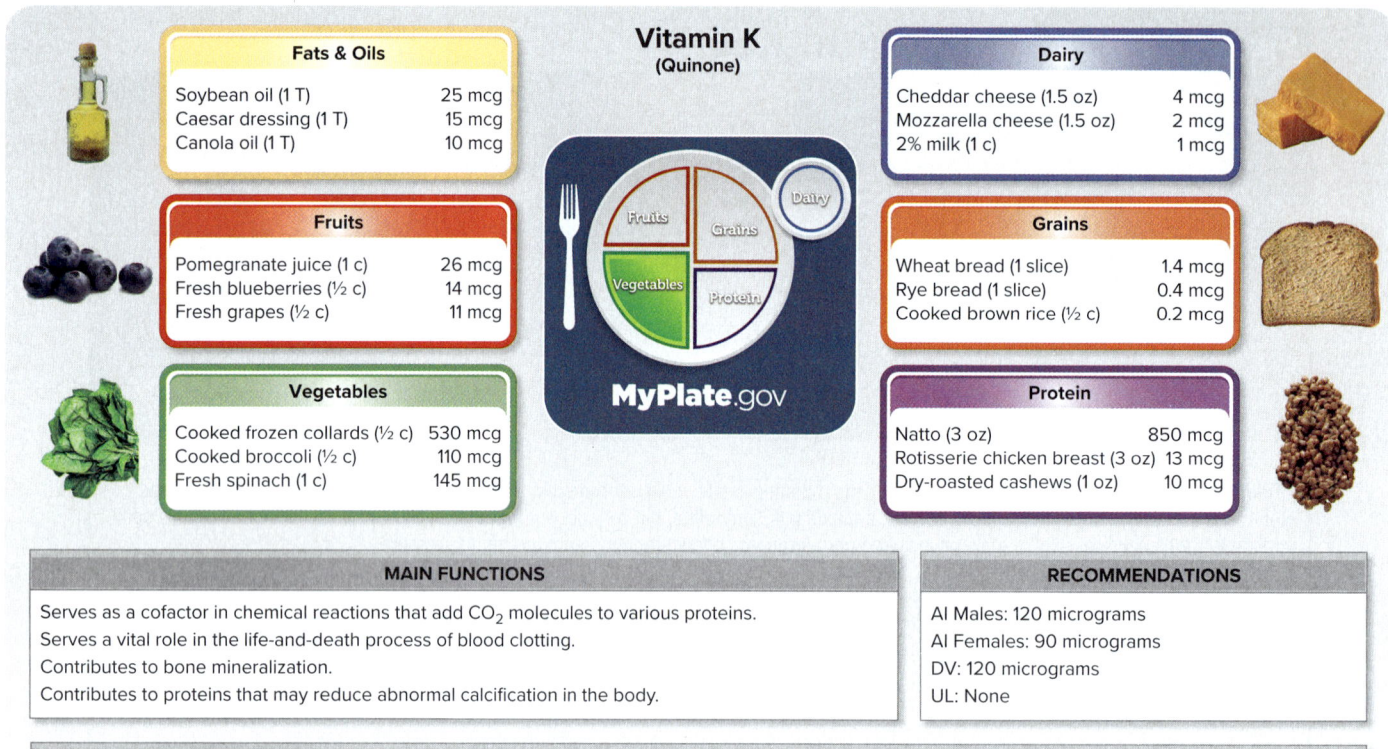

FIGURE 8-14 Food sources of vitamin K. The fill of the background color (none, 1/3, 2/3, or completely covered) within each food group on MyPlate indicates the average nutrient density for vitamin K in that group. The figure shows the vitamin K content of several foods in each food group. Overall, the richest sources of vitamin K are green, leafy vegetables. oil: Stockbyte/Getty Images; cheese: Brent Hofacker/Shutterstock; blueberries: photastic/Shutterstock; bread: Alex Cao/Photodisc/Getty Images; spinach: vvoennyy/123RF; natto: Alistair Forrester Shankie/E+/Getty Images; MyPlate: U.S. Department of Agriculture

Sources: Office of Dietary Supplements, Dietary Supplements Fact Sheets, available from https://ods.od.nih.gov/factsheets/list-all; USDA FoodData Central, available from https://fdc.nal.usda.gov.

As with other fat-soluble vitamins, absorption of vitamin K requires dietary fat and adequate liver and pancreatic secretions. Unlike other fat-soluble vitamins, though, not much vitamin K is stored in the body and excesses can be excreted via urine. Thus, a deficiency could develop rather quickly if dietary intake of this nutrient is insufficient, which can be a problem among older adults whose dietary patterns lack vegetables. However, because vitamin K is fairly widespread in foods and some can be synthesized by bacteria in the colon, deficiencies of this vitamin rarely occur.[26] No reports of toxicity have been published.

✓ CONCEPT CHECK 8.6

1. What is the role of vitamin K in blood clotting?
2. Identify two rich food sources of vitamin K.
3. Be sure to read the *Medicine Cabinet* feature in this section. Why is it important for people who take Coumadin to monitor their dietary intake of vitamin K?

Medicine Cabinet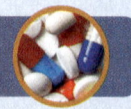

Anticoagulants

People who are prone to develop blood clots may take anticoagulants or *blood thinners*. One commonly prescribed anticoagulant is Coumadin® (warfarin). This medication inhibits vitamin K–dependent coagulation factors. When taking Coumadin or similar drugs, it is important to keep dietary intake of vitamin K consistent from day to day.

©Peter Dazeley/Photographer's Choice/Getty Images

Source: Hull RD, Garcia DA, Vasquez SR. Patient education: Warfarin (beyond the basics). UpToDate. Updated June 16, 2021. Accessed February 14, 2022. https://www.uptodate.com/contents/warfarin-beyond-the-basics/print

8.7 The Water-Soluble Vitamins

The next 10 sections of this chapter will explore the water-soluble vitamins. The B vitamins are thiamin, riboflavin, niacin, pantothenic acid, biotin, vitamin B-6, folate, and vitamin B-12. Choline is a related nutrient that has vitamin-like characteristics but currently is not classified as a vitamin. Vitamin C is also a water-soluble vitamin. The B vitamins often occur together in the same foods, so a lack of one B vitamin may mean other B vitamins are also low in a diet.

Regular consumption of good sources of these water-soluble vitamins are important. Most water-soluble vitamins are readily excreted from the body, with any excess generally ending up in the urine or stool and very little being stored. Because these vitamins dissolve in water, large amounts can be lost and destroyed during food processing and preparation. As emphasized earlier, vitamin content is best preserved by light cooking methods, such as stir-frying, steaming, and microwaving.

COENYZMES

Enzymes are catalysts for biochemical reactions in living organisms. A catalyst is a compound that speeds the rate of a reaction but is not altered by the reaction. Think about starting a fire manually. This process can be quite cumbersome, unless you have lighter fluid. Enzymes are like lighter fluid for chemical reactions. In fact, most of the chemical reactions in the body would not occur (or would occur at very slow rates) in the absence of enzyme catalysts. Enzymes are crucial players in antioxidant reactions, which help neutralize free radicals in the body. In Chapter 3, you learned that enzymes are necessary for the normal breakdown of carbohydrates, lipids, and proteins to yield energy. They also catalyze synthetic reactions, such as the assembly of triglycerides for storage in adipose tissue. These are the roles of just a few of the enzymes in the human body; thousands of other enzymes have been identified and studied!

The B vitamins function as **coenzymes,** small molecules that interact with enzymes to enable the enzymes to function. In essence, the coenzymes contribute to enzyme activity (Fig. 8-15).

As coenzymes, the B vitamins play many key roles in metabolism. The metabolic pathways used by carbohydrates, fats, and amino acids all require input from B vitamins. Because of their role in energy metabolism, needs for many B vitamins increase somewhat as energy expenditure increases. Still, this is not a major concern because this increase in energy expenditure is usually accompanied by a corresponding increase in food intake, which contributes more B vitamins to a diet. Many B vitamins are interdependent because they participate in the same processes (Fig. 8-16). B vitamin–deficiency symptoms typically occur in the brain and nervous system, skin, and

coenzyme An organic compound that combines with an inactive enzyme to form a catalytically active form. In this manner, coenzymes aid in enzyme function.

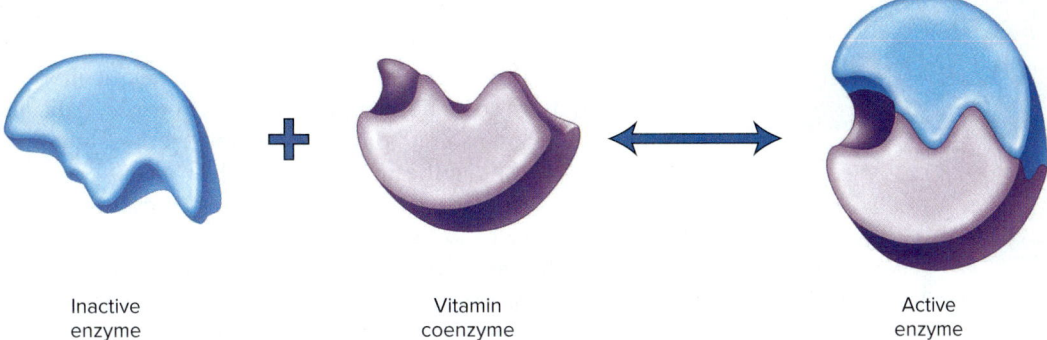

Inactive enzyme + Vitamin coenzyme ⇌ Active enzyme

FIGURE 8-15 Coenzymes, such as those formed from B vitamins, aid in the function of various enzymes. Without the coenzyme, the enzyme cannot function properly, and deficiency symptoms associated with the missing vitamin eventually appear. Health-food stores sell the coenzyme forms of some vitamins. These more expensive forms of vitamins are unnecessary. The body makes all the coenzymes it needs from vitamin precursors.

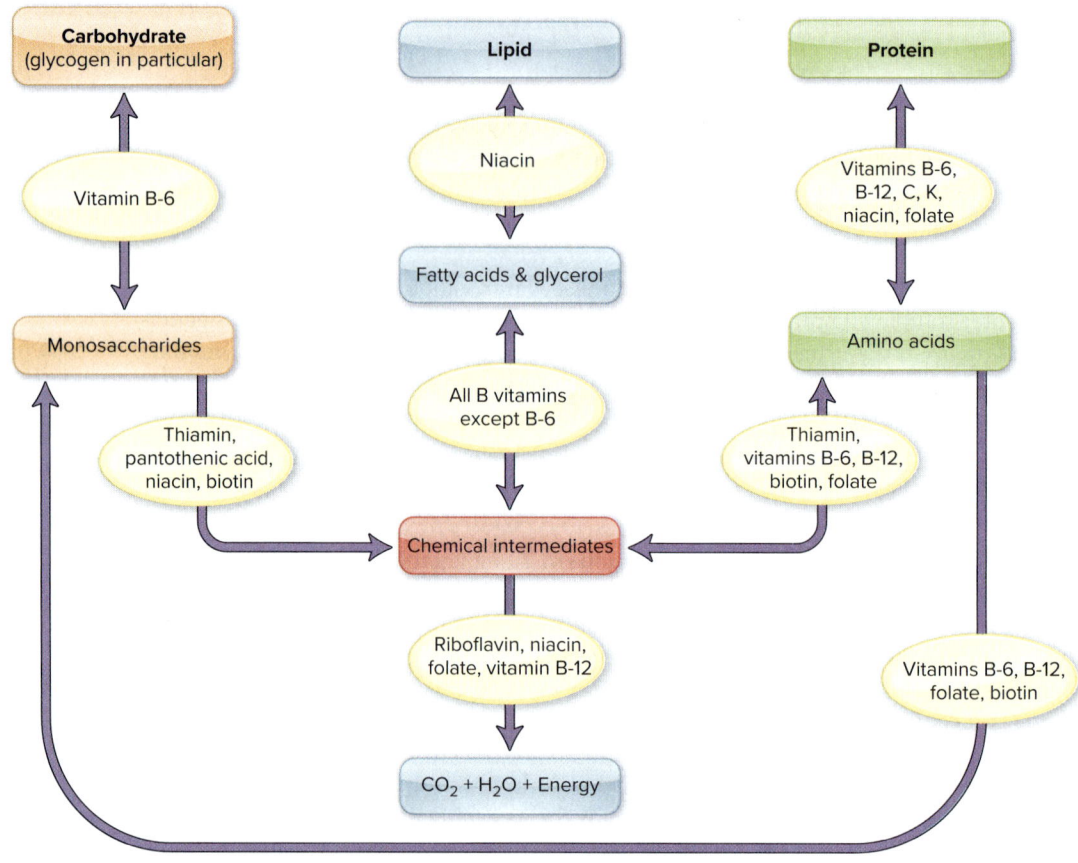

FIGURE 8-16 Examples of metabolic pathways for which B vitamins and other vitamins are essential. The metabolism of energy-yielding nutrients requires vitamin input.

gastrointestinal (GI) tract. Cells in these tissues are metabolically active, and those in the skin and GI tract are also constantly being replaced.

After being ingested, the B vitamins are first broken down from their active coenzyme forms into free vitamins in the stomach and small intestine. The vitamins are then absorbed, primarily in the small intestine. Typically, about 50% to 90% of the B vitamins in the diet are absorbed, which means that they have relatively high bioavailability. Once inside cells, the active coenzyme forms are resynthesized. There is no need to consume the coenzyme forms themselves. Some vitamins are sold in their coenzyme forms, but these are broken down during digestion, and we activate them when needed.

B VITAMINS IN THE TYPICAL DIETARY PATTERN

The nutritional health of most North Americans with regard to the B vitamins is adequate. Typical dietary patterns contain plentiful and varied natural sources of these vitamins. In addition, many common foods, especially ready-to-eat breakfast cereals, are fortified with one or more of the B vitamins. In some developing countries, however, deficiencies of the B vitamins are more common and the resulting deficiency diseases pose significant threats to public health.

The B vitamins in foods are vulnerable to losses during storage and preparation. Exposure to heat and UV light can damage some B vitamins. Also, because they are water soluble, some B vitamins leach out of foods into cooking water. On average, about 10% to 25% of these vitamins are lost from food during food processing and preparation. Quick cooking methods that minimize contact with water, such as stir-frying, steaming, and microwaving, best preserve B-vitamin content.

Because B vitamins are water soluble, very little is stored in the body and any excess that you consume ends up in the urine or stool. Thus, toxicities of B vitamins rarely

Rapid cooking of vegetables in minimal fluids reduces the vitamins lost during cooking. Steaming is one effective method. C Squared Studios/Photodisc/Getty Images

occur. On the other hand, the body's limited capacity to store B vitamins means you could develop a vitamin deficiency within a few days or weeks if your dietary intake is inadequate. Most Americans have good B-vitamin status, but marginal deficiencies of these vitamins may occur in some cases, especially among older adults who eat small amounts of food and in other people with inadequate dietary patterns. In the short run, such a marginal deficiency in most people likely leads only to fatigue or other unspecified physical effects. Although the long-term effects of such marginal deficiencies are yet unknown, increased risks of cardiovascular disease, cancers, and cataracts of the eye are suspected.

As you learn about the B vitamins in this chapter, notice that symptoms of B-vitamin deficiencies typically occur in the brain and nervous system, skin, and gastrointestinal (GI) tract. This is because cells in these tissues are very metabolically active and/or rapidly turned over. Thus, these tissues demand a steady supply of B vitamins to support energy metabolism. With rare exceptions, healthy adults do not develop severe B-vitamin-deficiency diseases from dietary inadequacy alone. The main exceptions are people with alcohol use disorders. The combination of extremely unbalanced eating patterns and alcohol-induced alterations of vitamin absorption and metabolism creates significant risks for serious nutrient deficiencies among people with alcohol use disorders.

B VITAMINS IN GRAINS

The process of refining grains, such as processing white flour from whole wheat, leads to the loss of B vitamins as well as other vitamins and minerals. When grains are milled to make refined products, seeds are crushed and the germ, bran, and husk layers are discarded, leaving just the starch-containing endosperm in the refined grains. This starch is used to make white flour, bread, and cereal products. Unfortunately, many nutrients are lost in the discarded germ, bran, and husk materials. To counteract these losses in the United States, bread and cereal products made from milled grains are enriched with four B vitamins (thiamin, riboflavin, niacin, and folic acid) and with the mineral iron.

Food enrichment was initiated by federal legislation in the 1930s to help combat nutrient deficiencies such as pellagra (niacin deficiency) and iron-deficiency **anemia.** Folate was included on the list of nutrients required to be added to refined grain products in 1998. However, not all nutrients lost in milling are added back through enrichment. Products made with refined flour remain lower in several nutrients, including vitamins E and B-6, potassium, magnesium, and fiber, than products made with whole grains (Fig. 8-17). This lower nutrient density is why nutrition experts and the *Dietary Guidelines* advocate daily consumption of whole grain products, such as brown rice, oats, whole-wheat bread, whole-grain cereals and crackers, and wild rice, rather than refined grain products. Remember the goal is for at least half of our total servings of grains each day come from whole grains.

anemia A decreased oxygen-carrying capacity of the blood. This can be caused by many factors, such as iron deficiency or blood loss.

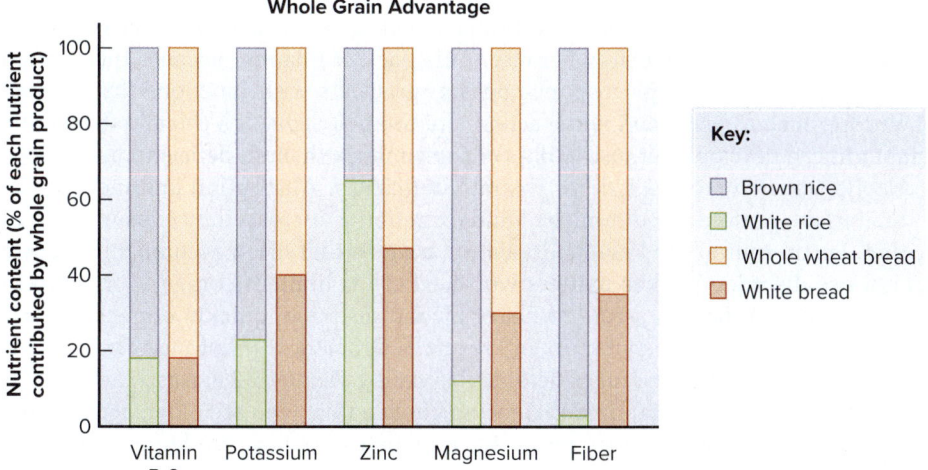

FIGURE 8-17 Comparison of the relative nutrient contents of refined versus whole grains. Nutrients are expressed as a percentage of the nutrient contribution of the whole-grain product.

The following sections focus on the B vitamins and trace minerals involved in energy metabolism.

> ### ✓ CONCEPT CHECK 8.7
>
> 1. What body organs or tissues are most likely to show symptoms if there is a deficiency of B vitamins and why?
> 2. Why are B vitamins lost when foods are cooked in water?
> 3. What group of people is at high risk of B-vitamin deficiency?
> 4. What happens during the refining of grains that causes a decrease in nutrient density?

8.8 Thiamin (Vitamin B-1)

FUNCTIONS OF THIAMIN

Thiamin was the first water-soluble vitamin to be discovered. One of its primary functions is to help release energy from carbohydrate. Its coenzyme form, thiamin pyrophosphate (TPP), participates in reactions in which carbon dioxide (CO_2) is released during the breakdown of carbohydrates and certain amino acids (see Fig. 8-16). These reactions are particularly important in the body's ATP-producing energy pathways. Thiamin also functions in chemical reactions that make RNA, DNA, and neurotransmitters.[27]

THIAMIN DEFICIENCY

beriberi The thiamin-deficiency disorder characterized by muscle weakness, loss of appetite, nerve degeneration, and sometimes edema.

Thiamin-deficiency disease is called **beriberi,** a word that means "I can't, I can't" in the Sri Lanka language of Sinhalese.[28] The symptoms include weakness, loss of appetite, irritability, nervous tingling throughout the body, poor arm and leg coordination, and deep muscle pain in the calves. This disease was described long before thiamin was discovered to be a vitamin in 1910. A person with beriberi often develops an enlarged heart and sometimes severe edema.

Beriberi is seen in areas where rice is a staple food and polished (white) rice is consumed rather than brown (whole grain) rice. In most parts of the world, even developing countries, white rice is preferred and is made by removing the bran and germ layer from brown rice. Removing the outer layer from rice during processing also removes most of its thiamin, so white rice is a poor source of thiamin. In the United States and Canada, thiamin is among the micronutrients added to white rice during enrichment to prevent widespread nutrient deficiencies.

Beriberi results when glucose, the primary fuel for brain and nerve cells, cannot be metabolized to release energy because of the lack of thiamin. Because the thiamin coenzyme participates in glucose metabolism, problems with functions that depend on glucose, such as brain and nerve action, are the first signs of a thiamin deficiency. Symptoms can develop after just 10 days of consuming a thiamin-deficient diet.

Alcohol abuse increases risk for thiamin deficiency. Absorption and metabolism of thiamin are profoundly diminished and excretion is increased by consumption of alcohol. Furthermore, the low-quality eating pattern that often accompanies severe alcohol use disorders makes matters worse. There is limited storage of thiamin in the body; several days in a row of heavy alcohol use may quickly deplete already diminished amounts of the vitamin and result in deficiency symptoms. The beriberi associated with alcohol use disorders is also called *Wernicke-Korsakoff syndrome.*[29] Other groups at risk of thiamin deficiency include adults who are older, are infected with human immunodeficiency virus, have diabetes, or have undergone bariatric surgery.

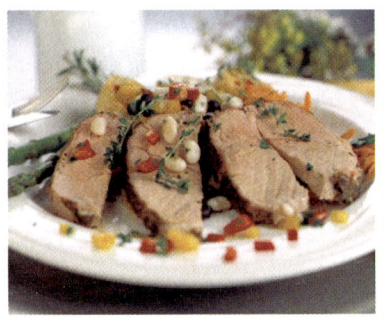

Pork is an excellent source of thiamin. **What foods would be good sources of thiamin for an individual who excludes pork from their dietary pattern for religious reasons?** Ingram Publishing/SuperStock

ASK THE RDN | Detox Diets

Dear RDN: *I put on 10 pounds last year, and I can't seem to shed the extra weight. Can a detox diet help me lose weight and get rid of toxic substances from my body?*

There is little consensus about the definition of a detoxification diet, but in general such plans are meant to assist the body's natural mechanisms to get rid of harmful toxins that arise from metabolism and from environmental exposures. When you look at the advocates of detox diets, it should raise a red flag that its praises are sung primarily by celebrities, tabloid magazines, and TV talk-show hosts who claim that detox diets induce weight loss, improve energy, and reduce risk of chronic diseases.

We are exposed to toxins every day. Some are produced by the body—such as the ammonia that arises from metabolism of amino acids. Many more are present in the foods we eat, the water we drink, and the air we breathe. Fortunately, the human body has several natural detoxification systems that convert harmful substances into water-soluble compounds that can be excreted via urine, sweat, bile, or feces.

Scientific evidence shows that the body's detoxification pathways are effective without any extra intervention. Popular culture detox diets promote extreme, uninformed, and nutritionally inadequate dietary practices. One of the most harmful regimens instructs dieters to subsist on a liquid diet of lemon juice, maple syrup, water, and cayenne pepper for a week or more. Some plans rely on herbal laxatives to purge the colon of waste materials. Others involve consuming up to 8 cups per day of juice made from organic fruits and vegetables. Such plans, while they may boost certain nutrients and phytochemicals, are extremely low in calories and protein.

Currently, there is no clinical evidence to support the benefits of these detox diets. Side effects such as fatigue, headaches, or decreased mental acuity are signs of low blood sugar. Taken to an extreme, prolonged fasts and nutritionally inadequate dietary patterns can lead to chemical imbalances, which could affect heart function.

In summary, an overly restrictive eating pattern is difficult to maintain and may end up decreasing lean mass and basal metabolic rate. Sustained weight loss requires a lifestyle change, not a quick fix! If weight loss is your goal, moderate calorie restriction combined with physical activity will support gradual and sustainable weight loss (see Chapter 7). B vitamins, antioxidant nutrients, phytochemicals (e.g., flavonoids), dietary fiber, and plenty of fluid are what the body requires to detoxify and flush harmful compounds from the body. The best prescription to support your body's detoxification pathways is to consume a dietary pattern rich in fruits, vegetables, and whole grains, and to emphasize plant sources of protein every day—not just for a few days a year.

Pure and simple,

Angela Collene, MS, RDN, LD

Senior Lecturer, The Ohio State University, Author of *Wardlaw's Contemporary Nutrition* and *Wardlaw's Contemporary Nutrition: A Functional Approach*

Source: Kavanagh MB. Examining popular detox diets—learn about their efficacy and safety for weight loss, their components, and potential adverse effects. *Today's Dietitian*. 2016 Oct;18(10):52.

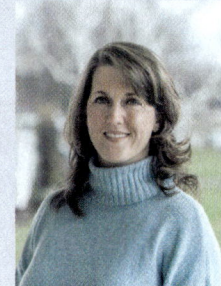
Tim Klontz

GETTING ENOUGH THIAMIN

Average daily intakes of thiamin for males exceed the RDA by 50% or more, and females generally meet the RDA.[26] Major sources of thiamin include pork products, whole grains, ready-to-eat breakfast cereals, enriched grains, green peas, milk, orange juice, organ meats, and dried beans. When considering the sections of MyPlate, the protein and grain groups contain the most foods that are nutrient-dense sources of thiamin (Fig. 8-18).

No toxicity has been observed from the use of oral thiamin supplements and thiamin is rapidly lost in the urine. Thus, no Upper Level (UL) has been set for thiamin.

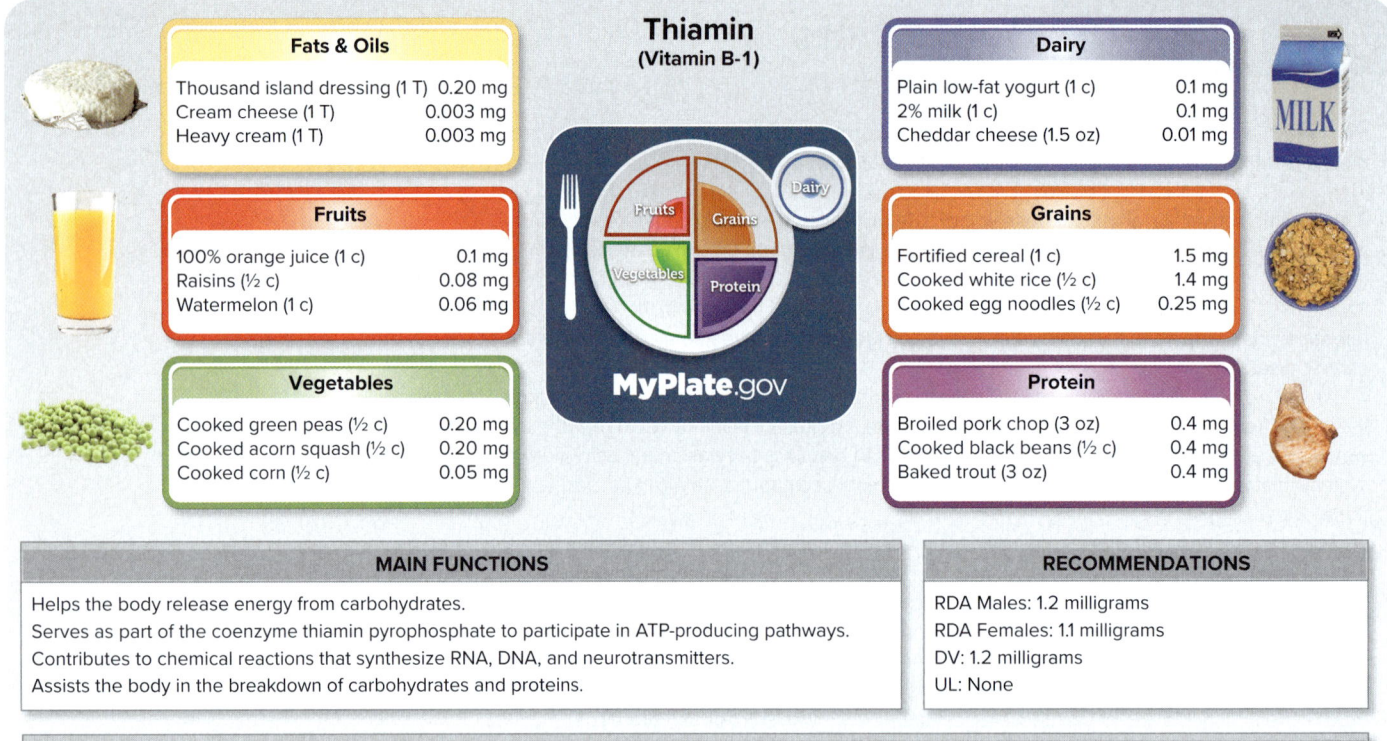

FIGURE 8-18 Food sources of thiamin. The fill of the background color (none, 1/3, 2/3, or completely covered) within each group on MyPlate indicates the average nutrient density for thiamin in that group. The figure shows thiamin content of several foods in each food group. Overall, the richest sources of thiamin are meats (especially pork), whole grains, and fortified breakfast cereals. cream cheese: Africa Studio/Shutterstock; milk: Hurst Photo/Shutterstock; juice: Sergei Vinogradov/seralexvi/123RF; cereal: Joe Belanger/iStock/Getty Images; peas: Ingram Publishing/SuperStock; pork chop: FoodCollection; MyPlate: U.S. Department of Agriculture

Sources: Office of Dietary Supplements, Dietary Supplements Fact Sheets, available from https://ods.od.nih.gov/factsheets/list-all; USDA FoodData Central, available from https://fdc.nal.usda.gov.

✓ CONCEPT CHECK 8.8

1. How is thiamin involved in energy metabolism?
2. What body organs or tissues are most likely to show symptoms if there is a deficiency of thiamin?
3. What group of people is at high risk of thiamin deficiency?
4. List three excellent sources of thiamin.

8.9 Riboflavin (Vitamin B-2)

FUNCTIONS OF RIBOFLAVIN

Riboflavin derives its name from its yellow color (*flavus* means "yellow" in Latin). The coenzyme forms of riboflavin, flavin adenine dinucleotide (FAD) and flavin mononucleotide (FMN), participate in many energy-yielding metabolic pathways, such as the breakdown of fatty acids (see Fig. 8-16). Some metabolism of vitamins and minerals also requires riboflavin. Indirectly, riboflavin also has an antioxidant role in the body through its support of the enzyme **glutathione peroxidase**.[30]

glutathione peroxidase An antioxidant enzyme system that requires selenium to convert certain free radicals (peroxides) into less harmful compounds (alcohols and water).

RIBOFLAVIN DEFICIENCY

Symptoms associated with riboflavin deficiency (**ariboflavinosis**) include inflammation of the mouth and tongue, **dermatitis,** various eye disorders, sensitivity to the sun, and confusion. Riboflavin deficiency typically would occur jointly with deficiencies of niacin, thiamin, and vitamin B-6 because these nutrients often occur in the same foods. **Glossitis** is characterized by pain and inflammation of the tongue; it can signal a deficiency of riboflavin, niacin, vitamin B-6, folate, or vitamin B-12. **Angular cheilitis,** also called cheilosis or angular stomatitis, is inflammation of the corners of the mouth that may cause painful cracking (Fig. 8-19). Both glossitis and angular cheilitis can be caused by other medical conditions; thus, further evaluation is required before diagnosing a nutrient deficiency. Such symptoms develop after approximately 2 months on a riboflavin-poor dietary pattern.

ariboflavinosis A deficiency disease resulting from a riboflavin deficiency; characterized by mouth sores, dermatitis, glossitis, and/or angular cheilitis.

dermatitis Condition that involves itchy, dry skin or a rash on swollen, reddened skin.

glossitis Inflammation and swelling of the tongue.

angular cheilitis Inflammation of the corners of the mouth with painful cracking; also called *cheilosis* or *angular stomatitis*.

GETTING ENOUGH RIBOFLAVIN

On average, daily intakes of riboflavin are slightly above the RDA.[26] As with thiamin, people with alcohol use disorders risk riboflavin deficiency because their eating patterns have low nutrient density. Although not common, others at risk for riboflavin deficiency are athletes who are vegetarian, individuals following a vegan eating plan, and females who are pregnant or lactating and their infants.

The grains, dairy, and protein groups of MyPlate contain the most nutrient-dense sources of riboflavin (Fig. 8-20). Naturally rich sources of riboflavin include milk and dairy products, meat, and eggs. Fortified breakfast cereals, enriched grains, asparagus, broccoli, and leafy green vegetables (e.g., spinach) are good vegetarian sources of riboflavin. Riboflavin is a relatively stable water-soluble vitamin; however, it is destroyed

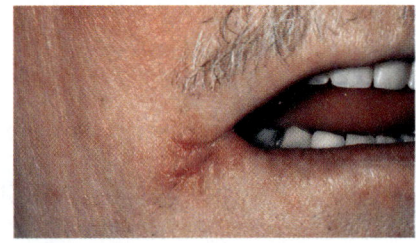

FIGURE 8-19 *Angular cheilitis*, also called *cheilosis* or *angular stomatitis*, causes painful cracks at the corners of the mouth. Dr. P. Marazzi/Science Photo Library/Science Source

---

CASE STUDY: Deficiency from a Vegan and Gluten-Free Diet?

Andrew has been following a vegan dietary pattern for about 1 year; therefore, he does not consume any animal products, including meat, fish, poultry, eggs, or dairy. Earlier this year, Andrew began experiencing gastrointestinal problems such as bloating, cramping, and occasional diarrhea. He read that these symptoms may be caused by the gluten in his dietary pattern, so he is now also avoiding gluten altogether by eliminating bread, cereals, pasta, and all other products made from enriched or whole wheat. Within a week of eliminating gluten, Andrew's gastrointestinal tract is feeling better, but his mouth and tongue have become very sore and inflamed. He also has developed sores and cracks at the corners of his mouth.

Answer the following questions related to Andrew's deficiencies.

1. What nutrients, including B vitamins, may be low or deficient in Andrew's vegan eating plan?
2. Why might the gluten in his dietary pattern be causing Andrew's gastrointestinal distress?
3. What nutrients may have been eliminated as a result of a gluten-free diet? (Refer back to discussion of the gluten-free diet in Section 3.11.)
4. What nutrient deficiency is most likely causing his problems around the mouth?
5. What food sources can be added to Andrew's vegan, gluten-free dietary pattern to alleviate his possible nutrient deficiencies?
6. Would a daily nutrient supplement be a possible remedy to avoid deficiencies? Why or why not?

Complete the Case Study. Responses to these questions can be provided by your instructor.

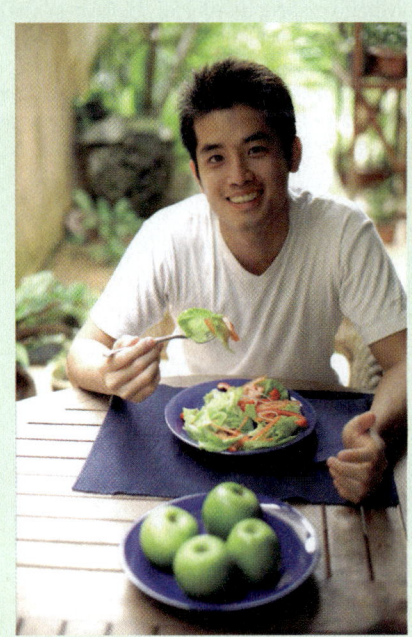

Andrew excludes animal products and gluten from his eating plan. Think about what nutrients may be low or missing from his dietary pattern. Asia Images Group/Shutterstock

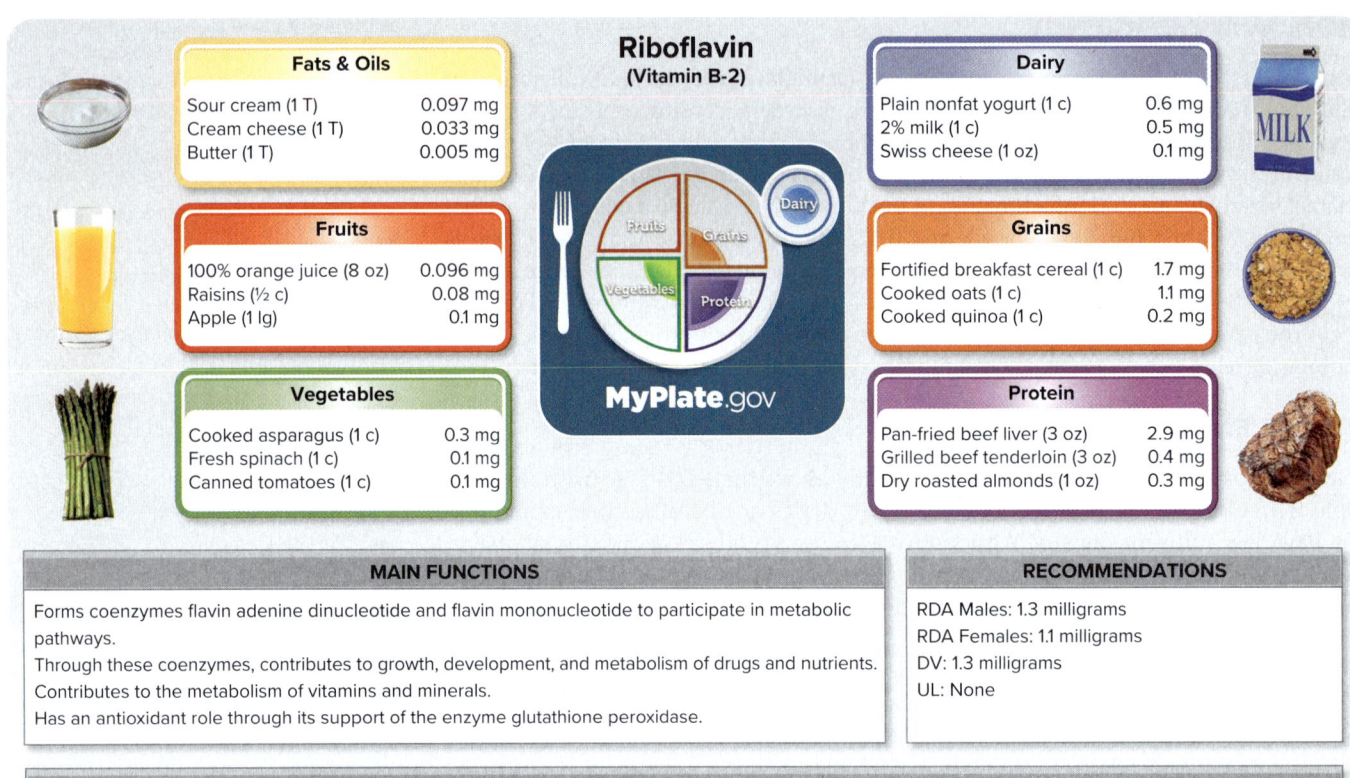

FIGURE 8-20 Food sources of riboflavin. The fill of the background color (none, 1/3, 2/3, or completely covered) within each group on MyPlate indicates the average nutrient density for riboflavin in that group. The figure shows riboflavin content of several foods in each food group. Overall, the richest sources of riboflavin are meats (especially liver), dairy products, and fortified breakfast cereals. Fruits are not particularly good sources of riboflavin.

sour cream: Oleksandra Naumenko/Shutterstock; milk: Hurst Photo/Shutterstock; juice: Sergei Vinogradov/seralexvi/123RF; cereal: Joe Belanger/iStock/Getty Images; asparagus: Burke Triolo Productions/Artville/Getty Images; beef: MaraZe/Shutterstock; MyPlate: U.S. Department of Agriculture

Sources: Office of Dietary Supplements, Dietary Supplements Fact Sheets, available from https://ods.od.nih.gov/factsheets/list-all; USDA FoodData Central, available from https://fdc.nal.usda.gov.

by light. Milk, therefore, is sold in paper or opaque plastic containers rather than clear glass to protect the riboflavin. In the United States, many meet the riboflavin recommendation by consuming three servings of dairy products each day. Riboflavin can also be produced by bacteria in the large intestine. More of this riboflavin is absorbed by the large intestine after consumption of vegetable-based foods compared to meat-based foods.

Ingestion of large doses of riboflavin has not been associated with any observable adverse symptoms, so no UL has been set. Because we excrete excess water-soluble vitamins in the urine, consuming dietary supplements or fortified foods (e.g., breakfast cereals) with more riboflavin than your body needs may impart a bright yellow color to your urine.

✓ CONCEPT CHECK 8.9

1. How is riboflavin involved in energy metabolism?
2. What body organs or tissues are most likely to show symptoms if there is a deficiency of riboflavin?
3. What types of foods are the best sources of riboflavin?

8.10 Niacin (Vitamin B-3)

FUNCTIONS OF NIACIN

Niacin functions in the body as one of two related compounds: nicotinic acid and nicotinamide. The coenzyme forms of niacin function in many cellular metabolic pathways. When you are generating energy (ATP) by burning carbohydrate and fat, a niacin coenzyme—nicotinamide dinucleotide (NAD) or nicotinamide dinucleotide phosphate (NADP)—is used. Anabolic pathways in the cell—those that make new compounds—also often use a niacin coenzyme. This is especially true for fatty-acid synthesis (see Fig. 8-16).[31]

One form of niacin, *nicotinic acid*, was previously prescribed in pharmacological doses to lower blood lipids including LDL cholesterol. However, research has revealed that niacin therapy does not lower risks for strokes, heart attacks, or overall mortality. Furthermore, use of pharmacological doses of niacin is associated with many adverse effects. Therefore, niacin is no longer recommended as a lipid-lowering therapy for prevention of heart attacks or strokes.[32]

NIACIN DEFICIENCY

Because niacin coenzymes function in over 200 enzymatic reactions, niacin deficiency causes widespread problems in the body. Early symptoms include poor appetite, weight loss, and weakness. The distinct group of niacin-deficiency symptoms is known as **pellagra,** which means "rough or painful skin." The symptoms of the disease are **dementia,** diarrhea, and dermatitis (especially on areas of skin exposed to the sun). Left untreated, death often results.

Pellagra is the only dietary deficiency disease ever to reach epidemic proportions in the United States. It became a major problem in the southeastern United States in the late 1800s and persisted until the 1930s, when standards of living and eating patterns improved. Pellagra was particularly prevalent among individuals with low socioeconomic status and among groups of people living in prisons and orphanages. At the time, most people assumed that pellagra was an infectious disease. However, Joseph Goldberger, a physician working with the U.S. Public Health Service, observed that pellagra was particularly prevalent in populations with eating patterns that were low in meat but high in corn-based products. He suspected pellagra was caused by a dietary deficiency. Although niacin was not identified as an essential nutrient until several years after his death, Dr. Goldberger was correct! Foods in the protein group are rich sources of niacin, whereas the niacin in corn is less bioavailable. (See *Roots* to learn how some populations figured out how to improve the bioavailability of niacin from corn.)[28] Today, pellagra is rare in Western societies and is typically only seen associated with chronic alcohol use disorders in conjunction with poverty and malnutrition and in those with rare inborn errors of metabolism.

GETTING ENOUGH NIACIN

The best natural food sources of niacin are found in the MyPlate protein group (Fig. 8-21). The grains group also makes a contribution to niacin intake due to enrichment and fortification. Major sources of niacin are tuna and other fish, poultry, peanuts, ready-to-eat cereals, beef, and asparagus. Coffee and tea also contribute some niacin to the dietary pattern. Niacin is heat stable; little is lost in cooking.

Besides obtaining niacin from food sources, humans can also synthesize some niacin from the essential amino acid tryptophan. In fact, endogenous synthesis of niacin from tryptophan can provide about half of the niacin we need each day. The process requires two other B vitamins (riboflavin and vitamin B-6), which function as coenzymes in this chemical conversion. Sixty milligrams of dietary tryptophan yield about 1 milligram of niacin.

pellagra Niacin-deficiency disease characterized by dementia, diarrhea, and dermatitis, and possibly leading to death.

dementia A general loss or decrease in mental function.

Roots

Nixtamalization

Archaeologists think maize (corn) was first domesticated in Mexico about 9000 years ago. It became a staple crop throughout much of Central, South, and North America. The native populations in this region developed a method, now called **nixtamalization,** to prepare corn. Nixtamalization is a food preparation process in which corn kernels are heated and soaked in an alkaline solution of water and calcium hydroxide (lime) or potassium hydroxide (lye). This culinary process removes the pericarp, which is the hard, outer layer surrounding the endosperm of the corn kernel (similar to the bran layer in a grain of wheat). The initial product is hominy, the softened endosperm of the original corn kernel. Hominy can be further processed and allowed to gelatinize to make masa (corn dough), which is important for culinary applications like making tortillas and tamales. The alkaline solution also makes corn safer to eat because it reduces harmful mycotoxins and kills some pathogens. Of great public health importance, nixtamalization improves the nutritional quality of corn because it breaks down hemicellulose, which increases the bioavailability of niacin.

Source: Orchardson E. What is nixtamalization? CIMMYT International Maize and Wheat Improvement Center. Published March 23, 2021. Accessed January 10, 2022. https://www.cimmyt.org/news/what-is-nixtamalization/

nixtamalization A culinary process in which whole maize (corn) kernels are soaked in a solution of water and calcium hydroxide (lime) or potassium hydroxide (lye) to make hominy and masa.

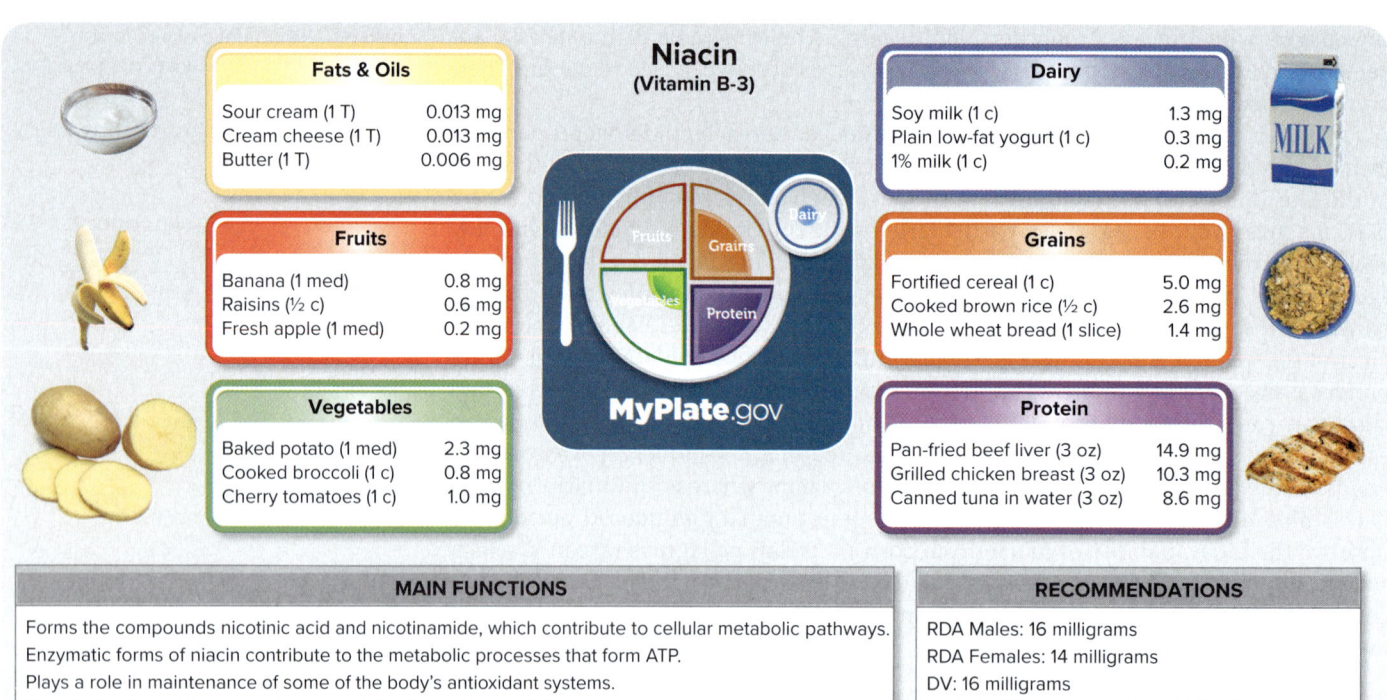

FIGURE 8-21 Food sources of niacin. The fill of the background color (none, 1/3, 2/3, or completely covered) within each group on MyPlate indicates the average nutrient density for niacin in that group. The figure shows niacin content of several foods in each food group. Overall, the richest sources of niacin are foods in the protein group and fortified breakfast cereals. Foods in the dairy group contain very little niacin, but the tryptophan in dairy foods can be converted into niacin. sour cream: Oleksandra Naumenko/Shutterstock; milk: Hurst Photo/Shutterstock; banana: lynx/iconotec.com/Glow Images; cereal: Joe Belanger/iStock/Getty Images; potatoes: Kaan Ates/E+/Getty Images; chicken: Nycshooter/Michael Krinke/E+/Getty Images; MyPlate: U.S. Department of Agriculture

Sources: Office of Dietary Supplements, Dietary Supplements Fact Sheets, available from https://ods.od.nih.gov/factsheets/list-all; USDA FoodData Central, available from https://fdc.nal.usda.gov.

Intakes of niacin by adults are about double the RDA, not including the contribution from tryptophan from protein-rich foods, such as meat, poultry, seafood, and dairy products.[26] Tables of food composition values also ignore tryptophan as a source of niacin. Nowadays, with better access to protein foods as well as enrichment of wheat flour and rice, niacin deficiency is extremely rare.

AVOIDING TOO MUCH NIACIN

The UL for niacin pertains only to the nicotinic acid form. Side effects include headache, itching, and increased blood flow to the skin because of blood vessel dilation (known as *niacin flush*). These symptoms are especially seen when intakes are above 100 milligrams per day. Besides these nuisances, long-term use of megadoses of niacin may damage the liver and increase the risk for diabetes. Megadoses of niacin are not recommended.

✓ CONCEPT CHECK 8.10

1. How is niacin involved in energy metabolism?
2. What are the three distinct signs of a niacin deficiency?
3. Which two MyPlate food groups provide many rich sources of niacin?
4. What is the relationship between tryptophan and niacin?

8.11 Pantothenic Acid (Vitamin B-5)

FUNCTIONS OF PANTOTHENIC ACID

Pantothenic acid is required for the synthesis of coenzyme A (CoA), a coenzyme in chemical reactions that release energy from carbohydrates, lipids, and protein. It is also used in the synthesis of fatty acids (see Fig. 8-16).[33]

PANTOTHENIC ACID DEFICIENCY

Pantothenic acid is so widespread in foods that a nutritional deficiency among healthy people with a varied eating pattern is unlikely. *Pantothen* means "from every side" in Greek. A deficiency of pantothenic acid might occur in alcohol use disorders along with a nutrient-deficient eating pattern. Signs of pantothenic acid deficiency include neurological problems, such as numbness and burning sensations in the hands and feet, and gastrointestinal distress. However, these symptoms would probably be hidden among deficiencies of thiamin, riboflavin, vitamin B-6, and folate, so the pantothenic acid deficiency might be unrecognizable.

GETTING ENOUGH PANTOTHENIC ACID

The Adequate Intake (AI) set for pantothenic acid is 5 milligrams per day for adults. Average consumption is well in excess of this amount. Pantothenic acid is found in every food group, but the richest sources are sunflower seeds, mushrooms, peanuts, and eggs (Fig. 8-22). Other rich sources are meat, milk, and many vegetables.

AVOIDING TOO MUCH PANTOTHENIC ACID

No observable toxicity is known for pantothenic acid, so no UL has been set. There have been some reports of individuals taking large doses of pantothenic acid supplements (e.g., 10 g/day) developing mild diarrhea and gastrointestinal distress.

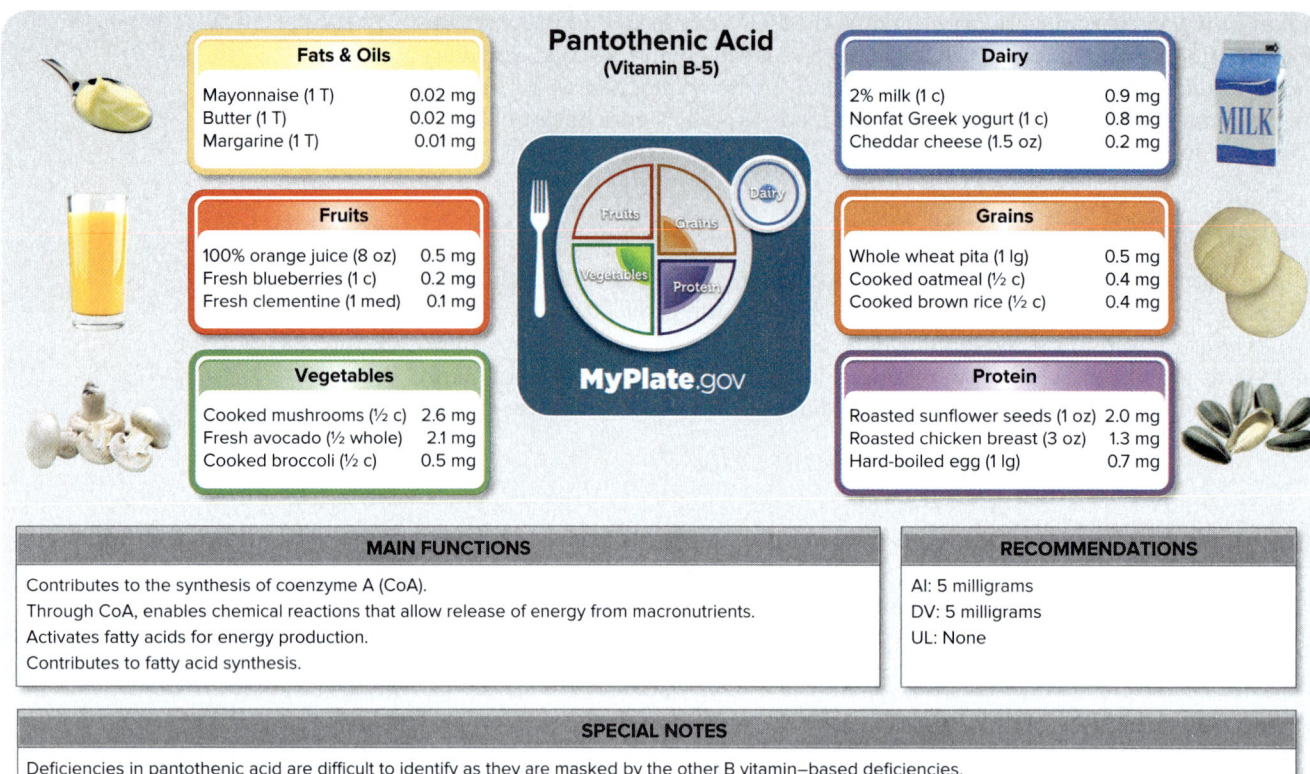

FIGURE 8-22 Food sources of pantothenic acid. The fill of the background color (none, 1/3, 2/3, or completely covered) within each group on MyPlate indicates the average nutrient density for pantothenic acid in that group. The figure shows the pantothenic acid content of several foods in each food group. Overall, fortified foods and foods rich in protein are the best sources of pantothenic acid. mayo: Iconotec/Alamy Stock Photo; milk: Hurst Photo/Shutterstock; juice: Sergei Vinogradov/seralexvi/123RF; pita bread: lynx/iconotec.com/Glowimages; mushrooms: Pixtal/age fotostock; seeds: JIANG HONGYAN/Shutterstock; MyPlate: U.S. Department of Agriculture

Sources: Office of Dietary Supplements, Dietary Supplements Fact Sheets, available from https://ods.od.nih.gov/factsheets/list-all; USDA FoodData Central, available from https://fdc.nal.usda.gov.

✓ CONCEPT CHECK 8.11

1. What is the role of pantothenic acid in energy metabolism?
2. List three rich food sources of pantothenic acid.

8.12 Vitamin B-6 (Pyridoxine)

FUNCTIONS OF VITAMIN B-6

Vitamin B-6 is known by its number, rather than its general name, and is a family of three structurally similar compounds. All can be converted into the active vitamin B-6 coenzyme, pyridoxal phosphate (PLP). The coenzyme forms of vitamin B-6 are needed for the activity of numerous enzymes involved in carbohydrate, protein, and lipid metabolism. One of the primary functions is as a coenzyme in over 100 chemical reactions that involve the metabolism of protein (see Fig. 8-16). The B-6 coenzyme, PLP, participates in reactions that allow the synthesis of nonessential (dispensable) amino acids by helping to split the nitrogen group ($-NH_2$) from an amino acid and making it available to another amino acid.

Vitamin B-6 also plays a role in **homocysteine** metabolism. Among the other important functions of vitamin B-6 are synthesis of neurotransmitters, such as serotonin and gamma aminobutyric acid (GABA); conversion of tryptophan to niacin; breakdown of stored glycogen to glucose; and synthesis of white blood cells and the heme portion of hemoglobin.[34]

homocysteine An amino acid that arises from the metabolism of methionine. Vitamin B-6, folate, vitamin B-12, and choline are required for its metabolism. Elevated levels are associated with an increased risk of cardiovascular disease.

VITAMIN B-6 DEFICIENCY

Because of the role of vitamin B-6 in hemoglobin synthesis and amino acid metabolism, a deficiency in vitamin B-6 affects multiple body systems, including the cardiovascular, immune, and nervous systems, as well as overall energy metabolism. Accordingly, vitamin B-6 deficiency results in widespread symptoms, including depression, vomiting, skin disorders, irritation of the nerves, anemia, and impaired immune response.

People with alcohol use disorders are susceptible to a vitamin B-6 deficiency. A metabolite formed in alcohol metabolism can displace the coenzyme form of vitamin B-6, increasing its tendency to be destroyed. In addition, alcohol decreases the absorption of vitamin B-6 and decreases the synthesis of its coenzyme form. Cirrhosis and hepatitis (both can accompany alcohol use disorders) also destroy healthy liver tissue. Thus, a cirrhotic liver cannot adequately metabolize vitamin B-6 or synthesize its coenzyme form.

GETTING ENOUGH VITAMIN B-6

With their ample consumption of animal products, the typical American dietary pattern exceeds the RDA for vitamin B-6.[26] There is some research to indicate that athletes may need slightly more vitamin B-6 than sedentary adults. The athlete's body processes large quantities of glycogen and protein, and the metabolism of these compounds requires vitamin B-6. However, unless athletes restrict their food intake, they are likely to consume plenty of this B vitamin.

Major sources of vitamin B-6 are animal products and fortified ready-to-eat breakfast cereals (Fig. 8-23). Other sources are vegetables and fruits such as potatoes,

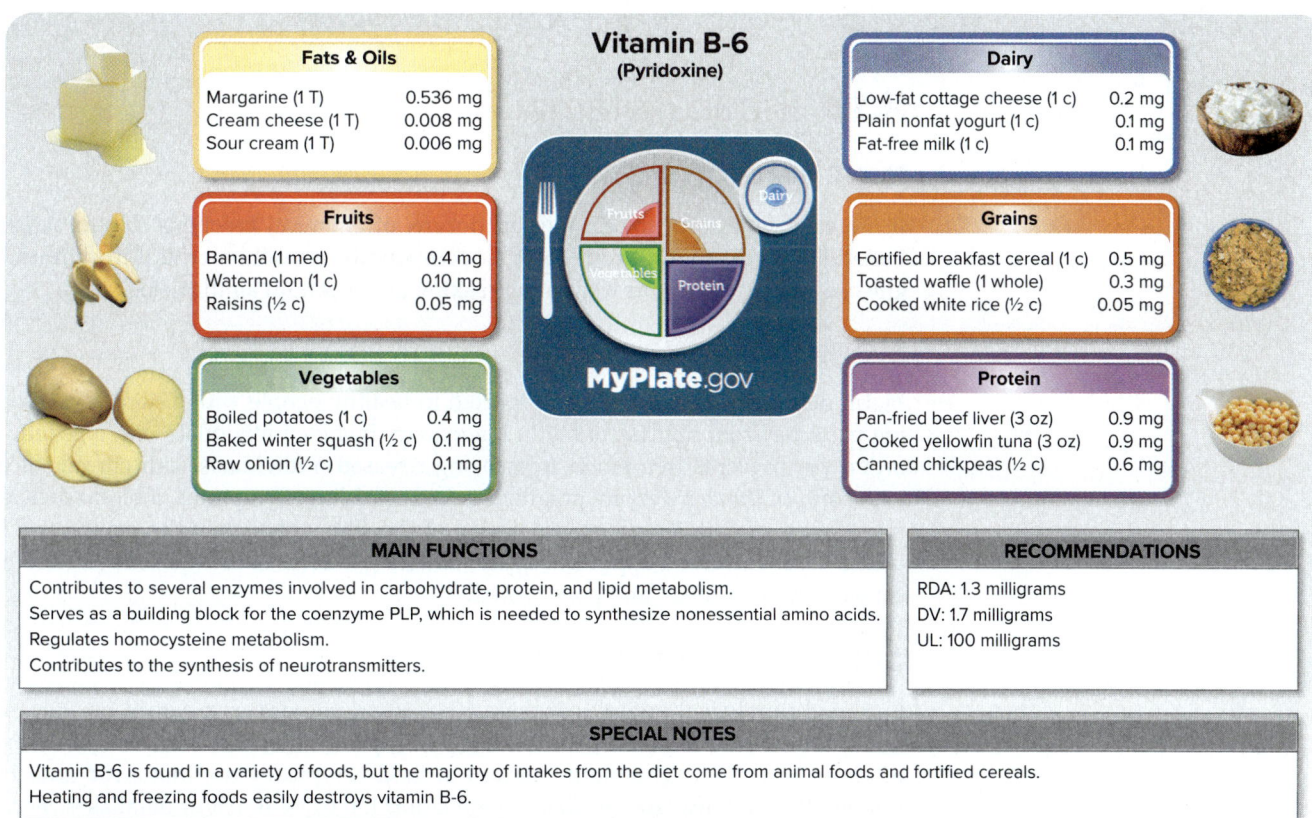

FIGURE 8-23 Food sources of vitamin B-6. The fill of the background color (none, 1/3, 2/3, or completely covered) within each group on MyPlate indicates the average nutrient density for vitamin B-6 in that group. The figure shows the vitamin B-6 content of several foods in each food group. Overall, the richest and most bioavailable sources of vitamin B-6 are animal sources of protein and fortified breakfast cereals. However, dairy foods are not a particularly good source of vitamin B-6. margarine: 2/James Worrell/Ocean/Corbis; rice: Oleksandra Naumenko/Shutterstock; banana: lynx/iconotec.com/Glow Images; cereal: Joe Belanger/iStock/Getty Images; potatoes: Kaan Ates/E+/Getty Images; chickpeas: Brett Stevens/Cultura/Getty Images; MyPlate: U.S. Department of Agriculture

Sources: Office of Dietary Supplements, Dietary Supplements Fact Sheets, available from https://ods.od.nih.gov/factsheets/list-all; USDA FoodData Central, available from https://fdc.nal.usda.gov.

spinach, bananas, and cantaloupes. Overall, the protein group of MyPlate offers most of the food sources of vitamin B-6, and animal sources and fortified grain products are the most reliable because the vitamin B-6 they contain is more absorbable than that in plant foods. Vitamin B-6 is rather unstable; heating and freezing can easily destroy it.

AVOIDING TOO MUCH VITAMIN B-6

Unlike most B vitamins, vitamin B-6 can accumulate to toxic levels in tissues, such as the muscles, liver, and red blood cells. The UL for vitamin B-6 is 100 milligrams per day, based on the risk of developing nerve damage. Studies have shown that intakes of 2 to 6 grams of vitamin B-6 per day for 2 or more months can lead to irreversible nerve damage. Symptoms of vitamin B-6 toxicity include walking difficulties and hand and foot tingling and numbness. Some nerve damage in individual sensory neurons is probably reversible, but damage to the ganglia (where many nerve fibers converge) appears to be permanent. Other effects of excessive vitamin B-6 intakes include painful, disfiguring skin lesions, photosensitivity, and gastrointestinal symptoms, such as nausea and heartburn. With 500-milligram tablets of vitamin B-6 available in health-food stores, taking a toxic dose is possible.

✓ **CONCEPT CHECK 8.12**

1. What is the role of vitamin B-6 in energy metabolism and other body functions?
2. Which MyPlate food group provides many nutrient-dense and bioavailable sources of vitamin B-6?
3. Are vitamin B-6 supplements safe? Why or why not?

8.13 Biotin (Vitamin B-7)

FUNCTIONS OF BIOTIN

In its coenzyme form, biotin aids in dozens of chemical reactions. Biotin assists in the addition of carbon dioxide to other compounds, a reaction critical in synthesizing glucose and fatty acids, as well as in breaking down certain amino acids.[35]

BIOTIN DEFICIENCY

Biotin deficiency has never been reported in healthy people with a normal mixed eating pattern. Groups at risk of biotin inadequacy include individuals with a genetic disorder that prevents free biotin from being released, individuals with chronic alcohol exposure, or females who are pregnant or breastfeeding. Symptoms of biotin deficiency include loss of hair, a scaly inflammation of the skin, changes in the tongue and lips, brittle nails, decreased appetite, nausea, vomiting, a form of anemia, depression, muscle pain and weakness, and poor growth.

GETTING ENOUGH BIOTIN

Our food supply is thought to provide 40 to 60 micrograms per person per day, more than the AI. Protein sources, such as egg yolks, peanuts, and cheese, are good sources of biotin (Fig. 8-24). The biotin content of food is typically not measured and therefore is often not available in food composition tables or nutrient databases. Because intestinal bacteria synthesize some biotin that you can absorb, a biotin deficiency is unlikely. Scientists are not sure how much of the bacteria-synthesized biotin in our intestines is absorbed, so we still need to consume biotin. If bacterial synthesis in the intestines is not sufficient, as in people who are missing a large part of the colon or who take antibiotics for many months, special attention must be paid to meeting biotin needs.

Biotin (Vitamin B-7)

Fats & Oils
- Sour cream (1 T) — 0.31 mcg
- Ranch dressing (1 T) — 0.03 mcg
- Margarine (1 T) — 0.02 mcg

Fruits
- Raisins (½ c) — 0.3 mcg
- Banana (1 med) — 0.3 mcg
- Strawberries (1 c) — 0.2 mcg

Vegetables
- Cooked sweet potato (1 med) — 3.5 mcg
- Cooked spinach (1 c) — 1 mcg
- Fresh broccoli (1 c) — 0.8 mcg

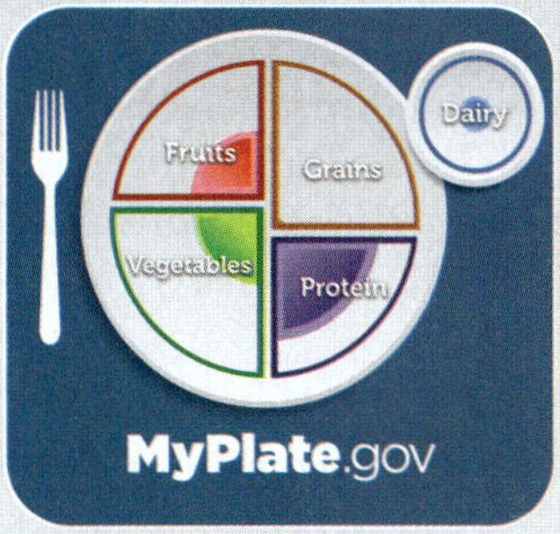

Dairy
- Cheddar cheese (1.5 oz) — 0.6 mcg
- 2% milk (1 c) — 0.3 mcg
- Plain yogurt (1 c) — 0.2 mcg

Grains
- Oatmeal (½ c) — 0.1 mcg
- Saltine crackers (1 c) — 0.1 mcg
- Whole wheat bread (1 slice) — 0.02 mcg

Protein
- Cooked egg (1 lg) — 10 mcg
- Canned salmon (3 oz) — 5 mcg
- Roasted sunflower seeds (1 oz) — 2 mcg

MAIN FUNCTIONS
- Aids in dozens of chemical reactions in the body.
- Contributes to development of coenzymes that aid in the synthesis of glucose and fatty acids.
- Related coenzymes also assist in the breakdown of certain amino acids.
- Plays a role in histone modification, thus contributing to gene regulation.

RECOMMENDATIONS
- AI: 30 micrograms
- DV: 30 micrograms
- UL: None

SPECIAL NOTES
- Biotin deficiencies are rare as the gut microbiota synthesize some biotin that the body can absorb.
- Biotin bioavailability is altered significantly in various foods due to the nutrient being bound to proteins; one such example is eggs.

FIGURE 8-24 Food sources of biotin. The fill of the background color (none, 1/3, 2/3, or completely covered) within each group on MyPlate indicates the average nutrient density for biotin in that group. The figure shows the biotin content of several foods in each food group. Overall, foods rich in protein are the best sources of biotin. Grains (even fortified varieties) contain very little biotin. sour cream: Oleksandra Naumenko/Shutterstock; cheese: Brent Hofacker/Shutterstock; raisins: lynx/iconotec/Glowimages; oatmeal: Olga Traskevych/123RF; sweet potatoes: lynx/iconotec.com/Glow Images; egg: Sven Kahns/McGraw-Hill; MyPlate: U.S. Department of Agriculture

Sources: Office of Dietary Supplements, Dietary Supplements Fact Sheets, available from https://ods.od.nih.gov/factsheets/list-all; USDA FoodData Central, available from https://fdc.nal.usda.gov.

Biotin's bioavailability varies significantly among foods based on the food's biotin–protein complex. In raw egg whites, biotin is bound to **avidin**, which inhibits absorption of the vitamin. Consuming many raw egg whites can eventually lead to biotin-deficiency disease. Cooking, however, denatures the protein avidin in eggs so it cannot bind biotin. In addition to food safety concerns, this is one of the important reasons to avoid consuming raw eggs.[36]

avidin A protein found in egg whites that binds to and decreases the bioavailability of biotin. Cooking denatures avidin.

AVOIDING TOO MUCH BIOTIN

Biotin appears relatively nontoxic. Thus, no UL for biotin has been set. Some reports suggest that high biotin intakes may cause false laboratory test results. These false results may lead to misdiagnosis and mistreatment of medical conditions.

✓ CONCEPT CHECK 8.13

1. What is the role of biotin in energy metabolism?
2. What are the signs and symptoms of biotin deficiency?
3. Which MyPlate food group contains the most nutrient-dense sources of biotin?
4. Why does consumption of raw eggs lead to biotin deficiency?

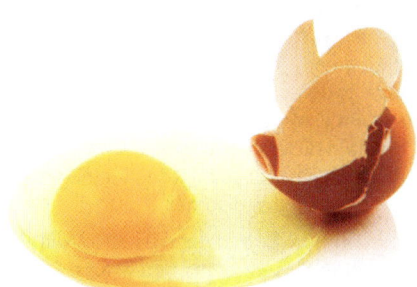

Eating a lot of raw eggs can lead to a biotin deficiency. Biotin is bound to avidin in raw egg whites, inhibiting its absorption. Cooking denatures avidin and releases biotin. sil63/Shutterstock

8.14 Folate (Vitamin B-9)

The term *folate* is used to describe a variety of forms of this B vitamin found in foods and in the body. *Folic acid* is the synthetic form added to fortified foods and present in supplements.

Folate recommendations for all but females of childbearing age are based on dietary folate equivalents (DFE). Synthetic folic acid, found in supplements and fortified foods, is more bioavailable than the folate that naturally occurs in food. The DFE unit takes into account these differences in bioavailability.

> 1 DFE = 1 microgram folate from food
> = 0.6 microgram folic acid from fortified food
> = 0.5 microgram folic acid from a supplement on an empty stomach

FUNCTIONS OF FOLATE

A key role of the folate coenzyme is to supply or accept single-carbon compounds in chemical reactions. In this role, folate coenzymes aid in the synthesis of DNA and metabolism of amino acids.[37] For example, folate works along with vitamin B-6 and vitamin B-12 to metabolize homocysteine. Folate also functions in the formation of neurotransmitters in the brain. Meeting the RDA for folate can improve symptoms of depression in some cases of mental illness.[38]

Research is also underway on the role of folate in cancer protection. Because folate aids in DNA synthesis, adequate folate status is important to maintain DNA integrity, including the control of certain cancer-promoting genes. Meeting the RDA for folate may be one way to reduce risk for some types of cancers. However, the influence of folate on cancer risk is complex; genetic variations in folate metabolism play a role and the nutrient may have different effects on different types of cancer.[39] Folic acid supplements are not recommended for cancer prevention or treatment, but food sources of folate are a safe way to meet the RDA.

FOLATE DEFICIENCY

One of the major results of a folate deficiency occurs in the early phases of red blood cell synthesis. With inadequate folate, immature red blood cells cannot divide because they cannot form new DNA. The cells grow progressively larger because they are still synthesizing protein and other cell parts to make new cells. When the time comes for the cells to divide, however, the amount of DNA is insufficient to form two nuclei. Thus, the red blood cells remain in a large immature form, have a large nucleus, and are known as **macrocytes** (also called *megaloblasts*). When fewer mature red blood cells are present, the blood's capacity to carry oxygen decreases, causing a condition known as **macrocytic anemia** (also called *megaloblastic anemia*) (Fig. 8-25).

Clinicians focus on red blood cells as an indicator of folate status because they are easy to collect and examine. Folate deficiency, however, disrupts cell division throughout the entire body. Other symptoms of folate deficiency are inflammation of the tongue, diarrhea, poor growth, mental confusion, depression, and problems with nerve function. Another result of folate deficiency is elevated blood homocysteine levels, which have been associated with cardiovascular disease and are considered an independent risk factor for atherosclerosis. Research is ongoing to examine the impact of folate (and other B vitamins) on cardiovascular disease risk.[40]

Maternal folate deficiency (along with a genetic abnormality related to folate metabolism) has been linked to the development of **neural tube defects** in the fetus. These defects include **spina bifida** (spinal cord or spinal fluid bulge through the back) and **anencephaly** (absence of a major portion of the brain). Adequate folate status is crucial for all females of childbearing age, pregnant or not, because the neural tube closes

---

macrocyte A large, immature red blood cell that results from the inability of the cell to divide normally; also called *megaloblast*.

macrocytic anemia Anemia characterized by the presence of abnormally large red blood cells; also called *megaloblastic anemia*.

neural tube defect A defect in the formation of the neural tube occurring during early fetal development. This type of defect results in various nervous system disorders, such as spina bifida. Folate deficiency in a female who is pregnant increases the risk that the fetus will develop this disorder.

spina bifida Birth defect resulting from improper closure of the neural tube during embryonic development. The spinal cord or fluid may bulge outside the spinal column.

anencephaly Birth defect characterized by the absence of some or all of the brain and skull.

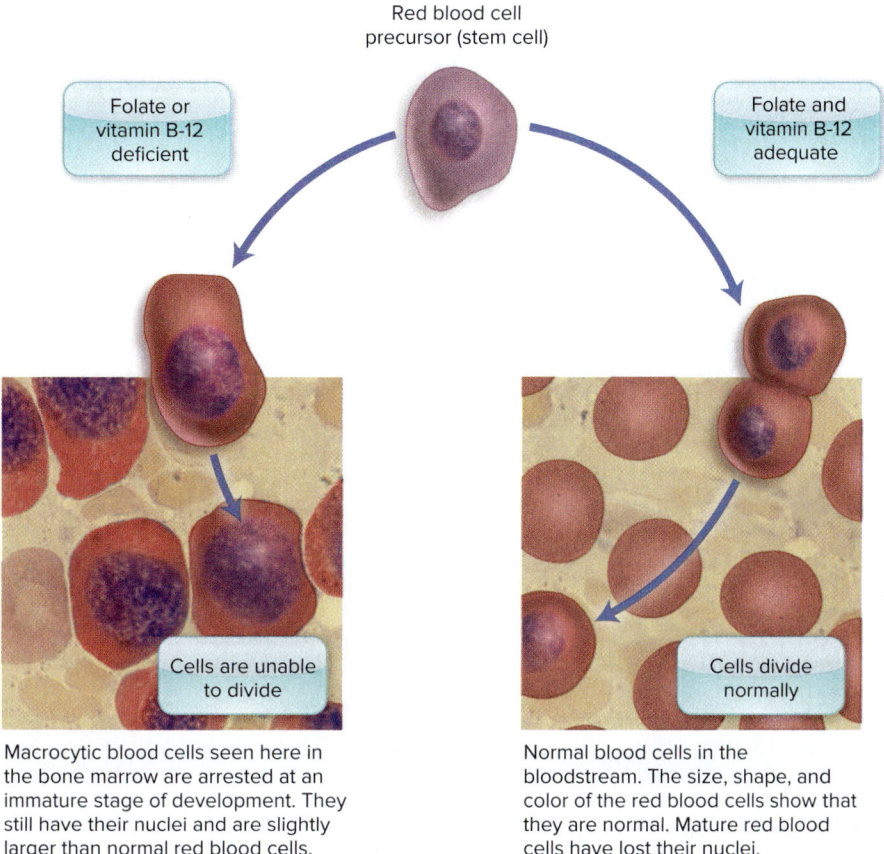

FIGURE 8-25 Macrocytic (megaloblastic) anemia occurs when red blood cells are unable to divide, leaving large, immature red blood cells. Either a folate or vitamin B-12 deficiency may cause this condition. Measurements of blood concentrations of both vitamins are taken to help determine the cause of the anemia.

within the first 28 days of pregnancy, which is earlier than many females are aware of a pregnancy. Research suggests that the risk for neural tube defects can be decreased by folate supplementation for mothers-to-be.[41]

As they age, some adults may be at risk for folate deficiency due to a combination of inadequate folate intake and decreased folate absorption. Perhaps these people fail to consume sufficient amounts of fruits and vegetables because of limited financial resources or physical problems, such as poor dental health. In addition, folate deficiencies often occur with alcohol use disorders, due mostly to inadequate intake and impaired absorption. Symptoms of a folate-related anemia can alert a primary care provider to the possibility of alcohol use disorders.

GETTING ENOUGH FOLATE

Folate's name is derived from the Latin word *folium,* which means foliage or leaves. Quite predictably, the richest sources of folate are green leafy vegetables. In addition, other vegetables, legumes, and organ meats are naturally rich sources of folate (Fig. 8-26). Enriched grains and fortified ready-to-eat breakfast cereals are important sources of folic acid for many adults.

Folate is susceptible to destruction by heat and oxygen. The vitamin C present in some food sources of folate, such as orange juice, helps to reduce folate destruction, but food processing and preparation destroy 50% to 90% of the folate in food. This underscores the importance of regularly eating fresh fruits and raw or lightly cooked vegetables.

Females who are pregnant need extra folate (a total of 600 micrograms dietary folate equivalent [DFE]) to accommodate the increased rates of cell division and DNA synthesis in their bodies and in the developing fetus. A healthy eating pattern can

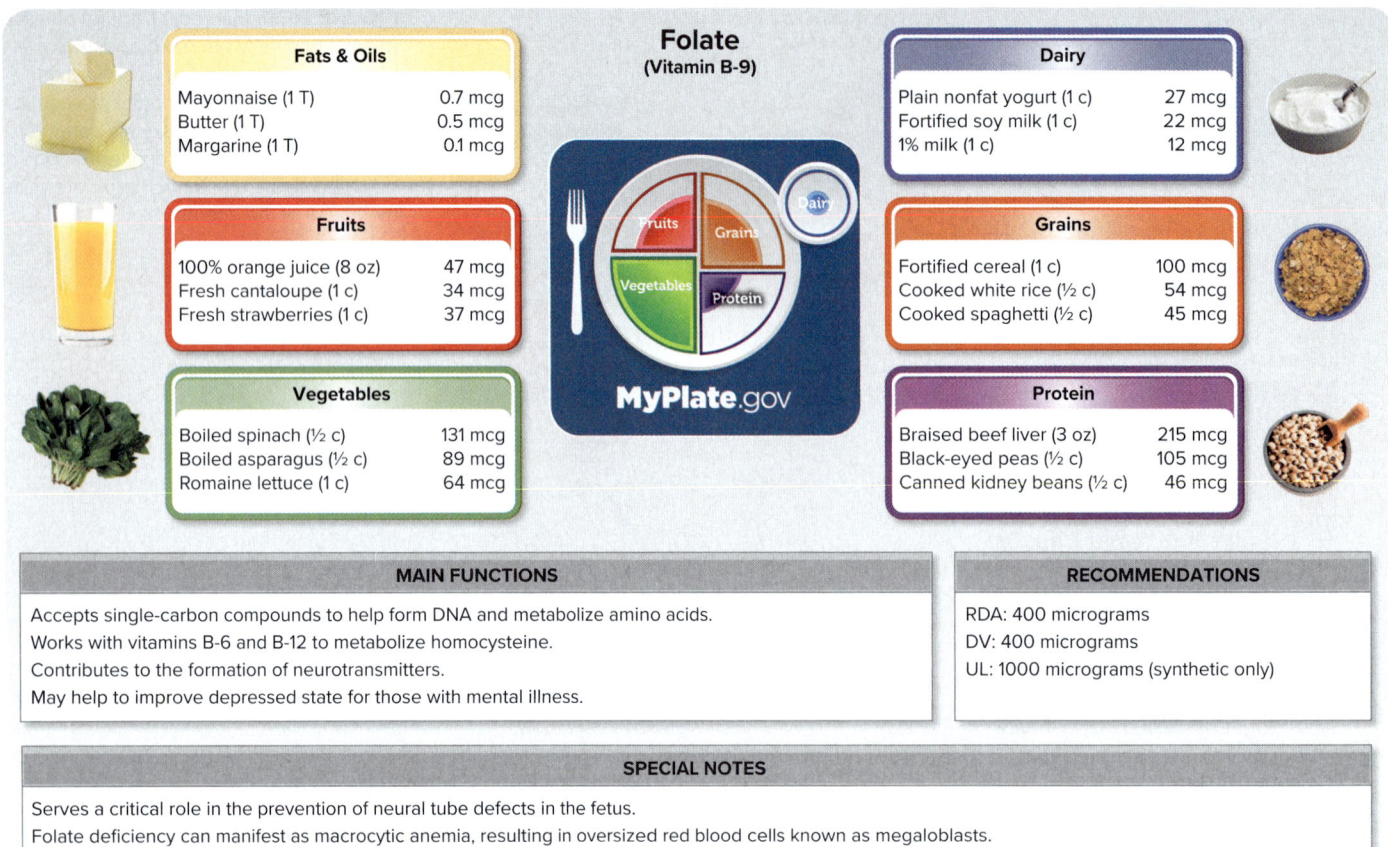

FIGURE 8-26 Food sources of folate. The fill of the background color (none, 1/3, 2/3, or completely covered) within each food group on MyPlate indicates the average nutrient density for folate in that group. The figure shows the folate content of several foods in each food group. Overall, the richest sources of folate are green, leafy vegetables and fortified grains. margarine: 2/James Worrell/Ocean/Corbis; Greek yogurt: Anastasios71/Shutterstock; juice: Sergei Vinogradov/seralexvi/123RF; cereal: Joe Belanger/iStock/Getty Images; spinach: Burke Triolo Productions/Artville/Getty Images; black-eyed peas: joannawnuk/123RF; MyPlate: U.S. Department of Agriculture

Sources: Office of Dietary Supplements, Dietary Supplements Fact Sheets, available from https://ods.od.nih.gov/factsheets/list-all; USDA FoodData Central, available from https://fdc.nal.usda.gov.

supply this much. Still, prenatal care often includes a specially formulated multivitamin and mineral supplement enriched with folic acid to meet the higher RDA during pregnancy.

In 1998, the FDA mandated the fortification of refined grain products with folate with the aim of reducing neural tube defects of the spine. With this program, average intakes have increased by about 200 micrograms per day. Including natural food sources, fortified foods, and dietary supplements, usual intakes of folate exceed the RDA.[26] Factors other than folate deficiency (e.g., genetics and environment) play a role in the development of neural tube defects, but studies have shown fortification of grain products with folic acid has decreased rates of neural tube defects in infants by an estimated 15% to 30% in the United States and up to 50% in other countries with higher background rates of neural tube defects.[42]

The folic acid enrichment of grains has also been accompanied by a noticeable decline in cardiovascular risk, especially risk for stroke, due to a drop in blood homocysteine levels among U.S. adults. Supplements of folic acid, vitamin B-6, and vitamin B-12 have been promoted to help lower homocysteine and decrease cardiac and stroke risk. This is only likely to be effective for individuals who start out with elevated homocysteine levels. Taking pharmacological doses of folate is not likely to benefit people who have blood homocysteine levels in the normal range.[43]

AVOIDING TOO MUCH FOLATE

The UL for folate only refers to synthetic folic acid because the absorption of the natural form of folate in food is limited. Some research indicates that too much folic acid could promote tumor development. Thus, even though folic acid fortification has been a public health success story for prevention of neural tube defects, there are concerns about the appropriate dose for the entire population.[44] In addition, large doses of folic acid can hide the signs of vitamin B-12 deficiency and therefore complicate its diagnosis. Specifically, regular consumption of large amounts of folate can prevent the appearance of an early warning sign of vitamin B-12 deficiency—enlarged red blood cells. For this reason, the FDA limits the amount of folic acid in supplements (for nonpregnant adults) to 400 micrograms.

✓ CONCEPT CHECK 8.14

1. Explain what happens to red blood cells in macrocytic anemia.
2. Why does the RDA for folate increase from 400 micrograms to 600 micrograms per day for females who are pregnant?

8.15 Vitamin B-12 (Cobalamin or Cyanocobalamin)

Vitamin B-12 is a unique vitamin. Its structure is the largest of all the vitamins, and it is the only vitamin that contains a mineral as part of its structure. Unlike most water-soluble vitamins, B-12 can be stored to a significant extent in the liver, so it takes many months of an eating pattern devoid of vitamin B-12 for a deficiency to occur. Vitamin B-12 is only naturally found in foods of animal origin.[45] Finally, the means by which the body absorbs vitamin B-12 is complex; a problem at any of several steps of digestion and absorption could lead to deficiency.

To illustrate the multistep process by which vitamin B-12 is absorbed, we will trace the path of a meal containing vitamin B-12 through the digestive tract (Fig. 8-27). In food, much of the vitamin B-12 is bound to protein and therefore cannot be absorbed. When food enters the mouth, **R-proteins** are secreted by the salivary glands. The bolus of food, including the R-proteins, travels down the esophagus to the stomach. Acid and enzymes present in the stomach release vitamin B-12 from food proteins, and the free vitamin B-12 then binds to R-protein. While food is in the stomach, the stomach cells release intrinsic factor, a protein-like compound. When the chyme reaches the duodenum, pancreatic enzymes release vitamin B-12 from R-proteins. The free vitamin B-12 then combines with intrinsic factor. The vitamin B-12–intrinsic factor complex travels the length of the small intestine to the ileum, where vitamin B-12 is finally absorbed.

If any of these steps fails or is altered, absorption of vitamin B-12 can drop to 1% to 2%. In these cases of malabsorption, the person usually takes monthly injections of vitamin B-12, uses nasal gels of the vitamin to bypass the need for intestinal absorption, or takes megadoses of a supplemental form (300 times the RDA). With this large dose, an adequate quantity of vitamin B-12 is able to cross the intestinal barrier via passive diffusion.

Most cases of vitamin B-12 deficiencies in healthy people result from defective absorption rather than from inadequate intakes. This is especially true for adults who are older. As we age, stomach acid production declines and our stomachs have a decreased ability to synthesize the intrinsic factor needed for adequate vitamin B-12 absorption.

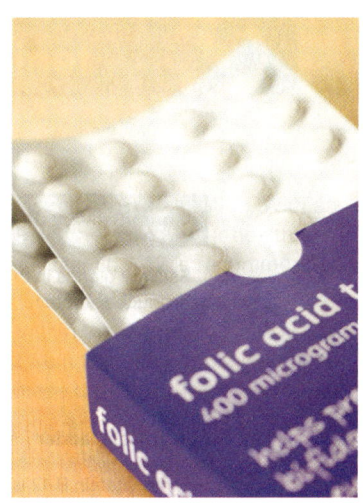

To lower the risk for neural tube defects, females of childbearing age should take a daily multivitamin and mineral supplement that contains 400 micrograms of folic acid. **How does the bioavailability of folic acid in supplements and fortified foods compare to the bioavailability of folate found naturally in foods?** BananaStock/Getty Images

R-proteins Proteins produced by the salivary glands that bind to free vitamin B-12 in the stomach and protect it from stomach acid.

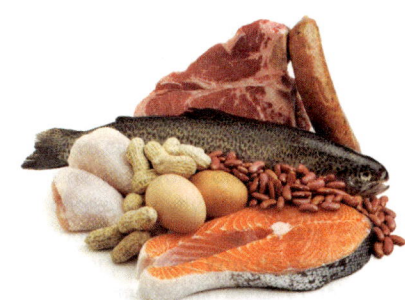

Vitamin B-12 is only naturally present in animal foods. With age, absorption of vitamin B-12 from food becomes less efficient, usually due to decreases in stomach acid production. D. Hurst/Alamy Stock Photo

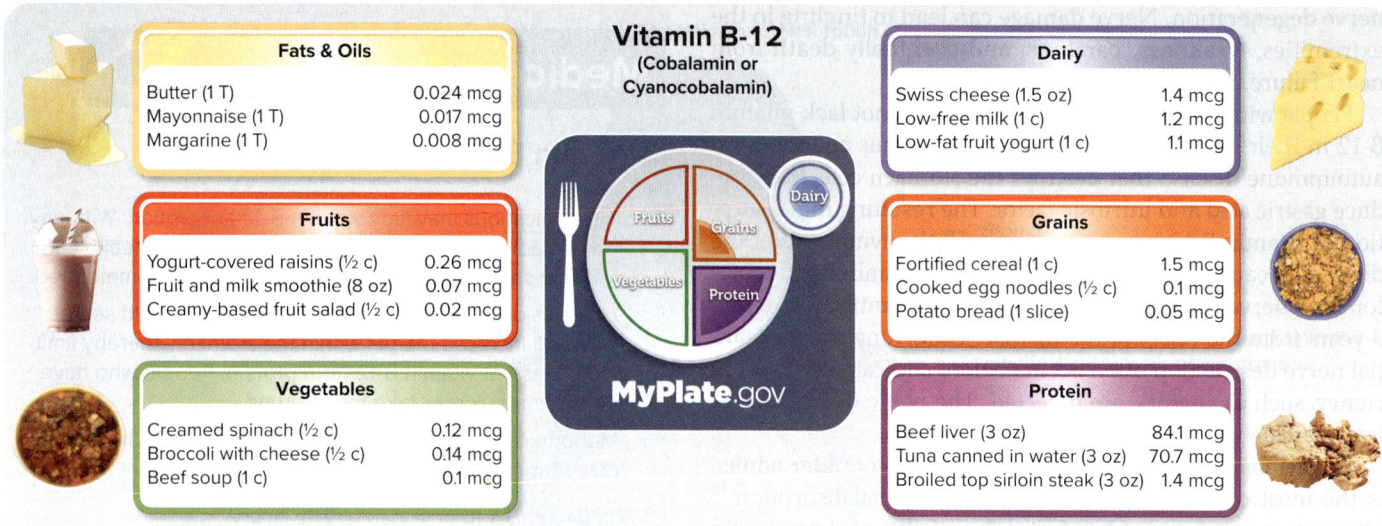

FIGURE 8-28 Food sources of vitamin B-12. The fill of the background color (none, 1/3, 2/3, or completely covered) within each food group on MyPlate indicates the average nutrient density for vitamin B-12 in that group. The figure shows the vitamin B-12 content of several foods in each food group. Overall, foods of animal origin and fortified grains are the richest sources of vitamin B-12. Except for fortified grains, foods of plant origin do not contain vitamin B-12. butter: 2/James Worrell/Ocean/Corbis; cheese: Comstock/Jupiter Images/Getty Images; smoothie: 5 second Studio/Shutterstock; cereal: Joe Belanger/iStock/Getty Images; soup: James Gathany/CDC; tuna: lynx/iconotec.com/Glow Images; MyPlate: U.S. Department of Agriculture

Sources: Office of Dietary Supplements, Dietary Supplements Fact Sheets, available from https://ods.od.nih.gov/factsheets/list-all; USDA FoodData Central, available from https://fdc.nal.usda.gov.

✓ CONCEPT CHECK 8.15

1. How does a vitamin B-12 deficiency lead to macrocytic anemia?
2. What role does vitamin B-12 play in the health of the brain and nervous system?
3. Identify two population groups that are at risk for vitamin B-12 deficiency. Explain why these people are at risk.
4. List three rich food sources of vitamin B-12.

8.16 Vitamin C (Ascorbic Acid)

FUNCTIONS OF VITAMIN C

Supporting Body Defenses. Vitamin C (also known as *ascorbic acid* or *ascorbate*) supports body defenses in two ways: It functions as an antioxidant, and it is necessary for the health of white blood cells.[48]

Vitamin C functions as an antioxidant because it can readily accept and donate electrons. These antioxidant properties are thought to reduce the formation of cancer-causing **nitrosamines** in the stomach. Vitamin C also aids in the reactivation of vitamin E after it has donated an electron to a free radical. Population studies suggest

nitrosamine A carcinogen formed from nitrates and breakdown products of amino acids; associated with cancer risk.

that the antioxidant properties of vitamin C may be effective in the prevention of certain cancers and cataracts. The extent to which vitamin C functions in the reduction of specific diseases is debatable based on the scientific studies to date.

As part of its antioxidant role, vitamin C assists the immune system. Vitamin C protects the body's cells from the harmful oxidants that are generated as part of the immune response. Beyond its antioxidant activity, vitamin C is vital for the proper function of the immune system because it promotes the proliferation of white blood cells. Recall that certain white blood cells use oxidation reactions to destroy pathogens.

Can taking vitamin C fend off the common cold? Numerous well-designed, double-blind studies have failed to show that vitamin C *prevents* colds. Nevertheless, vitamin C does appear to reduce the duration of symptoms by a day or so and to lessen the severity of the symptoms. For vitamin C to be effective, start taking it as soon as symptoms appear. Once the cold has taken hold, it is too late!

Formation of Body Proteins. The best understood function of vitamin C is its role in the synthesis of collagen. This protein is highly concentrated in connective tissue, bone, teeth, tendons, and blood vessels. Vitamin C is very important for wound healing; it strengthens structural tissues by increasing the cross-connections between amino acids found in collagen.

Formation of Other Compounds. Vitamin C has a specific function in the synthesis of numerous other compounds in the body. It is required for the synthesis of carnitine, a compound that transports fatty acids into the mitochondria so they can be used as fuel. In addition, it takes part in the formation of two neurotransmitters, serotonin and norepinephrine.

Absorption of Iron. Vitamin C enhances iron absorption by keeping iron in its most absorbable form, especially as the mineral travels through the alkaline environment of the small intestine. Consuming over 75 milligrams (the amount of vitamin C in one orange) of vitamin C at a meal significantly increases absorption of the iron consumed at that meal. Increasing intake of vitamin C–rich foods is beneficial for those with poor iron status or for those who choose to limit iron-rich food sources. Iron deficiency is the most common nutritional deficiency worldwide.

VITAMIN C DEFICIENCY

On long sea voyages before the mid-eighteenth century, half or more of sailing crews died due to scurvy, the vitamin C–deficiency disease. The symptoms of scurvy, which include bleeding gums, tooth loss, bruising, and scaly skin, illustrate the important function of vitamin C in the formation of connective tissue. Without vitamin C, the skin and blood vessels weaken and wounds will not heal. In 1740, the Englishman Dr. James Lind first showed that citrus fruits—two oranges and one lemon a day—could prevent the development of scurvy. Fifty years after Lind's discovery, daily rations for British sailors included limes (thus their nickname, *limeys*). Even after this discovery, scurvy continued to affect many people, including thousands who died during the American Civil War owing to inadequate intake of vitamin C. The important function of vitamin C in the formation of connective tissue is exemplified in the early symptoms of a deficiency: pinpoint hemorrhages under the skin (Fig. 8-29), bleeding gums, and joint pain.

GETTING ENOUGH VITAMIN C

Fresh, ripe fruits and vegetables are loaded with vitamin C. Besides the foods listed in Figure 8-30, other citrus fruits, papayas, cauliflower, and other vegetables pack a lot of vitamin C into a low-calorie package. Ready-to-eat breakfast cereals and potatoes are also good sources of vitamin C. Five to nine servings of fruits and vegetables can easily provide enough vitamin C to meet the RDA. The brighter the fruit or vegetable, the higher it tends to be in vitamin C. For example, a green pepper has 60 milligrams of vitamin C, and a red bell pepper provides 95 milligrams of vitamin C. Keep in mind, however, that

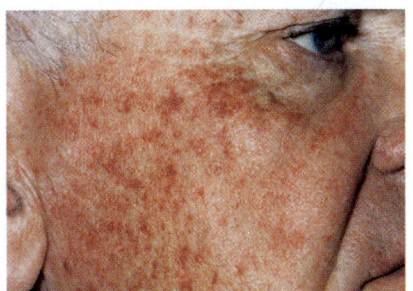

FIGURE 8-29 Pinpoint hemorrhages of the skin—an early symptom of scurvy. The spots on the skin are caused by slight bleeding. The person may experience poor wound healing. These are signs of defective collagen synthesis. Dr. P. Marazzi/Science Source

Vitamin C (Ascorbic Acid)

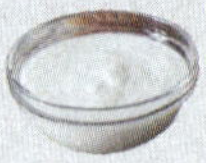

Fats & Oils
- Sour cream (1 T) — 0.13 mg
- Italian dressing (1 T) — 0.06 mg
- Margarine (1 T) — 0.01 mg

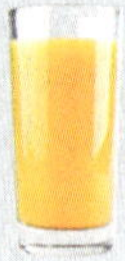

Fruits
- 100% orange juice (1 c) — 124 mg
- Kiwifruit (1 med) — 64 mg
- Fresh strawberries (½ c) — 49 mg

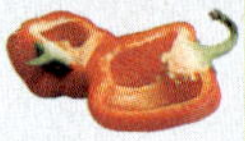

Vegetables
- Fresh red peppers (½ c) — 95 mg
- Cooked broccoli (½ c) — 51 mg
- Cooked Brussels sprouts (½ c) — 48 mg

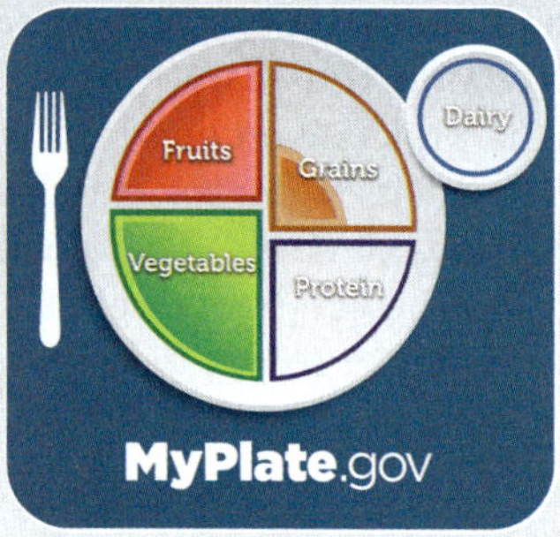

Dairy
- Cottage cheese with fruit (1 c) — 3.2 mg
- Nonfat buttermilk (1 c) — 2.4 mg
- Kefir (1 c) — 2.0 mg

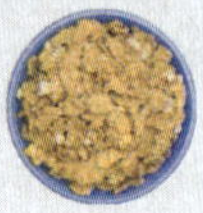

Grains
- Fortified cereal (1 c) — 8.9 mg
- Rye bread (1 slice) — 0.1 mg
- Wheat bread (1 slice) — 0.1 mg

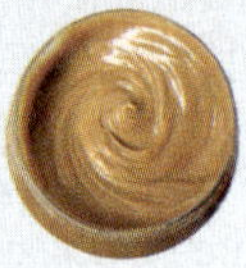

Protein
- Cooked chickpeas (½ c) — 1.07 mg
- Sunflower seed butter (2 T) — 0.86 mg
- Pistachios (1 oz) — 0.45 mg

MAIN FUNCTIONS
- Assists in formation of connective tissue, bone, teeth, tendons, and blood vessels.
- Serves as an antioxidant through acceptance and donation of electrons.
- Enhances the absorption of iron.
- Required for proper immune system functioning.

RECOMMENDATIONS
- RDA Adult Males: 90 milligrams
- RDA Adult Females: 75 milligrams
- DV: 90 milligrams
- UL: 2000 milligrams

SPECIAL NOTES
- Vitamin C deficiency is known as scurvy, which leads to bleeding gums, tooth loss, bruising, and scaly skin.
- Often, the brighter the fruit or vegetable, the higher the food is in vitamin C.

FIGURE 8-30 Food sources of vitamin C. The fill of the background color (none, 1/3, 2/3, or completely covered) within each food group on MyPlate indicates the average nutrient density for vitamin C in that group. The figure shows the vitamin C content of several foods in each food group. Overall, fruits and vegetables are the richest sources of vitamin C. Foods in the dairy and protein groups are poor sources of vitamin C. sour cream: Oleksandra Naumenko/Shutterstock; buttermilk: Nipaporn Panyacharoen/Shutterstock; juice: Sergei Vinogradov/seralexvi/123RF; cereal: Joe Belanger/iStock/Getty Images; peppers: lynx/iconotec.com/Glow Images; sunflower butter: D. Hurst/Alamy Stock Photo; MyPlate: U.S. Department of Agriculture

Sources: Office of Dietary Supplements, Dietary Supplements Fact Sheets, available from https://ods.od.nih.gov/factsheets/list-all; USDA FoodData Central, available from https://fdc.nal.usda.gov.

vitamin C is rapidly lost in processing and cooking as it is unstable in the presence of heat, iron, copper, or oxygen and is water soluble. Boiling fruits and vegetables can destroy much of the vitamin C or cause it to leach out of the food. Extended time on grocery store shelves or on your countertop at home will also decrease vitamin C content. Thus, you should consume fresh fruits and vegetables as soon after harvest as possible.

The RDA for vitamin C is 75 milligrams per day for adult females and 90 milligrams per day for adult males. According to the FDA's new food labeling rules, the Daily Value used on food and supplement labels is 90 milligrams. Tobacco users need to add an extra 35 milligrams per day to the RDA. The toxic by-products of cigarette smoke and the oxidizing agents found in tobacco products increase the need for the antioxidant action of vitamin C. Average daily consumption of vitamin C in the United States is in the range of approximately 70 to 80 milligrams, and at this level of intake, absorption efficiency is about 70% to 90%.

AVOIDING TOO MUCH VITAMIN C

The Upper Level (UL) of vitamin C is 2000 milligrams. Note that when vitamin C is consumed in large doses, the amount in excess of daily needs mostly ends up in the feces or urine. The kidneys start rapidly excreting vitamin C when intakes exceed 100 milligrams per day. As the amount ingested increases, absorption efficiency decreases precipitously—to approximately 50% with intake of 1000 milligrams per day. Regular consumption of more than 3000 milligrams per day may cause stomach inflammation and

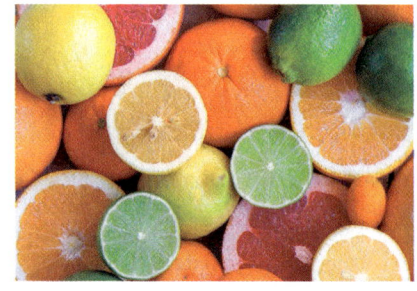

Citrus fruits are good sources of vitamin C. Maria Uspenskaya/Shutterstock

diarrhea. Even lower-dose supplement pills can cause some nausea and GI distress. Ingesting large amounts of vitamin C supplements is discouraged in people predisposed to kidney stones. Because vitamin C enhances the absorption of iron, vitamin C supplements are also not recommended for those who overabsorb iron or have excessive iron stores. High doses of vitamin C may interfere with medical tests for diabetes or blood in the feces. If you take vitamin C supplements at any dose, be sure to inform your primary care provider. Primary care providers may misdiagnose conditions if they do not realize the influence of large doses of vitamins on your medical test results.

✓ CONCEPT CHECK 8.16

1. How does the antioxidant role of vitamin C assist the immune system?
2. How do the signs of vitamin C deficiency relate to the many roles of the vitamin discussed in this chapter?
3. Why are fresh foods the best sources of vitamin C?

8.17 Choline: The Newest Vitamin?

Our knowledge of micronutrients continues to evolve. The first vitamin was isolated in 1913—barely a century ago—and within 25 years, all the vitamins we know to be essential in the human dietary pattern were identified. For choline, a water-soluble compound that is important for many aspects of human health, the story is still unfolding.

In 1998, the National Academy of Medicine recognized choline as an essential nutrient. When the Dietary Reference Intakes were released in 2000, only limited research on the dietary requirements for choline existed. One study of male volunteers showed decreased choline stores and liver damage when they were fed choline-deficient intravenous nutrition solutions. Based on this human study, plus laboratory animal studies, choline has been deemed essential and *vitamin-like*, but it is not yet classified as a vitamin.[49]

FUNCTIONS OF CHOLINE

Despite its lack of vitamin status, choline is needed by all cells and plays several important roles in the body.[49]

Cell Membrane Structure. Choline is a precursor for several phospholipids. Phosphatidylcholine (also known as *lecithin*) accounts for about half of the phospholipids in cell membranes. Recall from Chapter 5 that phospholipids contribute to the flexibility of cell membranes and allow for the presence of both water- and fat-soluble compounds in cell membranes. With its role in cell membrane structure, choline is important for the health of every cell and particularly for the health of brain tissue, where it is present in high levels.

Single-Carbon Metabolism. Choline is a precursor for betaine, a compound that participates in many chemical reactions that involve the transfer of single-carbon groups in metabolism. Important examples of metabolic pathways that involve the transfer of single-carbon groups include the synthesis of neurotransmitters, modifications of DNA during embryonic development, and the metabolism of homocysteine. As you learned in Section 8.12, high levels of homocysteine in the blood are related to increased risk of heart disease. Betaine and the B vitamin folate both donate single-carbon groups to convert homocysteine to another compound, thus reducing levels of homocysteine in the blood.

Some research suggests a potential role of adequate choline for the prevention of birth defects (e.g., neural tube defects).[50] Choline's purported role in prevention of birth defects is similar to that of folate. Both folate and choline are involved in formation of DNA during embryonic development. As you will read in Chapter 14, problems with DNA formation lead to birth defects. Indeed, animal studies show that maternal choline supplementation during critical stages of embryonic development can improve learning

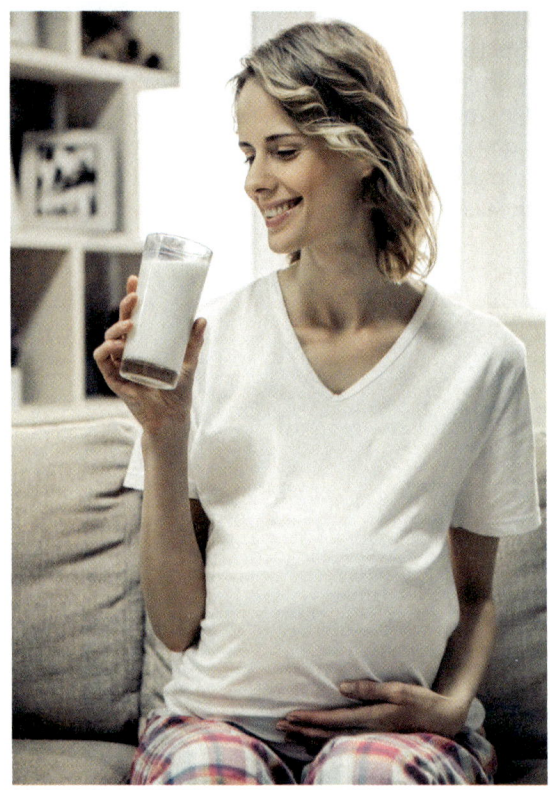

Choline is important for proper development of the fetal brain. Milk and other dairy products supply some choline. Vadim Guzhva/123RF

and memory in the offspring. In humans, as well, studies show that babies born to females with low choline intakes have four times higher rates of birth defects compared to babies born to females with high choline intakes. More recent studies, however, found no association between maternal blood concentrations of choline during pregnancy and risk of neural tube defects. More research is needed to determine whether choline supplementation would help prevent birth defects as has been demonstrated for folic acid.

Nerve Function and Brain Development. Choline is part of acetylcholine, a neurotransmitter associated with attention, learning, memory, muscle control, and many other functions. Sphingomyelin, a choline-containing phospholipid, is part of the myelin sheath that insulates nerve cells. As already mentioned, brain tissue is particularly high in choline. During pregnancy, the concentration of choline in amniotic fluid is high, supplying choline to the developing brain of the fetus. Animal studies demonstrate that choline deficiencies during pregnancy impair brain development, learning ability, and memory. The AI for choline is increased during pregnancy and breastfeeding to be available for proper brain development. Choline also may be useful for preventing or treating neurological disorders such as Alzheimer's disease.[51]

Lipid Transport. As part of phospholipids, choline is a component of lipoproteins, which carry lipids through the blood. Choline deficiency leads to decreased production of lipid transport proteins, such as very-low-density lipoproteins (VLDLs). The inability of the liver to export fat to the rest of the body can lead to a buildup of fat in the liver. A small amount of fat in the liver is normal, but excess fat leads to scarring of the liver tissue and eventual dysfunction. Fatty liver is a common cause of cirrhosis.

The roles of choline in lipid transport and homocysteine metabolism have implicated the nutrient in the prevention of cardiovascular disease. However, research has also raised some concerns about possible negative associations between dietary choline intake and increased cardiovascular disease risk. Recent findings have shown that oral supplements of phosphatidylcholine, along with choline from foods such as eggs, are metabolized by the intestinal microbiota to produce an atherosclerosis-promoting compound that has been associated with an increased risk of major adverse cardiovascular events.[52]

GETTING ENOUGH CHOLINE

Choline is widely distributed in foods (Fig. 8-31). Soybeans, egg yolks, beef, shiitake mushrooms, almonds, and peanuts are good sources. In the United States, most of our choline comes from eggs and other protein foods.[53] In addition to natural food sources, lecithin is often added to food products as an emulsifier during processing, so many other foods are sources of choline.

Eggs (with yolks) are by far the most nutrient-dense source of choline. One whole egg supplies about one-fourth of the daily choline needs in a 70 kcal package. Choline researchers suggest that an average of one egg per day would assist in achieving the AI for choline without raising risk for cardiovascular disease.

To some extent, choline also can be synthesized in the body by a process that involves other nutrients, such as folate and the amino acid methionine. If the body must synthesize choline to meet its needs, functional deficiencies of folate could result.

An AI for choline has been set for adults, but it is unknown whether a dietary supply is essential for infants or children. As noted, some choline can be synthesized in the body, but recent research indicates that synthesis by the body is not sufficient to meet the body's needs for choline. Nutrition surveys indicate that fewer than 10% of Americans meet the AI for choline.

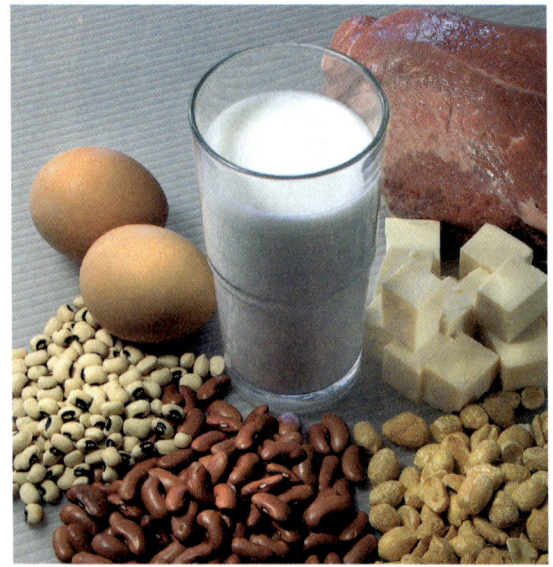

Eggs and other protein foods such as dry beans, meat, and dairy products are natural sources of choline. John Thoeming/McGraw Hill

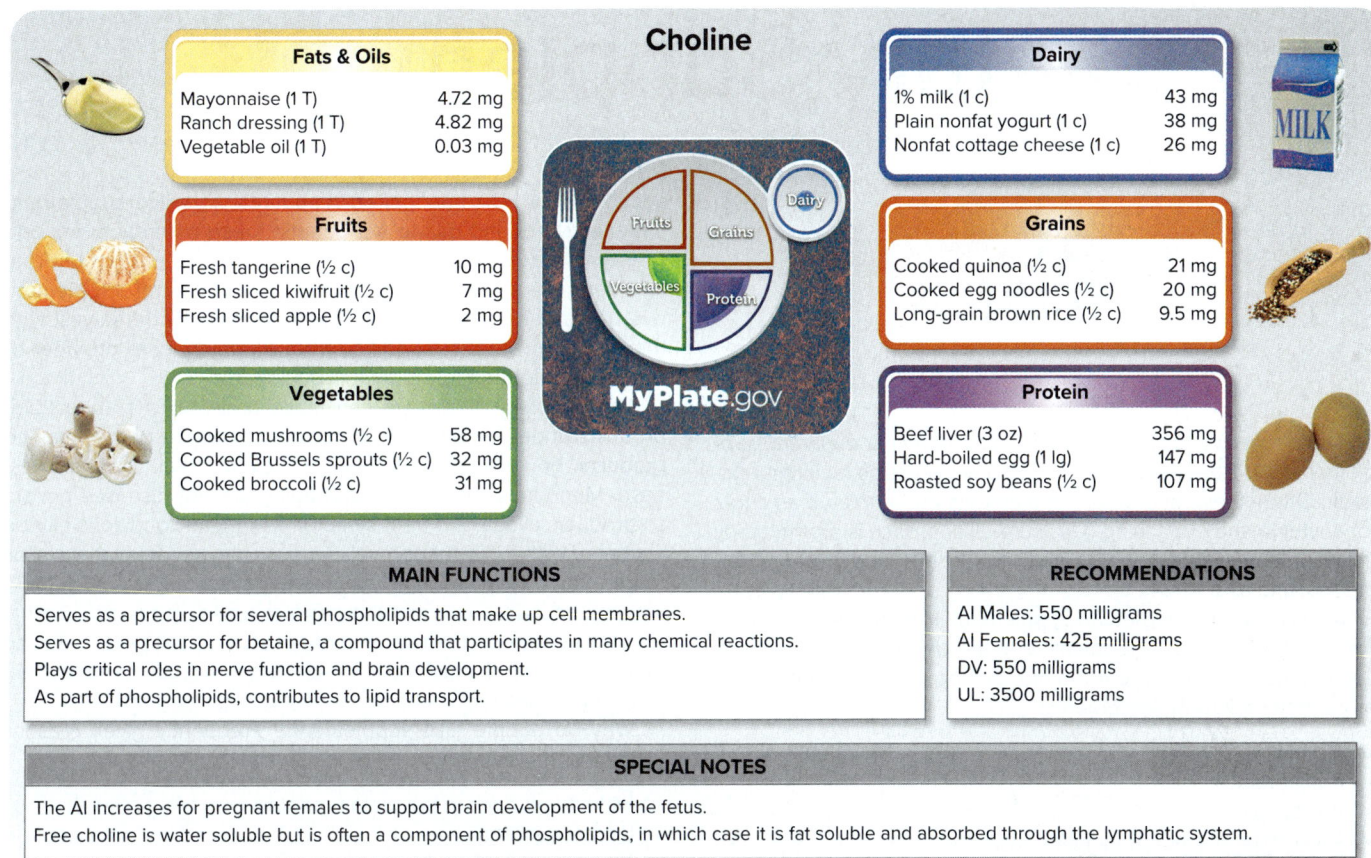

FIGURE 8-31 Food sources of choline. The fill of the background color (none, 1/3, 2/3, or completely covered) within each group on MyPlate indicates the average nutrient density for choline in that group. The figure shows the choline content of several foods compared in each food group. Overall, foods that are rich sources of protein are good sources of choline. Grains and fruits are, in general, poor sources of choline. mayonnaise: Iconotec/Alamy Stock Photo; milk: Hurst Photo/Shutterstock; tangerine: Jiang Hongyan/Shutterstock; quinoa: thunchanok tonuang/123RF; mushrooms: Pixtal/age fotostock; eggs: Vivian Thode/dancestrokes/123RF; MyPlate: U.S. Department of Agriculture

Sources: Office of Dietary Supplements, Dietary Supplements Fact Sheets, available from https://ods.od.nih.gov/factsheets/list-all; USDA FoodData Central, available from https://fdc.nal.usda.gov.

In addition, the AIs do not reflect wide genetic variation in individual choline requirements. Research suggests that at least half the population has genetic variations that increase dietary requirements for nutrients that serve in single-carbon metabolism, including choline and folate. Thus, even meeting the AI may not provide enough choline to support the body's needs for some people.[54]

The AI for choline increases during pregnancy (to 450 milligrams per day) and breastfeeding (to 550 milligrams per day) to support brain development of the fetus or infant. All prenatal vitamins do not contain choline; therefore, consumption of rich dietary sources of choline, such as eggs, is important for pregnant and breastfeeding females.[55]

AVOIDING TOO MUCH CHOLINE

The UL for adults is set at 3.5 grams per day. Routinely exceeding the UL will result in a fishy body odor and low blood pressure.

✓ CONCEPT CHECK 8.17

1. Describe three functions of choline in the human body.
2. List three foods you could include in your dietary pattern to ensure an adequate intake of choline.
3. Why is choline not considered a vitamin at this time?

8.18 Nutrition and Your Health: Dietary Supplements

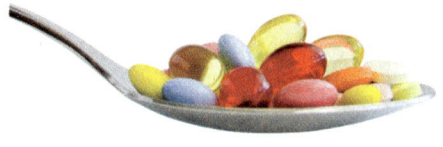

ma-k/Getty Images

The terms *dietary supplements* and *multivitamin and mineral supplement* (MVM) have been mentioned many times so far in this textbook. Often, these and other supplements are marketed as cures for anything and everything. This cure-all approach is promoted by the supplement industry and countless health-food stores, pharmacies, and supermarkets.

According to the Dietary Supplement Health and Education Act of 1994 (DSHEA), a supplement in the United States is a product intended to supplement the diet that bears or contains one or more of the following ingredients:

- A vitamin
- A mineral
- A probiotic
- An herb or another botanical
- An amino acid
- A dietary substance to supplement the diet, which could be an extract or a combination of the ingredients in this list

The definition is broad and covers a wide variety of nutritional substances. The use of dietary supplements is a common practice among individuals and generates about $35 billion annually for the industry in the United States (Fig. 8-32). Supplements can be sold without proof that they are safe and effective. Unless the FDA has evidence that a supplement is inherently dangerous or marketed with an illegal claim, it does not regulate such products closely (see the *Newsworthy Nutrition* in this section). The FDA has limited resources to police supplement manufacturers and has to act against these manufacturers one at a time. Thus, we cannot rely on the FDA to protect us from any dangers associated with vitamin and mineral supplement overuse and misuse. We bear that responsibility ourselves, with the help of professional advice from a primary care provider or registered dietitian nutritionist (RDN).

The supplement makers can make broad claims about their products under the *structure or function* provision of the law. The products, however, cannot claim to prevent, treat, or cure a disease. Menopause in females and aging are not diseases per se, so products alleging to treat symptoms of these conditions can be marketed without FDA approval. For example, a product that claims to treat hot flashes arising during menopause can be sold without any evidence to prove that the product works, but a product that claims to decrease the risk of cardiovascular disease by reducing blood cholesterol must have results from scientific studies that justify the claim.

Why do people take supplements? Frequently given reasons include to:

- Fill nutrient gaps in the dietary pattern.
- Increase energy.
- Maintain overall health.
- Prevent disease (cancer, osteoporosis, etc.).
- Reduce stress.
- Reduce susceptibility to health conditions (e.g., colds).

Who Should Take a Supplement?

Multivitamin and mineral supplements (MVMs) are popularly regarded as a simple backup plan or an insurance policy, even for people who consciously try to maintain a balanced dietary pattern. Users aim to prevent nutrient deficiencies or chronic diseases by filling any gaps between dietary intake and nutrient needs. However, evidence to support the widespread use of MVMs is lacking.[56] While there appears to be low risk of harm from consuming a balanced MVM that supplies no more than 100% of the Daily Value for the nutrients it contains, most studies indicate no discernible advantage. The National Institutes of Health, in its *State-of-the-Science Report,* concluded that the present evidence is insufficient to recommend either for or against the use of MVMs to prevent chronic disease.

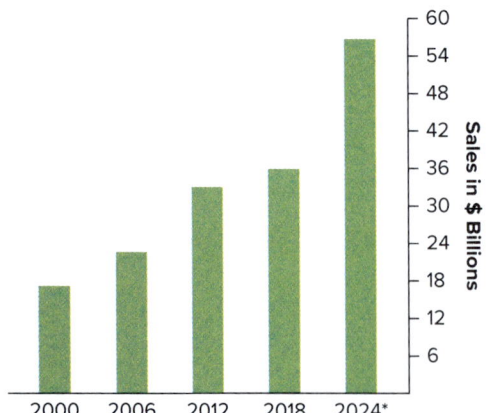

FIGURE 8-32 The dietary supplement industry is a growing multibillion-dollar business in the United States.
*Projected Sales

Top Five Dietary Supplements
1. Multivitamins
2. Vitamin D
3. Vitamin C
4. Protein
5. Calcium

Source: Council for Responsible Nutrition.

TABLE 8-5 ■ Who Is Most Likely to Benefit from Dietary Supplements?

Type of Supplement	Who May Benefit
Multivitamin/mineral supplement	People on restrictive diets (< 1200 kcal per day), vegans, vegetarians People with suboptimal diets (e.g., in cases of food insecurity or *picky* eaters) People with malabsorptive diseases People who take medications that interfere with nutrient absorption or metabolism Older adults (over 50 years of age) Females who are pregnant or of childbearing age
Various B vitamins	People who abuse alcohol
Folic acid	Females of childbearing age (especially during pregnancy and breastfeeding)
Vitamin B-12	Older adults Strict vegans
Vitamin C	People who use tobacco
Vitamin D	People with limited dairy intake (due to allergies or lactose intolerance) People with limited exposure to sunlight (e.g., all infants, many African Americans, and some older adults) Strict vegans
Vitamin E	People who follow diets low in fat (especially plant oils)
Vitamin K	Newborns
Calcium	Strict vegans Older adults with bone loss
Fluoride	Some older infants and children (as directed by a dentist)
Iron	Females with excessive bleeding during menstruation Females who are pregnant Strict vegans
Zinc	Strict vegans

Source: https://ods.od.nih.gov/factsheets/MVMS-HealthProfessional/

Do specific vitamin or mineral supplements provide any benefit? Only a few studies of vitamin and mineral supplements demonstrate beneficial effects for the prevention of deficiencies or chronic diseases. For example, females who are postmenopausal may benefit from taking calcium and vitamin D supplements to increase bone mineral density and decrease fracture risk. According to the *Dietary Guidelines,* dietary supplements should not replace regular food intake unless instructed by a health professional. Table 8-5 outlines the population groups that are most likely to benefit from taking dietary supplements.

While there may be moderate benefits of consuming dietary supplements for specific subgroups, uninformed use of supplements can be risky. Indeed, most cases of nutrient toxicity are a result of supplement use. High doses of one nutrient can affect absorption or metabolism of other nutrients. For example, excessive zinc intake can inhibit copper absorption, and large amounts of folate can mask signs and symptoms of a vitamin B-12 deficiency. In addition, some supplements can interfere with medications. For instance, high intakes of vitamin K or vitamin E alter the action of anticlotting medications, vitamin B-6 can offset the action of L-dopa (used in treating Parkinson's disease), and large doses of vitamin C might interfere with certain cancer therapy regimens.

For most adults, finding ways to incorporate the recommended servings of fruits, vegetables, and whole grains into the

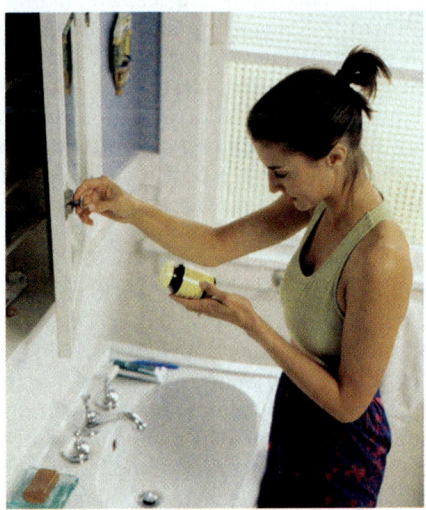

Believing that supplements provide the nutrition her body needs, Janice regularly takes numerous supplements while paying relatively little attention to daily food choices. **How would you explain to her that this practice may lead to health problems?** Ryan McVay/Photodisc/Getty Images

Newsworthy Nutrition

Increased emergency department visits for dietary supplement users

INTRODUCTION: Intake of dietary supplements, including herbs, vitamins, and mineral supplements, continues to increase in the United States, yet few studies have investigated the safety of these products. **OBJECTIVE:** The aim of this *cohort study* was to evaluate adverse events directly related to dietary supplement intake that resulted in emergency department visits. **METHODS:** Surveillance data were collected from 63 nationally representative emergency departments from 2004 to 2013. **RESULTS:** Over 23,000 emergency department visits per year were attributed to adverse events related to dietary supplement intake, resulting in 2154 hospitalizations annually. Of emergency department visits, 28% related to supplement use involving young adults (ages 20 to 34). After excluding dietary supplement intake by unsupervised children, 66% of supplement-related emergency department visits involved herbal or complementary nutritional products and 32% involved micronutrients. Herbals and complementary nutritional products for weight loss and enhanced energy were prevalent. These products resulted in complaints of heart palpitations, chest pain, or tachycardia. **CONCLUSION:** In light of the fact that the dietary supplement industry is not well regulated, supplement users must be extremely cautious and stay well informed of the potential health risks.

Source: Geller AI et al. Emergency department visits for adverse events related to dietary supplements. *N Engl J Med.* 2015 Oct 15;373(16): 1531-1540.

---

dietary pattern is the safest and healthiest way to ensure nutrient adequacy. Many of the health-promoting effects of foods cannot be found in a bottle. Few or no phytochemicals or fiber is present in most supplements. Multivitamin and mineral supplements also contain little calcium to keep the pill size small. Furthermore, the oxide forms of magnesium, zinc, and copper used in many supplements are not as well absorbed as forms found in foods. Overall, supplement use cannot fix an inadequate dietary pattern in all respects.

So, are vitamin-fortified foods healthier? A growing number of food and beverage manufacturers are adding vitamins, minerals, and even phytochemicals to foods and beverages to increase sales. Note that many of these items, such as cookies, candies, chips, and many snacks, are highly processed and energy dense. This marketing strategy seems to be working and has altered consumer purchasing behavior in favor of nutrient-fortified products. The fact is that added vitamins or minerals to highly processed foods does not compensate for empty calories, added sugars, and saturated fats in any product. Consumers should strive to obtain a dietary pattern rich in nutrients from whole nutritious foods, such as those provided in a plant-forward dietary pattern. Instead of vitamin water, grab your water bottle and an apple!

As illustrated in Figure 8-33, when it comes to improving nutrient intake, choose foods rich in vitamins and minerals before considering dietary supplements. First, you should assess your current dietary patterns. MyPlate is a tool consumers can use to plan a healthy dietary pattern. If nutrient gaps still remain, identify food sources that can help. For example, fortified, ready-to-eat breakfast cereals supply a variety of micronutrients, including vitamin E, folic acid, vitamin B-6, and highly absorbable forms of vitamin B-12. Other fortified foods, such as calcium-fortified orange juice, can also be helpful. Be aware of portion sizes of highly fortified foods, however, as multiple servings could lead to excessive intakes of some nutrients, such as vitamin A, iron, and synthetic folic acid. Last, if supplement use is desired, educate yourself and discuss it with your primary care provider or RDN.

Which Supplement Is Appropriate?

If, after consulting with your primary care provider or dietitian, you decide to take a multivitamin and mineral supplement, start by choosing a nationally recognized brand (from a supermarket or pharmacy) that contains about 100% of the Daily Values for the nutrients present. A multivitamin and mineral supplement should generally be taken with or just after meals to maximize absorption. Make sure also that intake from the total of this supplement, any other supplements used, and highly fortified foods (such as ready-to-eat breakfast cereals) provides no more than

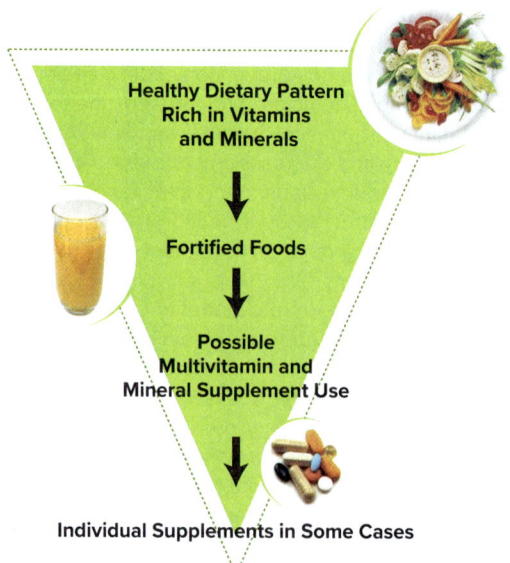

FIGURE 8-33 Supplement savvy—an approach to the use of nutrient supplements. Emphasizing a healthy dietary pattern rich in vitamins and minerals is always the first option. glass of orange juice: George Doyle/Stockbyte/Getty Images; plate of fresh vegetables: C Squared Studios/Photodisc/Getty Images; multi drugs: Don Wilkie/E+/Getty Images

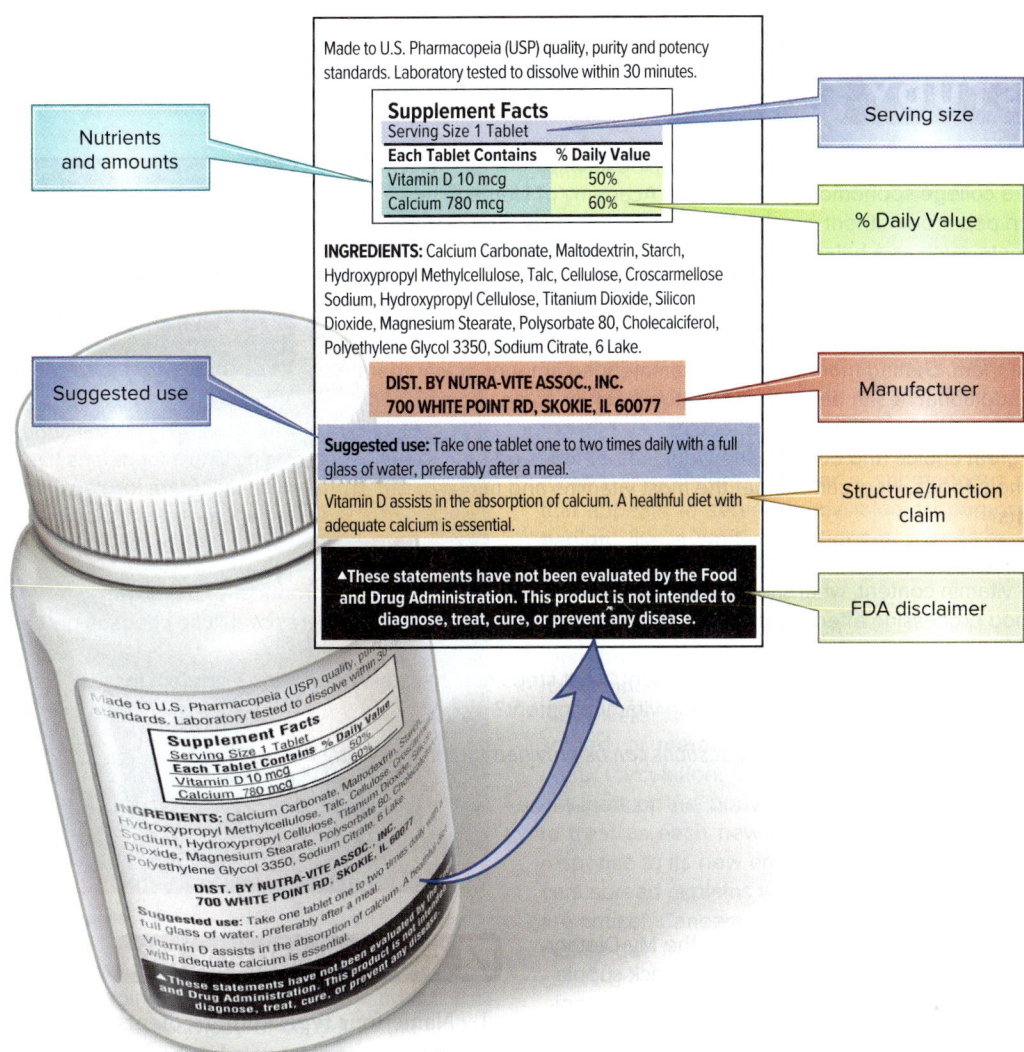

FIGURE 8-34 Nutrient supplements display a nutrition label different from that of foods. This Supplement Facts label must list the ingredient(s), amount(s) per serving, serving size, suggested use, and % Daily Value if one has been established. In addition, this label includes structure/function claims, which are not mandatory elements of the supplement label. When structure/function claims are made, however, the label also must include the FDA warning that these claims have not been evaluated by the agency.

the UL for each vitamin and mineral. This is especially important with regard to preformed vitamin A intake. Two exceptions are: (1) older adults should make sure any product used is low in iron or iron free to avoid possible iron overload; and (2) somewhat exceeding the Upper Level for vitamin D is likely a safe practice for adults. Read the labels carefully to be sure of what is being taken (Fig. 8-34).

Because research on a variety of nutrient supplements has revealed a lack of product quality, the FDA now requires supplement makers to test the identity, purity, strength, and composition of all their products. As an extra protection, select supplements that bear the logo of the U.S. Pharmacopeial Convention (USP). The USP is an independent, nonprofit group of scientists who review products for strength, quality, purity, packaging, labeling, speed of dissolution, and shelf-stability. The USP designation on a supplement label indicates that the product has been evaluated and meets professionally accepted standards of supplement quality. Other supplement testing organizations include NSF International, National Product Association (NPA), and ConsumerLab. Although these organizations do not guarantee that a product has therapeutic value, nor do they test each batch of supplements, their seals indicate that the product contains the amount of the active ingredient advertised on the label and is free from dangerous or toxic substances, such as bacteria, arsenic, or lead.

Another consideration in choosing a supplement is avoiding superfluous ingredients, such as added sugars, para-aminobenzoic acid (PABA), hesperidin complex, inositol, bee pollen, and lecithins. These are not needed in our dietary patterns. They are especially common in expensive supplements sold in health-food stores and online. In addition, use of l-tryptophan and high doses of beta-carotene or fish oils is discouraged. The National Institutes

Symptoms of Cancer

Many early cancer symptoms are overlooked and attributed to other potential problems (Fig. 8-36). If you have symptoms that do not get better after a few weeks, please see your primary care provider. Early diagnosis and treatment of cancer are critical. Note that cancer does not typically cause pain, so do not wait to feel pain before seeing a physician.

Routine screenings are important for early detection of cancer. The American Cancer Society publishes current cancer screening guidelines based upon expert recommendations and research. Families with genetic predispositions to cancer should consult their primary care provider to discuss enhanced and earlier surveillance.

Factors That Influence the Development of Cancer

Genetics, environment, and lifestyle are potent forces that influence the risk for developing cancer. Of cancers, 5% to 10% are thought to be inherited and 90% to 95% are related to environmental factors. Genetic predispositions to cancers are most prevalent in the colon, breast, and prostate cancers. Modifiable lifestyle and environmental exposures explain the huge variation in cancer rates from country to country. Excessive body fatness and dietary patterns account for over half of all environmentally related cancers.

Although we have little control over our genetic risk factors for cancer, we have tremendous influence over our lifestyle behaviors,

Symptoms of Cancer

Breast changes
- Lump or firm feeling in your breast or under your arm
- Nipple changes or discharge
- Skin that is itchy, red, scaly, dimpled, or puckered

Bladder changes
- Trouble urinating
- Pain when urinating
- Blood in the urine

Bleeding or bruising, for no known reason

Bowel changes
- Blood in the stools
- Changes in bowel habits

Cough or hoarseness that does not go away

Eating problems
- Pain after eating (heartburn or indigestion that doesn't go away)
- Trouble swallowing
- Belly pain
- Nausea and vomiting
- Appetite changes

Fatigue that is severe and lasts

Fever or night sweats for no known reason

Mouth changes
- A white or red patch on the tongue or in your mouth
- Bleeding, pain, or numbness in the lip or mouth

Neurological problems
- Headaches
- Seizures
- Vision changes
- Hearing changes
- Drooping of the face

Skin changes
- A flesh-colored lump that bleeds or turns scaly
- A new mole or a change in an existing mole
- A sore that does not heal
- Jaundice (yellowing of the skin and whites of the eyes)

Swelling or lumps anywhere such as in the neck, underarm, stomach, and groin

Weight gain or weight loss for no known reason

FIGURE 8-36 Early cancer symptoms.

Source: National Institutes of Health; National Cancer Institute. Symptoms of cancer. February 2019. Accessed November 7, 2021. https://www.cancer.gov/about-cancer/diagnosis-staging/symptoms

ASK THE RDN: Supplements and Immunity

Dear RDN: *There's much talk about the role of nutrition in supporting the immune system. Can I boost my immune system by taking supplements?*

Since 2020, there has been much buzz in the media about dietary supplements "boosting" the immune system; currently there is no evidence to support this statement. Unfortunately, social media influencers (often without any professional training) often push near-lethal doses of some vitamins, minerals, botanicals, herbs, and extracts. No supplements contain all the benefits provided by healthy foods, so supplements should not be used as substitutes for a healthy dietary pattern. Recall that megadose supplements (many times the RDA) can be harmful and are discouraged. In this chapter, you learned how the vitamins, minerals, phytochemicals, and probiotics in whole foods can help support your immune system over time. In addition to consuming nutritious dietary patterns, you should strive to obtain adequate sleep and engage in regular physical activity.

Recall in Chapter 3, you learned the human microbiome is comprised of organisms that impact human physiology and contribute to either the enhancement or impairment of metabolic and immune functions. Alterations in the intestinal microbial community play a major role in the immune system, thus resulting in enhancing human health or promoting disease. To help support our immune system, we should strive to include food sources rich in pre- and probiotics.

To your health,

Colleen Spees, PhD, MEd, RD, FAND, FAHA
Associate Professor, The Ohio State University College of Medicine, Author of *Wardlaw's Contemporary Nutrition* and *Wardlaw's Contemporary Nutrition: A Functional Approach*

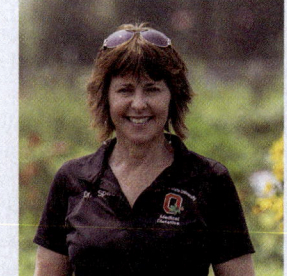
Wendy Pramik/The Ohio State University

especially with regard to smoking, alcohol intake, physical activity, UV exposure, and dietary patterns. Indeed, over one-third of all cancers are due to use of tobacco products. About half of the cancers of the mouth, pharynx, and larynx are associated with heavy use of alcohol. The combined use of both alcohol and tobacco products increases cancer risks higher than either alone.

BODY FATNESS LINKED TO CANCER RISK

An estimated one of every three cancer deaths in the United States is linked to excess body fat, suboptimal nutrition, and inadequate physical activity. Of these, excess body fat appears to have the greatest impact on cancer risk. This includes a greater risk for at least 13 different types of cancer.[60]

There are several ways excess body fat can influence cancer risk. Excess body fat stimulates secretion of hormones (insulin from the pancreas and estrogen from adipose cells) and other proteins that promote systemic inflammation and oxidative stress, which contribute to carcinogenesis.

A strong link exists between cancer risk and excess calories in the dietary pattern. In animal experiments, restricting total calorie intake to about 70% of usual intake results in significant reduction in tumor development, regardless of the macronutrient composition of the dietary pattern. Currently, calorie restriction appears to be an effective technique for preventing cancer in laboratory animals. While the data obtained from animal studies are interesting, understand that severe calorie restrictions are not feasible and sustainable for most individuals. In addition, once cancer is present, calorie restriction may no longer be helpful.

It is worth noting that there remains much confusion about the role of sugar in "feeding cancer." Although cancer cells consume more glucose than noncancerous cells, no research has proven that eating sugar will make your cancer more aggressive or grow faster. However, a high-sugar dietary pattern, over time, contributes to weight gain. Recall that obesity is strongly associated with an increased risk of developing several types of cancer.[61]

CANCER-FIGHTING FOODS

Research shows that foods of plant origin protect against a range of cancers. This could be due to a variety of nutrients, phytochemicals, and other plant compounds. Besides containing key vitamins and minerals, which strengthen our immune system, fruits, vegetables, nuts, and seeds are good sources of biologically active phytochemicals. Foods containing fiber are also linked to a reduced risk of cancer. Fiber is thought to speed up *gut transit time*, or the length of time it takes food to move through the digestive system.

Although no single food or food component can fully protect you against cancer, evidence clearly shows that dietary patterns that are rich in a variety of plant foods help to reduce the risk for many cancers. MyPlate is aimed at disease prevention. It is likely that consumption of a wide variety of plant-based foods and adequate physical activity result in a dose effect that, together, is more potent and protective than either in isolation.

Evidence-Based Recommendations for Cancer Prevention

Given the devastating toll of cancer treatment and lack of a definitive cure, efforts at prevention are of prime importance. Several health organizations have issued their own sets of dietary and lifestyle guidelines for cancer prevention and survivorship. Here, we present the most recent recommendations of the American Cancer Society, which are consistent with the recommendations of other cancer organizations.[62]

AMERICAN CANCER SOCIETY GUIDELINE FOR DIET AND PHYSICAL ACTIVITY FOR CANCER PREVENTION

1. Achieve and maintain a healthy body weight throughout life.
   - Keep body weight within the healthy range and avoid weight gain in adult life.
2. Be physically active.
   - Adults should engage in 150–300 min of moderate-intensity physical activity per week, or 75–150 min of vigorous-intensity physical activity, or an equivalent combination; achieving or exceeding the upper limit of 300 min is optimal.
   - Limit sedentary behavior, such as sitting, lying down, and watching television, and other forms of screen-based entertainment.
3. Follow a healthy eating pattern at all ages.
   - A healthy eating pattern includes:
     - Foods that are high in nutrients in amounts that help achieve and maintain a healthy body weight;
     - A variety of vegetables—dark green, red, and orange, fiber-rich legumes (beans and peas), and others;
     - Fruits, especially whole fruits with a variety of colors; and
     - Whole grains.
   - A healthy eating pattern limits or does not include:
     - Red and processed meats;
     - Sugar-sweetened beverages; or
     - Highly processed foods and refined grain products.
4. It is best not to drink alcohol.
   - People who do choose to drink alcohol should limit their consumption to no more than one drink per day for adult females and two drinks per day for adult males.

   Recommendation for Community Action
   - Public, private, and community organizations should work collaboratively at national, state, and local levels to develop, advocate for, and implement policy and environmental changes that increase access to affordable, nutritious foods; provide safe, enjoyable, and accessible opportunities for physical activity; and limit alcohol for all individuals.

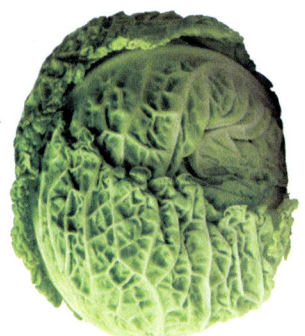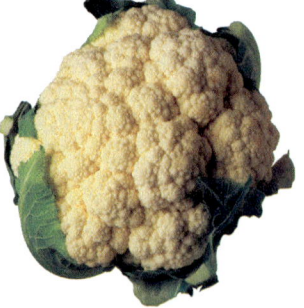

A dietary pattern that includes cruciferous vegetables, such as cabbage and cauliflower, is related to lower risk of developing cancer. **What components of these foods may support your body's defense against cancer?** C Squared Studios/Photodisc/Getty Images

Nutrition Concerns During Active Cancer Treatment

Eating and lifestyle changes can exert a powerful influence on the risk for developing cancer, but it is important to note that they are no substitute for preventive screening and appropriate medical care. Once cancer has developed, dietary and lifestyle changes will not be adequate to prevent cancer growth or metastasis. Nutrition concerns during active cancer treatment (chemotherapy, immunotherapy, radiation, surgery) vary depending on the site and stage of the cancer, but the overall goals of nutrition therapy are to minimize weight fluctuations and prevent nutrient deficiencies.

Weight loss, particularly loss of muscle mass, is a major concern during cancer treatment because malnutrition can interrupt treatment regimens and impede recovery. Common effects of cancer and/or cancer treatments include fatigue, mouth sores, dry mouth, taste abnormalities, nausea, and diarrhea—all of which can lead to inadequate food intake.

During active treatment, the most appropriate food choices are those that the patient with cancer craves and can tolerate. Although food choices vary widely based on each patient's individual symptoms, cool, nonacidic liquids and soft, mildly flavored foods are generally well accepted. Small, frequent meals and foods with high nutrient and calorie density should be emphasized to meet calorie and protein needs. Often, liquid nutritional supplements are warranted during this time. Because many patients with cancer are immunocompromised as a result of their treatment, safe food handling practices are extremely important. Individuals in active cancer treatment should seek the advice of an experienced RDN.

> To learn more about cancer, review these sources of credible cancer information on the Internet:
> American Cancer Society: www.cancer.org
> American Institute for Cancer Research: www.aicr.org
> National Cancer Institute: www.cancer.gov

✓ CONCEPT CHECK 8.19

1. List four symptoms of cancer.
2. Describe the top two modifiable risk factors associated with cancer risk.
3. What are the dietary and physical activity recommendations for cancer prevention?

CASE STUDY: Choosing Cancer Prevention Dietary and Physical Activity Patterns

Jaden is a 35-year-old nontraditional student who works the late shift at a popular bar and attends full-time classes during the day. Lately, Jaden has been unable to exercise as much as he would like, his consumption of highly processed convenience foods has increased, and he's experienced bouts of chronic constipation. Last week in his nutrition class, the instructor presented data on cancer risk and shared that trends in the onset of colorectal cancer have increased in those younger than age 50 and these individuals often present with more advanced disease. The instructor also shared some early signs and symptoms of colorectal cancer such as changes in bowel habits, rectal bleeding or blood in the stool, abdominal discomfort, weakness or fatigue, and unexplained weight loss. This class was a wake-up call for Jaden, and he committed to change his behaviors immediately to reduce his risk of cancer and other nutrition-related chronic diseases.

Answer the following questions related to Jaden's dietary and physical activity patterns.

1. What are the current cancer prevention physical activity recommendations?
2. How could Jaden increase his physical activity given his tight schedule?
3. What might be contributing to Jaden's chronic constipation?
4. What could Jaden do to improve his bowel habits?
5. List three changes Jaden could immediately implement to improve his adherence to the cancer prevention dietary recommendations.

Complete the Case Study. Responses to these questions can be provided by your instructor.

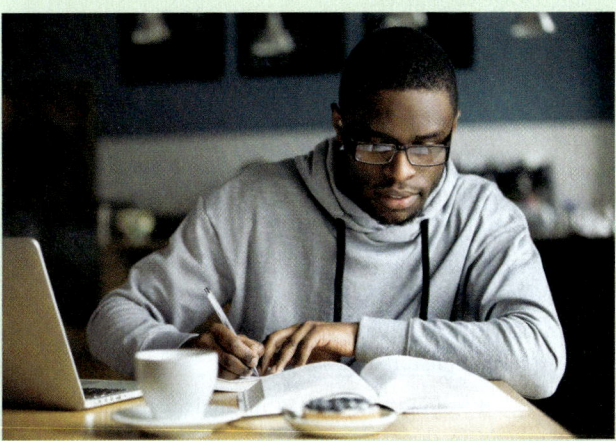

Jaden is concerned about the growing prevalence of colorectal cancer in younger adults. He is focused on improving his adherence to the evidence-based guidelines to reduce his personal risk. fizkes/Shutterstock

Summary (Numbers refer to numbered sections in the chapter)

8.1 Vitamins are organic substances required in small amounts in the dietary pattern for growth, function, and body maintenance. These can be categorized as fat soluble (vitamins A, D, E, and K) or water soluble (B vitamins and vitamin C). Vitamins cannot be synthesized by the body in adequate amounts to support health, and absence of a vitamin from the diet leads to the development of a deficiency disease. Fat-soluble vitamins require dietary fat for absorption and are carried by lipoproteins in the blood. Vitamin toxicity is most likely to occur from megadoses of fat-soluble vitamins because they are readily stored in the body. Intakes of water-soluble vitamins that exceed the storage ability of tissues are typically excreted in urine. Some vitamins are susceptible to destruction by light, heat, air, or alkalinity, or may be lost from foods in cooking water or fats.

8.2 Functional foods, such as oatmeal, provide health benefits beyond basic nutrition and often contain large amounts of plant-derived compounds known as phytochemicals. These nonessential compounds are what provides plants with their unique color, odor, and flavor. Rich sources of phytochemicals include fruits, vegetables, whole grains, beans, peas, lentils, herbs, spices, nuts, and seeds. Human consumption of phytochemicals are linked to numerous protective health benefits.

8.3 Vitamin A maintains the health of epithelial tissues and is also vitally important for normal vision. Vitamin A is found in its active forms in meats, fortified dairy products, fish, and eggs, and it can be derived from carotenoids in a variety of fruits and vegetables. Carotenoids are phytochemicals that can be converted into vitamin A in the body. Although carotenoids are not essential nutrients, some have health-promoting qualities for humans. In addition to their contribution to vitamin A intake, carotenoids are powerful antioxidants. The antioxidant abilities of several carotenoids are linked to prevention of macular degeneration, cataracts, cardiovascular disease, and cancer. Carotenoids are plentiful in dark-green and orange vegetables.

8.4 Vitamin D is both a hormone and a vitamin. Human skin synthesizes it using sunshine and a cholesterol-like substance. If we do not spend enough time in the sun, foods such as fish and fortified milk can supply the vitamin. The active hormone form of vitamin D helps regulate blood calcium in part by increasing calcium absorption from the intestine. Infants and children who do not get enough vitamin D may develop rickets, and adults with inadequate amounts in the body develop osteomalacia. Older people and infants often need a supplemental source. Toxicity may lead to calcification of soft tissue, weakness, and gastrointestinal disturbances.

8.5 Vitamin E functions primarily as an antioxidant and is found in plant oils. By donating electrons to electron-seeking, free-radical (oxidizing) compounds, it neutralizes them. This effect shields cell membranes and red blood cells from breakdown. Claims are made about the curative powers of vitamin E, but more information is needed before megadose vitamin E recommendations for healthy adults can be made with certainty.

8.6 Vitamin K is essential for blood clotting and imparts calcium-binding ability to various proteins, including those in bone. Some vitamin K absorbed each day comes from bacterial synthesis in the intestine, but most comes from foods, primarily green, leafy vegetables.

8.7 The B vitamins yield no energy directly, but they contribute to energy-yielding chemical reactions in the body by virtue of their coenzyme functions. B vitamins are highly bioavailable. North American diets are typically adequate in B vitamins except in cases of food insecurity, metabolic disorders, or alcoholism. Whole grains are more nutrient-dense sources of B vitamins (as well as other nutrients) than refined grains. Several B vitamins function as coenzymes in energy metabolism.

8.8 Thiamin's coenzyme form is involved in the metabolism of carbohydrates and proteins as well as the synthesis of RNA, DNA, and neurotransmitters. Rich food sources of thiamin include pork, enriched or fortified grain products, and milk. Beriberi, the thiamin-deficiency disease, leads to muscle weakness and nerve damage. Thiamin toxicity is unknown, and no UL has been set.

8.9 The coenzymes of riboflavin participate in the catabolism of fatty acids, metabolism of other vitamins and minerals, and antioxidant activity of glutathione peroxidase. Dairy products, enriched and fortified grain products, meat, and eggs are rich food sources of riboflavin. Symptoms of ariboflavinosis include glossitis and angular cheilitis. There is no evidence of toxicity with high doses of riboflavin; no UL has been set.

8.10 Niacin's coenzymes function in many synthetic reactions, especially fatty-acid synthesis. Rich food sources include seafood, poultry, meats, peanuts, and enriched or fortified grains. Pellagra, the disease of niacin deficiency, results in dermatitis, diarrhea, dementia, and, eventually, death. Megadoses of niacin may damage the liver and increase the risk for diabetes. Therefore, megadoses of niacin are not recommended.

8.11 Pantothenic acid functions as a coenzyme in reactions that yield energy from carbohydrates, lipids, and protein, as well as fatty-acid synthesis. It is widely distributed among foods, with sunflower seeds, mushrooms, peanuts, and eggs among the richest sources. A deficiency of pantothenic acid is unlikely, but symptoms would be similar to those seen with deficiencies of other B vitamins. There is no known toxicity and no UL for pantothenic acid.

8.12 Vitamin B-6 coenzymes activate many enzymes of carbohydrate, lipid, and, especially, protein metabolism. They also help synthesize neurotransmitters and participate in homocysteine metabolism. Rich food sources include animal products and enriched or fortified grain products, as well as some fruits and vegetables. A deficiency of vitamin B-6 leads to headaches, depression, gastrointestinal symptoms, skin disorders, nerve problems, anemia, and impaired immunity. Vitamin B-6 toxicity can result in nerve damage.

8.13 Biotin's coenzyme form aids in reactions that synthesize glucose and fatty acids and in the metabolism of amino acids. Egg yolks, peanuts, and cheese provide dietary biotin, but this vitamin is also synthesized by bacteria in the intestines. Consuming raw egg whites may lead to a biotin deficiency because avidin in egg whites binds biotin and reduces its bioavailability. Biotin deficiency can lead to inflammation of the skin and mouth, gastrointestinal symptoms, muscle pain and weakness, poor growth, and anemia. No UL has been set for biotin as no toxicity has ever been observed.

8.14 Folate plays an important role in DNA synthesis and homocysteine metabolism. Symptoms of a deficiency include generally poor cell division in various areas of the body, macrocytic anemia, tongue inflammation, diarrhea, and poor growth. Pregnancy puts high demands for folate on the body; deficiency during the first month of pregnancy can result in neural tube defects in offspring. A deficiency can also occur in people with alcoholism. Food sources are leafy vegetables, organ meats, and orange juice.

8.15 Vitamin B-12 is needed to metabolize folate and homocysteine, and to maintain the insulation surrounding nerves. Absorption of vitamin B-12 is a complex process that requires a salivary protein, adequate stomach acid production, and an intrinsic factor produced by the stomach. A deficiency, which results in anemia and nerve degeneration, most likely results from poor absorption of vitamin B-12 rather than poor dietary intake. Pernicious anemia is one condition that can impair vitamin B-12 absorption. Vitamin B-12 is found in foods of animal origin, fortified foods, and supplements.

8.16 Vitamin C is a potent antioxidant and also promotes the production of white blood cells to support immune function. In addition, vitamin C takes part in the synthesis of collagen, carnitine, and neurotransmitters, and it can modestly enhance iron absorption. A vitamin C deficiency results in scurvy, evidenced by pinpoint hemorrhages in the skin, bleeding gums, and joint pain. Smoking increases the possibility of vitamin C deficiency. Fresh fruits and vegetables, especially citrus fruits, are good sources. Vitamin C also modestly enhances iron absorption. A great amount of vitamin C is lost in storage and cooking. Deficiencies can occur in people with alcoholism and those whose diets lack sufficient fruits and vegetables.

8.17 Choline is an essential nutrient but is not classified as a vitamin. As a component of phospholipids, it is important for cell membrane structure, myelination of nerves, and lipid transport. Like folate, choline plays a role in single-carbon metabolism, which has implications for prevention of birth defects, cancer, and heart disease. Egg yolks, meats, dairy products, soybeans, and nuts are good food sources of choline.

8.18 To meet nutrient needs and prevent chronic disease, whole foods should be emphasized, but occasionally, dietary supplements may be necessary. For example, females of childbearing age, older adults, vegans, and people with malabsorptive diseases are most likely to benefit from dietary supplements. Consumers should educate themselves about possible benefits and risks and discuss concerns with their primary care provider.

The Dietary Supplement Health and Education Act of 1994 (DSHEA) is a federal statute that defines and regulates dietary supplements in the U.S.

8.19 Given the toll of cancer treatment and lack of a definitive cure, efforts at prevention are key. A variety of dietary changes will reduce your risk for cancer. Start by making sure that your dietary pattern is moderate in calories, added sugars, red and processed meats, alcohol, and highly processed foods. Increase consumption of a variety of colorful whole fruits and vegetables, and whole grains. In addition, keep a healthy body weight and be physically active.

Check Your Knowledge (Answers are available at the end of this question set)

1. Vitamins are classified as
   a. organic and inorganic.
   b. fat soluble and water soluble.
   c. essential and nonessential.
   d. elements and compounds.

2. A vitamin synthesized by bacteria in the intestine is
   a. A.
   b. D.
   c. E.
   d. K.

3. A deficiency of vitamin A can lead to the disease called
   a. xerophthalmia.
   b. osteomalacia.
   c. scurvy.
   d. pellagra.

4. Vitamin D is called the sunshine vitamin because
   a. it is available in orange juice.
   b. exposure to sunlight converts a precursor into vitamin D.
   c. it can be destroyed by exposure to sunlight.
   d. it is an ingredient in sunscreen.

5. Vitamin E functions as
   a. a coenzyme.
   b. a hormone.
   c. an antioxidant.
   d. a peroxide.

6. Bowed legs, an enlarged and misshapen head, and enlarged knee joints in children are all symptoms of
   a. rickets.
   b. xerophthalmia.
   c. osteoporosis.
   d. vitamin D toxicity.

7. A deficient intake of _____ has been shown to increase the risk of having a baby with a neural tube defect such as spina bifida.
   a. vitamin A
   b. vitamin C
   c. vitamin E
   d. folate

8. Vitamin C is necessary for the production of
   a. stomach acid.
   b. collagen.
   c. insulin.
   d. clotting factors.

9. B vitamins, including thiamin, riboflavin, and niacin, are called the *energy vitamins* because they
   a. can be broken down to provide energy.
   b. are ingredients in energy drinks such as Powerade.
   c. are part of coenzymes needed for release of energy from carbohydrates, fats, and proteins.
   d. are needed in large amounts by competitive athletes.

10. Noodles, spaghetti, and bread are made from wheat flour that is enriched with all of the following nutrients except
    a. vitamin B-6.
    b. thiamin.
    c. niacin.
    d. riboflavin.

11. Which of the B vitamins is sensitive to and can be degraded by light?
    a. Riboflavin
    b. Niacin
    c. Thiamin
    d. Pantothenic acid

12. Niacin can be synthesized in the body from the amino acid
    a. tyrosine.
    b. tryptophan.
    c. phenylalanine.
    d. glutamine.

13. Avidin, a component of raw egg whites, may decrease the absorption of
    a. biotin.
    b. thiamin.
    c. iron.
    d. riboflavin.

meta-analysis of prospective cohort studies. *Crit Rev Food Sci Nutr.* 2019;59(16):2697-2707. doi: 10.1080/10408398.2018.1511967

41. Peker E, Demir N, Tuncer O, et al. The levels of vitamin B12, folate and homocysteine in mothers and their babies with neural tube defects. *J Matern Fetal Neonatal Med.* 2016 Sep;29(18):2944-2948. doi: 10.3109/14767058.2015.1109620

42. Crider KS, Bailey LB, Berry RJ. Folic acid food fortification—its history, effect, concerns, and future directions. *Nutrients.* 2011 Mar;3(3):370-384. doi: 10.3390/nu3030370

43. Debreceni B, Debreceni L. The role of homocysteine-lowering B-vitamins in the primary prevention of cardiovascular disease. *Cardiovasc Ther.* 2014 Jun;32(3):130-138. doi: 10.1111/1755-5922.12064

44. Kim YI. Folate and cancer: a tale of Dr. Jekyll and Mr. Hyde? *Am J Clin Nutr.* 2018 Feb 1;107(2):139-142. doi: 10.1093/ajcn/nqx076

45. Vitamin B12 fact sheet for health professionals. National Institutes of Health, Office of Dietary Supplements. Updated Nov 12, 2023. Available at https://ods.od.nih.gov/factsheets/vitaminb12-Health Professional/l/. Accessed Nov 12, 2023.

46. Gwathmey KG, Grogan J. Nutritional neuropathies. *Muscle Nerve.* 2020 Jul;62(1):13-29. doi: 10.1002/mus.26783

47. Palmer S. Vitamin B12 and the vegan diet. *Today's Dietitian.* 2018 Apr;20(4):38.

48. Vitamin C fact sheet for health professionals. National Institutes of Health, Office of Dietary Supplements. Updated Nov 12, 2023. Available at https://ods.od.nih.gov/factsheets/vitaminc-HealthProfessional/l/. Accessed Nov 12, 2023.

49. Choline fact sheet for health professionals. National Institutes of Health, Office of Dietary Supplements. Updated Nov 12, 2023. Available at https://ods.od.nih.gov/factsheets/choline-HealthProfessional/l/. Accessed Nov 12, 2023.

50. Choline. Linus Pauling Institute, Oregon State University, Micronutrient Information Center. Updated January 2015. Accessed Nov 4, 2023. https://lpi.oregonstate.edu/mic/other-nutrients/choline#neural-tube-defects-prevention

51. Velazquez R, Winslow W, Mifflin MA. Choline as a prevention for Alzheimer's disease. *Aging* (Albany NY). 2020 Feb 9;12(3):2026-2027. doi: 10.18632/aging.102849

52. Meyer KA, Shea JW. Dietary choline and betaine and risk of CVD: a systematic review and meta-analysis of prospective studies. *Nutrients.* 2017 Jul 7;9(7):711. doi: 10.3390/nu9070711

53. Wallace TC, Fulgoni VL. Usual choline intakes are associated with egg and protein food consumption in the United States. *Nutrients.* 2017 Aug 5;9(8):839. doi: 10.3390/nu9080839

54. Zeisel SH, Klatt KC, Caudill MA. Choline. *Adv Nutr.* 2018 Jan 1;9(1):58-60. doi: 10.1093/advances/nmx004

55. Wallace TC, Blusztajn JK, Caudill MA, Klatt KC, Zeisel SH. Choline: the neurocognitive essential nutrient of interest to obstetricians and gynecologists. *J Diet Suppl.* 2020;17(6):733-752. doi: 10.1080/19390211.2019.1639875

56. Dietary supplement fact sheet for health professionals. National Institutes of Health, Office of Dietary Supplements. Updated Nov 12, 2023. Available at https://ods.od.nih.gov/factsheets/list-all/. Accessed Nov 12, 2023.

57. American Cancer Society, Cancer Statistics Center. Accessed November 7, 2021. https://cancerstatisticscenter.cancer.org/#!/

58. Cancer trends progress report. National Institutes of Health, National Cancer Institute. Updated July 2021. Accessed November 7, 2021. https://progressreport.cancer.gov/after/economic_burden

59. An update on cancer deaths in the United States. Centers for Disease Control & Prevention. Updated February 23, 2021. Accessed November 7, 2021. https://www.cdc.gov/cancer/dcpc/research/update-on-cancer-deaths/index.htm

60. Does body weight affect cancer risk? American Cancer Society. Updated June 9, 2020. Accessed November 7, 2023. https://www.cancer.org/cancer/cancer-causes/diet-physical-activity/body-weight-and-cancer-risk/effects.html

61. Common cancer myths and misconceptions. National Institutes of Health, National Cancer Institute. Updated August 22, 2018. Accessed November 7, 2023. https://www.cancer.gov/about-cancer/causes-prevention/risk/myths

62. Rock CL, Thomson C, Gansler T, et al. American Cancer Society guideline for diet and physical activity for cancer prevention. *CA A Cancer J Clin.* 2020:70;245-271. https://doi.org/10.3322/caac.21591

Design Element Credits: Fact Check/magnifying glass icon: McGraw Hill; Magnificent Microbiome background image: Alena Ohneva/Shutterstock; Sustainable Solutions icon: McGraw Hill; Roots icon: McGraw Hill; Medicine Cabinet icon: Peter Dazeley/Photographer's Choice/Getty Images

Chapter 9: Water and Minerals

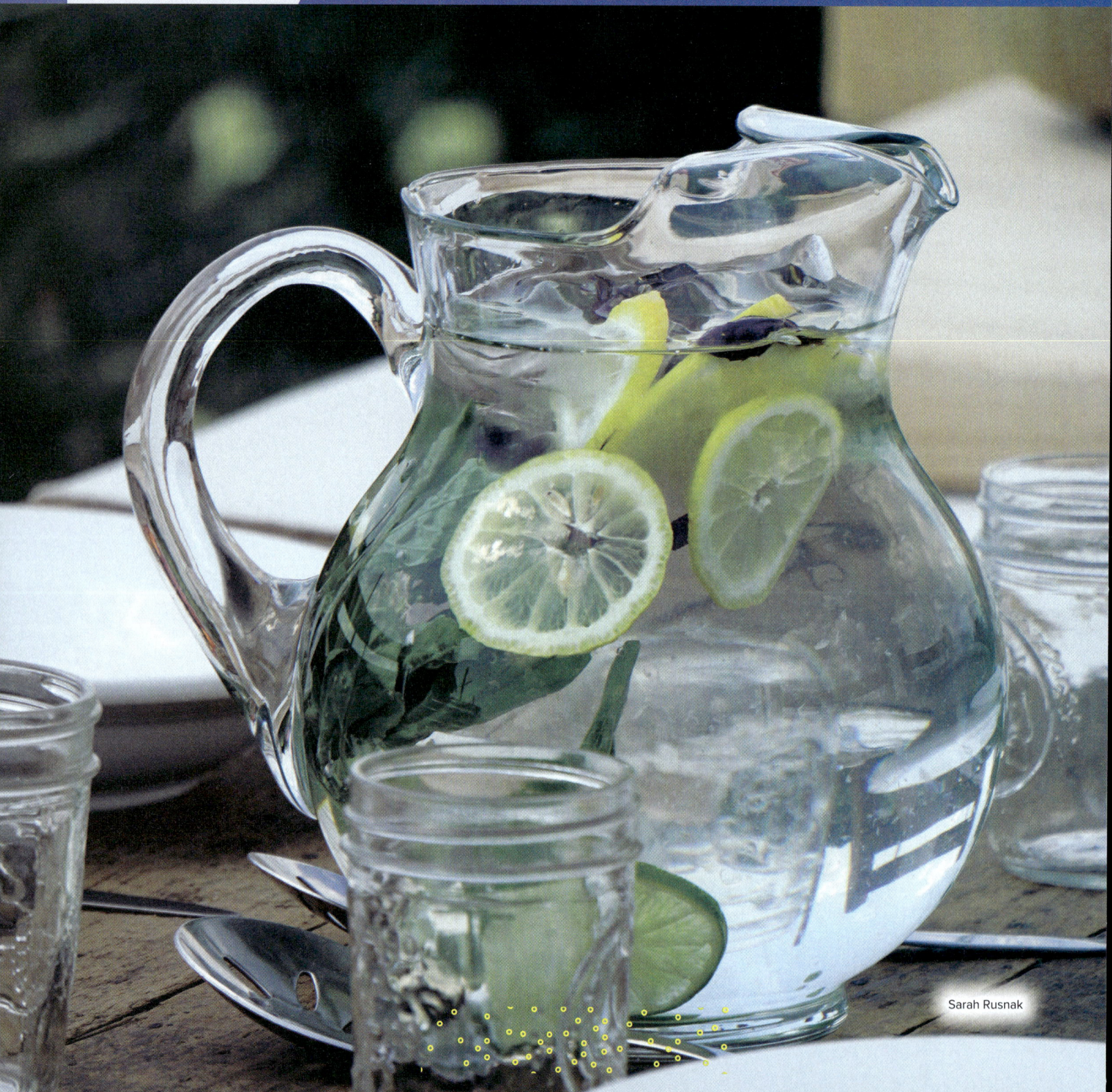

Sarah Rusnak

Student Learning Outcomes

Chapter 9 is designed to allow you to:

9.1 Understand the functions of water in the body, the regulation of fluid balance, and the health consequences of fluid imbalance, as well as list recommended intakes and sources of water.

9.2 Describe the general characteristics of the major and trace minerals, their absorption and storage, the dangers of mineral toxicities, and ways to preserve minerals in foods.

9.3 Describe the roles of sodium, potassium, and chloride in controlling fluid balance, acid–base balance, and nerve impulse transmission.

9.4 Describe the role of calcium, phosphorus, magnesium, and fluoride in body functions including bone health.

9.5 Describe the functions of the trace minerals including the role of iron in blood health, zinc in immune function, iodine in thyroid metabolism, and chromium in glucose metabolism.

9.6 List some of the best dietary sources for each major and trace mineral.

9.7 List the dietary requirements for each major and trace mineral, as well as the dangers of exceeding these recommendations.

9.8 Describe the signs and symptoms of mineral deficiency and conditions that lead to a deficiency.

9.9 Describe factors that can contribute to the development of hypertension and strategies to lower blood pressure.

9.10 Outline dietary and other lifestyle strategies to prevent osteoporosis.

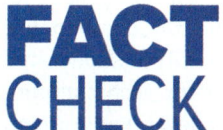

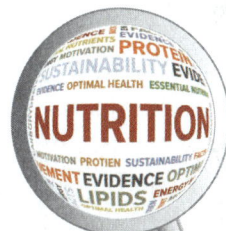

Can red meat be part of a healthy eating pattern?

Red meat refers to beef, pork, lamb, veal, goat, and game (e.g., venison). There are a few reasons you may want to limit your intake of red meats. First, red meat is a source of saturated fat. High intakes of saturated fat tend to increase blood levels of LDL cholesterol, which can increase your risk for cardiovascular disease. Second, high intakes of red meat are associated with an increased risk for several types of cancer. On the other hand, red meat is a good source of high-quality protein, vitamin B-6, vitamin B-12, iron, and zinc. While it is not necessary to eliminate red meat from your eating pattern, the American Institute for Cancer Research recommends limiting your intake of red meat to two to three servings per week. Choosing lower-fat cuts of meat (e.g., loin or round), trimming the fat from meat before cooking, and preparing meats with low-heat, slow-cooking methods can help you meet your dietary requirements for iron, zinc, and other nutrients without increasing your risk for chronic diseases. See Sections 9.9 and 9.10 to learn more about the roles of iron and zinc in human health.

Source: What's the beef with red meat? Harvard Health Publishing. Published February 1, 2020. Accessed November 12, 2023. https://www.health.harvard.edu/staying-healthy/whats-the-beef-with-red-meat

FIGURE 9-1 Where's the water? Although the percentages vary for males and females, the main constituent of the body is water. The percentage of water varies tremendously among tissues. For example, muscle is 73% water, adipose tissue is 10% to 20% water, and bone contains approximately 20% water. As the fat content of the body increases, the percentage of lean muscle decreases, and subsequently the percentage of body water decreases. When body composition measurements are performed on extremely lean athletes, the percentage of body water can be around 70%. Shutterstock

Healthy Male (170 pounds)	Healthy Female (130 pounds)
1 pound of glycogen (< 1%)	1 pound of glycogen (< 1%)
10 pounds of minerals (6%)	7 pounds of minerals (5%)
27 pounds of protein (16%)	17 pounds of protein (13%)
27 pounds of fat (16%)	32 pounds of fat (25%)
105 pounds of water (62%)	74 pounds of water (57%)

9.1 Water

Every cell, tissue, and organ contains some water. Overall, water makes up 50% to 70% of the human body (Fig. 9-1). Indeed, water is essential for life. Whereas humans can live for several weeks without food, we can survive for only a few days without water.

WATER BALANCE

Water is continuously lost from the body via several routes. To maintain proper function, fluid intake must balance fluid losses. Figure 9-2 illustrates the components of water intake and water output. The volumes of water intake and output shown in Figure 9-2 are estimates for an adult female. The volumes of water for each component may vary based on body size and composition, physical activity level, environmental conditions (e.g., ambient temperature and humidity), and dietary factors (e.g., intake of **diuretics,** such as caffeine and alcohol).

Water Intake. Body water comes from three sources: beverages, foods, and **metabolic water.**

Fluid intake in the form of beverages—including plain water, juice, coffee, tea, soft drinks, milk, and even alcoholic beverages—makes the biggest contribution to our total water needs. For the female in Figure 9-2, fluid intake adds up to about 9 cups per day.

Some water (about 2 cups per day) comes from foods. Many fruits and vegetables are more than 80% water—think of how refreshing a cool slice of watermelon is on a hot summer day! Meats contain at least 50% water. Even foods that seem very dry (e.g., grains) supply a small amount of water. The only foods that are practically devoid of water are fats and oils.

In addition, the body produces a variable amount of metabolic water each day as a by-product of the chemical reactions used to break down energy-yielding nutrients. For the individual shown in Figure 9-2, metabolic water amounts to 1.25 cups; however, the amount of metabolic water produced can double in physically active people.

Water Output. There are four routes by which water is lost from the body: urine, perspiration, respiration, and feces.

Urinary excretion of water accounts for the majority of water output. Over a 24-hour period, your kidneys filter approximately 600 cups of blood as your entire blood supply flows through your urinary system many times each day. Your kidneys can reabsorb as

diuretic A substance that increases urinary fluid excretion.

metabolic water Water formed as a by-product of carbohydrate, lipid, and protein metabolism.

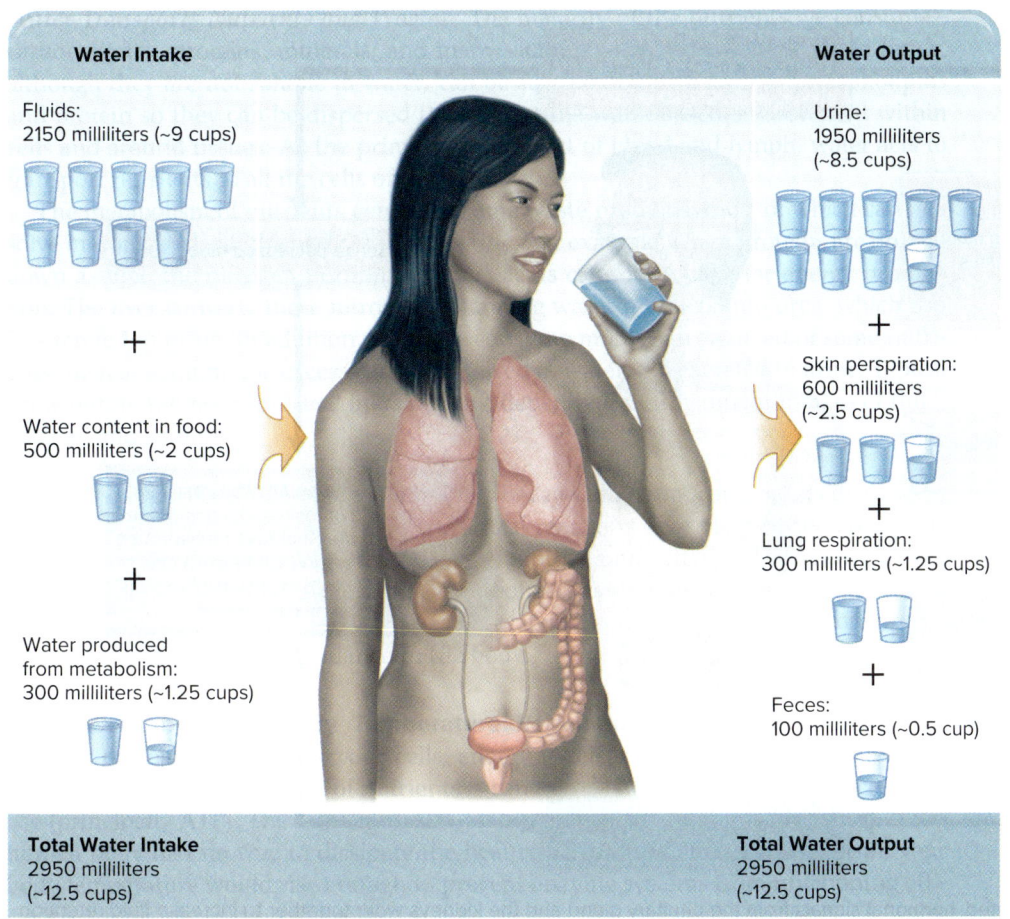

FIGURE 9-2 Estimate of water balance—intake versus output—in an adult female. We primarily maintain body fluids at an optimum amount by adjusting water intake to output. As you can see for this individual, most water comes from the liquids we consume. Some comes from the moisture in foods, and the remainder is manufactured during metabolism. Water output refers to water that is lost via urine, skin, lungs, and feces.

much as 99% of the water filtered each day. Average urinary water loss per day is approximately 1950 milliliters (about 8.5 cups), but it may vary based on intake of fluids, protein, and sodium (as intakes of protein or sodium increase, production of urine increases to rid the body of extra wastes). Because it can be measured, water lost via urine is also referred to as *sensible* water loss. At minimum, the removal of waste products requires at least 500 milliliters (2 cups) of urine production per day. Urine output consistently below this level is often a sign of chronic **dehydration** due to low fluid intake.

In addition to the sensible water lost via urine, the body loses water in ways that are not as noticeable and cannot be easily measured. Collectively, these routes of water loss are called *insensible* water losses. Some water is lost through the skin in the form of perspiration. On days of low physical activity, these losses amount to less than 1 liter. Under hot, humid conditions or with strenuous physical activity, losses can be much greater. Some water is also lost from the lungs in the form of water vapor in exhaled air. Last, a relatively small amount of water is lost daily in the feces. When we consider the large amount of water used to lubricate the digestive tract, the loss of only 100 milliliters (~0.5 cup) of water each day through the feces is remarkable. In addition to the variable amount of water ingested in the form of foods and fluids, about 8000 milliliters (~34 cups) of water enters the digestive tract daily through secretions from the mouth, stomach, intestine, pancreas, and other organs. The small intestine absorbs most of this water, while the colon takes up a lesser but important amount.

dehydration A harmful condition in which water intake is inadequate to replace losses.

Fluid Conservation. Despite its critical importance for human survival, water is not stored in your body. It is continually lost through respiration (lungs), perspiration (skin), and excretion (urine and feces). Through mechanisms that monitor blood pressure and the concentration of solutes in body fluids, your nervous, endocrine, digestive, and urinary systems work together elegantly to maintain fluid balance and support life.

FIGURE 9-4 As perspiration evaporates from the surface of the skin, heat is released into the environment. This cools the blood, which circulates back to the body, reducing body temperature.

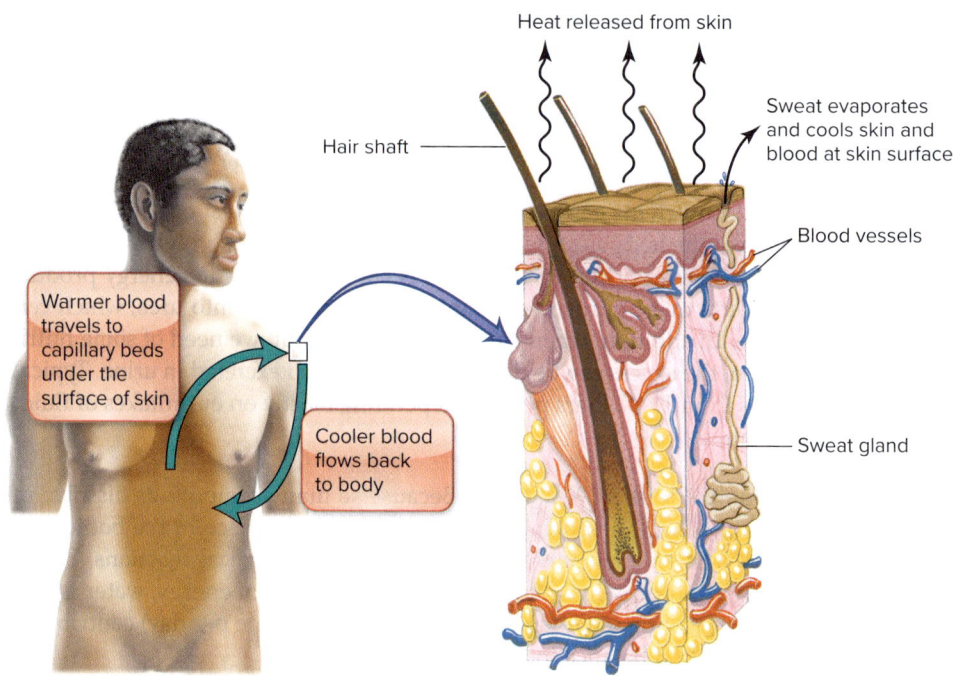

hemoconcentration Decrease in plasma volume, causing an increase in the concentration of red blood cells and other constituents of the blood.

WATER DEFICIENCY (DEHYDRATION)

Despite mechanisms that work to conserve water, fluid continues to be lost via the feces, skin, and lungs. Those losses must be replaced. In addition, there is a limit to how concentrated urine can become. Eventually, if fluid is not consumed, dehydration leads to impairments of physical and mental function.

By the time you lose just 1% to 2% of body weight in fluids, you will be thirsty and experience lack of appetite and **hemoconcentration** (Fig. 9-5). Even this small water deficit can cause you to feel tired and dizzy and to experience headaches. At a 4% loss of body weight from fluids, muscles lose significant strength and endurance, and central nervous system function is negatively affected (e.g., memory and reaction time are compromised and you become impatient). By the time body weight is reduced by 10% from fluid loss, heat tolerance is decreased and weakness results. Ultimately, dehydration will lead to kidney failure, coma, and death. Dehydration is a contributing factor to the development of heatstroke, a serious condition. Performing strenuous physical activity, including athletic training, in hot, humid conditions can lead to dehydration and the inability to regulate body temperature. Heart rate is increased and the skin becomes dry. Unassisted, an individual with heatstroke will become unconscious and die. Adequate fluid intake and, if possible, avoidance of physical activity in hot, humid conditions are the best ways to prevent heat illness.

Another potential consequence of inadequate fluid intake is kidney stones. When urine production is lower than about 500 milliliters (approximately 2 cups) per day, the urine is concentrated, increasing the risk of kidney stone formation in susceptible people (generally males). Kidney stones form from minerals and other substances that have precipitated out of the urine and accumulate in the kidney.

If you do not drink enough water, your brain communicates the need to drink by signaling thirst. In most cases, drinking fluids to quench your thirst will result in adequate hydration. However, the thirst mechanism can lag behind actual water loss during prolonged physical activity and illness (e.g., fever, vomiting, diarrhea). Older adults, as well, may need to be reminded to drink plenty of fluids because the thirst sensation tends to decline with age.

As you will learn in Chapter 10, athletes need to monitor fluid status. They should weigh themselves before and after training sessions to determine their rate of water loss

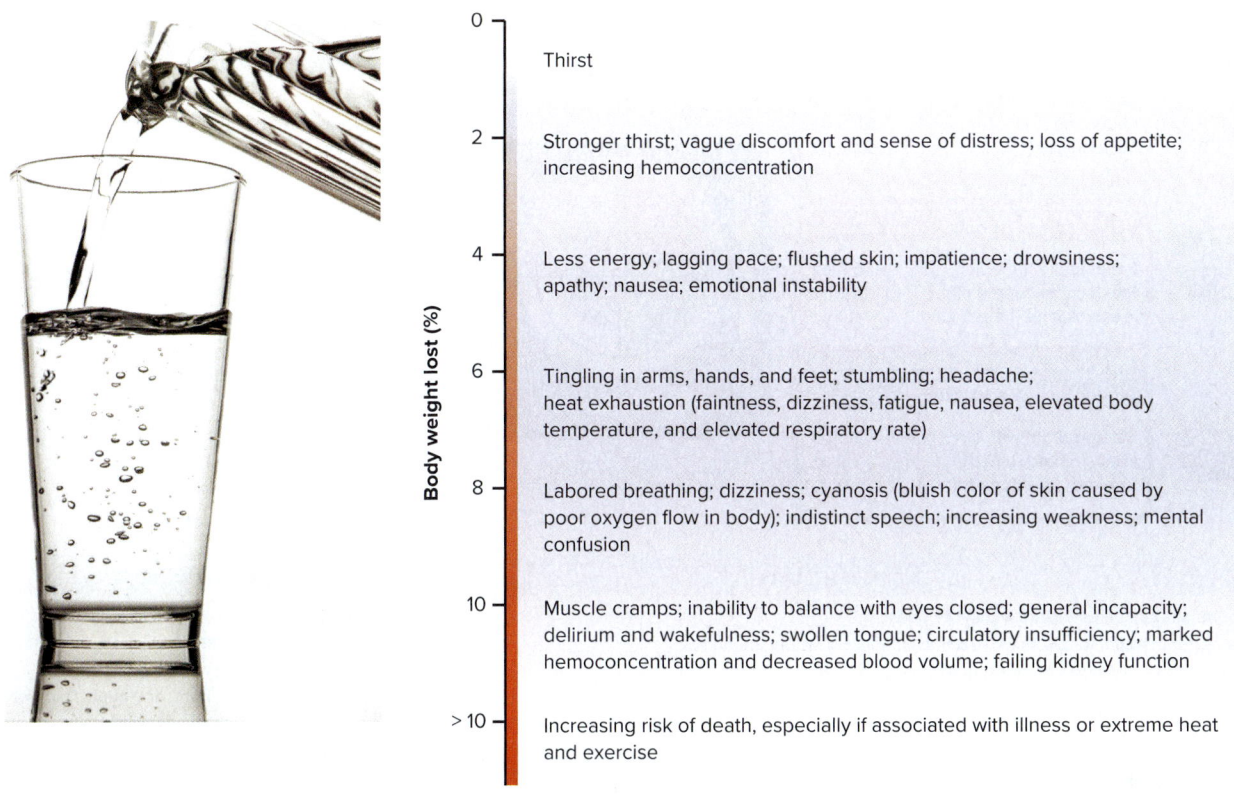

FIGURE 9-5 This list of dehydration effects ranges from thirst to risk of death, depending on the extent of water weight lost, shown on the left as a percentage. Holly Hildreth/McGraw Hill

and, thus, their water needs. A general guideline for athletes is to consume 2 to 3 cups of fluid for every pound lost through sweating during a workout.

The simplest way to determine if water intake is adequate is to observe urine color (Fig. 9-6). If hydration is adequate, urine should be clear or pale yellow (the color of lemonade). Concentrated urine is dark yellow (the color of apple juice). Urine color, however, can be influenced by consuming supplements (especially some B vitamins), medications, and certain foods. Lots of carotenoid-containing items (e.g., carrot juice, pumpkin, winter squash) can tint the urine orange. Too many fava beans or too much rhubarb will turn it dark brown. A reddish or pinkish urine results from eating too many beets or blackberries. Asparagus not only makes the urine smell like asparagus but can also turn it a bit green.

GETTING ENOUGH WATER

The Adequate Intake (AI) for *total* water is 2.7 liters (~11 cups) for adult females and 3.7 liters (~15 cups) for adult males. This total amount includes water from both fluids (i.e., beverages) and foods. Not considering the water we obtain from foods, adult females need to consume about 2.2 liters (~9 cups) of fluids and adult males need to consume about 3 liters (~13 cups) each day.

Figure 9-7 illustrates food sources of water. Besides beverages, which are nearly 100% water, fruits, vegetables, and dairy foods are good sources of water.

What Is the Difference Between Hard and Soft Water? In the United States, about 85% of homes have hard water.[1] **Hard water** contains relatively high levels of the minerals calcium and magnesium, whereas **soft water** contains much lower levels of dissolved minerals. Naturally occurring soft water is found in the Pacific North and Northwest, New England, South Atlantic–Gulf States, and Hawaii. Hard water can be converted

hard water Water that contains high levels of calcium and magnesium.

soft water Water that contains low levels of calcium and magnesium.

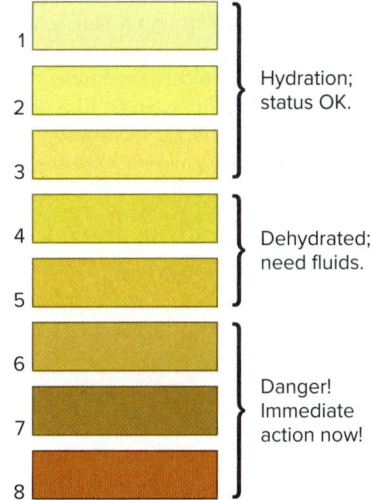

FIGURE 9-6 Monitoring the color of urine is a good gauge of hydration.

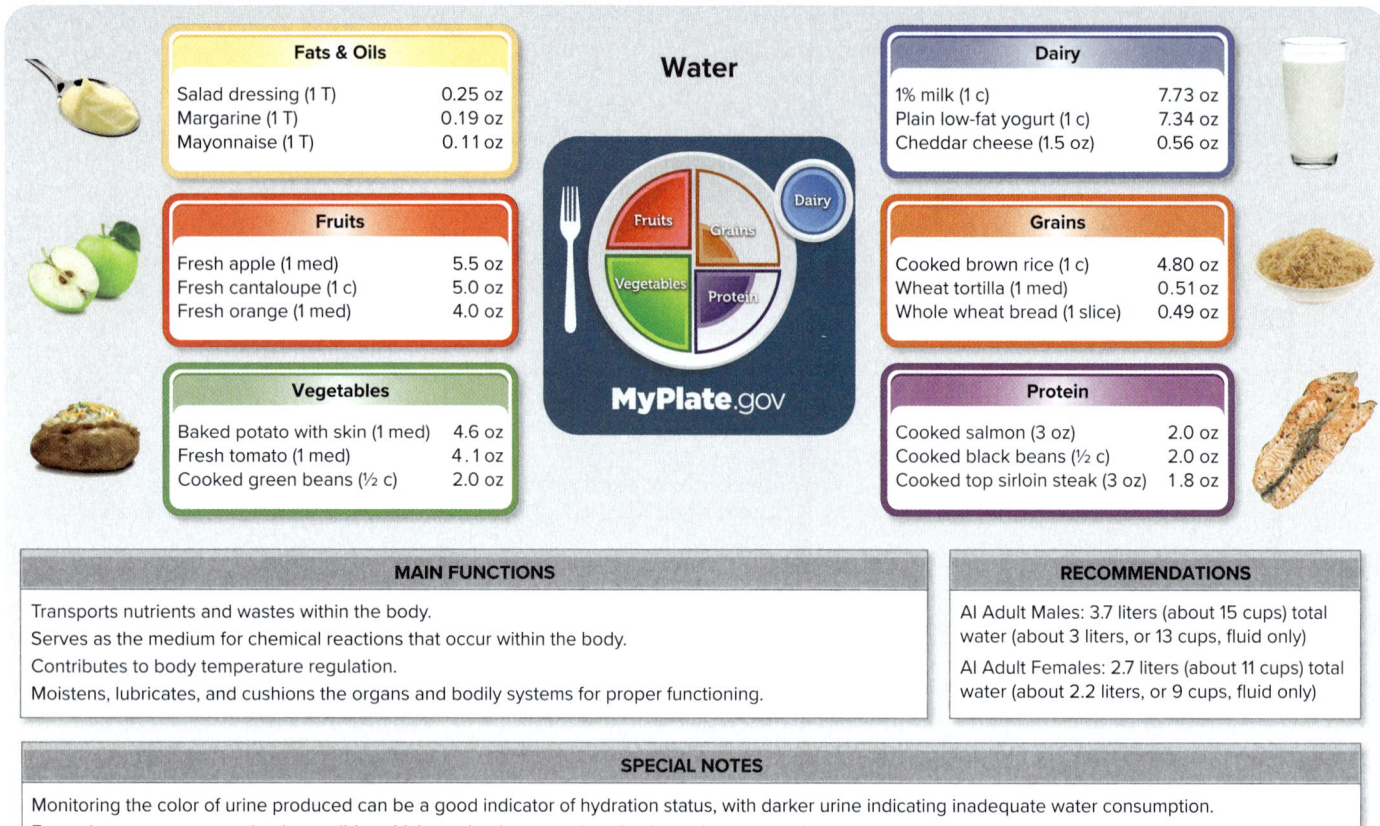

FIGURE 9-7 Sources, functions, and recommendations for water. On MyPlate, the fill of the background color (none, 1/3, 2/3, or completely covered) within each group on the plate indicates the average nutrient density for water in that group. Overall, the vegetables, fruits, dairy, and protein groups contain many foods that are nutrient-dense sources of water. Although not depicted on MyPlate, all beverages are nearly 100% water. Fats and oils, on the other hand, have almost no water. mayonnaise: Iconotec/Alamy Stock Photo; ripe green apple: Roman Samokhin/Shutterstock; baked potato: DNY59/E+/Getty Images; glass of milk: Nipaporn Panyacharoen/Shutterstock; brown rice: Yellow Cat/Shutterstock; salmon: Zoran Kolundzija/E+/Getty images; MyPlate: U.S. Department of Agriculture

Sources: Office of Dietary Supplements, Dietary Supplements Fact Sheets, available from https://ods.od.nih.gov/factsheets/list-all/; USDA FoodData Central, available from https://fdc.nal.usda.gov/

Water that comes out of your refrigerator dispenser or through a filter on your faucet typically runs through a charcoal (carbon) filter. The carbon attracts compounds present in tap water to remove off-flavors. Importantly, it does not remove fluoride, a mineral essential to help fight tooth decay.

into soft water through the use of a commercial water softener. As water travels through the water softener, calcium and magnesium exchange with sodium found in the water softener device. The water that exits the softener has a low calcium and magnesium content, but it contains a small amount of sodium (10 to 50 milligrams of sodium per 8 fluid ounces of water). The additional intake of sodium from soft water may be undesirable for people who need to limit sodium intake for reasons such as hypertension. The additional intake of calcium and magnesium afforded by consuming hard water would be more beneficial than increasing sodium intake through the use of softened water.

Is Bottled Water Healthier Than Tap Water? Bottled water is a popular alternative to tap water; in fact, Americans consume about 46 gallons of bottled water per person per year.[2] You will see a variety of terms used to describe bottled water. *Artesian water* must come from a confined aquifer. *Spring water* must flow naturally to the surface. *Mineral water* comes from a ground source that is naturally high in minerals, such as calcium and magnesium. *Purified water* is produced through an approved process such as distillation or reverse osmosis.[3] Some consumers choose bottled water simply because they prefer the taste. Many people choose bottled water because they believe it is less likely to be contaminated with pathogens or impurities than tap water. Much of the bottled water produced in the United States, however, is actually purified municipal tap water. There are some differences in water treatment methods: rather than using chlorine to disinfect water, most bottled water is treated with ozone, which does not impart a flavor to the water. The Environmental Protection Agency regulates and monitors public water supplies, while the Food and Drug Administration regulates bottled water, but the standards for quality and contaminant levels are identical for both.

Beyond the level of contaminants, there are some definite differences between bottled and tap water. As you'll learn in Section 9.14, a small amount of fluoride is added to municipal water supplies to prevent dental caries. Very few bottled water manufacturers add the mineral fluoride to the water. People who drink primarily bottled water should include regular tap water throughout the day in order to receive the benefits of fluoride. Trips to the drinking fountain or making coffee or tea with tap water should suffice.

The use of plastics may pose some threats to human health. Drinking water from a freshly washed or newly opened bottle is fine, but plastic, like the food we eat, has a shelf life. Over time, the chemicals that make up plastic break down and can make their way into the foods and beverages they are designed to protect. One example is **bisphenol A (BPA).** Since the 1950s, BPA has been used in food packaging, including cans and plastic containers. Unfortunately, this organic compound can leach into foods and liquids over time, especially when exposed to acidic or hot conditions. BPA is considered an **endocrine disruptor,** which means it can interfere with the body's own hormones. Temperature, acidity of the contents, the type of plastic (recycling code), and the age of the bottle all influence the stability of plastics. The age of the consumer makes a difference, too, as babies and young children are more vulnerable to low levels of toxins than adults. Concern over the impact of BPA on infant development led the FDA to ban BPA for use in baby bottles and sippy cups. However, BPA is still used in many types of food containers.

The United States has some of the cleanest, safest tap water in the world. For on-the-go hydration, the most environmentally friendly solution is to fill a reusable water bottle with tap water or home-filtered water (see *Sustainable Solutions* in this section). If you choose single-use bottled water, store your products safely and recycle your empty bottles. Figure 9-8 lists several guidelines to ensure the safety of the bottled water you drink.

Is Sparkling or Seltzer Water Harmful to Your Teeth? Sparkling or seltzer waters have become popular and healthier alternatives to sugar-sweetened sodas and diet sodas. Sparkling water is simply water with carbon dioxide pumped into it. This carbonated water becomes more acidic because the carbon dioxide turns into carbonic acid. Pure water has a neutral pH of 7, but seltzer or sparkling water has a pH between 3 and 4 and is acidic enough to erode tooth enamel. Beverages with a pH below 4 are considered erosive, whereas those with a pH of 2 to 3, including colas, are extremely erosive. Club soda and carbonated mineral waters, such as plain San Pellegrino® or Perrier®, are not erosive because the natural or added minerals raise the pH to about 5. In contrast, if citric acid, a component of many "flavors," is added to sparkling water, the pH drops. Unfortunately, the citric acid does not have to be listed separately on labels, making it difficult for consumers to know it is present. Because its acid content can soften tooth enamel, wait at least 30 minutes to brush your teeth after drinking sparkling water. To decrease the time acid is in contact with your teeth, drink sparkling water with food rather than sipping it all day. Because saliva is needed to neutralize acid, avoid sparkling water if you have a dry mouth.[4]

AVOIDING TOO MUCH WATER

Even though the kidneys of a healthy person can process up to 15 liters of urine per day, it is possible to drink too much water. As water intake increases moderately above the AI, kidneys process the excess fluid and excrete more dilute urine. However, if water intake far exceeds the kidneys' processing ability, overhydration and sodium dilution in the blood result. This condition is commonly known as **water intoxication** or, more accurately, **hyponatremia.** The kidneys are unable to excrete

bisphenol A (BPA) An organic compound used in the manufacture of plastics and resins, including some materials used to make food containers. BPA may leach into foods and be ingested by humans.

endocrine disruptor A natural or synthetic compound that can mimic and interfere with hormones in the body.

To find a list of brands of bottled water that contain fluoride, check out the website of the International Bottled Water Association at www.bottledwater.org/fluoride

water intoxication Potentially fatal condition that occurs with a high intake of water, which results in a severe dilution of the blood and other fluid compartments.

hyponatremia Dangerously low blood sodium level.

Sustainable Solutions

Bottled Water or Tap Water?

One of the big differences between bottled water and tap water is the way it is delivered. Tap water travels through pipes into your home, but bottled water requires extra packaging and more costly methods of transport and storage. The large quantity of plastic used to package more than a billion gallons of bottled water each year in the United States creates huge concerns related to energy use, recycling, and solid waste disposal. Instead of reaching for bottled water, consider a reusable water bottle, preferably stainless steel, with a wide mouth for easy cleaning (Fig. 9-8).

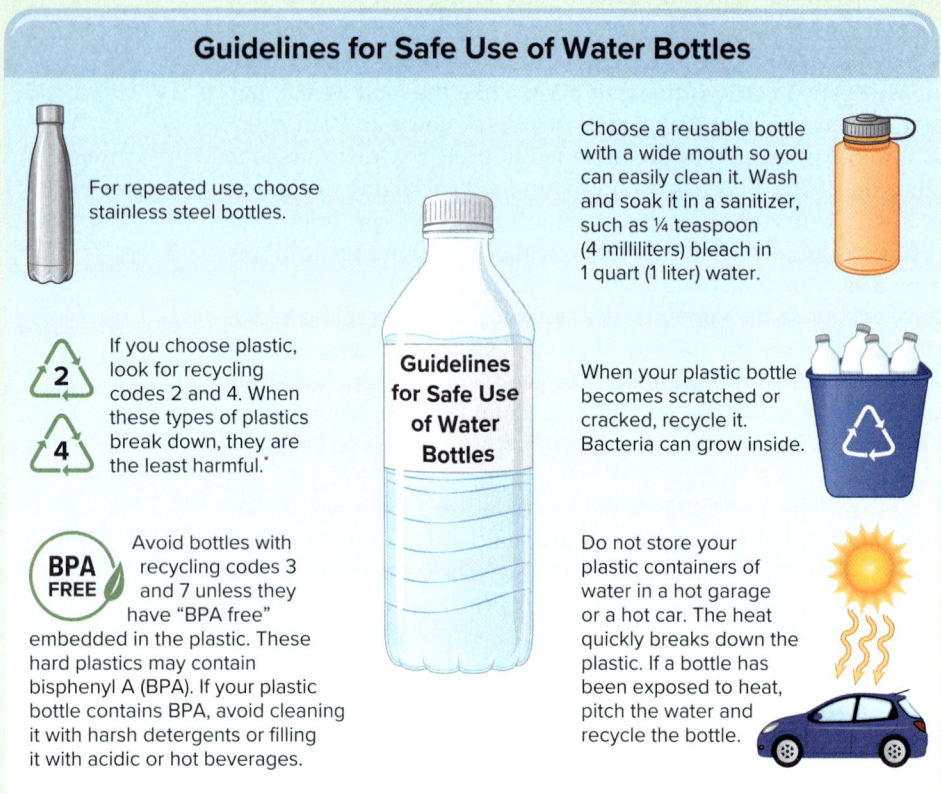

FIGURE 9-8 Following the guidelines listed here for the safe use of water bottles will protect the consumer from the ingestion of harmful plastics and microorganisms, while saving the environment from the pollution caused by disposable water bottles.

*Seaman G. Plastics by the numbers. *Eartheasy.* May 2, 2020. https://learn.eartheasy.com/articles/plastics-by-the-numbers

the excess fluid, so blood volume increases, which rapidly dilutes the blood. Tissues swell and body functions that rely on sodium and potassium are impaired. The heartbeat becomes irregular, allowing fluid to enter the lungs; the brain and nerves swell, causing severe headaches, confusion, seizure, and coma. Unless water is restricted and a concentrated salt solution is administered under close medical monitoring, the person will die.

Some mental health conditions (e.g., schizophrenia or other personality disorders) may cause a person to drink a large volume of water in a short period of time, but water intoxication can happen to healthy people, too. Endurance athletes who exercise for prolonged times and drink large volumes of plain water without replacing electrolytes are especially at risk for hyponatremia. Using sports drinks for hydration during endurance activities (see Chapter 10) will help replace the sodium along with the water lost in sweat.

✓ CONCEPT CHECK 9.1

1. List the components of water intake and water output.
2. Why is it significant that water is the *universal solvent*?
3. Describe how water regulates body temperature.
4. Provide two examples of water's role as a lubricant.
5. In your own words, describe the hormonal regulation of water balance (see Fig. 9-3).
6. What is the AI for total water for adult males? For adult females?
7. Which three MyPlate food groups supply the most water?
8. List the guidelines for the safe use of water bottles.
9. What are the consequences of water intoxication?

9.2 Minerals: Essential Elements for Health

While vitamins are compounds consisting of many elements (e.g., carbon, oxygen, and hydrogen), minerals are individual chemical elements. They cannot be broken down further. The mineral content of foods is sometimes called "ash" because it is all that remains after the whole food has been destroyed by high temperatures or chemical degradation. In humans, minerals make up about 4% of adult body weight (Fig. 9-9). A mineral is essential for humans if a dietary inadequacy of it results in a physiological or structural abnormality and its addition to the diet prevents such illness or reinstates normal health.

Minerals are categorized based on the amount we need per day. If we require greater than 100 milligrams (1/50 of a teaspoon) of a mineral per day, it is considered a major mineral. These include calcium, phosphorus, magnesium, sulfur, sodium, potassium,

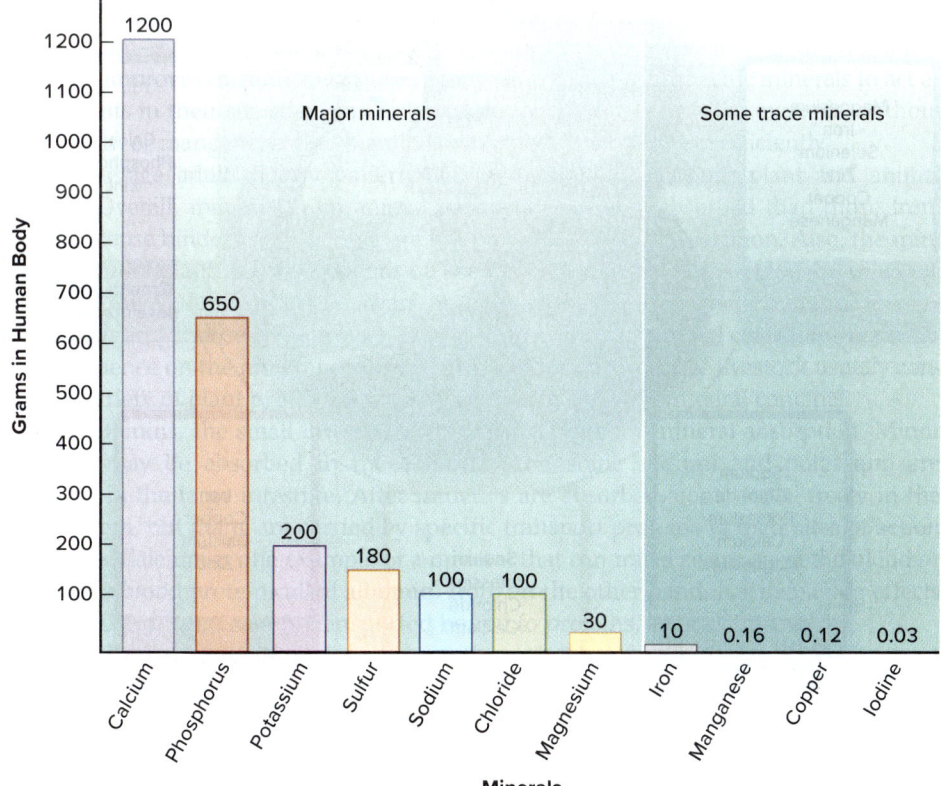

FIGURE 9-9 Approximate amounts of various minerals present in the average human body. Other trace minerals of nutritional importance not listed include chromium, fluoride, molybdenum, selenium, and zinc.

MINERAL TOXICITIES

Excessive mineral intake, especially of trace minerals such as iron and copper, can have toxic results. For many trace minerals, the gap between just enough and too much is small. Taking minerals in supplement form poses the biggest threat for mineral toxicity, whereas food sources are unlikely culprits. Mineral supplements exceeding current standards for mineral needs—especially those that supply more than 100% of the Daily Values on supplement labels—should be taken only under a primary care provider's supervision. The Daily Values for minerals are typically greater than our current standards (e.g., Recommended Dietary Allowances [RDA]). Unless you are under medical supervision for a diagnosed deficiency, your daily dose of minerals should not exceed the Upper Level.

The potential for toxicity is not the only reason to be cautious about the use of mineral supplements. Harmful interactions with other nutrients are possible. Furthermore, there is no guarantee of safety or purity for dietary supplements. Use of brands approved by the U.S. Pharmacopeial Convention (USP) lessens this risk.

PRESERVATION OF MINERALS IN FOODS

Good sources of minerals can be found in all food groups, especially grains and protein foods (Fig. 9-11). Minerals are found in plant and animal foods, but as you previously read, the bioavailability of minerals varies widely. Minerals are not typically lost from animal sources during processing, storage, or cooking; but for plant sources, significant amounts may be lost during food processing. When grains are refined, the minerals that are found in the bran are lost. The more refined a plant food, as in the case of white flour, the lower its mineral content. During the enrichment of refined grain products, iron is the only mineral added, whereas the magnesium, zinc, copper, selenium, and other minerals lost during refinement are not replaced. Following the recommendation of the MyPlate Plan to "make half your grains whole" will effectively improve the mineral content of an eating pattern.

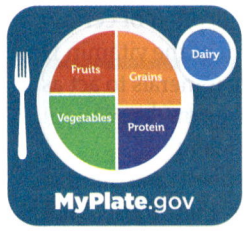

MyPlate:
Sources of Minerals

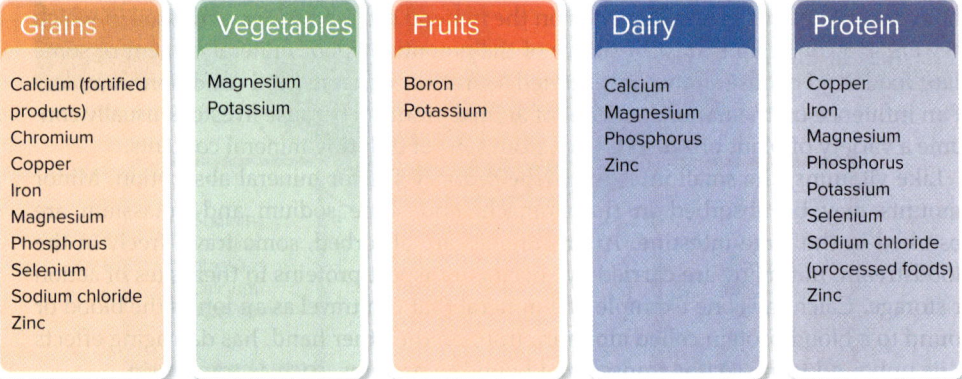

FIGURE 9-11 Certain groups of MyPlate are especially rich sources of various minerals. This is true for the minerals listed. Each mineral may also be found in other groups but in lower amounts. Other trace minerals are also present in moderate amounts in many groups. With regard to the grains group, whole grain varieties are the richest sources of most trace minerals listed.

Source: (MyPlate): U.S. Department of Agriculture

✓ CONCEPT CHECK 9.2

1. Are ultratrace minerals essential for humans? List three examples of ultratrace minerals.
2. Should people take individual mineral supplements? Why or why not?
3. Where are minerals stored in the body?

9.3 Sodium

Sodium (Na) is best known as one of the elements in common table salt. Salt is nutritionally important and was once a highly valued chemical compound! Historically, salt was treasured because of its ability to preserve foods. It was so valuable, it was used as a form of payment, and the word *salary* comes from the Latin word for salt. Salt is 40% sodium and 60% chloride by weight (the chemical symbol Na represents the Latin term *natrium*). One teaspoon of salt contains 2400 milligrams of sodium. Although salt was once difficult to find, it is now overly abundant in our food supply. Indeed, the majority of Americans exceed the recommendations for sodium intake, so reducing sodium in our dietary patterns is the focus of major public health campaigns.

AN OVERVIEW OF OSMOSIS

Before you learn about the functions of sodium, let's review a few common chemistry terms. A **solution** is a liquid mixture made of a solvent and one or more solutes. The **solvent** is the larger component of the solution. Often, water is the solvent. The **solute** is the minor component of the solution—the substance that is dissolved in the solvent. For example, in body fluids, sodium is the main solute dispersed in the extracellular fluid. When we talk about the **concentration** of a solution, we are describing how much of the solute is mixed into or dissolved in the solvent.

Each cell is surrounded by a cell membrane. Cell membranes are *semipermeable*, which means some substances can easily pass through but others cannot. Water can easily pass through the cell membrane, but many solutes are either too large or too polar to pass freely through it. Water found inside the cell membrane is part of the **intracellular fluid.** Intracellular fluid accounts for 63% of the fluid in the body. The remaining 37% of body fluid—**extracellular fluid**—is found in one of two extracellular spaces: (1) the fluid portion of blood (plasma) and lymph or (2) the fluid between cells (i.e., interstitial fluid).

The relative amounts of water in the intracellular and extracellular compartments are controlled by the concentration of ions in the intracellular or extracellular fluids. **Ions** are minerals that dissolve in water and are either positively (+) or negatively (−) charged. These charged ions allow the transfer of electrical current, so they are also called **electrolytes.** Four electrolytes predominate: sodium (Na^+) and chloride (Cl^-) are primarily found in the extracellular fluid, and potassium (K^+) and phosphate (PO_4^-) are the principal electrolytes in the intracellular fluid.

The term **osmosis** is used to describe the passage of water through a membrane from an area of lower electrolyte concentration to an area of higher electrolyte concentration. Where ions move, water follows passively. Under normal conditions, the concentration of electrolytes on either side of the cell membrane is controlled in such a way that the intracellular fluid and extracellular fluid are **isotonic.** Thus, water movement into and out of the cell is in equilibrium (Fig. 9-12). However, if the extracellular fluid is **hypertonic** (i.e., it has a higher concentration of electrolytes) compared to the intracellular fluid, water will be drawn out of the cell, leading to cell shrinkage. The opposite can also occur. When the extracellular fluid is **hypotonic** (i.e., it has a lower concentration of electrolytes) compared to the intracellular fluid, water will flow into the cell. If too much water flows in, the cell can burst, similar to filling a balloon with too much air.

solution Liquid mixture made of a solvent and a solute.

solvent A liquid substance in which other substances dissolve.

solute A substance that dissolves in a solvent to make a solution.

concentration The amount of a solute dissolved in a solvent; usually expressed as mass per unit of volume (e.g., milligrams per deciliter).

intracellular fluid Fluid contained within a cell; it represents about two-thirds of body fluid.

extracellular fluid Fluid found outside the cells; it represents about one-third of body fluid.

ion A positively or negatively charged atom.

electrolyte A mineral that separates into positively or negatively charged ions in water. Electrolytes are able to transmit an electrical current.

osmosis The passage of water through a membrane from a less concentrated compartment to a more concentrated compartment.

isotonic Having equal concentration of solutes.

hypertonic Having high concentration of solutes.

hypotonic Having low concentration of solutes.

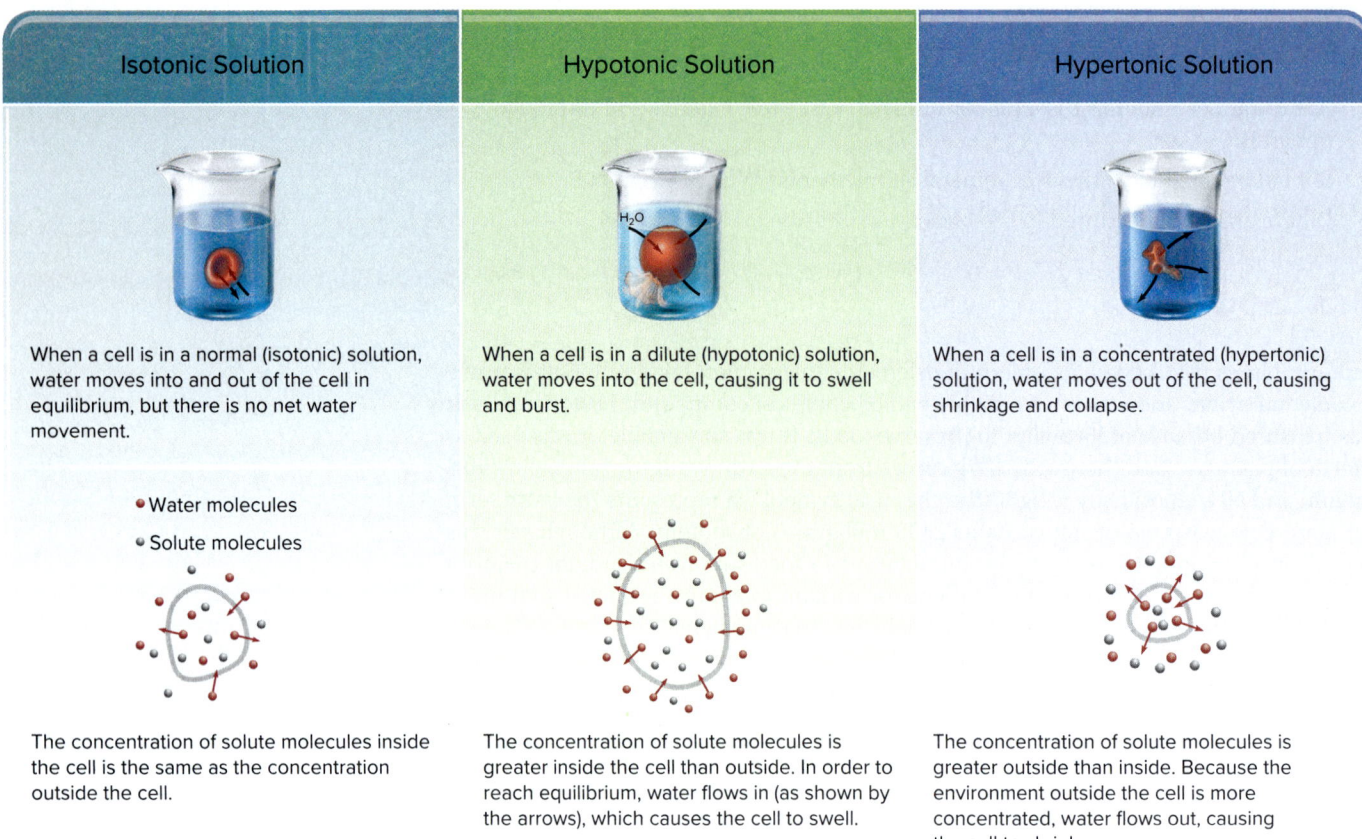

FIGURE 9-12 Effects of various ion concentrations in a fluid on human cells. This shows the process of osmosis. Fluid is shifting in and out of the red blood cell in response to changing ion concentrations in the fluid surrounding the cells.

The principle of osmosis is used by the digestive tract to absorb water from the colon. Water from beverages, foods, and intestinal tract secretions makes the contents of the intestinal tract high in water as it enters the colon from the small intestine. Cells that line the colon actively absorb sodium. Water follows sodium, which facilitates the efficient absorption of water from the large intestine into the bloodstream. As a result, daily water loss from feces is low—approximately 100 milliliters (~0.5 cup).

During illness, when large volumes of fluid are lost through vomiting and diarrhea, osmosis can lead to a life-threatening condition. As fluid is lost from the gastrointestinal tract, the extracellular fluid becomes more and more concentrated, or hypertonic to cells. Intracellular water exits the cells in an attempt to dilute the extracellular fluid, and cells shrink and lose their ability to function normally. In the heart, this imbalance can lead to a decreased ability of the heart to pump blood and, ultimately, to cardiac failure. Infants and older adults are particularly susceptible to the effects of severe dehydration.

FUNCTIONS OF SODIUM

Sodium is one of the electrolytes dissolved in body fluids. When sodium chloride (NaCl) is dissolved in water, the chemical bond holding the two atoms together breaks and the charged ions, Na^+ and Cl^-, are released. These electrolytes attract water. Indeed, the ability of sodium to dissolve in water and attract water molecules is the basis for sodium's functions in regulating fluid balance, nerve impulse conduction, muscle contractions, and the absorption of some nutrients.

Fluid balance is regulated by moving or actively pumping sodium ions where more water is needed. In human physiology, where sodium goes, water follows. Thus, if sodium is pumped out of a cell, water will flow out of the cell via osmosis. This mechanism is used in the large intestine to absorb water from the lumen of the intestine into the blood. Also in the GI tract, the movement of sodium is sometimes coupled with the transport of other nutrients, such as glucose. In the kidneys, the active pumping of sodium ions across cell membranes in the nephrons helps to regulate how much water is retained in the blood or excreted via urine.

Along with a few other minerals, sodium also plays a role in nerve impulse transmission. Sodium, potassium, chloride, and phosphate ions are found in different concentrations on either side of the cell membrane. In nerve cells, not only does this difference in concentration result in a *chemical* gradient across the cell membrane, but because these ions are charged, there is also an *electrical* gradient across the cell membrane. We can refer to the differences in both concentration and electrical charge across the nerve cell membrane as an **electrochemical gradient.** At rest, the nerve cell membrane is polarized—the inside of the nerve cell membrane has a slightly negative charge, whereas the outside of the nerve cell membrane has a slightly positive charge. When the nerve cell is in a resting state, this slight polarization of the cell membrane is maintained by the action of ion pumps. However, when the nerve cell is stimulated, the cell membrane becomes depolarized. Positively charged sodium ions rush into the cell. **Depolarization** of one part of the nerve cell membrane subsequently triggers the depolarization of an adjacent area of the membrane, such that an electrical signal is transmitted along the nerve cell and from one cell to the next. After the stimulus, ions are actively pumped across the nerve cell membrane to restore the normal electrolyte balance. Simply put, the transmission of nerve impulses along nerve cells depends on shifts in the concentrations of electrolyte minerals, such as sodium, across the nerve cell membrane.

Sodium also plays an important role in muscle contraction. Not only is sodium vital for the transmission of nerve impulses that signal muscles to contract, but sodium is also directly involved in the activation of muscle cells during muscle contraction. Alterations in blood electrolyte levels can cause muscle cramps in those who sweat profusely during exercise, and chronically low sodium levels have been shown to impair muscle function among older adults.[5]

electrochemical gradient A difference in both the concentration of solutes and the electrical charge across the cell membrane.

depolarization During nerve impulse transmission, the process in which the resting state of the nerve cell membrane (slightly negative charge inside the cell membrane) is temporarily disrupted.

SODIUM DEFICIENCY

A true deficiency of sodium, in which blood levels of this mineral are too low to maintain normal body functions, is called hyponatremia. Sodium deficiency is uncommon, however, because sodium is abundant in our food supply and our kidneys are very good at regulating sodium levels in the blood. If blood sodium is too low, sodium is secreted back into the blood as it flows through the kidneys, resulting in a decreased urine output. Conversely, if our blood sodium levels are too high, the excess sodium is filtered out by the kidneys and excreted into the urine. When this excess sodium is removed, water follows, resulting in greater urine output.

As described in Section 9.1, excessive water intake could dilute the blood, leading to hyponatremia (i.e., water toxicity). In combination with excessive perspiration or persistent vomiting or diarrhea, a low sodium intake may deplete the body of sodium. Whether due to excessive water intake, deficient sodium intake, or a combination of both, hyponatremia may result in muscle cramps, nausea, vomiting, dizziness, mental confusion, seizures, or a coma.

Perspiration contains about 1 gram of sodium per liter. When sweat losses exceed 2% to 3% of total body weight (or about 5 to 6 pounds), sodium losses should raise concern. Even then, adding salt to food or selecting some salty foods, such as soup or crackers, is sufficient to restore body sodium for most people. Athletes who perspire for hours during endurance activities need to consume sodium from electrolyte replacement or sports drinks during exercise to avoid hyponatremia (see Chapter 10).

GETTING ENOUGH SODIUM

Whole, unprocessed foods are naturally low in sodium. In fact, only about 12% of the sodium in our food supply is naturally present in foods. Another 11% of our sodium intake comes from salt added while cooking or at the table at home. The vast majority (77%) of the sodium in the typical American dietary pattern comes from salt added during food processing or preparation at restaurants (Fig. 9-13).

FIGURE 9-13 Most of the sodium in the typical American dietary pattern comes from the salt added to foods during processing.

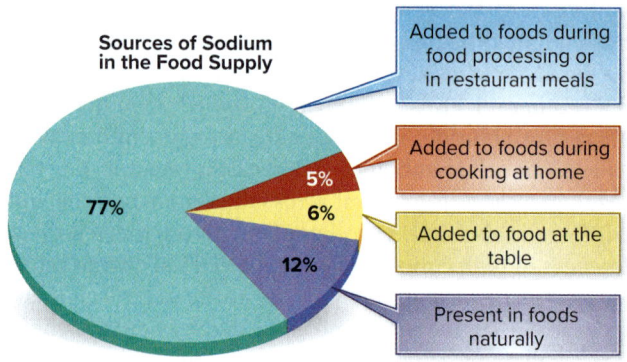

The AI for sodium is 1500 milligrams per day for individuals ages 14 and older. The sodium AI for children ages 9–13 decreased to 1200 milligrams. The AI is even lower for younger children (see Appendix F for a full list of DRIs). The average daily sodium intake of Americans (age 2 and older), however, is about 3400 milligrams![6]

Leading contributors of sodium in the typical American eating pattern include bread and rolls, pizza, sandwiches, cold cuts and cured meats, cheese, soups, burritos and tacos, savory snacks (chips, popcorn, pretzels, snack mixes, and crackers), chicken, and eggs and omelets (Fig. 9-14). When dietary sodium must be restricted,

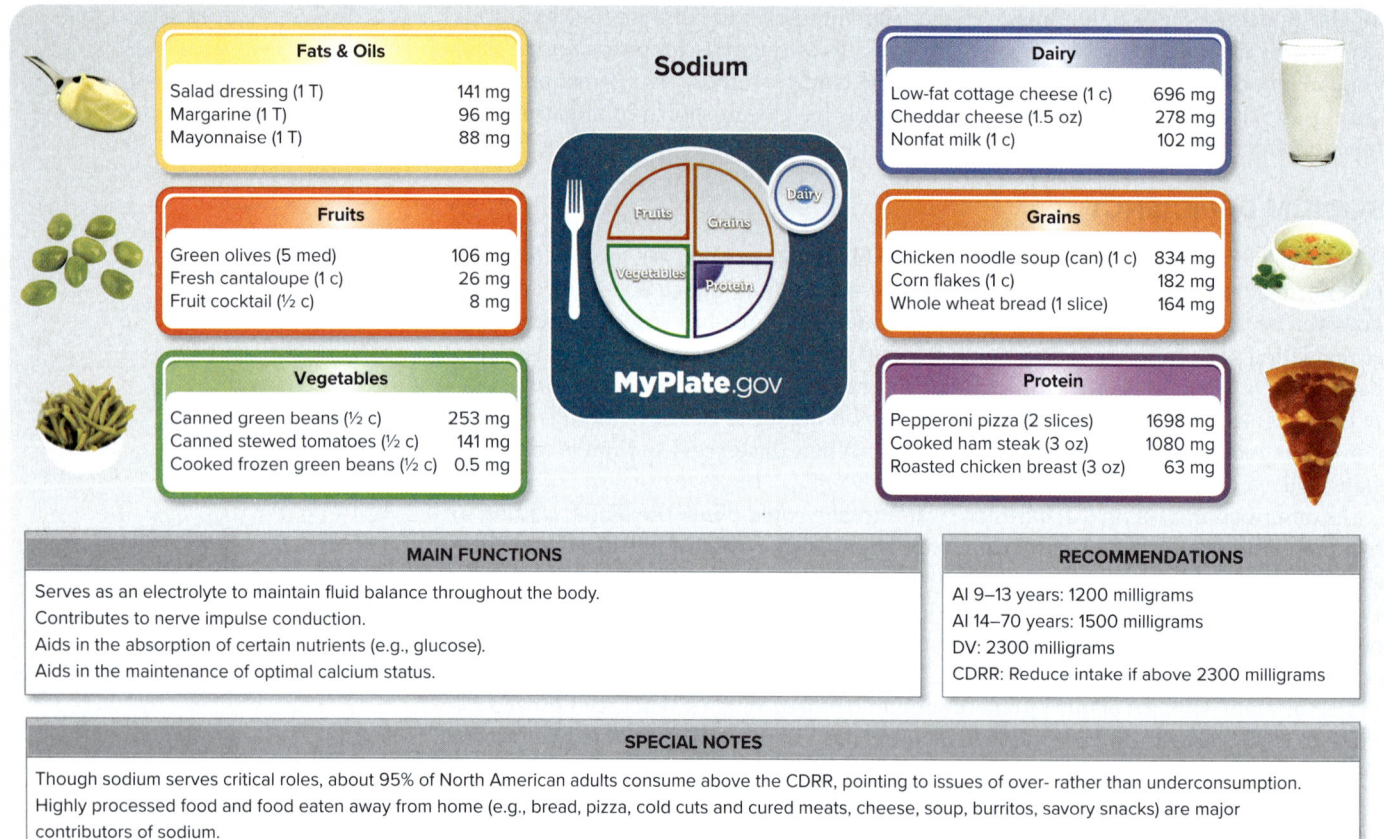

FIGURE 9-14 Food sources, functions, and recommendations for sodium. The fill of the background color (none, 1/3, 2/3, or completely covered) within each food group on MyPlate indicates the average nutrient density for sodium for *natural, unprocessed foods* in that group. The figure shows the sodium content of several natural and processed foods from each food group. Overall, the dairy group is the only food group that provides much sodium in its natural form. Food processing adds significant sodium to foods such as canned vegetables and cured meats. mayonnaise: Iconotec/Alamy Stock Photo; green olives: Iconotec/Glow Images; green beans: ncognet0/iStock/Getty Images; glass of milk: Nipaporn Panyacharoen/Shutterstock; chicken soup: ma-k/E+/Getty Images; pepperoni pizza slice: Burke/Triolo/Brand X Pictures/Getty Images; MyPlate: U.S. Department of Agriculture

Source: Office of Dietary Supplements, Dietary Supplements Fact Sheets, available from https://ods.od.nih.gov/factsheets/list-all/; USDA FoodData Central, available from https://fdc.nal.usda.gov/

it is important to check the sodium content listed on food labels to monitor sodium intake. The more you consume highly processed and restaurant foods, the higher your sodium intake will be. Conversely, you will have more control over your sodium intake if you prepare meals yourself and choose whole, unprocessed foods most of the time. If we ate only unprocessed foods and added no salt, we would consume about 500 milligrams of sodium per day.

AVOIDING TOO MUCH SODIUM

In 2019, a new DRI category, Chronic Disease Risk Reduction Intake (CDRR), was introduced for sodium. This new category is historic in that it is the first time that overuse of a nutrient is being tied to chronic disease. The CDRR recommendation for individuals ages 14 and older is to reduce sodium intakes if they are above 2300 mg per day. Reducing sodium intakes that exceed the CDRR is expected to reduce the risk for cardiovascular disease and high blood pressure within the healthy population.[6] It must be noted that the Daily Value (DV) of 2300 milligrams equals the CDRR for sodium. About 95% of adults in the United States exceed the CDRR.[7]

In general, your kidneys help you adapt to wide variations in daily sodium intakes, with today's sodium intake found in tomorrow's urine. However, approximately one-third of adults with normal blood pressure and at least half of adults with hypertension are *salt sensitive* or, more specifically, *sodium sensitive*.[8] For these individuals, changes in sodium intake have a profound effect on blood pressure. Among individuals who are sodium sensitive, lowering sodium intake to about 2000 milligrams per day can often decrease blood pressure. Females tend to be more salt-sensitive than males and salt sensitivity increases with age. Individuals with kidney disease, diabetes, and hypertension seem to be most salt-sensitive (see Section 9.17). Salt sensitivity is considered to be a risk factor for hypertension.

Besides its effects on blood pressure, reducing sodium intake may also help maintain a healthy calcium status, as sodium intake greater than about 2000 milligrams per day may cause calcium to be lost along with the sodium in the urine. Current research also links excessive sodium consumption to overweight and obesity. As salt intake increases, fluid intake also increases; if high-calorie beverages are chosen, weight gain may follow.[9]

Adopting a reduced-salt dietary pattern is a significant lifestyle change for most people because many typical food choices will have to be limited (Fig. 9-15). At first, foods may taste bland, but eventually, you will perceive more flavor as the taste receptors in the tongue become more sensitive to the salt content of foods. It takes 6 to 8 weeks to retrain your taste buds to sense sodium at a lower level. Slowly reducing sodium intake by substituting lemon juice, herbs, and spices will allow you to become accustomed to a dietary pattern that contains minimal amounts of salt. Many cookbooks and online sources offer excellent recipes for flavorful dishes that are lower in sodium.

In 2021, the Food and Drug Administration released new voluntary guidance for the food industry to reduce the sodium content of packaged foods. The goal is to reduce the usual sodium intake of Americans by 12%—from the current average of 3400 milligrams per day to about 3000 milligrams per day—over the next few years.[10] This target is still higher than the CDRR but would be an achievable improvement. In the past few decades, major public health campaigns to educate and motivate consumers to lower their intakes of sodium have been unsuccessful without the cooperation of the food industry. This modest reduction in average sodium intake across the population has the potential to reduce the incidence of heart disease and stroke by tens of thousands of cases per year and save billions of dollars on health care expenses.

Overall, to lower sodium intake, the *Dietary Guidelines* recommends cooking at home more often; using the Nutrition Facts label to choose products with less sodium, reduced sodium, or no added salt; and flavoring foods with herbs and spices

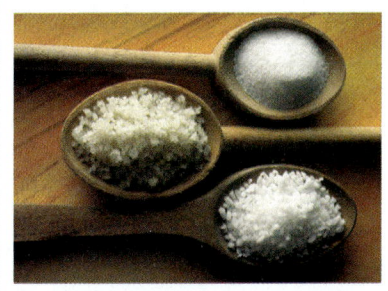

Table salt, kosher salt, sea salt—which one is best? Choosing the best salt really comes down to personal preference or what works best in a recipe.

- *Table salt* is typically mined from the earth and processed into fine grains. These fine, evenly shaped grains can be measured precisely when a recipe needs an exact amount of salt. Most of the table salt sold in North America is fortified with iodine, an essential nutrient for thyroid function.
- *Kosher salt*, also called coarse salt, is chunky and its large grains are easy to see when applying it by hand. It gets its name from its role in *koshering*, also known as curing or pickling.
- *Sea salt* is made through the evaporation of seawater. It is minimally processed, which gives it a coarser texture. It may contain traces of magnesium, calcium, and potassium, giving it some color and flavor variations. Flaky sea salt can be used as the last touch in dishes where the flakes of salt create tiny explosions of salty flavor. Although many consumers prefer the taste and texture of sea salt to table salt, when it comes to heart health, there is no significant difference in sodium or chloride content.

I. Rozenbaum & F. Cirou/PhotoAlto

instead of salt based on personal and cultural foodways.[7] Reducing your sodium intake while boosting your potassium intake by eating more fruits and vegetables might help you achieve even greater health benefits because potassium helps to *lower* your blood pressure. See *Ask the RDN* for more ideas about modifying your risk for hypertension.

ASK THE RDN Pass the Salt?

Dear RDN: *As a college student, do I need to be concerned about the amount of salt in my dietary pattern or are the limits just for older adults with high blood pressure?*

Since the 1970s, Americans have been told to limit their consumption of salt, more specifically sodium, to control blood pressure. For most Americans, this is a tough rule to follow because of our preference for salty foods. While experts have long agreed that consuming too much salt may be harmful, especially for individuals with high blood pressure, reducing your sodium intake has also been linked to reducing your risk of cardiovascular disease. The *Dietary Guidelines* defines too much as > 2300 milligrams of sodium per day, the amount in approximately 1 teaspoon of salt. The American Heart Association recommends 1500 milligrams per day for most adults, especially those with hypertension. The new CDRR for sodium recommends that individuals ages 14 and over should reduce sodium intake if it exceeds 2300 milligrams per day. The sodium CDRR for children ages 9 to 13 recommends a reduction in sodium intake if it exceeds 1800 milligrams. These recommendations seek to reduce the risk of cardiovascular disease and hypertension within the healthy population, including college students.

Remember, even though too much sodium can increase your risk for chronic diseases, it is still an essential nutrient that affects every body system, including the cardiovascular system. Indeed, too little sodium may pose serious health risks. The typical American, however, consumes around 3400 milligrams of sodium per day!

Current evidence links excessive sodium intake with high blood pressure. Most Americans, including college-age students, should reduce sodium intakes to < 2300 milligrams per day. To begin reducing overall sodium consumption, read food labels carefully and select foods low in sodium (140 milligrams or less per serving); consume more fresh meats and vegetables rather than highly processed varieties; choose low-sodium or no-salt-added nuts, seeds, and snacks; cook at home; and ask for low-sodium options in restaurants. Deli meats and cheeses are very high in sodium. The sodium in breads, pizza, crackers, and snack foods adds up quickly because we typically eat so much of them.

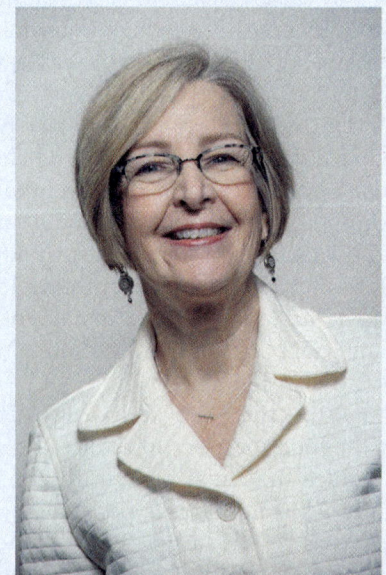
Monty Soungpradith/Open Image Studio LLC

Reducing sodium while eating foods rich in potassium, such as fruits and vegetables, might achieve greater health benefits than reducing sodium alone. Salt substitutes containing potassium chloride can be used to reduce sodium intake and increase potassium intake. This strategy will help lower blood pressure and prevent the adverse consequences of high blood pressure. Salt substitutes are sometimes called "lite" or low-sodium salt and can be used just like table salt. The additional potassium these products provide is usually fine; however, some people experience a bitter or metallic aftertaste. A quarter-teaspoon serving of one potassium chloride salt substitute contains about 800 milligrams of potassium, or about one-sixth of the daily recommended intake for potassium, which is 2,600 to 3,400 milligrams for adult females and males, respectively. Because of the potential for increases in blood potassium levels, salt substitutes can be dangerous for individuals with conditions such as kidney disease and for those taking certain medications such as ACE inhibitors and potassium-sparing diuretics. An alternative way to reduce sodium in your dietary pattern is to use herbs, spices, lemon juice, and flavored vinegars to season your food. You can find many salt-free herb blends at the grocery store. In sum, choosing fewer highly processed foods and preparing most of your meals at home will result in a healthy, yet achievable, sodium intake.

With just a dash of salt,

Anne M. Smith, PhD, RDN, LD

Associate Professor Emeritus, The Ohio State University, Author of *Wardlaw's Contemporary Nutrition* and *Wardlaw's Contemporary Nutrition: A Functional Approach*

Sources: Cobb LK, Anderson CAM, Elliot P, et al. Methodological issues in cohort studies that relate sodium intake to cardiovascular disease outcomes: a science advisory from the American Heart Association. *Circulation.* 2014 Mar 11;129(10):1173-1186. doi: 10.1161/CIR.0000000000000015; Greer RC, Marklund M, Anderson CAM, et al. Potassium-enriched salt substitutes as a means to lower blood pressure: benefits and risks. *Hypertension.* 2020 Feb;75(2):266-274. doi: 10.1161/HYPERTENSIONAHA.119.13241; Institute of Medicine (IOM). *Sodium Intake in Populations: Assessment of Evidence.* Washington, DC: National Academies Press; 2013; U.S. Food & Drug Administration. Sodium in your diet: use the Nutrition Facts label and reduce your intake. Food Facts. June 2021. https://www.fda.gov/food/nutrition-education-resources-materials/sodium-your-diet

✓ CONCEPT CHECK 9.3

1. Define *osmosis*.
2. Which organ regulates the amount of sodium in your blood?
3. Define *sodium sensitivity*.
4. Sodium is the only nutrient with a CDRR. What is the CDRR for sodium? Why is it important to keep your intake of sodium below the CDRR?
5. List three specific changes you could make to your dietary pattern to decrease your sodium intake.

9.4 Potassium

FUNCTIONS OF POTASSIUM

Potassium (K) performs many of the same functions as sodium, including water balance, nerve impulse transmission, and muscle contraction. (The chemical symbol K represents the Latin term *kalium*.) All membranes contain an energy-dependent pump that can transfer sodium from inside to outside the cell. When sodium (Na^+) is actively pumped out of the cell, potassium (K^+) enters the cell in an attempt to balance the loss of the positively charged sodium ions. That makes potassium the principal positively charged ion inside cells. Intracellular fluids contain 95% of the potassium in the body. Higher potassium intake is associated with *lower* rather than higher blood pressure values (Section 9.17).

POTASSIUM DEFICIENCY

Low blood potassium, also known as *hypokalemia*, is a life-threatening problem. Symptoms often include a loss of appetite, muscle cramps, confusion, and constipation. Eventually, the heart beats irregularly, decreasing its capacity to pump blood.

Hypokalemia could result from extremely low dietary potassium intake (i.e., prolonged undernutrition). However, it arises more commonly as a result of chronic diarrhea or vomiting or as a side effect of medications (e.g., diuretics or laxatives) that increase excretion of this mineral. Vulnerable populations include people with certain eating disorders (Chapter 11) or alcohol use disorders (Chapter 1). Other populations at increased risk for potassium deficiency include people on very-low-calorie diets and athletes who exercise for prolonged periods. In these situations, more potassium-rich foods should be consumed to compensate for potentially low body potassium. People who take potassium-wasting diuretics (water pills) for high blood pressure need to carefully monitor their dietary intake of this mineral. Increased intake of fruits and vegetables or potassium chloride supplements are typically prescribed by primary care providers.

GETTING ENOUGH POTASSIUM

Unprocessed foods, including fruits, vegetables, milk, whole grains, beans, peas, lentils, and meats, are rich sources of potassium (Fig. 9-15). An easy guide is to remember that the more processed your food, the higher it is in sodium and the lower it is in potassium. Major contributors of potassium to the adult dietary pattern include milk, potatoes, beef, coffee, tomatoes, and orange juice. Bananas are a popular fruit and an excellent source of potassium. Read more about them in the *Farm to Fork* feature in this section.

Potassium is efficiently absorbed from the small and large intestines—approximately 90% of what we consume gets absorbed—but typical American dietary patterns do not meet the AI for this mineral. The recently updated AIs for potassium are

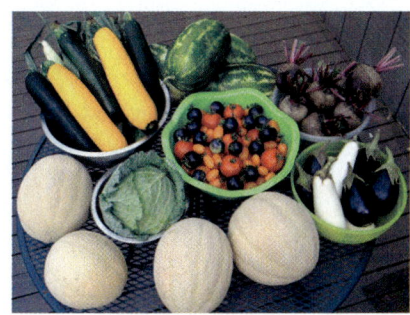

Fruits and vegetables are rich sources of potassium. Mary Jon Ludy/McGraw Hill

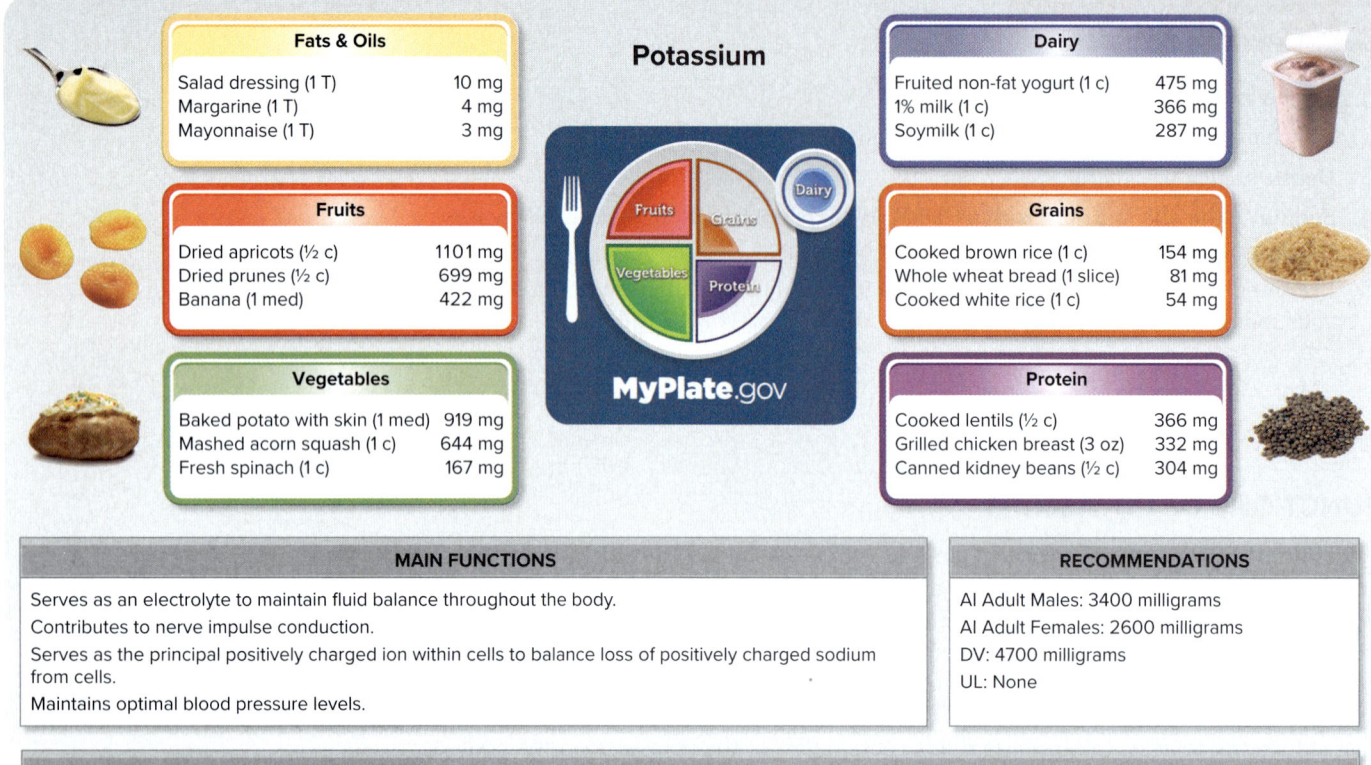

FIGURE 9-15 Food sources, functions, and recommendations for potassium. The fill of the background color (none, 1/3, 2/3, or completely covered) within each food group on MyPlate indicates the average nutrient density for potassium in that group. The figure shows the potassium content of several foods in each food group. Overall, the richest sources of potassium are unprocessed foods of plant origin, such as fruits, vegetables, and beans. mayonnaise: Iconotec/Alamy Stock Photo; dried apricots: lynx/iconotec/Glowimages; baked potato: DNY59/E+/Getty Images; yogurt in a container: Ingram Publishing/SuperStock; brown rice: Yellow Cat/Shutterstock; heap of lentils: asterix0597/E plus/Getty Images; MyPlate: U.S. Department of Agriculture

Source: Office of Dietary Supplements, Dietary Supplements Fact Sheets, available from https://ods.od.nih.gov/factsheets/list-all/; USDA FoodData Central, available from https://fdc.nal.usda.gov/

2600 milligrams per day for adult females and 3400 milligrams per day for adult males.[6] Many of us need to increase potassium intake, preferably by increasing fruit and vegetable intake.

According to the *Dietary Guidelines,* potassium is considered a dietary component of public health concern for the general U.S. population. This is because suboptimal intakes of potassium may contribute to cardiovascular disease and other health risks. To meet potassium recommendations, the *Dietary Guidelines* encourages individuals to increase intakes of vegetables, fruits, beans, whole grains, and dairy and fortified soy alternatives.

AVOIDING TOO MUCH POTASSIUM

At this time there is not sufficient research evidence to set a UL or CDRR for potassium. If the kidneys function normally, typical food intakes will not lead to potassium toxicity. When the kidneys function poorly, potassium increases in the blood, inhibiting heart function and leading to a slowed heartbeat. If left untreated, the heart eventually stops beating, resulting in a cardiac arrest and death. Therefore, in cases of kidney failure or kidney disease, close monitoring of the levels of potassium in blood and in the dietary pattern becomes critical. Experts suggest being cautious with potassium supplements.

✓ CONCEPT CHECK 9.4

1. List two functions of potassium in the body.
2. How is potassium intake related to blood pressure?
3. List three specific changes you could make to your dietary pattern to increase your potassium intake.

9.5 Chloride

FUNCTIONS OF CHLORIDE

Chloride (Cl) is a negative ion found primarily in the extracellular fluid. Along with sodium and potassium, chloride helps to regulate fluid balance in the body. In fact, chloride itself may be partially responsible for increases in blood pressure that accompany eating patterns high in salt.

Chloride ions are also a component of the acid produced in the stomach (hydrochloric acid) and are important for the overall maintenance of acid–base balance in the body. This electrolyte is used during immune responses as white blood cells attack foreign cells. In addition, nervous system function relies on the presence of chloride.

CHLORIDE DEFICIENCY

Low levels of chloride in the blood can lead to a disturbance of the body's acid–base balance. A chloride deficiency is unlikely, however, because our dietary salt intake is so high. Frequent and lengthy bouts of vomiting, if coupled with a nutrient-poor dietary pattern, can contribute to a deficiency because stomach secretions contain a lot of chloride. Individuals with bulimia nervosa or severe cases of gastroenteritis are at risk for chloride deficiency. In addition, low chloride levels could occur as a side effect of some medications, such as diuretics or laxatives.

GETTING ENOUGH CHLORIDE

When it comes to sources of chloride, it is important to make the distinction between the chloride ion, which is vital for body functions, and chlorine (Cl_2), which is a poisonous gas. Chlorine is used to disinfect municipal water supplies. A small amount of chlorine may remain in tap water, but the substance evaporates quickly. Municipal and well water supplies usually contain some chloride (leached from the earth) as well, but water does not represent a significant source of chloride.

A few fruits and vegetables, such as seaweed, celery, tomatoes, and olives, are naturally good sources of chloride. Most of our dietary chloride, however, comes from salt added to foods. Knowing a food's salt content allows for a close prediction of its chloride content. Salt is 60% chloride by weight.

Like sodium, chloride is efficiently absorbed. The AI for chloride (see box) is based on the 40:60 ratio of sodium to chloride in salt (1500 milligrams of sodium to 2300 milligrams of chloride).

FARM to FORK Bananas

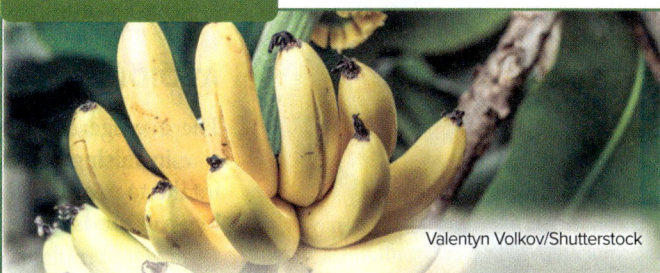
Valentyn Volkov/Shutterstock

Bananas are tasty and convenient sources of potassium. Bananas are the most consumed fruit in the United States—more than apples and oranges combined!

Grow
- Bananas grow on "banana palms," which are actually a perennial herb rather than a tree.
- Bananas do not grow from a seed but instead from a bulb or rhizome. After planting a banana palm in a subtropical environment, it can take up to 12 months to literally enjoy the fruits of your labor.
- Because bananas grow in tropical climates, they are not seasonal fruits but rather continue to grow all year long.

Shop
- There are two main categories of bananas. Plantains (or cooking bananas) are starchy, and Cavendish (or dessert bananas) are the sweet, yellow bananas most commonly sold at the supermarket.
- To get the most antioxidants from bananas, look beyond Cavendish bananas. Red bananas and niños, or Lady Fingers, provide greater vitamin C, potassium, calcium, manganese, carotenoids, and zinc than the common Cavendish.

Store
- Bananas continue to ripen after harvest and are often harvested when immature and green. These bananas ripen in 5 to 7 days at room temperature.
- Store ripe bananas in the refrigerator. Although their skins will turn brown, the flesh will stay fresher for days.
- Instead of throwing away overripe bananas, slice and freeze the fruit for use in smoothies or baked goods, or use a food dehydrator to make your own dried banana chips.

Prep
- Plantains are the main carbohydrate source for 20 million people globally. Harvested when green, plantains are skinned, then steamed, baked, or fried.
- In the Caribbean, fried plantains are a dietary staple. For a healthier recipe, try baked plantains. Use ripe plantains, spotted with brown or black spots, and slice after peeling. Coat a nonstick baking sheet with cooking spray and lay the plantains in rows. Cook at 450°F for 15 minutes, flipping them frequently.
- Celebrate bananas as the perfect on-the-go snack, lunch box treat, or sliced treat on top of cereal, yogurt, or whole wheat pancakes.

Source: Robinson J. Tropical fruits: make the most of eating globally. In *Eating on the Wild Side: The Missing Link to Optimum Health.* New York: Little, Brown & Co.; 2013.

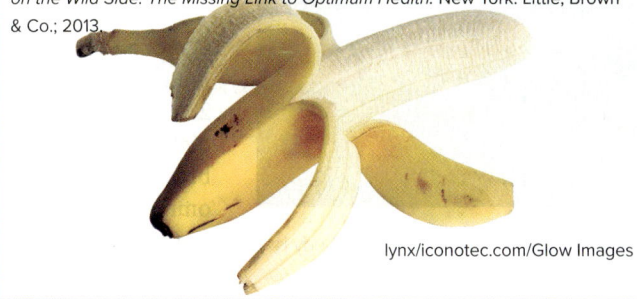
lynx/iconotec.com/Glow Images

Newsworthy Nutrition

Calcium supplements and cardiovascular disease risk

INTRODUCTION: Although several studies have shown a beneficial effect of calcium intake on cardiovascular effects, others have shown that calcium intake, especially from calcium supplements, is associated with increased mortality or the risk of heart attack and stroke. **OBJECTIVE:** The goal of this study was to explore the associations between calcium from dietary and supplemental intakes and cardiovascular disease (CVD) risks. **METHODS:** The study design was a *systematic review and meta-analysis* of 16 randomized controlled trials and 26 prospective cohort studies of dietary or supplemental intake of calcium, with or without vitamin D, and cardiovascular outcomes. Data was from PubMed, Cochrane Central, Scopus, and Web of Science, published up to March 2019. **RESULTS:** Results of cohort studies indicated that there were no associations between dietary calcium intakes and the risk of CVD, coronary heart disease (CHD), and stroke, for intakes ranging from 200 to 1500 mg/day. Results showed that calcium supplements, ranging from 1000 to 1400 mg/day, did not increase the risk of CVD and stroke; however, the risk of CHD increased by 20% and the risk of heart attack increased by 21% with the use of oral calcium supplements. **CONCLUSIONS:** Keeping in mind that very high calcium intakes are difficult if not impossible to achieve by dietary sources alone, the authors conclude that calcium intake from dietary sources does not increase the risk of CVD, and they suggest that adequate dietary calcium intakes are beneficial to cardiovascular protection. They conclude that calcium supplements might raise CHD risk, especially heart attack, and therefore the concerns regarding potential adverse cardiovascular risks are related to the use of calcium supplements.

Source: Yang C, Shi X, Xia H, et al. The evidence and controversy between dietary calcium intake and calcium supplementation and the risk of cardiovascular disease: a systematic review and meta-analysis of cohort studies and randomized controlled trials. *J Am Coll Nutr.* May-Jun 2020;39(4):352370. doi: 10.1080/07315724.2019.1649219

health and worsen cardiovascular health. One study found that a calcium intake beyond the RDA for elderly individuals, usually achieved by calcium supplements, did not provide any benefit for hip or lumbar spine bone mineral density in older adults.[17] The results of other studies, including the large Women's Health Initiative trial, have shown an increase in the rate of heart attacks and possibly stroke among older adults taking calcium supplements with or without vitamin D.[18] A recent meta-analysis of cohort studies and randomized controlled trials also determined that calcium supplements are linked to adverse cardiovascular events, especially heart attacks (see *Newsworthy Nutrition*).

On the positive side, another report from the Women's Health Initiative study indicates that long-term use of a daily calcium and vitamin D supplement that is close to the RDA results in a substantial reduction in the risk of hip fracture among postmenopausal females.[19] These authors also reported that this level of calcium and vitamin D supplementation did not result in an increase in other chronic diseases, including heart disease. The more positive effects of supplementation appear to happen when the level of total calcium and vitamin D intake is kept very close to the RDA. Therefore, taking 1000 milligrams of calcium carbonate or calcium citrate daily as a supplement in divided doses (about 500 milligrams per tablet) is probably safe in many instances.

So which is better: calcium from food or supplements? The National Osteoporosis Foundation and other experts agree that we should consume the recommended amounts of calcium and vitamin D from foods first and that more research is needed to better comprehend the benefits and risks associated with calcium and vitamin D supplementation. Modification of eating habits to include foods that are good sources of calcium appears to be the safest means to prevent osteoporosis without jeopardizing heart health. Foods that contain calcium also supply other vitamins, minerals, phytochemicals, and fats needed to support health. Problems associated with excessive consumption of calcium, such as constipation, are not likely when foods are the primary sources of calcium.

TABLE 9-2 ■ Calcium Supplement Comparisons

	Calcium Carbonate	Calcium Citrate
Calcium content	40%	21%
Forms	Tablets, chewable tablets, soft chews	Pills (can be quite large) Liquid (sometimes easier to tolerate)
Cost	Least expensive, most common form	Most expensive
Bioavailability and meal timing	Needs acidic environment in stomach, so take with acidic food or take with meals	Best absorbed; does not need acidic environment to be absorbed

In an effort to provide guidance for the public, the U.S. Preventive Services Task Force reviewed current research studies on the use of vitamin D and calcium supplements to prevent fractures and issued recommendations.[20] The recommendations apply to adults who live at home. They do not apply to those living in assisted living or skilled nursing facilities or who have been diagnosed with osteoporosis or vitamin D deficiency. The Task Force concluded that there is currently not enough evidence to determine if vitamin D and calcium supplementation, alone or combined, are beneficial or harmful for the prevention of fractures. See Section 9.18 for a summary of the conclusions of the Task Force.

Keeping in mind the recommendations just discussed, increasing calcium intake through the use of a calcium supplement may be beneficial if you have a milk allergy; do not like milk; are ovovegetarian, vegan, or lactose intolerant; or cannot incorporate enough calcium-containing foods into your dietary pattern.[21] Always look for a supplement with added vitamin D, as it enhances calcium uptake. This additional vitamin D typically does not add to the cost of the supplement. Table 9-2 compares the two most common forms of calcium supplements. Calcium carbonate should be taken with meals because it requires an acidic environment in the stomach to dissolve and maximize calcium absorption. Calcium citrate is indicated for people who cannot remember to take calcium carbonate with meals and for those who have low-acid stomach conditions, such as people who take acid-reducing medications for ulcers or reflux, or those who have had bariatric surgery.

Calcium supplements have side effects, including gas, bloating, or constipation. Distributing small-dose supplements throughout the day, taking them with meals, or even changing the supplement brand may alleviate some problems. Intake of calcium from supplements and/or food above 500 milligrams at any one time significantly reduces the percent absorbed.

With calcium supplements, interactions with other minerals are a concern. There is evidence that calcium supplements may decrease the absorption of zinc, iron, and other minerals. An effect of calcium supplementation on iron absorption is possible; however, this appears to be small over the long term. To be safe, people using a calcium supplement on a regular basis should notify their primary care provider of the practice. Calcium supplements can also interfere with the body's ability to absorb certain antibiotics. If your doctor prescribes antibiotics, especially tetracycline, be sure to talk with your pharmacist about the timing of your supplement, medication, and meals.

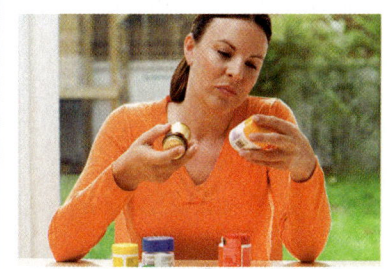

Tablet or liquid calcium supplements with the U.S. Pharmacopeia (USP) symbol are considered the safest. FDA has cautioned the public on the use of calcium supplements from dolomite, bone meal, coral, or oyster shell because of the potential for unhealthy levels of environmental contaminants, especially lead. **Why are supplements containing calcium citrate more desirable than those containing calcium carbonate?** Isadora Getty Buyou/Image Source

✓ CONCEPT CHECK 9.6

1. What percentage of calcium in the body is found in bones?
2. Beyond its role in bone health, what are some other critical functions of calcium?
3. What role does vitamin D play in calcium metabolism?
4. What factors reduce calcium absorption?

9.7 Phosphorus

FUNCTIONS OF PHOSPHORUS

Phosphorus (P) is the second most abundant mineral in the body. Approximately 85% of phosphorus is found as a component of hydroxyapatite crystals that provide the functional component of bone and teeth. The remaining 15% of phosphorus is in the soft tissues, blood, and extracellular fluid. Phosphorus is part of DNA and RNA, the genetic material present in every cell. Because DNA and RNA are responsible for protein synthesis, phosphorus is critical for cellular replication and growth. Phosphorus is also a primary component of adenosine triphosphate (ATP), the energy molecule that fuels body functions. Phosphorus is essential for the activation and deactivation of certain enzymes, and many of the B vitamins are functional only when a phosphate group is attached.

A major class of lipids, the **phospholipids,** also contains phosphorus. Recall that phospholipids are the principal structural component of cell membranes, making up approximately 60% of membranes. Cell membranes regulate the transport of nutrients and waste products into and out of cells. Phosphorus also serves as a buffer to maintain blood pH. Lastly, phosphorus (in the form of the phosphate ion) is the principal negatively charged ion in intracellular fluid and thus is essential for the maintenance of fluid balance.

phospholipid Any of a class of fat-related substances that contain phosphorus, fatty acids, and a nitrogen-containing component. Phospholipids are an essential part of every cell.

PHOSPHORUS DEFICIENCY

Deficiencies of phosphorus are unlikely in healthy adults because it is widespread in food and beverages and efficiently absorbed. If intakes of phosphorus are inadequate, the kidney compensates by increasing the reabsorption of phosphorus to prevent blood phosphorus levels from decreasing. Dietary phosphorus deficiency usually occurs only in cases of near-total starvation, including anorexia nervosa. Some health conditions, such as diabetes and alcohol use disorders, and use of certain medications, such as antacids and diuretics, can cause body phosphorus levels to fall. Marginal phosphorus status can be found in infants born preterm, individuals consuming a vegan dietary pattern, older people with nutrient-poor dietary patterns, and people with long-term bouts of diarrhea, as often occurs in Crohn's disease and celiac disease. Symptoms of phosphorus deficiency include loss of appetite, anemia, muscle weakness, bone pain, fragile bones, increased susceptibility to infection, numbness and tingling of the extremities, difficulty walking, and irregular breathing.[22]

GETTING ENOUGH PHOSPHORUS

Phosphorus is naturally abundant in many foods and beverages. Milk, cheese, meat, and bread provide most of the phosphorus in the adult dietary pattern. Nuts, fish, breakfast cereals, bran, and eggs are also good sources (Fig. 9-19). About 20% to 30% of dietary phosphorus comes from food additives, especially in baked goods, cheeses, processed meats, and many soft drinks (about 75 milligrams per 12 ounces). As a food additive, phosphorus is considered a GRAS (generally recognized as safe) substance, and its function is to increase water binding and taste. Phosphoric acid, which gives a tangy, sour taste, will also significantly lower the pH of a food or beverage, such as a soft drink that has a pH less than 3. Absorption of phosphorus is generally high, ranging from 55% to 80%. Phosphorus absorption from grains, however, is reduced because of the high phytic acid content. Vitamin D enhances phosphorus absorption.

The RDA for phosphorus is 700 milligrams for adults (Fig. 9.19). The recommendation is higher (1250 milligrams per day) for young people ages 9 to 18 years to support growth and development. Average daily adult consumption is about 1200 to 1600 milligrams.[15]

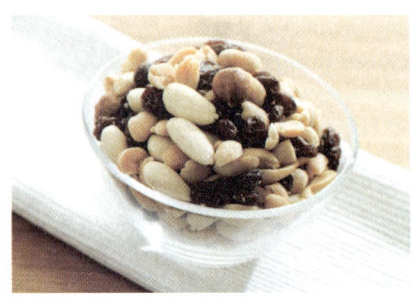

Trail mix is rich in phosphorus. imagebroker/Alamy Stock Photo

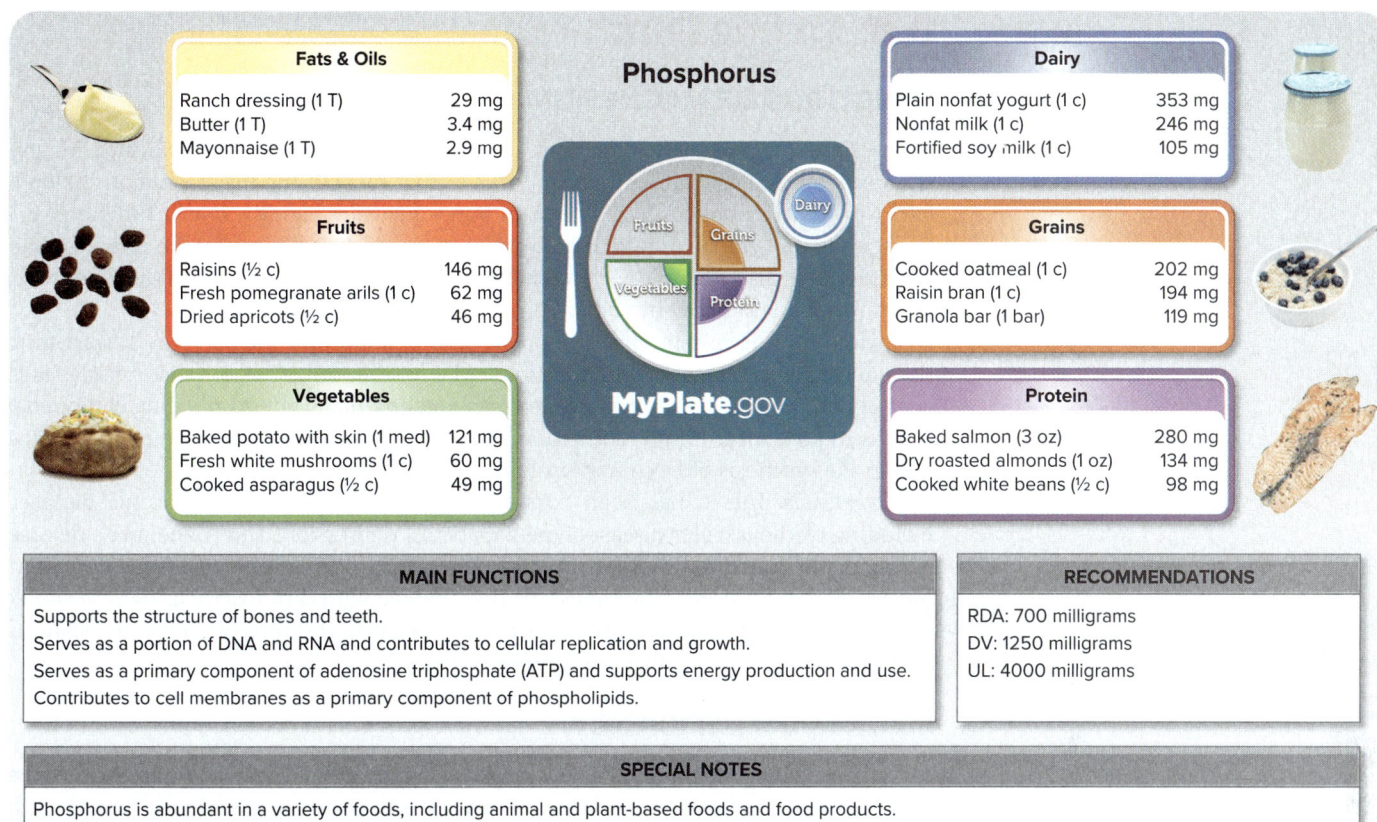

FIGURE 9-19 Food sources, functions, and recommendations for phosphorus. The fill of the background color (none, 1/3, 2/3, or completely covered) within each food group on MyPlate indicates the average nutrient density for phosphorus in that group. The figure shows the phosphorus content of several foods in each food group. Overall, the richest sources of phosphorus are dairy products and protein foods. mayonnaise: Iconotec/Alamy Stock Photo; raisins: lynx/iconotec/Glowimages; baked potato: DNY59/E+/Getty Images; two jars of yogurt: Foodcollection; oatmeal and blueberries: Lucy Stein/Image Source/Glow Images; salmon: Zoran Kolundzija/E+/Getty images; MyPlate: U.S. Department of Agriculture

Sources: Office of Dietary Supplements, Dietary Supplements Fact Sheets, available from https://ods.od.nih.gov/factsheets/list-all/; USDA FoodData Central, available from https://fdc.nal.usda.gov/

AVOIDING TOO MUCH PHOSPHORUS

The UL for phosphorus is 4000 milligrams per day for adults through age 70 and 3000 milligrams per day for those older than 70 years. Intakes greater than this can result in the mineralization of soft tissues. Phosphorus levels in the blood are regulated primarily by the kidneys, and these organs are particularly sensitive to phosphorus toxicity. High intakes can lead to serious problems in people with certain kidney diseases. In addition, a high phosphorus intake coupled with a low calcium intake can cause a chronic imbalance in the calcium-to-phosphorus ratio in the dietary pattern and contribute to bone loss. This situation most likely arises when the RDA for calcium is not met, as can occur in adolescents and adults who regularly substitute soft drinks for milk or otherwise underconsume calcium.

✓ CONCEPT CHECK 9.7

1. What effect does vitamin D have on phosphorus absorption?
2. What are the key functions of phosphorus beyond bone health?
3. Is a deficiency of phosphorus likely? Why or why not?
4. What are the primary food sources of phosphorus?
5. What are the risks of excess intake of phosphorus?

9.8 Magnesium

FUNCTIONS OF MAGNESIUM

Magnesium (Mg) has many functions, some of which are related to bone health. Magnesium is similar to calcium and phosphorus in that most of the magnesium in the body (60%) is found in bones. Magnesium in bones provides rigidity, and it functions as a storage site that can be drawn upon by other tissues when dietary intake is inadequate. Magnesium is also required for the synthesis of vitamin D in the liver. It also promotes resistance to tooth decay by stabilizing calcium in tooth enamel.

Beyond its role in bone health, magnesium is important for nerve and heart function, and aids in many enzyme reactions. Magnesium functions to relax muscles after contraction. Over 300 enzymes use magnesium, and many energy-yielding compounds in cells require magnesium to function properly (e.g., ATP). Magnesium plays a critical role in the synthesis of DNA and protein.[23]

Magnesium intake has been correlated to the risk for several chronic diseases, including cardiovascular disease, type 2 diabetes, depression, and Alzheimer's disease. For example, meeting the RDA for magnesium may decrease blood pressure by dilating arteries and prevent heart abnormalities. People with cardiovascular disease should closely monitor magnesium intake, especially because they are often on medications, such as diuretics, that reduce magnesium levels.[24]

MAGNESIUM DEFICIENCY

In humans, a magnesium deficiency causes an irregular heartbeat, sometimes accompanied by weakness, muscle pain, disorientation, and seizures. In terms of bone health, low magnesium levels disrupt the hormonal regulation of blood calcium by parathyroid hormone and affect the activity of vitamin D (review Fig. 9-16).[25] You might expect that magnesium deficiency would result in diminished bone mass, but to date, this has only been observed in animals. There is some evidence, however, that magnesium supplementation may improve bone density in postmenopausal females.

Magnesium deficiency develops very slowly. Not only is the mineral present in foods of both plant and animal origin, but the kidneys also are very efficient at retaining magnesium. Poor magnesium status is most commonly found among people with abnormal kidney function, whether as a result of kidney disease or as a side effect of certain diuretics. Alcohol use disorders also can increase the risk of deficiency because dietary intake may be poor and because alcohol increases magnesium excretion in the urine. The disorientation and weakness associated with alcohol use disorders closely resemble the behavior of people with low blood magnesium. In addition, people with malabsorptive diseases (e.g., Crohn's disease), heavy perspiration, or prolonged bouts of diarrhea or vomiting are susceptible to low blood levels of magnesium.

GETTING ENOUGH MAGNESIUM

Magnesium is found in the plant pigment chlorophyll, so rich sources of magnesium are plant products, such as squash, whole grains (e.g., wheat bran), beans, nuts, seeds, and broccoli (Fig. 9-20). Animal products (e.g., milk and meats) and chocolate supply some magnesium, although not as much as foods of plant origin. Another source of magnesium is hard tap water, which contains a high mineral content.

The RDA for magnesium varies by age and biological sex, based on the amount needed to offset daily losses (Fig 9-20).[26] On average, adult males consume approximately 340 milligrams daily, whereas adult females consume approximately 270 milligrams daily, suggesting that many of us should improve our intakes of magnesium-rich foods, such as whole-grain breads and cereals. The refined grain products that dominate the typical American dietary pattern are poor sources of this mineral because refining reduces the magnesium content by as much as 80%. This low value also reflects poor intake of green and other brightly colored vegetables. Speak to your primary care

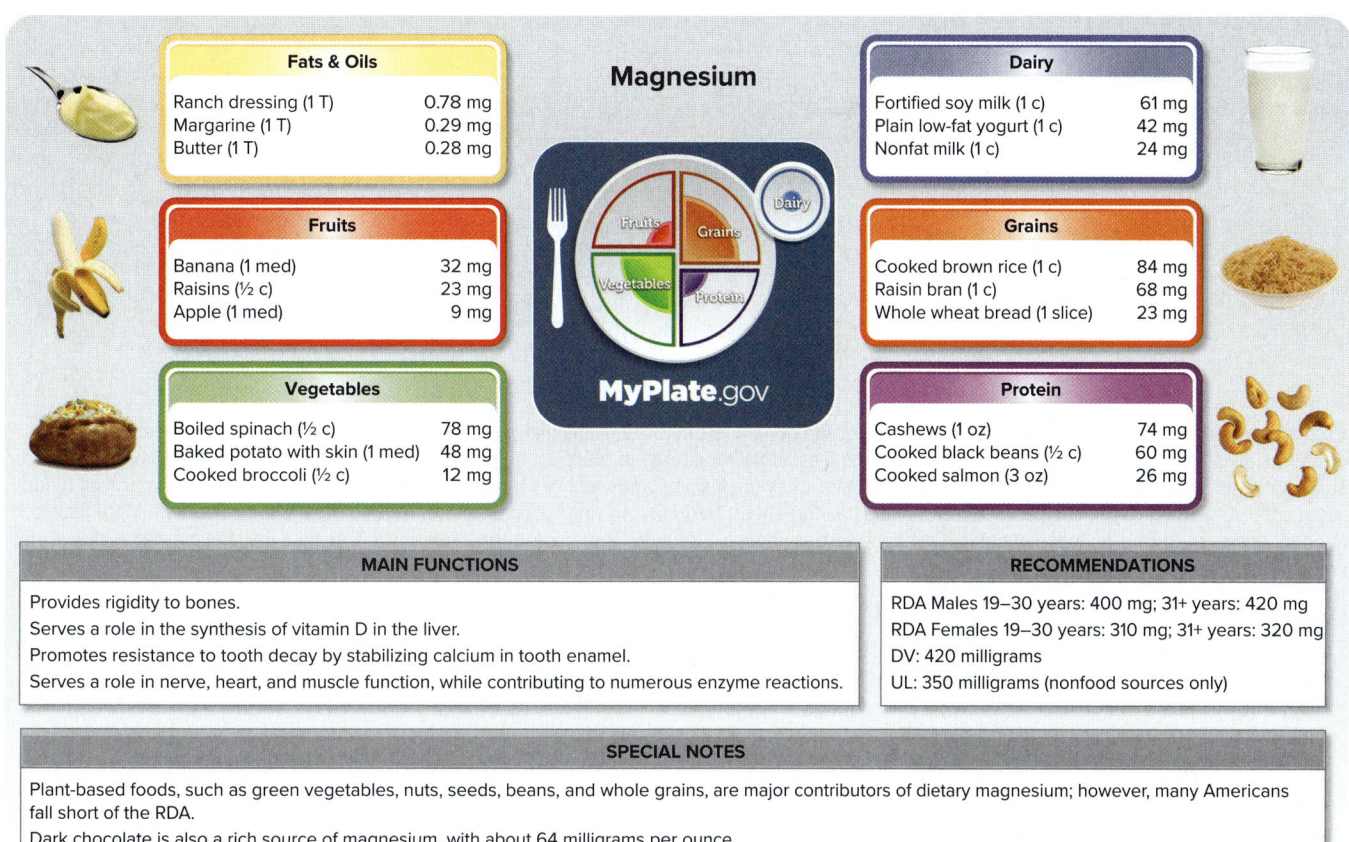

FIGURE 9-20 Food sources, functions, and recommendations for magnesium. The fill of the background color (none, 1/3, 2/3, or completely covered) within each food group on MyPlate indicates the average nutrient density for magnesium in that group. The figure shows the magnesium content of several foods in each food group. Overall, the richest sources of magnesium are vegetables and whole grains. mayonnaise: Iconotec/Alamy Stock Photo; banana: lynx/iconotec.com/Glow Images; baked potato: DNY59/E+/Getty Images; glass of milk: Nipaporn Panyacharoen/Shutterstock; brown rice in bowl: Yellow Cat/Shutterstock; cashew nuts: C Squared Studios/Photodisc/Getty Images; MyPlate: U.S. Department of Agriculture

Sources: Office of Dietary Supplements, Dietary Supplements Fact Sheets, available from https://ods.od.nih.gov/factsheets/list-all/; USDA FoodData Central, available from https://fdc.nal.usda.gov/

provider or an RDN if you are concerned about your magnesium intake. If dietary intake of magnesium is inadequate, a balanced multivitamin and mineral supplement containing approximately 100 milligrams of magnesium can help close the gap between intake and needs. Dietary patterns very high in phosphorus or fiber (phytate) limit intestinal absorption of magnesium, as do dietary patterns too low in protein.

AVOIDING TOO MUCH MAGNESIUM

The UL for magnesium intake is 350 milligrams per day, based on the risk of higher intakes causing diarrhea. This guideline refers only to *nonfood* sources such as antacids, laxatives, or supplements.[26] Food sources are not known to cause toxicity. Magnesium toxicity especially occurs in people who have kidney failure or who overuse over-the-counter medications that contain magnesium, such as certain antacids and laxatives (e.g., milk of magnesia). Older people are at particular risk, as kidney function may be compromised.

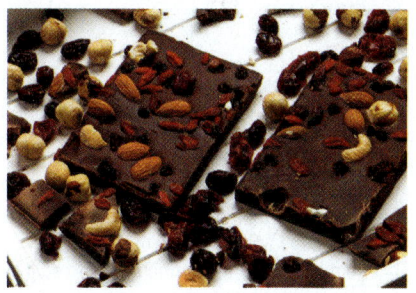

Magnesium is in good supply in the dark chocolate (64 milligrams in 1 ounce) and nuts (82 milligrams in 1 ounce of cashews) shown here. CDL Creative Studio/Shutterstock

✓ CONCEPT CHECK 9.8

1. List three functions of magnesium.
2. What are the primary food sources of magnesium?
3. Who is at greatest risk of developing a magnesium deficiency?
4. When is magnesium toxicity most likely to occur?

FARM to FORK Cashews

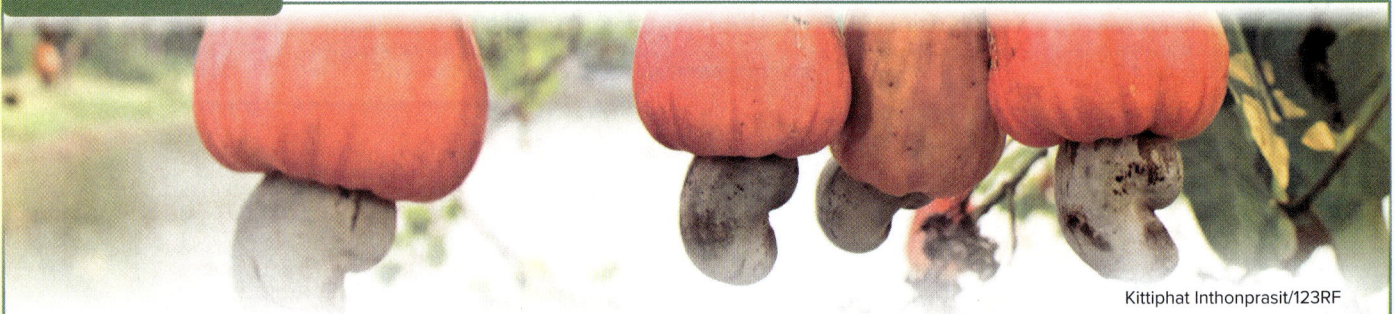

Kittiphat Inthonprasit/123RF

Cashews are rich in fiber, unsaturated fats, plant protein, and beneficial phytochemicals that may help reduce inflammation and protect us from disease. Cashews are also a good source of copper, a mineral essential for energy production, healthy brain development, and a strong immune system, and magnesium and manganese, important for bone health. They are low in sugar and have been linked to benefits like weight loss, improved blood sugar control to protect against type 2 diabetes, and a healthier heart through lowering blood pressure, triglycerides, and cholesterol. More research is needed, however, to confirm these benefits. Cashews are classified as tree nuts. Therefore, people allergic to tree nuts may have a higher risk of also being allergic to cashews.

Grow
- Cashews are the seeds of a tropical evergreen shrub cultivated in warm, humid climates and related to mango, pistachio, and poison ivy. The cashew seed hangs from the bottom of a cashew apple. Fresh cashew apples taste delicious but are highly perishable.
- The kidney-shaped cashew seed is harvested by hand and is encased in a hard shell with two layers. Between these two layers is a toxic resin, urushiol (also found in poison ivy), which can trigger a skin reaction.
- During processing, the cashew kernels are shelled and cooked to remove the toxic urushiol, and the resulting product is sold as "raw" cashews.

Shop
- Cashews are sold in bags or in bulk bins and may be salted, unsalted, or flavored.
- For the freshest cashews, make sure there is no evidence of moisture or insects and that the cashews are not shriveled. If buying in bulk, smell the cashews to ensure they are not rancid. Cashews sold in vacuum-packed jars or cans will stay fresh longest.
- Cashews sold as "roasted" have been cooked twice—once during the shelling process and then roasted to deepen the color and enhance the flavor, sometimes with salt. Dry-roasted nuts are cooked without any added oil.
- For the most nutritional benefits and to limit excess salt or added fats, consider choosing dry roasted or "raw" unsalted cashew varieties whenever possible.

Store
- Because cashews are high in unsaturated fatty acids, they are susceptible to oxidation and rancidity and should be stored in an airtight container to minimize air exposure.
- Refrigerate or freeze cashews in tightly sealed containers to help them last longer. Cashews can last up to 6 months in the refrigerator and up to 1 year in the freezer.

Prep
- Cashews can be eaten "raw" or roasted and are a portable snack. Whole cashews can be used in stir-fries, soups, salads, and stews. Asian and Indian cuisines frequently include whole or chopped cashews as a stir-fry ingredient and in curries.
- Owing to their creamy texture when blended, cashews are used to make several dairy alternatives. These include cashew milk, cream and cream sauces, cheese, mayonnaise, butter, and pesto.
- To make cashew butter, roast cashews at 330°F/165°C for 10 to 15 minutes, until golden in color and fragrant. After the nuts have cooled, blend them in a food processor until smooth (about 12 to 15 minutes). Cashew butter can be spread on toast, stirred into yogurt or oatmeal, or mixed with oats and dried fruit to make no-bake energy bites.
- To make dairy-free sour cream or cream cheese, soak cashews and blend them with apple cider vinegar or lemon juice. A probiotic can also be used to ferment the cream cheese (https://www.hummusapien.com/vegan-cashew-cream-cheese-recipe/).

Sources: Are cashews good for you? Nutrition, benefits, and downsides. *Healthline*. Updated June 10, 2020. https://www.healthline.com/nutrition/are-cashews-good-for-you Oliveira NN, Mothé CG, Mothé MC, de Oliveira LG. Cashew nut and cashew apple: a scientific and technological monitoring worldwide review. *J Food Sci Technol*. 2020 Jan;57(1):12-21. doi: 10.1007/s13197-019-04051-7

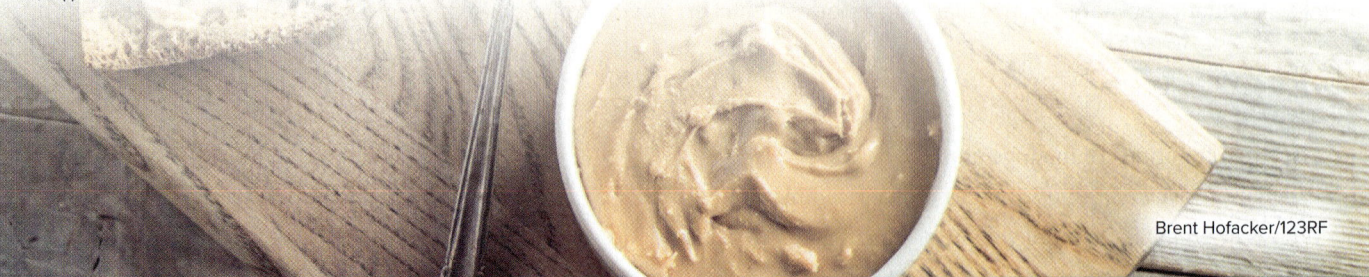

Brent Hofacker/123RF

9.9 Iron

Iron (Fe) is a trace mineral. The total amount of iron in the body is only 10 grams, which is about as heavy as 2 nickels. Even though we only need to eat small amounts of this trace mineral each day, iron has some mighty important functions.

FUNCTIONS OF IRON

Iron is part of the **hemoglobin** in red blood cells and **myoglobin** in muscle cells. Hemoglobin molecules in red blood cells transport oxygen (O_2) from the lungs to all the cells of the body and then transport carbon dioxide (CO_2) from cells back to the lungs for excretion. In addition, iron is used as part of many enzymes, some proteins, and compounds that cells use in energy production. Iron also is needed for brain and immune function, drug detoxification in the liver, and synthesis of collagen for bone health.[27]

IRON DEFICIENCY

Iron deficiency is the most common nutrient deficiency worldwide. Globally, about 40% of children and about 30% of females of reproductive age are anemic, and more than half of these cases are caused by iron deficiency.[28]

When neither the dietary pattern nor body stores can supply the iron needed for hemoglobin synthesis, the concentration of hemoglobin in red blood cells decreases. The percentage of blood made up of red blood cells **(hematocrit)** as well as the hemoglobin concentration in the blood are used to assess iron status. Other measures of iron status include the concentration of iron (serum iron) and iron-containing proteins in blood (**ferritin** or **transferrin**).

When hematocrit and hemoglobin fall, an iron deficiency is suspected. In a severe deficiency, hemoglobin and hematocrit fall so low that the amount of oxygen carried in the bloodstream is decreased. This condition is called *iron-deficiency anemia*.

Iron deficiency can be categorized into three stages:

- **Stage 1:** Iron stores become depleted, but no physiological impairment is observed.
- **Stage 2:** The amount of iron in transferrin is depleted; some physiological impairment occurs. Heme production is decreased, and the activities of enzymes that require iron as a cofactor are limited.
- **Stage 3** *(iron-deficiency anemia):* Red blood cells are small **(microcytic)**, pale **(hypochromic)**, and reduced in number; the oxygen-carrying capacity of red blood cells declines.

Clinical symptoms of iron-deficiency anemia are associated with the lack of oxygen getting to the tissues. An individual with iron-deficiency anemia may experience pale skin, fatigue upon exertion, poor temperature regulation (always feeling cold, especially toes and fingers), loss of appetite, and apathy. Poor iron stores may decrease learning ability, attention span, work performance, and immune status even before a person is anemic. Children with chronic anemia have abnormal cognitive development.

Note that many more people have an iron deficiency *without* anemia (stages 1 or 2) than have iron-deficiency anemia (stage 3). Their blood hemoglobin values are still normal, but they have no stores to draw from in times of pregnancy or illness, and basic functioning may be marginally impaired. That could mean anything from chronic fatigue to difficulties staying mentally alert.

It is important to understand that many conditions lead to an anemic state; iron-deficiency anemia is the most prevalent nutrient deficiency worldwide. About 10% of U.S. females and 2% of U.S. males have anemia. Over the past 20 years, the prevalence of anemia appears to be rising, most likely due to lower dietary iron intakes.[29] This appears most often in infancy, during the preschool years, and at puberty. Growth—with accompanying expansion of blood volume and muscle mass—increases iron needs, and some individuals are unable to consume enough iron to meet the body's requirements. Females are vulnerable to anemia during childbearing years

hemoglobin The iron-containing part of the red blood cell that carries oxygen to the cells and carbon dioxide away from the cells. The heme iron portion is also responsible for the red color of blood.

myoglobin Iron-containing protein that binds oxygen in muscle tissue.

hematocrit The percentage of blood made up of red blood cells.

ferritin A protein that stores iron and releases it in a controlled manner; acts as a buffer against iron deficiency and iron overload.

transferrin Iron-binding protein; controls the level of free iron in blood.

microcytic Small cell size.

hypochromic Pale in color (in reference to red blood cells), as could occur with inadequate hemoglobin content.

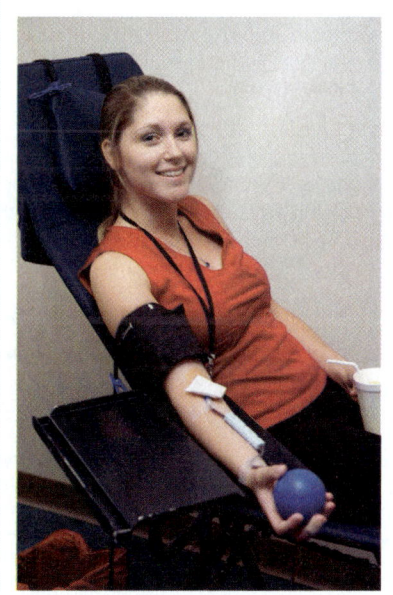

Red blood cells contain about two-thirds of the body's total iron supply. Each time blood is donated, about 10% of total blood volume is sacrificed, which removes about 7% of the body's iron supply. Over the next few weeks, the red blood cells will be replaced, so healthy people can usually donate blood two to four times a year without harmful consequences. **How do blood banks screen potential donors for anemia?**
David H. Lewis/E+/Getty Images

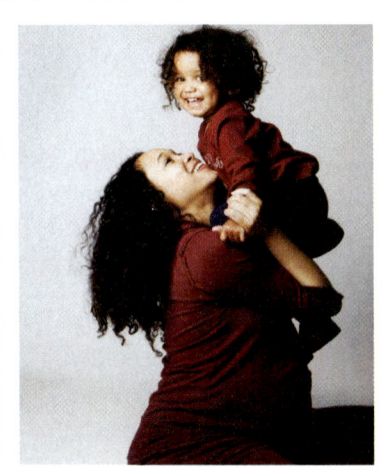

Iron deficiency is the most common nutrient deficiency. **Why are females who are pregnant and children of preschool age at risk for iron-deficiency anemia?** Tanya Constantine/Blend Images/Getty Images

heme iron Iron provided from animal tissues in the form of hemoglobin and myoglobin. Approximately 40% of the iron in meat, fish, and poultry is heme iron; it is readily absorbed.

nonheme iron Iron provided from plant sources, supplements, and animal tissues other than in the forms of hemoglobin and myoglobin. Nonheme iron is less efficiently absorbed than heme iron; absorption is closely dependent on body needs.

magnificent microbiome

Iron Bioavailability

Several *in vitro* (i.e., test-tube) studies have shown interactions between iron and the intestinal microbiota. The gut microbiota can favorably modify dietary nonheme iron, leading to an increase in iron availability. In addition, *Bifidobacteriaceae* can bind the iron present in the large intestine, which limits the formation of free radicals and thereby reduces the risk of colorectal cancer. On the negative side, high levels of iron in the intestine can promote the development of pathogenic microorganisms.

Source: Skrypnik K, Suliburska J. Association between the gut microbiota and mineral metabolism. *J Sci Food Agric*. 2018;98(7):2449-2460. doi: 10.1002/jsfa.8724

due to menstrual blood loss. Anemia is also found among females who are pregnant because blood volume expands during pregnancy and extra iron is needed to synthesize red blood cells for the mother and the fetus.[30] Iron-deficiency anemia can also be caused by blood loss from ulcers, colon cancer, or hemorrhoids. Endurance athletes may have increased iron requirements due to increased blood loss in feces and urine and chronic lysis of red blood cells in the feet due to the trauma of running. Additional risk factors for iron-deficiency anemia include inappropriately planned vegan dietary patterns, extreme dietary restrictions (e.g., eating disorders), and frequent blood donation.

To cure iron-deficiency anemia, a person needs to take iron supplements.[31] A primary care provider should also find the cause so that the anemia does not reoccur. Changes in the dietary pattern may *prevent* iron-deficiency anemia, but supplemental iron is the only reliable *cure* once it has developed. Supplements must be taken for 3 to 6 months or perhaps longer. Hemoglobin levels respond quickly to dietary changes and supplementation, but stopping supplements too soon means that iron stores (blood, bone marrow, etc.) will not be fully replenished. Remember, it takes longer than 1 month to become anemic, so it will take longer than 1 month to cure it.

ABSORPTION AND DISTRIBUTION OF IRON

Overall, iron absorption depends on the following factors: (1) the person's iron status; (2) its form in food; (3) the acidity of the GI tract; and (4) other dietary components consumed with iron-containing foods. Controlling iron levels in the body is important because there is a narrow gap between just enough and too much iron. As you've learned, too little iron can impair oxygen transport. To prevent deficiency, the human body highly conserves iron. Except for bleeding associated with menstruation, injury, or childbirth, body loss of iron is minimal. Approximately 90% is recovered and reused every day. On the other hand, too much iron in the body is also extremely damaging. It can accumulate in organs and promote oxidative damage. To avoid toxicity, iron absorption from the small intestine is tightly regulated.

The most important factor influencing iron absorption is the body's need for iron. Iron needs are increased during pregnancy and growth. At high altitudes, the lower oxygen concentration of the air causes an increase in the hemoglobin concentration of blood and thus an increase in iron needs.

The principal mechanism to regulate iron content in the body is tight control of absorption. High doses of iron can still be toxic, but absorption is carefully regulated under most conditions. In general, healthy people with adequate iron stores absorb between 5% and 15% of dietary iron, which is quite low compared to other nutrients. When iron stores are inadequate or needs are high due to growth or pregnancy, the main protein that carries iron (transferrin) more readily binds iron, shifting it from the intestinal cells into the bloodstream. Absorption efficiency in times of need can be as high as 50%. On the other hand, if iron stores are adequate and the iron-binding protein in the blood is fully saturated with iron, absorption from the intestinal cells is minimal—as low as 2%. The iron remains in the intestinal cells, and it will be excreted in the feces when those intestinal cells slough off, which occurs every 5 to 6 days.

Another major influence on iron absorption is the form of iron in the food. **Heme iron,** derived from hemoglobin and myoglobin, comprises 40% of the iron in meat, fish, and poultry (MFP). Absorption of heme iron ranges from about 15% to 35%. Almost nothing affects its absorption. **Nonheme iron,** on the other

TABLE 9-3 ■ Dietary Factors That Affect Nonheme Iron Absorption

Nonheme Enhancers	Nonheme Inhibitors
Vitamin C • Add marinara sauce to your spaghetti noodles. MFP (meat, fish, poultry) meat protein • Add some tuna to your snack of crackers.	Tannins (found in tea) • Drink tea between meals rather than with meals. (Does not apply to herbal tea.) Oxalates (spinach, rhubarb, and chard) Phytates (whole grains, bran, and soybean) Megadoses of calcium

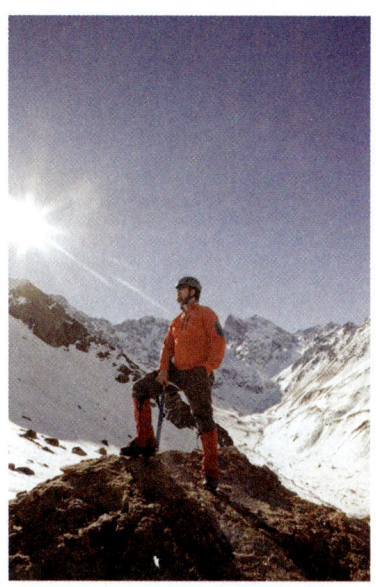

Micah is preparing for a hiking trip in the Rocky Mountains. To support optimal physical performance at high altitude, where the oxygen levels in the air are lower, his body must manufacture additional red blood cells to transport oxygen through his blood. **Design three meals or snacks Micah could eat to supply the nutrients that support healthy red blood cells.** REB Images/Getty Images

hand, is subject to many conditions that can either enhance or inhibit its absorption, which ranges from 2% to 8%. Table 9-3 summarizes dietary factors that affect the bioavailability of nonheme iron. Nonheme iron makes up 60% of the iron in MFP and 100% of the iron found in beans, peas, lentils, fruits, vegetables, grains, fortified foods, and supplements. Because most of our dietary iron is nonheme iron, our overall dietary iron absorption is 5% to 15%.[32]

Acidity also affects iron absorption: an acidic environment solubilizes iron and keeps it in a form that can be readily absorbed. Therefore, any medication or health condition that lowers acid production in the stomach can decrease iron absorption. For example, acid-reducing medications that people take to control heartburn or ulcers can impair iron absorption. Also, as people age, gastric acid secretion may decline. This puts older adults at risk for iron-deficiency anemia.[33]

Lastly, other micronutrients affect iron absorption and availability. Large doses of zinc or calcium can compete with iron for absorption in the small intestine. If you need to take an iron supplement, it is best to take it at least 2 hours before or after a calcium-rich meal or supplement. In contrast, vitamin C is a powerful enhancer of iron absorption. Doses of 75 milligrams of vitamin C can increase nonheme iron absorption by 4%—a lot for nonheme iron. If you want to get the most iron out of your dietary supplement, take it with a glass of orange juice. Research also indicates that adequate vitamin A and copper intakes promote good iron status due to their roles in iron absorption, transport, and metabolism.[32]

GETTING ENOUGH IRON

Lean meats and seafood are good sources of heme iron, the most bioavailable form. Leafy green vegetables (e.g., spinach) and legumes also provide iron, but the absorption of nonheme iron from these foods is relatively low. Some nonheme iron is naturally present in whole grains, but iron is added to milled grains and white rice during the enrichment process (Fig. 9-21). The major sources of iron in the adult eating pattern are red meats, ready-to-eat breakfast cereals, and enriched grains. Please note that milk and products made from milk are poor sources of iron. In fact, excessive consumption of cow's milk coupled with low meat intake can result in iron-deficiency anemia among young children.

The adult RDA is based on a 10% absorption rate to cover average losses of about 0.8 milligram per day. For females of reproductive age, menstrual losses are an average of about 1 gram of additional iron per day. Thus, iron is the only nutrient for which females have higher requirements than males. Most females do not consume the recommended 18 milligrams of iron daily. The average daily amount consumed by females is closer to 12 milligrams, while in males it is about 16 milligrams per day.[15] Females of reproductive age can close this gap between average daily intakes and needs by seeking out iron-fortified foods, such as ready-to-eat breakfast cereals that contain at least 50% of the DV. Use of a balanced multivitamin and mineral supplement containing up to 100% of the DV for iron is another option. Consuming more than the RDA for iron is not advised unless recommended by a primary care provider.

The iron added to foods and in most dietary supplements is nonheme iron.

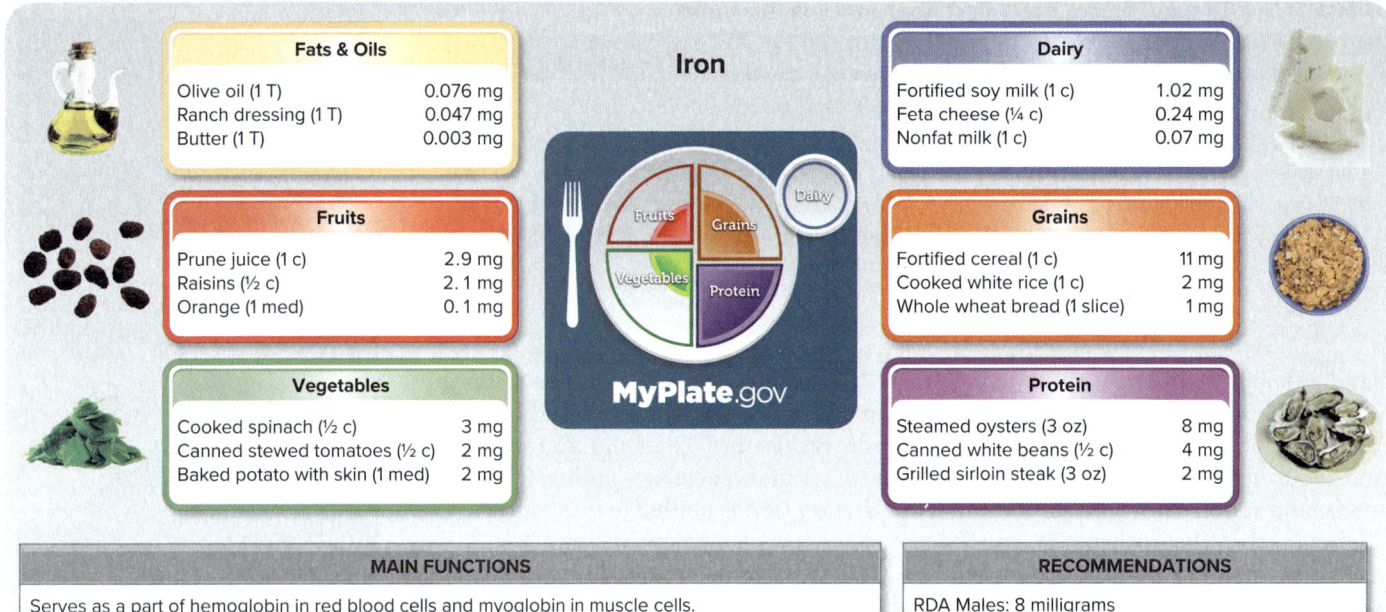

FIGURE 9-21 Food sources, functions, and recommendations for iron. The fill of the background color (none, 1/3, 2/3, or completely covered) within each food group on MyPlate indicates the average nutrient density for iron in that group. The figure shows the iron content of several foods in each food group. Overall, the richest sources of iron are meats, legumes, and fortified grain products. olive oil: Iconotec/Glow Images; raisins: lynx/iconotec/Glowimages; pile of spinach: Elena Elisseeva/Shutterstock; sheep's cheese (feta): Foodcollection; bowl of cereal: Joe Belanger/iStock/Getty Images; oyster plate: lynx/iconotec.com/Glow Images; MyPlate: U.S. Department of Agriculture

Sources: Office of Dietary Supplements, Dietary Supplements Fact Sheets, available from https://ods.od.nih.gov/factsheets/list-all/; USDA FoodData Central, available from https://fdc.nal.usda.gov/

AVOIDING TOO MUCH IRON

The UL for iron is 45 milligrams per day. Higher amounts can lead to stomach irritation. Although iron overload is not as common as iron deficiency, the consequences can be dire. Even a large single dose of 60 milligrams of iron can be life threatening to a 1-year-old. Children are the most likely victims of iron poisoning (acute toxicity) because supplements, which often look a lot like candy, may be easily accessible from kitchen counters and cabinets. The FDA requires that all iron supplements carry a warning about toxicity. Since the introduction of that warning label in the 1990s, cases of accidental iron poisoning among children have been greatly reduced.

Iron toxicity accompanies hereditary **hemochromatosis,** a genetic disease. It is associated with a substantial increase in iron absorption from both food and supplements. The harshest effects are seen in iron-storing organs such as the liver and heart. Some iron is deposited in the pancreas and muscles. Blood levels of iron remain high too, which increases the likelihood of infections and may promote cardiovascular disease.

Hereditary hemochromatosis occurs when a person carries two dysfunctional copies of a particular gene. People with one dysfunctional gene and one functional gene

hemochromatosis A disorder of iron metabolism characterized by increased iron absorption and deposition in the liver and heart. This eventually poisons the cells in those organs.

therapeutic phlebotomy Periodic blood removal, as a blood donation, for the purpose of ridding the body of excess iron.

(i.e., carriers) may also absorb too much dietary iron but not to the same extent as those with two dysfunctional genes. About 10% of people in the United States are carriers of hemochromatosis. Approximately 1 in 300 non-Hispanic whites in the United States has both hemochromatosis genes. The prevalence of hemochromatosis is lower in other racial and ethnic groups.[34] These numbers are high, considering that many primary care providers regard hemochromatosis as a rare disease and therefore do not routinely test for it.

Anyone who has a blood relative (including uncles, aunts, and cousins) who has hemochromatosis or is a carrier should be screened for iron overload. At your next visit to a primary care provider, ask for a transferrin saturation test to assess iron stores. A ferritin test may also be added to assess your stores. Hemochromatosis can go undetected until a person reaches age 50 to 60, so some experts recommend screening for anyone over the age of 20.

If the disease goes untreated, iron accumulates and serious health problems may result: arthritis, heart disease, diabetes, liver disease, gallbladder disease, some cancers, hypothyroidism, reproductive dysfunction, and depression. Even with iron overload, the person may have anemia due to damage to the bone marrow or liver. Treatment of hemochromatosis is relatively easy, but it must be monitored consistently. **Therapeutic phlebotomy** to remove excess iron is essential. One must be very careful about dietary choices. Few sources of heme iron should be eaten, and supplements with iron or vitamin C should be avoided. Highly fortified breakfast cereals must also be avoided.

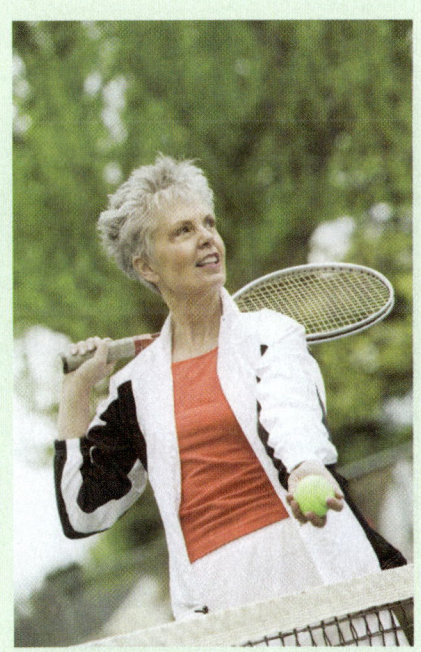

The FDA requires all dietary supplements with 30 milligrams or more of elemental iron to carry a warning label about accidental poisoning. **What are the risks of consuming too much iron?** Angela Collene

CASE STUDY Anemia

Anita is a 60-year-old female who prides herself on taking charge of her health. Her daily physical activities include walking her dog, playing tennis, or participating in a tai chi class at the senior center. She follows the *Dietary Guidelines,* choosing a variety of whole grains; eating at least five servings per day of fruits and vegetables; and keeping her saturated fat and sodium intakes to a minimum. She eats lean sources of protein, choosing poultry, fish, or vegetable sources of protein instead of red meat. She maintains a healthy body weight, has never had high blood pressure or high blood sugar, and does not take medications or supplements. Last week, she went to a blood drive at her church with the intent of donating blood, but she was turned away because her hematocrit (a measure of the percentage of red blood cells in the blood) was slightly below the requirements for donation. Anita was surprised because she has never had a problem donating blood before. The nurse told Anita that her low hematocrit level was indicative of anemia, which has many possible causes. As Anita thought about it, she realized that she had been feeling more tired than usual.

Answer the following questions related to Anita's anemia.

1. Iron deficiency is the most common form of anemia. What role does iron play in the health of red blood cells?
2. During their reproductive years, females are at increased risk for iron deficiency due to monthly menstrual losses. Most females reach menopause (cessation of menstrual periods) around the age of 50. Is it likely that Anita has low iron stores? Why or why not?
3. If Anita's anemia is due to iron deficiency, what dietary changes could Anita make to improve her iron status?
4. Folate deficiency (review Section 8.14) may lead to anemia. What role does folate play in the health of red blood cells?
5. Considering her dietary pattern, is it likely that Anita is deficient in folate? Why or why not?
6. Low vitamin B-12 (review Section 8.15) may result in anemia. What role does vitamin B-12 play in the health of red blood cells?
7. Suggest an explanation for why Anita may have low vitamin B-12 status even with adequate dietary intake of vitamin B-12.
8. If Anita is having trouble absorbing vitamin B-12, what dietary changes could Anita make to improve her vitamin B-12 status?

Anita has been feeling tired lately after playing tennis. How could her fatigue be related to her dietary pattern? Big Cheese Photo/SuperStock

Complete the Case Study. Responses to these questions can be provided by your instructor.

> ✓ **CONCEPT CHECK 9.9**
>
> 1. List three symptoms of iron deficiency. How do these symptoms relate to the roles of iron in the body?
> 2. What are *heme* and *nonheme* iron? What can you do to enhance your absorption of nonheme iron?
> 3. Why should a person with hemochromatosis avoid dietary supplements with vitamin C?

9.10 Zinc

Zinc (Zn) deficiency was first recognized in the early 1960s in Egypt and Iran, where it was linked to impaired growth and poor sexual development. Even though the zinc content of the diets of people in these areas was fairly high, absorption of the mineral was limited by the phytic acid in unleavened bread. Parasite infestation and the practice of eating clay and other parts of soil also contributed to the severe zinc deficiency.

FUNCTIONS OF ZINC

Approximately 200 enzymes require zinc as a cofactor for activity. Adequate zinc intake is necessary to support many physiological functions:

- DNA synthesis and function
- Protein metabolism, wound healing, and growth
- Development of bones and reproductive organs
- Storage, release, and function of insulin
- Cell membrane structure and function
- Component of **superoxide dismutase**, an enzyme that aids in the prevention of oxidative damage to cells (zinc, therefore, has an indirect antioxidant function)
- Immune function through white blood cell formation

It is important to note that although zinc is important for immune function, intakes in excess of the RDA do not provide any extra benefit toward immunity. In fact, chronic excessive intakes of zinc can actually depress immune function. Zinc supplementation may be useful to slow the progression of macular degeneration of the eye and reduce the risk of developing certain forms of cancer.[35]

ZINC DEFICIENCY

Symptoms of adult zinc deficiency include an acnelike rash, diarrhea, lack of appetite, delayed wound healing, impaired immunity, reduced or altered senses of taste and smell, and hair loss. In children and adolescents with zinc deficiency, growth, sexual development, and learning ability may also be impaired.

GETTING ENOUGH ZINC

Protein-rich diets, especially those that include many animal sources of protein, are high in zinc. The average adult consumes about 10 to 13 milligrams of zinc per day, about 80% of which is provided by meat, fish, poultry, fortified cereal, and dairy products (Fig. 9-22). There are no indications of moderate or severe zinc deficiencies in an otherwise healthy adult population. It is likely, however, that some Americans—especially children with food insecurity, vegans, and older people with alcohol use disorders—have marginal zinc status. Individuals who experience deterioration in taste sensation, recurring infections, poor growth, or depressed wound healing should have their zinc status checked.

superoxide dismutase Antioxidant enzyme system that converts certain free radicals (superoxide anions) into less damaging products (oxygen and hydrogen peroxide).

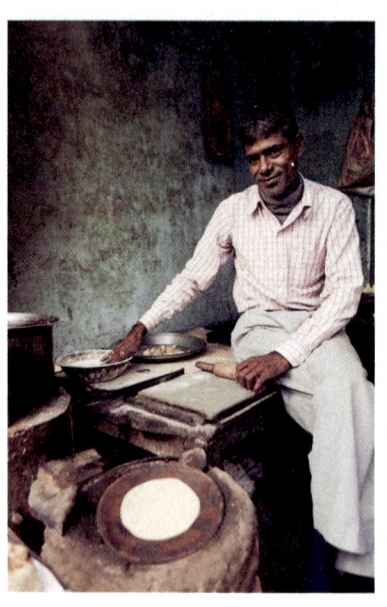

Zinc deficiency has been associated with the consumption of unleavened bread in Middle Eastern countries. **What is the name of the plant compound in grains that binds to zinc and decreases its bioavailability?** hadynyah/Vetta/Getty Images

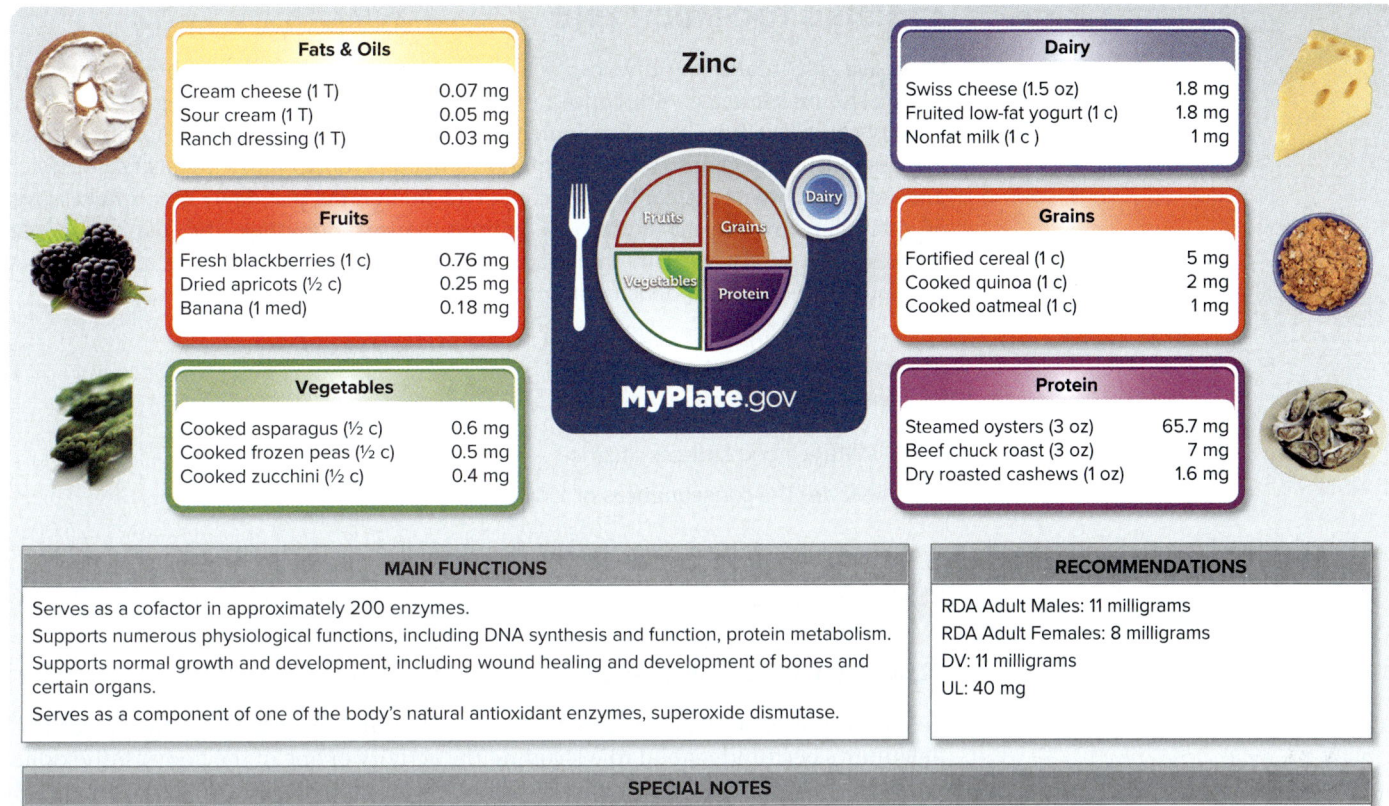

FIGURE 9-22 Food sources, functions, and recommendations for zinc. The fill of the background color (none, 1/3, 2/3, or completely covered) within each food group on MyPlate indicates the average nutrient density for zinc in that group. The figure shows the zinc content of several foods. Overall, the richest sources of zinc are in the protein group. bagel with cream cheese: Renee Comet/National Cancer Institute (NCI); fresh blackberries: Vitalina Rybakova/Shutterstock; asparagus: Ingram Publishing/SuperStock; wedge of Swiss cheese: Comstock/Jupiter Images/Getty Images; bowl of cereal: Joe Belanger/iStock/Getty Images; oyster plate: lynx/iconotec.com/Glow Images; MyPlate: Source: U.S. Department of Agriculture

Sources: Office of Dietary Supplements, Dietary Supplements Fact Sheets, available from https://ods.od.nih.gov/factsheets/list-all/; USDA FoodData Central, available from https://fdc.nal.usda.gov/

Overall, about 40% of dietary zinc is absorbed. Absorption efficiency depends on the body's need for zinc and the form of the mineral in foods. When zinc status is poor, absorption of the mineral increases. The zinc found in animal foods is better absorbed than that found in plants. Worldwide, however, most people rely on unfortified cereal grains (low in zinc) as their source of protein, calories, and zinc. Phytic acid in plant foods binds to zinc and limits its availability. Adding yeast to grains (leavening) breaks down phytic acid, increasing zinc bioavailability from leavened grain products. In populations that consume mainly unleavened bread, zinc deficiency can be a problem.

The form generally used in multivitamin and mineral supplements (zinc oxide) is not as well-absorbed as zinc found naturally in foods but still contributes to meeting zinc needs. High-dose calcium supplementation decreases zinc availability if taken too close to mealtime. Finally, zinc competes with copper and iron for absorption, and vice versa, when supplemental sources are consumed. Supplements with more than 100% of the Daily Value for individual minerals are not recommended without medical supervision.

AVOIDING TOO MUCH ZINC

Excessive zinc intake over time can lead to problems by interfering with copper metabolism. The interference with copper metabolism is the basis for setting the UL. Zinc toxicity can occur from zinc supplements and overconsumption of zinc-fortified foods. A person using megadose supplementation should be under close medical supervision and take a supplement containing copper (2 milligrams per day). Zinc intakes over 50 milligrams may result in diarrhea, cramps, nausea, vomiting, and loss of appetite. Intakes consistently over 300 milligrams per day can lead to depressed immune function and decreased high-density lipoproteins.

✓ CONCEPT CHECK 9.10

1. List three good sources of zinc.
2. What are the consequences of zinc deficiency?

9.11 Selenium

FUNCTIONS OF SELENIUM

Selenium (Se) is a trace mineral that exists in many absorbable chemical forms.[36] Selenium's best-understood role is aiding the activity of one of the body's antioxidant enzymes, glutathione peroxidase. Glutathione peroxidase converts potentially damaging peroxides (e.g., hydrogen peroxide) into water. As part of this antioxidant enzyme, selenium spares vitamin E and helps maintain cell membrane integrity. Selenium is also part of an enzyme that is essential for the activation of thyroid hormone.

SELENIUM DEFICIENCY

The selenium content of foods is strongly dependent on the selenium content of the soil where plants are raised or animals graze. Selenium deficiency symptoms in humans include muscle pain and wasting, and a certain form of heart damage. Also, due to its role in thyroid hormone metabolism, selenium deficiency may impair thyroid function, thereby limiting growth. In some locations, unless children and adults receive selenium supplements, they develop characteristic muscle and heart disorders associated with inadequate selenium intake.

Low blood levels of selenium have been linked to an increased incidence of some forms of cancer, specifically prostate cancer. Although selenium could prove to have a role in the prevention of cancers in those with low or marginal selenium stores, it is premature to recommend selenium supplementation for this purpose. The *Newsworthy Nutrition* in Chapter 8 discusses the SELECT trial and speaks to micronutrient supplementation for cancer prevention. Animal studies in this area are conflicting. Current studies examine the interaction of selenium and vitamin E on gene expression in some cancers.

GETTING ENOUGH SELENIUM

Overall, the major selenium contributors to the adult dietary pattern are animal and grain products. Fish, shellfish, meat (especially organ meats), and eggs are good animal sources of selenium (Fig. 9-23). Brazil nuts, as well as grains and seeds grown in soils containing selenium, are good plant sources. Some geographic regions with low-selenium soil in North America include the Northeast, Pacific, Southwest, and coastal plain of the Southeast in the United States, along with the north-central and eastern regions in Canada. If you consume a variety of foods from many geographic areas, it is

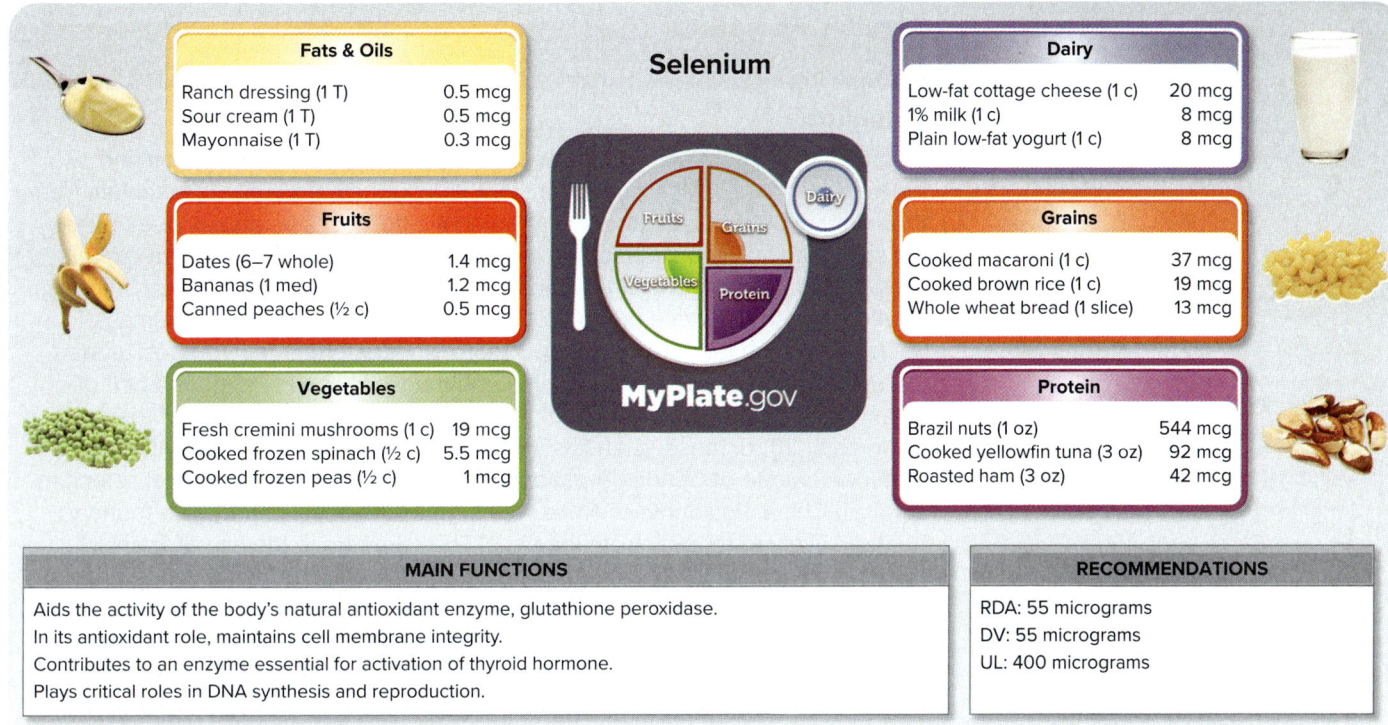

FIGURE 9-23 Food sources, functions, and recommendations for selenium. The fill of the background color (none, 1/3, 2/3, or completely covered) within each food group on MyPlate indicates the average nutrient density for selenium in that group. The figure shows the selenium content of several foods. Overall, the richest sources of selenium are found in the protein foods and grains groups. mayonnaise: Iconotec/Alamy Stock Photo; banana: lynx/iconotec.com/Glow Images; pile of peas: Ingram Publishing/SuperStock; glass of milk: Nipaporn Panyacharoen/Shutterstock; pile of pasta: olgaman/iStock/Getty Images; raw brazil nuts: 4kodiak/E plus/Getty Images; MyPlate: U.S. Department of Agriculture

Sources: Office of Dietary Supplements, Dietary Supplements Fact Sheets, available from https://ods.od.nih.gov/factsheets/list-all/; USDA FoodData Central, available from https://fdc.nal.usda.gov/

unlikely that your eating pattern is deficient in selenium. Garlic and onions can be rich sources of selenium because they have the ability to accumulate it from soil, which may increase their cancer-fighting potential.

The RDA for selenium is 55 micrograms per day for adults (Fig. 9-23). This intake maximizes the activity of selenium-dependent enzymes. On updated food and supplement labels, the Daily Value is also 55 micrograms. Most adults meet the RDA, consuming on average 115 micrograms each day.

AVOIDING TOO MUCH SELENIUM

High concentrations of selenium are rarely found in food, with the exception of Brazil nuts. Therefore, selenium toxicity has not been reported from eating food. Excessive selenium supplementation for an extended period has been shown to be toxic. The UL for selenium is 400 micrograms per day for adults. This is based on overt signs of selenium toxicity, such as hair loss, weakness, nausea, vomiting, and cirrhosis. Because Brazil nuts are such a concentrated source of selenium, you should not consume them every day, and when you do eat them, limit your portion size.

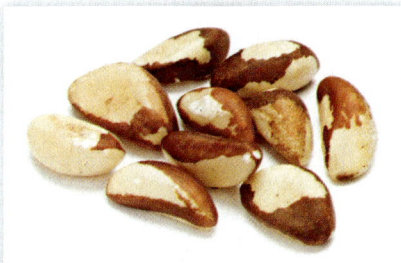

This portion of 10 Brazil nuts contains approximately 960 micrograms of selenium. **How does this compare to the UL for selenium?** 4kodiak/E plus/Getty Images

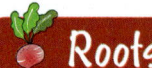

Roots

Selenium

Selenium is a potent antioxidant that strongly influences inflammation and immune responses. Most Americans obtain adequate amounts of selenium from their dietary patterns, but there are regional differences in intakes due to varying soil selenium levels that affect its concentration in vegetables. Yet globally, up to 1 billion people consume inadequate intakes of selenium, which is known to affect the severity of a number of viral infections in animals and humans. Such knowledge led an international team of researchers to hypothesize that the appearance of COVID-19 in China could possibly be linked to the belt of selenium deficiency that runs from the northeast to the southwest of the country. In early 2020, these scientists identified a link between the COVID-19 cure rate (percentage of COVID-19 patients declared "cured") and regional selenium status in China. Residents of areas with high levels of selenium were found to be more likely to recover from the virus. The cure rate in the city of Enshi in Hubei Province, which has the highest selenium intake in China, was almost three times higher than the average for all the other cities in Hubei Province. In contrast, the death rate from COVID-19 in Heilongjiang Province, which has a selenium intake among the lowest in the world (and where Keshan is located), was almost five times as high as the average of all the other provinces outside of Hubei. In addition, selenium status, measured by the amount of selenium in hair, was significantly associated with the COVID-19 cure rate. These links discovered between selenium status and COVID-19 are compelling but warrant a more thorough assessment that will take into account other possible factors such as age and underlying diseases.

Source: Zhang J, Taylor EW, Bennett K, Saad R, Rayman MP. Association between regional selenium status and reported outcome of COVID-19 cases in China. *Am J Clin Nutr. 2020* Jun 1;111(6):1297–1299. doi: 10.1093/ajcn/nqaa095

✓ CONCEPT CHECK 9.11

1. How does selenium participate in the body's antioxidant defenses?
2. What other functions does selenium play in the body?
3. What are the signs of a selenium deficiency?
4. What food groups are the best sources of selenium?
5. Are Brazil nuts bad for you? Why or why not?

9.12 Iodine

FUNCTIONS OF IODINE

Iodine is essential for brain development during gestation and early infancy and for the synthesis and function of thyroid hormones, which promote growth and development at critical stages and regulate metabolic rate throughout the lifespan.[37] The thyroid gland—part of your endocrine system—is a butterfly-shaped organ in the neck. The thyroid gland actively accumulates and traps iodine (I) from the bloodstream to support thyroid hormone synthesis. The synthesis of thyroid hormones also requires the amino acid tyrosine and selenium, which is part of the enzymes that convert the hormone to its active form.

IODINE DEFICIENCY

If a person's iodine intake is insufficient, the thyroid gland enlarges as it attempts to take up more iodine from the bloodstream. This eventually leads to **goiter.** Simple goiter is a painless condition but, if uncorrected, can lead to pressure on the trachea (windpipe), which may cause difficulty in breathing. Although consuming adequate iodine can prevent goiter formation, it does not significantly shrink a goiter once it has formed. Surgical removal may be required in severe cases.

If a female has an iodine-deficient eating pattern during the early months of her pregnancy, the fetus suffers iodine deficiency because the available iodine is used by the mother's body. As a result, the infant may experience a condition of stunted growth, a small head and brain, problems with speech and hearing, and intellectual disabilities that collectively are known as **congenital hypothyroidism** (formerly called *cretinism*). This condition appeared in North America before iodine fortification of table salt began. Today, congenital hypothyroidism still appears in some regions of Europe, Africa, Latin America, and Asia. Marginal iodine status still occurs even in developed countries, including the United States. Recent studies have shown a link between mild iodine deficiency during pregnancy and decreased cognitive performance in the offspring.[38,39] It is not clear whether iodine supplementation during pregnancy can prevent or correct these problems. Given that central nervous system development occurs in the early weeks of gestation, by the time a pregnancy is recognized, it may be too late.[40]

During World War I, males drafted into the military from areas such as the Great Lakes Region of the United States had a much higher rate of goiter compared to males from other areas of the country. The soil in the Great Lakes region has low iodine content. In the 1920s, a researcher in Ohio found that low doses of iodine given to children over a 4-year period could prevent goiter. This research eventually led to the iodization of salt, which began in the United States in 1924.[41] This was the first time a nutrient was purposely added to food to prevent a disease. Now, the World Health Organization recommends iodization of salt as the safest and most effective way to prevent iodine deficiency disorders.[42]

Globally, about 88% of households now have access to iodized salt. Despite tremendous progress toward universal salt iodization over the past 20 years, there are still at least 20 countries with insufficient iodine intake.[43] Whereas many nations, such as Canada, require iodine fortification of salt, some areas of Europe, such as northern Italy, have very low soil levels of iodine but have yet to adopt an iodine-fortification program. People in these areas, especially females, still suffer from goiter, as do people in areas of Latin America, the Indian subcontinent, Southeast Asia, and Africa. Eradication of iodine deficiency is still a goal of many health-related organizations worldwide.

GETTING ENOUGH IODINE

Seafood and seaweed are naturally rich sources of iodine because the mineral is present in seawater (Fig. 9-24). Dairy and grain products contribute significant amounts of iodine to the food supply because dairies use iodine as a sterilizing agent and bakeries use iodine as a dough conditioner. Iodine is also part of other food additives, such as food colorants. Iodized salt, however, is the main source of iodine in the typical American dietary pattern. In the United States, salt can be purchased either iodized or plain. Although processed foods are prepared with lots of salt, food processors usually do not use iodized salt. Sea salt and kosher salt are not typically iodized. Be sure to check the label to make sure you have a reliable source of iodine in your dietary pattern.

The RDA for iodine for adults is 150 micrograms per day. This is the same as the DV used on food and supplement labels. A half teaspoon of iodized salt (about 2 grams) meets the RDA for adults. The typical American dietary pattern supplies an estimated 190 to 300 micrograms of iodine daily. During pregnancy and lactation, however, the

goiter An enlargement of the thyroid gland; this is often caused by insufficient iodine in the dietary pattern.

congenital hypothyroidism A birth defect that impairs thyroid hormone synthesis. If untreated, this can lead to intellectual disability and stunting of growth.

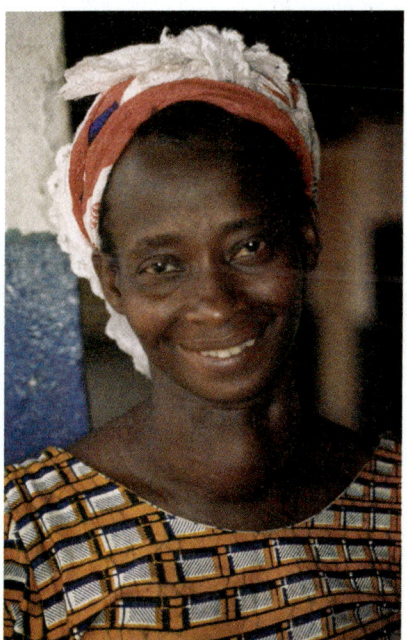

This individual has an enlargement of the thyroid gland (also known as goiter) caused by insufficient iodine in her dietary pattern. Adequate iodine intake during pregnancy is important to prevent congenital hypothyroidism in the infant. Scott Camazine/Science Source

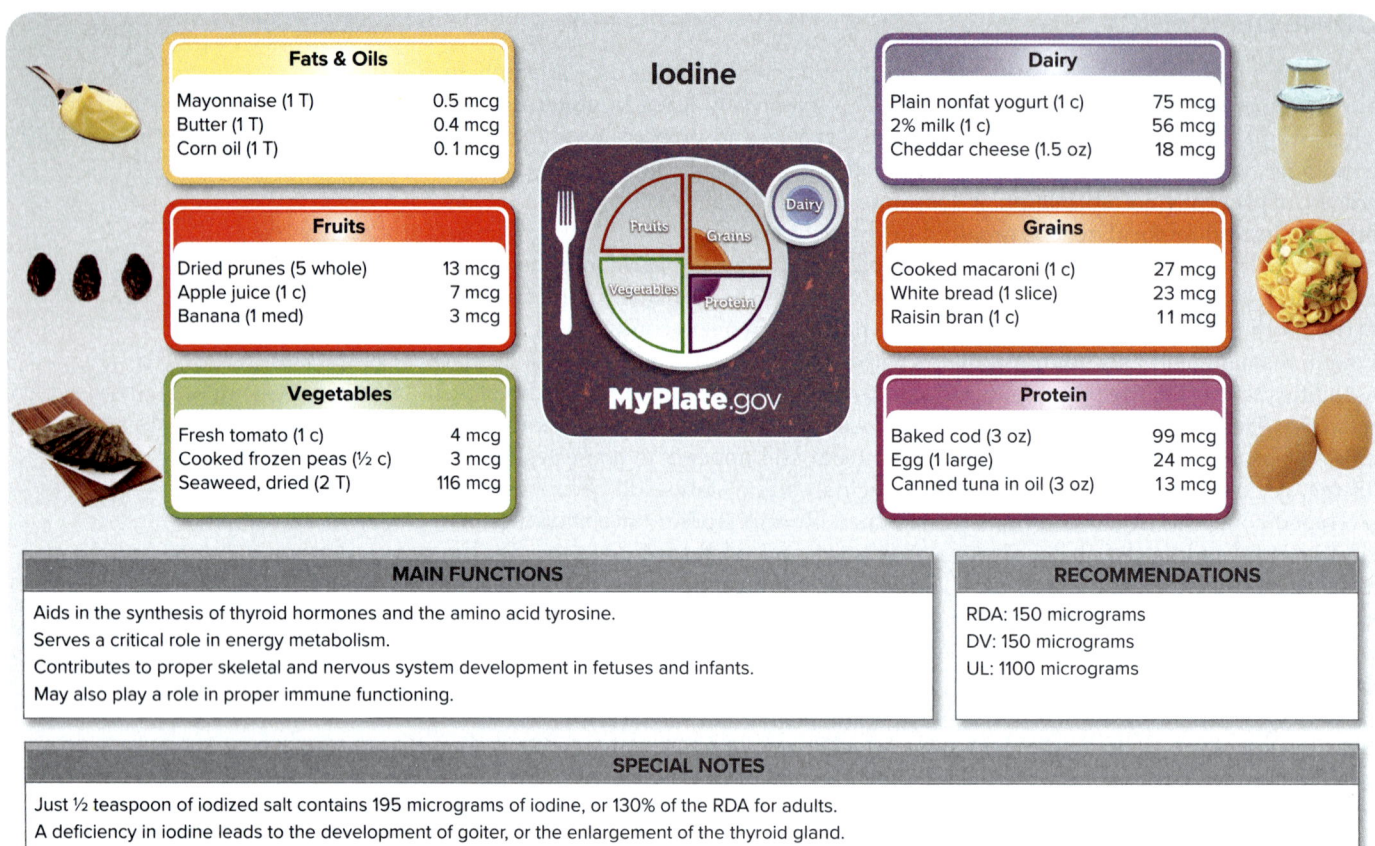

FIGURE 9-24 Food sources, functions, and recommendations for iodine. The fill of the background color (none, 1/3, 2/3, or completely covered) within each food group on MyPlate indicates the average nutrient density for iodine in that group. The figure shows the iodine content of several foods. Overall, the richest sources of iodine are iodized salt (added to foods in any group), seafood and seaweed, and dairy products. Fruits and vegetables other than seaweed are poor sources of iodine. mayonnaise: Iconotec/Alamy Stock Photo; three prunes: I. Rozenbaum & F. Cirou/PhotoAlto; dry seaweed: Hheinteh/123RF; two jars of yogurt: Foodcollection; pasta: tobi/123RF; eggs: clubfoto/E+/Getty Images; MyPlate: U.S. Department of Agriculture

Sources: Office of Dietary Supplements, Dietary Supplements Fact Sheets, available from https://ods.od.nih.gov/factsheets/list-all/; USDA FoodData Central, available from https://fdc.nal.usda.gov/

goitrogen A compound that interferes with the uptake or utilization of iodine by the thyroid gland. Food sources of goitrogens include sweet potatoes, broccoli, and soy products.

RDA for iodine increases significantly to support the growth and development of the offspring. Supplementation may be needed for some females to maintain adequate iodine status during pregnancy and lactation. There is also concern that individuals following a vegan dietary pattern may not consume enough iodine unless they use iodized salt.

There are some compounds called **goitrogens** in foods that may interfere with uptake or utilization of iodine by the thyroid gland. Dietary goitrogens are a chemically diverse group of compounds found naturally in some starchy vegetables (e.g., sweet potatoes, cassava, and corn), cruciferous vegetables (e.g., broccoli, cauliflower, and cabbage), fruits (e.g., strawberries, peaches, and pears), grains (e.g., millet), and soy products (e.g., tofu and edamame).[44] Most people do not need to restrict their intake of these nutritious fruits, vegetables, and grains. Cooking foods will denature most of these compounds. Furthermore, consuming a variety of different foods will limit the impact of any antinutrients on overall nutrient status.[45] The effect of consuming goitrogens on thyroid functioning is thought to depend on the quantity eaten and the overall iodine content of the diet. Moderate intake of these goitrogen-containing foods appears to have little, if any, impact on thyroid function. However, a high goitrogen intake coupled with a marginal iodine intake may lead to iodine deficiency and contribute to goiter (see *Newsworthy Nutrition*).[46,47] Individuals with existing thyroid conditions should seek

Newsworthy Nutrition

Goitrogens and iodine deficiency

INTRODUCTION: Worldwide, pregnant females and school-age children are disproportionately vulnerable to iodine deficiency. Goiter and iodine deficiency disorder continue to be major public health concerns in Ethiopia, despite the universal iodization of their salt. In addition to insufficient iodine intake, the consumption of other food items called goitrogens may interfere with the synthesis and function of thyroid hormone. **OBJECTIVE:** This study was designed to assess the association between iodine deficiency and the dietary pattern of school-age children in Ethiopia. **METHODS:** In this *cross-sectional study,* the Helen Keller international food-frequency questionnaire was used to measure the dietary patterns of 767 children aged 6 to 12 years in southwest Ethiopia. Using the World Health Organization threshold criteria, iodine deficiency was measured using urinary iodine concentration level and total goiter rate (TGR). Results were analyzed to identify dietary and sociodemographic factors that affected urinary iodine levels among children. **RESULTS:** Of the 767 children studied, the TGR was 16% with grade 1 and grade 2 goiter present in 12% and 4% of children, respectively. The total prevalence of iodine deficiency based on urinary iodine concentration was 58.8%, of which 13.7% was severe, 18.6% moderate, and 26.5% mild. Age and sex of the child, as well as consumption of taro root, millet, cabbage, Abyssinian cabbage, and banana, were significantly associated with urinary iodine level. Urinary iodine decreased as consumption of taro, cabbage, and millet increased. Taro root is high in phytate, which inhibits iodine absorption; cabbage and millet are associated with suppression of thyroid hormones. Children who consumed fish, Abyssinian cabbage, and banana more frequently had higher urinary iodine level. **CONCLUSION:** Iodine deficiency including the prevalence of goiter that exceeds the WHO threshold of 5% continues to be a public health problem in southwest Ethiopia. Both overconsumption of goitrogenic foods and underconsumption of iodine-rich foods were common and associated with lower urinary iodine level. Dietary counseling and the continuation of universal salt iodization are recommended as well as further research to answer the causal relationship between dietary pattern and iodine deficiency.

Source: Hassen HY, Beyene M, Ali JH. Dietary pattern and its association with iodine deficiency among school children in southwest Ethiopia; a cross-sectional study. *PLoS ONE.* 2019 Aug 13; 14(8):e0221106. doi: 10.1371/journal.pone.0221106

advice from a physician or registered dietitian nutritionist to determine if any dietary modifications are needed.

AVOIDING TOO MUCH IODINE

The UL for iodine is 1100 micrograms per day. When high amounts of iodine are consumed, thyroid hormone synthesis is inhibited, as in a deficiency. This can appear in people who eat a lot of seaweed because some seaweeds contain as much as 1% iodine by weight. Total iodine intake then can add up to 60 to 130 times the RDA.

✓ CONCEPT CHECK 9.12

1. What is the role of iodine in energy metabolism?
2. What are the effects of iodine deficiency?
3. Name three good food sources of iodine that you include in your dietary pattern.

9.13 Copper

Copper (Cu) and iron are similar in terms of food sources, absorption, and functions. Copper is a component of blood. In the body, it is found in the highest concentration in the liver, brain, heart, kidneys, and muscles. **Ceruloplasmin** is the name of the protein that carries most of the body's copper in the blood.

ceruloplasmin Copper-containing protein in the blood; functions in the transport of iron.

FUNCTIONS OF COPPER

Copper is a cofactor for many enzymes, including some involved in the body's antioxidant defenses. Copper serves as a cofactor for superoxide dismutase, an enzyme that defends the body against free-radical damage. Copper also has a role in the function of enzymes that create cross-links in connective tissue proteins, such as the collagen in bone. Another very important role of copper is as a cofactor in the last stage of energy metabolism, which converts the energy stored in carbohydrates, fats, and proteins into ATP.

Copper is important for blood health because of its role in making iron available for the formation of red blood cells. Copper is part of three different enzymes that assist in the transport of iron out of intestinal cells, through the blood, and to the bone marrow, where iron is incorporated into hemoglobin. Copper is also a cofactor for enzymes involved in blood clotting and blood lipoprotein metabolism. In addition, copper is needed for brain health through its role in enzymes involved in nerve myelination and neurotransmitter synthesis.[48]

A genetic disease called **Menkes syndrome** decreases the amount of copper available to the brain and nervous system. Babies born with Menkes syndrome suffer from nervous system disorders, weak muscle tone, and delays in physical and cognitive development. These symptoms are related to the lack of copper-containing enzymes that help to form nervous tissue and synthesize neurotransmitters. They usually do not live past the age of 3 years.

COPPER DEFICIENCY

Considering the many roles of copper, it is not surprising that copper deficiency affects so many different body systems. Symptoms of copper deficiency include a form of anemia, weakened immunity, bone loss, poor growth, and some forms of cardiovascular disease.

The groups most likely to develop copper deficiencies are infants who are born preterm and people recovering from intestinal surgery. A copper deficiency can also result from the overuse of zinc supplements because zinc and copper compete with each other for absorption.

Menkes syndrome An inherited X-linked recessive pattern disorder that affects copper levels in the body.

GETTING ENOUGH COPPER

Rich sources of copper include organ meats, shellfish, nuts and seeds, whole grain breads and cereals, and cocoa (Fig. 9-25). Milk and dairy products, fruits, and vegetables are generally poor sources of copper. Also, the form of copper typically found in multivitamin and mineral supplements (copper oxide) is not readily absorbed. It is best to rely on food sources to meet copper needs.

Copper absorption is highly variable; as copper intake increases, the mineral is absorbed less efficiently. Absorption takes place in the stomach and upper small intestine. Excess copper is not stored to a great extent, so when intake exceeds needs, the liver incorporates it into bile, which is excreted as part of the feces. Phytates, fiber, and excessive zinc and iron supplements may all interfere with copper absorption.

The copper status of adults appears to be good: The average daily adult intake is about 1.1 milligram for females and 1.3 milligrams for males.[15] However, sensitive laboratory tests to determine copper status are lacking.

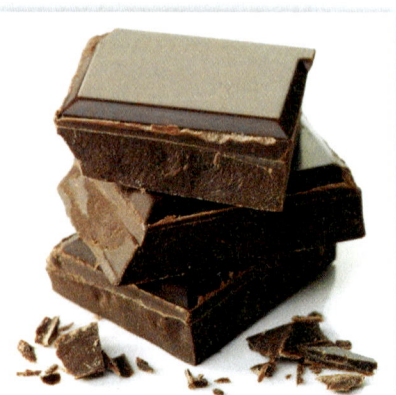

Dark chocolate is a rich source of copper. One ounce of dark chocolate candy provides about 500 micrograms of copper. **Has anyone ever suffered from copper toxicity because of eating too much chocolate?** Baiba Opule/Baibaz/123RF

AVOIDING TOO MUCH COPPER

A single dose of copper greater than 10 milligrams can cause toxicity. Consequences of copper toxicity include GI distress, vomiting blood, tarry feces, and damage to the liver

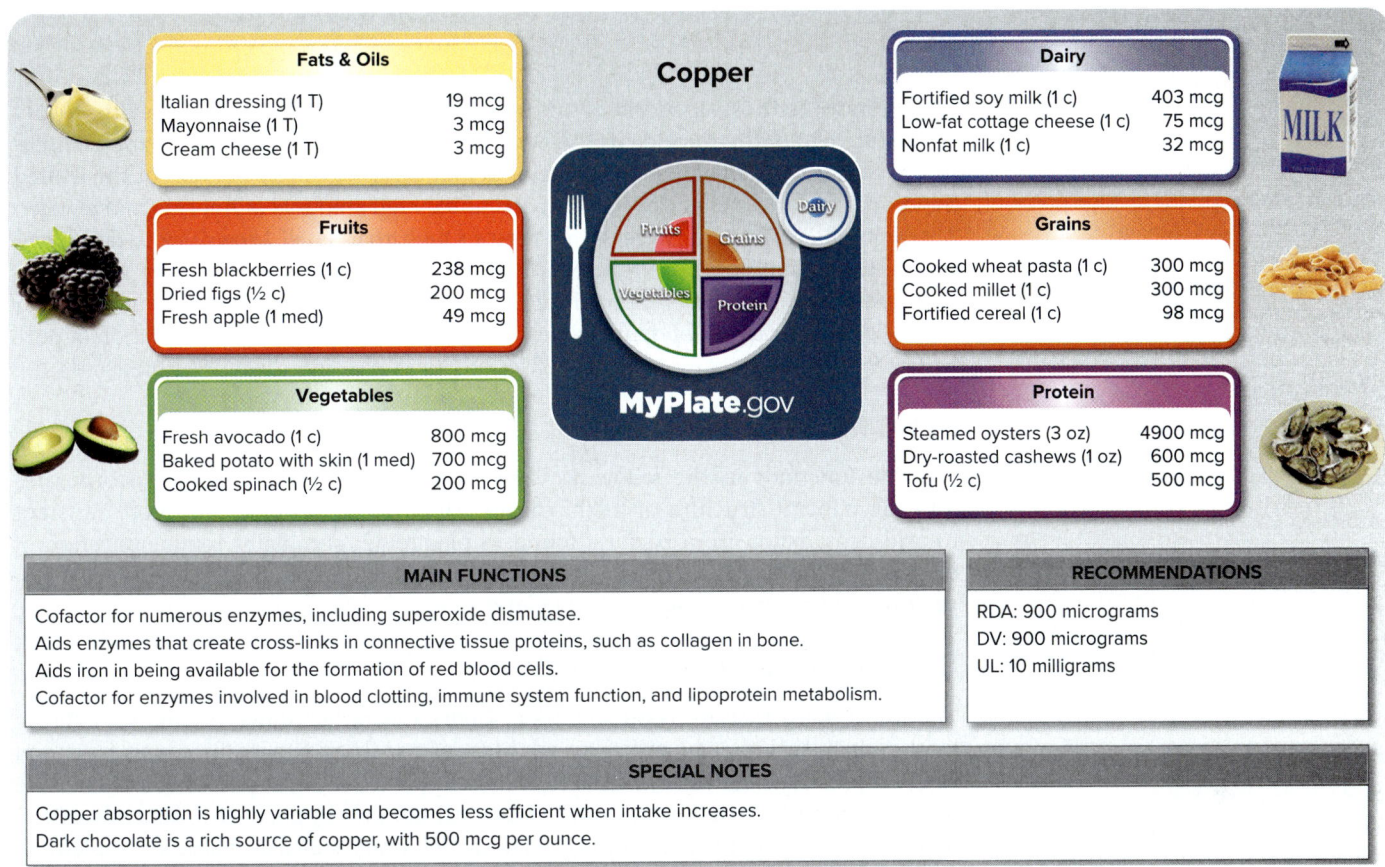

FIGURE 9-25 Food sources, functions, and recommendations for copper. The fill of the background color (none, 1/3, 2/3, or completely covered) within each food group on MyPlate indicates the average nutrient density for copper in that group. The figure shows the copper content of several foods in each food group. Overall, the richest sources of copper are found in the protein foods and grains groups. mayonnaise: Iconotec/Alamy Stock Photo; fresh blackberries: Vitalina Rybakova/Shutterstock; avocado: lynx/iconotec.com/Glow Images; milk: Hurst Photo/Shutterstock; wholemeal pasta: HandmadePictures/iStock/Getty Images; oyster plate: lynx/iconotec.com/Glow Images; MyPlate: U.S. Department of Agriculture

Sources: Office of Dietary Supplements, Dietary Supplements Fact Sheets, available from https://ods.od.nih.gov/factsheets/list-all/; USDA FoodData Central, available from https://fdc.nal.usda.gov/

and kidneys. Toxicity cannot occur with food, only supplements or excessive exposure to copper salts used in agriculture.

Wilson's disease is a rare genetic disease in which the liver cannot synthesize ceruloplasmin. In turn, copper accumulates in tissues, such as lungs and liver. People with Wilson's disease suffer damage to the liver and nervous system. A primary treatment for Wilson's disease is a vegan dietary pattern, as fruits and vegetables are low in copper.[49] Researchers are currently interested in how excess copper in the blood may influence the development of **Alzheimer's disease** and **Parkinson's disease**.[50]

Wilson's disease A genetic disorder that results in accumulation of copper in the tissues; characterized by damage to the liver, nervous system, and other organs.

Alzheimer's disease A progressive neurodegenerative disease that gradually impairs memory and thinking skills.

Parkinson's disease Disease that belongs to a group of conditions called motor system disorders, which are the result of the loss of dopamine-producing brain cells. The four primary symptoms are tremor, or trembling in hands, arms, legs, jaw, and face; rigidity, or stiffness of the limbs and trunk; bradykinesia, or slowness of movement; and postural instability, or impaired balance and coordination.

✓ CONCEPT CHECK 9.13

1. List three functions of copper.
2. Describe some interactions among iron, zinc, and copper in the body.
3. What changes to the dietary pattern will be required for a person with Wilson's disease?

9.14 Fluoride

The fluoride ion (F⁻) is the form of this trace mineral essential for human health. Nearly all (about 95%) of the fluoride in the body is found in the teeth and skeleton. Dentists in the early 1900s noticed a lower rate of dental caries (cavities) in areas of the United States, particularly the Southwest, that contained high amounts of fluoride in the water. The amounts of fluoride were sometimes so high that small brown spots developed on the teeth (mottling). Even though mottled teeth were discolored, they were resistant to dental caries. Experiments in the early 1940s showed that fluoride in the water decreased the incidence of dental caries by 20% to 80% in children. Fluoridation of public water supplies in many parts of the United States has since been instituted.[51]

> **Is your water supply fluoridated?**
> You can find information about fluoridation of water by searching https://nccd.cdc.gov/DOH_MWF/Default/Default.aspx. If your hometown isn't listed, contact your local government or water treatment facility.

> **Fluoride**
> AI: 3.1 to 3.8 milligrams
> UL:
> Young children: 1.3 to 2.2 milligrams
> > 9 years: 10 milligrams

FUNCTIONS OF FLUORIDE

Fluoride functions in the following ways to prevent dental caries: (1) incorporates into the mineral structure of teeth, causing them to be stronger and more resistant to acid degradation from bacteria found in plaque; (2) stimulates remineralization of enamel and inhibits tooth demineralization; and (3) has an antibacterial effect on acid-producing microorganisms found in plaque.

GETTING ENOUGH FLUORIDE

The list of foods that are good sources of fluoride is rather short: marine fish, clams, lobster, crab, shrimp, tea, and seaweed. Most of our fluoride actually comes from oral hygiene products and the fluoridated water supply. Numerous products are available to apply fluoride to teeth topically. These include gels applied at a dentist's office, toothpaste, and mouth rinses for everyday use. Fluoride is also available in supplement form, although use should be directed by a dentist or primary care provider. The most economical method of distributing fluoride is to add the mineral to the community's drinking water. When water fluoridation and fluoridated topical products are used in combination, the reductions in dental caries are additive.

In a few areas of the world, the fluoride content of groundwater is naturally high, but most groundwater supplies contain low levels of fluoride. In the 1950s, after researchers established a connection between fluoride and rates of dental caries, communities in the United States began adding fluoride to the municipal water supply to achieve a fluoride level of 0.7 to 1.2 milligrams per liter. (The lower levels are for communities in hotter climates, where total water consumption is higher.) About three-quarters of U.S. households have fluoridated water; these policies are made by individual municipalities.[52] Because most people now have ample access to oral hygiene products with fluoride, the level of water fluoridation has been lowered to just 0.7 milligram per liter.

The AI for fluoride for adults is 3.1 milligrams per day for adult females and 3.8 milligrams per day for adult males. This range of intake provides the benefits of resistance to dental caries without causing ill effects. As described, typical fluoridated water contains about 1 milligram per liter, which works out to about 0.25 milligram per cup. In communities without fluoridated water (e.g., those that rely on private well water), use of fluoride-containing oral hygiene products or dietary supplements is of heightened importance for combating dental decay.

Note that fluoride is generally not added to bottled water. Frequent use of bottled water or a household reverse osmosis water purification system significantly restricts fluoride intake. A refrigerator or Brita® filter does not remove fluoride.

AVOIDING TOO MUCH FLUORIDE

The UL for fluoride is set at 1.3 to 2.2 milligrams per day for young children and 10 milligrams per day for children over 9 years of age and adults, based on skeletal and tooth damage seen with higher doses. Children may develop **fluorosis** if they swallow large amounts of fluoride toothpaste as part of daily tooth care. Fluorosis leads to stained

fluorosis Discoloration of tooth enamel sometimes accompanied with pitting due to consuming a large amount of fluoride for an extended period.

and pitted teeth and can permanently damage teeth if it occurs during tooth development (first decade of life) (Fig. 9-26). Not swallowing toothpaste and limiting the amount used to "pea" size are the best ways to prevent this problem. In addition, children under 6 years should have tooth brushing supervised by an adult and should never use fluoride mouthwash. In adults, fluorosis is associated with hip fractures, weak or stiff joints, and chronic stomach inflammation.

There have been opponents to the fluoridation of public water supplies. Some people argue that water fluoridation standards were set at a time when much of the population did not have adequate access to fluoride-containing oral hygiene products, and therefore addition of fluoride to the water supply is no longer necessary. Other critics claim that chronic exposure to fluoridated water is linked to a variety of health ailments affecting the skeletal, nervous, or endocrine systems. At this time, there is little scientific evidence to support claims that water fluoridation at current levels has adverse health effects other than dental fluorosis. The recommendations for the level of water fluoridation aim to take advantage of the oral health benefits of fluoride while limiting unwanted health effects, including fluorosis. The CDC provides more information on fluoridation at https://www.cdc.gov/fluoridation/index.html.

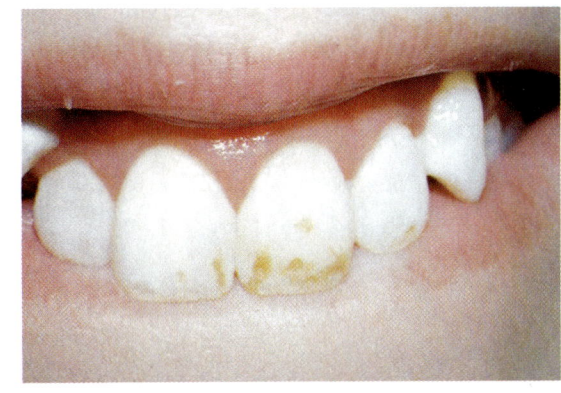

FIGURE 9-26 One sign of fluorosis is mottling (brown spots) on the teeth. Children can develop fluorosis as a result of swallowing large amounts of fluoride toothpaste. Paul Casamassimo, DDS, MS

✓ CONCEPT CHECK 9.14

1. How does fluoride help reduce the development of dental caries?
2. What are our primary sources of fluoride?
3. What are the risks of excessive fluoride intake?

9.15 Chromium

FUNCTIONS OF CHROMIUM

Chromium (Cr) enhances the function of insulin, so it is required for glucose uptake into cells. The mineral is involved in the metabolism of lipids and proteins as well, although the exact mechanisms are not known. Chromium supplements have been promoted for building muscle mass and for weight loss, but there is not much evidence to support these claims.[53]

CHROMIUM DEFICIENCY

A chromium deficiency is characterized by impaired blood glucose control and elevated blood cholesterol and triglycerides. Low or marginal chromium intakes may contribute to an increased risk for developing type 2 diabetes, but opinions are mixed on the true degree of this effect. Overt chromium deficiency appears in people maintained on intravenous nutrition solutions not supplemented with chromium and in children with malnutrition. Marginal deficiencies may go undetected because sensitive measures of chromium status are not available.

GETTING ENOUGH CHROMIUM

Specific data regarding the chromium content of various foods are scant. Meat and whole grain products, eggs, mushrooms, nuts, beer, and spices are relatively good sources of chromium. Brewer's yeast (used to make bread and some alcoholic beverages) is also a very good source.

> **Chromium**
> AI:
> Males (19 to 50 y): 35 micrograms
> Males (> 50 y): 30 micrograms
> Females (19 to 50 y): 25 micrograms
> Females (> 50 y): 20 micrograms
> DV: 35 micrograms
> UL: none

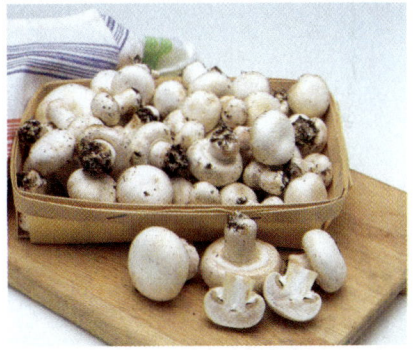

Mushrooms are a good source of chromium. Pixtal/age fotostock

Chromium absorption is quite low: only 0.4% to 2.5% of the amount consumed. Absorption is enhanced by vitamin C and niacin. Any unabsorbed chromium is excreted in the feces. Once absorbed, it is stored in the liver, spleen, soft tissue, and bone, and it is excreted via urine. Certain conditions can increase the loss of chromium in the urine: eating patterns high in simple sugars (more than 35% of total calories), serious infection, acute prolonged exercise, pregnancy and lactation, and major physical trauma. If chromium intakes are already low, these states potentially can lead to deficiency.

The Adequate Intake (AI) for chromium is based on the amount present in a balanced dietary pattern (see box). Average adult intakes in America are estimated at about 30 micrograms per day but could be somewhat higher.

No UL for chromium has been set because food sources of chromium have never caused toxicity of this mineral. Chromium toxicity, however, has been reported in people exposed to industrial waste and in painters who use art supplies with high chromium content. Liver damage and lung cancer can result. In general, aim for no more than the DV when taking any dietary supplements unless your primary care provider recommends otherwise.

✓ CONCEPT CHECK 9.15

1. How is chromium involved in carbohydrate metabolism?
2. What conditions can increase the loss of chromium in the urine?
3. Which foods are considered the best sources of chromium?

9.16 Other Trace Minerals

MANGANESE

The mineral manganese (Mn) is easily confused with magnesium (Mg). Not only are their names similar, but they also often substitute for each other in metabolic processes. As a participant in energy metabolism, manganese is required as a cofactor for the synthesis of glucose and the metabolism of some amino acids. Manganese is also needed by some enzymes, such as those used in free-radical metabolism (via superoxide dismutase). Manganese is also important in bone formation; 25% to 40% of the manganese in your body is stored in your bones.[54]

Manganese deficiency does not develop in humans unless individuals are fed intravenously with solutions lacking manganese. Animals on manganese-deficient diets suffer alterations in brain function, bone formation, and reproduction. If human dietary patterns were low in manganese, these symptoms would probably appear as well. As it happens, our need for manganese is low, and our eating patterns tend to be adequate in this trace mineral.

The AI for manganese is 1.8 to 2.3 milligrams to offset daily losses (see box). Average intakes fall within this range. The DV used on food and supplement labels is 2.3 milligrams. Good food sources of manganese include mollusks (e.g., mussels and clams), nuts, whole grains, legumes, and leafy green vegetables.

Manganese is toxic at high doses. Supplements are not recommended, as large doses can decrease the absorption of other minerals. People with low iron stores must avoid manganese supplements or risk worsening anemia. The UL is 11 milligrams per day. This value is based on the development of nerve damage. Miners who have inhaled dust fumes high in manganese experience symptoms that mimic Parkinson's disease, including cognitive and muscular dysfunction.

Manganese
AI:
Males: 2.3 milligrams
Females: 1.8 milligrams
DV: 2.3 milligrams
UL: 11 milligrams

MOLYBDENUM

Several human enzymes use molybdenum (Mo), including some involved in metabolism of amino acids that contain sulfur.[55] No molybdenum deficiency has been reported in people who consume food and beverages orally. Deficiency symptoms have appeared in people maintained on intravenous nutrition devoid of this trace mineral. Symptoms include increased heart and respiratory rates, night blindness, mental confusion, edema, and weakness.

Good food sources of molybdenum include milk and dairy products, beans, whole grains, and nuts. The RDA for molybdenum is 45 micrograms to offset daily losses. The DV used on food and supplement labels is 45 micrograms. Our daily intakes average 76 micrograms (for females) and 109 micrograms (for males).

The UL for molybdenum is 2000 micrograms per day. When consumed in high doses, molybdenum causes toxicity in laboratory animals, resulting in weight loss and decreased growth. Toxicity risk in humans is quite low.

> **Molybdenum**
> RDA: 45 micrograms
> DV: 45 micrograms
> UL: 2000 micrograms

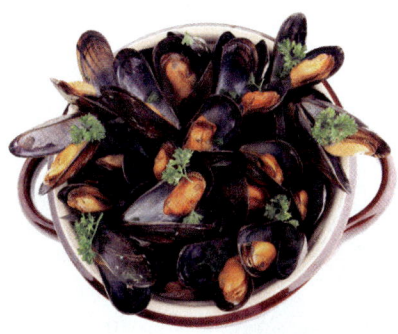

Mollusks are rich in manganese. A 3-ounce serving of steamed mussels provides 5.8 milligrams of manganese. margouillat/123RF

✓ CONCEPT CHECK 9.16

1. What are the primary functions of manganese and molybdenum in the metabolism of nutrients?
2. Which food groups provide the most manganese and molybdenum?

9.17 Nutrition and Your Health: Minerals and Hypertension

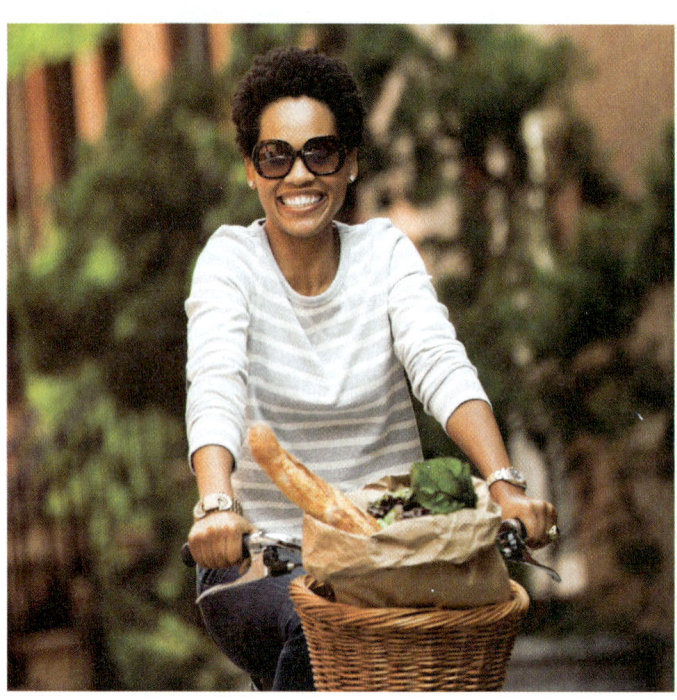
Sam Edwards/Caia Image/Glow Images

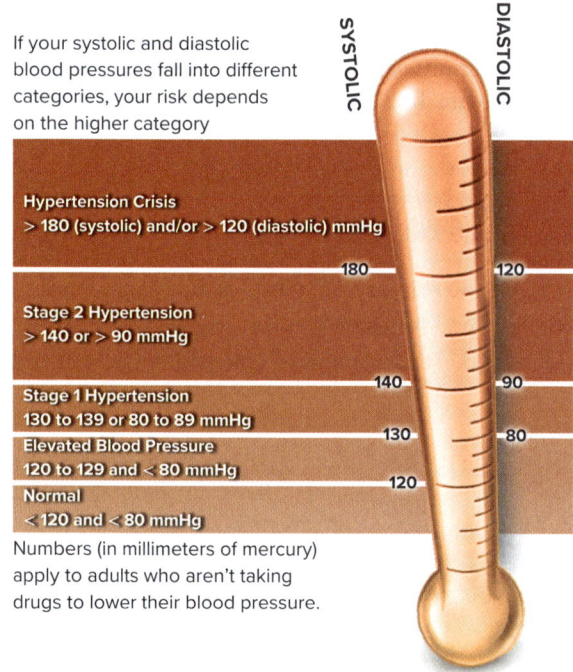

FIGURE 9-27 Guidelines for the detection of high blood pressure in adults. Values listed for each category are for systolic and diastolic, respectively. Hypertension is now defined as a systolic BP ≥ 130 mmHg or diastolic BP ≥ 80 mmHg.

In the United States, approximately 120 million adults have hypertension or take medicine to control their blood pressure. That's nearly half of all adults![56] Blood pressure is expressed by two numbers. The higher number represents **systolic blood pressure,** the pressure in the arteries when the heart muscle is contracting and pumping blood into the arteries. Optimal systolic blood pressure is less than 120 mmHg. The second value is **diastolic blood pressure,** the artery pressure when the heart is relaxed. Optimal diastolic blood pressure is less than 80 mmHg. Elevations in both systolic and diastolic blood pressure are strong predictors of disease.

The American College of Cardiology and American Heart Association revised the blood pressure (BP) guidelines in 2017 (Fig. 9-27).[57] These guidelines are intended to serve as a resource for health care providers and the general public while emphasizing the importance of earlier detection and treatment of this potentially deadly condition. Hypertension is defined as sustained systolic blood pressure exceeding 130 mmHg or diastolic blood pressure exceeding 80 mmHg. Most cases of hypertension (about 95%) have no clear-cut cause. Such cases are classified as **primary hypertension** (also known as *essential hypertension*). Kidney disease, sleep-disordered breathing (sleep apnea), and endocrine abnormalities lead to the other 5% of cases, classified as **secondary hypertension.**

Unless blood pressure is periodically measured, the development of hypertension is easily overlooked. By lowering the cutoff for hypertension, the new guidelines promote earlier detection and treatment to reduce the complications of hypertension.

Why Control Blood Pressure?

Because it usually does not cause symptoms, hypertension is described as a silent disorder. If left untreated, hypertension can lead to cardiovascular disease, kidney disease, strokes and related declines in brain function, poor blood circulation in the legs, problems with vision, and sudden death. These conditions are much more

systolic blood pressure The pressure in blood vessels when the heart beats, squeezing and pushing blood through the arteries to the rest of the body.

diastolic blood pressure The pressure in the arteries when the heart rests between beats and fills with blood and receives oxygen.

primary hypertension Systolic blood pressure of 130 mmHg or higher and/or diastolic blood pressure of 80 mmHg or higher with no identified cause; also called *essential hypertension*.

secondary hypertension Systolic blood pressure of 130 mmHg or higher and/or diastolic blood pressure of 80 mmHg or higher as a result of disease (e.g., kidney dysfunction or sleep apnea) or drug use.

likely to be found in individuals with hypertension than in people with normal blood pressure. Smoking and elevated blood lipoproteins make these diseases even more likely. Individuals with hypertension need to be diagnosed and treated as soon as possible, as the condition generally progresses to a more serious stage over time and even resists therapy if it persists for years. The benefits of controlling blood pressure were confirmed by the results of a recent randomized study of patients at high risk for cardiovascular events.[58] Decreasing the systolic blood pressure of these patients to less than 120 mmHg, as compared with less than 140 mmHg, resulted in lower rates of fatal and nonfatal major cardiovascular events and death from any cause.

Risk Factors for Hypertension

There are several nonmodifiable risk factors for hypertension:

- A *family history of hypertension* is a risk factor, especially if both parents have (or had) the condition. Some of the apparent heritability of hypertension may be due to sharing a common environment and common behaviors, but there are certainly genetic factors that affect blood pressure.
- *Advancing age* also increases your risk for hypertension. Some of this increase is caused by atherosclerosis. As plaque builds up in the arteries, the arteries become less flexible and cannot expand. When the blood vessels remain rigid, blood pressure remains high. Eventually, the plaque begins to make the problem worse by decreasing the blood supply to the kidneys, which decreases their ability to control blood volume and, in turn, blood pressure.
- There are *racial differences* in hypertension risk as well. Compared to other racial and ethnic groups, Black individuals have higher blood pressure measurements and tend to develop hypertension at a younger age.

Aside from those risk factors we cannot change, there are many modifiable risk factors for hypertension:[59,60]

- Overall, *obesity* is considered the leading lifestyle factor related to hypertension. Additional blood vessels develop to support excess body tissue in individuals who are overweight or obese, and these extra miles of blood vessels increase the workload for the heart and elevate blood pressure. As discussed in Section 4.7, obesity is also linked to insulin resistance, and elevated blood insulin levels tend to augment sodium retention. Obesity-related changes in hormones and inflammation may also accelerate atherosclerosis. A weight loss of as little as 10 to 15 pounds often can help treat hypertension.
- *Physical inactivity* is another lifestyle factor that increases the risk for hypertension. Adopting a physically active lifestyle can be especially impactful in combination with weight loss. If a person with obesity can engage in regular physical activity (at least 5 days per week for 30 to 60 minutes) and lose weight, blood pressure often returns to normal.
- *Excess alcohol intake* is responsible for about 10% of all cases of hypertension. When hypertension is caused by excessive alcohol intake, it is usually reversible. A sensible alcohol intake for people with hypertension is no more than two drinks per day for adult males and no more than one drink per day for adult females and all older adults.
- *Excess sodium intake* is related to hypertension. In general, increases in sodium intake are accompanied by increases in blood pressure because excess sodium leads to fluid retention by the kidneys. The corresponding increase in blood volume results in increased blood pressure. However, as described in Section 9.3, some individuals are especially sodium-sensitive. For sodium-sensitive individuals, blood pressure responds dramatically to changes in sodium intake.
- *Inadequate intakes of potassium, calcium, and magnesium* also increase the risk of hypertension, especially when combined with excessive sodium intake (see *Newsworthy Nutrition*).[61,62] All three of these minerals are important for healthy blood pressure because they help blood vessels relax. Studies show that altering the dietary pattern to include these minerals and be low in salt can decrease blood pressure within days,

Newsworthy Nutrition

DASH diet is associated with lower blood pressure among college students

INTRODUCTION: Although adverse health outcomes may not be observed until middle or older adulthood, hypertension develops early in life. Many studies show the positive impact of the DASH diet on blood pressure and other health parameters among middle-aged and older adults. However, the DASH diet has not been sufficiently studied among young adults. **OBJECTIVES:** In this *cross-sectional study,* the researchers wanted to determine if stricter adherence to a DASH diet was associated with lower blood pressure, lower visceral fat (i.e., fat deposited around the waist), and lower waist circumference. **METHODS:** A sample of 244 university students in Spain completed a food frequency questionnaire, 3-day food record, and a physical activity questionnaire. From the dietary data, researchers evaluated adherence to the DASH diet based on intakes of fruits, vegetables, nuts, legumes, whole grains, low-fat dairy products, sodium, sweets, and processed meats. Systolic and diastolic blood pressure, height, weight, waist circumference, hip circumference, and body fat were measured. **RESULTS:** Study participants with lower adherence to the DASH diet had higher intakes of total fat, saturated fat, cholesterol, and sodium. Study participants with higher adherence to the DASH diet had higher intakes of fiber, fruits, vegetables, legumes, nuts, low-fat dairy products, and whole grains, which yielded higher intakes of potassium, magnesium, and calcium. Higher adherence to the DASH diet was associated with lower systolic blood pressure, lower visceral fat, and lower waist circumference. **CONCLUSION:** This observational study showed that higher adherence to a DASH diet is linked with lower blood pressure, lower visceral fat, and lower waist circumference among young, college-age adults. This is important because health behaviors developed in young adulthood are likely to persist throughout life. Promoting a DASH dietary pattern to young adults has the potential to influence long-term cardiovascular health outcomes.

Source: Navarro-Prado S, Schmidt-RioValle J, Montero-Alonso MA, Fernández-Aparicio Á, González-Jiménez E. Stricter adherence to dietary approaches to stop hypertension (DASH) and its association with lower blood pressure, visceral fat, and waist circumference in university students. *Nutrients*. 2020 Mar 11;12(3):740. doi: 10.3390/nu12030740

especially among African Americans. The response is similar to that seen with commonly used medications.

- *Tobacco use* is linked to an increased risk of hypertension. Nicotine and other compounds in tobacco—in all forms—can damage the blood vessels and reduce the oxygen-carrying capacity of the blood.

Although most public health campaigns focus on controlling sodium intake, efforts to prevent hypertension should also focus on energy balance, physical activity, intake of minerals that can lower blood pressure, and reducing consumption of alcohol.

magnificent microbiome

Sodium, Microbiota, and Blood Pressure

The role of sodium in fluid balance is one mechanism by which lowering sodium intake may lower blood pressure. However, scientists are also learning about the effects of sodium on the gut microbiota. High sodium intakes may decrease the abundance of certain strains of bacteria that produce short-chain fatty acids (e.g., butyrate), which are associated with lower blood pressure in animal and human studies.

Source: Smiljanec K, Lennon SL. Sodium, hypertension, and the gut: does the gut microbiota go salty? *Am J Physiol Heart Circ Physiol.* 2019 Dec 1;317(6): H1173-H1182. Doi: 10.1152/ajpheart.00312.2019

TABLE 9-4 ■ What Is the DASH Diet?
The DASH diet is low in fat and sodium and rich in fruits, vegetables, and low-fat dairy products. Here is the breakdown:

Per Day	Per Week
6 to 8 servings of grains and grain products	—
4 to 5 servings of fruit	—
4 to 5 servings of vegetables	—
2 to 3 servings of low-fat or fat-free dairy products	—
2 or fewer servings of meats, poultry, and fish	4 to 5 servings of nuts, seeds, beans, peas, or lentils
2 to 3 servings of fats/oils	5 or fewer servings of sweets and added sugars

The DASH Diet

Considering the dietary risk factors outlined, researchers funded by the National Heart, Lung, and Blood Institute came up with Dietary Approaches to Stop Hypertension (DASH) (Table 9-4). The DASH diet is rich in calcium, potassium, and magnesium and low in salt. Compared to a standard MyPlate Plan, the DASH diet adds extra vegetables and fruits and emphasizes the consumption of plant sources of protein. The DASH diet also encourages two to three servings per day of low-fat or fat-free dairy products. In DASH studies, participants also consumed no more than 3 grams of sodium and no more than one to two alcoholic drinks per day. A DASH 2 dietary trial tested three daily sodium intakes (3300 milligrams, 2400 milligrams, and 1500 milligrams). Regardless of sodium intake, following the DASH diet improved blood pressure, but lowering sodium intake resulted in even greater reductions in

Medicine Cabinet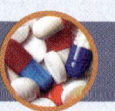

Blood Pressure Control

Diuretics are commonly prescribed to lower blood pressure. Diuretics cause the kidneys to excrete more urine but at the same time may increase urinary excretion of minerals and decrease blood levels of potassium, magnesium, and zinc. Those taking diuretics need to carefully monitor their dietary intake of these minerals, especially potassium, and increase their intake of fruits and vegetables or potassium chloride supplements as prescribed by primary care providers.

Examples:
- Hydrochlorothiazide (Microzide®)
- Chlorothiazide (Diuril®)

Beta-blockers decrease the heart's rate, as well as its workload and blood output.

Examples:
- Atenolol (Tenormin®)
- Metoprolol tartrate (Lopressor®)

ACE (angiotensin-converting enzyme) inhibitors cause the body to produce less angiotensin, which causes the blood vessels to relax and open up and thus lower blood pressure.

Examples:
- Captopril (Capoten®)
- Lisinopril (Prinivel®, Zestril®)

Source: Godman H. Best medications for hypertension. *U.S. News & World Report.* July 15, 2021. https://health.usnews.com/health-care/patient-advice/articles/best-medications-for-hypertension

Advice	Details	Drop in Systolic Blood Pressure
Lose excess weight	For every 20 pounds you lose (if BMI > 25)	5 points
Adopt a DASH eating plan	Eat a lower-fat diet rich in vegetables, fruits, and low-fat dairy foods	11 points
Exercise daily	Get 90–150 min/wk of aerobic activity (such as brisk walking)	5 to 8 points
Limit sodium	< 1500 mg/d is optimal goal but at least 1000 mg/d reduction in most adults	5 to 6 points
Enhance intake of dietary potassium	Consume 3500–5000 mg per day preferably from a dietary pattern rich in potassium	4 to 5 points
Limit alcohol	Have no more than 2 drinks per day for males, 1 drink per day for females (1 drink = 12 oz beer, 5 oz wine, or 1.5 oz 80-proof whiskey)	4 points

FIGURE 9-28 What works? If your blood pressure is high, here's how much lifestyle changes can lower it.

Source: 2017 Guideline for the Prevention, Detection, Evaluation, and Management of High Blood Pressure in Adults. https://www.acc.org/~/media/Non-Clinical/Files-PDFs-Excel-MS-Word-etc/Guidelines/2017/Guidelines_Made_Simple_2017_HBP.pdf

blood pressure.[63] Overall, the DASH diet is seen as a total dietary approach to treating hypertension.

The DASH diet was created over 20 years ago, and it has stood the test of time. Numerous studies have shown that it consistently lowers blood pressure in diverse populations with elevated blood pressure or hypertension.[61,62] Subsequent research has shown the DASH plan also improves blood glucose control, reduces blood lipids, reduces the risk of strokes, protects kidney health, supports bone health, slows the rate of cognitive decline throughout aging, and can assist with weight management.[64,65] A panel of health experts has named the DASH diet one of the best overall eating plans. The DASH diet tied with the Flexitarian diet for second place on the *U.S. News & World Report*'s 2023 Best Diets Overall list.[66]

Medications to Treat Hypertension

There are a variety of high blood pressure medications, otherwise known as antihypertensives. The different classes of these drugs are summarized in the *Medicine Cabinet* feature in this section. Diuretics, or "water pills," are one class that works to reduce blood volume (and therefore blood pressure) by increasing fluid output in the urine. Other medications act by slowing heart rate or by causing relaxation of the small muscles lining the blood vessels. A combination of two or more medications is commonly required to treat hypertension that does not respond to nutrition and lifestyle therapy.

Prevention of Hypertension

Many of the risk factors for hypertension and stroke are controllable, and appropriate lifestyle changes can reduce a person's risk (Fig. 9-28), depending on the severity of the hypertension. Experts recommend that those with hypertension lower blood pressure through diet and lifestyle changes before resorting to blood pressure medications.

✓ CONCEPT CHECK 9.17

1. What are the systolic and diastolic blood pressure values for the diagnosis of Stage 1 and Stage 2 hypertension?
2. Describe three similarities and three differences between the DASH diet and the dietary pattern recommended by MyPlate.
3. What lifestyle changes can help lower high blood pressure?

9.18 Nutrition and Your Health: Osteoporosis

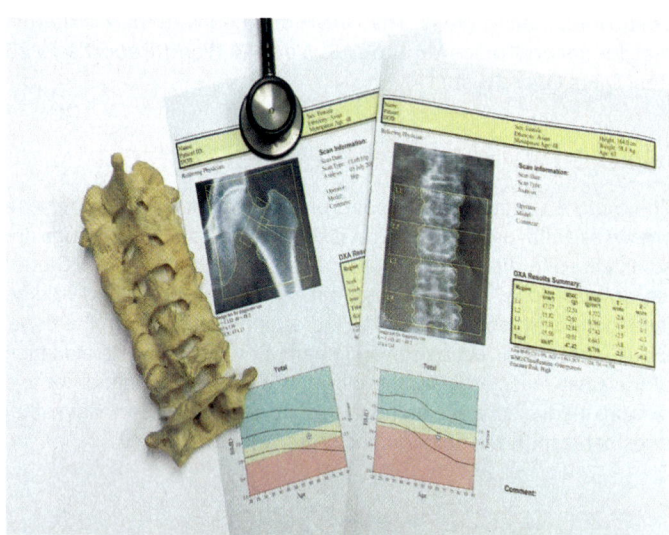

April KASA/123RF

There are two types of bone: *cortical bone* and *trabecular bone*:

- **Cortical bone** (80% of adult bone mass) is sometimes called dense or compact bone. The shafts of long bones (e.g., leg bone) and the outer portion of nearly all bones are composed of cortical bone, which functions to provide strength and stability. Microscopic openings in cortical bone allow blood vessels and nerves to pass through, supplying nutrients, oxygen, and hormones to bone cells.
- **Trabecular bone** (20% of adult bone mass) is predominant in the ends of long bones, vertebrae, rib cage, and flat bones of the pelvis. Like cortical bone, trabecular bone provides strength and structural stability. However, because it is spongy and less rigid, it also functions as a shock absorber. It has an open structure, which lightens the weight of bones. The latticelike matrix of trabecular bone has small cavities that can be filled with marrow or connective tissue.

Bone Growth and Remodeling

The growth, maintenance, and repair of both cortical bone and trabecular bone involve a complex relationship between the synthesis of new bone by the bone-building cells, **osteoblasts,** and the breakdown of bone by **osteoclasts.** The continual degradation and resynthesis of bone is termed **bone remodeling.** When you remodel a room, you tear down first and then you rebuild or add on. The same principle applies to bone. Osteoclasts break down or degrade small amounts of bone. This process is called **resorption.** In doing so, minerals embedded in the bone matrix, including calcium, phosphorus, and magnesium, are freed and released into the blood. Then, osteoblasts embed within the dissolved "resorption bay" provided by the osteoclasts. The osteoblasts take up free calcium and phosphorus and, along with collagen, form a complex mixture called hydroxyapatite. This mixture adds strength and structure to the bone.

Bone growth typically occurs in length and width during the first two decades of life. The rate of bone formation exceeds the rate of bone breakdown during infancy, childhood, and young adulthood. The majority of bone growth occurs before adulthood, although peak bone mass is usually achieved a few years before age 30. Genetics as well as nutrient intake, drugs, hormones, physical activity, and lifestyle choices will influence the age at which peak bone mass is achieved. People with a larger frame size and body weight will have a greater bone mass due to the additional stress on the bone associated with the extra weight.

The optimal situation throughout adulthood would be to maintain peak bone mass through an equal amount of bone resorption and resynthesis. However, after 30 years of age, bone resorption occurs at a faster rate than synthesis, resulting in a gradual loss of bone mass and a decrease in **bone mineral density.** Throughout midlife and older adulthood, this decrease in bone mass is normal and expected. Around menopause, which usually occurs around age 50, females go through a period of accelerated bone loss (1% to 3% of bone mass per year) due to declines in estrogen. Males also lose bone mass as they age, but the loss is more gradual (Fig. 9-29).

How do you know if your bones are healthy? What happens if your bone mass gets too low? And, starting today, what can you do to protect your bone health?

Bone Health Assessment

Before the 1990s, clinicians relied on X-rays to assess bone health. It is possible to detect problems with X-rays, but not until significant changes have taken place (e.g., loss of 30% or more of bone mass or presence of a fracture). Today, we have more sensitive tools that can quantitate bone mineral density and, subsequently, assess the likelihood of a person developing bone disease.

cortical bone The compact or dense bone found on the outer surfaces of bone.

trabecular bone The less dense, more open structure bone found in the inner layer of bones; also called *cancellous bone*.

osteoblast Bone cells that initiate the synthesis of new bone.

osteoclast Bone cells that break down bone and subsequently release bone minerals into the blood.

bone remodeling The chemical process by which bone is broken down and replaced by new bone.

resorption The process of losing substance. Bone resorption is part of the initial process for remodeling and growth.

bone mineral density A measure of the amount of the total mineral contained in a certain volume of bone, generally expressed as grams per cubic centimeter.

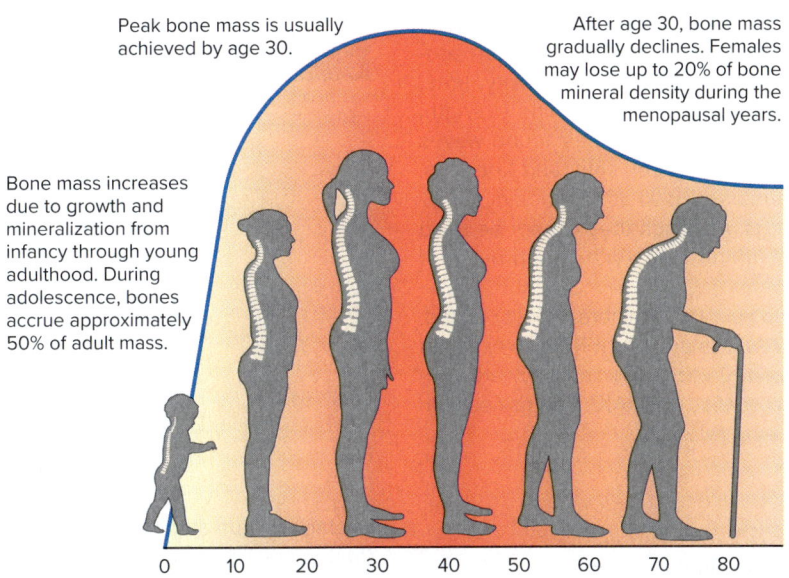

FIGURE 9-29 Through processes that are primarily regulated by hormones, bone mass changes across the lifespan. Dietary and other lifestyle behaviors during the growing years can influence peak bone mass, which affects the risk for osteopenia or osteoporosis during older adulthood.
Source: National Osteoporosis Foundation, *Healthy Bones for Life: Patient's Guide.* 2014. http://www.bonehealthandosteoporosis.org/wp-content/uploads/NOF-Health-Bones-For-Life-Patients-Guide.pdf

The most accurate way to assess bone health is the central **dual energy X-ray absorptiometry (DXA)** measurement of the hip and spine. The central DXA procedure is simple, painless, safe, and noninvasive, and generally takes less than 15 minutes. The ability of the bone to block the path of a low-level X-ray is used to determine bone mineral density. A very low dose of radiation is used for the DXA—about one-tenth of the exposure from a chest X-ray. The hip and spine are measured because these are the most common sites of fractures among older adults. From the DXA measurement of bone mineral density of the hip and spine, a T-score is generated, which compares the observed bone mineral density to that of a healthy, 30-year-old adult at peak bone mass. The T-score is interpreted as shown in Figure 9-30.[67]

Bone mineral density does not tell the whole story when it comes to bone health and fracture risk. In fact, as many as half of females who suffer from a hip fracture would not be diagnosed as having osteoporosis based on the T-score alone. Combining bone mineral density with other assessments of bone quality may facilitate the early identification of individuals who would benefit from interventions to protect bone health. For example, DXA equipment can be used to examine the shape and features of the vertebrae to detect prior compression fractures, which often go unnoticed but are highly predictive of future fracture risk. In addition, DXA equipment can be used to examine the architecture of the bones in the spine to score the health of the trabecular bone.[67]

When DXA measurements of the hip and spine are not feasible due to portability, expense, or severe obesity, several peripheral measurements of bone density can be used as screening methods at various sites on the body. Peripheral DXA uses the same technology as central DXA but scans only the ankle or wrist. Peripheral quantitative computed tomography (pQCT) generates

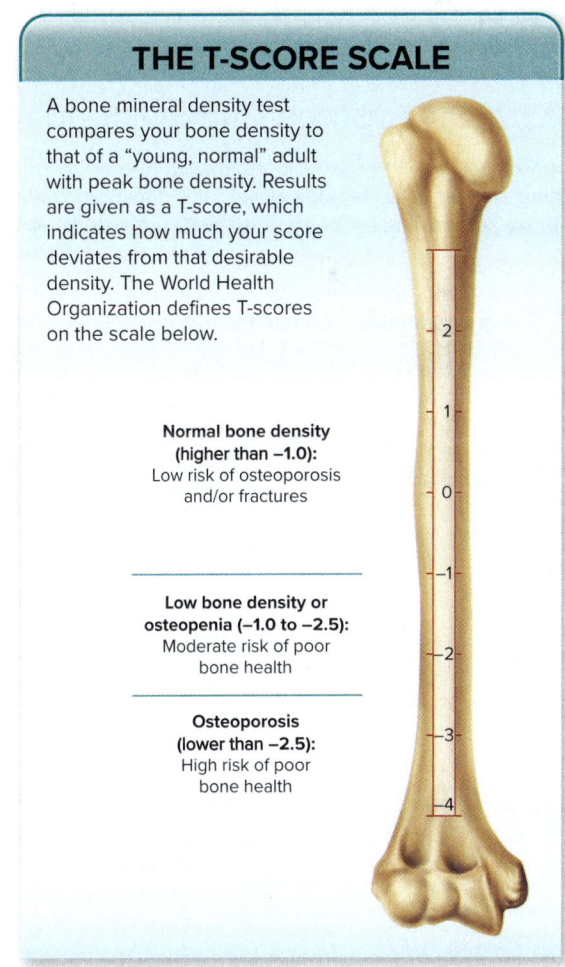

FIGURE 9-30 The classification for diagnosing osteoporosis is used by the World Health Organization.

dual energy x-ray absorptiometry (DXA) A scientific tool used to measure bone mineral density and body composition.

a three-dimensional scan of the radius in the arm or the tibia in the lower leg. It measures bone mineral density and can provide information on cortical and trabecular bone density, area, and thickness, as well as some measurements of bone strength. The quantitative ultrasound (QUS) technique uses sound waves to measure the density of bone in the heel, shin, and kneecap. These peripheral tests are sometimes used at health fairs, medical offices, and research settings. Although they cannot be used to diagnose disease, they can inform the health care provider if additional testing is warranted.[67]

Whether or not you have had your bone mineral density tested, you can use the Fracture Risk Assessment Tool (FRAX) to estimate your risk of fracture over the next 10 years. You can calculate your FRAX score online at https://frax.shef.ac.uk/FRAX/. This risk estimator takes into account the following factors:[68]

- Age
- Sex
- Weight status
- Personal and family history of fractures
- Smoking status
- Use of glucocorticoid medications
- Presence of rheumatoid arthritis and a variety of other disorders (e.g., endocrine conditions, malabsorptive disorders) that are strongly associated with osteoporosis
- Alcohol use
- Bone mineral density (if known)

Defining Osteoporosis and Osteopenia

Peak bone mass and the rate of bone loss during adulthood vary depending on genetics, biological sex, and lifestyle (Tables 9-5 and 9-6). A person whose peak bone mass at age 30 is below average will be at greater risk for fractures as bone mass declines later in life. Likewise, conditions that speed up bone loss can lead to deterioration of bone health. **Osteopenia** and osteoporosis are two terms that describe different degrees of bone loss. Osteopenia refers to moderately low bone mineral density, which may be a precursor to osteoporosis. Osteoporosis is a condition in which bones are porous, fragile, and susceptible to fracture as a result of severely low bone mineral density (Fig. 9-31).

The Bone Health and Osteoporosis Foundation (formerly the National Osteoporosis Foundation) sets the following criteria for diagnosis of osteoporosis:[67]

- T-score ≤ -2.5 for bone mineral density at the spine or hip.
- Hip fracture (regardless of bone mineral density).
- T-score between -1 and -2.5 plus a fracture of the vertebrae, proximal humerus, pelvis, or wrist.

osteopenia A bone disease defined by low mineral density.

TABLE 9-5 ■ Biological Factors Associated with Bone Status

Biological Factors	Effect on Bone Status
Sex	Females have lower bone mass and density than males.
Age	Bone loss often begins after age 30.
Race	Individuals of Caucasian or Asian heritage are at greater risk for poor bone health than individuals of African descent.
Frame size	People with "small bones" have a lower bone mass.
Estrogen	Females at menopause and beyond should consider use of current medical therapies to reduce bone loss linked to the fall in estrogen output.

TABLE 9-6 ■ Modifiable Lifestyle Factors Associated with Bone Status

Lifestyle Factors	Call to Action
Adequate dietary pattern containing an appropriate amount of nutrients	Follow the MyPlate Plan or the DASH diet with special emphasis on adequate amounts of fruits, vegetables, and low-fat and fat-free dairy products. Consider use of fortified foods (or supplements) to make up for specific nutrient shortfalls, such as vitamin D and calcium. If deficient, consult your primary care provider and a registered dietitian nutritionist (RDN).
Healthy body weight	Maintain a healthy body weight (BMI of 18.5–24.9) to support bone health.
Normal menses	During childbearing years, seek medical advice if menses cease for more than 3 months (such as in cases of anorexia nervosa or extreme athletic training).
Movements that create impact and muscle-loading forces on bone.	Perform weight-bearing activity as this contributes to bone maintenance, whereas bed rest and a sedentary lifestyle promote bone loss. Strength training, especially upper body, is helpful to bone maintenance.
Smoking	Smoking lowers estrogen synthesis in females. Cessation is advised. Passive exposure is a risk.
Medications	Some medications (e.g., thyroid hormone, cortisol, diuretics) stimulate urinary calcium excretion. Some medications (e.g., diuretics, cancer medications) stimulate urinary excretion of magnesium.
Excessive intake of protein, phosphorus, sodium, caffeine, wheat bran, or alcohol	Moderate intake of these dietary constituents is recommended. Problems primarily arise when excessive intakes of these nutrients are combined with inadequate calcium consumption. Excessive soft drink consumption is especially discouraged.
Inadequate UVB exposure	If sunlight exposure is limited (< 10 to 15 minutes per day without sunscreen), focus on food to meet current RDA for vitamin D. Consult your primary care provider before using vitamin D supplements.

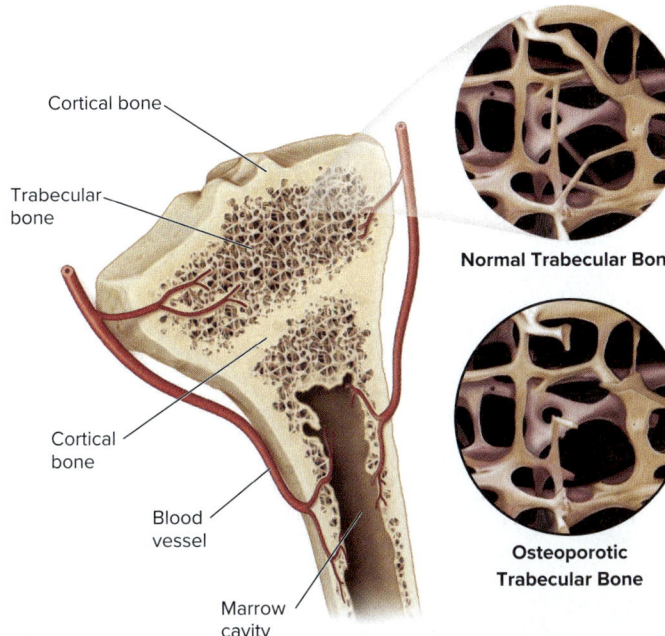

FIGURE 9-31 Normal and osteoporotic bone. Cortical bone forms the shafts of bones and their outer mineral covering. Trabecular bone supports the outer shell of cortical bone in various bones of the body. Note how the osteoporotic bone has much less trabecular bone. This leads to a more fragile bone and is not reversible to any major extent with current therapies.

- Fracture risk above the treatment threshold as determined by FRAX (≥ 20% estimated risk of major osteoporotic fracture or ≥ 3% estimated risk of hip fracture).

The Bone Health and Osteoporosis Foundation recommends DXA testing for the following groups of people:[67]
- All females age 65 and older and males age 70 and older.
- Younger postmenopausal females, females in the menopausal transition, and males (age 50 to 69) who have clinical risk factors for fracture.
- Adults who have a fracture at age 50 and older.
- Adults with a condition (e.g., rheumatoid arthritis) or taking a medication (e.g., glucocorticoids) associated with low bone mass or bone loss.

Osteoporosis is sometimes called a "silent" disease because it may cause no symptoms until a bone fracture occurs. Osteoporotic fractures can occur at any site, but they are most common in trabecular bone, where the rate of bone turnover is highest. Trabecular bone has an open, spongelike appearance; it is meant to be flexible and absorb shock. However, as bone loss occurs, the open spaces in the trabecular bone widen and the structure of the bones can break down. The bones at greatest risk for osteoporotic fractures are the trabecular-rich bones of the pelvis (6% of fractures), spine (23%), and ends of the long bones, such as the hip (17%) or wrist (13%).[69]

Among adults over age 50 in the United States, osteoporosis affects 18.4% of non-Hispanic Asian adults, 14.7% of Hispanic adults, 12.9% of non-Hispanic white adults, and 6.8% of non-Hispanic Black adults.[70] It is more common among females (80% of cases) than males for several reasons: Females tend to achieve lower peak bone mineral density, females experience drastic bone loss during menopause, and females tend to live longer than males.

There are two main types of osteoporosis: primary and secondary.[71] **Primary osteoporosis** is low bone mineral density that results from changes in bone metabolism caused by aging or imbalances in reproductive hormones; it is not associated with another chronic disease. **Secondary osteoporosis** is low bone mineral density that results from other chronic conditions that accelerate bone loss. For example, some genetic or endocrine disorders can affect bone metabolism, and some GI disorders can affect the absorption of bone-building nutrients. In addition, certain medications, such as glucocorticoids, which are commonly used to treat inflammation, affect bone health.

Primary osteoporosis can be further subdivided into type 1 and type 2 osteoporosis. **Type 1 osteoporosis,** also called *postmenopausal osteoporosis,* typically appears in females between 50 and 60 years of age. This type of osteoporosis is directly linked to decreased estrogen concentrations that occur at menopause. The osteoblasts require estrogen for maximal activity. After menopause, as estrogen decreases, osteoblast activity decreases while osteoclast activity remains high. The result is rapid bone loss. Type 1 osteoporosis most dramatically affects trabecular bone. Without intervention, a female can lose up to 20% of her bone density in the years following menopause (i.e., between ages 50 and 60) (Fig. 9-29).[72]

Type 2 osteoporosis, sometimes called *senile osteoporosis,* tends to be diagnosed later in life (70 to 75 years of age) and affects both males and females. Type 2 osteoporosis is a result of the breakdown of both cortical and trabecular bone. It is mostly due to age-related factors that affect the rate of bone turnover and the digestion and absorption of bone-building nutrients. Low dietary intake of bone-building nutrients compounds the problem.

Osteoporotic fractures—particularly of the hip and vertebrae—can be devastating. For example, 20% of patients who suffer a hip fracture will die within the first year after fracture.[73] For survivors, osteoporotic fractures often result in loss of mobility and the need for long-term care. Fewer than half of survivors will regain their pre-fracture levels of mobility and independence in activities of daily living (e.g., self-care, cooking, shopping). Subsequent fractures (or fear of fracture) can affect quality of life.[74]

Vertebral fractures, especially if there are several of them, can cause significant pain and **kyphosis,** which is a curvature in the upper spine (Fig. 9-32). Kyphosis is a major concern because the bending of the spine may decrease the volume of the chest cavity,

primary osteoporosis Low bone mineral density that results from changes in bone metabolism caused by aging or imbalances in reproductive hormones.

secondary osteoporosis Low bone mineral density that results from a chronic condition that accelerates bone loss.

type 1 osteoporosis Porous trabecular bone characterized by rapid bone demineralization following menopause.

type 2 osteoporosis Porous trabecular and cortical bone observed in males and females after the age of 70.

kyphosis Abnormally increased bending of the spine; commonly known as *dowager's hump.*

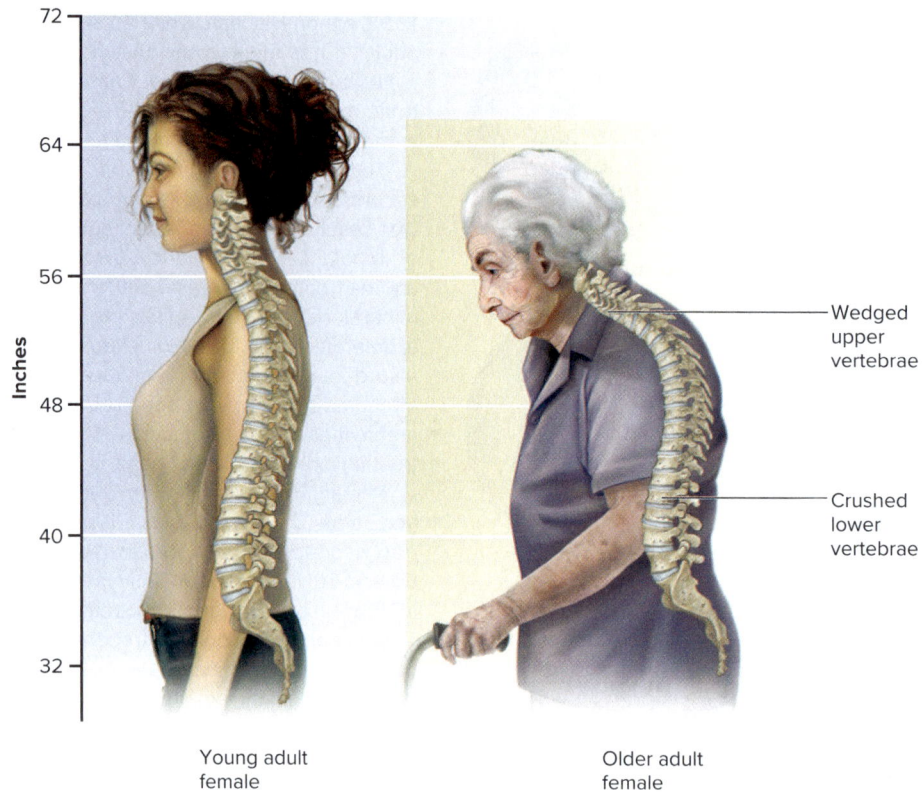

FIGURE 9-32 A young adult female with healthy bones and an older adult female with osteoporosis. Osteoporotic bones have less supportive structure, so osteoporosis generally leads to loss of height, distorted body shape, fractures, and possibly loss of teeth. Monitoring changes in adult height is one way to detect early evidence of osteoporosis. Kyphosis, or curvature of the upper spine, shown on the right, results from demineralization of the vertebrae. This can lead to both physical and emotional pain. Kyphosis occurs in both males and females.
Source: National Osteoporosis Foundation. *Healthy Bones for Life Patient's Guide.* 2014. https://cdn.nof.org/wp-content/uploads/NOF-Health-Bones-For-Life-Patients-Guide.pdf.

resulting in difficulty breathing, abdominal pain, decreased appetite, and premature satiety. Changes in mobility and physical function increase the risk of falling, and with decreased bone mineral density, the bones are more susceptible to fractures following a fall.

Prevention of Osteoporosis

Bone health is only partially (60% to 80%) determined by your genes.[75] This means you have some control over your bone health. The key to protecting yourself from osteoporosis in older adulthood is to build dense bones during the first 30 years of life and then limit the amount of bone loss in adulthood. People who achieve a higher peak bone mass early in life have higher calcium stores to draw upon during the older years. What dietary and other lifestyle modifications can you make to support your bone health?

Physical activity is a major contributor to bone health throughout life. Bones are very adaptable; when bones are exposed to physical stress, the process of bone remodeling leads to the synthesis of stronger, more dense bone tissue. Any exercise is beneficial, but weight-bearing activities and resistance exercises can particularly increase bone strength.[76] Conversely, a sedentary lifestyle leads to decreased bone strength. A striking example of this effect has been observed in astronauts, whose bone mineral density begins to decrease after only a few days in the weightless environment of space. The *Physical Activity Guidelines* specifically recommends that children and adolescents perform bone-strengthening activities at least 3 days per week. Examples of bone-strengthening activities include running, jumping, and lifting weights.[77]

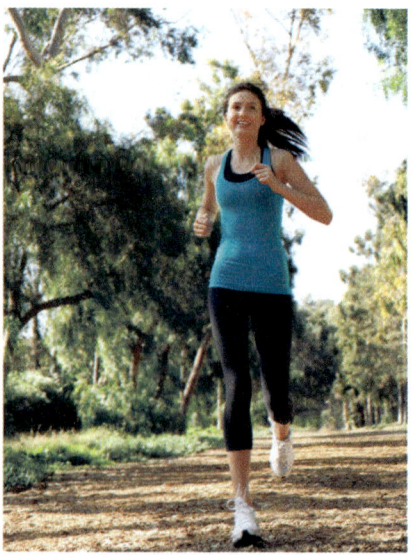

Weight-bearing physical activity, such as walking or running, is associated with increased bone density. Female athletes, however, must maintain an adequate energy intake to maintain estrogen levels, which stimulates bone formation. Derek E. Rothchild/Photodisc/Getty Images

The synthesis, maintenance, and repair of bone requires several key nutrients, including calcium, phosphorus, magnesium, and vitamin D. Other micronutrients that support bone health include vitamin C, vitamin K, and potassium. In addition, adequate protein must be consumed, especially during older adulthood, to reduce bone loss.[78] Epidemiological studies suggest that dietary patterns rich in fruits, vegetables, low-fat dairy products, and seafood are associated with higher bone mineral density and lower fracture risk.[79,75] Following the advice of the *Dietary Guidelines*, which emphasizes low-fat dairy products, seafood, and plenty of fruits and vegetables, will support your bone health throughout life.

Aim to meet your DRIs for nutrients using foods and beverages. Current evidence does not support the recommendation of dietary supplements alone as a strategy to prevent osteoporosis among community-dwelling adults (see box), but if your dietary pattern is habitually low in bone-building nutrients, supplementation can be useful to close the gap. Calcium and vitamin D supplements can be especially helpful for individuals who do not consume dairy products (whether due to food allergies, lactose intolerance, or personal preference), those who take medications known to compromise bone health, and females going through menopause. However, more is not better when it comes to calcium supplementation. Consult your primary care provider about supplementation if you are not able to meet your nutrient needs from foods and beverages.[75]

> *Vitamin D, Calcium, or Combined Supplementation for the Primary Prevention of Fractures in Community-Dwelling Adults* Task Force Conclusions:
>
> 1. Current evidence is insufficient to assess the balance of the benefits and harms of vitamin D and calcium supplementation, alone or combined, for the primary prevention of fractures in community-dwelling, asymptomatic males and premenopausal females.
> 2. Current evidence is insufficient to assess the balance of the benefits and harms of daily supplementation with doses greater than 400 IU (10 micrograms) of vitamin D and greater than 1000 mg of calcium for the primary prevention of fractures in community-dwelling, postmenopausal females.
> 3. The Task Force recommends against daily supplementation with 400 IU (10 micrograms) or less of vitamin D and 1000 mg or less of calcium for the primary prevention of fractures in community-dwelling, postmenopausal females. These recommendations do not apply to persons with a history of osteoporotic fractures, increased risk for falls, or a diagnosis of osteoporosis or vitamin D deficiency.
>
> Source: U.S. Preventive Services Task Force. Vitamin D, calcium, or combined supplementation for the primary prevention of fractures in community-dwelling adults: US Preventive Services Task Force Recommendation Statement. *JAMA*. 2018;319(15):1592-1599. doi: 10.1001/jama.2018.3185

Maintaining a healthy body weight across the lifespan is another nutrition-related strategy to reduce the risk of osteoporotic fractures. It is clear that low body weight is associated with lower bone mineral density. Part of this effect is probably due to lower mechanical loading of the bones. In other words, when the bones are not stressed as much by the weight of everyday activities, the osteoblasts are not stimulated as much to synthesize new bone tissue. Individuals with lower body weight also tend to have lower dietary intake, so the availability of bone-building nutrients may be inadequate to support bone health. Furthermore, low energy availability and lower levels of adipose tissue usually result in lower production of reproductive hormones, which compromises bone health.

For many years, clinicians assumed that higher body weight should be protective of bones because the increased mechanical stress of supporting a higher body weight should stimulate bone remodeling. However, research shows a surprising relationship between obesity and bone health. While higher BMI is associated with higher bone mineral density, this higher bone mineral density does not directly translate into a lower risk for fractures, particularly among individuals with upper body obesity (i.e., android body fat distribution). Common fracture sites differ for individuals with obesity, as well. Whereas individuals with low or normal BMI are more likely to suffer hip fractures, individuals with higher BMI are more likely to fracture the wrist or ankle.[80]

There are many possible explanations for this paradox. One is that individuals with obesity are more prone to falls. Another is that obesity is linked to chronic, low-grade inflammation, which accelerates bone resorption and inhibits bone synthesis. Endocrine abnormalities, such as insulin resistance and hyperparathyroidism, may also negatively impact bone metabolism. Of concern, recent increases in pediatric obesity are impacting the bone health of younger generations.[80] Overall, research on the relationship between obesity and bone health suggests that a BMI in the healthy or overweight range is associated with the most favorable bone health outcomes.

In Section 9.3, you learned about the benefits of limiting sodium intake for cardiovascular health. Some research shows that limiting sodium intake may be beneficial for bone health, too. Excessive

> **magnificent microbiome**
>
> **Gut–Bone Axis**
> There are several ways the gut microbiota may positively influence bone health. When microorganisms in the gut ferment dietary fiber, they produce short-chain fatty acids (e.g., butyrate), which can lower the pH in the intestine and promote the health of the cells that line the intestine. Both of these changes could promote the absorption of bone-building minerals, such as calcium and magnesium. Then, as these short-chain fatty acids are absorbed, they travel through the blood to the bones, where they may stimulate the osteoblasts (bone-building cells) and inhibit osteoclasts (bone-resorbing cells). A dietary pattern that is rich in dietary fiber or use of prebiotic or probiotic supplements may be useful in the prevention of osteoporosis.
>
> Source: Weaver CM. Diet, gut microbiome, and bone health. *Curr Osteoporos Rep*. 2015 Apr;13(2):125-130. doi: 10.1007/s11914-015-0257-0

sodium intake is linked to increased calcium excretion, which could limit bone mineralization, particularly if calcium intake is inadequate.[81] Other lifestyle modifications that can reduce fracture risk include limiting alcohol intake and quitting smoking.[72]

Treatment of Osteoporosis

Adults diagnosed with osteoporosis should first be counseled on risk factor reduction, and much of this advice echoes what you have just read about the prevention of osteoporosis. Exercise is a big part of risk factor reduction. Losses of muscle mass that commonly accompany aging contribute to bone loss and increase the risk of falling.[82] Exercises that improve muscle strength and balance are specifically recommended. The Bone Health and Osteoporosis Foundation recommends engaging in moderate-intensity, weight-bearing physical activity for at least 30 minutes on most days of the week. They also recommend performing resistance training (including 8 to 12 different muscle-strengthening activities that target all major muscle groups) on 2 to 3 days per week. Older adults with advanced osteoporosis or a history of fractures may need to take special precautions when it comes to high-impact activities, but some physical activity is better than none.[72]

In addition to the dietary advice recommended for prevention of osteoporosis, dietary supplements of calcium (1000 milligrams per day in divided doses) and vitamin D (25 to 50 micrograms per day) may be needed for adults with osteoporosis who are unable to meet the RDA with dietary sources. Vitamin D supplements are often recommended for individuals with low vitamin D levels.[69]

Because falls precede most osteoporotic fractures, patients will also be counseled on strategies to reduce the risk for falls. Physical activity is helpful for improving strength and balance, but other measures include wearing comfortable, supportive shoes; removing hazards (e.g., cords, loose rugs) from the home environment; and installing adequate lighting and handrails.[67]

Primary care providers have guidelines regarding pharmacological (drug) intervention for patients. These drugs are indicated for postmenopausal females and males over 50 who meet specific standards for the level of risk of future fracture and medical history.[83] Current medication options include **bisphosphonates** and parathyroid hormone. Females may also use calcium and hormone replacement therapy (see *Medicine Cabinet* for a list of osteoporosis medications).

Summary

The significance of osteoporosis as a personal and public health problem is intensifying as the population ages, not just in the United States, but worldwide.[84] Many of the risk factors for osteoporosis are modifiable. However, most people do not recognize that their choices during adolescence can have a profound impact on their bone health during adulthood. The time to make lifestyle changes, like ensuring adequate intakes of bone-building nutrients and engaging in weight-bearing physical activity, is now!

bisphosphonates Drugs that bind minerals and prevent osteoclast breakdown of bone. Examples are alendronate (Fosamax) and risedronate (Actonel).

Medicine Cabinet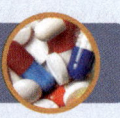

Types of Osteoporosis Medications

Antiresorptive agents are used to prevent bone loss and decrease the risk of bone fractures. They slow bone loss that occurs during the breakdown phase of the remodeling cycle. These medicines slow bone loss without affecting bone synthesis so that bone density can increase.

- Bisphosphonates
  - Alendronate (Fosamax® and Fosamax Plus D®)
  - Ibandronate (Boniva®)
  - Risedronate (Actonel®, Actonel® with Calcium, and Atelvia™)
  - Zoledronic acid (Reclast®)
- Calcitonin (Fortical® and Miacalcin®)
- Denosumab (Prolia®)
- Estrogen therapy
- Raloxifene (Evista®)
- Basedoxifene + estrogen (Duavee®)

Anabolic agents are used to increase the rate of bone formation and decrease the risk of fractures.

- Teriparatide (Forteo®)
- Abaloparatide (Tymlos)
- Romosozumab-aqqg (Evenity)

©Peter Dazeley/Photographer's Choice/Getty Images

✓ CONCEPT CHECK 9.18

1. Osteoporosis has been described as a pediatric disease with geriatric consequences. Explain what this means.
2. Explain why females have a higher risk of osteoporosis than males.
3. What is the most accurate test for bone density, and how is it done?
4. According to the Bone Health and Osteoporosis Foundation, who should have their bone density checked?
5. Describe one change you could make to your current lifestyle to decrease your risk for osteoporosis.

CASE STUDY: Worried About Bone Health

Grace, a 23-year-old female of Korean descent, is in her final year of nursing school in Boston. She also works 20 hours per week at a local pharmacy. Grace is worried after a phone call she just received from her father. While out on her walk yesterday, Grace's mother caught her foot on an uneven section of the sidewalk, fell, and broke her hip. The doctor diagnosed Grace's mother with osteoporosis, and the family is worried about the long recovery ahead. As a nursing student, Grace knows how devastating a hip fracture can be. She also knows that osteoporosis can run in families. Grace resolves to do whatever she can to learn about osteoporosis and strengthen her bones now.

She searches online and finds the Osteoporosis Risk Check at https://riskcheck.osteoporosis.foundation. The online tool from the International Osteoporosis Foundation focuses mainly on nonmodifiable risk factors for osteoporosis: age, family history, chronic conditions, and use of medications that can influence bone health. The site also highlights some modifiable risk factors: weight status, exposure to sunlight, physical activity level, intake of good food sources of calcium and vitamin D, and use of alcohol or tobacco products.

Grace is 5'4" and weighs 105 pounds. Currently, she does not have any chronic health conditions. She does not take any medications or dietary supplements. Grace wonders if her intakes of calcium and vitamin D are adequate. She cooks traditional Korean dishes for half of her meals but eats fast food or sandwiches for the rest. Her go-to beverages are water and unsweetened tea. She admits she has not been able to fit physical activity into her busy schedule lately. On weekends, she goes out with friends and may have a glass or two of wine. Grace does not smoke.

Answer the following questions about Grace's bone health.

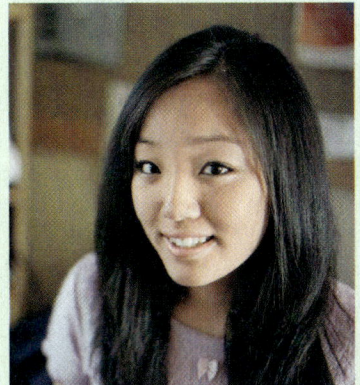

Grace is exploring ways she can decrease her risk for osteoporosis.
Dennis Wise/Digital Vision/Getty Images

1. Go to https://riskcheck.osteoporosis.foundation and fill out the risk assessment using Grace's information. Identify two nonmodifiable risk factors for Grace.
2. Identify two modifiable risk factors for Grace.
3. What are the environmental conditions that inhibit Grace from adequately synthesizing vitamin D? How can she overcome some of them?
4. What are some calcium and vitamin D sources in traditional Korean dishes? (See http://www.pbs.org/hiddenkorea/food.htm for information about traditional Korean food.)
5. Give Grace some tips to increase her calcium and vitamin D intake at fast-food restaurants without significantly increasing costs or calories.
6. Based on her current dietary pattern, do you think Grace should take any dietary supplements? If so, which one(s)?

Complete the Case Study. Responses to these questions can be provided by your instructor.

Summary (Numbers refer to numbered sections in the chapter)

9.1 Water constitutes 50% to 70% of the human body. Its unique chemical properties enable it to dissolve substances as well as serve as a medium for chemical reactions, temperature regulation, and lubrication. Water also helps regulate the acid–base balance in the body.

Daily water needs are estimated at 11 cups (9 cups from beverages) for adult females and 15 cups (13 cups from beverages) for adult males. Hormones participate in the process of fluid conservation. Receptors in the kidneys, blood vessels, and brain monitor blood pressure and solute concentration in the blood. Dehydration leads to kidney failure, coma, and death. The amount of water in the intracellular and extracellular compartments is controlled mainly by ion concentrations.

9.2 Minerals are categorized based on the amount we need per day. If we require greater than 100 milligrams of a mineral per day, it is considered a major mineral; otherwise it is considered a trace mineral. Many minerals are vital for sustaining life. For humans, animal products are the most bioavailable sources of most minerals. Supplements of minerals exceeding 100% of the Daily Values should be taken only under a primary care provider's supervision. Toxicity and nutrient interactions are especially likely if the Upper Level (when set) is exceeded on a long-term basis.

9.3 Sodium, the major positive ion found outside cells, is vital in fluid balance and nerve impulse transmission. The North American diet provides abundant sodium through processed foods and table salt. About one-third of the adult population is especially sodium-sensitive and at risk for developing hypertension from consuming excessive sodium.

9.4 Potassium, the major positive ion found inside cells, has a similar function to sodium. Milk, fruits, and vegetables are good sources. The kidneys closely regulate the amount of potassium in the blood, but if blood potassium gets either too low or too high, heart function can be negatively affected.

9.5 Chloride is the major negative ion found outside cells. It is important in digestion as part of stomach acid and in immune and nerve functions. Table salt supplies most of the chloride in our diets.

9.6 Calcium forms a part of bone structure and plays a role in blood clotting, muscle contraction, nerve transmission, and cell metabolism. Calcium absorption is enhanced by stomach acid and the active vitamin D hormone. Dairy products are important calcium sources, but many dairy alternatives (e.g., soy or almond milk) are available. Deficient calcium intake decreases bone mineralization, ultimately leading to osteopenia and osteoporosis.

9.7 Phosphorus aids enzyme function and forms part of key metabolic compounds, cell membranes, and bone. It is efficiently absorbed, and deficiencies are rare, although there is concern about possible poor intake by some older females. Good food sources include dairy products, bakery products, and meats.

9.8 Magnesium is a mineral found mostly in plant food sources. It is important for nerve and heart function and as an activator for many enzymes. Whole grain breads and cereals (bran portion), vegetables, nuts, seeds, milk, and meats are good food sources.

9.9 Iron absorption depends mainly on the form of iron present and the body's need for it. Heme iron from animal sources is better absorbed than the nonheme iron obtained primarily from plant sources. Consuming vitamin C or meat simultaneously with nonheme iron increases absorption. Iron operates mainly in synthesizing hemoglobin and myoglobin and in the action of the immune system. Females are at highest risk for developing iron deficiency, which decreases blood hemoglobin and hematocrit. When this condition is severe, iron-deficiency anemia develops. This decreases the amount of oxygen carried in the blood. Hemochromatosis is a genetic disorder that causes overabsorption and accumulation of iron, which can result in severe liver and heart damage.

9.10 Zinc aids in the action of up to 200 enzymes important for growth, development, cell membrane structure and function, immune function, antioxidant protection, wound healing, and taste. A zinc deficiency results in poor growth, loss of appetite, reduced sense of taste and smell, hair loss, and a persistent rash. Zinc is best absorbed from animal sources. The richest sources of zinc are oysters, shrimp, crab, and beef. Good plant sources are whole grains, peanuts, and beans.

9.11 An important role of selenium is decreasing the action of free-radical (oxidizing) compounds. In this way, selenium acts along with vitamin E in providing antioxidant protection. Muscle pain, muscle wasting, and a form of heart damage may result from a selenium deficiency. Meats, eggs, fish, and shellfish are good animal sources of selenium. Good plant sources include grains and seeds.

9.12 Iodine forms part of the thyroid hormones. A lack of dietary iodine results in the development of an enlarged thyroid gland or goiter. Iodized salt is a major food source.

9.13 Copper is important for iron metabolism, cross-linking of connective tissue, and other functions, such as enzymes that provide antioxidant protection. A copper deficiency can result in a form of anemia. Copper is found mainly in liver, seafood, cocoa, legumes, and whole grains.

9.14 Fluoride as part of regular dietary intake or toothpaste use makes teeth resistant to dental caries. Most North Americans receive the bulk of their fluoride from fluoridated water and oral hygiene products.

9.15 Chromium aids in the action of the hormone insulin. Chromium deficiency results in impaired blood glucose control. Egg yolks, meats, and whole grains are good sources of chromium.

9.16 Manganese and molybdenum are used by various enzymes. One enzyme that uses manganese provides antioxidant protection. Clear deficiencies in otherwise healthy people are rarely seen for these nutrients. Human needs for other trace minerals are so low that deficiencies are uncommon.

9.17 Hypertension is defined as sustained systolic blood pressure exceeding 130 mmHg or diastolic blood pressure exceeding 80 mmHg. Maintaining a healthy weight; limiting alcohol intake; exercising regularly; decreasing salt intake; and ensuring adequate potassium, magnesium, and calcium in the dietary pattern all can play a part in controlling blood pressure.

9.18 The gold standard of bone health assessment is central dual energy X-ray absorptiometry (DXA). Osteoporosis occurs when bones are porous and fragile due to low mineral density. Osteopenia is low bone mineral density that does not meet the diagnostic criteria of osteoporosis. Aside from bone fractures, osteoporosis causes kyphosis, pain, loss of mobility and independence, decreased lung capacity, fear of falling, and mortality. Type 1 osteoporosis is loss of trabecular bone that follows menopause. Type 2 osteoporosis is loss of cortical and trabecular bone that occurs in both males and females over age 60. Lifestyle modifications (e.g., consuming adequate dietary calcium, phosphorous, and vitamin D; exposure to UVB sunlight; and performing weight-bearing physical activity) are encouraged for prevention of osteoporosis. When lifestyle modifications are not enough, medications (e.g., antiresorptive drugs and hormone therapies) may be used to prevent bone loss, but they are not without side effects.

Check Your Knowledge

1. Dietary heme iron is derived from
   a. elemental iron in food.
   b. animal flesh.
   c. breakfast cereal.
   d. vegetables.

2. Chloride is
   a. a component of hydrochloric acid.
   b. an intracellular fluid ion.
   c. a positively charged ion.
   d. converted to chlorine in the intestinal tract.

3. Which of the following minerals are involved in fluid balance?
   a. Calcium and magnesium
   b. Copper and iron
   c. Selenium and zinc
   d. Sodium and potassium

4. In a situation where there is an insufficient intake of dietary iodine, the thyroid-stimulating hormone promotes the enlargement of the thyroid gland. This condition is called
   a. Graves' disease.
   b. goiter.
   c. hyperparathyroidism.
   d. congenital hypothyroidism.

5. Ninety-nine percent of the calcium in the body is found in
   a. intracellular fluid.
   b. bones and teeth.
   c. nerve cells.
   d. the liver.

6. A deficiency of _____ may lead to impaired glucose tolerance.
   a. iodine   c. chromium
   b. manganese   d. molybdenum

7. Which compartment contains the greatest amount of body fluid?
   a. Intracellular
   b. Extracellular
   c. They contain the same amount.

8. The primary function of sodium is to maintain
   a. bone mineral content.
   b. hemoglobin concentration.
   c. immune function.
   d. fluid distribution.

9. Hypertension is defined as a blood pressure greater than
   a. 110/60.   c. 130/80.
   b. 120/65.   d. 190/80.

10. Which of the following individuals are most likely to develop osteoporosis?
    a. Premenopausal female athletes
    b. Females taking estrogen replacement therapy
    c. Slender, inactive females who smoke
    d. Females who eat a lot of high-fat dairy products

Answer Key: 1. b (LO 9.6), 2. a (LO 9.3), 3. d (LO 9.3), 4. b (LO 9.8), 5. b (LO 9.4), 6. c (LO 9.5), 7. a (LO 9.1), 8. d (LO 9.3), 9. c (LO 9.9), 10. c (LO 9.10)

Study Questions (Numbers refer to Learning Outcomes)

1. Approximately how much water do you need each day to stay healthy? Identify at least two situations that increase the need for water. Then list three sources of water in the average person's dietary pattern. **(LO 9.1)**

2. Identify four factors that influence the bioavailability of minerals from food. **(LO 9.2)**

3. What is the relationship between sodium and water balance, and how is that relationship monitored as well as maintained in the body? **(LO 9.3)**

4. List three sources of dietary calcium. Identify two factors that negatively influence the absorption of calcium. Identify two factors that positively influence the absorption of calcium. **(LO 9.6)**

5. What is the UL for calcium and what is the advice regarding the use of calcium supplements? **(LO 9.7)**

6. List three roles of magnesium in the body. Identify two chronic diseases that may be affected by magnesium status. **(LO 9.4)**

7. Describe the symptoms of iron-deficiency anemia, and explain possible reasons they occur. **(LO 9.8)**

8. Iodization of salt is a successful public health effort that has reduced global rates of iodine deficiency disorders. However, public health authorities recommend limiting salt intake to reduce the risk of hypertension. Can these two public health strategies be compatible? Explain your response. **(LO 9.3, LO 9.5)**

9. Describe the functions of fluoride in the body. List three sources of fluoride. **(LO 9.4, 9.6)**

10. Explain the function of selenium in body defenses. **(LO 9.5)**

11. List three dietary strategies to lower blood pressure. **(LO 9.9)**

12. Describe two methods that can be used to assess bone density. What demographic groups should have bone density measured? **(LO 9.10)**

References

1. A look at hard water across the US. HomeWater 101. Accessed November 12, 2023. https://homewater101.com/articles/hard-water-across-us

2. Ridder M. Per capita consumption of bottled water in the U.S. 1999 to 2022. Statista. August 2, 2023. Accessed November 12, 2023. https://www.statista.com/statistics/183377/per-capita-consumption-of-bottled-water-in-the-us-since-1999/

3. Bottled water. International Bottled Water Association. Accessed November 12, 2023. https://bottledwater.org/types-of-water-bottled/

4. Dow C. Is your seltzer habit harming your teeth? *Nutrition Action Healthletter.* June 2018.

5. Fujisawa C, Umegaki H, Sugimoto T, et al. Mild hyponatremia is associated with low skeletal muscle mass, physical function impairment, and depressive mood in the elderly. *BMC Geriatr.* 2021;21(1):15. Published 2021 Jan 6. doi:10.1186/s12877-020-01955-4

6. National Academies of Sciences, Engineering, and Medicine. *Dietary Reference Intakes for Sodium and Potassium.* Washington (DC): The National Academies Press; 2019.

7. U.S. Department of Agriculture; U.S. Department of Health & Human Services. *Dietary Guidelines for Americans, 2020–2025.* 9th ed. December 2020; pp. 46–48.

8. Bailey MA, Dhaun N. Salt sensitivity: causes, consequences, and recent advances *Hypertension.* 2024;81(3):476-489. doi:10.1161/HYPERTENSIONAHA.123.17959

9. Grimes CA, Riddell LJ, Campbell KJ, Nowson CA. Dietary salt intake, sugar-sweetened beverage consumption, and obesity risk. *Pediatrics.* 2013 Jan;131(1):14-21. doi: 10.1542/peds.2012-1628

10. U.S. Food & Drug Administration. Sodium in your diet: Use the Nutrition Facts label and reduce your intake. *Food Facts.* June 2021. https://www.fda.gov/food/nutrition-education-resources-materials/sodium-your-diet

11. Cormick G, Ciapponi A, Cafferata ML, Cormick MS, Belizán JM. Calcium supplementation for prevention of primary hypertension. *Cochrane Database Syst Rev.* 2022 Jan 11;1(1):cd010037. doi: 10.1002/14651858.CD010037.pub4

12. Hofmeyr GJ, Lawrie TA, Atallah ÁN, Torloni MR. Calcium supplementation during pregnancy for preventing hypertensive disorders and related problems. *Cochrane Database Syst Rev.* 2018 Oct 1;10(10):CD001059. doi: 10.1002/14651858.CD001059.pub5

13. World Cancer Research Fund International. *Diet, Nutrition, Physical Activity and Cancer: A Global Perspective–The Third Expert Report.* World Cancer Research Fund International; 2018. https://www.wcrf.org/dietandcancer

14. Rodak K, Kokot I, Kratz EM. Caffeine as a factor influencing the functioning of the human body–friend or foe? *Nutrients.* 2021 Sep 2;13(9):3088. doi: 10.3390/nu13093088

15. USDA, Agricultural Research Service. Usual nutrient intake from food and beverages, by gender and age, *What We Eat in America,* NHANES 2017–March 2020 Prepandemic. Accessed November 17, 2023. http://www.ars.usda.gov/nea/bhnrc/fsrg

16. Li K, Wang X-F, Li D-Y, et al. The good, the bad, and the ugly of calcium supplementation: a review of calcium intake on human health. *Clin Interv Aging.* 2018 Nov 28;13:2443-2452. doi: 10.2147/CIA.S157523

17. Anderson JJB, Roggenkamp KJ, Suchindran CM. Calcium intakes and femoral and lumbar bone density of elderly U.S. men and women: National Health and Nutrition Examination Survey 2005–2006 analysis. *J Clin Endocrinol Metab.* 2012 Dec;97(12):4531-4539. doi: 10.1210/jc.2012–1407

18. Reid IR, Bristow SM, Bolland MJ. Cardiovascular complications of calcium supplements. *J Cell Biochem.* 2015 Apr;116(4):494-501. doi: 10.1002/jcb.25028

19. Prentice RL, Pettinger MB, Jackson RD, et al. Health risks and benefits from calcium and vitamin D supplementation: Women's Health Initiative clinical trial and cohort study. *Osteoporos Int.* 2013 Feb;24(2):567-580. doi: 10.1007/s00198-012-2224-2

20. Grossman DC, Curry SJ, Owens DK, et al.; U.S. Preventive Services Task Force. Vitamin D, calcium, or combined supplementation for the primary prevention of fractures in community-dwelling adults: US Preventive Services Task Force Recommendation Statement. *JAMA.* 2018 Apr 17;319(15):1592-1599. doi: 10.1001/jama.2018.3185

21. Calcium fact sheet for health professionals. National Institutes of Health, Office of Dietary Supplements. Updated October 6, 2022. https://ods.od.nih.gov/factsheets/Calcium-HealthProfessional/. Accessed November 17, 2023

22. Phosphorus fact sheet for health professionals. National Institutes of Health, Office of Dietary Supplements. Updated May 4, 2023. https://ods.od.nih.gov/factsheets/Phosphorus-HealthProfessional/

23. Magnesium fact sheet for health professionals. National Institutes of Health, Office of Dietary Supplements. Updated June 2, 2022. https://ods.od.nih.gov/factsheets/Magnesium-HealthProfessional/

24. Barbagallo M, Veronese N, Dominguez LJ. Magnesium in aging, health and diseases. *Nutrients.* 2021;13(2):463. Published 2021 Jan 30. doi:10.3390/nu13020463

25. Uwitonze AM, Razzaque MS. Role of magnesium in vitamin D activation and function. *J Am Osteopath Assoc.* 2018 Mar 1;118(3):181-189. doi: 10.7556/jaoa.2018.037

26. Institute of Medicine (US) Standing Committee on the Scientific Evaluation of Dietary Reference Intakes. *Dietary Reference Intakes for Calcium, Phosphorus, Magnesium, Vitamin D, and Fluoride.* National Academies Press (US); 1997.

27. Iron fact sheet for health professionals. National Institutes of Health, Office of Dietary Supplement. Updated June 15, 2023. Accessed November 18, 2023. https://ods.od.nih.gov/factsheets/Iron-HealthProfessional/

28. Safiri S, Kolahi AA, Noori M, et al. Burden of anemia and its underlying causes in 204 countries and territories, 1990–2019: results from the Global Burden of Disease Study 2019. *J Hematol Oncol.* 2021 Nov 4;14(1):185. doi: 10.1186/s13045-021-01202-2

29. Sun H, Weaver CM. Decreased iron intake parallels rising iron deficiency anemia and related mortality rates in the US population. *J Nutr.* 2021 Jul 1;151(7):1947-1955. doi: 10.1093/jn/nxab064

30. McDonagh M, Cantor A, Bougatsos C, Dana T, Blazina I. Routine iron supplementation and screening for iron deficiency anemia in pregnant women: a systematic review to update the U.S. Preventive Services Task Force recommendation. *Evidence Synthesis* No. 123. AHRQ Publication no. 13-05188-EF-1. Rockville, MD: Agency for Healthcare Research and Quality; 2015.

31. Pasricha SR, Tye-Din J, Muckenthaler MU, Swinkels DW. Iron deficiency. *Lancet.* 2021 Jan 16;397(10270):233-248. doi: 10.1016/S0140-6736(20)32594-0

32. Hurrell R, Egli I. Iron bioavailability and dietary reference values. *Am J Clin Nutr.* 2010 May;91(5):1461S-1467S. doi: 10.3945/ajcn.2010.28674F

33. Carabotti M, Annibale B, Lahner E. Common pitfalls in the management of patients with micronutrient deficiency: keep in mind the stomach. *Nutrients.* 2021 Jan 13;13(1):208. doi: 10.3390/nu13010208

34. Hereditary hemochromatosis. Centers for Disease Control and Prevention, Office of Genomics & Precision Health. Reviewed May 20, 2022. Accessed November 18, 2023. https://www.cdc.gov/genomics/disease/hemochromatosis.htm

35. Zinc fact sheet for health professionals. National Institutes of Health, Office of Dietary Supplements. Updated September 28, 2022. Accessed November 18, 2023. https://ods.od.nih.gov/factsheets/Zinc-HealthProfessional/

36. Selenium fact sheet for health professionals. National Institutes of Health, Office of Dietary Supplements. Updated March 26, 2021. Accessed November 18, 2023. https://ods.od.nih.gov/factsheets/Selenium-HealthProfessional/

37. Iodine fact sheet for health professionals. National Institutes of Health, Office of Dietary Supplements. Updated October 13, 2023. Accessed November 18, 2023. https://ods.od.nih.gov/factsheets/Iodine-HealthProfessional/

38. Bath SC, Steer CD, Golding J, Emmett P, Rayman MP. Effect of inadequate iodine status in UK pregnant women on cognitive outcomes in their children: results from the Avon Longitudinal Study of Parents and Children (ALSPAC). *Lancet.* 2013 Jul 27;382(9889):331-337. doi: 10.1016/S0140-6736(13)60436-5

39. Hynes KL, Otahal P, Hay I, Burgess JR. Mild iodine deficiency during pregnancy is associated with reduced educational outcomes in the offspring: 9-year follow-up of the gestational iodine cohort. *J Clin Endocrinol Metab.* 2013 May;98(5):1954-1962. doi: 10.1210/jc.2012-4249

40. Opazo MC, Coronado-Arrázola I, Vallejos OP, et al. The impact of the micronutrient iodine in health and diseases. *Crit Rev Food Sci Nutr.* 2022:62(6):1466-1479. doi: 10.1080/10408398.2020.1843398

41. Leung AM, Braverman LE, Pearce EN. History of U.S. iodine fortification and supplementation [published correction appears in *Nutrients.* 2017 Sep 5;9(9):976. doi: 103390/nu9090976]. *Nutrients.* 2012 Nov 13;4(11):1740-1746. doi: 10.3390/nu4111740

42. Iodization of salt for the prevention and control of iodine deficiency disorders. World Health Organization, E-Library of Evidence for Nutrition Actions (eLENA). Updated August 9, 2023. Accessed November 18, 2023. https://www.who.int/tools/elena/interventions/salt-iodization

43. Iodine Global Network. Annual Report 2022. Accessed November 18. Available at https://ign.org/app/uploads/2023/07/11736-IGN-%E2%80%93-Annual-Report-2022_FINAL4.pdf

44. Ershow AG, Skeaff SA, Merkel JM, Pehrsson PR. Development of databases on iodine in foods and dietary supplements. *Nutrients.* 2018 Jan 17;10(1):100. doi: 10.3390/nu10010100

45. Harris C. Thyroid disease and diet—nutrition plays a part in maintaining thyroid health. *Today's Dietitian.* 2012 July;14(7):40.

46. Gaitan E. Goitrogens in food and water. *Annu Rev Nutr.* 1990;10:21-39. doi: 10.1146/annurev.nu.10.070190.000321

47. Hassen HY, Beyene M, Ali JH. Dietary pattern and its association with iodine deficiency among school children in southwest Ethiopia; a cross-sectional study. *PLoS One.* 2019 Aug 13;14(8):e0221106. doi: 10.1371/journal.pone.0221106

48. Copper fact sheet for health professionals. National Institutes of Health, Office of Dietary Supplements. Updated October 18, 2022. Accessed November 18, 2023. https://ods.od.nih.gov/factsheets/Copper-HealthProfessional/

49. Wilson disease. National Institute of Diabetes and Digestive and Kidney Diseases. Reviewed November 2018. Accessed November 18, 2023. https://www.niddk.nih.gov/health-information/liver-disease/wilson-disease

50. Bandmann O, Weiss KH, Kaler SG. Wilson's disease and other neurological copper disorders. *Lancet Neurol.* 2015 Jan;14(1):103-113. doi: 10.1016/S1474-4422(14)70190-5

51. Rugg-Gunn AJ, Do L. Effectiveness of water fluoridation in caries prevention. *Community Dent Oral Epidemiol.* 2012 Oct;40 Suppl 2:55-64. doi: 10.1111/j.1600-0528.2012.00721.x

52. Water fluoridation basics. Centers for Disease Control and Prevention. Updated June 13, 2023. Accessed November 18, 2023. https://www.cdc.gov/fluoridation/basics/index.htm

53. Chromium fact sheet for health professionals. National Institutes of Health, Office of Dietary Supplements. Updated June 2, 2022. Accessed November 18, 2023. https://ods.od.nih.gov/factsheets/Chromium-HealthProfessional/

54. Manganese fact sheet for health professionals. National Institutes of Health, Office of Dietary Supplements. Updated March 29, 2021. Accessed November 18, 2023. https://ods.od.nih.gov/factsheets/Manganese-HealthProfessional/

55. Molybdenum fact sheet for health professionals. National Institutes of Health, Office of Dietary Supplements. Updated March 30, 2021. Accessed November 18, 2023. https://ods.od.nih.gov/factsheets/Molybdenum-HealthProfessional/

56. Facts about hypertension. Centers for Disease Control and Prevention. Updated July 6, 2023. Accessed November 18, 2023. https://www.cdc.gov/bloodpressure/facts.htm

57. Whelton PK, Carey RM, Aronow WS, et al. 2017 ACC/AHA/AAPA/ABC/ACPM/AGS/APhA/ASH/ASPC/NMA/PCNA guideline for the prevention, detection, evaluation, and management of high blood pressure in adults: A report of the American College of Cardiology/American Heart Association Task Force on Clinical Practice Guidelines. *J Am Coll Cardiol.* 2018 May 15;71(19):e127-e248. doi: 10.1016/j.jacc.2017.11.006

58. Wright JT Jr, Williamson JD, Whelton PK, et al.; SPRINT Research Group. A randomized trial of intensive versus standard blood-pressure control. *N Engl J Med.* 2015 Nov 26;373(22):2103-2116. doi: 10.1056/NEJMoa1511939

59. Beilin LJ, Puddey IB, Burke V. Lifestyle and hypertension. *Am J Hypertens.* 1999;12(9 Pt 1):934-945. doi:10.1016/s0895-7061(99)00057-6

60. Know your risk for high blood pressure. Centers for Disease Control and Prevention. Updated March 17, 2023. Accessed November 19, 2023. https://www.cdc.gov/bloodpressure/risk_factors.htm

61. McDonough AA, Veiras LC, Guevara CA, Ralph DL. Cardiovascular benefits associated with higher dietary K^+ vs. lower dietary Na^+: evidence from population and mechanistic studies. *Am J Physiol Endocrinol Metab.* 2017 Apr 1;312(4):E348-E356. doi: 10.1152/ajpendo.00453.2016

62. Steinberg D, Bennett GG, Svetkey L. The DASH diet, 20 years later. *JAMA.* 2017 Apr 18;317(15):1529-1530. doi: 10.1001/jama.2017.1628

63. Sacks FM, Svetkey LP, Vollmer WM, et al.; DASH-Sodium Collaborative Research Group. Effects on blood pressure of reduced dietary sodium and the Dietary Approaches to Stop Hypertension (DASH) diet. DASH–Sodium Collaborative Research Group. *N Engl J Med.* 2001 Jan 4;344(1):3-10. doi: 10.1056/NEJM200101043440101

64. Onwuzo C, Olukorode JO, Omokore OA, et al. DASH diet: a review of its scientifically proven hypertension reduction and health benefits. *Cureus.* 2023;15(9):e44692. Published 2023 Sep 4. doi:10.7759/cureus.44692

65. Aburto NJ, Ziolkovska A, Hooper L, Elliott P, Cappuccio FP, Meerpohl JJ. Effect of lower sodium intake on health: systematic review and meta-analyses. *BMJ.* 2013 Apr 3;346:f1326. doi: 10.1136/bmj.f1326

66. Best diets overall. *U.S. News & World Report.* 2023. Updated January 3, 2023. Accessed November 19, 2023. https://health.usnews.com/best-diet/best-diets-overall

67. National Osteoporosis Foundation. *Healthcare Professionals Toolkit.* Medtronic; 2019. https://www.bonesource.org/s/HCP-Toolkit-with-graphics.pdf

68. FRAX Fracture Risk Assessment Tool. Centre for Metabolic Bone Diseases. Accessed November 19, 2023. https://frax.shef.ac.uk/FRAX/

69. Camacho PM, Petak SM, Binkley N, et al. American Association of Clinical Endocrinologists/American College of Endocrinology Clinical Practice Guidelines for the diagnosis and treatment of postmenopausal osteoporosis—2020 update. *Endocr Pract.* 2020 May;26(Suppl 1):1-46. doi: 10.4158/GL-2020-0524SUPPL

70. Wambogo E, Sarafrazi N. Percentage of adults aged ≥ 50 years with osteoporosis, by race and Hispanic origin—United States, 2017–2018. *MMWR.* 2021 May 14;70(19):731. https://www.cdc.gov/mmwr/volumes/70/wr/pdfs/mm7019a5-H.pdf

71. South-Paul JE. Osteoporosis: part I. Evaluation and assessment. *Am Fam Physician.* 2001 Mar 1;63(5):897-904, 908.

72. National Osteoporosis Foundation. *Healthy Bones for Life: Patient's Guide.* 2014. https://www.bonehealthandosteoporosis.org/wp-content/uploads/NOF-Health-Bones-For-Life-Patients-Guide.pdf

73. Mundi S, Pindiprolu B, Simunovic N, Bhandari M. Similar mortality rates in hip fracture patients over the past 31 years. *Acta Orthop.* 2014 Feb;85(1):54-59. doi: 10.3109/17453674.2013.878831

74. Dyer SM, Crotty M, Fairhall N, et al.; Fragility Fracture Network (FFN) Rehabilitation Research Special Interest Group. A critical review of the long-term disability outcomes following hip fracture. *BMC Geriatr.* 2016 Sep 2;16(1):158. doi: 10.1186/s12877-016-0332-0

75. Weaver CM, Gordon CM, Janz KF, et al. The National Osteoporosis Foundation's position statement on peak bone mass development and lifestyle factors: a systematic review and implementation recommendations. *Osteoporos Int.* 2016 Apr;27(4):1281-1386. doi: 10.1007/s00198-015-3440-3

76. Carter NI, Hinton PS. Physical activity and bone health. *Mo. Med.* Jan-Feb 214;111(1): 59-64.

77. U.S. Department of Health and Human Services. *Physical Activity Guidelines for Americans,* 2nd edition. 2018. https://health.gov/sites/default/files/2019-09/Physical_Activity_Guidelines_2nd_edition.pdf

78. Shams-White MM, Chung M, Du M, et al. Dietary protein and bone health: a systematic review and meta-analysis from the National Osteoporosis Foundation. *Am J Clin Nutr.* 2017 Jun;105(6):1528-1543. doi: 10.3945/ajcn.116.145110

79. Sahni S, Mangano KM, McLean RR, Hannan MT, Kiel DP. Dietary approaches for bone health: lessons from the Framingham Osteoporosis Study. *Curr Osteoporos Rep.* 2015 Aug;13(4):245-255. doi: 10.1007/s11914-015-0272-1

80. Rinonapoli G, Pace V, Ruggiero C, et al. Obesity and bone: a complex relationship. *Int J Mol Sci.* 2021 Dec 20;22(24):13662. doi: 10.3390/ijms222413662

81. Fatahi S, Namazi N, Larijani B, Azadbakht L. The association of dietary and urinary sodium with bone mineral density and risk of osteoporosis: a systematic review and meta-analysis. *J Am Coll Nutr.* 2018 Aug:37(6): 522-532. doi: 10.1080/07315724.2018.1431161

82. Jeremiah MP, Unwin BK, Greenawald MH, Casiano VE. Diagnosis and management of osteoporosis. *Am Fam Physician.* 2015 Aug;92(4): 261-268.

83. Ishtiaq S, Fogelman I, Hampson G. Treatment of post-menopausal osteoporosis: beyond bisphosphonates. *J Endocrinol Invest.* 2015 Jan;38(1): 13-29. doi: 10.1007/s40618-014-0152-z

84. Pisani P, Renna MD, Conversano F, et al. Major osteoporotic fragility fractures: risk factor updates and societal impact. *World J Orthop.* 2016 Mar 18;7(3):171-181. doi: 10.5312/wjo.v7.i3.171

Design Element Credits: Fact Check/magnifying glass icon: McGraw Hill; Magnificent Microbiome background image: Alena Ohneva/Shutterstock; Sustainable Solutions icon: McGraw Hill; Roots icon: McGraw Hill; Medicine Cabinet icon: Peter Dazeley/Photographer's Choice/Getty Images

Chapter 10

Nutrition: Fitness and Sports

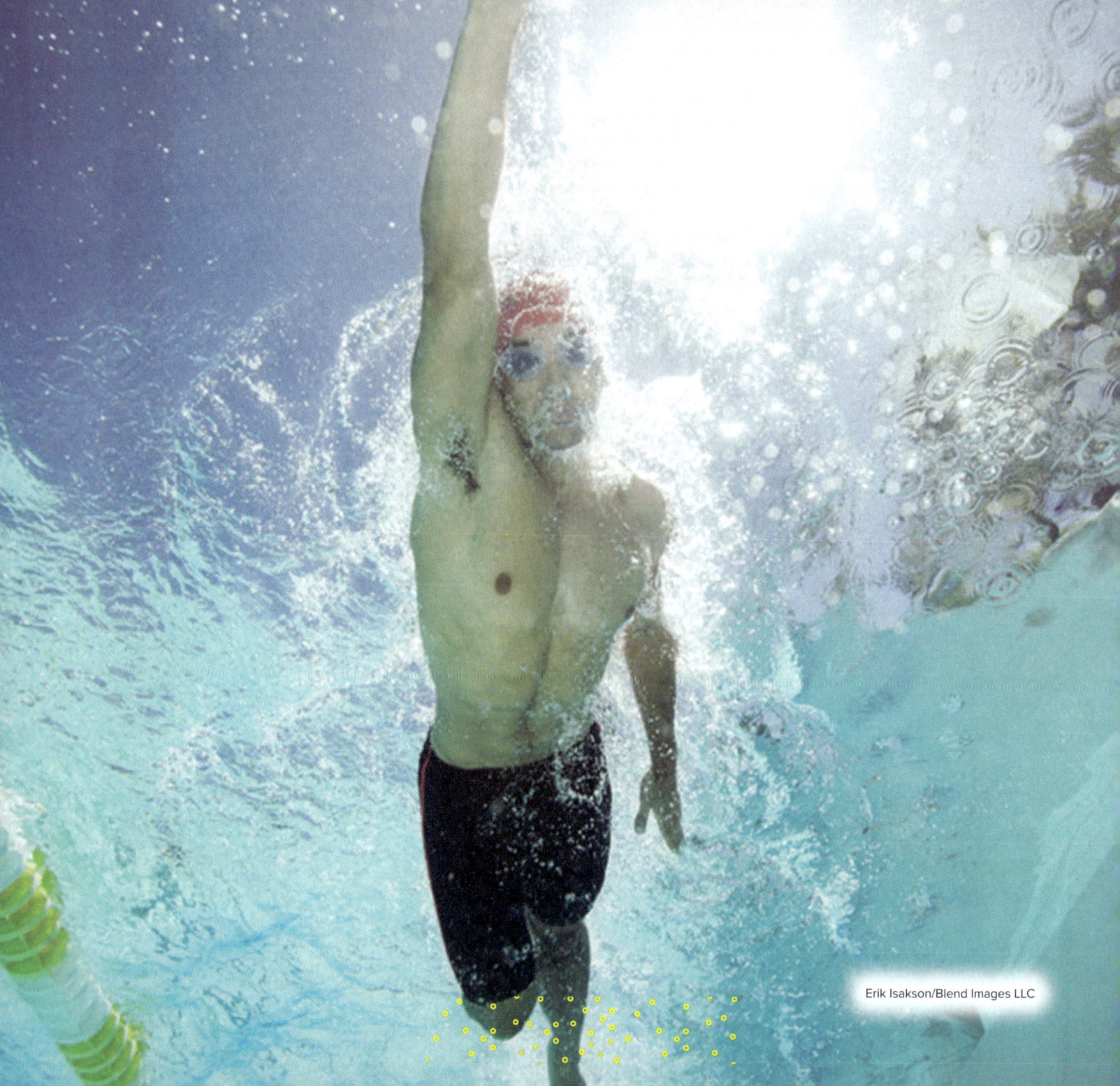

Erik Isakson/Blend Images LLC

Student Learning Outcomes

Chapter 10 is designed to allow you to:

10.1 List health-related outcomes of a physically active lifestyle.

10.2 List key components of a sound fitness regimen.

10.3 Describe the use of carbohydrates, fat, and protein to meet energy needs during various activities.

10.4 Differentiate between anaerobic and aerobic uses of glucose and identify advantages and disadvantages of each.

10.5 Explain how muscles and organs adapt to physical activity.

10.6 Describe how to estimate an athlete's nutrient requirements during various activities.

10.7 Examine optimal fluid status during physical activity and issues related to dehydration.

10.8 Describe how individuals can optimize performance by consuming foods and fluids before, during, and after physical activity.

10.9 List several ergogenic aids and describe their effects on an athlete's performance and health risks.

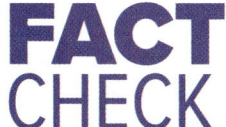

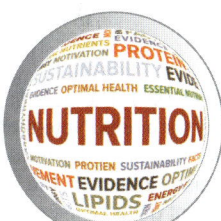

If I eat more protein, will I gain more muscle?

Most active individuals are seeking any advantage that might enhance performance. For this reason, individuals striving to improve their fitness are likely targets for nutrition quackery and misinformation. As you sort fact from fiction, be sure of this: long-term health promotion and maintenance should include adherence to the evidence-based dietary and physical activity guidelines. This includes protein recommendations. Indeed, making informed lifestyle choices can optimize many aspects of physical performance, from preventing fatigue to gaining muscle to optimizing recovery from workouts.

Although protein does impact muscle mass, the fact is the majority of college students meet their daily protein requirements through their dietary patterns. Protein intake beyond what is required equates to extra calories that active individuals do not need. It is best to time your protein intake in relation to your workouts. For instance, consuming ample protein before or immediately after a workout is important for muscle repair and recovery.

In this chapter, you will discover how all physical activity benefits both physical and mental health and how nutrients, including protein, relate to optimal physical performance. Visit Section 10.4 to read more about specific protein recommendations for various types of activity.

Source: Nestlé Nutrition.

10.2 Achieving and Maintaining Physical Fitness

Many of the recommendations that appear later in this chapter focus on enhancing the performance of highly competitive athletes; however, not many students are elite athletes. Furthermore, in a health profession, most clients are at a beginner or intermediate level of fitness. Certainly, proper nutrition supports physical performance at all levels. This section outlines how to get started with a plan to achieve physical fitness.

ASSESS YOUR CURRENT LEVEL OF FITNESS

Start by assessing your current level of fitness. In some cases, it is beneficial to seek medical advice before getting started. Males age 45 years or older and females age 55 years or older, anyone who has been inactive for many years, or those who have an existing health problem should discuss their fitness goals with their primary care provider before altering physical activity patterns.[3] Health concerns that may require medical evaluation before beginning a fitness program include obesity, cardiovascular disease (or family history), hypertension, diabetes (or family history), chest pains, shortness of breath, history of dizzy spells, respiratory ailments, osteoporosis, hypertension, or arthritis. If you are unsure, you can take the Physical Activity Readiness Questionnaire (PAR-Q), found at https://www.acsm.org/docs/default-source/files-for-resource-library/par-q-acsm.pdf. This tool can help you decide if you need to see your primary care provider first. Even if you do not have preexisting medical problems, enlisting the aid of a sports dietitian can help you to determine a safe starting point and establish realistic fitness goals.

ASSESS YOUR LEVEL OF PHYSICAL ACTIVITY

There are four levels of aerobic physical activity:[2]

1. *Inactive* means that you are not getting moderate- to vigorous-intensity activities beyond daily life activities.
2. *Insufficiently active* is engaging in some moderate- or vigorous-intensity physical activity but less than 150 minutes of moderate-intensity physical activity per week or 75 minutes of vigorous-intensity physical activity (or the equivalent in combination). This level is less than the target range for meeting the key physical guidelines for adults.
3. *Active* is doing the equivalent of 150 minutes to 300 minutes of moderate-intensity physical activity per week. This level meets the key guideline target range for adults.
4. *Highly active* means you are meeting the equivalent of more than 300 minutes of moderate-intensity physical activity per week. This level exceeds the key guideline target range for adults.

SET YOUR PHYSICAL ACTIVITY GOALS

For any behavior change, goal setting will enhance your success. Sports dietitians are trained professionals who can help you set reasonable physical activity goals based on your current level of fitness. A Board Certification as a Specialist in Sports Dietetics (CSSD) credential is the premier professional sports nutrition credential in the U.S. CSSDs are registered dietitian nutritionists (RDNs) who provide safe, effective, evidence-based nutrition services for health, fitness, and athletic performance.

Wearable fitness trackers that measure physical movement are now more accurate and less expensive than ever. These can help motivate you on your quest to become more physically active. Devices include pedometers that count steps and accelerometers that measure trunk or limb movement. Smartphone app accelerometers, such as wrist watches, have become the norm. Many of these devices use multi-sensor systems that measure steps, often paired with global positioning systems (GPS) that provide estimates of speed and distance. Many now include heart rate monitors and track intensity of movements. We should all strive for a lifespan approach to physical activity. This means we should try to be active for life. These devices may help reinforce positive behaviors for some people.[2]

PLAN YOUR PROGRAM

Although your goal may focus on just one aspect of fitness, such as being able to bench-press your body weight, a balanced fitness program will include various types of activities, such as aerobics, muscle- and bone-strengthening, balance training, flexibility, and more.

Many physical activity experts use the FITT-VP principle to design a fitness program. FITT-VP stands for frequency, intensity, time, type, volume, and progression of activity. Frequency (how often) refers to the number of sessions or bouts of physical activity per day or per week. Relative intensity (how hard) refers to the ease or difficulty with which an individual performs physical activity. Intensity is often categorized by very light, moderate, to vigorous intensity. Training time (how long) refers to the duration of time spent in the activity or the number of repetitions. Training type (what kind) refers to the mode or choice of activity. Volume (amount) refers to the quantity of the training load. Progression refers to the increase (or advancement) in activity over time. Table 10-1 summarizes the American College of Sports Medicine (ACSM) recommendations for planning a general fitness program.

Cardiorespiratory Endurance. As you learned earlier, *aerobic* means "with oxygen." Aerobic activity is intense enough and long enough to maintain or improve your cardiorespiratory fitness.[2] There are three components of aerobic activity: (1) *intensity*, or how hard a person works to complete the activity (usually described as moderate or vigorous); (2) *frequency*, or how often a person engages in aerobic activity; and (3) *duration*, or how long a person engages in the activity for one session. The ability to perform aerobic activity depends on the health of your heart and lungs and the organ systems that provide oxygen to the cells of the body. Aerobic activities usually form the backbone of a fitness program. Indeed, many of the benefits of fitness are direct effects of aerobic training.

Remember that heart rate is an estimate of workout intensity. You can take your pulse using the radial artery on your wrist or the carotid artery in your neck (Fig. 10-2). Medications, such as those for hypertension and other health conditions, may impact heart rate. If you have health concerns, a primary care provider can help to personalize your safe target heart rate zone.

Another way of determining the intensity of activities is the Rating of Perceived Exertion (RPE) Scale. This scale includes a range of 0 to 10, with each number corresponding to a subjective feeling of exertion. For

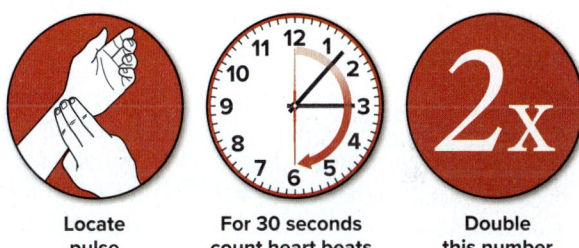

Measuring Your Heart Rate

Locate pulse | For 30 seconds count heart beats | Double this number

FIGURE 10-2 Tips to manually measure your own heart rate. PeopleImages/E+/Getty Images

TABLE 10-1 ■ Elements of a Well-Rounded Fitness Program

	Aerobic Fitness	Muscular Fitness	Flexibility
Frequency	3 to 5 days per week of moderate and vigorous activity	2 to 3 days per week	2 to 3 days per week, daily if possible
Intensity	Moderate (64% to 76% MHR[a]) or vigorous (77% to 93% MHR)	60% to 80% of 1 RM[b]	To point of tension
Time	30–60 min/day moderate activity or 20–60 min/day vigorous activity	No guideline established	10–30 seconds static stretching
Type	Involves major muscle groups	Involves major muscle groups and single plus multi-joint movements	Involves major muscles and tendons
Volume	Increasing per day until goal	8–12 reps for strength and power; 15–20 reps for muscular endurance	2–4 reps, 60 seconds of total stretching time
Progression	Gradual progression of any category. Start low and go slow.	Progression by adjusting resistance, repetitions, and/or frequency	Gradual progression increasing point of tension and repetitions

Source: American College of Sports Medicine Position Paper and CDC.

TABLE 10-2 ■ Finding Your Target Heart Rate. Maximum Heart Rate = 220 − Age

Training Zone	Goal	Target Heart Rate						
		Age 20	Age 30	Age 40	Age 50	Age 60	Age 70	Age 80
Maximum (90–100% effort)	Speed	180	171	162	153	144	135	126
Hard (80–90% effort)	Anaerobic, speed endurance	160	152	144	136	128	120	112
Moderate (70–80% effort)	Aerobic, fitness & power	140	133	126	119	112	105	98
Light (60–70% effort)	Aerobic endurance	120	114	108	102	96	90	84
Very light (50–60% effort)	Warm-up and recovery	100	95	90	85	80	75	70

Source: Adapted from OhioHealth.

Calculating Your Target Heart Rate

1. Determine your age-predicted maximum heart rate (MHR) by subtracting your age from 220:

For a 20-year-old person, MHR is calculated by using 220 − 20 (age) = 200 beats per minute (bpm).

2. At the initiation of an aerobic exercise program, aim for about 50% to 70% of MHR as a target heart rate (THR):

200 bpm × 0.5 (50%) = 100 bmp

200 bpm MHR × 0.7 (70%) = 140 bpm

As you progress and become more physically fit, you can work up to a higher THR (Table 10-2). For intermediate exercisers, 60% to 75% of MHR is recommended. For trained exercisers, 70% to 85% MHR is suitable.

example, the number 0 is "nothing at all" (e.g., sitting), and the number 10 is considered close to maximal effort or "very, very heavy" (e.g., all-out sprint; Fig. 10-3).

When using the 10-point RPE scale, the goal is to aim for a minimum rating of 4, which corresponds to the beginning of "somewhat hard." This is the point at which you begin to obtain significant benefits. If you are hovering around an RPE of 4, you should still be able to talk somewhat comfortably to a workout partner (talk test). Generally, if you are engaging in moderate-intensity aerobic activity, you should be able to talk, but not sing, during the activity. If you are engaging in vigorous-intensity activity, you probably cannot say more than a few words without pausing for a breath.[2]

Musculoskeletal Fitness. Muscles are strengthened by the principles of overload, adaptation, progression, and specificity. *Overload* indicates that a resistance is applied on a regular basis and manageable to handle. The muscles *adapt* to this new load and become stronger. Over time, *progression* is possible as the body adapts. These improvements in strength are *specific* to the overloaded muscles.[2] Muscle-strengthening activities include three components: (1) *intensity*, or how much force or weight is applied relative to how much you can lift; (2) *frequency*, or how often you engage in muscle-strengthening activities; and (3) *sets and repetitions*, or how many times you complete the muscle-strengthening activity. *Muscular endurance* refers to the ability of the muscle to perform repeated, submaximal contractions over time without becoming fatigued. An athlete training for muscular endurance may bench-press 80 to 100 pounds for several sets of 15 to 20 repetitions. Both muscular strength and endurance are important aspects of muscular fitness that relate to health for athletes of all levels. *Muscular power* combines strength with speed for explosive movements such as jumping or throwing. Power is a crucial aspect of muscular fitness for many athletes. Studies also show that developing muscular power can help to improve function and balance among older adults.

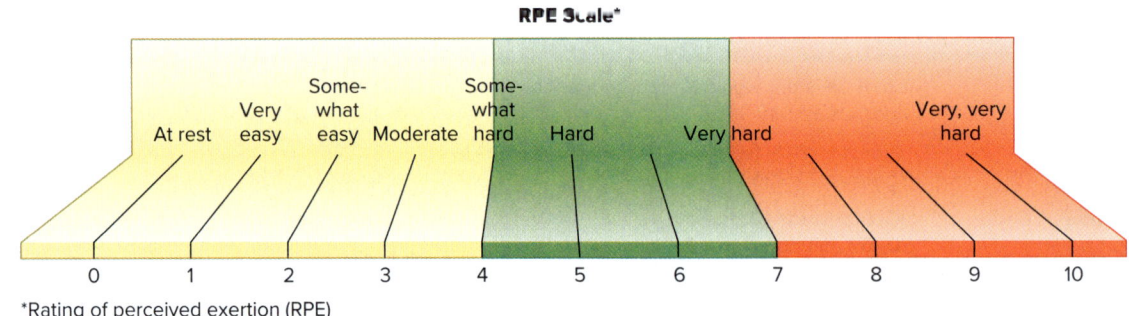

FIGURE 10-3 Rating of Perceived Exertion Scale. When engaging in physical activity, a rating of a 5 or 6 produces noticeable increases in breathing rate and heart rate. A level of 7 or 8 produces large increases in a person's breathing and heart rate.

Source: U.S. Department of Health & Human Services. *Physical Activity Guidelines for Americans*. 2nd ed. Washington, DC: U.S. Department of Health & Human Services; 2018. Accessed January 12, 2020. https://health.gov/sites/default/files/2019-09/Physical_Activity_Guidelines_2nd_edition.pdf

Overall, muscular fitness is developed by performing resistance training for all the major muscle groups of the body, including legs, hips, back, abdomen, chest, shoulders, and arms. This resistance may come from free weights (e.g., barbells), weight machines (e.g., leg press), or the weight of your own body (e.g., push-ups).

The *Physical Activity Guidelines* recommend including muscle-strengthening activities in your fitness program on at least 2 to 3 nonconsecutive days per week (Fig. 10-4). Taking a day or more to rest between bouts of resistance training or alternating groups of muscles is recommended to allow time for muscles to recover and increase in size.

To enhance muscle strength, 8 to 12 repetitions of each exercise should be performed to volitional fatigue. One set of 8 to 12 repetitions is effective at increasing muscular strength; limited evidence suggests that 2 or 3 sets are more effective.[2]

Bone-Strengthening Activities. Also referred to as *weight bearing* or *weight loading*, these activities produce force on the bones to promote bone growth and strength.[2] Jumping, running, brisk walking, and weight lifting are examples of bone-strengthening activities.

Balance Activities. These activities improve the ability to resist forces that cause falls while a person is stable or moving.[2]

Multicomponent Physical Activities. The concept of physical fitness includes cardiorespiratory endurance (aerobic power), musculoskeletal fitness, flexibility, balance, and speed of movement.[2] Dancing, tai chi, gardening, and sports are considered multicomponent physical activities.

Flexibility Activities. Flexibility is an often-overlooked aspect of physical health and tends to decline with age. Flexibility, often called stretching, refers to the ability to move a joint through its full range of motion. Poor flexibility is often linked to chronic pain, especially in the lower back. Contrary to popular belief, research studies do not clearly support a role of flexibility training in preventing injury or muscle soreness from aerobic or strength-training activities. However, gains in flexibility can improve balance and stability, thereby reducing risks of falls and injuries.

Warm-Up and Cool-Down. Be sure to plan for adequate warm-up and cool-down periods as part of your physical activity routine. Begin by warming up with low-intensity exercises, such as walking, slow jogging, or any low-intensity performance of the anticipated activity. This warms up your muscles so that muscle filaments slide over one another more easily, which increases range of motion and flexibility and decreases the risk of injury. It is also thought to lower cardiovascular risks, particularly among people who are not accustomed to regular exercise. During cool-down, slow down to low-intensity activity followed by stretching. The same physical activities performed during warm-up are appropriate. Although the cool-down does not actually prevent muscle soreness, it does reduce the dizziness or light-headedness that can occur with an abrupt end to a vigorous workout.

Getting Started. For sedentary people who are otherwise healthy, gradual **progression** toward meeting the *Physical Activity Guidelines* is recommended. During the first phase of a fitness program to promote health, you should begin to incorporate short periods of physical activity into your daily routine. This includes brisk walking, taking the stairs instead of the elevator, dancing, hiking, and other activities. A sensible goal is at least 30 to 60 minutes of this moderate type of physical activity on most (and preferably all)

Josie's Fitness Plan

Monday
Spinning class (45 min)
Stretching routine (20 min)

Tuesday
Walking (30 min)
Strength training (30 min)

Wednesday
Spinning class (45 min)
Stretching routine (20 min)

Thursday
Walking (30 min)
Strength training (30 min)

Friday
Yoga (30 min)

Saturday
Trail hiking (60 min)

Sunday
Rest

FIGURE 10-4 Sample fitness plan. Josie's fitness plan incorporates aerobic, strength, and flexibility exercises. John Lund/Sam Diephuis/Blend Images LLC

progression Incremental increase in frequency, intensity, and time spent in each type of physical activity over several weeks or months.

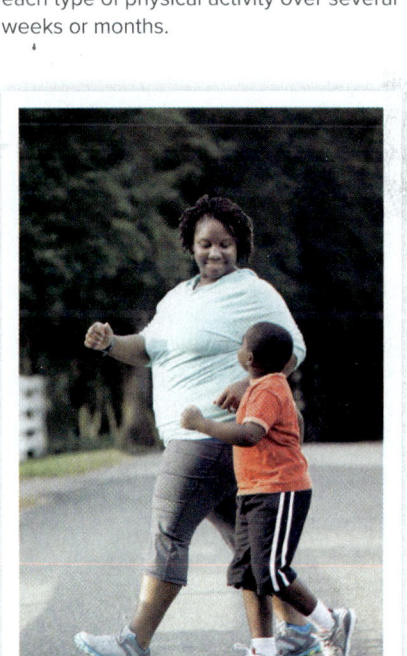

Good social support is a key to maintaining behavioral change. **Which friends or family members would help you achieve your fitness goals?** Ariel Skelley/Blend Images/Getty Images

magnificent microbiome

Exercise
Ongoing research confirms that exercise is associated with beneficial changes in gut microbial composition and metabolites independent of diet in both rodents and humans. Intense activities have also been linked to regulating oxidative stress and inflammatory responses in addition to improvements in metabolism and energy expenditure. Another reason the microbiome is truly magnificent!

Source: Mach N, Fuster-Botella D. Endurance exercise and gut microbiota: a review. *J Sport Health Sci.* 2017 Jun;6(2):179-197. doi: 10.1016/j.jshs.2016.05.001

---

days of the week. If there is not much time for activity, you can still obtain significant benefits from performing shorter sessions of increased intensity. Remember that any activity is better than no activity. Aim to move more and sit less!

Stick with It! Even after all the effort of assessing baseline fitness, setting goals, designing a program, and getting started, it turns out that maintaining a physical activity program may be the hardest part! To stick with a fitness program, experts recommend the following:

- Forgive occasional setbacks; focus on the long-term benefits to your health.
- Frequently revisit both short- and long-term goals.
- Include friends and family members for additional motivation.
- Reward yourself when achieving goals.
- Set aside a specific time each day for movement; set physical activity calendar appointments.
- Start slowly and progress incrementally.
- Vary your activities to keep it fresh; rotate indoor and outdoor activities.

✓ CONCEPT CHECK 10.2

1. List the four levels of aerobic physical activity.
2. Why is goal setting important for the success of a physical activity program?
3. Differentiate between muscular strength, muscular endurance, and muscular power.
4. Provide three tips for a person who needs help maintaining a fitness program.

10.3 Energy Sources for Active Muscles

Like other cells, muscle cells cannot directly use the energy released from breaking down glucose or triglycerides. Muscle cells need a specific form of energy for contraction. Body cells must first convert the chemical energy in carbohydrates, proteins, and fats into **adenosine triphosphate (ATP)**.

The chemical bonds between phosphates in ATP and related molecules are high-energy bonds. Using the energy obtained from food, cells make ATP from its breakdown product **adenosine diphosphate (ADP)** and a phosphate group (abbreviated P_i). Conversely, to release energy from ATP, cells partially break down the compound into ADP and P_i (Fig. 10-5). The released energy is used for many cell functions.

adenosine triphosphate (ATP) The main energy currency for cells. ATP energy is used to promote ion pumping, enzyme activity, and muscular contraction.

adenosine diphosphate (ADP) A breakdown product of ATP. ADP is synthesized into ATP using energy from foodstuffs and a phosphate group (abbreviated P_i).

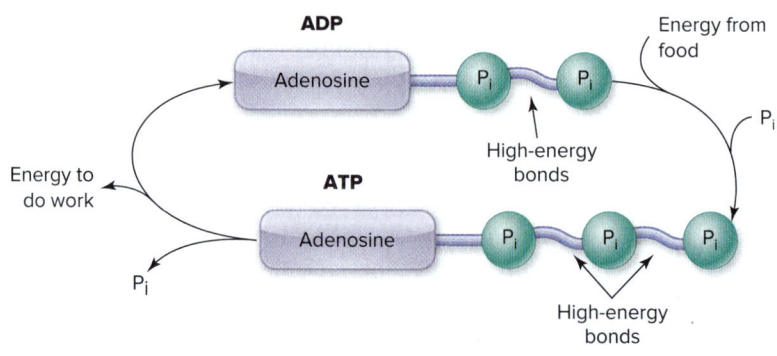

FIGURE 10-5 Food energy is stored in the chemical bonds between the phosphate groups in ATP. When a phosphate group (P_i) is cleaved from ATP, energy to perform work is released. The product of the breakdown of ATP is adenosine diphosphate (ADP).

ANAEROBIC METABOLISM SUPPLIES ENERGY FOR SHORT BURSTS OF INTENSE ACTIVITY

Stored ATP. Essentially, ATP is the immediate source of energy for body functions. The primary goal in the use of any fuel, whether carbohydrate, fat, or protein, is to make ATP. A resting muscle cell contains only a small amount of ATP that can be used immediately. This amount of ATP could keep the muscle working maximally for only about 2 seconds if no resupply of ATP were possible. Fortunately, the cells have various mechanisms to resupply ATP. Overall, cells must constantly and repeatedly use and then reform ATP, using a variety of energy sources.

Phosphocreatine. As soon as ATP stored in muscle cells begins to be used, another high-energy compound, **phosphocreatine (PCr),** is used to resupply ATP. An enzyme in the muscle cell is activated to split PCr into phosphate and **creatine** (Fig. 10-6). This releases energy that can be used to reform ATP from its breakdown products. If no other source of energy for ATP resupply were available, PCr could probably maintain maximal muscle contractions for about 15 seconds.

The main advantage of PCr is that it can be activated instantly and can replenish ATP at rates fast enough to meet the energy demands of the fastest and most powerful actions, including jumping, lifting, throwing, and sprinting. The disadvantage of PCr is that not much of it is made and stored in the muscles. Strength-training athletes sometimes use creatine supplements in an effort to increase PCr in muscles.

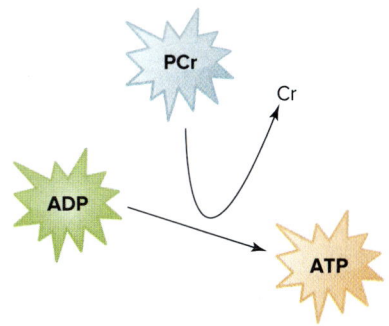

FIGURE 10-6 Phosphocreatine (PCr) reacts with ADP to yield ATP plus creatine (Cr).

phosphocreatine (PCr) A high-energy compound that can be used to reform ATP. It is used primarily during bursts of activity, such as lifting and jumping.

creatine An organic (i.e., carbon-containing) molecule in muscle cells that serves as part of a high-energy compound (termed *creatine phosphate or phosphocreatine*) capable of synthesizing ATP from ADP.

pyruvate A three-carbon compound formed during glucose metabolism; also called *pyruvic acid*.

lactate A chemical produced when cells break down carbohydrates for energy; also referred to as *lactic acid*.

Anaerobic Glucose Breakdown. Carbohydrates are an important fuel for muscles. The most useful form of carbohydrate fuel is the simple sugar glucose, available to all cells from the bloodstream. As you will recall, glucose is stored as glycogen in the liver and muscle cells. Blood glucose is maintained by the breakdown of liver glycogen. Breakdown of glycogen stored in a specific muscle also helps meet the carbohydrate demand of that muscle, but the actual amount of glycogen stored in muscle is limited (about 350 grams for all the muscles in the body yielding approximately 1400 kcal).

Whether oxygen is available or not, glucose can be broken down to a three-carbon compound called **pyruvate** (sometimes called pyruvic acid) in a pathway that releases some energy. However, when the oxygen supply in the muscle is limited (anaerobic conditions), glucose cannot be fully broken down. The pyruvate accumulates in the muscle and is converted to **lactate** (also called lactic acid). Some lactate may be used locally as fuel and the rest circulates through the bloodstream to the liver, where it can be converted back to glucose. Anaerobic metabolism provides a rapid (but less efficient) way to generate ATP compared to aerobic metabolism.

Only about 5% of the total amount of ATP that could be formed from complete breakdown of glucose is released through this anaerobic process (Fig. 10-7). The advantage of anaerobic glucose breakdown is that it is the fastest way to resupply ATP, other than PCr breakdown. It therefore provides most of the energy needed for events that require a quick burst of energy, ranging from about 30 seconds to 2 minutes. Examples of activities that primarily rely on anaerobic glucose breakdown include sprinting 400 meters or swimming 100 meters.

Before long, muscle cells release the accumulating lactate into the bloodstream. The liver (and the kidneys to some extent) takes up the lactate and resynthesizes it into glucose. Glucose can then reenter the bloodstream, where it is available for cell uptake and breakdown. Individuals vary in their ability to clear lactate from the muscles and recycle it. Physical training may improve the ability of the body to remove and recycle lactate.

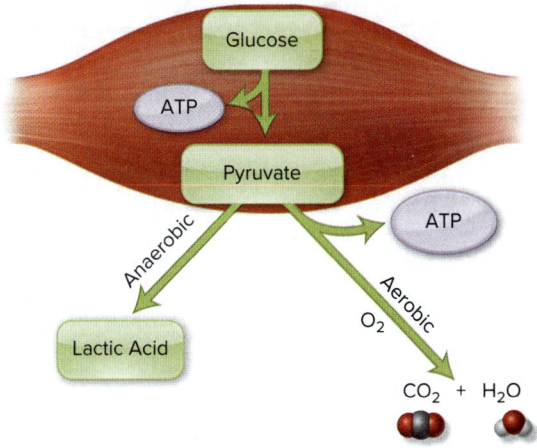

FIGURE 10-7 ATP yield from aerobic versus anaerobic glucose use.

AEROBIC METABOLISM FUELS PROLONGED, LOWER-INTENSITY ACTIVITY

Carbohydrates. If plenty of oxygen is available in the muscle (aerobic conditions), such as when the physical activity is of low to moderate intensity, the bulk of the pyruvate is shuttled to the mitochondria of the cell, where it is fully metabolized into carbon dioxide (CO_2) and water (H_2O) (Fig. 10-8). This aerobic breakdown of glucose yields approximately 95% of the ATP made from complete glucose metabolism (glucose → $CO_2 + H_2O$).

Aerobic glucose breakdown supplies more ATP than the anaerobic process, but it releases the energy more slowly. This slower rate of aerobic energy supply can be sustained for hours. One reason is that the products are carbon dioxide and water, not lactate. Aerobic glucose breakdown makes a major energy contribution to activities that last anywhere from 2 minutes to several hours. Examples of such activities include jogging or distance swimming (Table 10-3).

Endurance athletes sometimes reach a point in an event at which extreme physical and mental fatigue sets in; it feels impossible to stand up, let alone continue competing. Long-distance runners call this phenomenon *hitting the wall,* and cyclists sometimes refer to it as *bonking.* This occurs because muscle glycogen has been depleted and blood glucose has begun to decline during exercise, leading to deterioration of both physical and mental function. As discussed in more detail later, maximizing glycogen storage before physical activity, supplying carbohydrates during activity, and replenishing glycogen stores between events can help athletes avoid the game-stopping effects of glycogen depletion.

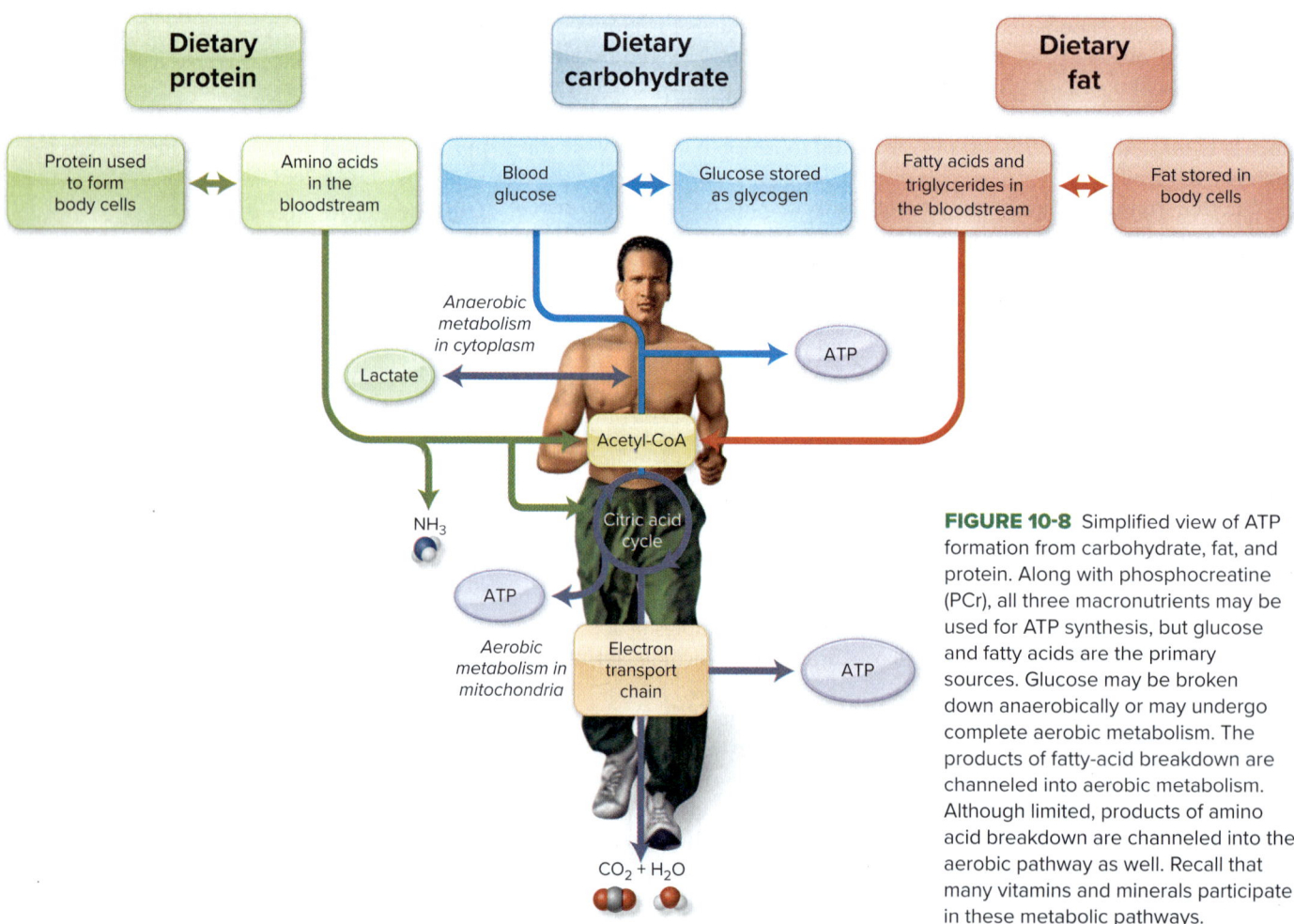

FIGURE 10-8 Simplified view of ATP formation from carbohydrate, fat, and protein. Along with phosphocreatine (PCr), all three macronutrients may be used for ATP synthesis, but glucose and fatty acids are the primary sources. Glucose may be broken down anaerobically or may undergo complete aerobic metabolism. The products of fatty-acid breakdown are channeled into aerobic metabolism. Although limited, products of amino acid breakdown are channeled into the aerobic pathway as well. Recall that many vitamins and minerals participate in these metabolic pathways.

TABLE 10-3 ■ Energy Sources Used by Resting and Working Muscle Cells

Energy Source*	When in Use	Activity
ATP	At all times	All types
Phosphocreatine (PCr)	All physical activity initially; short bursts up to 10 seconds	Throws, jumps, or 100- to 400-meter sprints
Carbohydrate (anaerobic)	High-intensity activity, especially lasting 30 seconds to 2 minutes	400-meter running sprint or 100-meter swimming sprint
Carbohydrate (aerobic)	Physical activity lasting 2 minutes to several hours; the higher the intensity, the greater the use	Basketball, distance swimming, jogging, power walking
Fat (aerobic)	Activities lasting more than a few minutes; greater amounts are used at lower intensities	Long-distance running or cycling; much of the fuel used in a 30-minute brisk walk
Protein (aerobic)	Low amount used during all activities; slightly more in endurance exercise, especially when carbohydrate fuel is depleted	Long-distance running

*At any given time, more than one source is used. The relative amount of use differs during various activities.

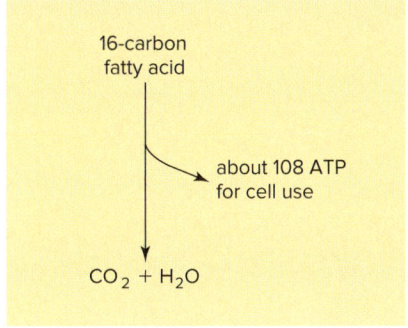

FIGURE 10-9 ATP yield from aerobic fatty-acid utilization.

Fat. When fat stores in body tissues begin to be broken down for energy, each triglyceride first yields three fatty acids (tri-) and a glycerol molecule (glyceride). The majority of the stored energy is found in fatty acids. During physical activity, fatty acids are released from various adipose tissue depots into the bloodstream and travel to the muscles, where they are taken into each cell and broken down aerobically to carbon dioxide and water (Fig. 10-9). Some of the fat stored in muscles (intramuscular triglycerides) also is used, especially as activity increases from a low to a moderate pace.

Fat is an advantageous fuel for muscles: We generally have plenty of it stored, and it is a concentrated source of energy. For a given weight of fuel, fat supplies more than twice as much energy as carbohydrate does. However, the ability of muscles to use fat for fuel depends on the intensity of the activity.

At rest or during light activity, nearly equal amounts of carbohydrate and fat are used to generate ATP. As activity intensifies (e.g., sprinting), anaerobic processes supply quick fuel, so the relative proportion of carbohydrates used for fuel increases. Except during endurance activities, very little protein is used for fuel.

During intense, brief exercise, muscles may not be able to use much fat. The reason for this is that some of the steps involved in fat breakdown cannot occur fast enough to meet the ATP demands of short-duration, high-intensity exercise. However, fat becomes a progressively more important energy source as duration increases, especially when physical activity remains at a low or moderate (aerobic) rate for more than 20 minutes.

For lengthy activities at a moderate pace (e.g., hiking), fat supplies about 70% to 90% of the energy required. Carbohydrate use is much less. As intensity increases, carbohydrate use goes up and fat use decreases. During a 5-mile run at a moderate pace, muscles use about a 50:50 ratio of fat to carbohydrate.[4] In comparison, for a sprint, the contribution of fat to resupply ATP is minimal. To summarize, remember that the only fast-paced (anaerobic) fuel we eat is carbohydrate; slow and steady (aerobic) activity uses fat in addition to carbohydrate.

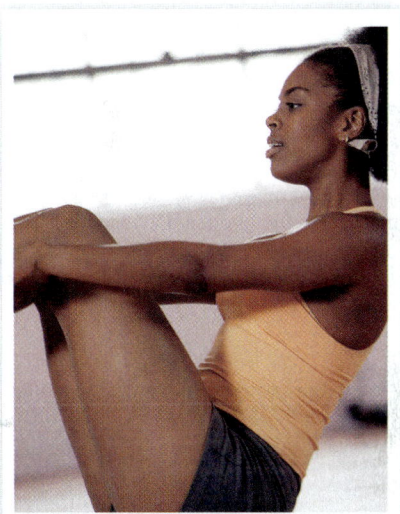

Fatty acids are recruited from all over the body, not necessarily from fat stored near the active muscles. This is why spot reducing does not work. Physical activity can tone the muscles near adipose tissue but does not preferentially use those stores. Comstock/Getty Images

Protein. Although amino acids derived from protein can be used to fuel muscles, their contribution is relatively small, compared with that of carbohydrate and fat. Most protein is reserved for building and repairing body tissues and for synthesizing important enzymes, hormones, and transporters. As a rough guide, only about 5% of the body's ATP comes from the metabolism of amino acids.[4]

During endurance activities, proteins can contribute importantly to energy needs, perhaps as much as 10% to 15%, especially as glycogen stores in the muscle are exhausted. Most of the energy supplied from protein comes from metabolism of the branched-chain amino acids: leucine, isoleucine, and valine. A healthy dietary pattern

Newsworthy Nutrition

Branched-chain amino acids impact health and lifespan in mice

Amino acids have long been advocated by the sports communities for their muscle-building benefits. Branched-chain amino acids (BCAAs) are a group of three essential amino acids: leucine, isoleucine, and valine, most commonly found in red meat and dairy. **INTRODUCTION:** Elevated BCAAs are associated with obesity and insulin resistance. While delivering muscle-building benefits, excessive consumption of BCAAs may reduce lifespan, negatively impact mood, and lead to weight gain. **OBJECTIVE:** The aim of this animal study was to evaluate the long-term effects of BCAA exposure on appetite, weight, mood, and lifespan. **METHODS:** Mice (312 male and female C57BL/6J) were fed dietary BCAAs in amounts of 200%, 50%, or 20% of the typical intakes throughout their life. **RESULTS:** Mice who were fed the highest amount of BCAAs increased their blood BCAA levels, which reduced serotonin levels in the brain. These levels of BCAA resulted in obesity and a shortened lifespan. **CONCLUSION:** The results of this study show that diets high in protein and low in carbohydrates had detrimental effects for health of mice in mid to late life, and also led to a shortened lifespan. Based on this information, athletes should vary protein sources in order to get a variety of essential amino acids through a healthy and balanced diet rich in fiber, vitamins, and minerals.

Source: Solon-Biet SM, Cogger VC, Pulpitel T, et al. Branched chain amino acids impact health and lifespan indirectly via amino acid balance and appetite control. *Nat Metab*. 2019 May;1(5):532-545. doi: 10.1038/s42255-019-0059-2

fat adaptation Manipulating the diet and physical training regimen so that muscles become more efficient at metabolizing fat as fuel during aerobic activity. Also known as *ketoadaptation*.

Marty started going to the gym about 8 weeks ago. At first, he noticed that he began huffing and puffing about 7 minutes into his basketball game. Now, however, he can play for about 25 minutes without tiring. **What is a possible explanation for this ability to work out longer?** Chrissy Walker/Realistic Reflections

provides ample branched-chain amino acids to supply this amount of fuel; protein or amino acid supplements are rarely needed (see *Newsworthy Nutrition*).

PHYSICAL TRAINING AFFECTS FUEL USE

As people start exercising regularly, they experience a training effect. Initially, these individuals might be able to engage in physical activity for 20 minutes before tiring. Months later, activities can be extended to an hour before they become fatigued. The training effect results from changes in the ability of exercising cells to use food fuel to generate ATP.

Almost immediately after a person begins a physical activity program, both aerobic and strength training improve the insulin sensitivity of cells. In other words, more glucose can be transported from the bloodstream into the cells, where it can be broken down either anaerobically or aerobically. Improved blood glucose management is an added benefit for preventing or treating metabolic syndrome or type 2 diabetes.

Endurance aerobic activities also increase the ability of muscles to store glycogen. This highly branched polymer of glucose can be broken down into individual glucose units when the energy needs of the cell are high or when blood glucose levels start to drop. Increasing glycogen storage will help to delay fatigue during prolonged activity.

Fat is a concentrated source of calories; complete oxidation of a long-chain fatty acid yields more than three times as much ATP as metabolism of glucose. Many endurance athletes attempt to train their muscles to readily use fat for fuel and thereby conserve muscle glycogen. Later in this chapter, you will learn more about this technique, known as **fat adaptation** or *ketoadaptation*.

Protein use becomes more efficient with training, too. Endurance training increases the ability of muscle cells to use branched-chain amino acids for fuel during prolonged activity. However, the ability to use carbohydrates and fats for fuel is also increased; as long as the diet is adequate in carbohydrates and fat, most protein is spared for muscle synthesis and repair.

In addition, training increases the number of mitochondria within muscle cells. Recall that mitochondria are the powerhouses of the cells; this is where glucose and fat are broken down aerobically to generate ATP. With more mitochondria, muscle cells can use carbohydrates and fat more efficiently.

Overall, the cardiovascular and respiratory systems become more efficient at providing oxygen to the cells of the body. Plasma volume increases shortly after a training program is started, and red blood cell volume eventually increases as well. The heart pumps more blood with each contraction. Training also increases the number of capillaries in muscles, which increases oxygen supply to the muscles. Meanwhile, lung capacity increases, so more oxygen is available. The increased supply of oxygen translates into more efficient aerobic metabolism of carbohydrates and fats. Through all these adaptations, physical training improves the ability of cells to convert food energy into fuel for physical activity.

✔ CONCEPT CHECK 10.3

1. Describe one process used to resupply ATP during a short, intense burst of activity, such as a 100-meter running sprint.
2. How does the ATP yield of anaerobic breakdown of glucose compare to that of aerobic breakdown of glucose?
3. Why is fat a useful source of energy during exercise? Name three types of activity during which fat supplies 50% or more of fuel.
4. Is protein a useful source of energy during physical activity? Why or why not?

10.4 Nutrient Recommendations for Active Adults and Athletes

Training and genetic makeup are two important determinants of physical performance. Although a healthy dietary pattern can't substitute for either factor, it can help to enhance and maximize performance. On the other hand, suboptimal dietary patterns can seriously reduce performance.[5] As highlighted in earlier chapters, the *Dietary Guidelines* notes several nutrients of public health concern given their inadequate consumption in the U.S. Active adults should consume nutrient-dense sources of dietary fiber, vitamin D, calcium, iron, and potassium for optimal performance.

CALORIES

The daily calorie needs of active adults are highly individualized: genetics, hormones, age, sex, height, weight, temperature, altitude, stress, physical health, medications, body composition, and training level influence energy expenditure. A small, female gymnast may need 2000 kcal daily to sustain her training regimen without losing body weight, whereas a large, muscular male football player may need 4000 kcal per day. Because athletic individuals are such a heterogeneous group, there is no perfect equation to estimate their daily calorie needs. Even for nonathletes, the Estimated Energy Requirement (EER) equation provides only a rough approximation. However, you can use the EER equation as a starting point and individualize recommendations based on trial and error.

An estimate of the calories required to sustain moderate activity is 3.5 to 7 kcal per minute. The calories required for sports training or competition, then, must be added to those used to carry on normal activities. For example, let's consider a 136-pound young female who requires 2275 kcal per day to fuel her low active normal activities. If she starts teaching two 45-minute dance classes each day, she will need about 400 extra kcal (a total of about 2700 kcal per day) to maintain her current body weight. If a very active adult experiences daily fatigue, the first consideration should be whether the individual is consuming enough food. Up to six meals per day may be needed, including one before each workout.

How can we know if an athlete is getting enough calories? Consulting with a sports dietitian would help answer this question. Estimating daily intake from a dietary intake log kept by the athlete is one way. Another option is to estimate the athlete's body fat percentage via body composition measures such as those detailed earlier (e.g., bioelectrical impedance analysis, DXA, etc.). Body fat should be the typical amount found for athletes in the specific sport practiced. The recommended body fat percentage for athletes varies based on the sex of the athlete and the sport itself. The best way to determine if an athlete is consuming enough calories is to monitor body weight changes over time. If body weight starts to fall unintentionally, calories should be increased; if weight rises and it is because of increases in body fat, the athlete should reduce calories or increase physical activity. Again, a sports dietitian is an excellent resource for estimating individual nutrient needs for athletes.

Body mass index (BMI) is not an appropriate surrogate for assessing body fat for athletes. Body composition assessments are preferred for determining body fatness. If assessments of body composition show that an athlete needs to reduce body fat or gain weight, a sports dietitian should be consulted to provide professional recommendations related to balancing dietary and physical activity patterns to achieve optimal performance status.

Historically, athletes who competed in sports with weight classes (e.g., wrestlers, boxers) would try to lose weight before a competition. Many of the methods used to cut weight are unhealthy and dangerous. It is important to remember that losing as little as 2% of body weight by dehydration can adversely affect physical and mental performance, especially in hot weather. A pattern of repeated weight loss of more than 5% of body weight by dehydration carries risk of kidney dysfunction and heat-related illness. Death is also a possibility.[6]

To discourage such unhealthy practices and prevent future deaths, the National Collegiate Athletic Association (NCAA) and many states have authorized physicians or athletic trainers to set safe weight and body fat content minimums in weight-class sports. Under current guidelines, athletes wishing to lose weight should slowly descend to the desired weight class by not losing more than 1.5% of body weight per week.[7]

relative energy deficiency in sport (RED-S) A syndrome of altered metabolism, immune function, and mental health caused by low energy availability in athletes, which may be due to unintentional failure to meet the high energy demands of sports or intentional restriction of energy intake to control weight.

Relative Energy Deficiency in Sport (RED-S). The concept of **relative energy deficiency in sport (RED-S)** addresses the full range of concerns to include amenorrhea (females), reduced testosterone levels and libido (males), suboptimal bone health, increased risk of illness and injuries, gastrointestinal disturbances, cardiovascular disease, impaired training capacity, and poor performance. The highest prevalence of low energy availability (LEA) involves weight-sensitive endurance sports. Athletes at greatest risk for disordered eating often follow misguided weight-loss programs and fail to recognize increased energy expenditure associated with training and competition. Treatment for these at-risk athletes includes increasing energy availability and often requires a comprehensive care team approach that includes a sports physician, sports dietitian, physiologist, and psychologist (Fig. 10-10).[8]

What is energy availability? Recall that you learned about energy balance in Chapter 7. Energy input comes from foods and beverages. Components of energy output include basal metabolism, physical activity, and the thermic effect of food. For athletes, the proportion of energy expenditure devoted to physical activity may be quite high. Energy availability is the amount of energy left after the demands of physical activity have been met. If the amount of energy supplied by the dietary pattern is insufficient to cover total energy needs (i.e., low energy availability), some basic metabolic functions will suffer.

CARBOHYDRATES

Anyone who exercises vigorously, especially for more than 1 hour per day on a regular basis, should adhere to an eating pattern that includes moderate to high amounts of carbohydrate. Numerous servings of varied grains, starchy vegetables, and fruits provide enough carbohydrate to maintain adequate liver and muscle glycogen stores.

Although it has been known for some time that the role of carbohydrate intake within (during) activity serves as an additional substrate for the muscle and the brain, there is now scientific evidence that carbohydrate consumption during physical activity provides additional performance benefits. Specifically, carbohydrate intake appears to

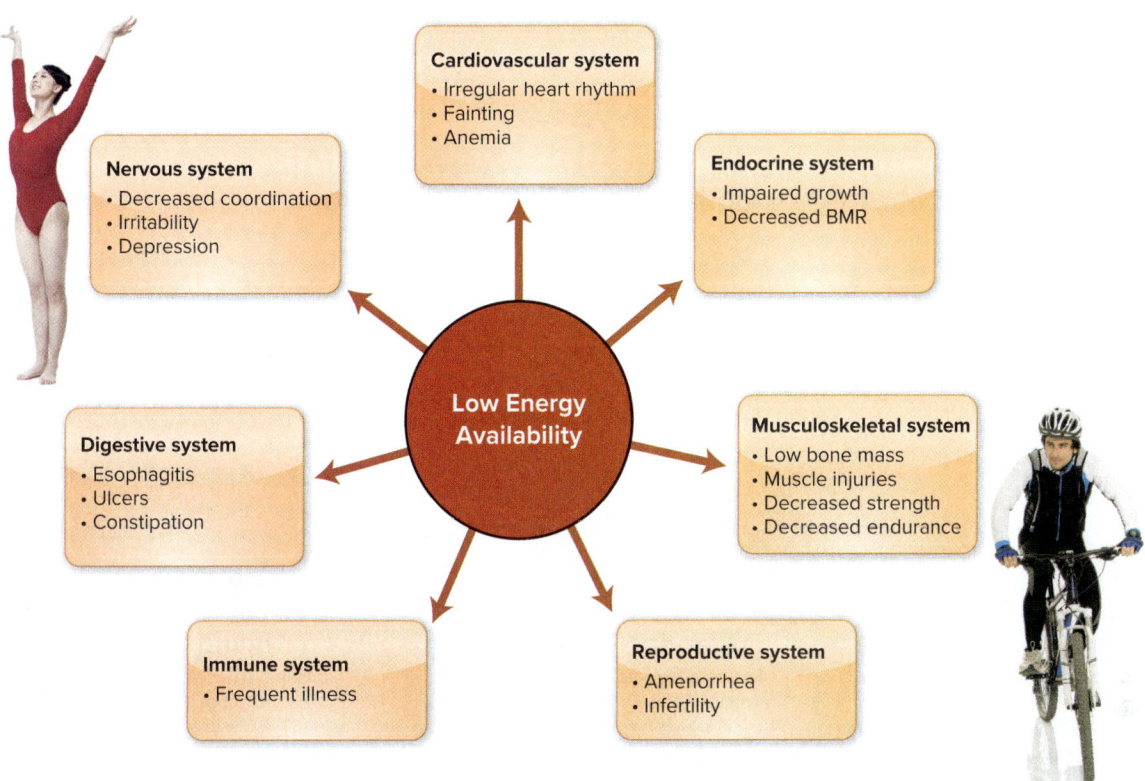

FIGURE 10-10 Relative energy deficiency in sport occurs when the athlete has low energy availability (with or without an eating disorder) that negatively impacts multiple body systems. Long-term health is at risk; thus, prevention and early treatment are crucial. Photos: (left) Lane Oatey/Blue Jean Images/Getty Images; (right) Aaron Amat/Shutterstock

stimulate areas of the brain that control both pacing and the reward system by enhancing communications with mouth and gut receptors. Termed *mouth sensing*, this may provide more rationale for frequent intakes of carbs during longer events.

Depletion of carbohydrate ranks just behind depletion of fluid and electrolytes as a major cause of fatigue and poor performance. Optimal carbohydrate intake depends on the size of the athlete and the type of physical activity. Recall that your weight in pounds divided by 2.2 converts your weight into kilograms. For light or skill-based sports, 3 to 5 grams of carbohydrate per kilogram of body weight will suffice (Fig. 10-11). For physical activity of moderate intensity, consume 5 to 7 grams of carbohydrate per kilogram. Athletes who train for several hours per day may need up to 12 grams of carbohydrates per kilogram of body weight, which may add up to over 800 grams per day. Attention to carbohydrate intake is especially important when performing multiple training bouts in one day (e.g., two-a-day swim practices) or heavy training on successive days (e.g., cross-country running).

Athletes should obtain at least 45% to 65% of their total energy needs from carbohydrate,[5] especially if activity duration is expected to exceed 2 hours and total caloric intake is about 3000 kcal per day or less. Eating patterns providing 4000 to 5000 kcal per day can be as low as 50% carbohydrate, as these will still provide sufficient carbohydrate (e.g., 500 to 600 grams or so per day).

Besides the total amount of carbohydrates, the *quality* of carbohydrates can certainly influence mental and physical performance. Sports dietitians emphasize the difference between a high-carbohydrate meal and a high-carbohydrate/high-fat meal. Before endurance events, such as marathons or triathlons, some athletes seek to increase their carbohydrate reserves by eating foods such as potato chips, French fries, banana cream pie, and pastries. Although such foods provide carbohydrate, they also contain a lot of saturated fat and are highly processed. Better high-fiber, high-carbohydrate

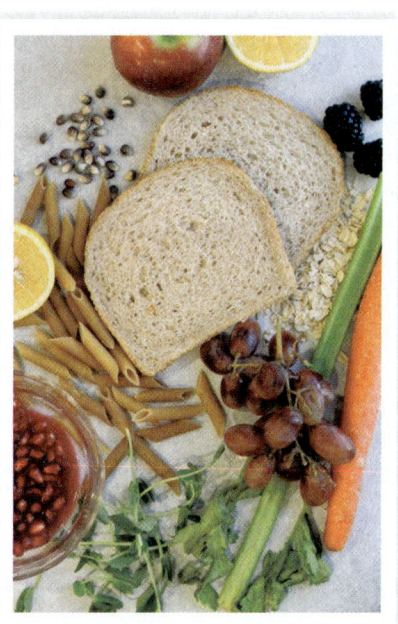

Fruits, vegetables, and whole grains should form the foundation of an athlete's dietary pattern. **What macronutrient contributes the majority of fuel from these food sources?** Alexis Joseph/McGraw Hill

Athlete's Nutritional Requirements

Carbohydrate	Total carbohydrate needs vary from athlete to athlete. In general, athletes should still thrive to consume 45–65% of total calories from carbohydrates. The higher the intensity, the more energy that is needed and the more carbohydrates that are needed for optimal performance and glycogen store replenishment.

Daily Carbohydrate Needs Relative to Exercise Intensity

Intensity	Low	Moderate	High	Extreme
Activity Type	Low intensity exercise	Moderate intensity exercise program for 1 hr	Moderate intensity exercise program for 1–3 hrs	Moderate intensity exercise program for 4–5 hrs
Carbohydrate Requirements	3–5 g/kg/day 210–350 g/day*	5–7 g/kg/day 350–490 g/day*	6–10 g/kg/day 420–700 g/day*	8–12 g/kg/day 560–840 g/day*

*Based on 70 kg (154 lb) body weight

Protein	Proteins are important to maintain muscle mass. Athletes should aim to consume about 1.2–2.0 g/kg of body weight per day to maintain and build muscle.

Quality
Focus on high-quality animal-based proteins or consume complementary plant-based proteins to provide you with all essential amino acids.

Quantity
Ensure adequate protein intake. For muscle building and maintenance, 1.2–2.0 g/kg of body weight is appropriate for most athletes.

Timing
Consume 0.3–0.4 g/kg of body weight of protein every 3–5 hrs to ensure adequate supply of amino acids for optimal muscle growth and maintenance.

Fat	Just like the general population, athletes require 20–35% of total calories from high quality fat sources. Fat is a dense source of energy and can help athletes reach their daily energy goals.

Fluids	Adequate fluid intake is crucial for athletic performance. Fluid needs depend on activity level and fluid losses during activity. For hydration assessment, use weight loss during activity, urine color, and thirst as indicators of hydration status.

Maintaining Adequate Hydration for Physical Activity

Before	It is recommended to drink 5–7 mL of fluid per kilogram of body weight 2–4 hrs before activity.
During	Avoid fluid losses of more than 2% of body weight to avoid dehydration.
After	For every pound lost during activity, it is recommended to drink 2–3 cups of fluids in the first 4–6 hrs after activity.

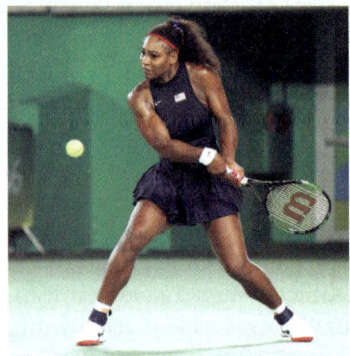

FIGURE 10-11 Nutrition recommendations for athletes. (photo): Leonard Zhukovsky/Shutterstock

dietary patterns are rich in whole grain pasta, brown rice, sweet potatoes, whole grain bread, fruit and 100% fruit juices, and various whole grain breakfast cereals.

See the *Farm to Fork* feature on carrots and beets to read about beet juice and athletic performance. Be sure to check the Nutrition Facts label for carbohydrate content (Table 10-4). Consuming a moderate amount of fiber during the final day of training is a good precaution to reduce the chances of bloating and intestinal gas during the next day's event. It is also essential to hydrate properly when consuming additional fiber.

FAT

A dietary pattern containing up to 20% to 35% of calories from fat is generally recommended for athletes (Fig. 10-11).[5] Rich sources of monounsaturated fat, such as olive and canola oil, should be emphasized, and saturated fat intake should be limited. Consuming ≤ 20% of energy intake from fat does not enhance performance, and extreme restriction of fat intake may limit the food range needed to meet overall health and performance goals.[5] At the other end of the spectrum, extremely high-fat, carbohydrate-restricted diets are not supported by the current evidence.

PROTEIN

Whether the recommended daily protein allowances for the general population, set at 0.8 g/kg, are appropriate for active adults remains a point of controversy.[9] For athletes, many experts recommend protein intake within the range of 1.2 to 2.0 grams of protein per kilogram of body weight, spacing modest amounts of high-quality protein (0.3 g/kg) after physical activity and throughout the day (Fig. 10-11).[5] Sports dietitians contend that the RDAs have been set to prevent deficiency among the general population not to optimize physical performance among athletes.[9]

The optimal protein intake for an athlete varies based on the athlete's activity and level of fitness. Athletes who are just beginning a strength-training program are likely to need the most protein to supply the building blocks for synthesis of new muscle tissue. Once the desired muscle mass is achieved, daily protein intake need not exceed 1.2 grams per kilogram of body weight. Some strength-training athletes tend to aim for excessive protein intakes, sometimes as high as 3 or 4 grams of protein per kilogram of body weight.[10] There remains conflicting evidence that protein intake above 2.0 grams per kilogram of body weight will benefit the athlete.[11] Protein intakes above this amount result in an increased use of amino acids for energy needs; no further increase in muscle protein synthesis is seen.

Unless an athlete follows a low-calorie diet, the recommended range of 1.2 to 2.0 grams of protein per kilogram of body weight can be met by eating a variety of foods. To illustrate, a 117-pound (53 kg) female performing moderate-intensity endurance activity can consume 64 grams of protein (53 × 1.2) during a single day by including 3 ounces of chicken (a small chicken breast), 3 ounces of tuna, and two glasses of low-fat milk. Similarly, a 170-pound (77 kg) male who aims to gain muscle mass through strength training needs to consume only 6 ounces of chicken (a large chicken breast), ½ cup of cooked beans, a 6-ounce can of tuna, and three glasses of low-fat milk to achieve an intake of 154 grams of protein (77 × 2.0) in a day. For both athletes, these calculations do not include the protein present in the grains or vegetables they will also eat. By simply meeting their calorie needs, many athletes easily meet their protein requirements.

FARM to FORK Carrots and Beets

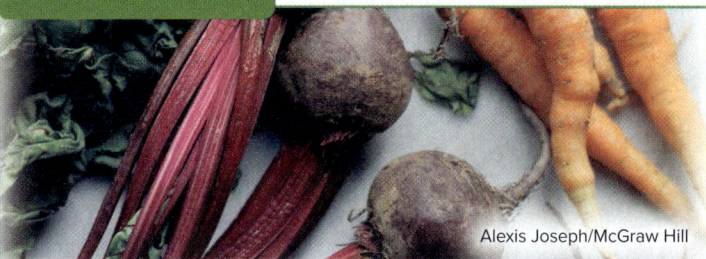

Alexis Joseph/McGraw Hill

Carrots and beets are root crops with a wide range of nutrients, flavors, and health-promoting benefits. Red beet juice has also been touted to enhance athletic performance.

Grow

- The wild ancestor of carrots was purple, but most carrots grown in the United States are orange, a good indicator of the nutrients and other phytochemicals they contain, especially beta-carotene. Farmers are again producing purple carrot varieties, which are sweeter and higher in beta-carotene and the purple pigments, anthocyanins.
- Red beets are high in betalins, phytochemicals that may reduce the risk of cancer and other diseases.

Shop

- For the freshest and sweetest carrots and beets, buy them with the green tops still attached. They will be at most only a few weeks old. Carrots and beets without tops can be several weeks to months old.
- Refrain from buying baby or frozen carrots. Baby carrots originate from misshapen mature carrots that have been whittled down to a smaller uniform size, and the remaining inner core is not as nutritious as the outer part that is discarded. The peeling, processing, and freeze/thaw cycle of frozen carrots destroys about half of their antioxidant value.
- The processing of beets into canned beets renders them more nutritious with more antioxidant value.

Store

- Cut the tops off of your fresh carrots so they retain their moisture. To protect carrots from the ethylene gas produced by other fruits and vegetables, store them in a sealed plastic bag in the refrigerator.
- Remove beet greens and store beet roots unwrapped in the crisper drawer of the refrigerator and use them within 2 weeks.

Prep

- Carrots and beets are more nutritious cooked. The heat breaks down cell walls and makes nutrients more bioavailable. Scrub carrots and beets, and cook them whole.
- Carrots can be sautéed or steamed to preserve more nutrients and sweetness. Eat carrots with oil or fat to allow best absorption of the fat-soluble beta-carotene, a precursor of vitamin A.
- Beets can be steamed, microwaved, or roasted. The skin helps retain the water-soluble nutrients while cooking and can be slipped off when cool. Beets will stain hands and surfaces, including wooden cutting boards. Use rubber gloves to avoid beet stains on your hands.
- Eating beets with mustard, horseradish, or vinegar will disguise their earthy flavor.

Source: Robinson J. The other root crops: carrots, beets and sweet potatoes. In: *Eating on the Wild Side: The Missing Link to Optimum Health.* New York: Little, Brown & Co.; 2013.

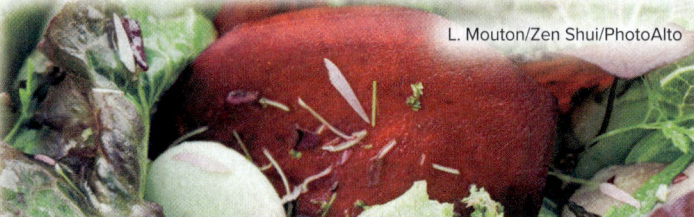

L. Mouton/Zen Shui/PhotoAlto

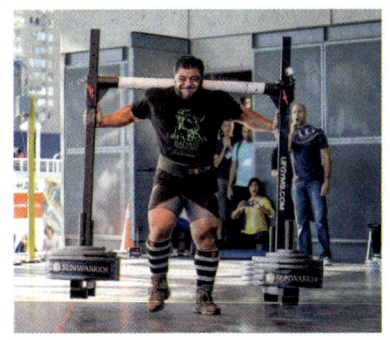

Do strength-trained athletes need to ingest tuna, chicken, and lean beef frequently to build muscle? Patrik Baboumian is a strongman competitor, former bodybuilder, and world record-holder who follows a vegan dietary pattern. The plant-based protein sources that built his 250-pound physique included beans, peas, lentils, nuts, seeds, and soy. David Cooper/Toronto Star/Getty Images

TABLE 10-4 ■ Carbohydrate-Rich Foods

Starches = 15 Grams Carbohydrate (80 kcal)	
Dry breakfast cereal,* ½–¾ cup	Baked potato, ¼ large
Cooked breakfast cereal, ½ cup	Bagel, ¼ (or 4 ounces)
Cooked rice, ⅓ cup	Bread, 1 slice
Cooked pasta, ⅓ cup	Pretzels, ¾ ounce
Cooked corn, ½ cup	Saltine crackers, 6
Cooked dry beans, ½ cup	Pancake, 4-inch diameter, 1
Vegetables = 5 Grams Carbohydrate (25 kcal)	
Cooked vegetables, ½ cup	Examples: carrots, green beans, broccoli, cauliflower, spinach, tomatoes, and vegetable juice
Raw vegetables, 1 cup	
Vegetable juice, ½ cup	
Fruits = 15 Grams Carbohydrate (60 kcal)	
Canned fruit or berries, ½ cup	Grapes, 17
100% fruit juice, ½ cup	Grapefruit, ½
Apple or orange, 1 small	Peach, 1
Banana, 1 small	Watermelon cubes, 1¼ cups
Dairy = 12 Grams Carbohydrate (100 to 150 kcal)	
Milk, 1 cup	Soy milk, 1 cup
Plain low-fat yogurt, ⅔ cup	
Sweets = 15 Grams Carbohydrate (variable kcal)	
Cake, 2-inch square	Ice cream, ½ cup
Cookies, 2 small	Sherbet, ½ cup

*The carbohydrate content of dry cereal varies widely. Check the labels of the ones you choose and adjust the serving size accordingly.

Source: Modified from Choose Your Foods: Food Lists for Diabetes by the American Diabetes Association and Academy of Nutrition and Dietetics, 2014.

Despite marketing claims, high-quality whole food proteins are superior to supplements for the maintenance, repair, and synthesis of muscle. The protein foods group comprises a broad group of foods from both animal and plant sources and includes several subgroups: meats, poultry, and eggs; seafood; and nuts, seeds, and soy products. Beans, peas, and lentils may be considered a part of the protein foods group as well.

The consumption of milk-based protein, especially after resistance training, is effective in increasing muscle strength and promotes positive results in body composition. Although supplements are usually expensive and unnecessary, many athletes choose to use protein powders (e.g., whey, casein, or soy) to add additional protein to their dietary patterns in hopes of achieving muscle protein synthesis. Whey protein is especially popular among strength-trained athletes. It is particularly rich in leucine, an essential branched-chain amino acid that has been shown in some studies to stimulate gains in muscle mass during strength training.[13] Yet experts still recommend that individuals attempt to meet their protein needs via whole foods, including plant-based proteins (see *Ask the RDN*).

Consuming excessive amounts of protein has drawbacks. It increases calcium loss somewhat in the urine. It also leads to increased urine production, which could increase dehydration. Excess animal protein also may lead to kidney stones in people with a history of this or other kidney problems. Last but not least, a dietary pattern that is so focused on animal protein may leave the athlete short on carbohydrates, leading to fatigue and poor athletic performance.

VITAMINS AND MINERALS

Compared to the needs of sedentary adults, vitamin and mineral needs for athletes are the same or slightly higher. At this time, there are not enough data to support separate Dietary Reference Intakes (DRIs) specific to athletes for any of the micronutrients. Athletes usually have high calorie intakes, so they tend to consume plenty of vitamins and minerals. An exception is athletes consuming low-calorie diets (1200 kcal or less), as seen with some female athletes participating in events in which maintaining a low

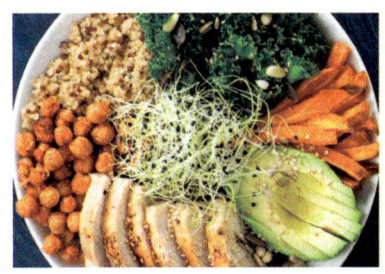

Researchers suggest a dose of at least 30 grams of protein per meal is ideal to promote muscle synthesis.[12] **How many sources of high-quality protein can you spot on this plate?** asife/Shutterstock

ASK THE RDN: The No-Meat Athlete

Dear RDN: For a variety of reasons, I am considering switching to a vegan eating pattern. However, I am a sprinter on the college women's swimming and diving team, and I want to make sure that a vegan diet would not affect my athletic performance. Can a "no-meat athlete" compete?

A well-planned plant-based diet can absolutely support optimal athletic performance. From better weight management to reduced risk for chronic diseases, vegan diets offer many health benefits. However, some nutrient needs may be difficult to meet with a plant-based diet. These include protein, iron, calcium, and vitamin B-12.

Protein intakes of athletes who follow a vegan dietary pattern, especially young females, are often low. You may need more than the RDA for protein because, first, you are an athlete and, second, the quality of plant proteins is generally lower than that of animal proteins. Those following a vegetarian or vegan dietary pattern should aim for 1.4 to 2.0 grams per kilogram of body weight. If you consume adequate calories, you can meet your protein needs without protein or amino acid supplements, but the *quality* of your protein matters. Be sure to consume a variety of plant proteins (legumes, grains, nuts) throughout the day to obtain all of the essential amino acids.

Iron delivers oxygen to exercising muscles and helps to convert food fuel into ATP—two processes that impact athletic performance. Iron needs can be difficult to meet even with omnivorous diets, so iron intake deserves special attention. Remember that plant (nonheme) sources of iron are not as well absorbed as animal (heme) sources, but foods with vitamin C can boost absorption of nonheme iron. Have your iron status checked periodically. If your iron stores are low, discuss options with your primary care provider or registered dietitian nutritionist (RDN).

Lean female athletes place themselves at risk for early osteoporosis if their dietary patterns are low in calcium (and vitamin D). A vegan eating pattern eliminates animal products, including dairy foods, which are excellent sources of these bone-building nutrients.

A deficiency of vitamin B-12 could also affect red blood cell health and possibly nerve function. Unlike iron and calcium, there are no plant-based alternatives for vitamin B-12. Use of fortified foods and/or dietary supplements will be crucial to meeting your vitamin B-12 needs.

One more concern is that this highly restrictive dietary change—even though it seems like a healthful choice—could promote disordered eating behaviors. As you move toward a plant-based dietary pattern, make sure your overall energy intake is adequate to support your needs for competitive training. If your weight drops too low, it could significantly affect your athletic performance and long-term bone health.

Start slowly and follow these general recommendations: begin your day with a bowl of fortified whole grain breakfast cereal. Check the label for brands of cereal that provide at least 20% of the DV for iron and vitamin B-12. Top your cereal with a fortified soy alternative (or another fortified alternative) that provides at least one-third of the DV for calcium. Also include calcium-fortified dairy alternatives as a substitute whenever you would have chosen dairy products. Enjoy a glass of calcium-fortified 100% orange juice with breakfast to enhance absorption of iron from your cereal. Throughout the day, be sure to choose plentiful and varied sources of plant proteins, including legumes, nuts, seeds, and whole grains. Try soy and quinoa, two versatile plant proteins that contain all essential amino acids. Last, monitor changes in your weight and performance. If your calorie intake is too low, consider incorporating more nuts, nut butters, avocados, and hummus into your meals and snacks, as these are energy-dense sources of healthy fats.

These are just a few basic ideas to help you remain healthy and compete at your highest level. To tailor your food intake to your specific needs, seek the expert advice of your team's sports dietitian at your university health center.

To your record-breaking success!

Angela Collene, MS, RDN, LD

Senior Lecturer, The Ohio State University, Author of *Wardlaw's Contemporary Nutrition* and *Wardlaw's Contemporary Nutrition: A Functional Approach*

Source: Rogerson D. Vegan diets: practical advice for athletes and exercisers. *J Int Soc Sports Nutr.* 2017 Sep 13;14:36. doi: 10.1186/s12970-017-0192-9

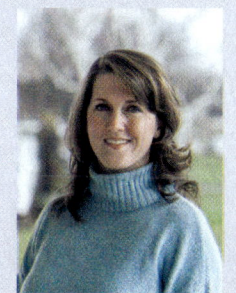
Tim Klontz

---

body weight is crucial. These eating patterns may not meet B vitamin and other micronutrient needs. Athletes who follow a vegan dietary pattern may also fall short on some nutrients. In these cases, consuming fortified foods, such as ready-to-eat breakfast cereals, or a balanced multivitamin and mineral supplement may be recommended. You can discuss options with a sports dietitian or your primary care provider. Vegetarian athletes, also discussed later in this chapter, are encouraged to consume generous amounts of fruits, vegetables, whole grains, and plant proteins (nuts, seeds, soy products, etc.) that contribute adequate fiber, phytochemicals, antioxidants, and other nutrients.

B Vitamins Support Energy Metabolism and Red Blood Cell Health. Recall that coenzyme forms of B vitamins facilitate chemical reactions that generate ATP from carbohydrates, proteins, and fats. Some B vitamins are involved in processes that build and repair tissue. Although no separate DRIs have been set, athletes may need more than the current RDA for some B vitamins, such as riboflavin and vitamin B-6.

Furthermore, physical performance is highly dependent on the availability of oxygen to active muscles. Folate, vitamin B-6, and vitamin B-12 are involved in the formation of healthy red blood cells, which transport oxygen to all body tissues.

As you can imagine, an inadequate supply of B vitamins could impair an athlete's physical performance. Yet deficiencies of B vitamins are not very common. As athletes consume greater quantities of food to meet their increased calorie needs, they typically consume enough B vitamins from food sources to support energy metabolism and red blood cell health. Taking more than the RDA for B vitamins is not likely to enhance performance.

On the other hand, for a person with a diagnosed vitamin or mineral deficiency, supplementation could improve athletic performance. At-risk populations include athletes who are vegan or older (vitamin B-12), female athletes of childbearing age (folate), and any athlete who restricts dietary intake to control body weight (variety of micronutrients). In these cases, fortified foods or a balanced multivitamin and mineral supplement may be beneficial to overall health and athletic performance.

Antioxidants May Prevent Oxidative Damage. Physical activity leads to increased production of free radicals. The presence of some free radicals in muscle tissue is actually beneficial for muscle contraction and adaptation to exercise. However, excessive free radicals can lead to fatigue and cell damage.

Athletes' needs for antioxidants such as vitamin E and vitamin C may be somewhat greater because of the potential protection these nutrients provide. However, there is evidence that antioxidant system activity increases in the body as training progresses. The use of large doses of antioxidants is not currently an accepted part of the dietary guidance for athletes. Food groups rich in antioxidants, include vegetables, fruits, and grains.[5]

Optimal Iron Status Improves Performance. Iron is involved in red blood cell production, oxygen transport, and energy production, so a deficiency of this mineral can noticeably detract from optimal athletic performance. Some of the consequences of iron deficiency include weakness, fatigue, and decreased work capacity. The potential causes for iron deficiency in athletes vary.[14] As in the general population, female athletes are most susceptible to low iron status due to monthly menstrual losses. Restrictive eating plans, such as low-calorie and vegan eating plans, are likely to be lower in iron. Distance runners should pay special attention to iron intake because their intense workouts may lead to gastrointestinal bleeding.

A less-threatening concern is **sports anemia.** At the start of an endurance training regimen, plasma volume expands, but the synthesis of additional red blood cells is slower to increase. This results in a temporary dilution of the blood; even if iron stores are adequate, blood iron tests may appear low. Sports anemia is not detrimental to performance, but it is hard to differentiate between sports anemia and true anemia. If iron status is low and not replenished, iron-deficiency anemia can markedly impair endurance performance.

Although true iron-deficiency anemia (a depressed blood hemoglobin level) is not that common among athletes, some studies suggest that iron deficiency without anemia may have a negative impact on physical activity and performance. Recall that iron deficiency occurs long before anemia is detected clinically. As body stores of iron are depleted, body processes that use iron, such as energy-yielding reactions, are impaired.

It is a good idea for athletes (especially females who are premenopausal) to have their iron status checked at the beginning of a training season and at least once midseason.[14] Current evidence suggests that as many as half of female athletes may be iron deficient. To identify iron deficiency without anemia among athletes, many experts advocate serum ferritin testing. Ferritin is an iron transport protein; low serum ferritin levels indicate low iron stores even before red blood cell health is affected.

Any blood test indicating low iron status—sports anemia or not—warrants follow-up. A primary care provider will need to determine the cause of iron depletion. Whatever the cause, once depleted, iron stores can take months to replenish. Dietary sources are typically not enough to correct iron-deficiency anemia; supplementation (under a primary

sports anemia Exercise-induced iron-deficiency anemia caused by plasma volume expansion, low hemoglobin synthesis, or increased destruction of red blood cells.

care provider's supervision only) is required. Athletes must be especially careful to meet iron needs because preventing iron deficiency is a lot simpler than treating it.

Knowing that iron is required for red blood cell synthesis, athletes may be tempted to self-prescribe iron supplements in an attempt to boost the oxygen-carrying capacity of the blood. However, indiscriminate use of iron supplements for people with normal hemoglobin and serum ferritin levels is never advised.[14] Research does not support a benefit of iron supplementation on athletic performance for athletes with normal iron status. Furthermore, liver damage and increased rates of heart disease and some forms of cancer are possible consequences of iron toxicity. A safer alternative would be to have iron status checked periodically. In addition, monitor dietary patterns to become aware of usual iron intakes. If dietary iron intake is low, incorporate more food sources of heme iron and pair nonheme sources with vitamin C to enhance absorption. Avoid drinking tea or iced tea with meals because this may inhibit iron absorption. The decision to use an iron supplement is best left to a primary care provider.

Calcium Intake Is Important, Especially in Females. Athletes, especially females trying to lose weight by restricting their intake of dairy products, can have marginal or low dietary intakes of calcium. This practice compromises bone health. Of still greater concern are female athletes who have stopped menstruating because their arduous training and low body fat interfere with the normal secretion of reproductive hormones. Female athletes who do not menstruate regularly are more likely to suffer **stress fractures** during training and will be susceptible to bone injuries throughout life. The negative impacts of low dietary calcium intake and irregular menses in female athletes outweigh the benefits of weight-bearing activities on bone density. Increasing energy intake to restore body weight and body fat stores is important to correct hormonal imbalances and prevent further bone loss.

Female athletes whose menstrual cycles become irregular should consult a primary care provider or sports dietitian. Decreasing the amount of training or increasing energy intake and body weight often restores regular menstrual cycles. If irregular menstrual cycles persist, severe bone loss (much of which is not reversible) and osteoporosis can result. Extra calcium in the diet does not necessarily compensate for these damaging effects of menstrual irregularities, but inadequate dietary calcium can make matters worse.

Vitamin D Status. Recent studies have documented a relationship between vitamin D status and injury prevention, improved neuromuscular function, enhanced muscle size, decreased inflammation, and reduced risk of stress fractures. Athletes who live at latitudes above the 35th parallel or who predominantly train indoors are at higher risk for vitamin D deficiency. Although vitamin D status is important for athletes and nonathletes alike, current data do not support vitamin D as an **ergogenic aid.** More data are needed to elucidate the role of vitamin D in athletics. Those who have a history of stress fractures, joint or overtraining injuries, or muscle pain and weakness should consult their primary care provider or sports dietitian.

FLUID

Fluid needs for an average adult are about 12 cups per day for females and 16 cups per day for males. These estimates include the fluids consumed from both eating and drinking. Most adults typically obtain about 20% of their water needs from the foods they consume. Adjusting for this, females need about 9 cups per day and males about 13 cups per day to replenish daily water losses.

Athletes generally need even more water to regulate body temperature. Heat production in contracting muscles can rise 15 to 20 times above that of resting muscles. Unless this heat is quickly dissipated, heat exhaustion, heat cramps, and potentially fatal heatstroke may ensue.

Fluid and electrolyte needs vary widely, based on differences in genetics, body mass, environmental conditions, level of training, and event duration. Because fluid needs

stress fracture A fracture that occurs from repeated jarring of a bone. Common sites include bones of the foot and shins.

ergogenic aid A mechanical, nutritional, psychological, pharmacological, or physiological substance or treatment intended to directly improve exercise performance.

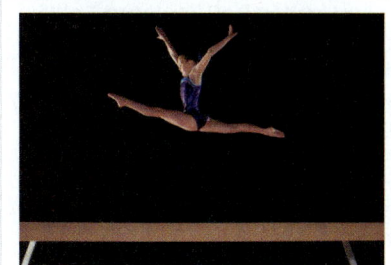

Weight-restricted athletes should make sure they are consuming enough calcium, protein, and other essential nutrients. Juice Images Ltd/Getty Images

are highly individualized and dynamic, it is difficult to make general recommendations for fluid replacement.[5] Thirst is actually a poor indicator of hydration status. The fact is that thirst is a late sign of dehydration. An athlete who drinks only when thirsty may take 48 hours to replenish fluid losses. After several days of training, an athlete relying only on thirst can build up a fluid debt that will impair performance. An athlete should consume enough fluid to prevent short-term (i.e., fluid-related) changes in body weight. The American College of Sports Medicine recommends losing *no more than 2%* of body weight during physical activity, especially in hot weather.[5] A football player wearing equipment in hot weather can lose this much within 30 minutes. However, it is important to remember this advice even when sweating can go unnoticed, such as when swimming or during the winter.

To determine fluid needs, athletes should first calculate 2% of their body weight. Next, it is useful to know the body's hourly sweat rate, which can be calculated by comparing weight loss during the activity to the amount of fluid consumed. This will require some self-monitoring of pre- and post-workout weight and fluid intake during workouts. For reference, sweat rates during prolonged activities can range from 1.5 to 10 cups (300 to 2400 mL) per hour.[5] If weight change cannot be monitored, urine color is another measure of hydration status. Urine color should be no more yellow than lemonade.

FLUID BEFORE, DURING, AND AFTER ACTIVITY

The fluid plan that suits most athletes needs to be tailored to meet the athlete's tolerance and experience, opportunities for drinking fluids throughout activities, and consumption of other nutrients (e.g., carbohydrate) in liquid form. The following fluid-replacement approach for before, during, and after workouts can meet an athlete's fluid needs in most cases.[5]

- Drink 5 to 7 mL/kg of body weight (about 1.5 to 2 cups for a 150-pound male) of water in the 2 to 4 hours before exercise.
- During sustained events, athletes should consume fluid to prevent dehydration (losses of > 2% body weight). The best plan is to determine individual rate of fluid losses during training and plan accordingly. For example, football players wearing equipment for two-a-day practices during the heat of August may need even more than 800 milliliters per hour to prevent dehydration. In many cases, athletes, especially children and teenagers, need to be reminded to consume fluids during physical activity.
- Within 4 to 6 hours after exercise, about 2 to 3 cups of fluid should be consumed for every pound lost. It is important that weight be restored before the next exercise period. Skipping fluids before or during events will almost certainly impair performance.

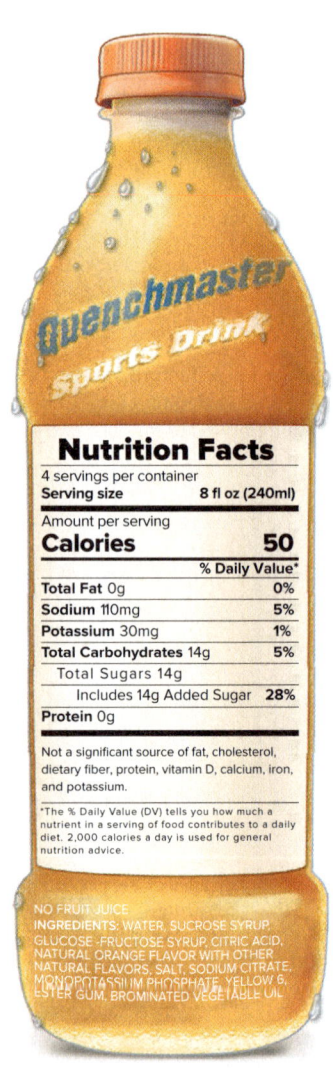

FIGURE 10-12 Most sports drinks for fluid and electrolyte replacement typically contain added sugars plus sodium and potassium. The various sugars in this product total 14 grams of carbohydrates per cup (240 mL) serving. Sports drinks typically contain about 6% to 8% sugar. Drinks with a sugar content above 8% to 10%, such as soft drinks or fruit juices, may cause gastrointestinal distress, may fail to empty from the stomach rapidly, and are not recommended for fluid repletion during sport.

Sports Drinks. For sports that require less than 60 minutes of continuous exertion, the primary concern is replacing the water lost in sweat. When continuous exercise extends beyond 60 minutes, electrolyte (especially sodium) and carbohydrate replacement becomes increasingly important.

Use of sports drinks (Fig. 10-12) during long bouts of continuous exercise—especially in hot weather—offers several advantages for athletes:

- *Water* increases blood volume to allow for efficient cooling and transport of fuels and waste products to and from cells.
- *Carbohydrates* supply glucose to muscles as they become depleted of glycogen and also add flavor, which encourages athletes to drink.
- *Electrolytes* in sports drinks help to maintain blood volume, enhance the absorption of water and carbohydrate from the intestine, and stimulate thirst.

TABLE 10-5 ■ Caffeine, Calorie, and Sugar Content of Popular Energy Drinks

Energy Drink	Serving	Caffeine (mg)	Energy (kcal)	Sugars (g)
Bang Energy®	16 fl oz	300	0	0
Monster Energy®	16 fl oz	164	233	54
Monster Ultra®	16 fl oz	144	24	7
Red Bull®	8.4 fl oz	75	112	27
Red Bull Sugar Free®	8.4 fl oz	76	13	0

Source: USDA FoodData Central.

Overall, the decision to use a sports drink hinges primarily on the duration, type, and intensity of the activity. As the projected duration of continuous activity approaches 60 minutes or longer, the advantages of sports drinks over plain water emerge.[15] However, athletes should experiment with sports drinks during practice, instead of trying them for the first time during competition. Also, both athletes and nonathletes should recognize that sports drinks can be a source of excess added sugars and calories that may result in undesired weight gain.

Energy Drinks. The popularity of caffeine-containing energy drinks has surged in recent years. Some studies show that caffeine may improve athletic performance during endurance events (e.g., cycling) or sports that require a high level of mental alertness (e.g., archery). However, excessive caffeine consumption can lead to shakiness, nervousness, anxiety, nausea, irregular heart rate, elevated blood pressure, and insomnia. Chronic intakes of energy drinks can lead to fatigue and headaches. The high added-sugar content in energy drinks also can lead to weight gain. In addition, the diuretic effect of caffeine may not support optimal hydration, particularly for athletes who are not accustomed to caffeine. Compare the caffeine and calorie contents of several top-selling energy drinks in Table 10-5.

Alcohol. Excessive alcohol consumption, consistent with binge drinking patterns, is observed among some athletes, particularly in team sports. Besides the nonnutritive calorie load of alcohol (7 kcal/g), alcohol has negative effects on performance and recovery from physical activity. A solid body of evidence cautions against consumption of alcohol before, during, or after physical activities.

Heat-Related Illness. As environmental temperature rises above 95°F (35°C), virtually all body heat is lost through the evaporation of sweat from the skin. As humidity rises, especially above 75%, evaporation slows and sweating is insufficient to cool the body. The result is rapid fatigue, increased work for the heart, and difficulty with prolonged exertion. Heat-related injuries—heat exhaustion, heat cramps, and heatstroke—can be deadly (Fig. 10-13). To decrease the risk of developing heat-related injuries, watch for rapid body-weight changes (2% or more of body weight), replace lost fluids, and avoid exercising under extremely hot, humid conditions.

Water Intoxication. It is also possible for some athletes to drink so much water that they develop water intoxication. Dilution of the electrolytes in the blood (i.e., hyponatremia) causes cardiovascular and neurological problems and can lead to death. Symptoms of hyponatremia include bloating, puffiness, weight gain, nausea, vomiting, headache, confusion, delirium, seizures, respiratory distress, loss of consciousness, and possibly death.

FIGURE 10-13 Heat-related illness chart showing symptoms and recommended actions. Warning Signs and Symptoms of Heat-Related Illness, CDC.

HEAT-RELATED ILLNESSES

WHAT TO LOOK FOR	WHAT TO DO
HEATSTROKE	
• High body temperature (103°F or higher) • Hot, red, dry, or damp skin • Fast, strong pulse • Headache • Dizziness • Nausea • Confusion • Losing consciousness (passing out)	• Call 911 right away—heatstroke is a medical emergency. • Move the person to a cooler place. • Help lower the person's temperature with cool cloths or a cool bath. • Do not give the person anything to drink.
HEAT EXHAUSTION	
• Heavy sweating • Cold, pale, and clammy skin • Fast, weak pulse • Nausea or vomiting • Muscle cramps • Tiredness or weakness • Dizziness • Headache • Fainting (passing out)	• Move to a cool place. • Loosen your clothes. • Put cool, wet cloths on your body or take a cool bath. • Sip water. **Get medical help right away if:** • You are throwing up. • Your symptoms get worse. • Your symptoms last longer than 1 hour.
HEAT CRAMPS	
• Heavy sweating during intense exercise • Muscle pain or spasms	• Stop physical activity and move to a cool place. • Drink water or a sports drink. • Wait for cramps to go away before you do any more physical activity. **Get medical help right away if:** • Cramps last longer than 1 hour. • You're on a low-sodium diet. • You have heart problems.
SUNBURN	
• Painful, red, and warm skin • Blisters on the skin	• Stay out of the sun until your sunburn heals. • Put cool cloths on sunburned areas or take a cool bath. • Put moisturizing lotion on sunburned areas. • Do not break blisters.
HEAT RASH	
• Red clusters of small blisters that look like pimples on the skin (usually on the neck, chest, or groin or in elbow creases)	• Stay in a cool, dry place. • Keep the rash dry. • Use powder (like baby powder) to soothe the rash.

✓ CONCEPT CHECK 10.4

1. What does it mean to *cut weight* before a competition? How might this affect physical performance?
2. Greta, a point guard on the women's basketball team, complains of chronic fatigue. Describe three nutritional concerns you would investigate.
3. During one day of preseason training for football, David loses 7 pounds as a result of sweat losses. How much fluid should he drink to rehydrate after practice?

10.5 Recommendations for Endurance, Strength, and Power Athletes

You have learned about ways in which nutrient needs can be universally affected by participation in sports. The definition of sports, however, is broad, and each individual is unique. Endurance athletes, who need to fuel activity that lasts several hours, should take a different approach to nutrition than strength and power athletes, who focus on gains in muscle mass. In this section, we present specific nutrition strategies for endurance, strength, and power athletes.

ENDURANCE ATHLETES: STRATEGIES TO DELAY OR PREVENT FATIGUE

The overarching goal for endurance athletes is to consume adequate carbohydrates and fluids. Before the event, endurance athletes should focus on maximizing muscle and liver glycogen stores, which will later be used to fuel muscles and maintain blood glucose. During an event, the goal is to prevent dehydration and glycogen depletion, as both of these conditions lead to fatigue and detract from physical performance. After an event, muscle glycogen stores need to be replenished, damaged muscle tissue must be repaired, and hydration should be restored.[10]

Maximize Glycogen Stores Before the Event. For athletes who compete in continuous, intense aerobic events lasting more than 60 to 90 minutes (or in shorter events taking place more than once within a 24-hour period), a regimen of **carbohydrate loading** can maximize the amount of energy stored in the form of muscle glycogen for the event. In one regimen, during the week prior to the event, the athlete gradually reduces the intensity and duration of exercise (*tapering*) while increasing the percentage of total calories supplied by carbohydrates. Shorter carbohydrate-loading regimens (e.g., 1 or 2 days before an event) may also be effective.

For example, consider the carbohydrate-loading schedule of a 25-year-old male preparing for a marathon. His typical calorie needs are about 3500 kcal per day. Six days before competition, he completes a final, hard workout of 60 minutes. On that day, carbohydrates contribute 45% to 50% of his total calorie intake. As he goes through the rest of the week, the duration of his workouts decreases to 40 minutes and then to about 20 minutes by the end of the week. Meanwhile, he increases the amount of carbohydrate in his eating plan to reach 70% to 80% of total calorie intake as the week continues (Table 10-6). Total calorie intake should decrease as exercise time decreases throughout the week. On the final day before competition, he rests while maintaining the high carbohydrate intake.

This carbohydrate-loading technique usually increases muscle glycogen stores by 50% to 90% over typical conditions (i.e., when dietary carbohydrate constitutes only about 50% of total calorie intake).[5] A potential disadvantage of carbohydrate loading is that additional water (about 3 grams) is incorporated into the muscles along with each gram of glycogen. This additional water weight and related muscle stiffness detract from their sports performance. Currently, expert advice is shifting away from such regimented carbohydrate loading in favor of supplying carbohydrates during the event (along with a consistent dietary pattern high in carbohydrate).

Even if an endurance athlete chooses not to practice a strict carbohydrate-loading regimen, a meal should be eaten 1 to 4 hours before an endurance event to top off muscle and liver glycogen stores, prevent hunger during the event, and provide extra

carbohydrate loading A process in which a high-carbohydrate diet is consumed for several days before an athletic event while tapering exercise duration in an attempt to increase muscle glycogen stores.

Carbohydrate Loading May Be Beneficial for These Activities
- Marathons
- Long-distance swimming
- Cross-country skiing
- 30-kilometer runs
- Triathlons
- Tournament-play basketball
- Cycling time trials

TABLE 10-6 ■ Sample Carbohydrate-Loading Regimen

Days Before Competition	6	5	4	3	2	1
Physical activity time (minutes)	60	40	40	20	20	Rest
Carbohydrate intake (grams)	450	450	450	600	600	600

TABLE 10-7 ■ High-Carbohydrate Pre-event Meals

Breakfast	
Cheerios®, ¾ cup	748 kcal
Reduced-fat milk, 1 cup	110 grams (59%) carbohydrate
Blueberry muffin, 1	
Orange juice, 4 ounces	
or	
Low-fat fruit yogurt, 1 cup	541 kcal
Plain bagel, ½	92 grams (68%) carbohydrate
Apple juice, 4 ounces	
Peanut butter (for bagel), 1 tbsp	
Lunch or Dinner	
Broiled chicken, 3 ounces	709 kcal
Rice, 1½ cups	116 grams (64%) carbohydrate
Steamed zucchini, 1 cup	
Low-fat chocolate milk, 1 cup	
Jello®, ½ cup	
or	
Spaghetti noodles, 2 cups	709 kcal
Spaghetti sauce, 1 cup	132 grams (66%) carbohydrate
Reduced-fat milk, 1½ cups	
Green beans, 1 cup	

With regard to the timing of pre-activity meals, a general guide is to allow 4 hours for a big meal (about 1200 kcal), 3 hours for a moderate meal (about 800 to 900 kcal), 2 hours for a light meal (about 400 to 600 kcal), and an hour or less for a snack (about 300 kcal).

fluid. A pre-event meal should consist primarily of carbohydrate, contain moderate fat or fiber, and include high-quality protein (Table 10-7). The longer the period before an event, the larger the meal can be because there will be more time available for digestion.

Carbohydrate-rich food choices for a pre-event meal include spaghetti, muffins, bagels, pancakes with fresh fruit topping, oatmeal with fruit, a baked potato topped with a small amount of low-fat cheese, toasted bread with jam, bananas, or low-sugar breakfast cereals with reduced-fat milk. Avoid fatty or fried foods such as sausage, bacon, sauces, and gravies. Athletes should experiment with the size, timing, and composition of pre-event meals during training to determine what is best tolerated.

Fat Adaptation. An alternative approach in training, known as fat adaptation, is becoming more popular among endurance athletes. Of all the energy-yielding nutrients, carbohydrates are utilized most rapidly to fuel exercising muscles. When athletes are following a high-carbohydrate dietary pattern or practice carbohydrate loading before an endurance event, they ensure that muscle and liver glycogen will be available to muscles throughout the race. Even after carbohydrate loading, however, the total amount of energy available from muscle glycogen is limited to approximately 2050 kcal.[4]

In comparison, the supply of energy from triglycerides stored in the muscle and adipose tissue is virtually limitless (about 72,500 kcal). Recall that, depending on intensity, about half of the energy for endurance events comes from fat. The metabolism of fat for energy occurs more slowly, but it provides more than twice as many calories per gram as carbohydrates or protein.

With fat adaptation, rather than following a traditional high-carbohydrate dietary pattern (about 65% of calories from carbohydrates and about 20% from fat) during the days leading up to an event, endurance athletes replace much of the carbohydrates with fat. For example, a high-fat training eating plan might consist of just 25% of calories from carbohydrate with 60% to 70% of calories from fat. The rationale is that high-carbohydrate dietary patterns, especially those with many simple sugars and refined grains, boost insulin secretion, which inhibits the breakdown of fat. By lowering carbohydrates and increasing the fat content of the diet, the cells will adapt to greater use of fat for fuel. If the athlete uses more fat for fuel during an endurance event, muscle glycogen might be spared so that those stored carbohydrates would be available for a burst of speed at the end of the race.

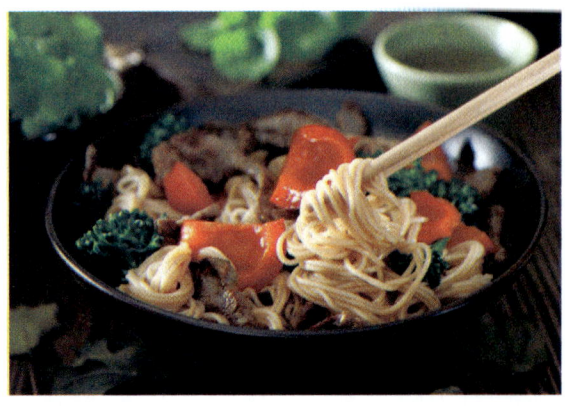

Pre-event meals may require a higher proportion of grains than suggested by MyPlate to boost carbohydrate content. Choose starchy vegetables and grain-based snacks to help top off glycogen stores. Cobraphotography/Shutterstock

Research comparing the effects of high-carbohydrate or high-fat training diets on athletic performance has yielded mixed results. One possible explanation is that the muscles of fat-adapted athletes are able to break down more fat for fuel during physical activity at low or moderate intensities, but the low carbohydrate intake depletes glycogen stores, so higher-intensity activity is impaired. More information can be found at https://www.sportsdietitians.com.au.

At this time, there is not enough consistent evidence to support a recommendation for high-fat diets for athletes. Although high-fat diets can lead to more fat oxidation and lower rates of muscle glycogen utilization, no improvements in overall performance are reported. Current evidence does support a performance-enhancing effect of carbohydrate ingestion before and during physical activity. To avoid compromising training performance, athletes exercising at a moderate to high intensity or engaging in competition should include quality carbohydrates in their dietary pattern that matches their training and body composition goals.

Replenish Fuel During the Event. For continuous sporting events longer than 60 minutes, consumption of carbohydrates and electrolytes, along with adequate fluids, during activity can improve athletic performance. Prolonged exercise depletes muscle glycogen stores and may transiently lower blood glucose, leading to physical and mental fatigue. One way to avoid *hitting the wall* is to maintain normal blood glucose concentrations by carbohydrate feedings during the activity.

A general guideline for endurance events is to consume 30 to 60 grams of carbohydrate per hour. A trend in sports nutrition is to use multiple sources of carbohydrates (e.g., glucose, fructose, and maltodextrin) with different routes and rates of absorption to maximize the supply of glucose to cells and lessen the risk of gastrointestinal distress.[5]

Compared to carbohydrates, fat is more slowly digested, absorbed, and metabolized. Thus, although fat serves as fuel during prolonged aerobic activity, consumption of fat during activity is unlikely to improve athletic performance and is likely to cause gastrointestinal distress.

Sports drinks are a good source of carbohydrate calories during continuous endurance events lasting over 60 minutes. Sports drinks usually contain about 14 grams of carbohydrate per 8-ounce serving. They supply the necessary fluid, electrolytes, and carbohydrates to keep athletes performing at their best in endurance or ultra-endurance events.

As an alternative to sports drinks, carbohydrate gels or chews are formulated with one or more sugars or starches to rapidly supply about 25 grams of carbohydrate per serving (Table 10-8). In addition, they provide electrolytes to replenish those lost in sweat. Some of these products also may contain certain amino acids, vitamins, caffeine, or herbal ingredients. An advantage of gels compared to energy bars or sports drinks is they are convenient to carry.

Popular energy bars typically provide about 180 to 250 kcal and anywhere from 2 to 45 grams of carbohydrate. If a bar is chosen, look for one with about 40 grams of carbohydrate and no more than 10 grams of protein, 4 grams of fat, and 5 grams of fiber.

TABLE 10-8 ■ Energy and Macronutrient Content of Popular Energy Bars, Gels, and Chews

	Serving (oz)	Energy (kcal)	Carb (g)	Fiber (g)	Protein (g)	Fat (g)
Energy Bars						
Atkins® (chocolate coconut)	1.41	170	19	9	4	12
Clif® Bar (crunchy peanut butter)	2.4	260	40	4	11	7
KIND® (dark chocolate cherry cashew)	1.41	160	22	6	4	10
Luna® (lemon zest)	1.69	190	28	3	8	6
Larabar® (banana bread)	1.59	200	24	4	5	10
Gels & Chews						
Clif® Shot (vanilla)	1.1	100	25	0	0	0
GU™ Energy Gel (lemon sublime)	1.1	100	23	0	0	0
Huma Chia Energy Gel® (strawberry)	1.52	100	22	2	1	0.5
PowerBar® Gel (strawberry banana)	1.44	110	27	0	0	0

Overall, choosing energy bars is preferable to choosing candy bars and packaged desserts. An additional concern is that micronutrient toxicity (e.g., vitamin A) might occur if numerous bars are eaten in a day, as many are highly fortified.

Source: Nutrition bars: healthy or hype? Nourish by WebMD. 2002. https://www.webmd.com/diet/features/nutrition-bars-healthy-hype#3

The bars are fortified with vitamins and minerals in amounts ranging from about 50% to 100% of the RDA. Outside of sporting events, some people use energy bars as a quick and convenient meal or snack. Keep in mind that energy bars contain a concentrated source of calories. Whole foods are always preferred for snacking.

Check the label on all of these products to gauge the amount of gel or bar that provides 30 to 60 grams of carbohydrate per hour. In addition, remember that any carbohydrate-containing food must be accompanied by fluid to ensure adequate hydration. At a minimum, one serving of any of these products will cost at least $1, and some brands with all natural or organic ingredients cost as much as $5. Are sports drinks, energy bars, and gels worth the price? Critics suggest that these products are essentially the nutritional equivalent of a cup of low-fat yogurt and a piece of fruit (Table 10-8). For an athlete on a tight budget, a small bag of graham crackers or jelly beans could just as easily provide a quick shot of glucose during a race. With a little bit of time and an Internet connection, you can even find recipes to make your own sports drinks and energy bars at home for a fraction of the cost of name-brand products.

Replenish Glycogen and Fluid After Physical Activity. After prolonged aerobic activities, muscle and liver glycogen stores will be depleted. To rapidly restore glycogen stores, carbohydrate-rich foods providing approximately 1.0 to 1.2 grams of carbohydrate per kilogram of body weight should be consumed shortly after continuous (endurance) physical activity. Immediately after exercise is when glycogen synthesis is greatest because the muscles are insulin-sensitive at this point. Foods such as fruit, fruit juice, bread, or a sports drink contribute to rapid restoration of glycogen stores.

Although carbohydrate intake is the most important factor for replenishing glycogen after endurance activities, adding an appropriate amount of high-quality protein during recovery can be helpful for stimulating glucose uptake and repairing damaged muscle tissue. The current recommendation for protein after endurance exercise is 0.25 to 0.3 gram of protein per kilogram of body weight.

Fluid and electrolyte (i.e., sodium and potassium) intake is another essential component of recovery for an endurance athlete, especially if two workouts a day are performed or if the environment is hot and humid. Specialized recovery drinks containing carbohydrates, amino acids, and electrolytes are available, but if food and fluid intake is sufficient to restore weight loss, it generally will also supply enough electrolytes to meet needs during recovery from endurance activities.

STRENGTH AND POWER ATHLETES: STRATEGIES TO ENHANCE MUSCLE GAIN

Strength training—improving the maximal force that can be exerted by the muscle—should be part of any well-rounded physical activity program. Resistance training may utilize free weights, specialized weight machines, or one's own body weight. As previously mentioned, a workout typically includes 8 to 12 different muscle-strengthening activities that target all the major muscle groups of the body. Most of the people you see lifting weights in the gym are probably performing several sets of 8 to 12 repetitions each, lifting about 50% of the maximum weight they could lift (1 repetition maximum [RM]). This type of workout improves muscular endurance, which is an important part of muscular fitness for overall health. However, to truly build muscular strength, athletes need to work against greater resistance (around 80% of 1 RM) over fewer repetitions. For a few athletes, such as those who participate in weight-lifting or body-building competitions, muscular strength is the focus of training.

Muscular power combines strength with speed, improving the ability to apply force quickly. Examples of power sports include middle-distance running, gridiron football, rowing, and swimming. In reality, many sports and everyday activities involve muscular power: jumping for a rebound in basketball, delivering a roundhouse kick to an opponent in martial arts, or driving the ball down the fairway in a round of golf are examples of muscular power in sports.

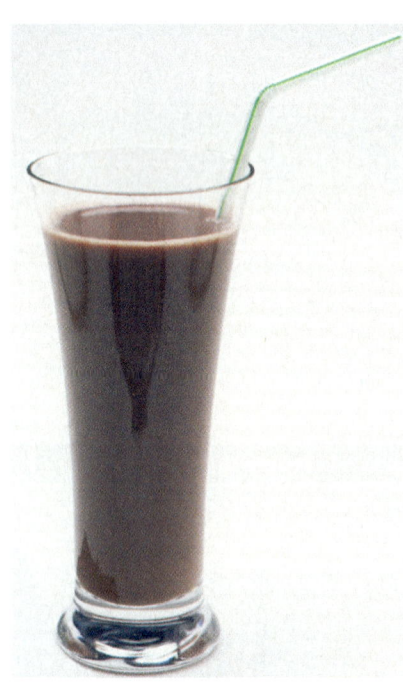

Low-fat chocolate milk is the go-to recovery drink for many athletes. This 1-cup serving of low-fat chocolate milk is a tasty vehicle for 25 grams of carbohydrate and 9 grams of protein. Pixtal/SuperStock

For strength and power athletes, calorie needs will be higher due to the additional lean mass and high-volume training routines of these athletes. Recall that the primary types of fuel for strength and power moves are phosphocreatine (PCr) and carbohydrates for the brief bursts of activity, with fat providing energy during the resting stages. Although very little protein is used as fuel during resistance activities, there will be some extra emphasis on protein intake in the recovery phase.[5] Low-fat chocolate milk is a great option to replenish the body!

Strength and power athletes tend to be extremely focused on consuming adequate protein to support muscle protein synthesis. Strength-training athletes in the early phases of training do have the highest estimated protein needs of any athletes. Once desired muscle mass has been achieved, however, protein requirements for maintenance of muscular strength decrease slightly. Meeting these recommendations for protein intake optimizes muscle protein synthesis, but consuming more than the recommended range of protein intake does not appear to offer advantage and could be detrimental. Recall that excess amino acids are used as fuel or stored as fat; they do not directly translate into increased muscular strength.

Before and During Strength and Power Training, Focus on Calories, Carbohydrates, and Fluids. Adequate hydration supports optimal athletic performance; strength and power athletes are no exception. Checking the urine color or urine specific gravity is a good indication of fluid status. If an athlete is poorly hydrated before an event, water or a sports drink should be sufficient to restore hydration.

Similar to nutrition strategies for endurance athletes, adequate carbohydrate ingestion in the days leading up to and hours immediately before physical activity has been shown to enhance performance for strength and power events, too. Athletes who perform many repetitions with moderate resistance will use more of their muscle glycogen stores than athletes who perform fewer repetitions with high resistance. Overall, research has shown that consuming approximately 4 to 7 grams of carbohydrates per kilogram of body weight per day is appropriate for strength and power training. The optimal rate of carbohydrate ingestion before and during resistance activities has not yet been established, but some research indicates that 1 to 4 grams of carbohydrate per kilogram of body weight in a pre-event meal or beverage will enhance work capacity during resistance workouts.

In strength and power sports, many athletes also use creatine supplements to increase levels of phosphocreatine in muscles. Recall that phosphocreatine is used to resupply ATP during short, intense bursts of activity. When phosphocreatine stores are increased, muscle glycogen may be preserved.[5]

Focus on achieving adequate hydration and maximizing muscle glycogen before activities because there may not be an opportunity to replenish fluids and carbohydrates during strength or power competitions. During extended training sessions, however, supplying fluids and carbohydrates will enhance both physical and mental performance.

While a few experts advocate ingesting protein before or during a resistance workout in an effort to promote muscle protein synthesis, the bulk of evidence points to emphasizing protein during the recovery period for optimal performance.

For athletes (and adults in general), fat intake should fall into the range of 20% to 35% of overall calorie intake. If fat intake is above 35% of total calories, replacing the excess fat with carbohydrates would have a favorable effect on protein balance. This is because insulin, secreted in response to glucose in the blood, triggers uptake of amino acids by cells, which provides materials for protein synthesis within the cells.

After Strength and Power Activities, Consuming Carbohydrates and Protein Promotes Recovery. Those first few hours after resistance training, according to many researchers, are the best time to provide carbohydrates and protein to replenish muscle glycogen and promote muscle repair and synthesis. Right after exercise, the cells are insulin sensitive, so they rapidly take up glucose from the blood and store it as

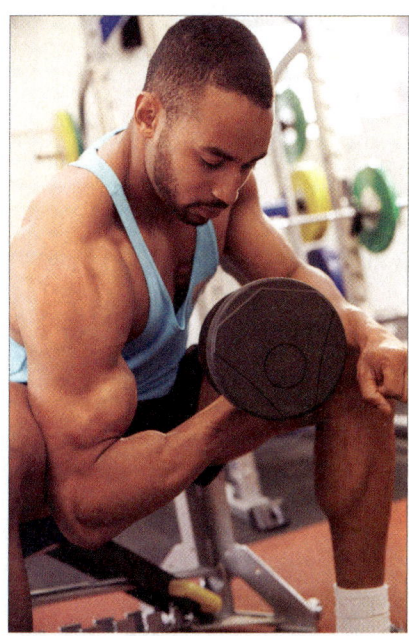

A special nutrition issue that concerns some strength-trained athletes is **body dysmorphic disorder.** In this disorder, individuals see themselves as being too thin, even though they are more muscular than average. People who have dysmorphia may practice disordered eating behaviors or use steroids to achieve high levels of muscularity. Shutterstock

body dysmorphic disorder (BDD) A psychiatric condition defined as a preoccupation with a perceived defect or flaw in one's physical appearance that is either not noticeable or only slightly observable by others; formally known as *dysmorphophobia*.

Many power athletes utilize a training technique called **periodization,** in which physical stresses on the body change throughout the year:

- Early in the training season, athletes work on building aerobic endurance.
- After gains in aerobic capacity have been achieved, the focus shifts to building strength, power, and sport-specific skills.
- During the competitive season, daily workouts are scaled back, but activity is intense and of long duration on game days.
- In the off-season, athletes continue to work out to stay in shape, but the volume is certainly lower than it was in season.

Athletes taking part in periodized training will use the full spectrum of energy systems we have discussed. Nutrition recommendations should also be periodized to match such dynamic training plans.[9]

periodization Cycling the volume, intensity, and activities of workouts throughout the training season.

glycogen. To promote muscle protein synthesis along with glycogen restoration, many experts recommend intakes at the upper end of the range (e.g., 1.2 to 1.5 grams of carbohydrates per kilogram of body weight) shortly after training.[5] The presence of certain amino acids further stimulates insulin secretion to enhance the uptake of glucose and synthesis of glycogen.

To promote gains in muscle mass, many experts recommend 0.25 to 0.30 gram of high-quality protein per kilogram of body weight within the first 1 or 2 hours after exercise to maximize protein synthesis.[10] Novice strength-training athletes who are seeking to gain muscle mass have the highest requirements for protein. With advanced training, the rate of protein turnover during exercise decreases. Therefore, well-trained strength athletes require less protein to repair and maintain muscles than their untrained counterparts. Some amino acids (e.g., leucine) may stimulate the metabolic pathways that lead to synthesis of muscle protein. The process of muscle protein synthesis not only requires amino acids as building blocks, of course, but also depends on carbohydrate as a source of energy.

Overall, recovery from resistance training requires a combination (approximately 3:1 ratio) of carbohydrates and high-quality protein. For a 154-pound (70 kg) athlete, this corresponds to about 70 grams of carbohydrate and 23 grams of protein in each 2-hour interval. Table 10-9 provides several options for recovery meals for athletes.

TAILORED SPORTS NUTRITION

Nutritional strategies have the potential to optimize athletic performance. Here, we have presented several generalized guidelines to plan nutritionally adequate dietary patterns that optimize energy stores, ensure hydration, and give athletes a competitive edge. We have stressed the importance of a food-first philosophy for carbohydrates and fluids pre-event, within-event, and between-events activity, as well as protein for muscle recovery. Above all, recognize that each athlete is unique. Remember that genetics can impact nutrition requirements. Each type of activity demands its own set of energy sources. Sports vary in training regimens, duration, and opportunities to acquire nourishment before, during, and between events. Even within a particular sport, each player's position has its own physical demands, which can alter nutritional needs.[13] Finally, personal taste preferences and gastrointestinal tolerance will dictate adherence to any nutrition plan. As you pursue your own physical activity pattern, start with your solid foundation of knowledge about nutrient needs, but be attentive to your concerns, be adaptable, and always continue to learn.

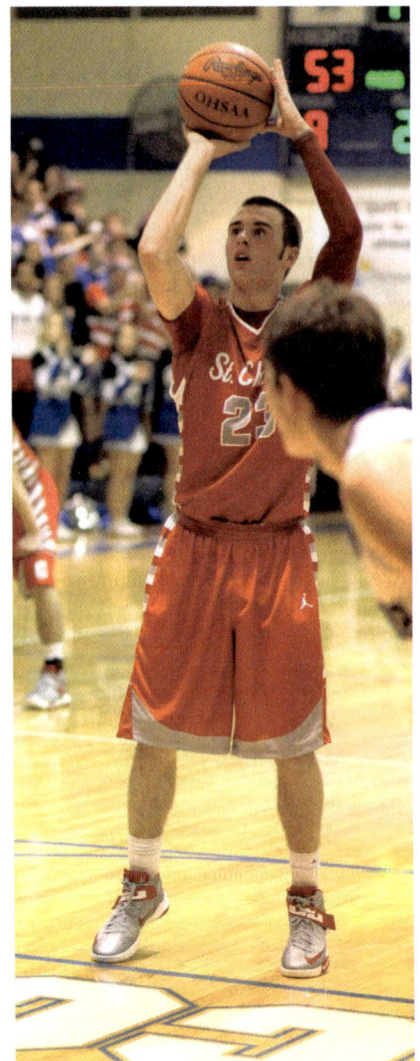

Athletes are subject to all the same nutritional challenges as the general public: overreliance on convenience foods, abundance of nutrition misinformation, temptations to eat out of boredom or for emotional comfort.

Furthermore, they must adapt to the seasonal demands of their sport and maintain exhausting training and travel schedules. *George Postalakis*

TABLE 10-9 ■ Sample Recovery Meals

Option 1: 491 kcal, 69 grams carbohydrate, 31 grams protein, 10 grams fat
  Bagel, 1 regular
  Deli turkey, 1 ounce
  Mozzarella cheese, 1 ounce
  Low-fat milk, 1 cup

Option 2: 571 kcal, 81 grams carbohydrate, 38 grams protein, 12 grams fat
  Low-fat flavored Greek yogurt, 16 ounces
  Banana, 1 medium

Option 3: (plant-based): 289 kcal, 52 grams carbohydrate, 13 grams protein, 4 grams fat
  Chickpeas, ½ cup
  Quinoa, ½ cup
  Tomatoes, ⅔ cup canned

CASE STUDY: Planning a Training Diet

Michael is a 6-foot, 185-pound male who is training for a 10K run coming up in 3 weeks. He has read a lot about sports nutrition and especially about the importance of eating more carbohydrates while in training. He also has been struggling to keep his weight in a range that he feels contributes to better speed and endurance. Consequently, he is also trying to eat as little fat as possible. Unfortunately, over the past week, his workouts in the afternoon have not met his expectations. His run times are slower, and he shows signs of fatigue after just 20 minutes into his training program.

His breakfast yesterday was a large bagel with cream cheese and orange juice. For lunch, he had a small salad with fat-free dressing, a large plate of pasta with marinara sauce and broccoli, and a diet soft drink. For dinner, he had a small broiled chicken breast, a cup of rice, some carrots, and iced tea. Later, he snacked on fat-free pretzels.

1. Is a high-carbohydrate dietary pattern a good idea during Michael's training?
2. Are there any important components missing in Michael's dietary pattern and could they be contributing to his fatigue?
3. Describe some changes that should be made in Michael's eating pattern, including specific foods that should be emphasized.
4. How should fluid needs be met during Michael's workouts?
5. Should Michael focus on fueling his body before, during, or after workouts?

Complete the Case Study. Responses to these questions can be provided by your instructor.

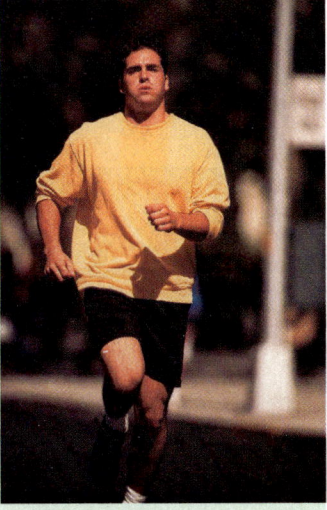

Michael, a senior studying engineering, is wise to seek nutrition advice in preparing for his first 10K. Comstock/Getty Images

✓ CONCEPT CHECK 10.5

1. Which nutrient(s) should be emphasized in a pre-event meal for an endurance athlete? Provide an example of a suitable pre-event meal for a long-distance cyclist.
2. What is carbohydrate loading? List three sports for which carbohydrate loading could enhance performance.
3. Why is a combination of carbohydrate and protein recommended for recovery after resistance training? Suggest a suitable recovery meal.

10.6 Nutrition and Your Health: Ergogenic Aids and Athletic Performance

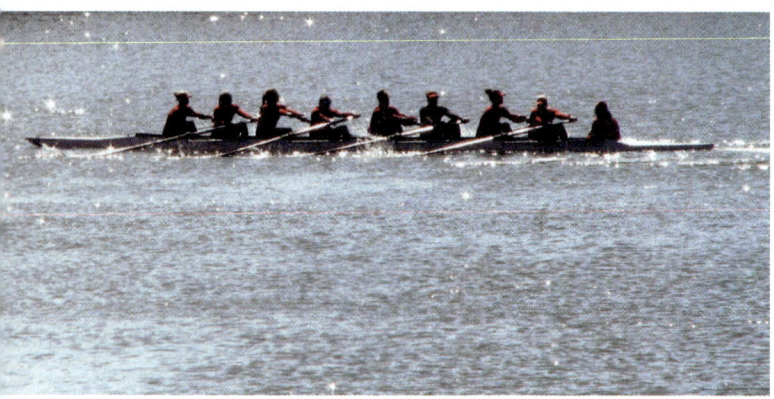

Elite athletes should be encouraged to gain the competitive edge with proper rest, fluids, stress reduction, and healthy dietary patterns versus opting for ergogenic aids and unnecessary supplementation. Colleen Spees

Extreme diet manipulation to improve athletic performance is not a recent innovation. Today's athletes are as likely as their predecessors to experiment with any substance that promises a competitive advantage. The U.S. sports nutrition supplement market now exceeds $11 billion, accounting for more than 35% of the global market. Caffeine, creatine, nitrate/beetroot juice, beta-alanine, and bicarbonate are just some of the substances used by athletes in hopes of gaining an ergogenic edge.[16]

Based on what is known, today's athletes can benefit from scientific evidence documenting the ergogenic properties of a few dietary substances. These ergogenic aids include sufficient water and electrolytes, adequate carbohydrates, and a balanced and varied dietary pattern consistent with MyPlate. Protein and amino acid supplements are often not needed as the vast majority of athletes can easily meet their protein needs from a food-first approach. In general, nutrient supplements should only be used to meet a specific dietary shortcoming, such as an inadequate iron intake. Beyond the proven benefits of the nutrition strategies presented in this chapter, Table 10-10 provides a list of well-studied ergogenic aids.

Dietary supplements rumored to enhance athletic performance require careful evaluation and monitoring. Overall, there is little scientific evidence to support the efficacy of many substances that are touted as performance-enhancing aids. Of these, many are useless, and some are dangerous enough to promote organ damage (Table 10-11). The liver and kidneys are particularly susceptible to damage because these organs help detoxify harmful compounds.[17] Athletes should be skeptical of any substance until its ergogenic effect is scientifically validated. The Food and Drug Administration (FDA) has a limited ability to regulate these dietary supplements, and the manufacturing processes for dietary supplements are not as tightly regulated by the FDA as they are for prescription drugs.

National Collegiate Athletic Association (NCAA) and Nutrition Supplements

The NCAA has developed lists of permissible and nonpermissible nutritional supplements for athletic departments to provide to student athletes. The NCAA has issued a warning advising students to discuss their use of *any* dietary supplement with their team medical staff to avoid unknowingly ingesting banned substances. Following are a few key examples:

Select Permissible Nutritional Supplements
- Carbohydrate boosters
- Electrolyte/carbohydrate replacement drinks
- Energy bars
- Vitamins and minerals

Select Nonpermissible Drug Classes
- Alcohol and beta blockers (rifle only)
- Anabolic agents
- Beta-2 agonists
- Cannabinoids
- Diuretics and masking agents
- Growth factor, related substances, and mimetics
- Hormone and metabolic modulators (anti-estrogens)
- Narcotics
- Peptide hormones
- Stimulants

For a complete explanation of the NCAA's rules regarding dietary supplements, see www.ncaa.org.

Sports Food
- *Electrolyte supplements* may be used for rehydration or hydration by replacing electrolytes lost in sweat.
- *Liquid meals* may provide a quick and convenient source of carbohydrate, protein, and nutrients when eating whole food is not practical.
- *Protein supplements* may provide a quick and convenient source of easily digested, high-quality protein.
- *Sports drinks* may be used for hydration and fueling strategies for longer or high-quality training sessions or longer races.
- *Sports gels/confectionery* may be used for fueling strategies during longer training sessions and races.

Source: International Association of Athletics Federations Consensus Statement 2019: Nutrition for Athletics.

TABLE 10-10 ■ Commonly Used Supplements for Athletes

Substance	Purported Benefits	Potential Risks
Antioxidants	Decreased levels of free radicals	Increased risk of cancers for certain supplements, nutrient-specific toxicities
Beta-alanine	Increased muscle carnosine, a protein that neutralizes acidic compounds that contribute to muscle fatigue during high-intensity activity	Flushing and feelings of "pins and needles"
Beta-hydroxy beta-methylbutyric acid (HMB)	Decreased muscle damage; speeds up recovery from intense physical activity	Itching, abdominal pain, and constipation
Branched-chain amino acids (BCAA)	Increased energy delivered to muscles during activity to increase muscle size and strength	Increased levels of ammonia in the blood, fatigue, loss of motor coordination, digestive discomfort, nausea, vomiting, and diarrhea
Caffeine	Increased vigilance and mental alertness; improved endurance; reduced perception of fatigue; enhanced lipolysis and fat oxidation	High doses may cause insomnia, nervousness, restlessness, digestive discomfort, nausea, vomiting, rapid heart rate, increased respirations, tremors, delirium, convulsions, and increased urination
Calcium	Maintains strength of bones and teeth	High doses may cause digestive discomfort, kidney stones, and heart problems
Collagen/Gelatin	Alleviate joint pain	Digestive discomfort, constipation, anorexia, and skin itching
Creatine	Increased lean mass; improved short-term performance; aid in muscle recovery; delay in muscle fatigue	Possible heat intolerance, fever, dehydration, reduced blood volume, electrolyte imbalances, digestive discomfort, and muscle cramping
Curcumin/Turmeric	Muscle repair, decreased soreness, and decreased inflammation	Digestive discomfort, constipation, indigestion, diarrhea, abdominal distension, acid reflux, nausea, and vomiting
Fish oil	Decreased muscle soreness	Fish burps, heartburn, acid reflux, nausea, diarrhea, and skin rash
Iron	Overcome deficiency that can lead to fatigue and irritability	High doses can cause digestive discomfort, nausea, vomiting, constipation, and diarrhea
Magnesium	Support testosterone production	Digestive discomfort, nausea, vomiting, and diarrhea
Nitric oxide boosters (arginine, beetroot juice, citrulline)	Improved blood flow to muscles and enhanced performance by improving oxygen consumption to deliver nutrients to muscles	Drop in blood pressure, dizziness, lightheadedness, and loss of balance
Probiotics	Improved gut health with mental and physical benefits	Digestive discomfort, rash, itching; infections in certain high-risk individuals
Protein powder	Provide necessary protein in absence of whole foods, increased lean mass production	High doses can cause nausea, thirst, bloating, cramps, diarrhea, reduced appetite, and fatigue; overreliance on supplements over food can increase potential for poor intakes of other key nutrients
Ketones	Support fat burning	Shakiness and abnormal heartbeat
Sodium bicarbonate (baking soda)	Neutralize acidic compounds that contribute to muscle fatigue	Digestive discomfort, diarrhea, and vomiting
Tart cherry	Reduced stress on the body from heavy bouts of training	Digestive discomfort and diarrhea
Vitamin D	Increased skeletal muscle function, decreased recovery time, improved power, and support of testosterone production	High doses can cause toxicities, leading to weakness, fatigue, sleepiness, headaches, loss of appetite, dry mouth, metallic taste, digestive discomfort, weight loss, and seizures
Vitamins and minerals	Provide necessary nutrition in absence of a balanced diet	Potential for nutrient-specific toxicity and related side effects (e.g., nausea, vomiting, organ damage); overreliance on supplements over food can increase potential for poor intakes of other key nutrients

Sources: Adapted from Natural Medicines Comprehensive Database (http://naturaldatabase.therapeuticresearch.com) and Dietary Supplements for Exercise and Athletic Performance, National Institutes of Health, Office of Dietary Supplements (https://ods.od.nih.gov/factsheets/ExerciseAndAthleticPerformance-Consumer).

TABLE 10-11 ■ Dangerous, Banned, or Illegal Substances and Practices

Substance/Practice	Purported Use	Risks
Alcohol and beta blockers	Decrease anxiety and allow for muscle relaxation	Changes in blood sugar, symptoms of heart failure
Anabolic agents (e.g., testosterone)	Increase muscle mass and strength	Liver cysts; increased risk of heart disease, hypertension, reproductive dysfunction; depression, sleep disturbances, mood swings
Anti-estrogens (e.g., anastrozole)	Improved physique, reduced estrogen and maximized testosterone production, masked signs of anabolic steroid use	Weakness, headaches, sweating, stomach pain, nausea/vomiting, poor appetite, weight gain, joint/bone/muscle pain, mood changes, depression
Beta-2 agonists (e.g., bambuterol)	Increased muscle strength, power; improved lung function	Chest pain, dizziness, dry mouth, headache, changes in blood pressure, muscle cramps, rapid heartbeat
Blood doping	Enhanced aerobic capacity by increasing red blood cells	Blood thickening that strains heart
Diuretics and masking agents (e.g., furosemide)	Rapid weight loss and masked presence of other banned substances	Rapid depletion of electrolytes, fatigue, dizziness, or muscle cramps
Gene doping	Increased muscle mass, fat burning, and endurance	Fatal immune responses, blood thickening, death
Illicit drugs	Relaxation, stress relief, pain management	Increased heart rate, dizziness, slowed reaction time, overdose, death
Local anesthetics	Pain management and injury recovery	Delayed recovery, worsening of injuries, damage to muscle or tendons
Peptide hormones and analogues (e.g., growth hormone)	Increased muscle mass and fat metabolism	Uncontrolled growth of the heart and other internal organs; death
Stimulants (e.g., caffeine, ephedrine)	Increased muscle strength and power, promote mental alertness, weight loss	Heart palpitations, anxiety, and death

Source: NCAA Banned Drugs List (http://www.ncaa.org/2018-19-ncaa-banned-drugs-list)

Some supplements contain substances that will cause athletes to test positive for various banned substances. For instance, creatine is not a substance banned by the National Collegiate Athletic Association (NCAA) because it is classified as a nutritional supplement. However, positive drug tests have occurred with some creatine supplements because they may contain other nonpermissible substances banned by the NCAA. Studies consistently show that many supplements do not contain the substance and/or the amount listed on the label. Not only must athletes determine whether there is evidence that a dietary supplement is safe and effective, but they must also question if the dietary supplement contains what it is supposed to contain.

Even substances whose ergogenic effects have been supported by scientific evidence should be used with extreme caution, as the testing conditions may not match those of the intended use. Careful judgment should be exercised when it comes to using the appropriate dose of supplements or using multiple types of supplements concurrently.[18]

Rather than waiting for a magic bullet to enhance performance, athletes are advised to concentrate their efforts on improving their training routines and sport techniques while adhering to a well-balanced dietary pattern embracing whole foods as described in this chapter.

✓ CONCEPT CHECK 10.6

1. What are some risks associated with commonly used ergogenic aids?
2. Name two permissible and two nonpermissible ergogenic aids.

Summary (Numbers refer to numbered sections in the chapter)

10.1 A gradual increase in regular physical activity is recommended for all persons. Key benefits include improvements in cardiovascular health, gastrointestinal function, blood glucose regulation, mental health, quality of life, sleep patterns; reduced risk of cancers; enhanced muscle mass and bone strength.

10.2 The *Physical Activity Guidelines for Americans* advises adults to do 150 to 300 minutes of moderate-intensity or 75 to 150 minutes of vigorous-intensity aerobic physical activity per week. In addition, adults should perform muscle-strengthening activities and flexibility activities at least twice per week. Workouts should allow time for warm-up exercises to increase blood flow and warm the muscles and then end with cool-down exercises, including stretching. Ultimately, any movement is better than no movement.

10.3 Human metabolic pathways extract chemical energy from carbohydrate, fat, and protein to yield ATP. Phosphocreatine is a high-energy compound that can be used to resupply ATP during short, intense activities. The mix of macronutrients used for fuel depends on the intensity and duration of activity: short-term, intense activities primarily use carbohydrate for fuel, whereas low- or moderate-intensity endurance activities use more fat for fuel. Protein makes a minor contribution as a fuel source.

10.4 To support physical activity, athletes require 3.5 to 7 kcal per minute of activity above energy needs for a moderately active person. Monitoring weight changes over time is a good way to assess the adequacy of energy intake. Athletes should obtain energy from a varied dietary pattern that includes sources of carbohydrates (3 to 12 grams of carbohydrate per kilogram of body weight), protein (1.2 to 2.0 grams of protein per kilogram, depending on the type of training), and fat (up to 35% of energy, focusing on vegetable oils instead of solid fats). The increased overall food intake of athletes typically furnishes adequate vitamins and minerals. Some micronutrients of concern are iron and calcium, especially for females. Athletes should drink fluid before, during, and after physical activity (approximately 2 to 3 cups per pound lost). Sports drinks may help replace fluid, electrolytes, and carbohydrates lost during continuous workouts that last beyond 60 minutes.

10.5 Endurance athletes can delay or prevent fatigue by consuming enough fluids, electrolytes, and carbohydrates before, during, and after events. In addition, protein in the post-activity period will aid muscle recovery. In addition to these strategies to maintain hydration and muscle glycogen stores, athletes who train to develop strength or power should place special emphasis on protein during the recovery period.

10.6 Athletes can benefit from ergogenic properties of sufficient water, electrolytes, and carbohydrates, and a balanced and varied dietary pattern consistent with the *Dietary Guidelines* and MyPlate. Although some ergogenic aids may be useful for enhancing athletic performance, extreme caution should be practiced as many ergogenic aids are dangerous. Protein and amino acid supplements are not necessary because athletes almost always meet protein needs from whole foods.

Check Your Knowledge (Answers are available at the end of this question set)

1. An energy-rich compound, phosphocreatine (PCr), is found in _____ tissue.
   a. adipose
   b. muscle
   c. liver
   d. kidney

2. A physical activity program for healthy adults should include
   a. aerobic activities 5 days per week.
   b. strength-training activities 2 to 3 days per week.
   c. stretching exercises 2 to 3 days per week.
   d. all of these.

3. During a strength-training regimen, athletes should consume approximately _____ grams of protein per kilogram body weight.
   a. 0.5 to 0.7
   b. 0.8
   c. 1.2 to 2
   d. 2 to 2.5

4. Which of these foods is the best choice for carbohydrate loading before endurance events?
   a. Potato chips
   b. French fries
   c. High-fiber cereal
   d. Rice

5. As the body adapts to regular exercise, the *training effect* results in
   a. decreased blood flow to muscles.
   b. increased lactate production.
   c. decreased muscle triglyceride content.
   d. decreased resting heart rate.

6. A physically active lifestyle leads to
   a. increased bone strength.
   b. decreased risk of colon cancer.
   c. reduced anxiety and depression.
   d. all of these.

7. Approximately how many cups of fluid are required to replace each pound of weight lost during an athletic event or workout?
   a. 0.5 to 0.75 cup
   b. 1 to 1.5 cups
   c. 2 to 3 cups
   d. 4 to 5 cups

8. The benefit of a sports drink is to provide
   a. water to hydrate.
   b. electrolytes to enhance water absorption in the intestine and maintain blood volume.
   c. carbohydrate for energy.
   d. all of these.

9. Compared to anaerobic glucose metabolism, aerobic glucose metabolism produces more
   a. lactate.
   b. ATP.
   c. phosphocreatine.
   d. fatty acids.

10. Caffeine is used as an ergogenic aid by some athletes because it is thought to
    a. decrease fatigue.
    b. decrease lactate.
    c. serve as an energy source.
    d. increase muscle mass and strength.

Answer Key: 1. b (LO 10.3), 2. d (LO 10.2), 3. c (LO 10.6), 4. d (LO 10.8), 5. d (LO 10.5), 6. d (LO 10.1), 7. c (LO 10.7), 8. d (LO 10.7), 9. b (LO 10.7), 10. a (LO 10.9)

Study Questions (Numbers refer to Learning Outcomes)

1. How does greater physical fitness contribute to better overall health? **(LO 10.1)**

2. You have set a goal to increase muscle mass and decrease body fat. Plan a weekly fitness regimen using the FITT-VP principle. **(LO 10.2)**

3. How are carbohydrates, fat, and protein used to supply energy during a 100-meter sprint? During a weight-lifting session? During a 3-mile walk? **(LO 10.3)**

4. What is the difference between anaerobic and aerobic activities? Explain why aerobic metabolism is increased by a regular fitness routine. **(LO 10.4)**

5. Is fat from adipose tissue used as an energy source during physical activity? If so, when? **(LO 10.5)**

6. What are some typical measures used to assess whether an athlete's calorie intake is adequate? **(LO 10.6)**

7. List five nutrients of specific concern for athletes and the appropriate food sources from which these nutrients can be obtained. **(LO 10.6)**

8. Your neighbor is planning to run a 5-kilometer race. Summarize for her what you have learned about fluid intake before, during, and after the event. **(LO 10.7)**

9. You plan to participate in a half-marathon. What are general guidelines you should consider for macronutrients and fluids before, during, and after the event? **(LO 10.8)**

10. Should competitive athletes take amino acid supplements? Why or why not? **(LO 10.9)**

References

1. Centers for Disease Control and Prevention. *Active People, Healthy Nation: At a Glance.* Accessed November 2, 2023. Washington, DC. https://www.cdc.gov/physicalactivity/downloads/Active_People_Healthy_Nation_at-a-glance_082018_508.pdf

2. U.S. Department of Health & Human Services. *Physical Activity Guidelines for Americans.* 2nd ed. Washington, DC: U.S. Department of Health & Human Services; 2018. Accessed November 12, 2023. http://www.health.gov/paguidelines

3. Continuing education: courses approved by ACE. ACE Fitness. Accessed November 16, 2023. https://www.acefitness.org/continuing-education/ace-approved-courses/

4. Melzer K. Carbohydrate and fat utilization during rest and physical activity. *Clin Nutr ESPEN.* 2011 Apr;6(2):e45-e52. doi: 10.1016/j.eclnm.2011.01.005

5. Thomas DT, Erdman KA, Burke LM. Position of the Academy of Nutrition and Dietetics, Dietitians of Canada, and the American College of Sports Medicine: nutrition and athletic performance. *J Acad Nutr Diet.* 2016 Mar;116(3):501-528. doi: 10.1016/j.jand.2015.12.006

6. McDermott BP, Anderson SA, Armstrong LE, et al. National Athletic Trainers' Association position statement: fluid replacement for the physically active. *J Athl Train.* 2017 Sep;52(9):877-895. doi: 10.4085/1062-6050-52.9.02

7. National Collegiate Athletic Association (NCAA). *2019–20 and 2020–21 NCAA Wrestling Rules.* August 2019. Accessed November 10, 2023. http://www.ncaapublications.com/productdownloads/WR20.pdf

8. Daily JP, Stumbo JR. Female athlete triad. *Prim Care.* 2018 Dec;45(4):615-624. doi: 10.1016/j.pop.2018.07.004

9. U.S. Department of Agriculture; U.S. Department of Health & Human Services. *Dietary Guidelines for Americans, 2020–2025.* 9th ed. December 2020. https://DietaryGuidelines.gov

10. Antonio J, Ellerbroek A, Silver T, et al. A high protein diet (3.4 g/kg/d) combined with a heavy resistance training program improves body composition in healthy trained men and women—a follow-up investigation. *J Int Soc Sports Nutr.* 2015 Oct 20;12:39. doi: 10.1186/s12970-015-0100-0

11. Jäger R, Kerksick CM, Campbell BI, et al. International Society of Sports Nutrition position stand: protein and exercise. *J Int Soc Sports Nutr.* 2017 Jun 20;14:20. doi: 10.1186/s12970-017-0177-8

12. Patterson RE, Laughlin GA, LaCroix AZ, et al. Intermittent fasting and human metabolic health. *J Acad Nutr Diet.* 2015 Aug;115(8):1203-1212. doi: 10.1016/j.jand.2015.02.018

13. Loenneke JP, Loprinzi PD, Murphy CH, Phillips SM. Per meal dose and frequency of protein consumption is associated with lean mass and muscle performance. *Clin Nutr.* 2016 Dec;35(6):1506-1511. doi: 10.1016/j.clnu.2016.04.002

14. Iron fact sheet for health professionals. National Institutes of Health, Office of Dietary Supplements. Accessed November 10, 2023. https://ods.od.nih.gov/factsheets/Iron-HealthProfessional
15. Sawka MN, Burke LM, Eichner ER, Maughan RJ, Montain SJ, Stachenfeld NS; American College of Sports Medicine. American College of Sports Medicine position stand. Exercise and fluid replacement. *Med Sci Sports Exerc.* 2007 Feb;39(2):377-390. doi: 10.1249/mss.0b013e31802ca597
16. Ergogenic aids. U.S. Department of Agriculture, National Agricultural Library. Accessed November 10, 2023. https://www.nal.usda.gov/fnic/ergogenic-aids
17. Burke LM, Castell LM, Casa DJ, et al. International Association of Athletics Federations Consensus Statement 2019: nutrition for athletics. *Int J Sport Nutr Exerc Metab.* 2019 Mar 1;29(2):73-84. doi: 10.1123/ijsnem.2019-0065
18. Nutrition for athletes. U.S. Department of Agriculture, National Agricultural Library. Accessed November 2, 2023. https://www.nal.usda.gov/fnic/nutrition-athletes

Design Element Credits: Fact Check/magnifying glass icon: McGraw Hill; Magnificent Microbiome background image: Alena Ohneva/Shutterstock; Sustainable Solutions icon: McGraw Hill; Roots icon: McGraw Hill; Medicine Cabinet icon: Peter Dazeley/Photographer's Choice/Getty Images

Chapter 11: Eating Disorders

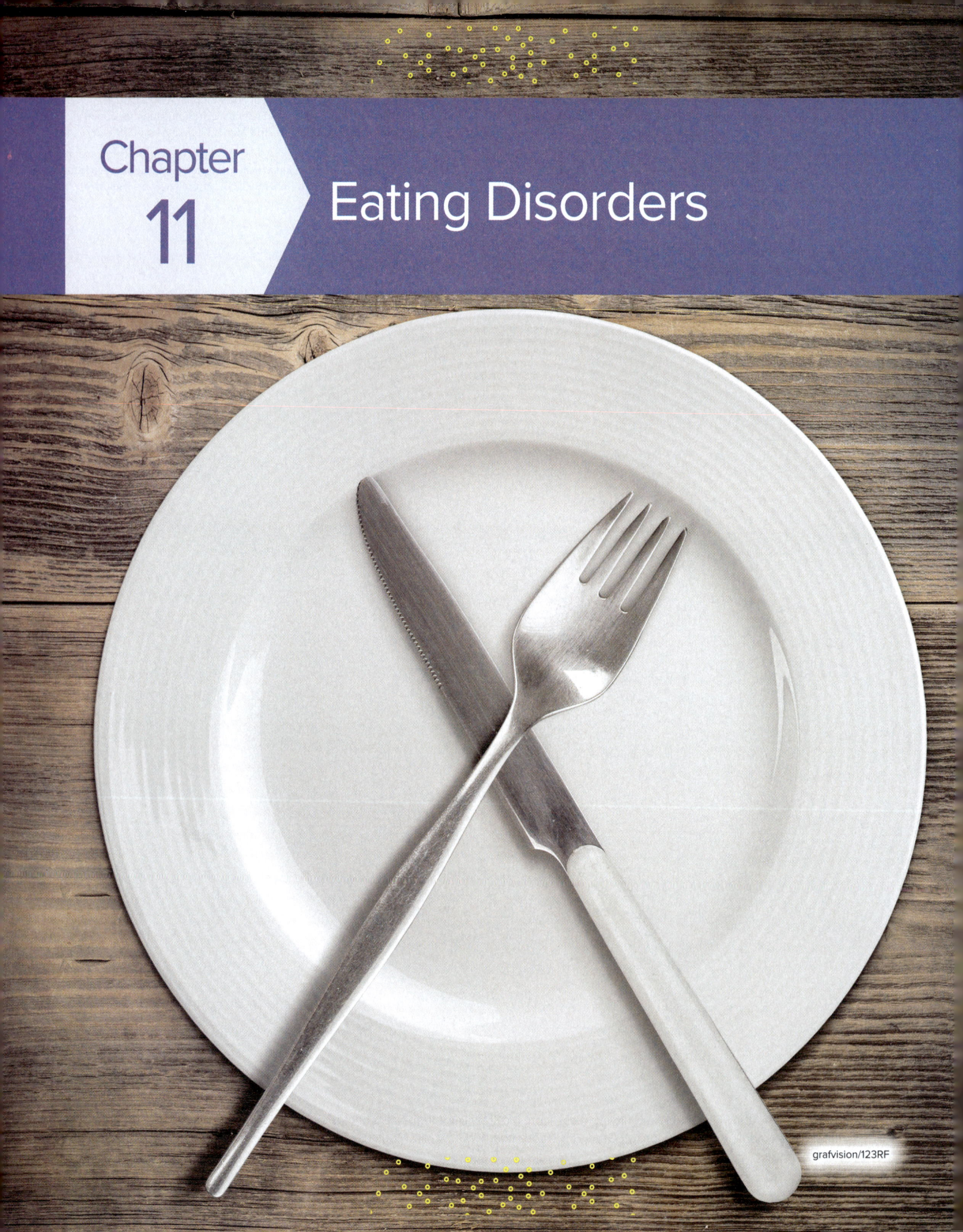

grafvision/123RF

Student Learning Outcomes

Chapter 11 is designed to allow you to:

11.1 Contrast healthy attitudes toward uses of food with behavior patterns that could lead to unhealthy uses of food.

11.2 Describe current hypotheses about the origins of eating disorders.

11.3 List physical and mental characteristics of anorexia nervosa, and outline current best practices for its treatment.

11.4 List physical and mental characteristics of bulimia nervosa, and outline current best practices for its treatment.

11.5 List physical and mental characteristics of binge eating disorder, and outline current best practices for its treatment.

11.6 Describe pica and other specified feeding and eating disorders.

11.7 Discuss other patterns of disordered eating that are seen in clinical practice, but are not formally diagnosed as eating disorders.

11.8 Describe strategies to reduce the development of eating disorders.

FACT CHECK

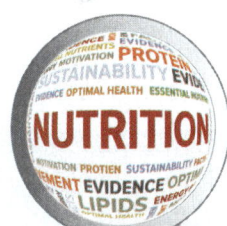

Do eating disorders only affect privileged white women?

In *Nine Truths about Eating Disorders,* The Academy of Eating Disorders promotes awareness that *eating disorders affect people of all genders, ages, races, ethnicities, body shapes and weights, sexual orientations, and socioeconomic statuses.*

Historically, research data indicated that white females were at the highest risk of eating disorders. Researchers proposed that white women were more likely to internalize the *thin ideal* and more likely to experience high levels of body dissatisfaction compared with individuals of other races, ethnicities, or genders. However, these findings may be related to a lack of research on eating disorders in males or minority populations or inequities in diagnosis or access to treatment.

Today's increased globalization and the wide reach of social media mean that diverse audiences are exposed to similar messages that equate thinness with beauty and success. Recent research indicates that the prevalence of eating disorders is similar across racial and ethnic groups. Recognition of eating disorders among males is increasing. Although sociocultural factors can influence individuals in diverse ways, eating disorders do not discriminate. See Section 11.1 for a deeper discussion of the changing face of eating disorders.

Source: Cheng ZH, Perko VL, Fuller-Marashi L, Gau JM, Stice E. Ethnic differences in eating disorder prevalence, risk factors, and predictive effects of risk factors among young women. *Eat Behav.* 2019 Jan;32:23-30. doi: 10.1016/j.eatbeh.2018.11.004

neurotransmitter A compound made by a nerve cell that allows for communication between it and other cells.

endorphins Natural body tranquilizers that function in pain reduction and may be involved in the feeding response.

disordered eating Mild and short-term changes in eating patterns that occur in relation to a stressful event, an illness, or a desire to modify one's dietary pattern for a variety of health and personal appearance reasons.

eating disorder Severe alterations in eating patterns linked to physiological changes. The alterations are associated with food restriction, binge eating, inappropriate compensatory behaviors, and fluctuations in weight. They also involve a number of emotional and cognitive changes that affect the way a person perceives and experiences their body.

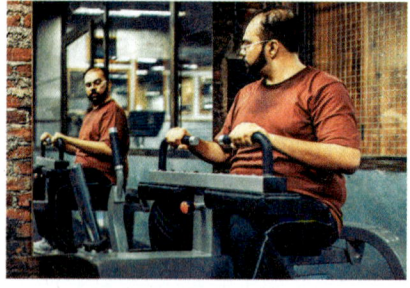

In a study about weight bias conducted by researchers at Yale University, nearly half of survey respondents said they would rather give up 1 year of life than live with obesity. GC Shutter/Getty Images

Source: Schwartz MB, Vartanian LR, Nosek BA, Brownell KD. The influence of one's own body weight on implicit and explicit anti-fat bias. *Obesity* (Silver Spring). 2006 Mar;14(3):440-447. doi: 10.1038/oby.2006.58

11.1 From Healthy to Disordered Eating Habits

FOOD: MORE THAN JUST A SOURCE OF NUTRIENTS

Eating serves an extraordinary number of physiological, psychological, social, and cultural purposes. As infants, we associate milk with security and warmth, so the breast or bottle becomes a source of comfort. Throughout life, eating practices may take on religious meanings; signify bonds within families and ethnic or racial groups; and provide a way to demonstrate affection, concern, prestige, or class values. Within the family, preparing and sharing food may be a means of expressing love.

Our enjoyment of food is both a biological and a psychological phenomenon. Indeed, eating can stimulate the release of certain **neurotransmitters** (e.g., serotonin) and natural opioids (including **endorphins**), which produce a sense of calm and euphoria in the human body. Yet, for some people, the experience of eating becomes dysfunctional. Individual variations in the structure of the brain or the function of hormones and neurotransmitters can disrupt the way a person experiences hunger or satiety, leading to chaotic eating patterns. Some individuals perceive increased anxiety or physical discomfort from eating, which leads them to turn away from food. For others, impulsivity may underlie behaviors that lead to loss of control around eating.

Adjacent to our internal experiences of eating, there are many external pressures that affect eating behaviors. Early in life, we form perceptions of *acceptable* and *unacceptable* body types. Television programs, billboard and Internet advertisements, video games, magazines, movies, and social media (see *Newsworthy Nutrition* in this section) suggest that an ultraslim body will bring happiness, love, admiration, and success. It can be difficult to resist comparing your body to what the popular media portrays as *ideal*. Individuals may also internalize the weight biases of others. Carelessly worded comments about body weight or body size from a family member, medical professional, or coach may unduly influence a person's sense of worth. In response to social pressures, some individuals engage in a pathological pursuit of weight control or weight loss. Dietary restrictions can morph into a pattern of **disordered eating** or a clinically recognized **eating disorder.**

EATING BEHAVIORS EXIST ON A SPECTRUM

At its best, eating is characterized by positive, comfortable, and flexible experiences with food.[1] Healthy eaters consume a variety of foods from all food groups and do not adhere to strict food rules or medically unnecessary dietary restrictions. Rather than relying on external cues or calorie counting apps, they pay attention to and trust their own internal signals of hunger and satiety to know when to eat and when to stop eating. Knowledge of health and nutrition informs their food choices, but healthy eaters also acknowledge the importance of the pleasure of eating; guilt and shame have no place in a healthy eating experience.

With disordered eating, this healthy relationship with food deteriorates. Disordered eating refers to short-term, mild changes in eating patterns that occur in response to a stressful event, an illness, or even a desire to modify food intake for a variety of health and personal appearance reasons. The problem may be no more than a bad habit, a style of eating adapted from friends or family members, or an aspect of preparing for athletic competition. While disordered eating can lead to weight fluctuations or nutrient deficiencies, it rarely requires in-depth professional attention.

If disordered eating becomes sustained or distressing, starts to interfere with everyday activities, or is linked to negative physiological changes, then it may be diagnosed as an eating disorder. Eating disorders involve physiological changes associated with food restriction, binge eating, purging, and/or fluctuations in weight. They also involve feelings of distress or extreme concern about body shape or weight. Eating disorders are not just a phase and will not go away on their own; they require professional treatment.

A recent analysis estimated the average tangible costs of treatment in the United States to be $11,808 per individual with an eating disorder.[2] For individuals with severe disorders, a few months of inpatient treatment could cost as much as $180,000. There are costs to society, as well, such as lost productivity of individuals with eating disorders and their caregivers. Timely treatment is costly but crucial. If left untreated, eating disorders can be fatal.

ORIGINS OF EATING DISORDERS

Given the common practice of dieting, it can sometimes be difficult to draw a definitive line between disordered eating and an eating disorder. Indeed, many eating disorders start with a simple diet. Eating disorders are not due to a failure of willpower; rather, they are biologically based, treatable medical illnesses with serious medical and psychological consequences.

People who have an eating disorder can experience a wide range of health complications, including heart conditions and kidney failure, which may lead to death. Thus, it is important to recognize the signs of eating disorders and treat them early. The three main types of eating disorders are **anorexia nervosa, bulimia nervosa,** and **binge eating disorder.** Although it is convenient to label patients with a clear-cut diagnosis, the various types of eating disorders share common features. Furthermore, many individuals who do not meet the criteria for an eating disorder diagnosis may experience physical and psychological impairments and would benefit from professional treatment.

Specific criteria from the *Diagnostic and Statistical Manual of Mental Disorders, 5th Edition, Text Revision (DSM-5-TR)*, are used by clinicians to diagnose eating disorders. As you read about the different eating disorders in this chapter, look for the relevant diagnostic criteria in Tables 11-1, 11-2, and 11-3. Keep in mind that individuals may exhibit a few symptoms of eating disorders but not enough to warrant a formal diagnosis. These people may be classified as having **subthreshold eating disorders.** Also, some people may migrate from one disorder to another over time.[3] Still, appreciating the differences between the disorders helps us to understand the various approaches to prevention and treatment.

Over the years, researchers have theorized that dysfunctional family interactions, especially between parents and adolescents, precipitate eating disorders. Historically, controlling parents were thought to cause anorexia nervosa, while unstructured, neglectful family relationships were implicated in the development of bulimia nervosa.[4] While unhealthy family relationships may lead to some emotional distress, there is little scientific evidence that family functioning is a primary cause for eating disorders. In fact, insinuating that the family has caused a person's eating disorder leads to feelings of guilt and shame within the family that may actually hinder efforts at treatment.[5]

Scientists now recognize that genes bear much of the blame for eating disorders.[6] Twin studies have shown that when one of a set of identical twins (i.e., who develop from a single fertilized egg, so they have the same genome) has an eating disorder, it is more likely that the other twin will also have an eating disorder—more likely than in sets of fraternal twins. Genetic factors appear to account for an estimated 50% to 83% of the overall risk of developing an eating disorder.

A variety of genes could be involved in the development of eating disorders, including those responsible for the synthesis of hormones and neurotransmitters involved in weight regulation and eating behaviors (review Section 7.4). In about 80% of cases, eating disorders co-occur with other psychological disorders, such as anxiety disorders, clinical depression, and substance use disorders.[7] It appears that genes influence the brain biology that determines how we perceive ourselves and respond to food stimuli or stress. In response to environmental triggers, some individuals may resort to self-destructive coping mechanisms, including disordered eating.

Because stressful life events may precipitate an eating disorder in genetically predisposed individuals, there is a strong association between eating disorders and

anorexia nervosa An eating disorder characterized by extreme restriction of energy intake relative to requirements, leading to significantly low body weight.

bulimia nervosa An eating disorder characterized by recurrent episodes of binge eating followed by inappropriate compensatory behaviors to prevent weight gain.

binge eating disorder An eating disorder characterized by recurrent episodes of binge eating that are associated with marked distress and lack of control over behavior, but not followed by inappropriate compensatory behaviors to prevent weight gain.

subthreshold eating disorder A clinically recognized eating disorder that meets some, but not all, of the criteria for diagnosis of anorexia nervosa, bulimia nervosa, or binge eating disorder.

psychiatric genetics The study of the role of genes in the development of mental health disorders.

genome-wide association study (GWAS) Research technique in which the genomes of many human subjects are scanned to identify common genes that are associated with a particular trait or disease.

> 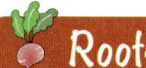 **Roots**
>
> ### Genetics and Eating Disorders
>
> **Psychiatric genetics** is a young but rapidly advancing field that explores the genetic traits that underlie mental illnesses. Decades ago, researchers noted the heritability of eating disorders through twin studies. Now, modern technology offers the ability to conduct **genome-wide association studies (GWAS),** in which researchers can identify correlations between specific genes and personality traits (e.g., neuroticism), mental health outcomes (e.g., anorexia nervosa), as well as anthropometric traits (e.g., obesity) and metabolic characteristics (e.g., hormones that regulate appetite).
>
> Eating disorders are difficult to treat and have a high rate of recurrence. Knowing more about the genetic underpinnings of mental health disorders may eventually help clinicians find better treatment options. Genetic factors also help to explain why it is common for individuals with eating disorders to cross over from one disorder to another and why there is a high co-occurrence of eating disorders with other mental illnesses, such as major depression, addictions, and obsessive-compulsive disorder. In a field where there is a history of blaming parents for the development of eating disorders, psychiatric genetics also helps families to understand that they are not to blame for a child's eating disorder diagnosis. The development of eating disorders results from a complex interplay between our genes and our environment. Genes may increase an individual's vulnerability to a mental health condition, but they do not guarantee it will develop.
>
> So far, GWAS of eating disorders have focused on anorexia nervosa. More than 130 genes have been associated with the development of anorexia nervosa. Research is now expanding to explore the genetics of bulimia nervosa, binge eating disorder, and other eating disorders.
>
> Sources: Bulik CM, Blake L, Austin J. Genetics of eating disorders: what the clinician needs to know. *Psychiatr Clin North Am.* 2019 Mar;42(1):59-73. doi: 10.1016/j.psc.2018.10.007
>
> Watson HJ, Palmos AB, Hunjan A, Baker JH, Yilmaz Z, Davies HL. Genetics of eating disorders in the genome-wide era. *Psychol Med.* 2021 Oct;51(13):2287-2297. doi: 10.1017/S0033291720005474

a history of trauma or abuse. In fact, a history of physical and sexual abuse is about twice as common among people with eating disorders compared to the population as a whole.[8] Other stressful life events, such as wartime military service, the death of a loved one, or constant social pressures to achieve thinness, are potential triggers for eating disorders.

In addition to genetics, researchers are studying epigenetics as it relates to the development of eating disorders.[9] Some studies suggest that maternal stress or hormone levels during pregnancy can predict the future development of an eating disorder in their children by affecting how the child's genes function.[10]

Overall, genes may set the stage for the development of an eating disorder, but environmental factors also play a role. Identifying specific genes or epigenetic markers linked to eating disorders eventually could help in tailoring prevention and treatment efforts for at-risk individuals. However, the counseling that is part of current therapy will still be of value.

THE CHANGING FACE OF EATING DISORDERS

If you were asked to paint a picture of a person with an eating disorder, who would you depict? The predominant stereotype is that eating disorders typically affect young, white females of middle or upper socioeconomic status. However, the face of eating disorders is changing.

Examining the **lifetime prevalence** of various eating disorders, females do outnumber males by about 12 to 1 for anorexia nervosa, by about 6 to 1 for bulimia nervosa, and by about 3 to 1 for binge eating disorder.[11] Perhaps social pressures can account for part of this disparity: in the media, females are held to standards of unnatural thinness, whereas the image conveyed for males is big and muscular. Among males, exercise status and sexual orientation are factors that particularly influence the development of anorexia and bulimia.[12] Among males, athletes are more prone than nonathletes to develop these eating disorders, especially those who participate in sports that require weight classes (e.g., boxers, wrestlers, and jockeys) or where judging is partly based on aesthetics (e.g., ice skating, diving, or dancing).[13] Perhaps due to stigma and shame, males with eating disorders are less likely to seek treatment.[14] When they do seek treatment, eating disorders are underdiagnosed among males, which may reflect cognitive biases of health care professionals, too.[15]

lifetime prevalence The proportion of a population that has had a disease, disorder, or condition at some point during life.

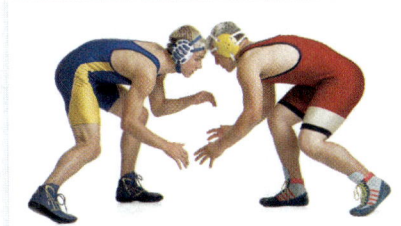

Individuals who participate in sports with weight classes, such as wrestling, may engage in disordered eating behaviors to gain a competitive advantage over other athletes in a lower weight class. **How do eating disorders impact sports performance?** Rubberball/Getty Images

Eating disorders typically develop during adolescence or young adulthood. Adolescence is a period of turbulent sexual and social tensions. At this time of life, teenagers establish their own identities. While declaring independence, they often seek acceptance and support from peers and parents and react strongly to how they think others perceive them. At the same time, their bodies are changing, and much of the change is beyond their control. This is a time when extreme dieting practices may take root. It is alarming that eating disorders are being diagnosed at earlier ages.[16] Note that calorie restriction is not always evidenced as weight loss; stunting (failure to grow in height) and delayed sexual maturation also could be signs of eating disorders among children and adolescents.

While much of the focus has been on youth, middle-aged and older adults are not immune to the devastating effects of eating disorders. Although eating disorders rarely make their first appearance late in adulthood, it may not be until later in adulthood that people who have suffered from eating disorders for years finally seek treatment. Furthermore, some adults who had recovered may relapse into former disordered eating practices. Research reveals that disordered eating behaviors and **body dissatisfaction** are quite common among older females. In one study, binge eating was reported by 3.5% of a community-based sample of females over age 50; purging behaviors, such as excessive exercise, were employed by 7.8% of the surveyed population.[17] Negative body image can have a dramatic impact on self-esteem and overall quality of life at any age.

body dissatisfaction Negative thoughts or attitudes about one's own body that may arise from a perceived gap between one's own physical appearance and one's ideal of attractiveness.

Until recently, most researchers have reported that eating disorders primarily affect middle- and upper-class white females. Now, studies show greater similarities in the rates of body dissatisfaction and disordered eating behaviors across ethnic and cultural groups. Perhaps minorities with eating disorders have been less likely to seek help in the past due to fear of shame or stigma, lack of resources, or language barriers. Also, health care workers may have been less likely to diagnose non-whites as having eating disorders. Previously, non-white cultures appeared to be more accepting of larger body shapes, but mainstream pressures for thinness now cut across cultural lines.

Individuals (particularly adolescents) who identify as lesbian, gay, bisexual, transgender, or queer (LGBTQ+) are at higher risk for disordered eating or eating disorders compared with those who identify as heterosexual and cisgender.[18] This may be due to higher levels of stress, stigma, and discrimination. Regardless of sexual orientation or gender identity, body dissatisfaction increases the risk for eating disorders. Among LGBTQ+ individuals, body dissatisfaction may extend beyond concerns about body weight to include gender dysphoria. Disordered eating behaviors may be used as a way to gain control over the body, to align with a particular gender.[19] Furthermore, LGBTQ+ individuals may be less likely to seek treatment for eating concerns due to fear of being outed or a history of negative experiences within the health care system.

Do you know someone who is at risk for an eating disorder? If so, suggest that the person seek a professional evaluation because the sooner treatment begins, the better the chances for recovery.[20] Figure 11-1 shows the SCOFF questionnaire, a

The SCOFF questions

Do you make yourself **S**ick because you feel uncomfortably full?

Do you worry that you have lost **C**ontrol over how much you eat?

Have you recently lost more than **O**ne stone (14 pounds) in a 3-month period?

Do you believe yourself to be **F**at when others say you are too thin?

Would you say that **F**ood dominates your life?

FIGURE 11-1 The SCOFF questionnaire is a simple screening tool that can be used to identify individuals at risk for eating disorders. Answering yes to more than one of these questions warrants follow-up with a mental health professional.

Source: Morgan JF, Reid F, Lacey JH. The SCOFF questionnaire: assessment of a new screening tool for eating disorders. *BMJ*. 1999;319(7223):1467-1468. doi: 10.1136/bmj.319.7223.1467

simple screening tool that can be helpful for identifying individuals at risk for eating disorders.[21] However, do not try to diagnose eating disorders in your friends or family members. Only a trained professional can exclude other possible diseases and correctly diagnose an eating disorder. Once an eating disorder is diagnosed, immediate treatment is advisable. As a friend, the best you can do is to encourage an affected person to seek professional help. Such help is commonly available at student health centers and student guidance/counseling facilities on college campuses.

Newsworthy Nutrition

Social media use and body dissatisfaction among college-age females

INTRODUCTION: Body dissatisfaction may lead to depression, restrictive dieting, and disordered eating behaviors. Previous research has shown a relationship between body dissatisfaction and exposure to traditional forms of media, such as print and television content. Social media may be especially problematic because it is used frequently and it facilitates social comparisons. However, the relationship between social media use and body dissatisfaction has not been adequately assessed. **OBJECTIVE:** In this cross-sectional study, the researchers aimed to assess the relationships among social media use (e.g., Facebook, Twitter, and Instagram), body dissatisfaction, and negative affect (i.e., depression). **METHODS:** The researchers used a technique called ecological model assessment, in which they contacted subjects in their natural setting on their own schedule. This method has been used to overcome the limitations of retroactive assessments, which may be inaccurate and underestimate social media use. A sample of 30 college students who identified as female at Missouri State University were contacted through their smartphones five times per day for 6 days (1 practice day and 5 test days) to answer a series of questions about social media use (including time spent on social media as well as number of sites visited), mood (the Positive and Negative Affect Schedule-Expanded Form), and body image (the Body Image States Scale). Each assessment took approximately 5 minutes to complete. **RESULTS:** Number of sites visited, but not time spent on social media, was a predictor of body dissatisfaction. Social media use (time spent and number of sites visited) also predicted general negative affect, sadness, and guilt. **CONCLUSION:** This observational study showed that social media use, unlike other forms of media, predicts negative affect and body dissatisfaction. Specifically, consistent messaging about unrealistic body weight or shape across several sites may reinforce body dissatisfaction. This information may assist in the development of media literacy interventions to modify the use of social media and improve and/or develop coping skills. Future studies may employ similar assessment techniques in a larger, more diverse population and should examine the bidirectionality of the relationships between depression or body dissatisfaction and social media use.

Source: Bennett BL, Whisenhunt BL, Hudson DL, et al. Examining the impact of social media on mood and body dissatisfaction using ecological momentary assessment. *J Am Coll Health*. 2020 Jul;68(5):502-508. doi: 10.1080/07448481.2019.1583236

✓ CONCEPT CHECK 11.1

1. Differentiate between disordered eating and an eating disorder.
2. Describe how genetics and environment interact in the development of eating disorders.
3. Why are eating disorders more common among adolescents than other age groups?

11.2 Anorexia Nervosa

Anorexia nervosa is an eating disorder characterized by extreme weight loss, an irrational fear of weight gain, and a distorted body image. These three criteria are outlined in Table 11-1 and described in detail in this section. Anorexia nervosa affects an estimated 0.8% of American adults (0.12% of males and 1.42% of females) at some point during their lives.[11]

First, people with anorexia nervosa severely restrict energy intake relative to requirements. The term *anorexia* implies a loss of appetite; however, a denial of one's appetite more accurately describes the behavior of people with anorexia nervosa. Low energy intake leads to a body weight that is significantly less than expected when compared to others of the same age, sex, stage of physical development, and activity level. Please note there is no defined threshold for BMI for the diagnosis of anorexia nervosa. While low body weight (i.e., less than 85% of expected body weight for a given age and sex or BMI of less than 17) may indicate anorexia nervosa, a variety of other medical conditions could also result in low body weight.

The second key criterion for diagnosis of anorexia nervosa involves an intense fear of gaining weight or becoming overweight or obese. Some individuals with eating disorders may deny fear of weight gain, so persistent behaviors that interfere with weight gain are also included in this criterion. To be diagnosed with anorexia nervosa, an individual must have experienced fear of weight gain or practiced behaviors to prevent weight gain at least 75% of the days in the last 3 months.

Third, as depicted in the photo on this page, individuals with anorexia nervosa have a distorted body image. The term *nervosa* refers to an unhealthy obsession. Individuals with anorexia nervosa may irrationally believe they are fat, despite their thin physique. Some people with anorexia nervosa realize they are thin but continue to be haunted by certain areas of their bodies that they believe to be fat (such as thighs, buttocks, and stomach). Even though extremely low body weight results in severe health effects, as described later in this section, people with anorexia nervosa do not acknowledge the problem. They may persist in efforts at weight loss and try to thwart the efforts of family members and medical professionals to increase their body weight to a healthy level.

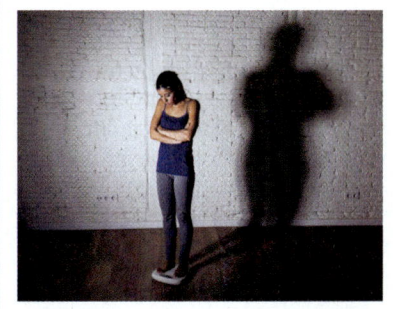

For people with eating disorders, the difference between the real and desired body images may be too difficult to accept. **See the website womenshealth.gov/body-image to learn more about body image.** Ocusfocus/123RF

There are two subtypes of anorexia nervosa: a *restricting type* and a *binge eating/purging type*. All individuals with anorexia nervosa severely restrict their calorie intake to achieve or maintain a low body weight; those with the binge eating/purging type of anorexia nervosa also engage in episodes of binge eating followed by **compensatory behaviors** to rid the body of calories. The difference between bulimia nervosa and anorexia nervosa of the binge eating/purging subtype is that individuals with anorexia nervosa go through long periods of dietary restriction and have low body weight (e.g., BMI < 17), whereas individuals with bulimia tend to have normal or high BMI. Although individuals with bulimia nervosa may engage in periods of fasting, they do not restrict intake as severely or for as long as individuals with anorexia nervosa.

compensatory behaviors Actions taken to rid the body of excess calories and/or to alleviate guilt or anxiety associated with a binge. Examples include purging (i.e., self-induced vomiting or abusing laxatives), fasting, or excessive exercise.

TABLE 11-1 ■ Diagnostic Criteria for Anorexia Nervosa

A. Extreme dietary restriction that leads to significantly low body weight
B. Overwhelming distress about weight gain (or avoidance of behaviors that may lead to weight gain) despite having a low body weight
C. Disturbed perception of one's own body weight or shape, overemphasis on body weight or shape in determining self-worth, or failure to recognize the dangers of extremely low body weight

Source: American Psychiatric Association. *Diagnostic and Statistical Manual for Mental Disorders*, 5th edition. American Psychiatric Association; 2022.

COMMON BEHAVIORS OF ANOREXIA NERVOSA

Individuals who develop anorexia nervosa share some common traits. Take a young female, for example, who is described by parents and teachers as responsible, meticulous, and obedient. She holds herself to high standards of performance and appearance. She is competitive and perfectionistic. At home, she may not allow clutter in her bedroom. Clinicians note that after a physical examination, she folds her examination gown very carefully and cleans up the examination room before leaving. As mentioned, both genetic and environmental factors contribute to both our self-perception and our responses to stress. These obsessive personality traits—rigidity and perfectionism—are related to the same brain biology that predicts the development of eating disorders.

Anorexia nervosa may begin as a simple attempt to lose weight. A comment from a well-meaning friend, relative, or coach suggesting that the person seems to be gaining weight or is too fat may be all that is needed. The stress of having to maintain a certain weight to look attractive or perform better can also lead to disordered eating. Abusive experiences, a difficult breakup, or the stress of leaving home for college are examples of triggers for extreme dieting. Changing one's appearance might be viewed as a way to avoid future conflict or ensure success in a new situation.

Still, losing weight does not help people deal with anger, grief, anxiety, or depression. If these psychological issues are not addressed, individuals may intensify efforts to lose weight rather than work through unresolved psychological concerns. At first, dieting becomes the life focus. Such persons may derive a sense of achievement from their "success" at controlling body weight or perceive improvements in other areas of their lives. What began as a diet leads to very abnormal self-perceptions and eating habits, such as cutting a pea in half before eating it.

Extreme dieting is the most important predictor of an eating disorder. (Adolescents expressing concern about their weight should be advised to focus on physical activity, which does not appear to impart a risk for subsequent problems.) Once dieting begins, a person developing anorexia nervosa does not stop. As the disorder progresses, the range of foods eaten may narrow; the list of "safe foods" shortens, whereas the list of "unsafe foods" gets longer. Abnormal habits include hiding and storing food or spreading food around a plate to make it look as if much has been eaten. A person with anorexia nervosa may cook a large meal and watch others eat it while refusing to eat anything or may insist on having different meals from the rest of the family. Frequent weighing and body checking—such as measuring the width of the thigh—are common.[22]

As mentioned, among some people with anorexia nervosa, disordered eating behaviors may eventually include bingeing on large amounts of food in a short time and/or inappropriate behaviors to compensate for the large number of calories consumed. Covered further in Section 11.3, compensatory behaviors (sometimes called *purging*) include vomiting, using laxatives or diuretics, and excessive exercise. Thus, people with anorexia nervosa may exist in a state of continuous semistarvation or may alternate between periods of starvation and periods of bingeing and purging.

A state of semistarvation can cause depression, irritability, and hostility. Individuals with anorexia may be excessively critical of themselves and usually withdraw from family and friends. Despite a strong drive for perfection, performance in school, sports, and work begins to deteriorate. (See Section 11.8 for a glimpse of the inner turmoil of a person with anorexia nervosa.)

Ultimately, a person with anorexia nervosa eats fewer calories than are required to maintain a healthy body weight. This can vary considerably from person to person, but 600 to 800 kcal daily is not unusual. In place of food, the person may consume up to 20 cans of diet soft drinks and chew many pieces of sugarless gum each day.

PHYSICAL EFFECTS OF ANOREXIA NERVOSA

The state of semistarvation disturbs many body systems as it forces the body to conserve energy stores as much as possible. Many of the following complications can be reversed

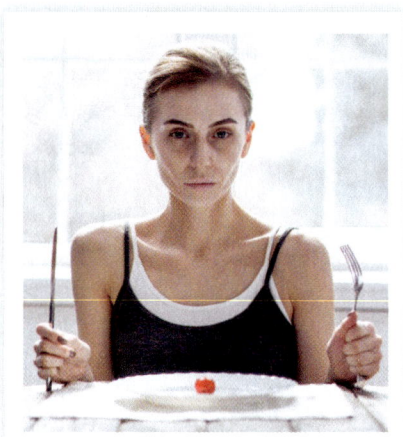

Extreme dietary rules severely limit nutritional intake among people with anorexia nervosa. **What happens to a person's basal metabolic rate (BMR) when calorie intake is severely restricted?** zinkevych/123RF

A disturbing Internet trend is the attempt to promote eating disorders as a way of life. Some individuals with eating disorders have personified their illness into a role model named *Ana*, who tells them what to eat and mocks them when they don't lose weight. Similarly, pro-*Mia* sites provide tips and encouragement for people with bulimia (e.g., how to induce vomiting and cover up evidence of compensatory behaviors). Pro-Ana and pro-Mia websites reject the serious health risks of eating disorders and instead dispense unsafe *thinspiration* to vulnerable individuals.[23]

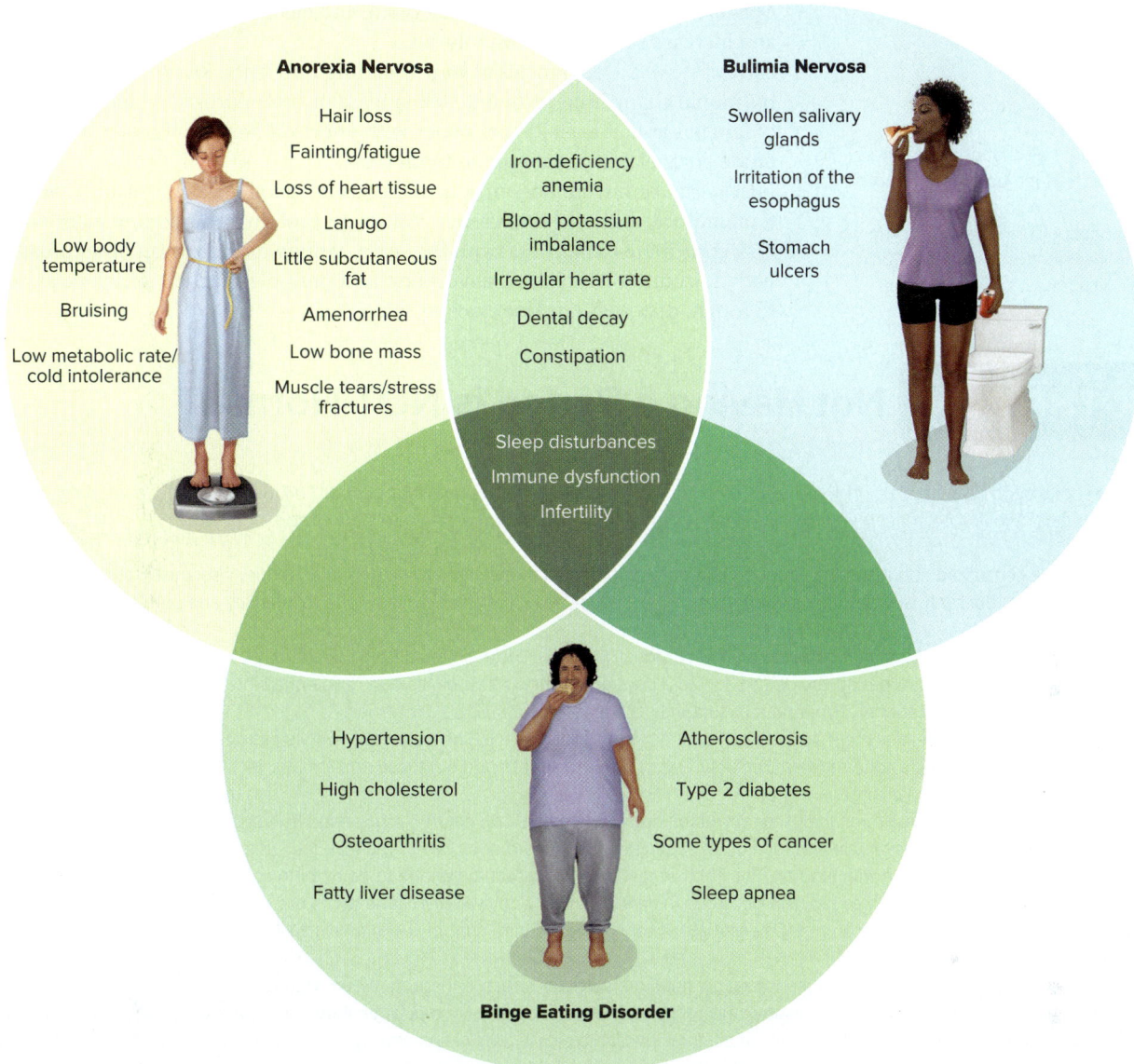

FIGURE 11-2 Physical effects of eating disorders. Although this figure contains many potential consequences, it is not an exhaustive list. Some of these physical effects can also serve as warning signs that a problem exists.

by restoring body weight to a healthy level, provided the duration of the semistarvation has not been too long.[24] (Many of these are illustrated in Figure 11-2.)

- *Cardiovascular system:* Loss of heart tissue, changes in blood electrolyte levels, and impaired red blood cell health contribute to fatigue, weakness, and fainting. Heart rhythm disturbances are a leading cause of death in people with anorexia nervosa.
- *Nervous system:* Changes in brain size, blood flow to the brain, and neurotransmitter synthesis affect cognitive function and mood.
- *Immune system:* Low white blood cell count increases susceptibility to illness.
- *Endocrine system:* Decreased synthesis of thyroid hormones slows the metabolic rate. Decreased production of sex hormones contributes to **amenorrhea** and infertility. The loss of menstrual periods may be the first sign of endocrine abnormalities among females (see *Ask the RDN* in this section).
- *Digestive system:* Changes in gastrointestinal function lead to abnormal feelings of fullness or bloating after eating. Chronic use of laxatives may lead to decreases in bowel motility. Impaired swallowing ability due to loss of muscle tissue in the pharynx increases the risk for aspiration of food and liquids into the lungs.

amenorrhea Absence of menstrual periods in a female of reproductive age.

- *Muscular system:* Atrophy of muscle tissue and electrolyte imbalances weaken muscles and increase susceptibility to injuries.
- *Skeletal system:* Deficiencies of bone-building nutrients, loss of muscle mass, and hormonal changes contribute to osteopenia or osteoporosis, which is evident in 85% of females and at least 25% of males with anorexia nervosa. Frequent vomiting may erode enamel and contribute to tooth loss.
- *Integumentary system:* Loss of subcutaneous fat leads to easy bruising, lowered body temperature, and cold intolerance. Although protein and micronutrient deficiencies may contribute to hair loss from the scalp, **lanugo** may grow on other areas of the body to counter heat loss. Dehydration and multiple nutrient deficiencies contribute to rough, dry, scaly, and/or cracked skin.

lanugo Downlike hair that appears after a person has lost much body fat through semistarvation. The hair stands erect and traps air, acting as insulation for the body to compensate for the relative lack of body fat, which usually functions as insulation.

ASK THE RDN — Not Having a Period is NOT Normal

Dear RDN: *I have been diligently tracking my weight on a daily basis since my first year in high school. I am happy that I can keep my weight just under 100 pounds. Should I be concerned that I have not had my period since starting college 2 years ago?*

Yes, you should be concerned about missing your period! Contrary to popular belief, not having a regular period, also known as amenorrhea, is not normal. It also means your body isn't producing enough estrogen, and low levels of estrogen may lead to infertility and premature osteoporosis or other health conditions.

So, what *is* a *normal* period? Well, that depends on the individual. A normal cycle, counted from the first day of your last period to the first day of the next period, is 25 to 35 days. A period can be as short as 2 days or as long as a week. If you're someone who has had 3-day periods since you began menstruating, that's normal. If your pattern suddenly changes, you should be concerned.

There are some medical conditions that may prevent or affect menstruation, including polycystic ovary syndrome (see Section 14.1), pelvic inflammatory disease, and genetic abnormalities. See your health care provider to rule out these possibilities. Most likely, the loss of your period is the result of a nutrition or lifestyle change.

Now let's talk birth control. If you're on the pill or any other kind of hormonal birth control, your period isn't a *real* period. Birth control has varying concentrations of synthetic female hormones. The absence of these hormones (when you take the sugar pills in your pack) induces a period. You cannot heal amenorrhea with birth control. For that reason, it is not recommended to be on birth control to regain a natural period, especially if you're recovering from an eating disorder. Keep in mind that your body will need time to restore its metabolic function, hormone levels, and natural set point where your body can freely menstruate. After coming off birth control, it can take anywhere from 3 to 6 months for your true period to normalize.

There are four factors that typically affect menstruation: nutrition, exercise, stress, and sleep. When we underfuel our bodies and/or over-exercise, menstruation takes a back seat. Your body can't focus on your reproductive system when it doesn't have enough energy to maintain vital functions, like breathing and heartbeat. Normal menstrual function typically requires an energy intake of about 30 kcal per kilogram of body weight (or about 13 to 14 kcal per pound), but every body has its own threshold to menstruate. Undernourishment—eating too few calories and/or consuming a suboptimal dietary pattern—can cause your period to stop. If low energy availability is the cause, slowly increasing caloric intake and eating a wider variety of foods should help induce a period. Seek the help of an RDN who specializes in eating disorders to help guide you through the process.

Respect your own body's threshold for exercise. If you love to run but suspect you may be putting too much stress on your body, perhaps alternate running days with other activities or decrease your mileage. If you're in a high-stress phase of life where you're dealing with anxiety, school demands, and working extra hours, intense exercise may place more demands on your body. Practicing meditation or yoga, taking walks, visiting with friends, or engaging in low-intensity physical activity would be wise choices until things settle down. Exercise in a way that's appropriate for *your* body and respect rest days.

If nutrition and exercise are not to blame for missed periods, stress could be the issue. When you're under significant stress, your body releases stress hormones, such as cortisol. When this happens, it's best to slow down and work on self-care and activities that bring you joy and relaxation.

Last, but certainly not least, a lack of sleep is one of the most overlooked factors when it comes to your health. Research suggests that sleep dysregulation may suppress reproductive hormones and affect frequency of periods. If you struggle to get at least 7 hours of sleep each night, create a nighttime routine that facilitates more quality sleep.

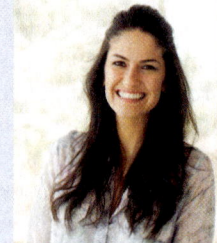
Raul Velasco

Menstruation matters—period.

Alexis Joseph, MS, RD, LD
Dietitian, Founder of Hummusapien, Co-owner of Alchemy Brands
Source: Daily JP, Stumbo JR. Female athlete triad. *Prim Care.* 2018 Dec;45(4):615-624. doi: 10.1016/j.pop.2018.07.004

Many of the psychological and physical problems associated with anorexia nervosa arise from insufficient calorie intake, as well as deficiencies of nutrients such as thiamin, calcium, and iron. A person with this disorder is psychologically and physically ill and needs immediate professional help.

About one-third of those with anorexia nervosa recover within 10 years, and about two-thirds recover within 20 years, yet many will struggle with the disease throughout life.[25] Among all psychiatric diseases, anorexia nervosa has the highest mortality rate—about six times higher than the general population.[26] Common causes of death among those with anorexia nervosa include heart ailments, infections, or suicide. The longer someone lives with this eating disorder, the poorer the chances for complete recovery. A young patient with a brief illness and a supportive family has a better outlook than an older patient with a long history of disordered eating and no family support. Overall, prompt treatment and close long-term follow-up improve the chances of a successful recovery.

TREATMENT FOR THE PERSON WITH ANOREXIA NERVOSA

People with anorexia often sink into shells of isolation and fear. They deny that a problem exists. Frequently, their friends and family members meet with them to confront the problem in a loving way. This is called an *intervention*. They present evidence of the problem and encourage immediate treatment.

Treatment requires a multidisciplinary team of experienced professionals (e.g., physicians, psychiatrists, psychologists, registered dietitian nutritionists [RDNs], nurses, occupational therapists, and social workers). An ideal setting is an eating disorders clinic in a medical center. Outpatient therapy generally begins first. This may be extended to 3 to 5 days per week. Day hospitalization (6 to 12 hours per day) is another option. Total hospitalization is necessary once a person falls below 75% of expected weight (i.e., how much an individual would weigh at a healthy BMI), experiences medical problems, and/or exhibits severe psychological problems or suicidal risk. Still, even in the most skilled hands at the finest facilities, efforts may fail. This tells us that the prevention of anorexia nervosa is of utmost importance.[27]

The health care team must gain the cooperation and trust of the client and work together to restore body weight, correct medical complications, and treat mental illness. However, an individual who has been barely existing in a state of semistarvation cannot focus on much besides food. Dreams and even morbid thoughts about food will interfere with therapy until the person regains sufficient weight. Outcomes are best among younger patients with earlier treatment, but the typical duration of anorexia nervosa is about 10 years.[28]

Nutrition Therapy. The ultimate goal of nutrition therapy for anorexia nervosa is to restore body weight to a healthy range. The individual must increase oral food intake and gain enough weight to raise the metabolic rate to normal and reverse as many physical signs of the disease as possible. The refeeding plan is designed first to minimize or stop any further weight loss. Then, the focus shifts to restoring appropriate eating behaviors. After this, the expectation can be switched to gaining weight; 2 to 3 pounds per week is appropriate. Tube and/or intravenous (IV) feeding is used only if immediate renourishment is required, as this can frighten the person and cause the person to distrust medical staff.

Individuals with anorexia nervosa need considerable reassurance during the refeeding process because of uncomfortable and unfamiliar effects—such as bloating and increased body temperature. These symptoms occur because of starvation-related changes in GI tract function and will usually resolve over time, but they can be frightening for the person recovering from anorexia. Rapid changes in electrolytes and minerals in the blood associated with refeeding—especially potassium, phosphorus, and magnesium—can be dangerous. Therefore, monitoring blood levels of these minerals is of critical importance during the process of incorporating more food into the dietary pattern.

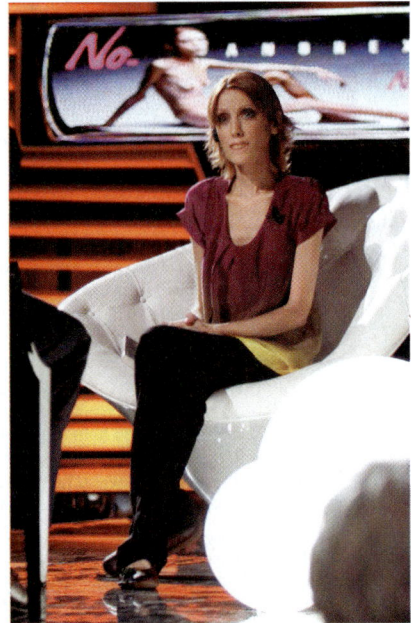

In 2010, the death of French fashion model Isabelle Caro increased awareness of the serious nature of anorexia nervosa. After surviving a coma related to her disorder, she resolved to speak out against dieting in the fashion industry. She posed for a controversial billboard ad under the words *No Anorexia*. She also authored a book about her 15-year struggle with an eating disorder and was interviewed for *National Geographic's Taboo: Beauty* documentary. Sadly, she died from complications of her disorder at age 28, before the documentary ever aired. Ernesto Ruscio/Getty Images

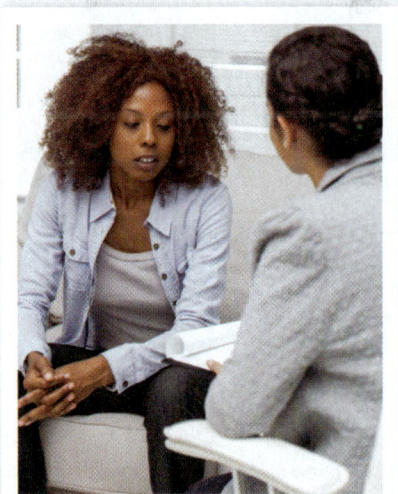

Early treatment for an eating disorder, such as anorexia nervosa, improves chances of success. **What resources are available on your campus for students who are living with eating disorders?** wavebreakmedia/Shutterstock

In addition to helping the person with anorexia nervosa reach and maintain adequate body weight and nutrient status, the RDN provides accurate nutrition information throughout the treatment, promotes a healthy attitude toward food, and helps the person learn to eat in response to natural hunger and satiety cues. The RDN educates the client on healthy and adequate food choices that promote weight gain to achieve a BMI of 20 or more for adults or BMI-for-age between the 25th and 85th percentile for children (see Section 15.1). For children and adolescents, additional energy needs for growth must be considered.

As noted, nutrient deficiencies are commonly observed in patients with anorexia nervosa. As treatment progresses, the health care team will work with the patient to fully restore nutritional status. A multivitamin and mineral supplement will be added, as well as enough calcium to raise intake to about 1500 milligrams per day. Bone loss will not likely be completely restored, even if nutrition is adequate. Adolescent patients, in particular, may have missed a critical time for accrual of bone mass or gains in height. However, supplementation with calcium and vitamin D is still necessary to prevent further bone loss.

Despite their extreme need for nutritional intervention, surrendering control overeating can be scary and frustrating for individuals with anorexia nervosa. These patients may be very resistant to therapy and fearful of weight gain. They may try to disguise their weight loss by wearing many layers of clothes, putting coins in their pockets, or drinking many glasses of water before stepping on the scale. Excessive physical activity may also impede weight gain. At many treatment centers, moderate bed rest is used in the early stages of treatment to help promote weight gain. Overall, experienced professional help is the key to effectively treating anorexia nervosa.[29]

Psychological Therapy. Once the immediate physical problems of anorexia nervosa are addressed, the focus of treatment shifts to the underlying emotional problems that preceded the eating disorder. If therapists can discover the psychological conflicts that triggered the disorder, they can develop more effective treatment strategies. Education about the medical consequences of semistarvation also may be helpful. A key aspect of psychological treatment is showing affected individuals how to regain control of other facets of their lives and cope with difficult situations. As eating evolves into a normal routine, they can turn to previously neglected activities.

Family-based treatment (usually 6 to 12 months) is the preferred method of psychological treatment for anorexia nervosa among *adolescents*.[30] Importantly, family-based treatment for anorexia nervosa absolves parents of blame for the eating disorder. Early treatment focuses on ways the family can help the person with anorexia achieve a healthy body weight. Eventually, responsibility for eating and weight control will be transferred back to the patient. Beyond eating behaviors, family-based treatment for anorexia nervosa also helps the patient establish healthy relationships with parents and other family members.

At this time, there is not enough evidence to promote one particular type of psychological therapy over another for *adults* with anorexia nervosa. Therapists may use **cognitive behavioral therapy,** which involves helping the person confront and change irrational beliefs about body image, eating, relationships, and weight. However, after subsisting in a starved state for months or years, the brain chemistry of a person with anorexia nervosa is so altered that attempts at cognitive restructuring are usually not effective in the early stages of treatment. Underlying issues that may have triggered the eating disorder, such as sexual abuse, also must be identified and addressed by the therapist. Guided self-help groups for people with eating disorders, as well as their families and friends, represent additional nonthreatening first steps into treatment.

Refeeding the Microbiota

Beneficial gut microbes produce compounds that regulate mood, appetite, and gastrointestinal symptoms. Among individuals with anorexia nervosa, beneficial probiotic microorganisms are reduced in number and activity, both before and after nutritional rehabilitation. To induce weight gain, the refeeding protocol for treatment of individuals with anorexia nervosa must include high-fat foods. However, food sources of probiotics (e.g., yogurt and other fermented foods) and prebiotics (e.g., fruits, vegetables, and whole grains) can also help the beneficial microorganisms in the GI tract to flourish and potentially improve physical and mental health outcomes for individuals in recovery for eating disorders.

Source: Ruusunen A, Rocks T, Jacka F, Loughman A. The gut microbiome in anorexia nervosa: relevance for nutritional rehabilitation. *Psychopharmacology (Berl).* 2019 May;236(5):1545-1558. doi: 10.1007/s00213-018-5159-2

---

family-based treatment An intensive outpatient treatment approach for eating disorders that involves the family and teaches the patient how to manage eating and other behaviors in their home environment; also called the *Maudsley method*.

cognitive behavioral therapy Psychological therapy in which the person's assumptions about dieting, body weight, and related issues are confronted. New ways of thinking are explored and then practiced by the person. In this way, an individual can learn new ways to control disordered eating behaviors and related life stress.

Pharmacological Therapy. There are no medications approved by the U.S. Food and Drug Administration (FDA) specifically for the treatment of anorexia nervosa. Rather, *food* is the treatment of choice for people with this disorder. Generally, medications are not effective in managing the primary symptoms of anorexia nervosa. Fluoxetine (Prozac®) and related medications may stabilize recovery once 85% of expected body weight has been attained. These medications work by prolonging serotonin activity in the brain, which in turn regulates mood and feelings of satiety. A variety of other pharmacological agents, such as olanzapine (Zyprexa®), may have some role in treating mood changes, anxiety, or psychotic symptoms associated with anorexia nervosa, but they have limited value unless weight gain is also achieved.[31]

With professional help, many people with anorexia nervosa can regain a balanced dietary pattern. Although they may not be totally cured, recovering individuals no longer depend on unusual eating habits to cope with daily problems. They recover a sense of normalcy in their lives. Recovery can be a long process, and longer follow-up is associated with better outcomes. About one-third of individuals with anorexia nervosa recover within 4 years, and about one-half recover within 10 years.[25] No universal approach exists because each case is unique. Establishing a strong relationship with either a therapist or another supportive person is especially important to recovery. As they learn alternative coping mechanisms, individuals with anorexia nervosa can relinquish dysfunctional relationships with food and instead develop healthy personal relationships.

✓ CONCEPT CHECK 11.2

1. Identify the three diagnostic criteria for anorexia nervosa.
2. List five physical effects of anorexia nervosa.
3. Describe elements of nutritional, psychological, and pharmacological therapy for anorexia nervosa.

11.3 Bulimia Nervosa

Literally translated, *bulimia* means ravenous (oxlike) hunger. This eating disorder is characterized by recurrent episodes of binge eating followed by some type of compensatory behavior to prevent weight gain (see Table 11-2). As with anorexia nervosa, individuals with bulimia nervosa overvalue body weight and shape.

Binge eating is defined as consuming an abnormally large amount of food within a short time period (e.g., 2 hours). Notably, binges are characterized by a lack of control over the food consumed. Compensatory behaviors (also known as *purging*) used to rid the body of excess calories consumed during a binge may include vomiting; misuse of laxatives, diuretics, enemas, or other prescription medications (e.g., insulin); or excessive exercise. For a diagnosis of bulimia nervosa, binge eating followed by inappropriate compensatory behaviors must take place at least once per week over a period of 3 months or more.[32]

binge eating Consuming an abnormally large amount of food within a short time period (e.g., 2 hours).

TABLE 11-2 ■ Diagnostic Criteria for Bulimia Nervosa

A. Repeated binge eating, characterized by:
   1. Eating a large amount of food in a short period of time (e.g., within 2 hours)
   2. Experiencing a loss of control overeating during binges

B. Binge-compensate cycles occur at least one time per week for 3 months
C. Undue influence of body weight or shape on self-evaluation
D. Behaviors are distinct from the binge eating/purging subtype of anorexia nervosa

Source: American Psychiatric Association. *Diagnostic and Statistical Manual for Mental Disorders*, 5th edition. American Psychiatric Association; 2022.

It is likely that many people with bulimic behaviors are never diagnosed. People with bulimia nervosa lead secret lives, hiding their abnormal eating habits. Moreover, it can be difficult to recognize the disorder based on appearance because people with bulimia nervosa are usually at or slightly above normal weight. By rough estimate, bulimia nervosa affects about 0.28% of U.S. adults (0.08% of males and 0.46% of females) at some point during their lives.[11] However, most diagnoses of bulimia nervosa rely on self-reports, so the disorder may be much more widespread than commonly thought.

COMMON BEHAVIORS OF BULIMIA NERVOSA

Bulimia nervosa involves episodes of binge eating followed by various means to rid the body of excess calories. Susceptible people often have genetic factors and lifestyle patterns that predispose them to becoming overweight, and many have tried multiple weight-reduction diets in the past. A person with bulimia nervosa may think of food constantly; however, unlike a person with anorexia nervosa, whose behavior is primarily characterized as restrictive, a person with bulimia nervosa turns toward food in critical situations. Also, unlike those with anorexia nervosa, people with bulimia nervosa recognize their behavior as abnormal.

For food intake to qualify as a binge, an atypically large amount of food must be consumed in a short time and the person must exhibit a lack of control over the behavior. Among individuals with bulimia nervosa, bingeing often alternates with attempts to rigidly restrict food intake. Elaborate food rules are common, such as avoiding all sweets. Thus, eating just one cookie or doughnut may cause an individual with this disorder to feel as though a rule has been broken. At that point, in the mind of a person with bulimia, the objectionable food must be eliminated.

Most commonly, individuals with bulimia nervosa consume cakes, cookies, ice cream, and other high-carbohydrate convenience foods during binges because these foods can be purged relatively easily and comfortably by vomiting. In a single binge, foods supplying 3000 kcal or more may be eaten. Compensatory behaviors follow in hopes that no weight will be gained; however, even when vomiting follows a binge, up to 75% of the calories taken in are still absorbed, inevitably causing some weight gain.[33] When laxatives or enemas are used, about 90% of the calories are absorbed, as laxatives act in the large intestine, beyond the point of most nutrient absorption.[34] The belief that purging soon after bingeing will prevent excessive calorie absorption and weight gain is a misconception.

Binge-compensate cycles may be practiced daily, weekly, or across longer intervals. A specific time of day often is set aside. Most binge eating occurs at night, when other people are less likely to interrupt, and usually lasts from 30 minutes to 2 hours. A binge can be triggered by stress, boredom, loneliness, depression, or any combination thereof. It often follows a period of calorie restriction and thus may be linked to intense hunger or cravings. A binge is not at all like normal eating; once begun, it seems to propel itself. The person not only loses control but generally does not even taste or enjoy food during a binge. This separates the practice from overeating.

At the onset of bulimia nervosa, some individuals may induce vomiting by placing their fingers deep into the mouth to trigger the gag reflex. They may bite down on their fingers inadvertently, resulting in bite marks and scars around the knuckles. These marks on the knuckles, known as **Russell's sign,** are a characteristic sign of this disorder (Fig. 11-3). Once the disease is established, however, a person may be able to vomit simply by contracting the abdominal muscles. Vomiting may also occur spontaneously.

Another way a person with bulimia may attempt to compensate for a binge is by engaging in excessive exercise to expend a large amount of calories. In this practice, referred to as *debting,* individuals try to estimate the amount of calories eaten during a binge and then work out to burn off the excess calories. Exercise is considered excessive when it is done at inappropriate times or in inappropriate settings, or when a person does it despite injury or other medical complications.

Bingeing and purging (via vomiting) were evident in pre-Christian Roman times but were practiced in a group setting. The eating disorder bulimia nervosa is generally practiced in private. It was first described in the medical literature in 1979.

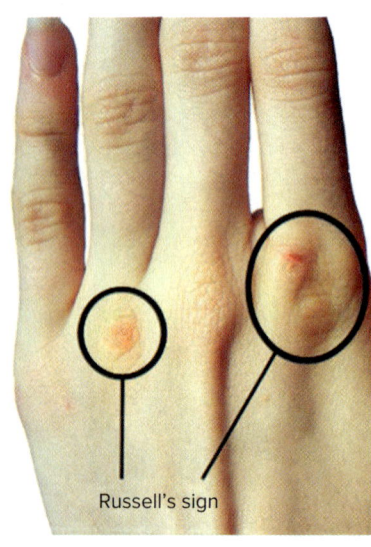

FIGURE 11-3 Russell's sign may indicate bulimia nervosa. It may appear as abrasions, calluses, or scars on the knuckles caused by trauma from the teeth while using the fingers to trigger the gag reflex to induce vomiting. Science Source

Russell's sign Evidence of abrasion that appears on the knuckles of a person who repeatedly induces vomiting by using the fingers to trigger the gag reflex in the back of the throat; named after the psychiatrist who first identified bulimia nervosa.

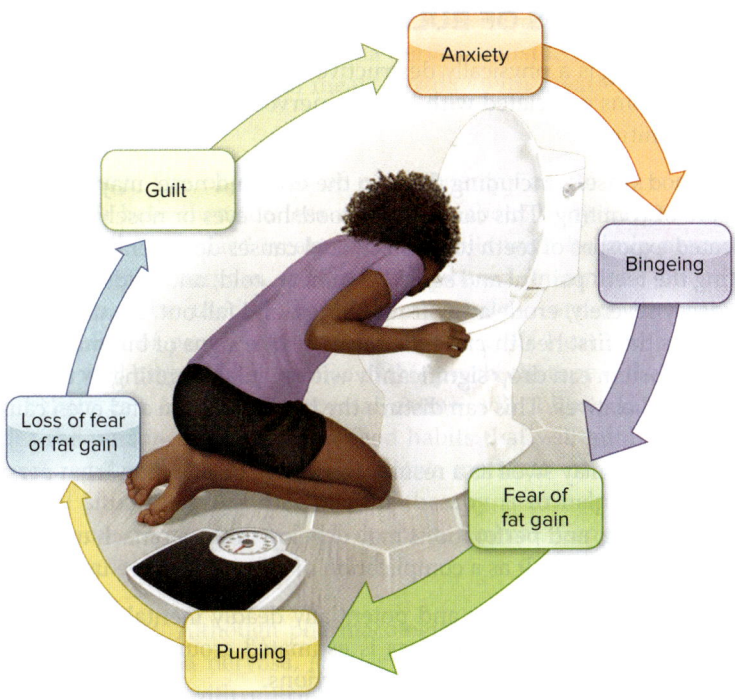

FIGURE 11-4 Bulimia nervosa's vicious cycle of obsession.

People with bulimia nervosa are not proud of their behavior. After a binge, they usually feel guilty and depressed. Over time, they experience low self-esteem, feel hopeless about their situation, and are caught in a vicious cycle of obsession (Fig. 11-4).[35] Compulsive lying, shoplifting to obtain food, and drug abuse can further intensify these feelings. A person discovered in the act of bingeing by a friend or family member may lash out and order the intruder to leave. People with bulimia nervosa gradually distance themselves from others, spending more time preoccupied by and engaging in bingeing and compensating.

Because individuals with bulimia nervosa attempt to hide their behaviors, it may be difficult to identify them early in the disease process, when treatment is likely to be most effective. An early warning sign of bulimia is frequent trips to the bathroom during or after meals. The noise of the bathroom fan or running water may be used to cover the sounds of vomiting. Despite efforts to disguise the behavior with air fresheners, mouthwash, or breath mints, there may be a lingering odor of vomit. Be suspicious of packages or receipts for laxatives, diuretics, diet pills, or enemas. People who use exercise to compensate for binges are usually preoccupied with their workout schedule or might seem extremely distressed when they are unable to work out. If you suspect someone is falling victim to bulimia nervosa, encourage the individual to get professional help. Early intervention can prevent some of the serious physical health effects described in the next section.[22]

As introduced in Section 11.1, eating disorders frequently co-occur with other mental health disorders. Disorders that commonly co-occur with bulimia nervosa include depression, anxiety, posttraumatic stress, and substance abuse.[36] Many people with bulimia nervosa report a history of sexual abuse. They appear competent to outsiders, while they actually feel out of control, ashamed, and frustrated.

Some experts have suggested that bulimia may actually arise from an inability to control responses to impulse and desire. Besides struggling to control impulses related to eating, other impulsive behaviors may include stealing, increased sexual activity, drug and alcohol abuse, self-mutilation, or attempted suicide.[35] The impulsive and risky nature of alcohol, tobacco, and other drug use is consistent with some behavioral traits of bulimia nervosa, which may be related to disruptions in neuroendocrine pathways. Clinicians working with individuals with eating disorders should be on the lookout for substance abuse; the coexistence of eating disorders with substance use greatly increases health risks, especially for adolescents.[37]

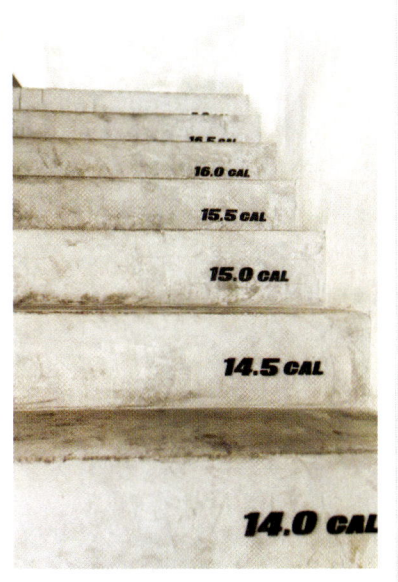

Excessive exercise can be one component of bulimia if it is used as a way to offset the calorie intake from a binge. **How can you tell if exercise is *excessive*?**
ronnarong/123RF

11.4 Binge Eating Disorder

First officially described in 1994, binge eating disorder is a growing, complex, and serious problem. Generally, binge eating disorder can be defined as binge eating episodes not accompanied by compensatory behaviors (as seen in bulimia nervosa) at least one time per week, on average, for at least 3 months. The diagnostic criteria for binge eating disorder are listed in Table 11-3.

The number of cases of binge eating disorder is greater than that of either anorexia nervosa or bulimia nervosa. While anorexia and bulimia disproportionately affect females, about 40% of people with binge eating disorder are males.[40] For adults, the lifetime prevalence of binge eating disorder is estimated to be about 0.85% (1.25% for females and about 0.42% for males).[11] However, many more people in the general population are likely to have less severe forms of the disorder that do not meet all the criteria described in Table 11-3. This disorder is most common among individuals with severe obesity and those with a history of yo-yo dieting, although obesity is not a criterion for having binge eating disorder. The average age of onset is around 25 years.[11]

Like anorexia and bulimia, binge eating disorder seems to arise when a person with a genetic predisposition for the disorder is faced with an environmental trigger, such as emotional stress. Individuals with binge eating disorder may have disruptions in neurotransmitter function or altered activity in the part of the brain that responds to rewarding stimuli.[9] There is a strong association between binge eating disorder and other psychological disorders, especially anxiety, depression, and addiction.[8,41]

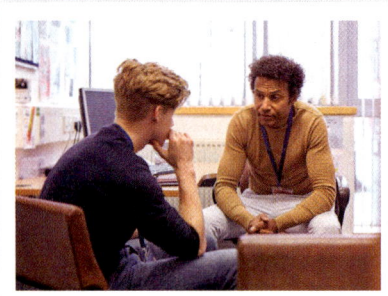

Approximately 40% of college-age adults (49% of females and 30% of males) exhibit some degree of binge eating. **What resources are available to help students who are struggling with eating disorders at your school?** Mark Bowden/123RF

Source: Lipson SK, Sonneville KR. Eating disorder symptoms among undergraduate and graduate students at 12 U.S. colleges and universities. *Eat Behav.* 2017 Jan;24:81-88. doi: 10.1016/j.eatbeh.2016.12.003

COMMON BEHAVIORS OF BINGE EATING DISORDER

As described in Section 11.3, a binge refers to the uncontrolled consumption of an unusually large amount of food within a discrete period of time. A binge can include any food, but most often consists of foods that carry the social stigma of *junk* or *bad* foods—ice cream, cookies, potato chips, and similar snack foods. During binges, food is eaten without regard to biological need and often in a recurrent, ritualized fashion. Unlike those with bulimia nervosa, people with binge eating disorder do not attempt to purge the excess calories.

Binge eating is usually triggered by negative emotions, such as stress, anxiety, loneliness, grief, or anger.[40] In fact, almost half of individuals with severe binge eating disorder exhibit clinical depression. Often, people with binge eating disorder have not

TABLE 11-3 ■ **Diagnostic Criteria for Binge Eating Disorder**

A. Recurrent binge eating, characterized by:
  1. Eating a large amount of food in a short period of time (e.g., within 2 hours)
  2. Experiencing a loss of control overeating during binges

B. Episodes of binge eating are associated with at least three of the following:
  1. Rapid rate of eating
  2. Continuing to eat beyond feelings of fullness
  3. Overeating in the absence of hunger
  4. Eating alone to avoid embarrassment
  5. Feelings of self-disgust, depression, or guilt after overeating

C. Extreme distress about binge eating
D. Binges occur at least one time per week for 3 months.
E. Behaviors are distinct from bulimia nervosa and anorexia nervosa.

Source: American Psychiatric Association, *Diagnostic and Statistical Manual for Mental Disorders*, 5th edition. American Psychiatric Association; 2022.

learned to express or appropriately deal with their feelings, so they turn to food to cope with stress or meet emotional needs. Those who regularly practice binge eating may have grown up nurturing others instead of themselves, avoiding their own feelings, and taking little time for themselves. Unfortunately, unresolved conflicts and unmet emotional needs will resurface. To make matters worse, binge eating itself brings added feelings of guilt, embarrassment, and shame.

Typically, binge eaters isolate themselves and eat large quantities of a favorite food—such as a whole pizza in one sitting—when an emotional setback occurs. Other people with this disorder consume excess calories by eating continuously over an extended period of time. For instance, someone with a stressful or frustrating job might come home every night and graze until bedtime.

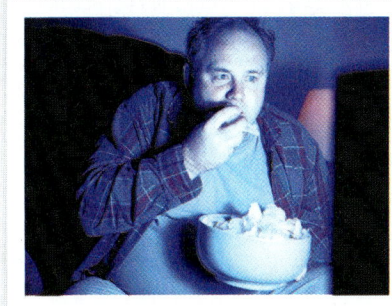

Some experts describe binge eating disorder as an addiction to food. **What are some similarities between binge eating and other addictive behaviors, such as smoking or gambling?** Ryan McVay/Photodisc/Getty Images

Many people with binge eating disorder have struggled to lose weight throughout their lives. As noted in Section 7.5, overly restrictive diets can lead to hunger and a sense of deprivation that trigger binge eating. People with binge eating disorder tend to perceive themselves as hungry more often than normal. During periods when little food is eaten, they get very hungry and obsessive about food. Restricting favorite foods, such as chocolate, leads to feelings of deprivation. When these individuals finally give themselves permission to eat a forbidden food or loosen up a rigid meal plan, they feel driven to eat in a compulsive, uncontrolled way. People with binge eating disorder usually began this cycle of strict dieting alternating with binge eating during adolescence or in their early twenties and have had little success with traditional weight-control programs.

PHYSICAL EFFECTS OF BINGE EATING DISORDER

Although obesity is not among the criteria for diagnosis of binge eating disorder, individuals with binge eating disorder are three to six times more likely to have a BMI in the obese range compared to those without the disorder.[42] The physical effects of the disorder stem from the comorbid conditions of obesity (Fig. 11-2).[40] The most deadly physical effects are listed here:

- Hypertension from excess body weight and high sodium intake
- Elevated cholesterol levels, which contribute to atherosclerosis (binge eating may have a more severe effect on blood lipids than overeating by grazing throughout the day because large meals are linked to high insulin and high triglycerides)
- Cardiovascular disease, which contributes to deaths from heart attacks and strokes
- Type 2 diabetes, which is strongly linked to obesity

TREATMENT FOR THE PERSON WITH BINGE EATING DISORDER

Many participants in organized weight-control programs engage in binge eating.[42] This means RDNs and others who lead weight-management programs may be the first to identify binge eating disorder among their clients. As with anorexia and bulimia, binge eating disorder truly is a psychological problem with nutritional consequences. The success of traditional weight-loss therapies for people with binge eating disorder has been poor because these approaches fail to address the underlying psychological causes of the disorder. While people with binge eating disorder will likely benefit from increased nutrition knowledge, treatment must also address psychological needs. Unless they find a way to manage or overcome negative emotions that underlie eating behaviors, the success of attempts to improve food choices and increase physical activity will be short lived.

The primary goal of treatment for people with binge eating disorder is to decrease and eventually eliminate episodes of binge eating. Losing excess body weight, alleviating comorbid conditions of obesity, and improving psychological disturbances are secondary goals of therapy.[43]

Psychological Therapy. Similar to treatments for bulimia nervosa, there is growing evidence that cognitive behavioral therapy techniques and emotion regulation skills training are useful for overcoming binge eating disorder.[44] Many people with binge eating disorder may experience difficulty in identifying personal emotional needs and expressing emotions. This problem is a common predisposing factor in binge eating, so communication issues should be addressed during treatment. Binge eaters often must be helped to recognize their buried emotions in anxiety-producing situations and then encouraged to share them with their therapist or therapy group. Learning simple but appropriate phrases to say to oneself can help stop bingeing when the desire is strong. Even if negative situations cannot be changed, people must learn how to adapt to and bear with them effectively—not through self-destructive binge eating behaviors.

Cognitive behavioral therapy can be delivered in many forms. One-on-one sessions with a therapist and group therapy are the most common methods. Self-help groups such as Overeaters Anonymous® also have value. Their treatment philosophy, which parallels that of Alcoholics Anonymous®, is to create an environment of encouragement and accountability to overcome this eating disorder. Recently, even web-based adaptations of cognitive behavioral therapy have proved to be useful.[44]

Although psychological therapy has been valuable for correcting binge eating behavior, it is not always successful at inducing weight loss among those who are overweight or obese and who may have one or more other health issues related to obesity. Thus, nutrition therapy is an important part of treatment for binge eating disorder.[43]

Nutrition Therapy. Once effective coping mechanisms are learned, the RDN can educate the patient on developing normal eating patterns and making healthful food choices. First, those with binge eating disorder must learn to eat in response to hunger—a biological signal—rather than in response to emotional needs or external factors (such as the time of day, boredom, or the simple presence of food). Counselors often direct binge eaters to record their perceptions of physical hunger throughout the day and at the beginning and end of every meal. Individuals with binge eating disorder must learn to respond to a prescribed amount of fullness at each meal.

Individuals recovering from binge eating disorder should initially avoid weight-loss diets because feelings of food deprivation can trigger binge eating. Even if exposure to favorite binge foods is limited in the early stages of treatment, many experts feel that learning to eat all foods—but in moderation—is an effective long-term goal for people with binge eating disorder. This practice can prevent the feelings of desperation and deprivation that come from limiting particular foods.

Pharmacological Therapy. Psychological and nutritional therapies are useful tools to treat binge eating disorder, but they are not 100% effective. Thus, there is growing interest in drug therapy.[43] The first drug to be approved for the treatment of binge eating disorder is lisdexamfetamine dimesylate (Vyvanse®), a stimulant that has been used to treat attention deficit hyperactivity disorder. Some antidepressants (e.g., fluoxetine [Prozac®] and duloxetine [Cymbalta®]) and antiseizure medications (e.g., topiramate [Topamax®]) are successful in reducing binge eating. Despite their usefulness for reducing binge eating, these medications still may not induce significant weight loss. Orlistat (Xenical®) and phentermine (Adipex-P®), discussed in Section 7.9, can assist with weight-loss efforts after binge eating is under control. Other weight-loss medications (e.g., semaglutide) are currently being studied for use in the treatment of binge eating disorder.[45]

Given the similarities between binge eating and other addictive behaviors, medications used to treat substance abuse (e.g., naltrexone) are being studied for use among patients with binge eating disorder. Another novel therapy that is currently being studied is Namenda®, which is used in patients with Alzheimer's disease.

Overall, people who have binge eating disorder are usually unsuccessful in controlling it on their own. Furthermore, unrecognized binge eating disorder will undermine the success of weight-loss therapies among many individuals who do seek professional help for weight loss. Health professionals can screen weight-loss clients for binge eating disorder by asking questions about eating patterns, feelings of loss of control overeating behaviors, and feelings of guilt after eating, and then refer affected individuals to appropriate treatments.

✓ CONCEPT CHECK 11.4

1. What distinguishes binge eating disorder from bulimia nervosa?
2. List at least three health effects that may result from binge eating disorder.
3. Why do people with binge eating disorder have little success in traditional weight-loss programs?

CASE STUDY: Eating Disorders—Steps to Recovery

At age 16, Sarah suddenly became self-conscious about her body when her peers teased her about being overweight. She began exercising with online workout videos for an hour each day and found that she had success in losing weight; this was the beginning of her obsession with being thin. Next, Sarah turned to eating less food to lose even more weight and began eliminating certain foods from her eating pattern, such as candy and meat. She increased her water and vegetable intake and chewed sugarless gum to curb her appetite. Once she began dieting, it felt impossible to stop. She enjoyed having a high degree of self-control over her body. Still, Sarah became obsessed with food, even staring at others while they were eating a meal. She occasionally cooked large meals and then refused to eat all but a few bites. By the time Sarah was 19 years old and 5 feet 6 inches tall, her weight had dropped from 150 to 105 pounds. Her family was concerned about her weight status, demanding that she go to her primary care provider for an evaluation. Sarah was not happy about this idea because she worried the doctors would force her to eat and gain back unwanted weight, but she believed that her family would stop pestering her if she went. Sarah did not think she had a problem; she thought she was still grotesquely overweight. She did notice, however, that she always felt cold and was concerned that she had not menstruated in a year.

1. Sarah appears to have an eating disorder. Which eating disorder best describes her behavior?
2. List the behaviors that Sarah developed between ages 16 and 19 that are signs of the development of this eating disorder.
3. What physical symptoms of this disorder does Sarah have (review Fig. 11-2)?
4. Outline the therapies you think the primary care provider will recommend for Sarah. Where could she go for the therapy she needs? Which types of professionals would be involved?
5. Do you think Sarah has developed any vitamin or mineral deficiencies? Which ones would be most likely? How could these deficiencies be treated?
6. What is the likelihood that she will fully recover from her condition?

Complete the Case Study. Responses to these questions can be provided by your instructor.

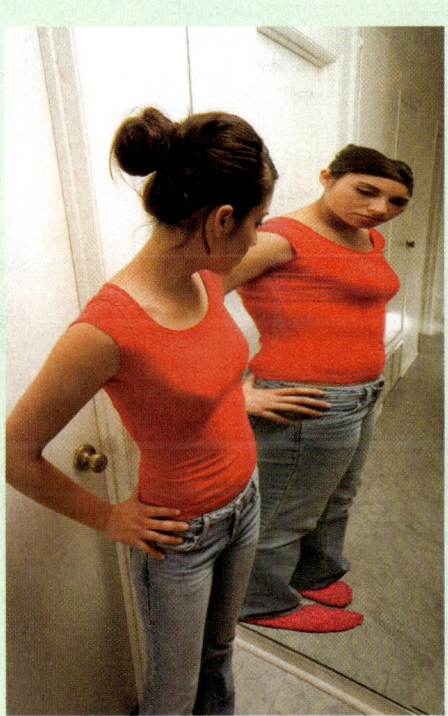

Individuals with eating disorders have a distorted body image. Even though she had lost significant weight, Sarah still believed she was overweight. Ted Foxx/Alamy Stock Photo

11.5 Other Eating Disorders

Besides those already covered, there are several lesser-known types of eating disorders. Some of these, such as **pica, rumination disorder,** and **avoidant/restrictive food intake disorder (ARFID),** are distinct eating disorders with their own sets of diagnostic criteria. Others fall under the *DSM-5-TR* category of *Other Specified Feeding or Eating Disorders*, which encompasses several disorders that do not meet all of the criteria for diagnosis of anorexia, bulimia, or binge eating disorder.

PICA

Pica is a disorder in which a person persistently eats nonnutritive, nonfood substances over a period of at least 1 month. A few examples of nonfood substances ingested by people with pica are clay, dirt, ice, chalk, or wood. Pica could lead to serious health consequences, including microbial infections, poisoning from toxins present in the nonfood material, gastrointestinal blockages, or nutrient deficiencies (in cases when nonfood substances displace nutritive foods in the dietary pattern).[46] Pica tends to co-occur with other mental disorders, such as **autism spectrum disorder (ASD)** or obsessive-compulsive disorder.

RUMINATION DISORDER

Rumination disorder is classified as both a functional gastrointestinal disorder and a mental health disorder. Individuals with rumination disorder experience frequent, effortless regurgitation of undigested food from the stomach within a few minutes of completing a meal. Regurgitation is not accompanied by nausea, the regurgitated food still tastes pleasant, and the individual may continue to chew the undigested food, swallow it, or spit it out. It can occur at any age, but most commonly presents during childhood and tends to occur alongside other mental health disorders, such as depression or anxiety. If left untreated, rumination disorder could lead to esophageal and dental damage, weight loss, electrolyte imbalances, and malnutrition.[47]

AVOIDANT/RESTRICTIVE FOOD INTAKE DISORDER

Avoidant/restrictive food intake disorder (ARFID), which was defined as a distinct eating disorder for the first time in *DSM-5,* most often occurs in the pediatric population and may be mistaken for extreme picky eating (see Section 15.4). However, ARFID is far more pathological than picky eating. Like anorexia nervosa, it is characterized by severe dietary restriction that results in weight loss or failure to grow as expected, as well as multiple nutrient deficiencies. In some cases, the individual may need to rely on tube or intravenous feeding to meet nutritional needs. Unlike anorexia nervosa, however, this disorder is not related to body image or weight concerns. Rather, it seems to be rooted in anxiety, which may or may not be centered around food.[48] Some individuals with ARFID may have experienced a frightening episode of choking or an allergic reaction. Others may be reacting to tension in the home environment. It also tends to co-occur with ASD.[49]

OTHER SPECIFIED FEEDING OR EATING DISORDERS

Subthreshold Eating Disorders. Individuals who meet some but not all of the criteria for diagnosis with anorexia nervosa, bulimia nervosa, or binge eating disorder may fall into one of five subthreshold classifications.[22]

- **Atypical anorexia nervosa** describes a person who meets most of the criteria for diagnosis of anorexia nervosa but whose weight is still within a normal range. This could occur if a person who is (or was) overweight has just begun severely restricting calories. Despite significant weight loss, BMI may still fall within the healthy range of 18.5 to 24.9.

---

pica A disorder characterized by eating nonfood items, such as dirt, laundry starch, or clay.

rumination disorder An eating disorder and functional gastrointestinal disorder in which undigested food is regurgitated shortly after a meal, rechewed, then swallowed or spit out; also called *regurgitation syndrome.*

avoidant/restrictive food intake disorder (ARFID) Eating disorder characterized by failure to meet energy or nutrient needs, resulting in significant weight loss, nutritional deficiencies, or dependence on tube or intravenous feeding; the eating disturbance is not explained by lack of available food, a medical problem, or another eating disorder.

autism spectrum disorder (ASD) A disorder of neurological development characterized by problems with social interaction, verbal and nonverbal communication, and/or unusual, repetitive, or limited activities and interests.

atypical anorexia nervosa A subthreshold eating disorder in which a person meets most of the criteria for diagnosis of anorexia nervosa, except BMI is within a normal range.

- **Bulimia nervosa of low frequency** is a subthreshold eating disorder in which the individual meets most of the criteria for diagnosis of bulimia nervosa, except episodes of binge eating and compensatory behaviors occur less than once per week.
- **Bulimia nervosa of limited duration** is a subthreshold eating disorder in which the individual meets most of the criteria for diagnosis of bulimia nervosa, except binge-compensate cycles have been taking place for less than 3 months.
- **Binge eating disorder of low frequency** is a subthreshold eating disorder in which the individual meets most of the criteria for diagnosis of binge eating disorder, except episodes of binge eating occur less than once per week.
- **Binge eating disorder of limited duration** is a subthreshold eating disorder in which the individual meets most of the criteria for diagnosis of binge eating disorder, except episodes of binge eating have been taking place for less than 3 months.

Subthreshold eating disorders are more prevalent than anorexia nervosa, bulimia nervosa, and binge eating disorder. Like those with full-syndrome eating disorders, individuals with subthreshold eating disorders are at increased risk for physical and mental health impairments, including suicide. Furthermore, subthreshold disorders may progress to full-syndrome eating disorders, particularly bulimia nervosa and binge eating disorder.[50] Early detection and treatment of subthreshold eating disorders could prevent significant morbidity and mortality.

Purging Disorder. **Purging disorder** is the name given to the behavior of people who repeatedly purge (i.e., vomit) to promote weight loss even in the absence of binge eating.[51] This disorder is related to body dissatisfaction, anxiety, and depression. The physical effects of purging disorder are the same as those of bulimia nervosa and include dental problems, mouth sores, damage to the esophagus, constipation, dehydration, electrolyte imbalances, and overall malnutrition.

Night Eating Syndrome. **Night eating syndrome** is characterized by recurrent episodes of night eating, manifested by eating after awakening from sleep or by excessive food consumption after the evening meal. With night eating syndrome, the person is fully aware of and able to recall the behavior, which results in marked distress.[52] This eating disorder should not be confused with *sleep-related eating disorder*, a sleep disorder (like sleepwalking) in which individuals have only partial or no memory of nocturnal food intake.

Although night eating syndrome was first observed among patients with obesity, it also occurs among people within a healthy BMI range. It has been estimated to occur in 1.5% of the general population and in 8.9% of patients treated in obesity clinics; it tends to co-occur with other disorders. Some typical signs and symptoms of night eating syndrome include:

- Not feeling hungry in the morning and delaying the first meal until several hours after waking
- Overeating in the evening with more than 25% of daily food intake consumed after dinner
- Difficulty falling asleep and needing to eat something to help fall asleep faster
- Waking at least once during the night with a need to eat to be able to fall asleep again
- Feelings of guilt and shame regarding eating behaviors
- Feeling depressed, especially at night

Research shows that the circadian rhythm (your body's 24-hour clock) of food intake appears to be disturbed in night eating syndrome. Studies have also shown that night eating syndrome is prevalent among outpatients with sleep apnea, restless leg syndrome, or some psychiatric conditions. Behavioral changes, such as establishing and monitoring the sleep-wake schedule and doing regular physical activity, can help. Symptoms are significantly improved with use of the antidepressant sertraline (Zoloft®).

---

bulimia nervosa of low frequency A subthreshold eating disorder in which a person meets all of the criteria for diagnosis of bulimia nervosa, except the frequency of binge-compensate cycles is less than once per week.

bulimia nervosa of limited duration A subthreshold eating disorder in which a person meets all of the criteria for diagnosis of bulimia nervosa, except the duration of the disordered eating behavior is less than 3 months.

binge eating disorder of low frequency A subthreshold eating disorder in which a person meets all of the criteria for diagnosis of binge eating disorder, except the frequency of binges is less than once per week.

binge eating disorder of limited duration A subthreshold eating disorder in which a person meets all of the criteria for diagnosis of binge eating disorder, except the duration of the disordered eating behavior is less than 3 months.

purging disorder An eating disorder characterized by repeated purging (e.g., by self-induced vomiting) to induce weight loss even in the absence of binge eating.

night eating syndrome An eating disorder characterized by consumption of a large volume of food in the late evening and nocturnal awakenings with ingestion of food.

> ✓ **CONCEPT CHECK 11.5**
>
> 1. List three ways pica could harm health.
> 2. How is ARFID different from anorexia nervosa?
> 3. Describe three different cases in which a person would be diagnosed with subthreshold eating disorders.
> 4. How is purging disorder similar to bulimia nervosa? How do these two disorders differ?
> 5. List three characteristics of night eating syndrome.

11.6 Additional Disordered Eating Patterns

There are several other patterns of disordered eating that have not yet been classified by *DSM-5-TR*, but health care providers report encountering them in clinical practice. Continued research will be required to set standardized diagnostic criteria and establish evidence-based treatments.

ORTHOREXIA NERVOSA

As you have learned about nutrition in this course, you may have changed some of your own food choices. A shift toward a healthier dietary pattern can help with weight management and prevention of disease. However, when strict food rules begin to interfere with everyday life, they can become pathological. Some people worry excessively about the availability of food they permit themselves to eat. The definition and rules about *healthy* or *proper* eating may vary from one individual to another. Some individuals may be focused on reducing fat intake. Others may attempt to eliminate all sources of added sugars. Still others may define the quality of food based on how or where it was grown or produced.

orthorexia nervosa A proposed psychological disorder characterized by an obsession with proper or healthful eating.

Although not currently classified as an eating disorder, **orthorexia nervosa** describes a condition in which healthful eating becomes an obsession.[53,54] The term comes from Greek words meaning *straight or proper appetite*. Unlike cases of anorexia or bulimia, orthorexia does not usually originate in the drive for thinness. Rather, a desire for perfection or purity lies at the heart of orthorexia. Low body weight may be a consequence of orthorexia nervosa, but it is not the underlying motivation for orthorexic behaviors. Such extreme dietary perfectionism may be related to obsessive-compulsive disorder,[55] but individuals with obsessive-compulsive disorder try to ignore or suppress intrusive thoughts or behaviors, whereas individuals with orthorexia nervosa embrace their obsessive thoughts about food and eating.[56]

Recently, an international panel of experts met to propose diagnostic criteria for orthorexia nervosa.[56] These proposed criteria include:

- A preoccupation with eating behaviors and strict food rules that interferes with normal activities of living (e.g., work, school) and social function.
- Experiencing emotional distress or anxiety when confronted with forbidden foods or when unable to adhere to self-imposed dietary rules.
- Self-evaluation is unduly influenced by adherence to self-imposed dietary rules.
- The disturbance in eating habits leads to a caloric deficit and/or nutrient deficiencies that affect physical and mental health.

As experts continue to debate about the inclusion of orthorexia nervosa in the next edition of the *DSM*, clinicians are calling for clear diagnostic criteria and evidence-based treatment guidelines to help their patients overcome this harmful pattern of disordered eating.

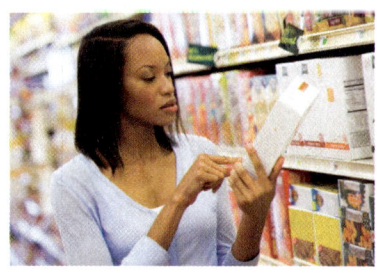

Orthorexia has been described as an unhealthy obsession with healthy eating. **At what point does a healthy concern about eating turn into a pattern of disordered eating?**
Cathy Yeulet/Hemera/Getty Images

BODY DYSMORPHIC DISORDER

Body dysmorphic disorder is a psychological condition in which a person fixates on and has negative thoughts about a perceived flaw in their physical appearance.[13,57] Some individuals with this disorder perceive themselves as *too thin*, rather than too fat, and are preoccupied with strict weightlifting and diet regimens to achieve a high level of muscularity. Among teenage and young adult males, in particular, body dissatisfaction may lead to disordered eating and exercise practices. In the popular press, such behaviors are sometimes called *reverse anorexia* or *bigorexia*.

In cases of BDD, numerous hours are devoted to working out at the gym; planning and eating meals that fit into a certain macronutrient ratio; and keeping meticulous records of exercise, body measurements, and food intake. The dietary practices (e.g., high-volume eating, protein intakes of up to 5 grams per kilogram of body weight), and use of unproven ergogenic aids or anabolic steroids can result in physical impairment. Such exercise and eating routines also interfere with social, occupational, and recreational activities. People with BDD may steer clear of social contact or eating with others because it may interfere with their strict diet and workout plans, and they may avoid being seen without clothes because of distress over appearing too thin. Some experts support recognition of BDD as a distinct eating disorder because of its many similarities with anorexia nervosa and a tendency for people with BDD to cross over to other forms of eating disorders over time.

EATING DISORDERS AND DIABETES

Individuals with diabetes—especially adolescents and young adults—are at heightened risk for eating disorders.[58,59] As you learned in Chapter 4, when insulin is absent or when cells are insulin resistant, cells are unable to use glucose for energy. Weight loss occurs because carbohydrate calories essentially are wasted. After a person starts insulin or insulin-sensitizing therapy, cells are able to utilize glucose and store fat, so weight gain is a common side effect. Individuals with diabetes may also become overwhelmed by a constant focus on achieving perfect numbers: not just body weight but also blood glucose measurements, insulin dosages, calories, carbohydrates, and perhaps physical activity.

Research shows that disordered eating behaviors are twice as common among patients with type 1 diabetes as in those without disease.[60] Approximately one in three teens with type 1 diabetes admits to intentionally skipping doses of insulin to induce weight loss.[61] This practice, colloquially dubbed *diabulimia*, can lead to severe hyperglycemia and its myriad consequences, which include eye damage, kidney damage, diabetic coma, or death. On the other hand, about one in five teens with type 1 diabetes uses overdoses of insulin to compensate for episodes of binge eating, a practice that could lead to dangerously low levels of blood sugar. Among adolescents with type 2 diabetes, up to 25% show signs of binge eating disorder.[62] For youth with diabetes, evidence of poor blood sugar control, frequently missed clinic visits, and the presence of depression can be warning signs of eating disorders.[63]

DISORDERED EATING AND BINGE DRINKING

A pattern of inappropriate compensatory behaviors to avoid weight gain from consuming alcohol—informally called *drunkorexia*—has recently gained recognition in the media and medical literature. This pattern of disordered eating involves compensatory behaviors (e.g., calorie restriction, self-induced vomiting, or excessive exercise) used to offset the calories consumed during episodes of binge drinking. These compensatory behaviors may occur before or after binge drinking. Recall from Chapter 1, binge drinking is defined as consuming four or more drinks (females) or five or more drinks (males) within a 2-hour period.

As with the other patterns of disordered eating described in this section, drunkorexia has not yet been recognized as a distinct eating disorder, nor does it have standard diagnostic criteria. However, several researchers have proposed defining drunkorexia in much the same way *DSM-5-TR* defines bulimia nervosa: a pattern of binge drinking accompanied by inappropriate compensatory mechanisms to rid the body of excess calories that occurs at least once per week for at least 3 months.[64] In light of its similarities with bulimia nervosa, some experts suggest this pattern should be named *alcoholimia*.

Researchers have just begun to examine the etiology of drunkorexia. Like binge eating, binge drinking may be a maladaptive coping mechanism that occurs in response to extreme stress, grief, or traumatic life events. Body dissatisfaction and fear of weight gain also play a role. The behaviors appear to be more common among females than males and are practiced mainly by adolescents and young adults. Reported motivations for these behaviors include both avoidance of weight gain and rapid induction of intoxication.[65]

The physical effects of drunkorexia could be severe. Malnutrition could result from repeated episodes of calorie restriction. Dehydration and electrolyte imbalances induced by vomiting or laxative abuse can threaten heart function. Overlapping these disordered behaviors with binge drinking can only intensify the dangerous effects of excessive alcohol. In the short term, this could include impaired judgment, increased risk of accidents, or alcohol poisoning. Repeated over time, these behaviors can harm relationships, diminish work or academic performance, and damage the liver and nervous system. Likewise, by altering the absorption, metabolism, and excretion of nutrients, heavy drinking may worsen the effects of malnutrition. Indeed, the combination of disordered eating and binge drinking is a double-edged sword.

✓ CONCEPT CHECK 11.6

1. How would you distinguish between healthy eating and orthorexia?
2. How is body dysmorphic disorder similar to anorexia nervosa? How is it different?
3. For an individual with type 1 diabetes, what are the long-term harmful effects of misusing insulin to prevent weight gain?

11.7 Prevention of Eating Disorders

A key to developing and maintaining healthful eating behavior is to realize that some concern about eating, health, and weight is normal. It is also normal to experience variations in what we eat, how we feel, and even how much we weigh. For example, it is common to experience some minimal weight change (up to 2 to 3 pounds) throughout the day and even more over the course of a week. A large weight fluctuation or ongoing weight gain or weight loss is more likely to indicate a problem. If you notice a significant change in your eating habits, how you feel, or your body weight, it is a good idea to consult your primary care provider. Treating physical and emotional problems early helps lead you to peace of mind and good health.

Many people begin to form opinions about food, nutrition, health, weight, and body image prior to or during puberty. Parents, friends, and professionals working with children and young adults should consider the following advice for preventing eating disorders:

- Discourage restrictive dieting and meal skipping. Fasting is also discouraged (except for religious occasions).
- Provide information about normal changes that occur during puberty.
- Correct myths about nutrition, healthy body weight, and approaches to weight loss.
- Carefully phrase any weight-related recommendations and comments.
- Do not overemphasize numbers on a scale. Instead, teach the basics of proper nutrition and regular physical activity in school and at home.
- Encourage normal expression of disruptive emotions.
- Encourage children to eat when they are hungry and stop eating when they are full.
- Provide adolescents with an appropriate, but not unlimited, degree of independence, choice, responsibility, and self-accountability for their actions.
- Increase self-acceptance and appreciation of the power and pleasure emerging from one's body.

These websites provide further information on eating disorders:
- Academy for Eating Disorders, www.aedweb.org
- The National Eating Disorders Association, www.nationaleatingdisorders.org
- National Institute of Mental Health's concise review of eating disorders, https://www.nimh.nih.gov/health/topics/eating-disorders

- Enhance tolerance for diversity in body weight and shape.
- Build respectful environments and supportive relationships.
- Encourage coaches to be sensitive to weight and body-image issues among athletes.
- Emphasize that thinness is not necessarily associated with better athletic performance.
- Support programs for eating disorder screening and prevention at high schools and colleges.

Our society as a whole can benefit from a fresh focus on nutritious food practices and a healthful outlook toward food and body weight (see *Farm to Fork* in this section). Not only is treatment of eating disorders far more difficult than prevention, but these disorders also have devastating effects on the entire family[66,67] and society as a whole.[68] For this reason, caregivers and health care professionals must emphasize the importance of an overall healthful dietary pattern that focuses on moderation, as opposed to restriction and perfection.

Overall, the challenge facing many Americans is achieving a healthy body weight without excessive dieting. A growing number of health professionals support a nondiet approach to weight management. This means adopting and maintaining sensible eating habits, a physically active lifestyle, and realistic and positive attitudes and emotions while practicing creative ways to handle stress. Certain cultural ideals of beauty can trigger eating disorders; increased acceptance of diverse shapes and sizes can help to reduce the pressures predisposing some people to various types of disordered eating behavior. For example, the Health at Every Size® approach aims to fight discrimination against individuals based on body shape and size and asserts that each person should be free to find their natural weight. Females who combine careers and motherhood are saying that they have more important things to worry about. Trendsetters in the fashion industry are tolerating more curves. We cannot change the genes that predispose people to eating disorders (at least not yet!), but we can make a difference in the environmental triggers that set these devastating disorders in motion.

✓ CONCEPT CHECK 11.7

1. Why is prevention of eating disorders so important?
2. Mr. Thomas, a high school health teacher, wants to try to prevent young adults from falling into the discouraging traps of anorexia nervosa and bulimia nervosa. What are some of the topics and issues he should discuss with students in his health classes?

FARM to FORK Apples

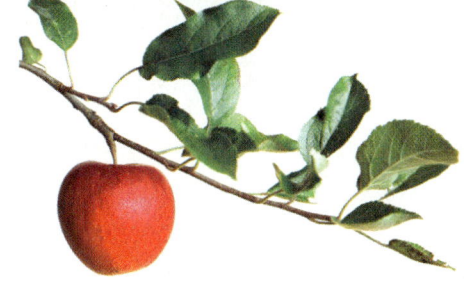

hans slegers/twixx/123RF

An apple a day keeps the doctor away? Evidence does support this old adage! With more than 7000 varieties to choose from, apples offer a range of colors, flavors, and phytochemicals.

Grow
- Small apples (< 2 inches in diameter) are called crabapples. These are quite tart, but they are edible and actually contain more phytochemicals than larger apples.
- Apple trees can be grown from seeds, but the end product can be unpredictable. To ensure a desirable harvest, plant a 2- or 3-year-old tree from a nursery.

Shop
- Common varieties with high phytochemical content include Cortland, Fuji, Granny Smith, and Honeycrisp. For the best phytochemical content, shop for varieties such as Haralson, Liberty, Northern Spy, and Ozark Gold at farmers' markets or specialty stores.
- Among the red apples, look for those with deep red color on all sides. This is an indication that the apples were exposed to lots of sunlight while growing. Sun exposure increases the phytochemical content of the fruit.
- To get the most nutrients and phytochemicals, whole fruit is a better choice than fruit juice, but if you do shop for apple juice, choose a cloudy bottle. Filtering juice removes many healthy phytochemicals. If you hold the bottle up to the light, the juice should not be see-through and there should be some sediment at the bottom.

Store
- Store apples in the refrigerator, preferably in the crisper drawer, set to high humidity. These will last about 10 times longer than apples stored at room temperature.
- Apples harvested early in the season (July and August) can be stored for just 2 or 3 weeks before spoiling, but apples harvested late in the season (September, October, and November) store well for several months.

Prep
- Don't throw the skin in the compost bin! Many nutrients and phytochemicals are concentrated in the apple's skin. If you are concerned about pesticide residues, scrubbing the fruit under running water is a good way to remove most pesticide residues. If you can afford them, organic apples would be a great choice for reducing pesticide exposure.
- Apple skins can be puréed in a food processor and incorporated into recipes for baked treats and applesauce.
- To prevent sliced apples from browning, sprinkle with lemon juice. The citric acid inhibits the oxidase enzymes that cause browning.
- What can you do with crabapples? These small, tart fruits are excellent for use in making jams and jellies or sauces to cook with meats.

Source: Robinson J. Apples: from potent medicine to mild-mannered clones. In: *Eating on the Wild Side: The Missing Link to Optimum Health.* New York: Little, Brown & Co.; 2013.

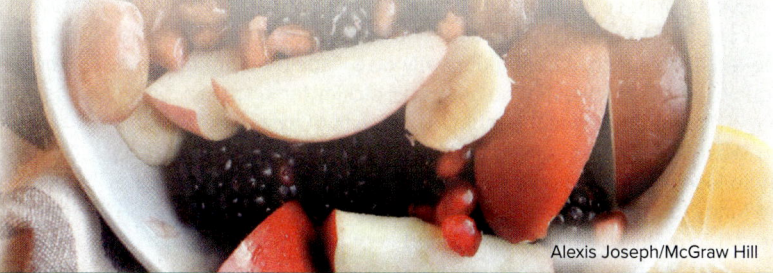

Alexis Joseph/McGraw Hill

11.8 Nutrition and Your Health: Eating Disorder Reflections

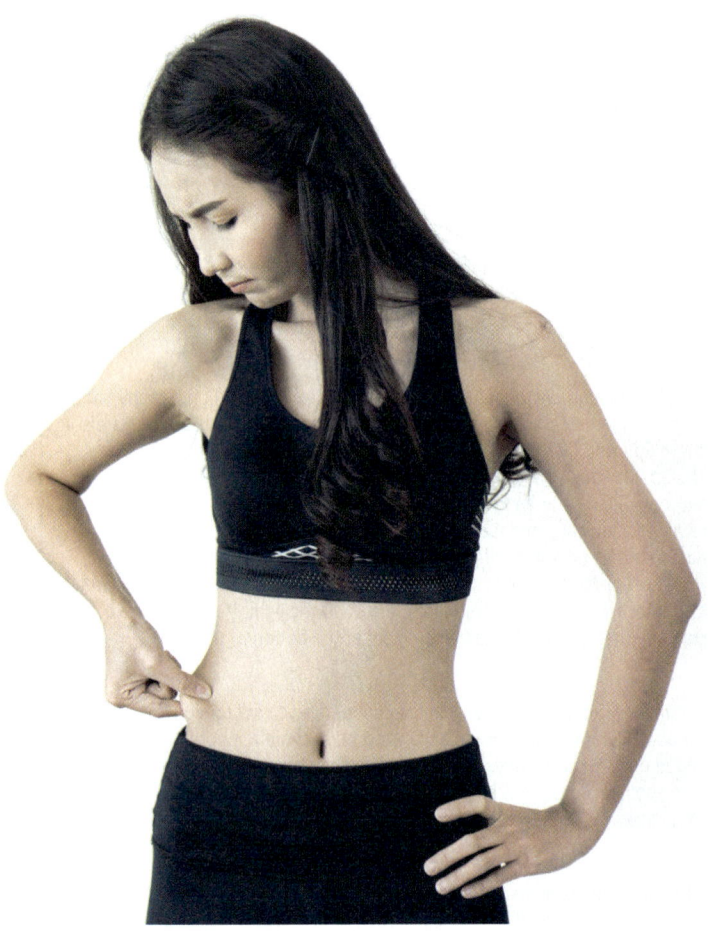
eggeeggjiew/123RF

Reflections from a Woman with Anorexia Nervosa

It was the spring of my first year of high school, and I had just turned 15 years old. I was determined to land a leading role in the upcoming high school musical, *West Side Story*. I thought I should lose some weight to appear more attractive to the student director, Shawn, so I decided to give up *junk* food. The next day, my friend Sandra looked at my lunch, spread out neatly on a napkin before me, and squawked, "Dill pickles?! Who brings dill pickles for lunch in a Ziploc bag?" The other girls at the table fell into a fit of hysterics. "Casting for *West Side Story* is coming up," I said, "and I gave up *junk* food to try to lose a few extra pounds." One of my friends thought it would be funny to give me one M&M—just to smell. Aren't they funny? So I put it in a little plastic container and kept it in my backpack as a reminder. Every once in a while, I did smell it.

For the next few weeks, there were times when I would find myself cracking open the refrigerator door and just staring at what I knew to be a deliciously crunchy, crisp, and cold Kit Kat® bar in the dairy bin. I didn't eat it, though. At the mall, my friends Bridgette and Nora wanted to stop and get a cinnamon bun. They chided me, but I didn't budge. The cinnamon bun smelled so good. But as I sat opposite them in the food court and watched them overdramatize its ooey-gooey goodness, I felt a sense of pride that I could make a decision and stick with it. I could see that they were jealous of my willpower.

When Easter came around, I took a look at the contents of the Easter basket my mom insisted on preparing and turned up my nose at it. I had proven to myself that I could resist temptation … why stop now?

After the musical, I started running with my friend Laura. She was getting in shape for the next season of field hockey. After school, we met in the locker room, changed out of our school clothes, and out we went. The running helped. Every morning, just after going to the bathroom and before getting any breakfast, I would pop onto the scale in my mom's bathroom. One hundred and fifteen pounds and still going. At 5 feet 7 inches, that wasn't too bad.

Cheese and butter had made it to the *no* list by the time I was 16 and down to 105 pounds. Fat-free was my mantra. For my sixteenth birthday, my friends threw a little surprise party for me. Nora, knowing I would put up a fight, made me a cake. "It's your birthday! You can have a piece of cake!" I politely said no, that I would cut it for everyone else, but I really didn't want any. They pestered me, and Nora started to feel offended, so finally I took a few bites, so she wouldn't burst into tears. It had been so long since I'd had so much sugar. I felt bloated and sick. I ate nothing for the rest of the day and only six saltines, an apple, and two stalks of celery the next day. Those foods were on the *yes* list. Salads also were okay but only with salt and vinegar. I told my parents that the dissections in biology class had given me a distaste for meat, but really, I just didn't want all those calories. For a while, I craved food day and night, but slowly, I was getting better and better at holding my ground.

By my senior year, I was skipping lunches altogether, opting instead to hang out in the library and read over my AP bio text. "Where were you at lunch today?" Bridgette would ask later. "Oh, I had some reading to do. The AP exam is going to be tough." At 100 pounds, I was getting closer to finding out what *tough* really meant.

Even though Laura moved out of state, I didn't give up on exercising. Now, my mom's stair stepper in the basement was my favorite. I'd take my biology notes, prop them up in front of me, and step-step-step until I had burned 400 kcal. I felt so efficient knowing that I could multitask. Sometimes I'd exercise twice a day. As senior year wore on, though, it got harder and harder to get up in the morning and put on my tennis shoes. And then one morning, in the shower, I just collapsed under the stream of hot water.

I ended up in this hospital bed with an IV in my arm. At 92 pounds, my body was starving. As it turns out, if you don't give your body enough fuel, you start to cannibalize yourself, in a sense. My body had been so hungry, my muscles had been wasting away, and the episode in the shower was due to a problem with my heart. It's a problem I have created … not my parents or my distant group of friends … only me. My mom was there, next to me, caressing the arm with the IV tube, putting her whole life on hold because of me. Isn't this what I'd wanted—to be in control of my own destiny?

Where do I go from here?

Thoughts of a Woman with Bulimia Nervosa

I am wide awake and immediately out of bed. I think back to the night before when I made a new list of what I wanted to get done. My husband is not far behind me on his way into the bathroom to get ready for work. Maybe I can sneak onto the scale before he notices me. I am already in my private world. I am overjoyed when the scale says that I am the same weight as I was the night before, and I can feel that slightly hungry feeling. Maybe it will stop today, maybe today everything will change. What were the projects I wanted to do?

We eat the same breakfast, except that I take no butter on my toast, no cream in my coffee, and never take seconds (until he gets out the door). Today, I am going to be really good, which means eating certain predetermined portions of food and not taking one more bite than I think I am allowed. I am careful to see that I don't take more than he does. I can feel the tension building. I wish he'd hurry up and leave, so I can get going!

As soon as he shuts the door, I try to involve myself with one of the myriad responsibilities on my list. But I hate them all! I just want to crawl into a hole. I don't want to do anything. I'd rather eat. I am alone, I am nervous, I am no good, I always do everything wrong anyway. I am not in control, I can't make it through the day—I know it. It has been the same for so long.

I remember the starchy cereal I ate for breakfast. I am back into the bathroom and onto the scale. It measures the same, but I don't want to stay the same! I want to be thinner! I look in the mirror. I think my thighs are ugly and deformed looking. I see a lumpy, clumsy, pear-shaped wimp. I feel frustrated, trapped in this body, and I don't know what to do about it.

I float to the refrigerator knowing exactly what is inside. I begin with last night's brownies. I always begin with the sweets. At first I try to make it look like nothing is missing, but my appetite is huge and I resolve to make another batch of brownies to replace the one I'm devouring. I know there is half of a bag of cookies in the trash, thrown out the night before, and I dig them out and polish them off. I drink some milk so my vomiting will be smoother. I like the full feeling I get after downing a big glass. I get out six pieces of bread and toast one side in the broiler, turn them over and cover them with butter and put them under the broiler again till they are bubbling. I take all six pieces on a plate to the television and go back for a bowl of cereal and a banana. Before the last toast is finished, I am already preparing the next batch of six more pieces. I might have another brownie or five from the new batch, and a couple large bowlfuls of ice cream, yogurt, or cottage cheese. My stomach is stretched into

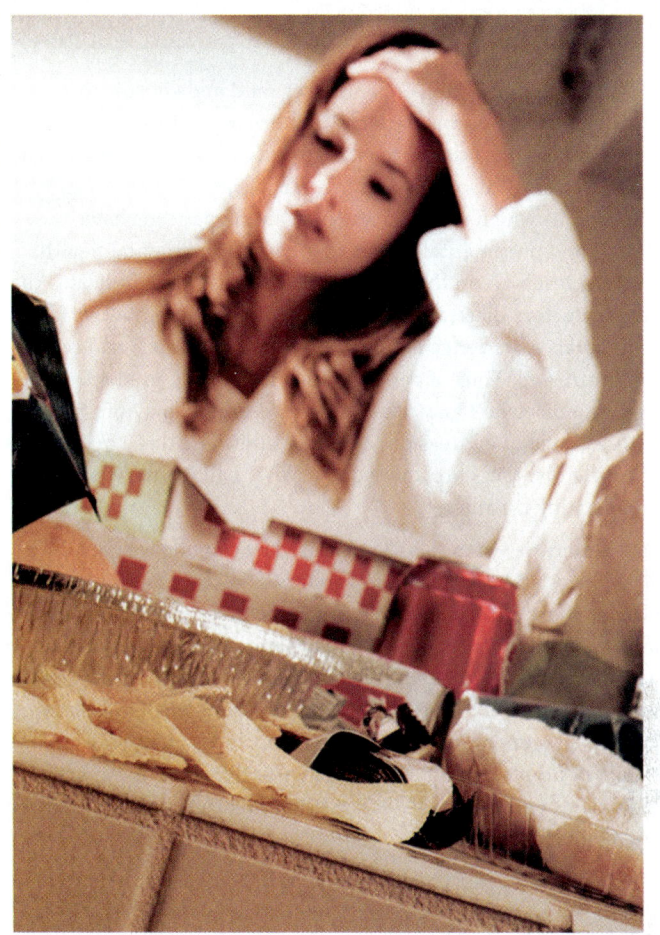

Bulimic episodes add to the despair felt in this disorder. **What are some strategies recommended by clinicians to develop normal eating habits?** Corbis/VCG/Getty Images

a huge ball below my rib cage. I know I'll have to go into the bathroom soon, but I want to postpone it. I am in never-never land. I am waiting, feeling the pressure, pacing the floor in and out of rooms. Time is passing. Time is passing. It is almost time.

I wander aimlessly through the living room and kitchen once more, tidying, making the whole house neat and put back together. Finally, I make the turn into the bathroom. I brace my feet, pull my hair back and stick my finger down my throat, stroking twice. I get up a huge gush of food. Three times, four, and another stream of partially digested food. I can see everything come back. I am glad to see those brownies, because they are SO fattening. The rhythm of the emptying is broken and my head is beginning to hurt. I stand up feeling dizzy, empty, and weak.

The whole episode has taken about an hour.

Source: Hall L and Cohn L. *Bulimia—A Guide to Recovery*, Gurze Books: Carlsbad, CA. Pages xvii–xviii. Copyright ©2011 by Gurze Books. All rights reserved. Reprinted with permission.

✓ CONCEPT CHECK 11.8

1. Which of the diagnostic criteria can you identify in the narrative about the young person with anorexia nervosa?

2. What are the defining characteristics of a binge? Are these characteristics evident in the narrative about the person with bulimia nervosa?

Summary (Numbers refer to numbered sections in the chapter)

11.1 Disordered eating encompasses mild and short-term changes in eating patterns that occur as a result of life stress, illness, or a desire to change body weight. When carried to the extreme, disordered eating may progress to an eating disorder, in which severe changes in eating patterns have lasting and detrimental effects on physical and mental health. Current research on the origins of eating disorders indicates that genetic factors dictate brain biology, which affects how certain individuals experience eating, perceive their bodies, and respond to life stresses. Thus, a person who is genetically predisposed to eating disorders may use disordered eating behaviors to cope with feelings of depression, anger, or guilt. The three main types of eating disorders are anorexia nervosa, bulimia nervosa, and binge eating disorder.

11.2 Anorexia nervosa is characterized by extreme weight loss, a distorted body image, and an irrational fear of weight gain and obesity. Weight loss is achieved primarily by severely restricting food intake. Physical consequences include a profound decrease in body weight and body fat, heart irregularities, iron-deficiency anemia, impaired immunity, digestive dysfunction, and loss of menstrual periods. Treatment of anorexia nervosa includes increasing food intake to support weight gain. Family-based treatment can help individuals with anorexia nervosa establish healthy eating behaviors and body image.

11.3 The disordered eating patterns of individuals with bulimia nervosa involve recurrent binge eating followed by compensatory behaviors. Binge eating is consuming an abnormally large amount of food within a short time period. A person with bulimia nervosa experiences a lack of control over bingeing behaviors and feels extremely distressed after a binge. Inappropriate compensatory behaviors used to rid the body of excess calories include vomiting or misusing laxatives, diuretics, or enemas. Alternatively, fasting and excessive exercise may be used. Vomiting as a means of purging is especially destructive to the body; it can cause severe tooth decay, stomach ulcers, irritation of the esophagus, low blood potassium, and other problems. Treatment of bulimia nervosa includes psychological and nutritional counseling. Prozac® is the only FDA-approved medication for the treatment of bulimia nervosa, but other antidepressants and antiseizure medications are sometimes prescribed.

11.4 Binge eating disorder is the most widespread eating disorder and affects males and females nearly equally. It is characterized by recurrent episodes of bingeing, which cause marked distress, but are not followed by compensatory behaviors. The health effects that stem from binge eating disorder are comorbid conditions of obesity, including hypertension, high blood cholesterol, cardiovascular disease, and type 2 diabetes. Treatment involves cognitive behavioral therapy and nutrition counseling. Vyvanse® is the only FDA-approved drug for the treatment of binge eating disorder. Antidepressants and other medications may also be useful.

11.5 Pica is an eating disorder in which a person persistently ingests nonnutritive, nonfood items such as clay, dirt, or ice. Individuals with rumination disorder regurgitate recently eaten food, and then rechew, swallow, or spit out the food. Avoidant/restrictive food intake disorder (ARFID) is characterized by extremely low food intake that leads to weight loss or failure to grow, as well as multiple nutrient deficiencies. Individuals with ARFID do not restrict dietary intake as a means to control body weight, but rather as a means to cope with fear or anxiety. Subthreshold eating disorders (e.g., atypical anorexia nervosa, bulimia nervosa of low frequency or limited duration, or binge eating disorder of low frequency or limited duration) describe the behaviors of individuals who meet some but not all of the criteria for diagnosis of anorexia nervosa, bulimia nervosa, or binge eating disorder. People with purging disorder practice purging behaviors to achieve weight loss, but they do not exhibit the binge eating behaviors typical of bulimia nervosa. Individuals with night eating syndrome consume more than 25% of their daily food intake after dinner, may have difficulty falling asleep without eating, and wake up at least once during the night to consume food.

11.6 Several additional disordered eating patterns that are not currently classified as eating disorders include orthorexia nervosa, body dysmorphic disorder, diabulimia, and drunkorexia. Orthorexia nervosa refers to an obsession with healthy eating such that overly restrictive food choices reduce the quality of life and cause physical harm. Some individuals with body dysmorphic disorder view themselves as less muscular than desired and resort to patterns of disordered eating and obsessive exercise to achieve a muscular body shape. Individuals with type 1 diabetes are at increased risk for disordered behaviors, such as the misuse of diabetes medication to regulate body weight. Some people with type 1 diabetes skip doses of insulin to induce weight loss but then suffer the consequences of hyperglycemia. Alternatively, overdoses of insulin or glucose-lowering medications could be used to counter the effects of a binge. This practice could result in hypoglycemia. Drunkorexia refers to the use of compensatory behaviors (e.g., caloric restriction, self-induced vomiting, excessive exercise) to counter the calories consumed while binge drinking.

11.7 Prevention of eating disorders is crucial because treatments are expensive, lengthy, and not 100% effective. Encouraging healthy attitudes about eating and exercise from a young age will aid in preventing the development of eating disorders. Those who work closely with children and young adults should encourage acceptance of diversity in body sizes and carefully phrase comments about body weight. Helping children to develop healthy ways to cope with emotions is also important.

11.8 Anorexia nervosa and bulimia nervosa are both biologically based disorders that are characterized by undue influence of body weight or shape on one's self-evaluation. The coping mechanisms (i.e., extreme dietary restriction versus binge-compensate cycles) used by people with these disorders can vary considerably.

Check Your Knowledge (Answers are available at the end of this question set)

1. For 3 weeks leading up to her friend's wedding, Teresa skipped meals and restricted her food intake to 800 kcal per day so that she could fit into her bridesmaid dress. After the wedding, she resumed eating 2200 kcal per day. This is an example of
   a. disordered eating.
   b. an eating disorder.
   c. size acceptance.
   d. body dysmorphic disorder.

2. Factors that could contribute to the development of eating disorders include
   a. genetics.
   b. social pressures to be thin.
   c. sexual abuse.
   d. all of these.

3. The most likely long-term health consequence of anorexia nervosa is
   a. fractures resulting from bone loss.
   b. atherosclerotic heart disease.
   c. esophageal ulcers.
   d. cancer.

4. A serious health consequence related to low estrogen levels among females of reproductive age is
   a. low energy availability.
   b. low basal metabolic rate.
   c. low bone mineral density.
   d. insomnia.

5. Cuts or calloused on the fingers or knuckles caused by using the fingers to trigger the gag reflex are known as
   a. lanugo.
   b. parotid signs.
   c. Russell's sign.
   d. Barrett's esophagus.

6. The *most life-threatening* health risk from frequent vomiting due to bulimia nervosa is
   a. a drop in blood potassium.
   b. constipation.
   c. weight gain.
   d. swollen salivary glands.

7. Binge eating disorder can be characterized as
   a. bingeing accompanied by purging.
   b. an obsession with healthy eating.
   c. eating to avoid feeling and dealing with emotional pain.
   d. the early phase of bulimia nervosa.

8. Night eating syndrome is characterized by
   a. eating dinner but no breakfast or lunch.
   b. the need to eat to fall asleep.
   c. waking at night to purge by vomiting.
   d. consuming all of the daily calories at night.

9. From the following list, select the potential dangers of *drunkorexia*.
   a. Electrolyte imbalances
   b. Nutrient deficiencies
   c. Alcohol poisoning
   d. All of these

10. If you were assigned to speak to a group of middle school students about healthy eating, which message would be best?
    a. Ask students to sort various snack ideas into *good* or *bad* groups.
    b. Illustrate how many minutes of exercise are needed to burn the calories in various snacks.
    c. Advise kids to restrict favorite treats (e.g., ice cream), except as a reward for reaching a goal, such as getting a good grade on a test.
    d. Emphasize that students should eat when they are hungry and stop eating when they are full.

Answer Key: 1. a (LO 11.1), 2. d (LO 11.2), 3. a (LO 11.3), 4. c (LO 11.3), 5. c (LO 11.4), 6. a (LO 11.4), 7. c (LO 11.5), 8. b (LO 11.6), 9. d (LO 11.7), 10. d (LO 11.8)

Study Questions (Numbers refer to Learning Outcomes)

1. A friend asks you if it is okay to "cleanse" the body by only drinking fruit juice for a week. Based on your knowledge of nutrition, what is your response? **(LO 11.1)**

2. Provide an example of the way social or cultural factors may contribute to the development of eating disorders. **(LO 11.2)**

3. Describe some differences between the types and rates of eating disorders among males and females. What contributes to these disparities? **(LO 11.2)**

4. What are the typical characteristics of a person with anorexia nervosa? What may influence a person to begin rigid, self-imposed dietary patterns? **(LO 11.3)**

5. Define binge eating. How does binge eating differ from overeating? **(LO 11.4)**

6. How does binge eating disorder differ from bulimia nervosa? Describe factors that contribute to the development of binge eating disorder. **(LO 11.5)**

7. What medications are currently used in the treatment of anorexia nervosa, bulimia nervosa, and binge eating disorder? **(LOs 11.3–11.5)**

8. Choose one of the subthreshold eating disorders and create a case description of a client with that disorder. **(LO 11.6)**

9. What is orthorexia nervosa? How may social media contribute to this pattern of disordered eating? **(LO 11.7)**

10. Provide two recommendations to reduce the problem of eating disorders in our society. **(LO 11.8)**

References

1. Satter E. *Secrets of Feeding a Healthy Family: How to Eat, How to Raise Good Eaters, How to Cook.* 2nd ed. Kelcy Press; 2008.

2. Streatfeild J, Hickson J, Austin SB, et al. Social and economic cost of eating disorders in the United States: evidence to inform policy action. *Int J Eat Disord.* 2021 May;54(5):851-868. doi: 10.1002/eat.23486

3. Miskovic-Wheatley J, Bryant E, Ong SH, et al. Eating disorder outcomes: findings from a rapid review of over a decade of research. *J Eat Disord.* 2023;11(1):85. Published 2023 May 30. doi:10.1186/s40337-023-00801-3

4. Marks A. The evolution of our understanding and treatment of eating disorders over the past 50 years. *J Clin Psychol.* 2019 Aug;75(8):1380-1391. doi: 10.1002/jclp.22782

5. le Grange D, Lock J, Loeb K, Nicholls D. Academy for Eating Disorders position paper: the role of the family in eating disorders. *Int J Eat Disord.* 2010 Jan;43(1):1-5. doi: 10.1002/eat.20751

6. Klump KL, Bulik CM, Kaye WH, Treasure J, Tyson E. Academy for Eating Disorders position paper: eating disorders are serious mental illnesses. *Int J Eat Disord.* 2009 Mar;42(2):97-103. doi: 10.1002/eat.20589

7. Steinglass JE, Berner LA, Attia E. Cognitive neuroscience of eating disorders. *Psychiatr Clin North Am.* 2019 Mar;42(1):75-91. doi: 10.1016/j.psc.2018.10.008

8. Mitchison D, Hay PJ. The epidemiology of eating disorders: genetic, environmental, and societal factors. *Clin Epidemiol.* 2014 Feb 17;6:89-97. doi: 10.2147/CLEP.S40841

9. Campbell IC, Mill J, Uher R, Schmidt U. Eating disorders, gene-environment interactions and epigenetics. *Neurosci Biobehav Rev.* 2011 Jan;35(3):784-793. doi: 10.1016/j.neubiorev.2010.09.012

10. Rivera HM, Christiansen KJ, Sullivan EL. The role of maternal obesity in the risk of neuropsychiatric disorders. *Front Neurosci.* 2015 Jun 18;9:194. doi: 10.3389/fnins.2015.00194

11. Udo T, Grilo CM. Prevalence and correlates of DSM-5-defined eating disorders in a nationally representative sample of U.S. adults. *Biol Psychiatry.* 2018 Sep 1;84(5):345-354. doi: 10.1016/j.biopsych.2018.03.014

12. Limbers CA, Cohen LA, Gray BA. Eating disorders in adolescent and young adult males: prevalence, diagnosis, and treatment strategies. *Adolesc Health Med Ther.* 2018 Aug 10;9:111-116. doi: 10.2147/AHMT.S147480

13. Mitchison D, Mond J. Epidemiology of eating disorders, eating disordered behaviour, and body image disturbance in males: a narrative review. *J Eat Disord.* 2015 May 23;3:20. doi: 10.1186/s40337-015-0058-y

14. Coffino JA, Udo T, Grilo CM. Rates of help-seeking in US adults with lifetime DSM-5 eating disorders: prevalence across diagnoses and differences by sex and ethnicity/race. *Mayo Clin Proc.* 2019 Aug;94(8):1415-1426. doi: 10.1016/j.mayocp.2019.02.030

15. Sim L. Our eating disorders blind spot: sex and ethnic/racial disparities in help-seeking for eating disorders. *Mayo Clin Proc.* 2019 Aug;94(8):1398-1400. doi: 10.1016/j.mayocp.2019.06.006

16. Campbell K, Peebles R. Eating disorders in children and adolescents: state of the art review. *Pediatrics.* 2014 Sep;134(3):582-592. doi: 10.1542/peds.2014-0194

17. Luca A, Luca M, Calandra C. Eating disorders in late-life. *Aging Dis.* 2014 Feb 5;6(1):48-55. doi: 10.14336/AD.2014.0124

18. Parker LL, Harriger JA. Eating disorders and disordered eating behaviors in the LGBT population: a review of the literature. *J Eat Disord.* 2020 Oct 16;8:51. doi:10.1186/s40337-020-00327-y

19. Joy P, White M, Jones S. Exploring the influence of gender dysphoria in eating disorders among gender diverse individuals [published online ahead of print, 2022 Mar 1]. *Nutr Diet.* 2022;10.1111/1747-0080.12727. doi: 10.1111/1747-0080.12727

20. Kalindjian N, Hirot F, Stona AC, Huas C, Godart N. Early detection of eating disorders: a scoping review [published correction appears in *Eat Weight Disord.* 2022 Feb;27(1):403]. *Eat Weight Disord.* 2022;27(1):21-68. doi: 10.1007/s40519-021-01164-x

21. Morgan JF, Reid F, Lacey JH. The SCOFF questionnaire: a new screening tool for eating disorders. *West J Med.* 2000 Mar;172(3):164-165. doi: 10.1136/ewjm.172.3.164

22. Rowe E. Early detection of eating disorders in general practice. *Aust Fam Physician.* 2017 Nov;46(11):833-838. PMID: 29101919

23. Mento C, Silvestri MC, Muscatello MRA, et al. Psychological impact of pro-anorexia and pro-eating disorder websites on adolescent females: a systematic review. *Int J Environ Res Public Health.* 2021;18(4):2186. Published 2021 Feb 23. doi:10.3390/ijerph18042186

24. Mehler PS, Brown C. Anorexia nervosa—medical complications. *J Eat Disord.* 2015 Mar;3:11. doi: 10.1186/s40337-015-0040-8

25. Eddy KT, Tabri N, Thomas JJ, et al. Recovery from anorexia nervosa and bulimia nervosa at 22-year follow-up. *J Clin Psychiatry.* 2017 Feb;78(2):184-189. doi: 10.4088/JCP.15m10393

26. van Eeden AE, van Hoeken D, Hoek HW. Incidence, prevalence and mortality of anorexia nervosa and bulimia nervosa. *Curr Opin Psychiatry.* 2021 Nov 1;34(6):515-524. doi: 10.1097/YCO.0000000000000739

27. Ozier AD, Henry BW; American Dietetic Association. Position of the American Dietetic Association: nutrition intervention in the treatment of eating disorders. *J Am Diet Assoc.* 2011 Aug;111(8):1236-1241. doi: 10.1016/j.jada.2011.06.016

28. Treasure J, Duarte TA, Schmidt U. Eating disorders. *Lancet.* 2020 Mar 14;395(10227):899-911. doi: 10.1016/S0140-6736(20)30059-3

29. Zipfel S, Giel KE, Bulik CM, Hay P, Schmidt U. Anorexia nervosa: etiology, assessment, and treatment. *Lancet Psychiatry.* 2015 Dec;2(12):1099-1111. doi: 10.1016/S2215-0366(15)00356-9

30. Lock J. Updates on treatments for adolescent anorexia nervosa. *Child Adolesc Psychiatr Clin N Am.* 2019 Oct;28(4):523-535. doi: 10.1016/j.chc.2019.05.001

31. Marvanova M, Gramith K. Role of antidepressants in the treatment of adults with anorexia nervosa. *Ment Health Clin.* 2018 Apr 26;8(3):127-137. doi: 10.9740/mhc.2018.05.127

32. Nitsch A, Dlugosz H, Gibson D, Mehler PS. Medical complications of bulimia nervosa. *Cleve Clin J Med.* 2021 Jun 2;88(6):333-343. doi: 10.3949/ccjm.88a.20168

33. Kaye WH, Weltzin TE, Hsu LK, McConaha CW, Bolton B. Amount of calories retained after binge eating and vomiting. *Am J Psychiatry.* 1993 Jun;150(6):969-971. doi: 10.1176/ajp.150.6.969

34. Bo-Linn GW, Santa Ana CA, Morawski SG, Fordtran JS. Purging and calorie absorption in bulimic patients and normal women. *Ann Intern Med.* 1983 Jul;99(1):14-17. doi: 10.7326/0003-4819-99-1-14

35. Wade TD. Recent research on bulimia nervosa. *Psychiatr Clin North Am.* 2019 Mar;42(1):21-32. doi: 10.1016/j.psc.2018.10.002

36. Ruchkin V, Isaksson J, Schwab-Stone M, Stickley A. Prevalence and early risk factors for bulimia nervosa symptoms in inner-city youth: gender and ethnicity perspectives. *J Eat Disord.* 2021 Oct 21;9(1):136. doi: 10.1186/s40337-021-00479-5

37. Mann AP, Accurso EC, Stiles-Shields C, et al. Factors associated with substance use in adolescents with eating disorders. *J Adolesc Health.* 2014 Aug;55(2):182-187. doi: 10.1016/j.jadohealth.2014.01.015

38. Carcieri E. How a pattern of regular eating can help eating disorder recovery. Verywell Mind. Updated November 23, 2020. Accessed

March 4, 2022. https://www.verywellmind.com/regular-eating-for-eating-disorder-recovery-4109419

39. Gorrell S, Le Grange D. Update on treatments for adolescent bulimia nervosa. *Child Adolesc Psychiatr Clin N Am.* 2019 Oct;28(4):537-547. doi: 10.1016/j.chc.2019.05.002

40. Guerdjikova AI, Mori N, Casuto LS, McElroy SL. Update on binge eating disorder. *Med Clin North Am.* 2019 Jul;103(4):669-680. doi: 10.1016/j.mcna.2019.02.003

41. Guerdjikova AI, Mori N, Casuto LS, McElroy SL. Binge eating disorder. *Psychiatr Clin North Am.* 2017 Jun;40(2):255-266. doi: 10.1016/j.psc.2017.01.003

42. McCuen-Wurst C, Ruggieri M, Allison KC. Disordered eating and obesity: associations between binge-eating disorder, night-eating syndrome, and weight-related comorbidities. *Ann N Y Acad Sci.* 2018 Jan;1411(1):96-105. doi: 10.1111/nyas.13467

43. Brownley KA, Peat CM, La Via M, Bulik CM. Pharmacological approaches to the management of binge eating disorder. *Drugs.* 2015 Jan;75(1):9-32. doi: 10.1007/s40265-014-0327-0

44. Hilbert A. Psychological and medical treatments for binge-eating disorder: A research update. *Physiol Behav.* 2023;269:114267. doi:10.1016/j.physbeh.2023.114267

45. Richards J, Bang N, Ratliff EL, et al. Successful treatment of binge eating disorder with the GLP-1 agonist semaglutide: a retrospective cohort study. *Obes Pillars.* 2023;7:100080. Published 2023 Jul 20. doi:10.1016/j.obpill.2023.100080

46. Miao D, Young SL, Golden CD. A meta-analysis of pica and micronutrient status. *Am J Hum Biol.* Jan-Feb 2015;27(1):84-93. doi: 10.1002/ajhb.22598

47. Kusnik A, Vaqar S. Rumination disorder. In: *StatPearls.* Treasure Island (FL): StatPearls Publishing; November 11, 2021.

48. Norris ML, Spettigue WJ, Katzman DK. Update on eating disorders: current perspectives on avoidant/restrictive food intake disorder in children and youth. *Neuropsychiatr Dis Treat.* 2016 Jan 19;12:213-218. doi: 10.2147/NDT.S82538

49. Bourne L, Mandy W, Bryant-Waugh R. Avoidant/restrictive food intake disorder and severe food selectivity in children and young people with autism: a scoping review. *Dev Med Child Neurol.* 2022 Jun;64(6):691-700. doi: 10.1111/dmcn.15139

50. Stice E, Marti CN, Rohde P. Prevalence, incidence, impairment, and course of the proposed DSM-5 eating disorder diagnoses in an 8-year prospective community study of young women. *J Abnorm Psychol.* 2013 May;122(2):445-457. doi: 10.1037/a0030679

51. Murray SB, Anderson LK. Deconstructing "atypical" eating disorders: an overview of emerging eating disorder phenotypes. *Curr Psychiatry Rep.* 2015 Nov;17(11):86. doi: 10.1007/s11920-015-0624-7

52. Allison KC, Spaeth A, Hopkins CM. Sleep and eating disorders. *Curr Psychiatry Rep.* 2016 Oct;18(10):92. doi: 10.1007/s11920-016-0728-8

53. Dunn TM, Bratman S. On orthorexia nervosa: a review of the literature and proposed diagnostic criteria. *Eat Behav.* 2016 Apr;21:11-17. doi: 10.1016/j.eatbeh.2015.12.006

54. Dennett C. Understanding orthorexia. *Today's Dietitian.* 2018 Feb;20(2):24.

55. Zagaria A, Vacca M, Cerolini S, Ballesio A, Lombardo C. Associations between orthorexia, disordered eating, and obsessive-compulsive symptoms: a systematic review and meta-analysis. *Int J Eat Disord.* 2022 Mar;55(3):295-312. doi: 10.1002/eat.23654

56. Donini LM, Barrada JR, Barthels F, et al. A consensus document on definition and diagnostic criteria for orthorexia nervosa [published correction appears in *Eat Weight Disord.* 2023 Sep 16;28(1):76]. *Eat Weight Disord.* 2022;27(8):3695-3711. doi:10.1007/s40519-022-01512-5

57. Baghurst T. Muscle dysmorphia and male body image: signs and symptoms. *SCAN's Pulse.* 2017;36(1):5-7.

58. Colton PA, Olmsted MP, Daneman D, et al. Eating disorders in girls and women with type 1 diabetes: a longitudinal study of prevalence, onset, remission, and recurrence. *Diabetes Care.* 2015 Jul;38(7):1212-1217. doi: 10.2337/dc14-2646

59. Clery P, Stahl D, Ismail K, Treasure J, Kan C. Systematic review and meta-analysis of the efficacy of interventions for people with type 1 diabetes mellitus and disordered eating. *Diabet Med.* 2017 Dec;34(912):1667-1675. doi: 10.1111/dme.13509

60. Staite E, Zaremba N, Macdonald P, et al. "Diabulimia" through the lens of social media: a qualitative review and analysis of online blogs by people with type 1 diabetes mellitus and eating disorders. *Diabet Med.* 2018 Oct;35(10):1329-1336. doi: 10.1111/dme.13700

61. Wisting L, Skrivarhaug T, Dahl-Jørgensen K, Rø Ø. Prevalence of disturbed eating behavior and associated symptoms of anxiety and depression among adult males and females with type 1 diabetes. *J Eat Disord.* 2018 Sep 11;6:28. doi: 10.1186/s40337-018-0209-z

62. Wilfley D, Berkowitz R, Goebel-Fabbri A, et al.; TODAY Study Group. Binge eating, mood, and quality of life in youth with type 2 diabetes: baseline data from the TODAY study. *Diabetes Care.* 2011 Apr;34(4):858-860. doi: 10.2337/dc10-1704

63. Cecilia-Costa R, Volkening LK, Laffel LM. Factors associated with disordered eating behaviours in adolescents with type 1 diabetes. *Diabet Med.* 2019 Aug;36(8):1020-1027. doi: 10.1111/dme.13890

64. Thompson-Memmer C, Glassman T, Diehr A. Drunkorexia: a new term and diagnostic criteria. *J Am Coll Health.* 2019 Oct;67(7):620-626. doi: 10.1080/07448481.2018.1500470

65. Laghi F, Pompili S, Bianchi D, Lonigro A, Baiocco R. Psychological characteristics and eating attitudes in adolescents with drunkorexia behavior: an exploratory study. *Eat Weight Disord.* 2020 Jun;25(3):709-718. doi: 10.1007/s40519-019-00675-y

66. Fox JR, Dean M, Whittlesea A. The experience of caring for or living with an individual with an eating disorder: a meta-synthesis of qualitative studies. *Clin Psychol Psychother.* 2017 Jan;24(1):103-125. doi: 10.1002/cpp.1984

67. Maon I, Horesh D, Gvion Y. Siblings of individuals with eating disorders: a review of the literature. *Front Psychiatry.* 2020 Jun 30;11:604. doi: 10.3389/fpsyt.2020.00604

68. Schwartz MB, Vartanian LR, Nosek BA, Brownell KD. The influence of one's own body weight on implicit and explicit anti-fat bias. *Obesity (Silver Spring).* 2006 Mar;14(3):440-447. doi: 10.1038/oby.2006.58

Design Element Credits: Fact Check/magnifying glass icon: McGraw Hill; Magnificent Microbiome background image: Alena Ohneva/Shutterstock; Sustainable Solutions icon: McGraw Hill; Roots icon: McGraw Hill; Medicine Cabinet icon: Peter Dazeley/Photographer's Choice/Getty Images

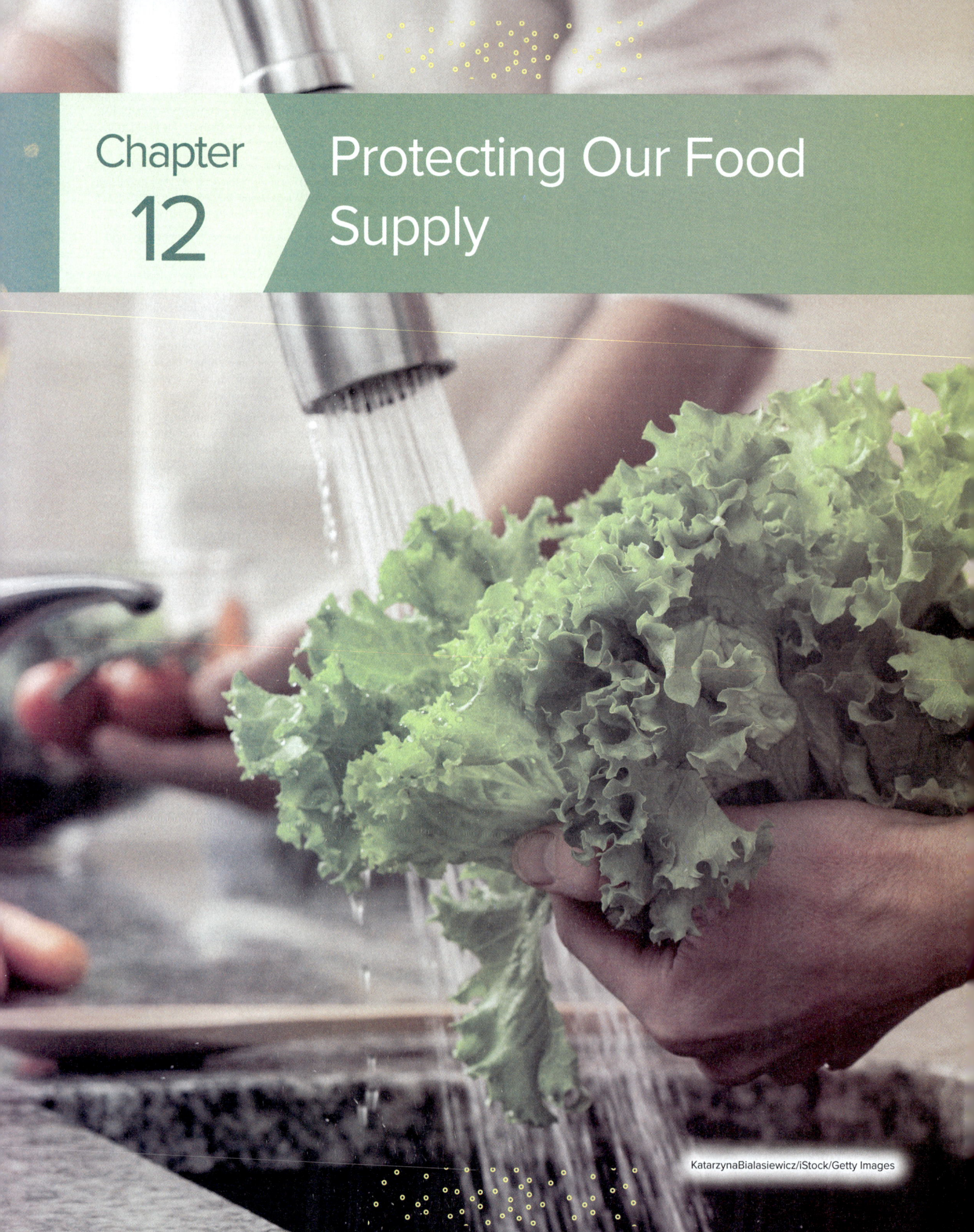

Chapter 12: Protecting Our Food Supply

KatarzynaBialasiewicz/iStock/Getty Images

Student Learning Outcomes

Chapter 12 is designed to allow you to:

12.1 Describe the effects of conventional and sustainable agriculture on our food choices, including the use of organic farming and food biotechnology; explain the benefits of locally grown foods and community-supported agriculture.

12.2 Outline the reasons behind pesticide use, the possible long-term health implications, and their safety limits.

12.3 List types and common sources of viruses, bacteria, fungi, and parasites that can make their way into food; compare and contrast food preservation methods.

12.4 Identify the foodborne illnesses caused by bacteria, viruses, and parasites.

12.5 Describe the main reasons for using chemical additives in foods, the general classes of additives, and the functions of each class; identify natural substances in foods that can cause illness and the consequences of their ingestion.

12.6 Describe the procedures that can be used to limit the risk of foodborne illness.

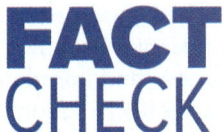

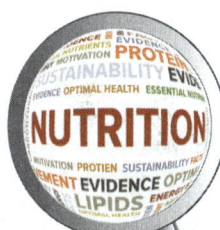

Are organic products worth the extra cost?

In 1940, a British author and Olympic athlete, Lord Northbourne, coined the term *organic farming* and, thus, began the organic movement. After famine led to widespread hunger, Norman Borlaug, an Iowa agronomist, used man-made pesticides, fertilizers, and crossbred crops to save countless lives. This movement led to the Green Revolution and earned Borlaug the Nobel Prize in 1970. Yet it wasn't until 1990 when the U.S. Congress officially defined the term *organic* and established a national certification that sparked an organic bonanza that continues today.

Yet there remains much controversy among the pro- and anti-conventional growing groups. Consumers may choose to eat organic foods for a variety of reasons. Some are trying to decrease their synthetic pesticide exposure and protect the environment. Organic produce typically carries fewer pesticide residues than conventional produce; however, the residues on both organic and nonorganic produce are tested annually by the USDA and remain well below government safety thresholds. Cautious consumers may consider organic as a wise choice for vulnerable populations (e.g., young children, seniors) and opt for organic foods to encourage environmentally friendly sustainable agriculture practices.

Organic produce is more expensive than conventionally grown alternatives. Consumers should turn toward the science to help guide their decision whether to pay more for organic or purchase conventionally grown food. Read more about the nutrient content and cost considerations of both types of food production strategies in Section 12.1.

12.1 Food Production Choices

During the last century, agriculture—the production of food and livestock—has seen tremendous rises in productivity as a result of human labor being replaced by automated technologies, selective animal and plant breeding, and synthetic fertilizers and pesticides. At one time, nearly everyone was involved in food production. Today, less than 1% in the United States are now involved in farming.[1,2] The majority of large farms are in the Americas, whereas smaller farms are predominate in Asia.

Numerous advances in agricultural sciences are affecting our food supply; of particular note are organic food production, food biotechnology, and **sustainable agriculture.** Many of these new developments in agriculture are aimed at reducing the overall **carbon footprint** (carbon dioxide and methane emissions) generated as crops move from the farm to the fork.

Food production is an efficient process. The world is currently producing enough food to feed the global population. Sadly, approximately ⅓ of annual global human food production gets lost or wasted. **Food waste** losses account for about $680 billion in industrialized countries and $310 billion in developing countries. Annually, consumers in more affluent countries waste almost as much food as the entire net food production of sub-Saharan Africa.[3] This chapter's *Ask the RDN* delves into the issue of food waste.

ORGANIC FOODS

The production of **organic foods** relies on farming practices such as **biological pest management,** composting, manure application, and crop rotation to maintain healthy soil, water, crops, and animals. In contrast, synthetic pesticides, fertilizers, and hormones; antibiotics; sewage sludge (used as fertilizer); genetic engineering; and irradiation are not permitted in the production of organic foods. However, many synthetic substances and natural pesticides may be used in organic crop production. See the U.S. Organic Regulations at https://www.ams.usda.gov/grades-standards/organic-standards for more information. Additionally, organic meat, poultry, eggs, and dairy products must come from animals allowed to graze outdoors and consume only organic feed.

Interest in personal and environmental health has contributed to the increasing availability and sales of organic foods. Organic foods are increasingly available in supermarkets, specialty stores, farmers' markets, and restaurants.[4] Consumers can select organic fruits, vegetables, grains, dairy products, meats, eggs, and many processed foods, including sauces and condiments, breakfast cereals, cookies, and snack chips. Direct marketing of farm products through farmers' markets is a growing sales outlet for organic products nationwide. According to the Organic Trade Association, U.S. sales of organic foods exceed $50 billion annually.[5] Canada's organic food and beverage market has also tripled, reaching $6.5 billion annually. Despite this rapid growth, only 5.8% of foods sold are organic.[6] Organic foods, because they cost more to grow and produce, are more expensive than comparable conventional foods.

The USDA's organic program provides a framework for stakeholders on how crops, orchards, and animals can be grown and raised in compliance with the USDA organic standards.[7] The green and white organic symbol (Fig 12-1), displayed on packaging or as a label on produce, is a marketing symbol, and those using it pay a fee and must be able to provide documentation that products and ingredients have been grown or raised according to USDA organic standards. The symbol is not meant to provide any information regarding nutrition, food safety, or health of the crop, animals, ingredients, or product.

Products labeled *100% organic* may only contain organically produced ingredients and processing aids, excluding water and salt. No other ingredients or additives are permitted. Foods made from multiple ingredients (e.g., breakfast cereal) can be labeled as *organic* if at least 95% of their ingredients (by weight) meet organic standards. The term *made with organic ingredients* can be used if at least 70% of the ingredients are organic.

---

sustainable agriculture Agricultural system that provides a secure living for farm families; maintains the natural environment and resources; supports the rural community; and offers respect and fair treatment to all involved, from farm workers to consumers to the animals raised for food.

carbon footprint The greenhouse gas emissions caused by an organization, event, product, or individual.

food waste Food that is edible or fit for consumption which is being discarded as plate waste by consumers and by retailers due to color or appearance.

organic food Food grown without use of pesticides, synthetic fertilizers, sewage sludge, genetically modified organisms, antibiotics, hormones, or ionizing radiation.

biological pest management Control of agricultural pests by using natural predators, parasites, or pathogens. For example, ladybugs can be used to control an aphid infestation.

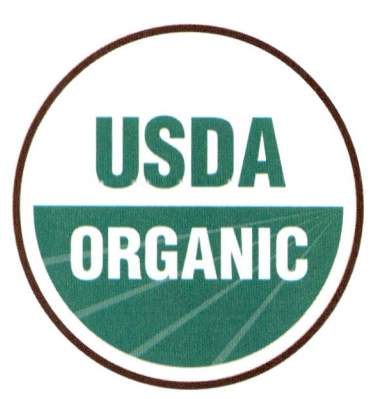

FIGURE 12-1 The USDA organic seal identifies organic foods grown on USDA-certified organic farms. The Organic Foods Production Act of 1990 established standards for the production of foods that bear this seal. Foods labeled and marketed as organic must be grown on farms that are certified by the USDA. USDA

Small organic producers and farmers with sales less than $5000 per year are exempt from the certification regulation.[8] Some farmers use organic production methods but choose not to be USDA certified. Their foods cannot be labeled as organic, but many of these farmers market and sell to those seeking organic foods.

There has been an increase in USDA support and funding for research, cost-share assistance, and other organic food programs since national organic standards were implemented. The organic food market grew exponentially in 2009, when the USDA offered $50 million in new funding to encourage greater production of organic food in the United States. With the additional financial support for farmers and ranchers, the number of USDA-certified organic operations in the United States increased to over 28,200 out of a global total of over 44,900. Because most stores now offer organic products, consumers have the opportunity to compare products and prices. Increased availability and use of coupons, the proliferation of private-label and store brands of organic products, and better-value products offered by major organic brands all have contributed to increased sales.

Organic Foods and Health. Some consumers believe that eating organic food will improve the overall nutritional quality of their dietary intake. In terms of nutritional quality, a large study examined half a century of scientific evidence about the nutrient content of organic and conventional foods. The researchers concluded that organic and conventional foods are not significantly different in their nutrient content or nutritional value.[9] At this time, it is not scientifically justified to recommend organic foods over conventional foods based on nutrient content alone: both can meet nutritional needs. Produce has its highest vitamin and phytochemical content when it is harvested at peak ripeness. To maximize the nutrient content of your produce, either grow your own, buy it locally at a farmers' market, or use canned or frozen fruits and vegetables because they are harvested close to ripeness. A healthy dose of common sense also is important; an *organic* label does not change a less healthy food into a more healthy food. For example, organic potato chips have the same calorie and fat content as conventional potato chips. Our health is affected by many factors including dietary patterns, physical activity, genetics, lifestyle choices, stress levels, tobacco and alcohol use, socioeconomic status, and health care access.

One concern raised about organic foods is that food safety may be jeopardized because animal manures used for fertilizers may contaminate food with pathogens. Although reports of outbreaks of foodborne illness linked to organically grown foods have been increasing, research has not shown that certified organic food has higher contamination with bacterial pathogens. To avoid exposure to potential pathogens, consumers should carefully wash or scrub all produce—organic and conventional—under running water. This safe food-handling practice is critical for individuals with depressed immune systems.

Unlike the term *organic*, the term *natural* is not regulated by any federal agency. Products labeled as "natural" are generally those derived from natural ingredients, such as a plant source, which retain their native properties in the finished product. Meat or poultry labeled "natural" is expected to be minimally processed and contain no artificial flavoring, coloring, chemical preservative, or other artificial or synthetic ingredients. Unfortunately, few regulations are in place to ensure adherence to the policies, and there is debate over what constitutes *minimally processed*. Although all organic products fit this definition of natural, not all natural products are necessarily organic. Also, many "natural" products, such as manure and arsenic, are detrimental to health and harmful if ingested.

FOOD BIOTECHNOLOGY

The ability of humans to modify natural resources has enabled us to improve the production and yield of many important foods. Traditional **biotechnology** is almost as old as agriculture itself. The first farmer to improve stocks by selectively breeding the best bull with the best cows was implementing biotechnology. The first baker to use yeast to make bread rise took advantage of biotechnology.

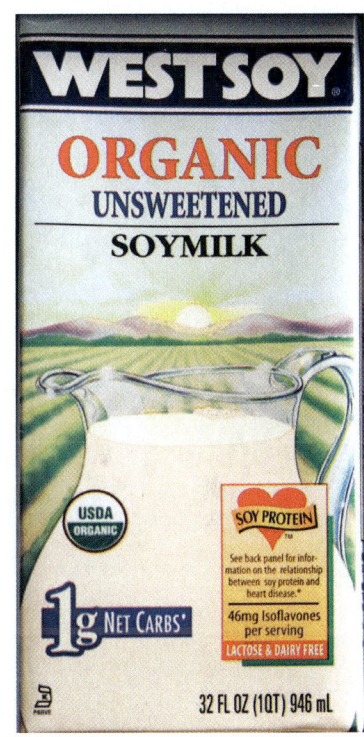

USDA organic products have strict production and labeling requirements. Organic products must be: (1) produced without excluded methods (e.g., genetic engineering, ionizing radiation, or sewage sludge); (2) produced using allowed substances; and (3) overseen by a USDA National Organic Program–accredited certifying agent, following all USDA organic regulations. Andrew Resek/McGraw Hill

biotechnology A collection of processes that involves the use of biological systems for altering and, ideally, improving the characteristics of plants, animals, and other forms of life.

genetic engineering Manipulation of the genetic makeup of any organism with recombinant DNA technology. This includes DNA insertion, deletion, modification, or replacement. Also referred to as *gene editing* or *genetic editing*.

genetically modified organism (GMO) Organisms such as plants, animals, or microorganisms in which the genetic material has been altered by mating or natural recombination.

By the 1930s, biotechnology made possible the selective breeding of improved plant hybrids. As a result, corn production in the United States quickly doubled. Through similar methods, agricultural wheat was crossed with wild grasses to confer more desirable properties, such as greater yield, increased resistance to mildew and bacterial diseases, and tolerance to salt or adverse climatic conditions. Another type of biotechnology uses hormones rather than breeding. In the last decade, Canadian salmon have been treated with a hormone that allows them to mature three times faster than normal—without changing the fish in any other way. In general terms, biotechnology can be understood as the use of living things—plants, animals, bacteria—to manufacture novel products.

Biotechnology used in agriculture includes several methods that directly modify products. It differs from traditional methods because it directly changes some of the genetic material (DNA) of organisms to improve characteristics. Crossbreeding of plants or animals is no longer the only tool. Development of **genetic engineering** began in the 1970s. The field now features a wide range of cell and subcell techniques for the synthesis and placement of genetic material into organisms. In comparison to modern biotechnology, conventional breeding is inefficient and has inconsistent results; biotechnology uses genetic material more precisely. Scientists select the traits they desire and genetically engineer or introduce the gene that produces that trait into plants or animals. The new organisms are called **genetically modified organisms (GMOs).** Only a few types of GMO crops are currently grown in the United States. Soybeans, corn, sugar beets, canola, and cotton make up the largest percentage of these crops.

The primary category where biotechnology is applied is the addition of a unique characteristic, called an *input trait,* to a crop. These enhanced input traits include herbicide (weed killer) tolerance, insect and virus protection, and tolerance to environmental stressors such as drought. Other categories are value-added *output traits,* such as plant oils with increased levels of omega-3 fatty acids, and crops that produce pharmaceuticals. Scientists have engineered plants that thrive with fewer pesticides, potatoes that can be stored longer, and apples that do not turn brown when cut or sliced. In addition, biotechnology allows scientists to create fruits and grains with greater amounts of nutrients such as beta-carotene (e.g., *golden rice*) and vitamins E and C. Biotechnology is being used cautiously and conservatively, so the benefits are subtle. The ultimate benefits, however, could be significant in developing countries given the technology, training, and access.

Few consumers realize that over 90% of corn and soybeans produced in the United States have been genetically engineered to either resist certain insects, thereby reducing pesticide use, or survive when sprayed with herbicides that kill surrounding weeds.[8] Papaya and sugar beet plants have been genetically engineered for viral resistance. Corn has been genetically altered by inserting a gene from the bacterium *Bacillus thuringiensis,* usually referred to as the *Bt gene,* into corn DNA (Fig. 12-2). The gene allows the corn plant to make a protein lethal to predator caterpillars that destroy the crop. The Bt protein in the corn is present in low concentrations with no effect on humans; it is digested along with the other proteins in corn. In fact, for many years, organic farmers have used the Bt bacteria directly on plants to destroy pests without changing the DNA of the plant.

The U.S. Food and Drug Administration (FDA) and the National Academy of Sciences are confident that approved varieties of genetically engineered foods are safe to consume.[10] The USDA has established the National Bioengineered Food Disclosure Standard (NBFDS) to provide a mandatory disclosure standard, by which uniform information for bioengineered foods is provided to consumers. This standard defines *bioengineering* to mean any food (1) that contains genetic material that has been modified through in vitro recombinant DNA techniques and (2) for which the modification could not otherwise be obtained through conventional breeding or is not found in nature. The rule makes no mention of whether crops produced use other gene-editing techniques. Figure 12-3 displays the USDA labels that appear on foods meeting the definition.[11]

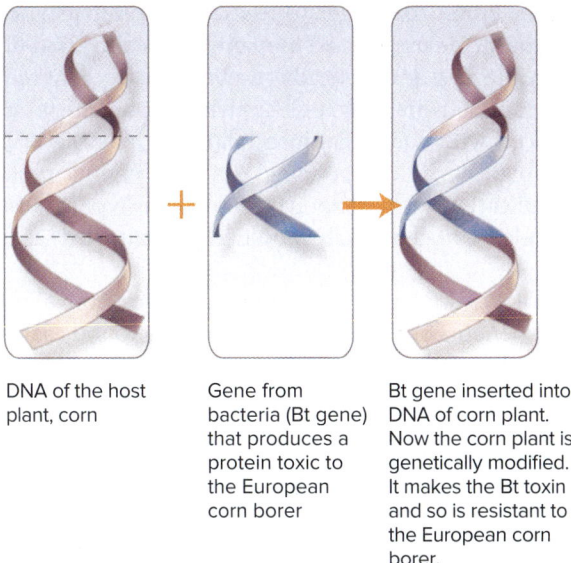

| DNA of the host plant, corn | Gene from bacteria (Bt gene) that produces a protein toxic to the European corn borer | Bt gene inserted into DNA of corn plant. Now the corn plant is genetically modified. It makes the Bt toxin and so is resistant to the European corn borer. |

FIGURE 12-2 Biotechnology involves various techniques for transferring foreign DNA into an organism. In this diagram, a sample of DNA is cleaved out of a larger DNA fragment and inserted into the DNA of a host cell. Thus, the host cell contains new genetic information, with the potential of providing the cell with new capabilities. For corn, this could mean resistance to the European corn borer, a plant predator that feeds on corn and attacks hundreds of crops.

New breeding techniques (NBTs) now genetically modify both crops and animals more precisely. Using these technologies, experts can enhance, silence, insert, or remove target characteristics. CRISPR-Cas9 (Clustered Regulatory Interspaced Short Palindromic Repeats) is a powerful gene-editing technique.[12] It is a natural bacterial defense system that scientists have reprogrammed to precisely target and edit DNA. CRISPR uses a molecular scissors that snips away or inserts specific traits found naturally in the species. At any given time, there are hundreds of CRISPR crops in development with advantageous traits. NBTs and other gene-editing techniques offer advantages over traditional transgenic methods. NBTs have allowed product engineering that has been quickly approved by regulatory systems, including a non-browning Arctic® apple.

Public response to use of biotechnology remains mixed.[13] The biggest debate in the United States surrounds the potential environmental hazards of introducing genes from

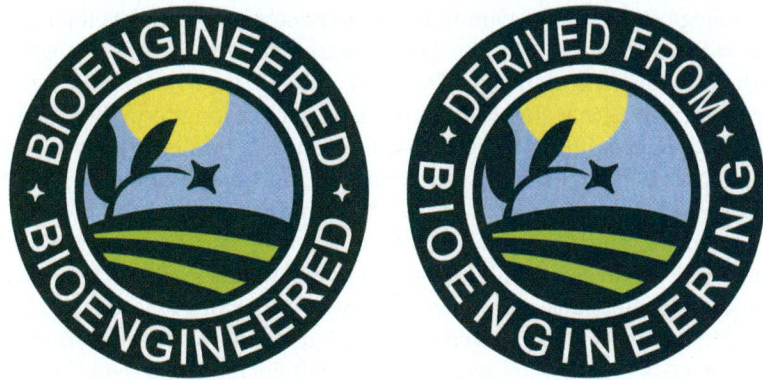

FIGURE 12-3 Retail food products that are bioengineered or contain bioengineered ingredients will carry one of these bioengineered labels. Regulated entities have several disclosure options: text, symbol, electronic or digital link, and/or text message. A phone number or web address is available to small food manufacturers or for small and very small packages. United States Department of Agriculture

one species to another. Some challengers of these transgenic technologies even question the reduction in pesticide use that accompanies the cultivation of genetically modified crops. Although the use of genetically modified crops may reduce the need for environmentally harmful activities, such as applying pesticides to crops, critics point out that seeds produced with additional insecticide, such as the Bt protein, may lead to insect resistance to the toxic compound. Use of traditional pesticides has always required prudent application, in part to avoid the same type of insect resistance. In addition, accidental release of genetically modified animals, such as fish, may go on to harm wild varieties.

A global analysis of 147 studies of biotechnology crops over a 20-year period confirmed the significant benefits of biotech crops. The study found that, on average, GMO technology has reduced chemical pesticide use by over 35%, increased crop yield by over 20%, and increased farmer profits by almost 70%.[14]

SUSTAINABLE AGRICULTURE

Conventional agriculture focuses on maximizing production through the use of large acreages, powerful machines, chemicals to control pests, and synthetic fertilizers to boost growth. A culture of sustainability has emerged, however, including a clear trend for sustainable food choices manufactured in an environmentally responsible way. Sustainable agriculture is an integrated system of plant and animal production that promises, over the long term, to have the following results:

- Satisfy human food needs.
- Enhance environmental quality.
- Efficiently use nonrenewable resources.
- Sustain the economic viability of farm operations.
- Enhance the quality of life for farmers and society as a whole.

In areas such as South America, successful sustainable practices have increased productivity. Sustainable farming practices include the following:

- *Crop rotation,* which protects the soil by reducing nutrient depletion of the soil.
- *Intercropping,* or the growing of two or more crops in proximity, which encourages plants to thrive in varying soil characteristics.
- *Step farming,* also known as *terrace farming,* which increases productivity by enabling planting on hillsides by terracing slopes to hold water for a long duration and retain the topsoil more effectively.

Sustainable Living and Eating. Adhering to a *lifestyle of health and sustainability* (LOHAS) describes a growing demographic group focused on sustainable living. Many of today's college students are joining this market segment and developing behaviors associated with social responsibility. These consumers are driving changes in many areas, including the food industry. The food industry has responded with a move toward *green* initiatives that should be sustainable for the long term. Slow Food USA is an example of a nonprofit group dedicated to creating a framework for a deeper environmental connection to our food and aiming to inspire and empower Americans to build a food system that is sustainable, healthy, and delicious.

Eating sustainably includes reducing the amount of food we waste in an effort to save money and resources.[15] While the global population is growing and resources are becoming scarce, Americans are throwing away an enormous amount of food.[16] Along with all that uneaten food go wasted resources, including water, fertilizer, farmland, and energy. See *Ask the RDN* on wasted food, which includes the food waste hierarchy that can be used to manage food surplus and food waste.[17]

Sustainable Seafood. Seafood choices become more complex when we consider the issue of overfishing and protecting endangered species of fish.[18] An *overfished* species is a population whose survival is jeopardized due to harvesting at a rate that exceeds the

ASK THE RDN: Food Waste

Dear RDN: I've heard that food waste is a global crisis. What can I do, individually, to help solve the problem?

Food loss and waste are undermining the sustainability of our food systems. This is because cultivating, transporting, processing, and storing food is incredibly resource intensive, accounting for 70% of freshwater use and one-third of global greenhouse gas emissions. It is estimated that one-third of global food production is wasted, and in the United States, the estimated range of food waste is 30–40% of the food supply. Additionally, when food waste enters the landfill, it creates methane gas (CH_4), which is a greenhouse gas that is 28 times more potent than carbon dioxide. In fact, if food waste were a country, it would be the third-largest greenhouse gas–emitting country in the world, behind the United States and China.

Reducing food loss and waste is a global priority that even the United Nations' Sustainable Development Goals (SDGs) recognize: SDG 12 (12.3) aims to reduce global food loss and waste by 50% by 2030. Cutting food waste in half can help meet hunger, climate, and economic goals by ensuring more food makes it to plates and not landfills. Perishable foods like fruits and vegetables are the most wasted foods in low-, middle-, and high-income countries but for varying reasons. In low- and middle-income countries, food loss is more typical, meaning that most food is lost before it reaches consumers due to a lack of technologies such as cold storage and transportation. Conversely, in high-income countries, food waste is more common, meaning that most food is wasted in retail, restaurants, and consumer household settings.

The good news is that reducing food loss and waste can be simple. Below are seven ways to start reducing food waste today.

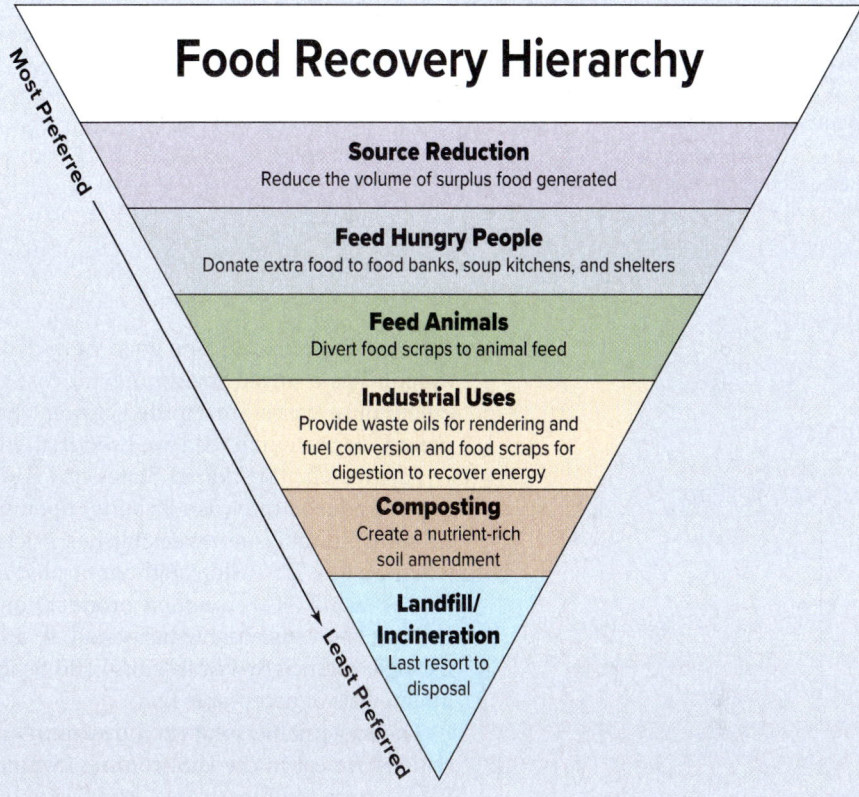

EPA Food Recovery Hierarchy.
Environmental Protection Agency, Food Recovery Hierarchy, Retrived from https://www.epa.gov/sustainable-management-food/food-recovery-hierarchy

1. **Plan ahead and buy only what you need:** Shopping or ordering food with meals in mind can help reduce impulse purchases, leading to a more efficient use of the food we purchase.
2. **Love your leftovers:** Leftovers are inevitable, but wasting them doesn't have to be. Be sure to eat your leftovers by planning ahead.
3. **Understand dates posted on product labels:** Contrary to popular belief, few foods contain expiration dates (infant foods are the exception). Most foods contain "best by," "sell by," or "best if used by" dates. These dates are indicative of quality, not safety. Most often, food is perfectly safe to eat after these dates. Check www.stilltasty.com for a free shelf-life guide for nearly every food product.
4. **Store produce properly:** Some fruits and vegetables give off natural gases, which expedite the natural ripening process of neighboring fruits. Refer to the *Farm to Fork* features in this book and consult a fruit and vegetable storing guide to determine the best possible place to store your produce. See https://fruitsandveggies.org/stories/storage-101/ for more information.
5. **Learn to love your freezer:** Frozen foods are a great option for extending the shelf life of food. Frozen bananas or berries make great additions to smoothies. Additionally, purchasing frozen foods can also be cost saving, as they are often less expensive and just as nutritious as their fresh counterparts.
6. **Donate it:** If faced with large amounts of leftover food, such as uneaten and safe leftovers from a catered event, these foods can often be donated to local food pantries for hungry neighbors. Check with www.ampleharvest.org to locate a food pantry near you.
7. **Compost:** While reducing the amount of wasted food is preferred to composting, composting is a great alternative to tossing food in the landfill. Composting food helps prevent the methane gas emissions that occur when it enters landfills. Compost is also a nutrient-rich soil improvement, which helps improve the productivity of gardens.

Cheers to a healthier and more sustainable food system,

Chris Vogliano PhD, RDN

Food Systems Technical Advisor, USAID Advancing Nutrition, Co-founder, Food + Planet (www.foodandplanet.org)

Sources: 15 quick tips for reducing food waste and becoming a food hero. food and Agriculture Organization of the United Nations. September 29, 2020. Accessed January 20, 2022. https://www.fao.org/fao-stories/article/en/c/1309609/

Flanagan K, Robertson K, Hanson C. Waste: setting a global action agenda. World Resources Institute. August 28, 2019. Accessed January 20, 2022. https://www.wri.org/research/reducing-food-loss-and-waste-setting-global-action-agenda

Food loss and waste. U.S. Food & Drug Administration. Updated November 19, 2021. Accessed January 20, 2022. https://www.fda.gov/food/consumers/food-loss-and-waste

Food waste FAQs. U.S. Department of Agriculture. Accessed January 20, 2022. https://www.usda.gov/foodlossandwaste/faqs

Tips to reduce food waste. U.S. Food & Drug Administration. Accessed January 20, 2022. https://www.fda.gov/food/consumers/tips-reduce-food-waste

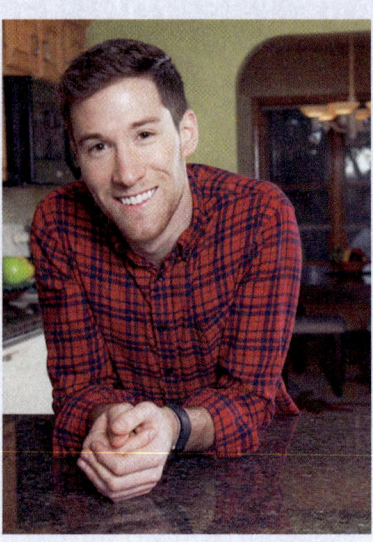

Melissa Olson

replenishing of stock. The good news is that fish production, whether farmed or wild caught, has a lower environmental cost compared to the production of meats. Fewer greenhouse gases are emitted, fewer chemicals and antibiotics are used, and fewer pounds of protein in feed are used than in beef, pork, or poultry production.

Fortunately, the United States has rigorous standards and closely monitors its fishing and aquaculture (fish farming) operations. The National Oceanic and Atmospheric Administration Fisheries establishes strict fishing catch levels in U.S. waters. As a result, when we buy U.S. wild-caught or farmed fish, we are making a sustainable choice. Look for the words "U.S. seafood product" on fish labels to ensure that the fish or shellfish has been sustainably harvested. In addition, groups such as the Natural Resources Defense Council (www.nrdc.org) and Seafood Watch (www.seafoodwatch.org) regularly update lists of acceptable fish.

The sustainable solution, however, is not that simple, with over 70% to 85% of the seafood we eat in the U.S. coming from international sources.[19] About half of this seafood is from Southeast Asia, and a significant portion of the seafood caught by American fishermen is exported overseas for processing and then reimported back to the U.S.

U.S. adults also have a limited seafood palate, with only 10 species making up 74% of the seafood we eat.[20] Fortunately, four of the most popular fish/seafood—shrimp, salmon, tilapia, and pangasius (a genus of catfish)—are largely raised by certified and sustainable aquaculture operations. For example, salmon must be farmed to supply two-thirds of the 400 million tons of salmon that Americans consume annually.[21] While many consumers perceive that wild-caught fish are the more environmentally friendly variety, many unregulated wild-caught fishing harvests have reached their peak capacity and are threatening future global seafood supplies. While sustainable seafood sourcing remains complex, both farmed and wild-caught fish can be healthy, sustainable, and economical choices.

LOCALLY GROWN FOODS

Consumers are demanding increased transparency in the food supply, and local food helps answer questions about where food comes from and how it was grown. *Glocalization* refers to the interaction between globalization that adapts to unique local needs and conditions. As consumers become more concerned and attentive to the global supply chain, retailers are responding. The *locally grown* label addresses consumer desires for fresh, safe products that also support small, local farmers and help the environment. Local products typically provide fresher options, do not have the added costs of long transportation, and thus use less fossil fuel. Food-service establishments

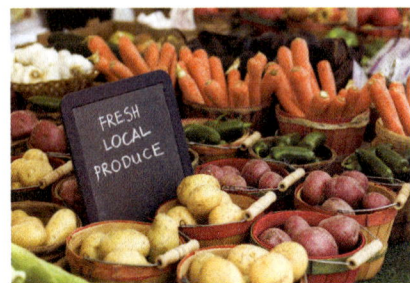

The locavore movement is based on the assumption that local products are more nutritious and taste better, and it encourages consumers to buy from farmers' markets or produce their own food. Arina P Habich/Shutterstock

are also placing greater emphasis on supporting local producers, encouraging a farm-to-fork approach.

Typically, consumers have had access to locally grown farm-fresh produce at farmers' markets. These markets are also an integral part of the way that urban communities are linked to farms and continue to gain popularity. There are almost 8600 farmers' markets listed in the USDA's *National Farmers Market Directory*. Visit https://www.ams.usda.gov/local-food-directories/farmersmarkets to find a farmers' market near you.

A **locavore** is defined as someone who eats food grown or produced locally or within a certain radius from home, such as 50, 100, or 150 miles. The locavore movement has gained prominence due to consumers' food-safety concerns and the search for local, sustainable foods. It also encourages consumers to buy from farmers' markets or produce their own food, with the argument that fresh, local products are more nutritious and taste better.

There is no evidence, however, that locally grown products are safer. Although many small producers have proper food-safety practices, they often lack the expensive food-safety audits that are more common among big producers. Food-safety auditors evaluate evidence of insects on produce, sanitation practices, and similar food-safety criteria. Undetected foodborne illness outbreaks are more likely with *local* products delivered in small quantities and sold in a small area. Local products are not necessarily pesticide free and may not be cheaper, given that smaller growers lack the economic advantages of bigger growers.

Unlike organic products, there are no federal regulations specifying the meaning of *locally grown*. Searchable databases and mapping resources such as MarketMaker (https://foodmarketmaker.com) are available to connect growers with buyers, restaurants with distributors, and consumers with local farmers' markets. These tools make it easier for people to find and sell locally grown foods. Positive attitudes toward organic, local, and sustainable food production practices are on the rise and appear to be increasing the conversations around the quality of dietary patterns. For example, a study of college students in Minnesota showed that students who put a high importance on alternative food production methods had a higher-quality dietary pattern. They consumed more fruits and vegetables and dietary fiber, fewer added sugars and sugar-sweetened drinks, and less fat.[22]

locavore Someone who eat locally grown food whenever possible.

hydroponics This type of agriculture involves growing plants in a nutrient solution root medium in a controlled, soilless environment.

COMMUNITY-SUPPORTED AGRICULTURE

Consumers are not only taking comfort in knowing where their food comes from but also are becoming interested in community connections with local and regional farmers. Stemming from the interest in locally grown food, there is growing national support for local food collaboratives and community-supported agriculture (CSA). CSA programs involve a partnership between local food producers and consumers. During each growing season, CSA farmers offer a share of foods to individuals, families, or companies that have pledged support to the CSA either financially and/or by working for the CSA.

Another example of a farm–community partnership is the National Farm to School Network, a nonprofit effort to connect farmers with nearby school (K–12) cafeterias. The objectives of this program are to serve healthy meals in school cafeterias; improve student nutrition; provide agriculture, health, and nutrition education opportunities; and support local and regional farmers. Since 1997, this program has grown from only 6 local programs to over 42,500 in all 50 states (or 42% of U.S. schools), incorporating the local bounty into their menus.[23] Administrators of the program have found that if children can meet the farmer who actually grew the food, they are much more likely to eat it.

✓ CONCEPT CHECK 12.1

1. What are the basic requirements for foods to be labeled as *organic*?
2. What two characteristics define a food as *bioengineered* according to the National Bioengineered Food Disclosure Standard (NBFDS)?
3. What is the definition of *sustainable agriculture*?

 Sustainable Solutions

Hydroponics

The sustainable practice of **hydroponics** is an alternative agricultural practice that involves growing plants in soilless and nutrient-rich root media in a variety of controlled environments, including gutters, pipes, and other space-saving and inexpensive containers. The benefits of hydroponics include rapid plant growth with greater yields, reduced food and water waste, plants free of weeds and soil-borne diseases, and the flexibility to farm in small spaces—perfect for students and urban dwellers! While we acknowledge that hydroponic farming is not meant to replace traditional farming techniques, it is a piece of the puzzle of finding sustainable solutions in a changing ecosystem.

12.2 Environmental Contaminants in Food

It typically takes multiple steps to get food from the farm or fishery to the table. We call these steps the food production chain (Fig. 12-4). Contamination can occur at any point along the supply chain—during production, processing, distribution, or preparation.

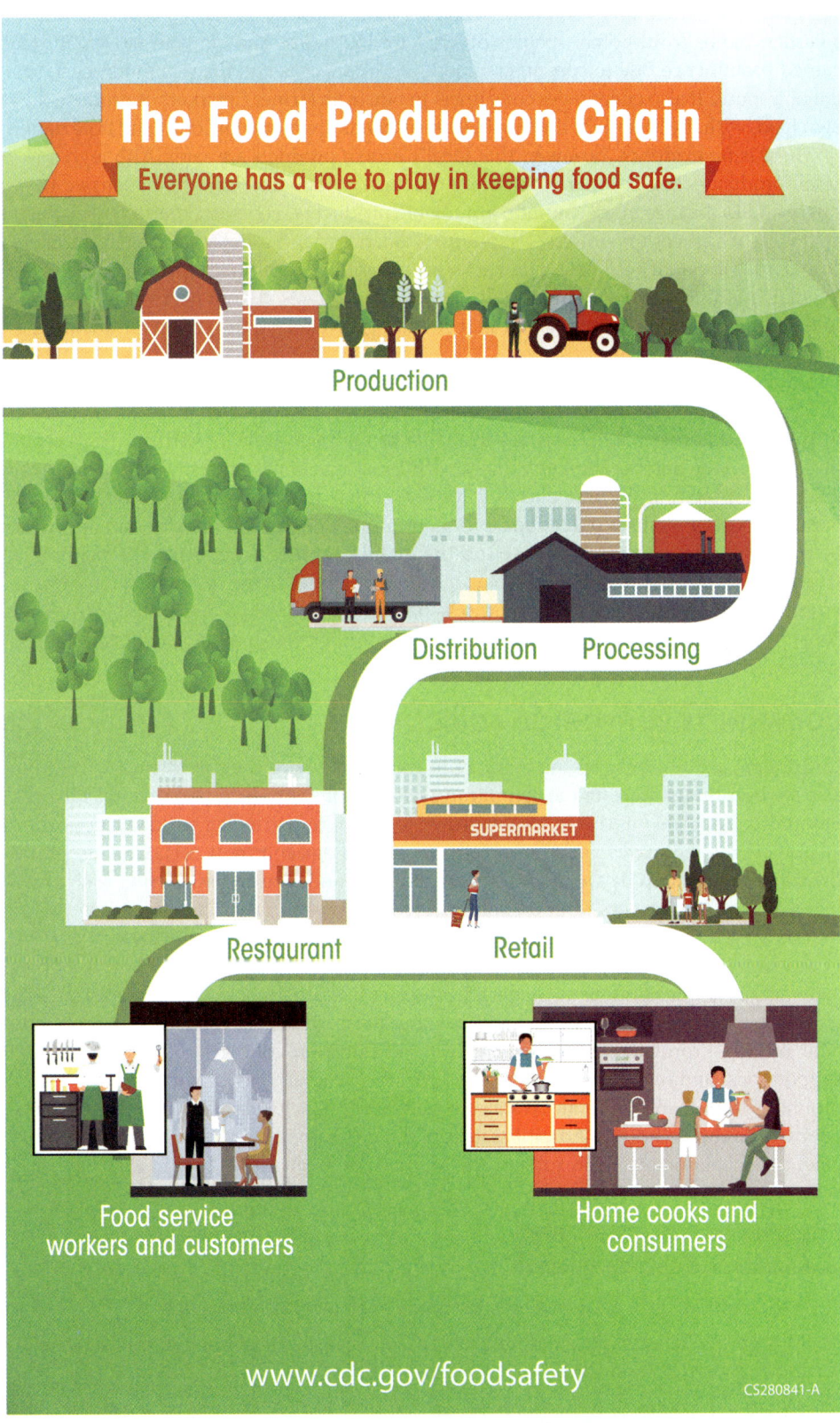

FIGURE 12-4 Food production chain. Along the food production chain, food may be mishandled. Once contamination occurs, further mishandling can make a foodborne illness more likely. How Food Gets Contaminated—The Food Production Chain. CDC

TABLE 12-1 ■ Potential Environmental Contaminants in Our Food Supply

Chemical Substance	Sources	Toxic Effects	Preventive Measures
Acrylamide	Fried foods rich in carbohydrate cooked at high temperatures for extended periods	Known carcinogen for laboratory animals; not been proven to be carcinogenic in humans	Limit intake of deep-fat-fried foods rich in carbohydrate.
Bisphenol A (BPA)	Leaching of BPA from plastic food and beverage packages	Reproductive and developmental defects in animals	Use BPA-free products. Do not microwave plastic containers. Avoid plastic packaging with recycle codes 3 and 7.
Cadmium	Plants grown in soil rich in cadmium. Clams, shellfish, tobacco smoke. Occupational exposure	Kidney disease. Liver disease. Bone deformities. Lung disease (when inhaled)	Consume a wide variety of foods, including seafood sources.
Dioxin	Trash-burning incinerators. Fat from animals exposed to dioxin via water or soil	Abnormal reproduction and fetal/infant development. Immune suppression. Cancer in laboratory animals	Pay attention to warnings of dioxin risks. Consume a variety of fish from diverse water sources.
Lead	Contaminated water. Lead-based paint chips and dust in older homes. Occupational exposure. Galvanized or tin containers or leaded glass. Some solder in copper pipes. Mexican pottery. Some imported herbal remedies. Leaded glass decanters	Anemia. Kidney disease. Nervous system damage (fatigue and changes in behavior). Learning impairments in childhood	Avoid paint chips and related dust in older homes. Meet iron and calcium needs. Use glass, plastic, or waxed paper containers. Let water run 1 to 2 minutes if off for more than 2 hours. Use cold water for cooking. Do not soften drinking water. Do not store alcohol in leaded glass.
Mercury	Swordfish, shark, king mackerel, and tilefish. Fresh and canned albacore tuna is also a possible source (chunk light tuna is very low in mercury)	Reduced fetal/child development. Birth defects. Toxic to nervous system	Avoid affected food. Females who are pregnant or breastfeeding and young children should avoid. Two to three fish meals per week is appropriate for females who are pregnant (or nursing) if different types of fish are eaten.
Polychlorinated biphenyls (PCBs)	Fish from the Great Lakes and Hudson River Valley. Farmed salmon are a possible source	Cancer in laboratory animals. Potential for liver, immune, and reproductive disorders	Pay attention to warnings of PCB contamination. Choose a variety of fish from diverse water sources.
Urethane	Alcoholic beverages such as sherry, bourbon, sake, and fruit brandies	Cancer in laboratory animals	Avoid typical sources.

Source: Adapted from NIH US Library of Medicine TOXNET.

A variety of environmental contaminants can be found in foods. Aside from pesticide residues, other potential contaminants are listed in Table 12-1. An approach to minimize exposure to environmental contaminants includes following safe food-handing procedures and consuming a wide variety of foods in moderation.

WHAT IS A PESTICIDE?

Federal law defines a pesticide as any substance or mixture of substances intended to prevent, destroy, repel, or mitigate any pest. The built-in toxic properties of pesticides lead to the possibility that other, nontarget organisms, including humans, might also be harmed. The term *pesticide* tends to be used as a generic reference to many types of products, including insecticides (to kill insects), herbicides (to kill weeds), rodenticides (to kill rodents), and fungicides (to control fungi, mold, and mildew). A pesticide product may be chemical or bacterial, natural or synthetic.

For agriculture, the Environmental Protection Agency (EPA) allows about 10,000 pesticides to be used, containing about 375 active ingredients. The EPA reports that

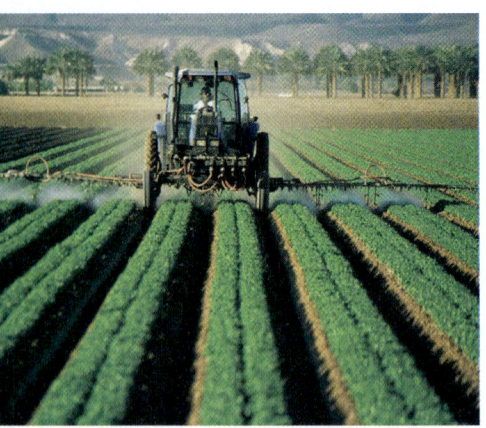

There are risks and benefits associated with pesticide use. The greatest short-term risk is in rural communities, where exposure is more direct. Jeff Vanuga/USDA Natural Resources Conservation Service

over 1.2 billion pounds of agricultural pesticide are used annually, with herbicides being the most widely used type.

Once a pesticide is applied, it can turn up in a number of unintended and unwanted places. It may be carried in the air and dust by wind currents, remain in the soil attached to soil particles, be taken up by organisms in the soil, decompose to other compounds, be taken up by plant roots, enter the groundwater, or invade aquatic habitats. Each is a route to the food chain; some are more direct than others. Another concern is that pesticides are the probable cause of *massive colony collapse disorder* (CCD). CCD occurs when bees disappear from the colony and then die off en masse. This has been an ongoing concern and is a critical issue for our food supply because one-third of all foods and beverages come from crops pollinated by honeybees.

WHY USE PESTICIDES?

Pesticides used in food production yield both beneficial and unwanted effects. Most health authorities believe that the benefits far outweigh the risks. Pesticides help ensure a safe and adequate food supply and help make foods available at reasonable cost. Nevertheless, many consumers consider organic foods safer than conventional foods based on the lack of pesticide use.

The primary reason for using pesticides is economic: the use of agricultural chemicals increases production and lowers the cost of food, at least in the short run. Many farmers believe that it would be impossible to stay in business without pesticides.

VALUE OF HERBICIDES, INSECTICIDES, AND FUNGICIDES IN U.S. CROP PRODUCTION

In the U.S., pesticides save approximately $60 billion on crops that otherwise would be lost to pest destruction. This is a net return of $6.50 for every $1.00 that growers spent on pesticides and their application.[24] Farmers also rely more on pesticides to produce cosmetically attractive fruits and vegetables.

Most concern about pesticide residues in food appropriately focuses on long-term toxicity because the amounts of residue present, if any, are extremely small. These low concentrations found in foods are not known to produce adverse effects in the short term, although harm has been caused by high amounts that result from accidents or misuse. For humans, pesticides pose a danger mainly in their cumulative effects, so their threats to health are difficult to determine. The contamination of underground water supplies and destruction of wildlife habitats indicate that pesticide use should be reduced. The U.S. federal government and many farmers are working toward that end. The use of biotechnology to reduce pesticide use is one alternative.

REGULATION OF PESTICIDES

The responsibility for ensuring that residues of pesticides in foods are below amounts that pose a danger to health is shared by the FDA, the EPA, and the Food Safety and Inspection Service (FSIS) of the USDA in the United States. Table 12-2 lists the roles of various food protection agencies. The FDA is responsible for enforcing pesticide tolerances in all foods except meat, poultry, and certain egg products, which are monitored by the USDA. A newly proposed pesticide must be tested extensively, perhaps over 10 years or more, before it is approved for use. The EPA must decide that the pesticide causes no unreasonable adverse effects on people and the environment and that benefits of use outweigh the risks. The FDA tests thousands of raw products each year for pesticide residues. Note that a pesticide residue is considered illegal in this case if it has not been approved for use on the crop in question or if the amount used exceeds the allowed tolerance.

HOW SAFE ARE PESTICIDES?

The USDA Pesticide Data Program collects data on pesticide residues in food, particularly foods most likely consumed by infants and children. For the most recent samples tested, nearly 99% of all samples tested had residues below the tolerances established by the

TABLE 12-2 ■ **Agencies Responsible for Monitoring the U.S. Food Supply***

Agency	Responsibilities
U.S. Department of Agriculture (USDA) Food Safety and Inspection Service (FSIS) www.fsis.usda.gov	The FSIS ensures that the nation's commercial supply of meat, poultry, and egg products is safe, wholesome, and correctly labeled and packaged.
Food and Drug Administration (FDA) www.fda.gov	Protects consumers against impure, unsafe, and fraudulently labeled products. Sets standards for specific foods. The FDA Center for Food Safety and Applied Nutrition (CFSAN) regulates foods other than the meat, poultry, and egg products regulated by the FSIS.
Centers for Disease Control and Prevention (CDC) National Outbreak Reporting System (NORS) https://wwwn.cdc.gov/norsdashboard	Leads federal efforts to gather data on foodborne illnesses, investigate foodborne illnesses and outbreaks, and monitor the effectiveness of prevention and control efforts in reducing foodborne illnesses. Plays a key role in building state and local health department capacity to support foodborne disease surveillance and outbreak response.
Environmental Protection Agency (EPA) www.epa.gov	Regulates pesticides. Establishes water-quality standards.
National Marine Fisheries Service or NOAA Fisheries www.nmfs.noaa.gov	Domestic and international conservation and management of living marine resources. Voluntary seafood inspection program; can use official mark to show federal inspection.
Bureau of Alcohol, Tobacco, Firearms and Explosives (ATF) www.atf.gov	Enforces laws on alcoholic beverages.
State and local governments www.FoodSafety.gov	Regulate milk safety. Monitor food industry within their borders. Inspect food-related establishments.

*Government agencies responsible for monitoring food safety in Canada and the specific laws followed can be found at http://www.inspection.gc.ca.

EPA, with 42.5% having no detectable pesticide residues. These findings are consistent with previous evidence showing that, in general, pesticide residues in food are well below EPA tolerances, confirming the safety of the food supply relative to pesticide residues. Visit the EPA website (https://www.epa.gov) for more information about pesticides and food.

Dangers from exposure to pesticides through food depend on how potent the chemical toxin is, how concentrated it is in the food, how much and how frequently it is eaten, and the consumer's resistance or susceptibility to the substance. Pesticide applicators, farm workers, and farmers are at greatest risk for negative effects associated with pesticide exposure. As part of the FDA's Total Diet Study (TDS), typical foods are analyzed for elements, pesticides, and industrial chemicals four times per year. Specific foods are also analyzed for mercury. For rural counties in the U.S., the incidence of lymph, genital, brain, and digestive-tract cancers increases with higher-than-average pesticide exposure. Respiratory cancer cases increase with greater insecticide use. In general, when comparing cancer incidence and death rates in rural and urban America, new cases of cancers of the lung, colon, and cervix as well as death rates from lung, colorectal, prostate, and cervical cancers have been higher in rural America.[25]

What about glyphosate? Glyphosate, the herbicide in Roundup®, is used frequently to kill certain weeds and grasses by blocking an enzyme essential for the plant's growth. According to the EPA, glyphosate is safe for humans if used according to the label. Pets may be at risk of digestive or intestinal issues if they touch or consume plants that have just been sprayed. Because this topic is quite controversial, the EPA requires management measures to help farmers and growers target pesticide sprays to intended pests, protect pollinators, and reduce the weed resistance to glyphosate.[26] To stay current on glyphosate, see https://www.fda.gov/food/pesticides/questions-and-answers-glyphosate.

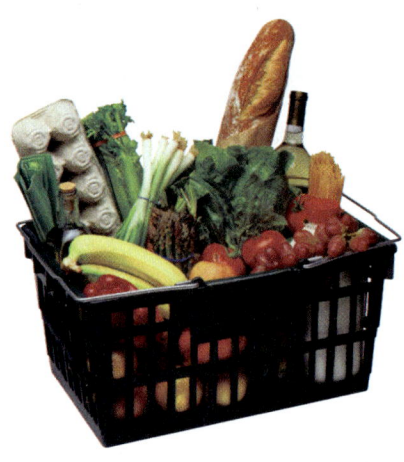

The FDA's yearly evaluation of a market basket of typical foods shows that pesticide residues are minimal in the vast majority of foods. C Squared Studios/Photodisc/Getty Images

Interestingly, research shows that the cancer risk from pesticide residues is hundreds of times less than the risk from eating such common foods as peanut butter, brown mustard, and basil. Recall that plants naturally manufacture toxic substances to defend themselves against insects, birds, and grazing animals (including humans). When plants are stressed or damaged, they produce even more of these toxins. Because of this, many foods contain naturally occurring chemicals considered toxic, and some possibly carcinogenic.

PERSONAL ACTION

The FDA and other scientific organizations report that the hazards of pesticides are extremely low and in the short run are much less dangerous than the hazards of foodborne illness that arise in our own kitchens. We can encourage farmers to use fewer pesticides to reduce exposure to our foods and water supplies, but we will have to settle for produce that is not perfect in appearance or that has been grown with the aid of biotechnology. Additional advice for limiting exposure to pesticides is found in Table 12-3. Choosing organic produce is one way to reduce your exposure to synthetic pesticides. One study found that people who report they "often or always" buy organic produce had significantly less insecticides in their urine samples, even though they reported eating 70% more servings of fruits and vegetables per day than adults reporting they "rarely or never" purchase organic produce.[27]

Each year, the Environmental Working Group (EWG) releases the *Dirty Dozen* and *Clean 15* lists of food they claim are most/least likely to contain pesticide residues. Recently researchers have discovered that the list makes some claims that are not based on scientific evidence. More importantly, the USDA and FDA have released reports showing that both organic food and conventional food are safe when handled appropriately and that such independent lists appear to be inducing fear and reducing consumer produce intake. According to these data, 99% of residues on the tested produce, if present at all, were well below safe threshold levels set by the EPA. In addition, 50% of foods sampled had no detectable residues at all. Fortunately, we have decades of high-quality nutrition studies documenting the numerous health benefits of consuming a dietary pattern rich in plant-based products. The Pesticide Residue Calculator (https://www.safefruitsandveggies.com/pesticide-calculator) shows that a child could eat over 180 servings of strawberries per day and still remain below the known harmful pesticide residue levels. To reduce the risk of foodborne illness and remove most pesticide residues, concerned consumers should simply wash their fruits and vegetables.

TABLE 12-3 ■ What You Can Do to Reduce Exposure to Pesticides

WASH: Wash and scrub all fresh fruits and vegetables thoroughly under running water to remove bacteria and soil. Running water has an abrasive effect that soaking does not. This will help remove bacteria and traces of chemicals from the surface of fruits and vegetables and dirt from crevices. Antibacterial washing products are not necessary.

PEEL AND TRIM: Peel fruits and vegetables when possible to reduce dirt, bacteria, and pesticides. Discard outer leaves of leafy vegetables. Trim fat from meat and skin from poultry and fish because some pesticides are fat soluble and can accumulate in the fatty tissues of animals.

SELECT A VARIETY: Eat a wide variety of foods from different sources to provide a better mix of nutrients and reduce your likelihood of exposure to a single pesticide.

CHOOSE ORGANIC: Choose organically grown foods to reduce exposure to synthetic pesticides, but keep in mind that organic regulations allow for natural pesticides.

USE INSECT REPELLENTS SAFELY: Read the label for pesticide safety information and apply insect repellents safely.

Source: Adapted from U.S. Environmental Protection Agency. See https://www.epa.gov/pesticide-incidents/pesticide-safety-tips for more pesticide safety tips.

ENVIRONMENTAL CONTAMINANTS IN FISH

The presence of the environmental contaminants mercury and polychlorinated biphenyls (PCBs) in fish has caused some confusion regarding the risks and benefits of fish consumption. In our previous discussion of the benefits of omega-3 fatty acids, it was recommended that we include cold-water fatty fish, such as salmon or tuna, in our eating pattern two times a week (up to 12 oz per week for adults).[28] Conversely, you may have heard recommendations to eat less fish because they are a source of environmental contaminants. Balancing the benefits and risks of consuming fish is tricky, and not all experts agree. Advice from the FDA and EPA indicates that salmon is safe to eat, even during pregnancy, because it is low in mercury.

Mercury and PCBs are by-products of industrial processes and accumulate in fish tissue. PCBs were banned from use in 1979, but environmental levels have been decreasing very slowly and therefore still persist in our food supply, especially in seafood. The contaminants become more concentrated in bigger fish as they eat smaller, contaminated fish. Fish are of primary concern because they are the only predators we eat regularly. The National Academy of Medicine, Food and Agriculture Organization, FDA, and EPA all have issued similar guidelines for fish consumption. These groups advise females who are pregnant to eat up to 12 ounces of low-mercury fish per week and to avoid the four highest-mercury fish, which are swordfish, shark, tilefish, and king mackerel. For other adults, the basic recommendation is to "eat fish" but to vary the source to reduce the risk of chronic exposure to the same contaminants.

U.S. adults typically do not eat enough fish to cause concern about high intakes of environmental contaminants. On average, we consume less than 5 ounces of seafood per week. Around 80% of that is shrimp, canned tuna, salmon, and whitefish, which are relatively low in environmental contaminants.[29] Most adults would benefit from eating more fish—a rich source of omega-3 fatty acids. Research shows that the risk of dying from heart disease is about 50% greater among people who do not eat fish compared to those who eat two servings of fatty fish each week.[30] Overall, it appears that the benefits of consuming fish twice per week outweigh the potential risks. Females who are pregnant should follow the FDA/EPA guidelines, and the rest of us should eat a variety of types of fish, focusing on the smaller, fatty fish at the bottom of the food chain.

AGROTERRORISM

Agroterrorism is the deliberate introduction of harmful agents, biological and otherwise, into the food supply chain with the intent of causing actual or perceived damage. The potential target areas for agroterrorism are typically farm animals and livestock, plant crops, and the food processing, distribution, and retailing system. In response to acts of terrorism in 2001, the U.S. Congress passed the Public Health Security and Bioterrorism Preparedness and Response Act

---

FARM to FORK — Melons

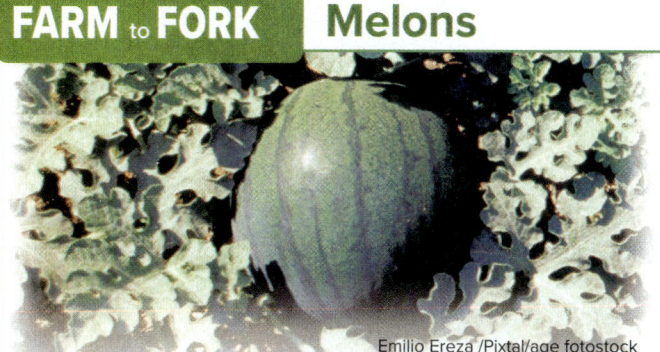

Emilio Ereza /Pixtal/age fotostock

Americans eat, on average, 26 pounds of melons a year, making them one of our favorite fruits. They are about 95% water, so they are a great source of fluid but a diluted source of other nutrients. Most contain a reasonable amount of vitamin C and are a juicy, low-calorie treat. Honeydew and casaba melons are the sweetest melons but also the least nutritious.

Grow
- Most melons available in the summer are grown in the U.S. The majority of melons sold in spring, fall, and winter have been imported from Mexico.
- Seedless watermelons are the most popular, making up 50% of the world market.
- Watermelons can grow in your backyard garden when daytime temperatures are between 70°F and 90°F and nighttime temperatures stay above 60°F.

Shop
- Fully ripe melons with deep-colored flesh are the most nutritious and delicious. The darker the red flesh of watermelons, the greater the lycopene content, whereas deep orange cantaloupe flesh is higher in overall carotenoid content.
- Melons presectioned into halves, quarters, or wedges are typically fresh and allow you to see the inside color before you buy them.
- Small watermelons are more nutritious than the large varieties.
- To find a ripe watermelon, look for one that has lost its gloss, has a yellow *ground spot*, and has a deep sound when you thump it.
- A ripe cantaloupe will have a slight depression or *innie* at its stem end.

Store
- Storing a watermelon at room temperature for a few days will increase its antioxidant value.
- Eat ripe cantaloupes as soon as possible. They will keep for up to 5 days in the drawer of the refrigerator.

Prep
- Scrub the outside of melons to remove any harmful bacteria on the outside. Although cantaloupes are virtually free of pesticides, they can harbor more bacteria because of their *netted* surface and therefore need vigorous rinsing.
- Once you have sliced open a melon, cover uneaten portions and refrigerate to inhibit the growth of bacteria. Eat within a day or two of slicing.

Source: Robinson J. Melons: light in flavor and nutrition. In: *Eating on the Wild Side: The Missing Link in Optimum Health*. New York: Little, Brown & Co.; 2013.

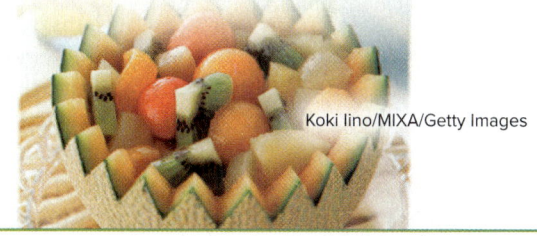

Koki Iino/MIXA/Getty Images

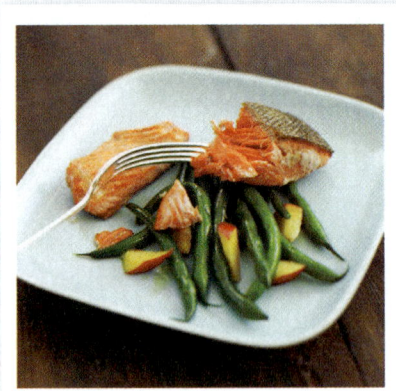

This wild Alaskan salmon is a top choice among types of fish based on its high nutritional value and low mercury levels. **What types of fish have the highest levels of mercury?**
Thomas Barwick/Digital Vision/Getty Images

(Bioterrorism Act). The Food Safety Modernization Act (FSMA) followed in 2011, giving the FDA increased power to monitor and control food in the United States. Although the United States has not been the victim of an agroterrorism attack, there remain potential vulnerabilities within our agricultural and food processing systems. The goals of the Bioterrorism Act and FSMA include the establishment of a process for regulators, scientists, and public health officials to improve the defensive position of the agriculture industry and to reduce the threat of agroterrorism.[31]

✓ CONCEPT CHECK 12.2

1. What are the benefits of pesticide use?
2. What agencies regulate the use of pesticides?
3. What environmental contaminants can be found in fish, and which fish are most likely to contain these toxins?
4. What can you do to reduce your exposure to pesticides?

12.3 Food Preservation and Safety

During the early stages of urbanization, contaminated water and food, especially milk, were responsible for large outbreaks of devastating human diseases. These experiences led to the development of procedures for purifying water, treating sewage, and **pasteurizing** milk. Since that time, safe water and milk have become more universally available, yet not always accessible. The greatest health risk from food today is contamination of a variety of foods by **viruses** and **bacteria** and, to a lesser extent, by various forms of **fungi** and **parasites.** These microorganisms can all cause **foodborne illness.** The Centers for Disease Control and Prevention (CDC) estimates that foodborne illness affects about one in six Americans each year. We generally have a safe food supply, but there are occasional instances of foodborne illnesses.

Microbial contamination of food is, by far, the more important issue for our short-term health. Adults are also concerned about health risks from chemicals such as food additives, although they cause only 5% of all cases of foodborne illness in the U.S.[32]

EFFECTS OF FOODBORNE ILLNESS

According to the CDC, foodborne illnesses cause nearly 48 million illnesses, 128,000 hospitalizations, and 3000 deaths in the United States each year.[33,34] The numbers of foodborne disease outbreaks by state are shown in Figure 12-5. Those most susceptible to foodborne illness include the following:

- Infants and children
- Older adults
- Those with liver disease, diabetes, **human immunodeficiency virus (HIV),** or cancer
- Patients recovering from surgery
- Females who are pregnant
- People taking immunosuppressant agents

Some bouts of foodborne illness, especially when coupled with ongoing health problems, are lengthy and lead to food allergies, seizures, blood poisoning (from **toxins** or microorganisms in the bloodstream), or other illnesses. Foodborne illnesses often result from the unsafe handling of food at home, so we each bear some responsibility for preventing them.[35,36] You cannot usually tell that a particular food contains harmful microorganisms by taste, smell, or sight; therefore, you might not even suspect that food has caused your distress. In fact, your last case of diarrhea may have been caused by foodborne illness.

pasteurizing The process of heating food products to kill pathogenic microorganisms and reduce the total number of bacteria.

virus One of the smallest known types of infectious agents, many of which cause disease in humans. A virus is essentially a piece of genetic material surrounded by a coat of protein. Viruses do not metabolize, grow, or move by themselves. They reproduce only with the aid of a living cellular host.

bacteria Single-cell microorganisms; some produce poisonous toxins, which cause illness in humans. Bacteria can be carried by water, animals, and people. They survive on skin, clothes, and hair and thrive in foods at room temperature. Some can live without oxygen and survive by means of spore formation.

fungi Simple parasitic life forms, including molds, mildews, yeasts, and mushrooms. They live on dead or decaying organic matter. Fungi can grow as single cells, like yeast, or as a multicellular colony, as seen with molds.

parasite An organism that lives in or on another organism and derives nourishment from it.

foodborne illness Sickness caused by the ingestion of food containing harmful substances.

human immunodeficiency virus (HIV) A virus that attacks cells that fight infection, making a person more susceptible to infections and diseases.

toxins Poisonous compounds produced by an organism that can cause disease.

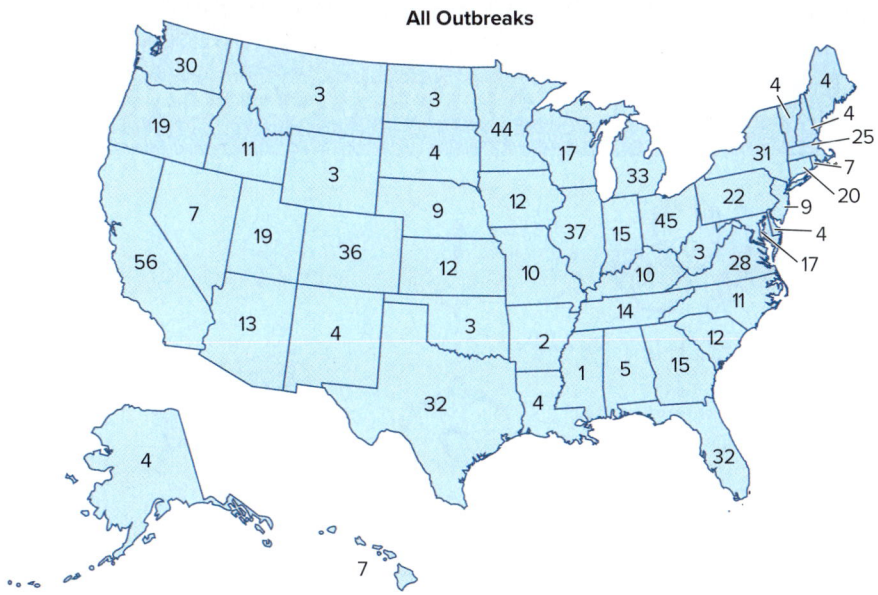

FIGURE 12-5 Foodborne disease outbreaks, 2021. The numbers on the map represent the number of confirmed outbreaks in each state in 1 year.

Source: https://wwwn.cdc.gov/norsdashboard/

PUBLIC HEALTH AND SAFETY

In response to the significant, largely preventable, public health risks of foodborne illness, the FDA Food Safety Modernization Act strengthened the food-safety system, enabling the FDA to better protect public health. It allows the FDA to focus on prevention of food-safety problems before they occur. The law provides new tools for inspection and compliance and for holding imported foods to the same standards as domestic foods.[37] The law directs the FDA to build a national food-safety system that is integrated and in partnership with state and local authorities. Several government agencies are at work on problems regarding food safety (Table 12-2). In addition, the CDC established the National Outbreak Reporting System (NORS) to alert the public of outbreaks (Fig. 12-6). Of course, the work of these agencies does not substitute for individual safety efforts.

WHY IS FOODBORNE ILLNESS SO COMMON?

Foodborne illness is carried or transmitted to people by food. Most foodborne illnesses are transmitted through food in which microorganisms are able to grow rapidly. Unfortunately, this includes many of the foods we eat every day, such as meats, eggs, and dairy products. See this chapter's *Newsworthy Nutrition* for risk of consuming unpasteurized milk.

The U.S. food industry tries whenever possible to prolong the shelf life of food products; however, a longer shelf life allows more time for bacteria in foods to multiply. Some bacteria even grow at refrigeration temperatures. Partially cooked—and some fully cooked—products pose a greater risk because refrigerated storage may only slow, not prevent, bacterial growth. Furthermore, we now know that in addition to providing a good growth medium for microorganisms, food (especially seafood) is also a carrier of many microorganisms.

The following consumer, environmental, and industry trends have increased the risk of contracting foodborne illness:

- Greater consumption of raw or undercooked animal products
- More foods prepared in kitchens outside the home
- Consumption of more imported ready-to-eat foods
- Centralized food production where food is prepared off-site for distribution
- Increased use of antibiotics in animal feeds

Microorganisms are able to grow rapidly in foods that are:
- generally moist.
- rich in protein.
- have a neutral or slightly acidic pH.

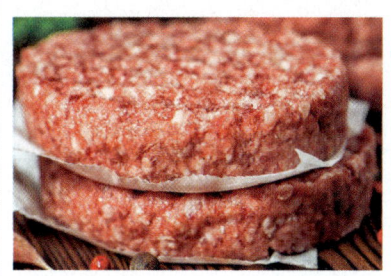

Restaurants that choose to serve raw or undercooked foods of animal origin are required to have a consumer advisory on the menu warning customers of the health risks of consuming such foods. Think of a recent outbreak of foodborne illness you heard about in the news. **What foods were implicated?** Olga Khomyakova/alisali/123RF

FIGURE 12-6 Learning from outbreaks. An investigation into a foodborne outbreak is complex and goes through a series of steps, many occurring simultaneously.

Source: Centers for Disease Control and Prevention, Steps in a Foodborne Outbreak Investigation, Retrieved from https://www.cdc.gov/foodsafety/outbreaks/investigating-outbreaks/investigations/index.html

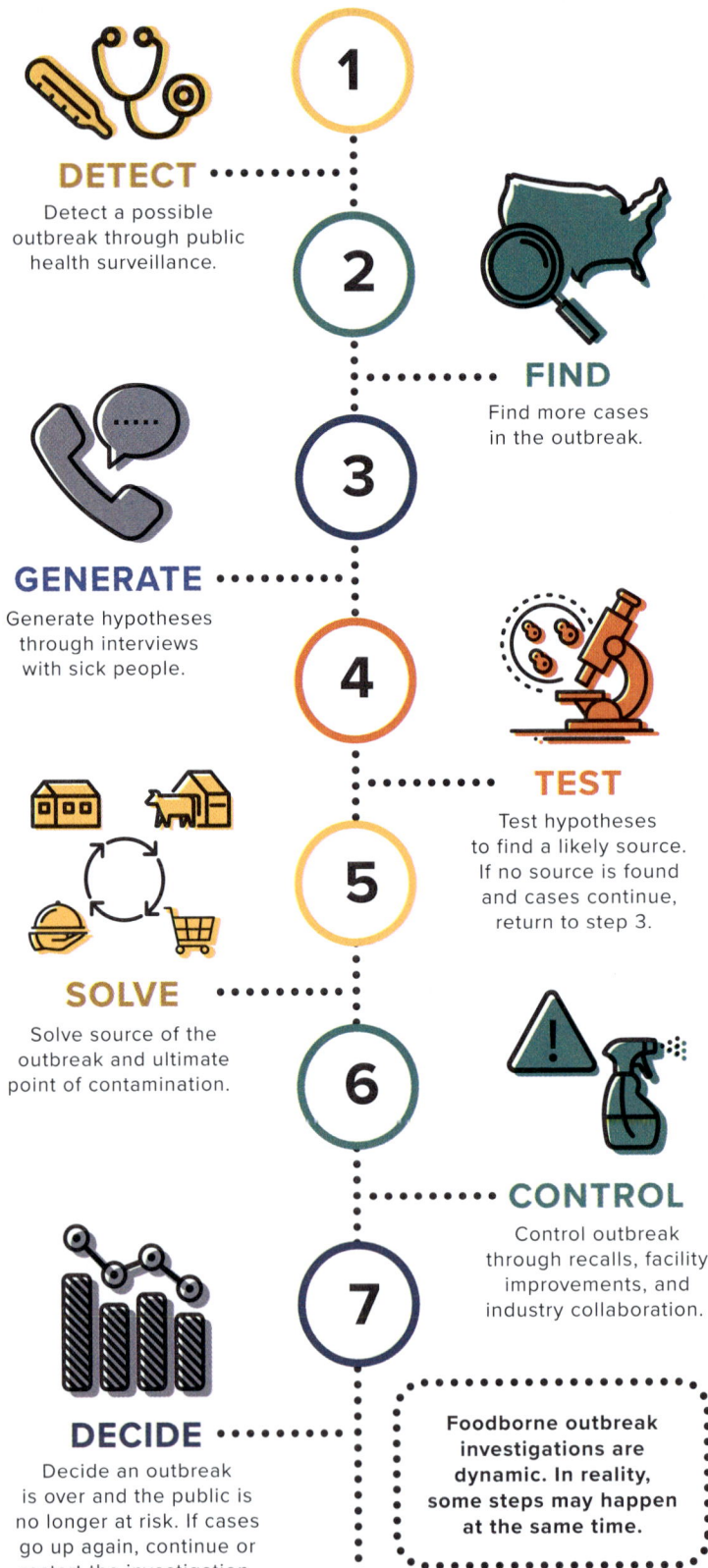

STEPS IN A FOODBORNE OUTBREAK INVESTIGATION

1. DETECT — Detect a possible outbreak through public health surveillance.

2. FIND — Find more cases in the outbreak.

3. GENERATE — Generate hypotheses through interviews with sick people.

4. TEST — Test hypotheses to find a likely source. If no source is found and cases continue, return to step 3.

5. SOLVE — Solve source of the outbreak and ultimate point of contamination.

6. CONTROL — Control outbreak through recalls, facility improvements, and industry collaboration.

7. DECIDE — Decide an outbreak is over and the public is no longer at risk. If cases go up again, continue or restart the investigation.

Foodborne outbreak investigations are dynamic. In reality, some steps may happen at the same time.

- More medications used that suppress the ability to combat foodborne infectious agents
- Increased number of severe storms and natural disasters resulting in power outages and contamination of water supplies
- Shipping of foods between multiple locations in the supply chain

With the high number of two-income families in the U.S., many people look for convenient and easy-to-prepare foods. Many grocery stores provide an alternative to cooking at home by offering a variety of prepared foods from the meat departments, salad bars, and bakeries. Supermarkets offer take-home meal kits or entrées that can be served immediately or reheated. The foods are usually prepared in central kitchens or processing plants and shipped to individual stores. This centralization of food production by the food processing and restaurant industry increases the risk of foodborne illness. If a food product is contaminated in a central processing plant, consumers over a wide area can experience foodborne illness. For example, in 1994 a contaminated ice cream mix used in a Schwan's® ice cream plant resulted in 224,000 suspected cases of *Salmonella* bacterial infections. The contamination was caused by an ice cream pre-mix that had been delivered to Schwan's in a truck that had not been properly washed after carrying raw, unpasteurized eggs.

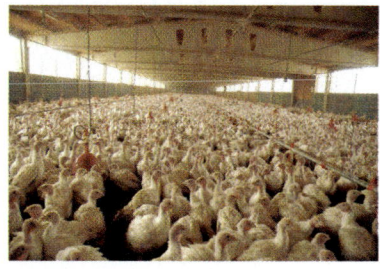

Antibiotics may be given to animals to prevent disease and increase feed efficiency. When antibiotics are used, a withdrawal period is required to ensure birds are free from any residues prior to slaughter. The USDA's Food Safety and Inspection Service randomly samples animals at slaughter to test for residues. Ingram Publishing/SuperStock

Greater consumption of ready-to-eat foods imported from foreign countries is another cause of increased foodborne illness in the U.S. Almost 20% of all food consumed in the U.S. is imported, including approximately 95% of fish and shellfish, 50% of fresh fruits, and 20% of fresh vegetables. Due to this increase, U.S. authorities are reexamining inspection procedures for these imports. For example, a 2012 outbreak of *Listeria* was caused by contaminated ricotta cheese imported from Italy.

The use of antibiotics in animal feeds has also had an impact on outbreaks and the severity of cases of foodborne illness. It is good to know that animals pass the antibiotics through their systems before they are slaughtered and that animal products to be used for human consumption are tested for antibiotics. The real danger from such widespread use of antibiotics is that it encourages the development of antibiotic-resistant strains of bacteria. In other words, the animals may be a reservoir of pathogens that can grow even when exposed to typical antibiotic medicines. This issue of resistant bacteria in food-producing animals is receiving considerable attention by scientists. The CDC encourages the judicious use of antibiotics in humans and animals because both uses contribute to the emergence, persistence, and spread of antibiotic-resistant bacteria. The good news is the significant decrease in the amount of antibiotics sold over the years without an increase in animal health issues or food safety problems. The FDA reports that sales and distribution of medically important antibiotics for use in U.S. livestock decreased by 33% from 2016 through 2017, and by 43% since sales peaked in 2015.[38]

Every decade, the list of microorganisms suspected of causing foodborne illness gets longer. One reason more cases of foodborne disease are reported now is that health care providers are more likely to suspect foodborne contaminants as a cause of illness.

FOOD PRESERVATION—PAST, PRESENT, AND FUTURE

For centuries, salt, sugar, smoke, fermentation, and drying have been used to preserve food. Ancient Romans used sulfites to disinfect wine containers and preserve wine. In the age of exploration, European adventurers traveling to the New World salted their meat to preserve it. Most preserving methods work on the principle of decreasing water content (Table 12-4). Bacteria need abundant stores of water to grow; yeasts and molds can grow with less water, but some is still necessary. Decreasing the water content of some high-moisture foods, however, causes them to lose essential characteristics. Fermentation is an ancient preservation method using selected bacteria or yeast to ferment or pickle foods, thereby producing pickles, sauerkraut, yogurt, and wine from

TABLE 12-4 ■ Food Preservation Techniques

Historic Methods	
Salt, sugar	These bind and reduce the water available to microorganisms.
Smoke	Heat kills microbes; chemicals in the smoke act as preservatives; water evaporates through drying.
Fermentation	Bacteria and yeast make acids and alcohol; minimizes growth of other bacteria and yeast.
Drying	Evaporates water.
Modern Methods	
Pasteurization	Moderately high (62°C to 100°C [144°F to 212°F]) temperatures are used for about 15 to 30 minutes to inactivate certain enzymes and kill microorganisms, especially in milk.
Refrigeration	Household refrigeration (typically at or below 40°F) slows down the deteriorative effects of microorganisms and enzymes.
Freezing	Freezing stops the growth of microorganisms, which do not grow when the temperature of the food is below 14°F (−10°C).
Canning	Food is heated in containers to a temperature that destroys microorganisms. Heating also causes air to be driven out of the container, forming a vacuum seal that prevents air and microorganisms from getting back into the product.
Chemical preservation	Preservation is usually based on the combined or synergistic activity of several additives. Certain preservatives have been used for centuries and include salt, sugar, acids, alcohols, and components of smoke. Some other chemicals used include sulfur dioxide, benzoic acid, sorbic acid, and formic acid.
Food irradiation	Radiation energy passes through food and controls growth of insects, bacteria, fungi, and parasites by breaking chemical bonds, destroying cell walls and cell membranes, and breaking down DNA.
Sterilization: Aseptic processing	Food and package are sterilized separately before the food enters the package.
Sterilization: Ultra-high temperature processing	Food is sterilized by heating it above 275°F (135°C) for 2 to 5 seconds.

magnificent microbiome

Fermented Foods

Fermentation can result in foods that contain live, probiotic organisms. The fermented foods that deliver the most beneficial bacteria to the gastrointestinal tract are kefir and yogurt. These dairy products have probiotic capabilities and have been associated with reduced inflammation and improved gut health. Most cheeses as well as nonheated kimchi and sauerkraut, kombucha, and miso also provide large numbers of live probiotic bacteria. Pickles that are fermented with salt, not vinegar, contain probiotics and are found in the refrigerated section of the grocery store. The live organisms in many other fermented foods, including sourdough bread and canned fermented vegetables such as sauerkraut, are destroyed by heat treatment. Beer and wine are also fermented, but the microbes used are filtered out of the finished product. Consume at least one serving of fermented foods daily to support your gut health. When adding fermented foods to your meals, remember to mix them in at the end to avoid destroying the beneficial probiotics with heat.

cucumbers, cabbage, milk, and grape juice, respectively. Check out the *Magnificent Microbiome* feature to see how these fermented foods provide a source of probiotics in the GI tract.

Today, we can add pasteurization, cooking, sterilization, refrigeration, freezing, canning, chemical preservation, and food **irradiation** to the list of food preservation techniques. Two specific methods of food sterilization, **aseptic processing** and **ultra-high temperature (UHT) processing,** are especially useful for liquid foods, such as fruit juices. With aseptic packaging and UHT processing, boxes of sterile milk, smoothies, and juices can remain unrefrigerated on supermarket shelves, free of microbial growth, for many years.

Food irradiation is an FDA-approved preservation technique that has dramatically improved food safety because it takes minimal doses of radiation to control pathogens such as *E. coli* O157:H7 and *Salmonella*. Irradiation is approved for use with eggs (still in the shell), seeds, meats, spices, dry vegetable seasonings, and fresh fruits and vegetables. The **radiation** energy used does not

Newsworthy Nutrition

Foodborne illness outbreaks linked to unpasteurized milk

INTRODUCTION: The consumption of raw, unpasteurized milk in the U.S. poses a persistent public health challenge, leading to an elevated risk of transmitting pathogens and causing outbreaks of illness. **OBJECTIVE:** The aim of this study was to identify the number of foodborne illness outbreaks linked to unpasteurized milk and identify the states in which they were reported. **METHODS:** In this *cross-sectional study,* researchers reviewed outbreaks of foodborne illness reported to the Foodborne Disease Outbreak Surveillance System of the Centers for Disease Control and Prevention (CDC) where the implicated source was reported to be unpasteurized milk. For each outbreak, a comparative analysis of the number of outbreaks and associated illnesses across state jurisdictions was conducted, categorizing them based on states permitting the sales of unpasteurized milk versus those that did not. **RESULTS:** Between 2013 and 2018, there were 75 outbreaks resulting in 675 illnesses linked to unpasteurized milk consumption, with 48% of these cases occurring in individuals aged 0 to 19 years. Of the 74 single-state outbreaks, 78% took place in states where the sale of unpasteurized milk was explicitly permitted. When compared to jurisdictions where retail sales were prohibited (n = 24), those allowing sales (n = 27) were estimated to have 3.2 times more outbreaks (95% CI 1.4–7.6). Among these, jurisdictions permitting retail store sales (n = 14) had 3.6 times more outbreaks (95% CI 1.3–9.6) compared to those allowing sales on-farm only (n = 13). **CONCLUSION:** This study reinforces previous findings that state laws facilitating increased access to unpasteurized milk are linked to a higher incidence of outbreak-associated illnesses and outbreaks.

Source: Koski L, Kisselburg, H, Landsman L, et al. Foodborne illness outbreaks linked to unpasteurised milk and relationship to changes in state laws—United States, 1998-2018. *Epidemiol Infect.* 2022;150:E183. doi:10.1017/S0950268822001649

irradiation A process in which radiation energy is applied to foods, creating compounds (free radicals) within the food that destroy cell membranes, break down DNA, link proteins, limit enzyme activity, and alter a variety of other proteins and cell functions of microorganisms that can lead to food spoilage. This process does not make the food radioactive.

aseptic processing A method by which food and container are separately and simultaneously sterilized; it allows manufacturers to produce boxes of milk that can be stored at room temperature.

ultra-high temperature (UHT) processing Method of sterilizing food by heating it above 275°F (135°C) for 2 to 5 seconds. Also called *ultra-heat treatment.*

FIGURE 12-7 The Radura® international label denotes prior irradiation of the food product. tatadonets/123RF

radiation Literally, energy that is emitted from a center in all directions. Various forms of radiation energy include X rays and ultraviolet rays from the sun.

make the food radioactive. The energy essentially passes through the food, as in microwave cooking, and no radioactive residues are left behind.

Irradiated food, except for dried seasonings, must be labeled with the international food irradiation symbol, the Radura (Fig. 12-7), and a statement that the product has been treated by irradiation. Some consumers have expressed concern that irradiation destroys nutrient content or makes food radioactive, but extensive studies confirm that irradiation does not compromise nutritional quality or noticeably change the taste, texture, or appearance of food. Keep in mind that even when foods, especially meats, have been irradiated, it is still important to follow basic food-safety procedures, as later contamination during food preparation is possible.

✓ CONCEPT CHECK 12.3

1. What lifestyle changes have made foodborne illness so common today?
2. Choose three agencies that bear some responsibility for monitoring the safety of our food supply and describe their specific roles.
3. What food preservation techniques have been used for centuries?
4. What is the UHT technique, and what types of foods are preserved with this process?
5. Why is irradiation considered a safe technique to preserve food?

12.4 Foodborne Illness Caused by Microorganisms

Most cases of foodborne illness are caused by specific viruses, bacteria, and parasites. The most common foodborn parasites are protozoa, roundworms, and tapeworms. Prions—proteins involved in maintaining nerve cell function—can also turn infectious and lead to diseases such as bovine spongiform encephalopathy, better known as mad cow disease. Although highly preventable, foodborne illnesses result in a significant number of illnesses, hospitalizations, and deaths each year (Fig. 12-8).

BACTERIA

Bacteria are single-cell organisms found in the food we eat, the water we drink, and the air we breathe. Many types of bacteria cause foodborne illness, including *Bacillus, Campylobacter, Clostridium, Escherichia, Listeria, Salmonella,* and *Staphylococcus,* and *Vibrio* (Fig. 12-9). Bacteria are everywhere: each teaspoon of soil contains up to a billion bacteria. Luckily, only a small number of all bacteria types pose a threat.

Bacteria can cause foodborne illness in three ways:

1. **Foodborne infection.** Foodborne bacteria directly invade the intestinal wall.
2. **Toxin-mediated infection.** Foodborne bacteria produce a harmful toxin as they colonize the GI tract.
3. **Foodborne intoxication.** Bacteria secrete a toxin into food before it is eaten, which causes harm to humans after the food is ingested.

The main way to distinguish an infectious route from an intoxication is time: if symptoms appear in 4 hours or less, it is an intoxication. *Salmonella,* for example, causes an infection because the bacteria cause the illness. *Clostridium botulinum, Staphylococcus aureus,* and *Bacillus cereus* produce toxins and therefore cause illness from intoxication. In addition, whereas most strains of *E. coli* are harmless, *E. coli* O157:H7 and O104:H4 produce a toxin that can cause severe illness, including severe bloody diarrhea and the potentially fatal kidney complication known as **hemolytic uremic syndrome (HUS).** Between 2009 and 2018, the FDA and CDC identified 40 foodborne outbreaks of toxin-producing *E. coli* infections in the U.S. that were confirmed or suspected to be linked to leafy greens. As a result of these recurrences, the FDA has developed the Leafy Greens Action STEC (Shiga toxin–producing *E. coli*) Plan to advance work in the prevention, response, and addressing of knowledge gaps in this area (https://www.fda.gov/food/foodborne-pathogens/2020-leafy-greens-stec-action-plan).

Bacterial foodborne illnesses typically cause gastrointestinal symptoms such as vomiting, diarrhea, and abdominal cramps. *Salmonella, Listeria, E. coli* O157:H7 and O104:H4, and *Campylobacter* are the bacterial foodborne illnesses of particular interest because

hemolytic uremic syndrome (HUS) Disease characterized by anemia caused by destruction of red blood cells (hemolytic), acute kidney failure (uremic), and a low platelet count.

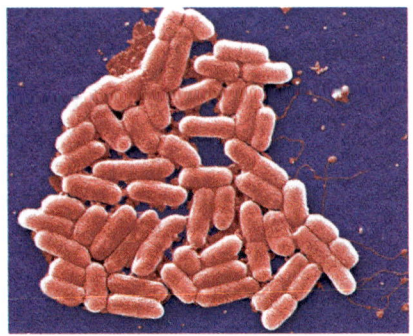

An electron micrograph of *E. coli* bacteria, strain O157:H7, magnified 6836×. Although most strains of *E. coli* are harmless and live in the intestines of healthy humans and animals, this strain produces a toxin that causes severe illness. Janice Haney Carr/CDC

TOP FIVE ANNUAL GERMS CAUSING ILLNESS, HOSPITALIZATIONS, AND DEATHS

48 MILLION ILLNESSES	128,000 HOSPITALIZATIONS	3,000 DEATHS
1. Norovirus	1. *Salmonella* (non-typhoidal)	1. *Salmonella* (non-typhoidal)
2. *Salmonella* (non-typhoidal)	2. Norovirus	2. *Toxoplasma gondii*
3. *Clostridium perfringens*	3. *Campylobacter*	3. *Listeria* monocytogenes
4. *Campylobacter*	4. *Toxoplasma gondii*	4. Norovirus
5. *Staphylococcus aureus*	5. *E. coli* O157	5. *Campylobacter*

FIGURE 12-8 Causes and prevalence of foodborne illnesses
Source: CDC.

Bacterial Causes of Foodborne Illnesses

Bacillus Cereus

Sources: Meats, stew, gravies, vanilla sauce

Onset: 10–16 hours
Duration: 24–48 hours

Symptoms:
- Abdominal cramps
- Diarrhea
- Nausea

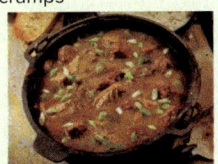

Campylobacter Jejuni

Sources: Raw and undercooked poultry, unpasteurized milk, contaminated water

Onset: 2–5 days
Duration: 2–10 days

Symptoms:
- Abdominal cramps
- Fever
- Diarrhea
- Vomiting

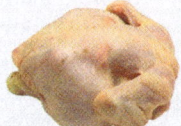

Clostridium Botulinum

Sources: Improperly canned foods, fermented fish, baked potatoes in aluminum foil

Onset: 12–72 hours
Duration: days to weeks

Symptoms:
- Muscle weakness
- Vision changes
- Swallowing difficulty
- Diarrhea
- Vomiting
- Respiratory failure

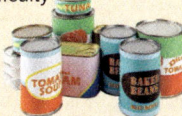

Clostridium Perfringens

Sources: Meats, poultry, gravies, dried or precooked foods, time and/or temperature-abused foods

Onset: 8–16 hours
Duration: 24 hours

Symptoms:
- Abdominal cramps
- Diarrhea

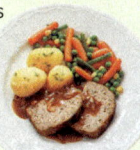

Escherichia Coli

Sources: Undercooked beef, unpasteurized milk or juice, raw fruits and vegetables, contaminated water

Onset: 1–8 days
Duration: 5–10 days

Symptoms:
- Abdominal pain
- Diarrhea (often bloody)
- Vomiting
- Can lead to kidney failure

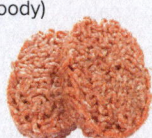

Listeria Monocytogenes

Sources: Unpasteurized milk, soft cheeses made with unpasteurized milk, ready-to-eat deli meats

Onset: 9–48 hours*
Duration: days to weeks

Symptoms:
- Muscle aches
- Fever
- Diarrhea
- Nausea
- Flu-like symptoms during pregnancy

Salmonella Species

Sources: Eggs, poultry, meats, unpasteurized milk or juice, cheese, contaminated raw fruits or vegetables

Onset: 6–48 hours
Duration: 4–7 days

Symptoms:
- Abdominal cramps
- Fever
- Diarrhea
- Vomiting

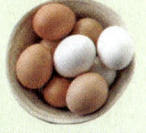

Shigella Species

Sources: Raw produce, contaminated water, foods contaminated by infected handlers due to poor hygiene

Onset: 4–7 days
Duration: 24–48 hours

Symptoms:
- Abdominal cramps
- Fever
- Diarrhea (may contain blood and mucous)

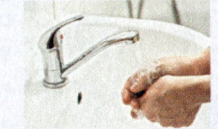

Staphylococcus Aureus

Sources: Improperly refrigerated meats, potato and egg salads, cream pastries

Onset: 1–6 hours
Duration: 24–48 hours

Symptoms:
- Abdominal cramps
- Fever may be present
- Diarrhea
- Nausea
- Vomiting

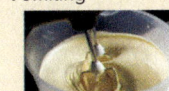

Vibrio Parahaemolyticus

Sources: Undercooked or raw seafood, such as shellfish

Onset: 4–96 hours
Duration: 2–5 days

Symptoms:
- Abdominal cramps
- Fever
- Diarrhea
- Nausea
- Vomiting

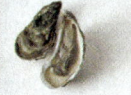

*For gastrointestinal symptoms; 2–6 weeks for invasive disease

FIGURE 12-9 Bacterial causes of foodborne illness. chicken and sausage gumbo: LauriPatterson/E+/Getty Images; chicken: Pixtal/AGE Fotostock; food cans: sockagphoto/Shutterstock; sliced roasted meat loaf: foodandmore/123RF; chopped steak: page frederique/Shutterstock; soft cheese: scol22/iStock/Getty Images; bowl of eggs: MaraZe/Shutterstock; hand washing: Shutterstock/Lubo Ivanko; mixer: Daria_vg/Shutterstock; open oyster: Isabelle Rozenbaum & Frederic Cirou/Photo Alto
Source: FDA at https://www.fda.gov/food/consumers/what-you-need-know-about-foodborne-illnesses

they are the ones most often associated with death. *E. coli* O157:H7 and O104:H4 have caused deaths when HUS has developed. Listeriosis is of particular concern for females who are pregnant because they are about 20 times more likely to get this infection than other healthy adults. Listeriosis can cause preterm birth, spontaneous abortion, or stillbirth because the *Listeria* bacteria can cross the placenta and infect the fetus.

Effects of Temperature: The Danger Zone. To proliferate, bacteria require nutrients, water, and warmth. Most grow best in **danger zone** temperatures of 40°F to 140°F (4.4°C to 60°C, Fig. 12-10). Pathogenic bacteria typically do not multiply when food is held at temperatures above 140°F (60°C) or stored at safe refrigeration temperatures, 32°F to 40°F (0°C to 4.4°C). One important exception is *Listeria* bacteria, which can multiply at refrigeration temperatures. Also note that high temperatures can kill toxin-producing bacteria, but any toxin produced in the food will not be inactivated by high temperatures. Most pathogenic bacteria also require oxygen for growth, but *Clostridium botulinum* and *Clostridium perfringens* grow only in anaerobic (oxygen-free) environments, such as those found in tightly sealed cans and jars. Food acidity can affect bacterial growth, too. Although most bacteria do not grow well in acidic environments, some, such as disease-causing *E. coli,* can grow in acidic foods, such as fruit juice.

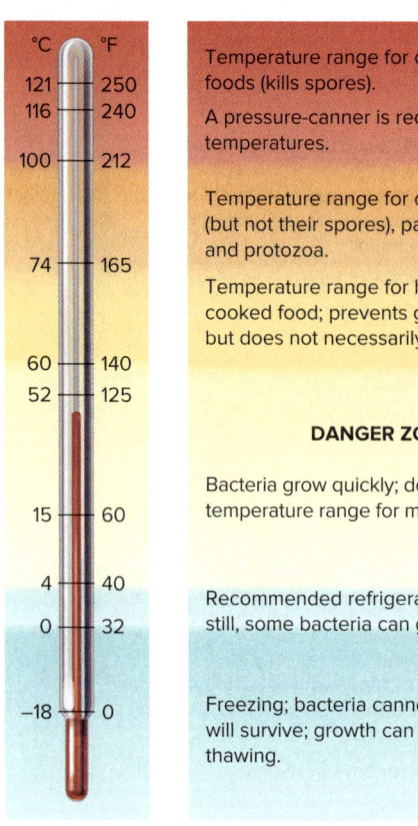

FIGURE 12-10 Effects of temperature on microbes that cause foodborne illness.
Source: USDA Food Safety and Inspection Service, Safe Minimum Internal Temperature Chart, www.fsis.usda.gov

danger zone Temperature range (40°F to 140°F) where bacteria grow most rapidly.

VIRUSES

Viruses, like bacteria, are widely dispersed in nature. Unlike bacteria, however, viruses can reproduce only after invading body cells, such as those that line the intestines. Experts speculate that about 67% of foodborne illness cases go undiagnosed because they result from viral causes, and there is no easy way to test for these pathogens.[39] Figure 12-11 describes the

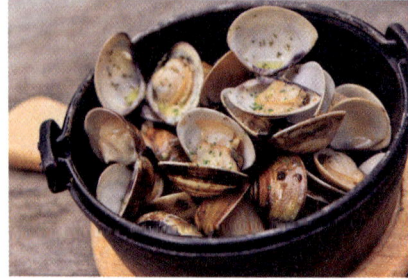

Raw shellfish, especially bivalves (e.g., oysters and clams), present a particular risk related to foodborne viral disease. These animals filter-feed, a process that concentrates viruses, bacteria, and toxins present in the water as it is filtered for food. Adequate cooking of shellfish will kill viruses and bacteria, but toxins may not be affected. It is important to buy shellfish from reliable sources that have harvested these foods from safe areas. Rcom Hdjuin/duybox/123RF

Viral Causes of Foodborne Illnesses

Hepatitis A Virus	Norovirus (Norwalk and Norwalk-like Viruses), Human Rotavirua
Sources: Raw produce, contaminated drinking water, undercooked foods and cooked foods not reheated after contact with infected handler, shellfish from contaminated waters	**Sources:** Raw produce, contaminated drinking water, undercooked foods and cooked foods not reheated after contact with infected handler, shellfish from contaminated waters
Onset: 15–50 days	**Onset:** 12–48 hours
Duration: 2–12 weeks	**Duration:** 12–60 hours
Symptoms: • Diarrhea • Dark urine • Jaundice • Flu-like symptoms	**Symptoms:** • Abdominal cramps • Fever • Diarrhea • Nausea • Vomiting

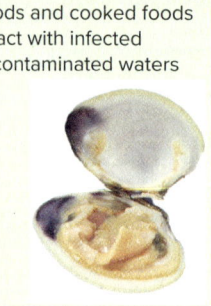
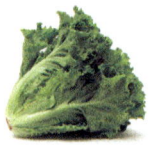

FIGURE 12-11 Viral causes of foodborne illness. open clam: Comstock/Stockbyte/Getty Images; fresh lettuce: JIANG HONGYAN/Shutterstock
Source: FDA at https://www.fda.gov/food/consumers/what-you-need-know-about-foodborne-illnesses

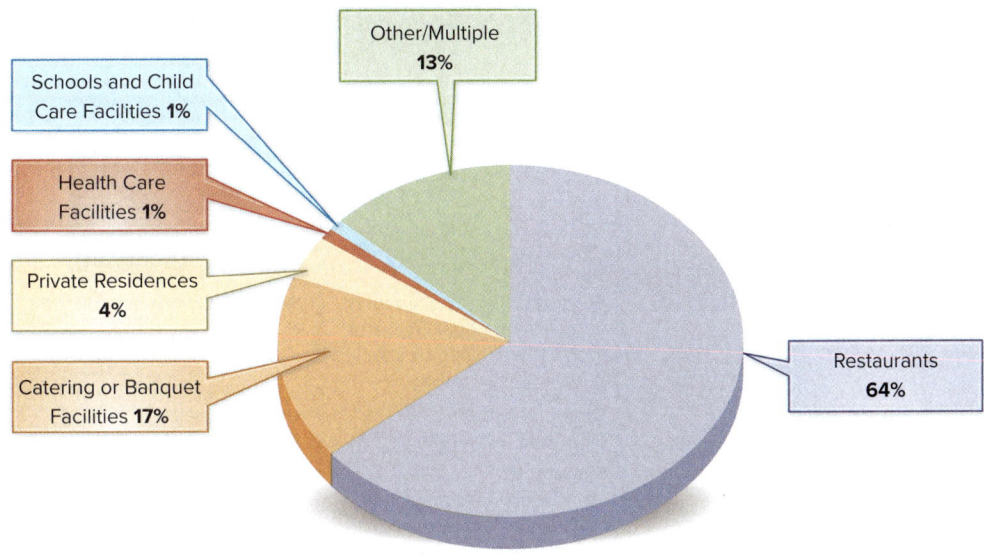

FIGURE 12-12 Settings of norovirus outbreaks from food contamination in the United States.
Source: Adapted from CDC, available at https://www.cdc.gov/vitalsigns/norovirus/index.html

two most common viral causes of foodborne illness, norovirus and hepatitis A, along with typical food sources and symptoms and outbreaks of the illnesses they cause.

Norovirus is the leading cause of foodborne illness, causing almost 60% of illnesses in the U.S. annually.[40] The origin of its name came from Norwalk, Ohio, where the virus was first isolated after a 1968 outbreak. Each year, norovirus results in almost 2.3 million outpatient clinic visits, 465,000 emergency department visits, and 800 deaths, mainly in young children and seniors. This virus is also responsible for over 90% of the diarrheal disease outbreaks on cruise ships, and almost 1 million pediatric medical care visits annually. It causes an illness commonly misdiagnosed as the *stomach flu*. These microorganisms are hardy and can survive freezing and relatively high temperatures, as well as chlorination up to 10 parts per million. The most commonly reported norovirus outbreaks from food contamination are at restaurants (Fig. 12-12).

PARASITES

Figure 12-13 describes common parasites and typical food sources and symptoms of the illnesses they cause. Parasitic infections spread via person-to-person contact and contaminated food, water, and soil. Parasites live in or on another organism, known as the host, from which they absorb nutrients. Humans may serve as hosts to parasites. These tiny ravagers rob millions of people around the globe of their health and, in some cases, their lives. Those hardest hit live in tropical countries where poor sanitation fosters the growth of parasites. The more than 93 foodborne parasites known to affect humans include mainly **protozoa,** such as *Cryptosporidium* and *Cyclospora,* and **helminths,** such as tapeworms and the roundworm *Trichinella spiralis.*

magnificent microbiome

Norovirus

Norovirus researchers are looking to the gut microbiome for some answers. Early animal studies have uncovered that some cells in the biome enhance norovirus replication and provide a safe haven that allows some people to remain contagious for weeks, even after symptoms dissipate. Scientists are investigating ways to manipulate the gut environment or microbiome itself to stimulate the immune system in ways that could shut down norovirus infection.

Source: Grau KR, Zhu S, Peterson ST, et al. The intestinal regionalization of acute norovirus infection is regulated by the microbiota via bile acid-mediated priming of type III interferon. *Nat Microbiol.* 2020 Jan;5(1):84-92. doi: 10.1038/s41564-019-0602-7

protozoa (singular, protozoan) One-celled animals that are more complex than bacteria. Disease-causing protozoa can be spread through food and water.

helminth Parasitic worm that can contaminate food, water, feces, animals, and other substances.

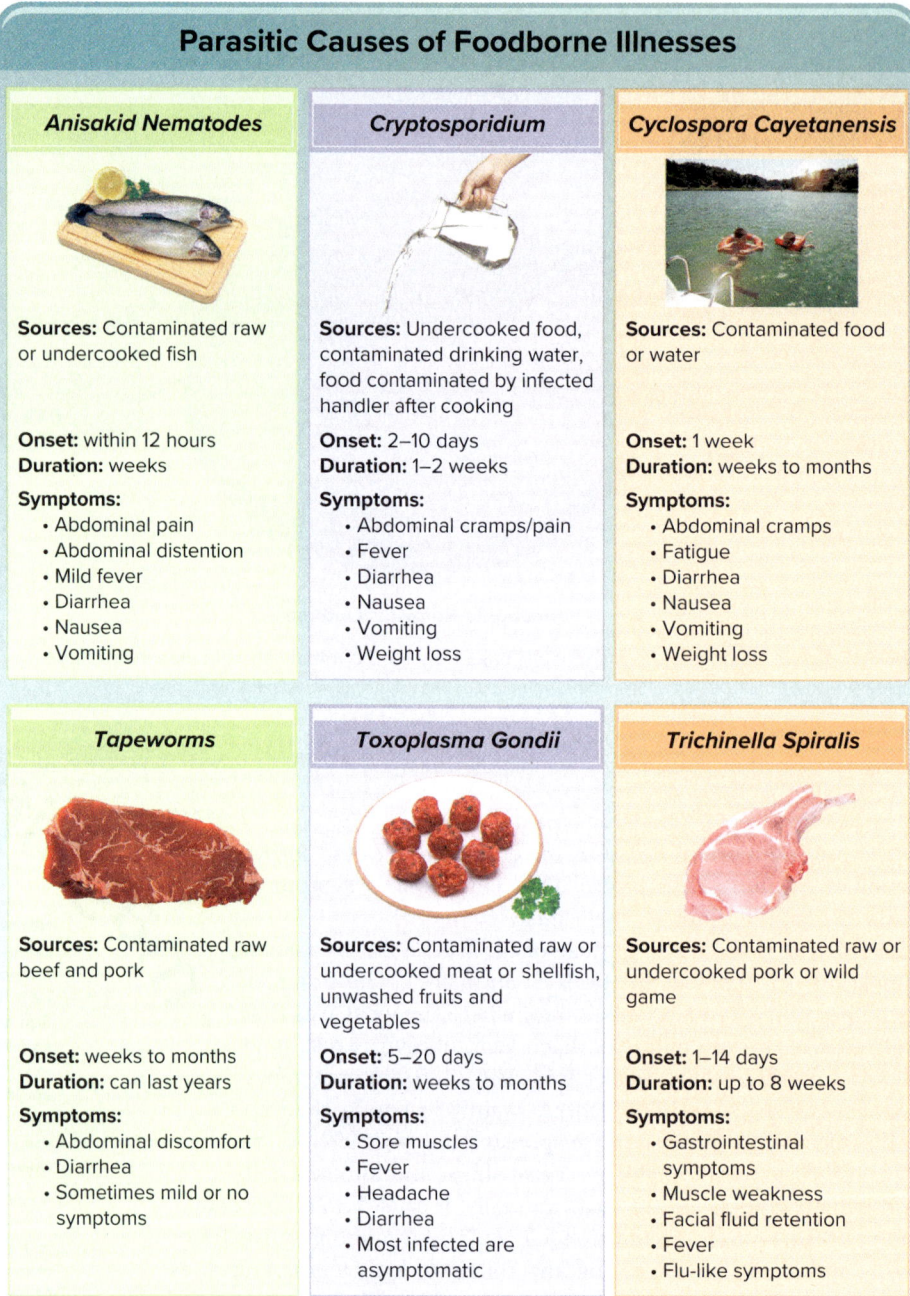

FIGURE 12-13 Parasitic causes of foodborne illness. sea trout: Pixtal/AGE Fotostock; pouring water: cloud7days/123RF; kids swimming: pio3/Shutterstock; raw striploin steak: Island Images/Alamy Stock Photo; meatballs: Pixtal/AGE Fotostock; raw pork chop: Yotrak Butda/123RF
Source: Adapted from CDC, available at https://www.cdc.gov/parasites/az/index.html#t

✓ CONCEPT CHECK 12.4

1. What is the temperature *danger zone* in which bacteria can grow rapidly?
2. What type of microorganisms pose the greatest risk for foodborne illness?
3. What is the setting for the most norovirus outbreaks from contaminated food?

12.5 Food Additives

By the time you see a food item on the market shelf, it usually contains substances added to make it taste better, increase its nutrient content or shelf life, or make it easier to process. Yet other substances may have accidentally found their way into the foods you buy. All of these extraneous substances are known as **additives,** and, although some may be beneficial, others, such as sulfites, may be harmful for some people. All purposefully added substances must be evaluated by the FDA. To evaluate the safety of an additive, the FDA considers: (1) the substance composition and properties; (2) typical amount consumed; (3) immediate and long-term effects on health; and (4) a variety of safety factors.

Food additives are classified into two types: **direct food additives** (intentionally added to foods) and **indirect food additives** (incidentally added as contaminants). Both types of agents are regulated by the FDA in the United States. Currently, more than 3950 different substances are directly added to foods.[41] As many as 3200 other substances enter foods as indirect contaminants. This includes substances that may reasonably be expected to enter food through contact with processing equipment or packaging materials.

WHY ARE FOOD ADDITIVES USED?

Most additives are used to reduce food spoilage. Common food additives serve the general function of **preservatives,** which can extend the shelf life of some foods. For example, antioxidants (e.g., vitamin E and sulfites) prevent discoloration caused by exposure to oxygen and enzymes. Antimicrobial additives (e.g., potassium sorbate) retard the growth of microbes in food products. Table 12-5 describes common food additives in detail.

additives Substances added to foods, either intentionally or incidentally.

direct food additives Additives knowingly (intentionally) incorporated into food products by manufacturers.

indirect food additives Additives that appear in food products incidentally, from environmental contamination of food ingredients or during the manufacturing process.

preservatives Compounds that extend the shelf life of foods by inhibiting microbial growth or minimizing the destructive effect of oxygen and metals.

TABLE 12-5 ■ **Types of Food Additives—Sources and Related Health Concerns**

Food Additive Class	Attributes	Health Risks
Acidic or alkaline agents, such as citric acid, calcium lactate, and sodium hydroxide	Acids inhibit mold growth, lessen discoloration and rancidity, and reduce botulism risk. Alkaline agents improve flavor by neutralizing acids.	No known health risks when used properly.
Anticaking and free-flow agents, such as calcium silicate	Absorb moisture to keep table salt and powdered food products free-flowing.	No known health risks when used properly.
Antimicrobial agents, such as salt and sodium benzoate	Inhibit mold and fungal growth.	Salt increases the risk of developing hypertension. No known health risks from other agents when used properly.
Antioxidants, such as BHA (butylated hydroxyanisole), BHT (butylated hydroxytoluene), vitamin E, vitamin C, and sulfites	Delay food discolorations from oxygen exposure, reduce rancidity, maintain the color of meats, prevent the formation of cancer-causing nitrosamines.	Approximately 10% of people have a sulfite intolerance. Symptoms include difficulty breathing, hives, diarrhea, abdominal pain, and dizziness.
Color additives, such as tartrazine	Make foods more visually appealing.	Tartrazine (Yellow Dye No. 5) can cause allergic symptoms. FDA requires synthetic colors to be listed on labels.
Curing and pickling agents, such as salt, nitrates, and nitrites	Nitrates and nitrites act as preservatives, especially to prevent the growth of *Clostridium botulinum*, often used in conjunction with salt.	Salt increases the risk of developing hypertension. Nitrate and nitrite consumption has been associated with synthesis of nitrosamines linked to cancer risk.
Emulsifiers, such as monoglycerides and lecithins	Suspend fat in water to improve uniformity, smoothness, and body of foods.	No known health risks when used properly.
Fat replacements, such as maltodextrins, emulsifiers, fiber, modified food starch, and engineered fats	Limit calorie content of foods by replacing some of the fat content.	Generally no known health risks when used properly. Possible loss of fat-soluble vitamins and GI distress.
Flavor and flavoring agents, such as natural and artificial flavors, sugar, and corn syrup	Impart more or improve flavor of foods.	Sugar and corn syrup can increase risk for dental caries and weight gain. No known health risks for flavoring agents when used properly.

(continued)

TABLE 12-5 ■ Types of Food Additives—Sources and Related Health Concerns (continued)

Food Additive Class	Attributes	Health Risks
Flavor enhancers, such as monosodium glutamate (MSG) and salt	Help bring out the natural flavor of foods.	MSG sensitivity can cause flushing, chest pain, facial pressure, dizziness, sweating, rapid heart rate, nausea, vomiting, increase in blood pressure, and headache.
Humectants, such as glycerol, propylene glycol, and sorbitol	Retain more moisture, texture, and fresh flavor in foods.	No known health risk when used properly.
Leavening agents, such as yeast, baking powder, and baking soda	Introduce carbon dioxide into food products.	No known health risk when used properly.
Maturing and bleaching agents, such as bromates, peroxides, and ammonium chloride	Shorten the time needed for maturation of flour.	No known health risk when used properly.
Nonnutritive sweeteners	Sweeten foods without adding more than a few calories.	Moderate use considered safe (except for people with phenylketonuria [PKU]).
Nutrient supplements, such as vitamin A, vitamin D, and iodine	Enhance the nutrient content of foods such as margarine, milk, and ready-to-eat breakfast cereals.	No known health risk if intake does not exceed the Upper Level for a particular nutrient.
Sequestrants, such as EDTA and citric acid	Bind free ions to prevent them from causing rancidity in products containing fat.	No known health risk when used properly.
Stabilizers and thickeners, such as pectins, gums, gelatins, and agars	Impart a smooth texture and uniform color and flavor to foods; prevent evaporation and deterioration of flavorings in foods.	No known health risk when used properly.

Source: Adapted from FDA, available at https://www.fda.gov/Food/IngredientsPackagingLabeling/FoodAdditivesIngredients/ucm094211.htm

sequestrants Compounds that bind free metal ions. By so doing, they reduce the ability of ions to cause rancidity in foods containing fat.

Additives are also used to reduce food spoilage caused by the activity of some enzymes that leads to undesirable changes in color and flavor in foods. This type of food spoilage occurs when enzymes in a food react to oxygen—for example, when apple and peach slices darken or turn rust colored as they are exposed to air. Antioxidants are a type of preservative that slows the action of oxygen-requiring enzymes on food surfaces. These preservatives include vitamins E and C and a variety of sulfites. Sugar, salt, and corn syrup are, by far, the most widely used additives in the U.S.[42]

Without the use of some food additives, it would be impossible to produce massive quantities of foods and safely distribute them nationwide or worldwide, as is now done. Despite consumer concerns about the safety of food additives, many have been extensively studied and proven safe when the FDA guidelines for their use are followed.

THE GRAS LIST

The Federal Food, Drug, and Cosmetic Act requires that any substance that is intentionally added to food is subject to review and approval by the FDA before it is used. Substances are exempted from review if they are generally recognized by qualified experts as having been adequately shown to be safe under the conditions of their intended use. In 1958, all food additives used in the United States and considered safe at that time were put on a generally recognized as safe (GRAS) list. The U.S. Congress established the GRAS list because it believed manufacturers did not need to prove the safety of substances that had been used for a long time and were already generally recognized as safe.

A substance can be removed from the GRAS list if the FDA can prove that it does *not* belong on the list. A few substances, such as cyclamates, failed the review process and were removed from the list. Red Dye No. 3 was removed because it was found to be linked to cancer. Many chemicals on the GRAS list have not yet been rigorously tested, primarily because of expense and because they have long histories of use without evidence of toxicity or their chemical characteristics do not suggest that they are potential health hazards. Substances may be added to the GRAS list if there are enough data to establish that the substance is safe under the conditions of its intended use.

In the past, the American Heart Association (AHA) and other experts have questioned the appropriateness of the GRAS listing for salt. They have suggested that sodium, one of the two components of salt, has negative health consequences and therefore does not meet the *safe* requirement of the GRAS. The AHA has advocated for the FDA to amend the GRAS listing for sodium chloride in an effort to reduce sodium content in processed foods. Hearing these concerns, the FDA issued a ruling that formalized the documentation of GRAS determinations and notifications. This ruling strengthened the oversight of food ingredients and included the consideration of both research results and expert opinion when making final determinations.[43]

SYNTHETIC CHEMICALS

Although human endeavors contribute some toxins to foods, such as synthetic pesticides and industrial chemicals, nature's poisons are often even more potent and widespread. Nothing about a natural product makes it inherently safer than a synthetic product. Many synthetic products are laboratory copies of chemicals that also occur in nature. Some cancer researchers estimate that we ingest at least 10,000 times more (by weight) natural toxins produced by plants than we do synthetic pesticide residues. Plants produce these toxins to protect themselves from predators and disease-causing organisms. Some of these plant toxins are the beneficial phytochemicals we have already discussed. This comparison does not make synthetic chemicals any less toxic, but it does put them in perspective.

Last, toxicity is related to dosage. Consider vitamin E, often added to food to prevent rancidity of fats. This chemical is safe when used within certain limits. However, high doses have been associated with health problems, such as interfering with vitamin K activity in the body. Thus, even well-known, commonly used chemicals can be toxic in some circumstances and at high concentrations.

TESTS OF FOOD ADDITIVES FOR SAFETY

Food additives are tested by the FDA for safety on at least two animal species, usually rats and mice. Scientists determine the highest dose of the additive that produces no *observable effects* in the animals. These doses are proportionately much higher than humans ever consume. The maximum dosage that produced no observable effects is then divided by at least 100 to establish a conservative margin of safety for human use. This 100-fold margin is used because it is assumed that we are at least 10 times more sensitive to food additives than laboratory animals and that any one person might be 10 times more sensitive than another. This conservative estimate essentially ensures that the food additive in question will cause no harmful health effects in humans.

One important exception applies to the procedure for testing direct food additives: if an additive is shown to cause cancer, even though only in high doses, no margin of safety is allowed. The food additive cannot be used because it would violate the **Delaney Clause.** This clause prohibits intentionally adding to foods a compound introduced after 1958 that causes cancer at any level of exposure. Evidence for cancer could come from either laboratory animal or human studies. A few exceptions to this clause, including the curing and pickling agents, nitrites and nitrates, are allowed.

Indirect food additives are another matter. The FDA cannot ban various industrial chemicals, pesticide residues, and mold toxins from foods, even though some of these contaminants increase cancer risk. These products are not purposely added to foods. The FDA sets an acceptable level for these substances. An incidental substance found in a food cannot contribute to more than one cancer case during the lifetimes of 1 million people. If a higher risk exists, the amount of the compound in a food must be reduced until the guideline is met.

In general, if you consume a variety of foods in moderation, the chances of food additives jeopardizing your health are minimal. Pay attention to your body. If you suspect an

Delaney Clause A clause to the 1958 Food Additives Amendment of the Pure Food and Drug Act in the United States that prevents the intentional (direct) addition to foods of a compound shown to cause cancer in laboratory animals or humans.

intolerance or a sensitivity, consult your health care provider for further evaluation. In the short run, you are more likely to experience foodborne illness due to the microbial contamination of food than from consuming additives.

APPROVAL FOR A NEW FOOD ADDITIVE

Before a new food additive can be added to foods, the FDA must approve its use. Besides rigorously testing an additive to establish its safety margins, manufacturers must give the FDA information that: (1) identifies the new additive; (2) gives its chemical composition; (3) states how it is manufactured; and (4) specifies laboratory methods used to measure its presence in the food supply at the amount of intended use.

Manufacturers must also offer proof that the additive will accomplish its intended purpose in a food, that it is safe, and that it is to be used in no higher amount than needed. Additives cannot be used to hide defective food ingredients, such as rancid oils; to deceive customers; or to replace good manufacturing practices. A manufacturer must establish that the ingredient is necessary for producing a specific food product.

Worldwide Differences in Approval. Despite these guidelines, many activists and public health watchdogs are not satisfied with the FDA procedures for regulating and monitoring the safety of food additives. These groups have urged the FDA and food manufacturers to stop the use of various chemicals until their safety can be more fully determined. A major incentive for these requests is the fact that many of the chemicals used in the United States are illegal to use as food additives in the countries of the European Union (EU) and others such as Brazil, Canada, India, and Japan.

Worldwide, there are differences in the approaches countries take to the approval of food additives. A key difference is that other countries do not rely on a GRAS list of compounds. An element that distinguishes the approach of the European Union (EU) from that of the United States is what the EU calls the *precautionary principle*. The EU believes that protective action or *precaution* should be taken when substantial, credible evidence of danger to human or environmental health is available, despite continuing scientific uncertainty. In contrast, the FDA's approach is that *proof of harm* must be demonstrated before regulatory action is taken. FDA approval is also unique in that when making determinations about additive safety, the FDA often relies on studies performed by the companies seeking approval.

As an example, the artificial colors Red Dye No. 40 and Yellow Dyes No. 5 and No. 6 are allowed in the United States but have been taken off the market in the United Kingdom. In the rest of Europe, products that contain these dyes must carry labels warning of their potential adverse effect on children's attention and behavior. These differences stem from varying conclusions made by authorities in the United States and Europe.[44] The study found that artificial colors or a sodium benzoate preservative (or both) resulted in increased hyperactivity in children. The study persuaded British authorities to ban use of these dyes as food additives, whereas the EU chose to require warning labels on products that contain them. In the United States, the colors remain in use because the FDA found the study inconclusive based on the fact that it examined effects of a mixture of additives rather than individual colorings.

Several large companies and retailers have policies voluntarily barring some approved additives from their products. The sandwich chain Subway voluntarily discontinued the use of the approved dough conditioner azodicarbonamide, whose breakdown product, urethane, raised health concerns. If you are concerned about the additives in your food sources, you can easily avoid most of them by consuming unprocessed whole foods such as produce, lean meats, whole grains, and low-fat dairy. However, no evidence shows that this will necessarily make you healthier, nor can you avoid all additives. Because some additives are used even in whole foods, it amounts to a personal decision.

NATURAL SUBSTANCES IN FOODS THAT CAN CAUSE ILLNESS

Foods contain a variety of naturally occurring substances that can cause illness. Table 12-6 shows some of the more important examples and the problems they can cause.

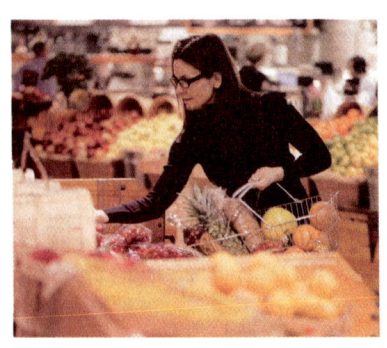

Your choice to consume fresh rather than processed foods will lower your intake of food additives. **Where can you usually find fresh produce, lean meats, and low-fat dairy in a grocery store?** Rob Melnychuk/Photodisc/Getty Images

TABLE 12-6 ■ Examples of Naturally Occurring Food Toxins

Substance	Source	Effect
Avidin	Raw egg whites (cooking destroys avidin)	Binds biotin and limits absorption
Mushroom toxins	Some species of mushrooms such as the jack-o'-lantern	Stomach upset, dizziness, hallucinations, and other neurological symptoms. Some varieties can cause liver and kidney failure, coma, and even death
Oxalic acid	Spinach, strawberries, sesame seeds	Binds calcium and iron in the foods and so limits absorption
Safrole	Sassafras, mace, and nutmeg	Cancer risk when consumed in high doses
Senna or comfrey	Herbal teas	Diarrhea and liver damage
Solanine (green spots on potato skins)	Potato shoots and flesh when stressed by exposure to light or pests	Inhibits the action of neurotransmitters
Tetrodotoxin	Puffer fish	Causes respiratory paralysis
Thiaminase	Raw fish, clams, and mussels	Destroys the vitamin thiamin

Source: Adapted from CDC. Available at https://www.cdc.gov/biomonitoring/nutritional_indicators.html

People have coexisted for centuries with these naturally occurring substances and have learned to avoid some of them and limit intake of others. They pose little health risk because we have developed cooking and food preparation methods to limit the potency of harmful substances, such as thiaminase. Spices are used in such small amounts that health risks do not result. Farmers know potatoes must be stored in the dark so that solanine will not be synthesized. Nevertheless, it is important to understand that some potentially harmful chemicals in foods occur naturally.

IS CAFFEINE A CAUSE FOR CONCERN?

Why all the controversy over a cup of coffee? Researchers have spent a great deal of time on the study of caffeine, the substance of greatest concern in the favorite beverage of many. Caffeine is found naturally in the leaves, seeds, or fruits of more than 60 plants, including coffee beans, cacao beans, kola nuts, guarana berries, and tea. Caffeine is a stimulant found as a natural or added ingredient in many beverages and chocolate. On average, we consume 64% of our caffeine intake as coffee, 16% as tea, 18% as soft drinks, and less than 1% from energy drinks (Fig. 12-14). For teenagers and young adults, this ratio is often relatively higher for soft drinks and lower for coffee.

Caffeine is not often consumed by itself. With the popularity of trendy coffee shops that serve everything from mocha java to flavored lattes, it is difficult to separate the effects of caffeine intake from those of cream, sugar, alternative sweeteners, and flavorings. Although a 6-ounce cup of black coffee contains just 2 kcal, adding cream and sugar increases the calorie count significantly. Adding just one small creamer package of half-and-half will give you an extra 20 kcal; liquid nondairy creamer adds 20 kcal; and 1 teaspoon of sugar adds about 16 kcal. So what is the health-conscious coffee drinker to think? Let us explore the myths and facts of caffeine intake.

Caffeine does not accumulate in the body and is normally excreted within several hours following consumption. Caffeine stimulates the central nervous system and can cause anxiety, increased heart rate, insomnia, increased urination (possibly resulting in dehydration), diarrhea, and gastrointestinal upset in high doses. Those with ulcers or heartburn may experience irritation because caffeine relaxes the lower esophageal sphincter and increases acid production. Those who have anxiety or panic attacks may find that caffeine worsens their symptoms. Some people need only a little caffeine to feel such effects, and the threshold for children is likely even lower than that for adults.

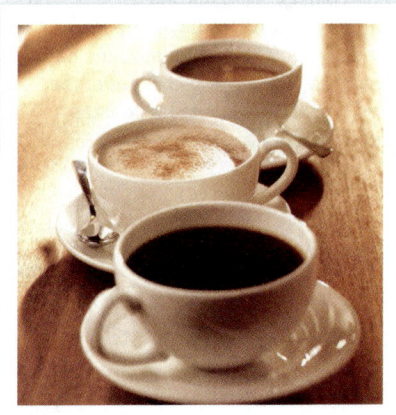

Because gourmet coffee drinks are consumed several times a day, it is difficult to separate the effects of caffeine from those of cream, sugar, chocolate, and other flavorings. **Do you know how many calories are in the typical gourmet coffee beverage?** Ingram Publishing/SuperStock

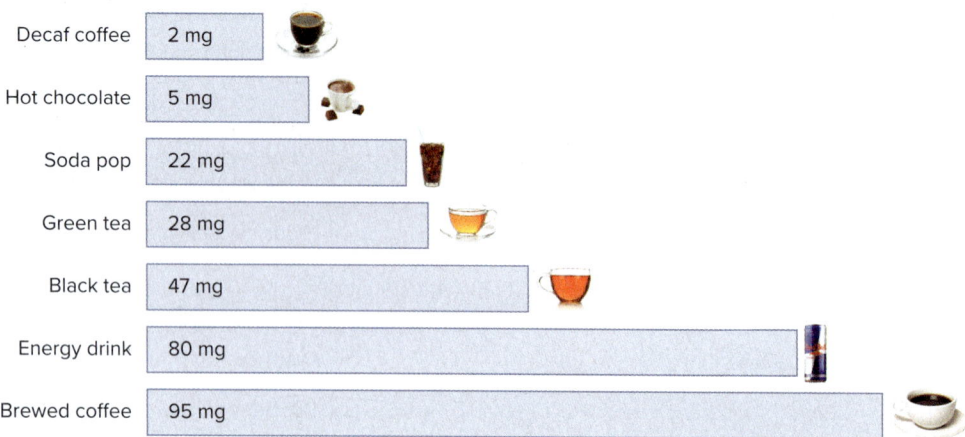

FIGURE 12-14 Amount of caffeine per cup of beverages. For the coffee and tea products, the range varies due to product brand, brewing method, plant variety, and other preparation methods.

Sources: https://www.cspinet.org/eating-healthy/ingredients-of-concern/caffeine-chart; decaf coffee: Davydenko Yuliia/Shutterstock; hot chocolate: Nelea33/Shutterstock; soda pop: Dave Thompson/Shutterstock; green tea: Evgeny Dubinchuk/Shutterstock; black tea: Evgeny Karandaev/Shutterstock; energy drink: monticello/Shutterstock; brewed coffee: pikselstock/Shutterstock

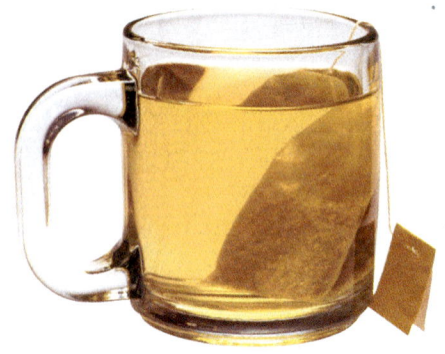

If drinking tea, opt out of using tea in trendy plastic tea bags. Micro- and nanoplastic particles have been found in tea steeped in these plastic tea bags compared to tea brewed in paper tea bags or in a reusable loose-leaf tea infuser. John A. Rizzo/Photodisc/Getty Images

Withdrawal symptoms are also real. Former coffee drinkers may experience headache, nausea, and depression for a short time after discontinuing use. These symptoms can be expected to peak at 20 to 50 hours following the last intake of caffeine. Withdrawal symptoms often occur for those trying to quit as little as a cup of coffee per day. Slow tapering of use over a few days is recommended to avoid these problems.

Are there more serious consequences of consuming caffeine regularly? Although it has been hypothesized that caffeine consumption can lead to certain types of cancer, the association of caffeine with cancer has not been established in the literature. In fact, regular coffee consumption has been linked to a decreased risk of head and neck, colorectal, breast, prostate, endometrial, and liver cancers.[45]

Heavy coffee consumption does increase blood pressure for a short period of time, and coffee consumption has been linked to increased LDL-cholesterol and triglycerides in the blood. This association was found to be caused specifically by cafestol and kahweol, two oils in ground coffee. However, filtered and instant coffees do not contain the harmful oils. It is prudent, though, to limit the amount of coffee in general, especially from French coffee presses and from espresso, as these beverages are not filtered.

Heavy caffeine use does mildly increase the amount of calcium excreted in urine. For this reason, it is important that heavy coffee drinkers ensure their overall dietary patterns contain adequate calcium sources. Females are thought to be at higher risk for a variety of deleterious effects with caffeine consumption, including miscarriages, osteoporosis, and birth defects in their offspring. Some studies show a higher likelihood for miscarriages in females consuming more than five 8-ounce cups of coffee per day (about 500 milligrams of caffeine). The position of the American College of Obstetricians and Gynecologists is that moderate caffeine intake—less than 200 milligrams a day—won't increase the risk of miscarriage, preterm birth, or birth defects.[46,47]

In contrast to these potential harmful effects of caffeine, coffee consumption is effective for treating migraines, likely effective for improving mental alertness, and possibly effective for improving memory, pain, Parkinson's disease, athletic performance, and glucose metabolism in diabetes.[48] Swedish scientists recently found that females ages 40 to 83 who consumed more than a cup of coffee per day for 10 years had a 22% to 25% lower risk of stroke.

Though the debate over caffeine will likely continue as long as adults drink coffee, research does not support many old misconceptions about caffeine. These studies are reinforcing the idea of moderation. A prudent dose of caffeine is 200 to 300 milligrams (about 2 to 3 cups of regular, brewed coffee) per day.

Roots

Variety is the SPICE of life

Have you ever heard the saying, *Variety is the spice of life*? Indeed, a variety of spices, such as those portrayed, contribute in many ways to our dietary patterns. From enhancing flavor and aroma to increasing taste and color, herbs and spices have been shown to confer antioxidant, antimicrobial, and anti-inflammatory effects impacting health.

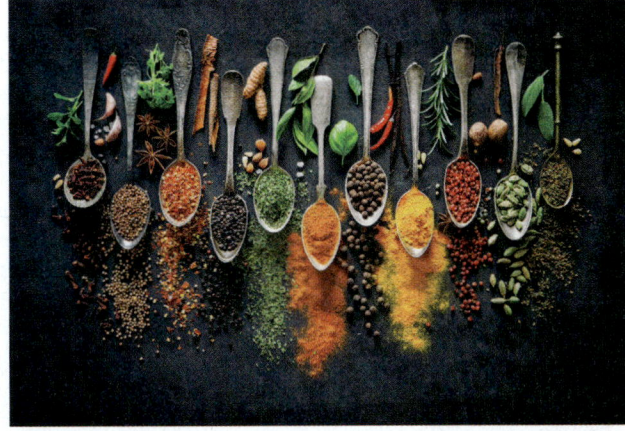

Alexander Raths/123RF

The FDA defines spices as aromatic vegetable substances, in the whole, broken, or ground form, whose significant function in food is seasoning rather than nutrition. For centuries, spices have been used in culinary, religious, and medicinal settings. Spices originate from across the globe and are derived from bark, seeds, roots, fruits, berries, or flowers. Yet spices also pose a risk of foodborne illness from contaminated spices. In turn, the FDA has been addressing spice safety on several fronts, including implementation of the Food Safety and Modernization Act (FSMA) to establish preventive controls in the food supply chain, for both domestically produced and imported food.

Source: U.S. Food & Drug Administration, Center for Food Safety and Applied Nutrition. Compliance Policy Guide: CPG Sec 525.750 Spices—Definitions. October 1980. Updated August 24, 2018. https://www.fda.gov/regulatory-information/search-fda-guidance-documents/cpg-sec-525750-spices-definitions

✓ CONCEPT CHECK 12.5

1. Choose three common food additives and state their purpose in food production.
2. What is the *GRAS* list?
3. What is the purpose of the *Delaney Clause*?
4. What is the typical caffeine content of 8-ounce cups of coffee and tea?
5. What are some of the negative effects of excess caffeine on the body?

12.6 Nutrition and Your Health: Preventing Foodborne Illness

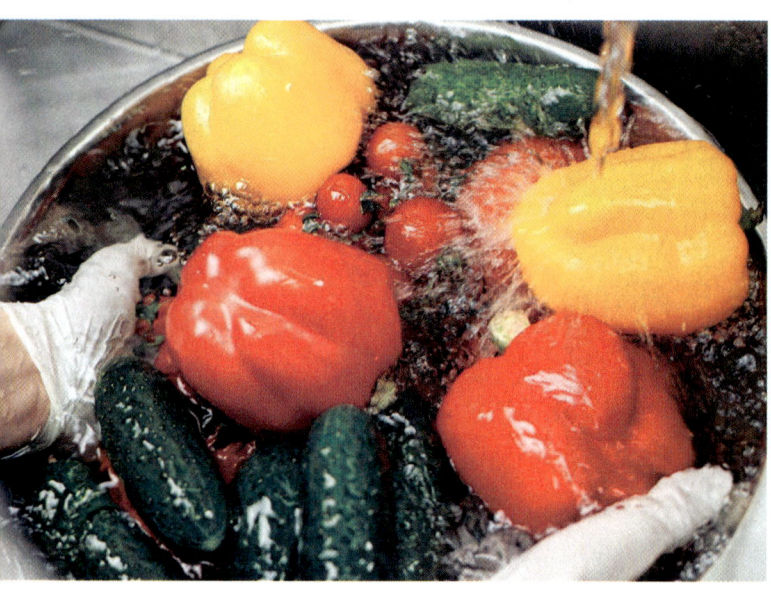

Denys Kovtun/Alamy Stock Photo

You can greatly reduce the risk of foodborne illness by following some important recommendations. When it comes to keeping food safe, keep those four main topics of clean, separate, cook, and chill in mind. These guidelines are detailed below to keep you safe!

Four Steps to Food Safety
1. Clean—wash hands and surfaces often.
2. Separate—don't cross-contaminate.
3. Cook—cook to proper temperatures.
4. Chill—refrigerate promptly.

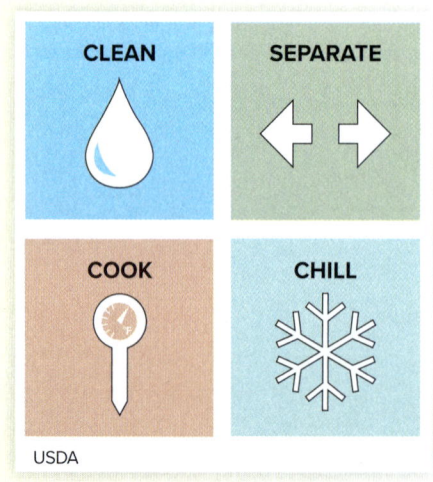

USDA

Clean

- Thoroughly wash your hands for 20 to 30 seconds with warm, soapy water before and after handling food. This practice is especially important when handling raw meat, fish, poultry, and eggs; after using the bathroom; after playing with pets; or after changing diapers. The *Four F's* of contamination include *fingers, foods, feces, and flies.*
- Make sure counters, cutting boards, dishes, and other equipment are thoroughly washed, rinsed, sanitized, and air-dried before use. Be especially careful to use hot, soapy water to wash surfaces and equipment that come in contact with raw meat, fish, poultry, and eggs as soon as possible to remove *Salmonella* bacteria that may be present. Otherwise, bacteria on the surfaces will infect the next foods that come in contact with the surface, a process called **cross-contamination.** In addition, replace sponges and wash kitchen towels frequently. Microwaving sponges for 60 seconds or washing them in the dishwasher helps rid them of live bacteria.
- If possible, cut foods to be eaten raw on a clean cutting board reserved for that purpose. Then clean this cutting board using hot, soapy water. If the same board must be used for both meat and other foods, cut any potentially contaminated items, such as meat, last. After cutting the meat, wash the cutting board thoroughly. The FDA recommends cutting boards with unmarred surfaces made of easy-to-clean, nonporous materials, such as plastic, marble, or glass. Wooden boards should be made of a nonabsorbent hardwood, such as oak, maple, or bamboo, and have no obvious seams or cracks. Recently, bamboo has become popular for cutting boards because its dense wood resists knife scarring and water penetration, leaving bacteria without a place to multiply. Keep a separate wooden cutting board for chopping produce and slicing bread to prevent cross-contamination. Furthermore, the FDA recommends that all cutting boards be replaced when they become streaked with hard-to-clean grooves or cuts, which may harbor bacteria. In addition, cutting boards should be sanitized once a week in a dilute bleach solution. Flood the board with the solution, let it sit for a few minutes, then rinse thoroughly.
- Carefully wash fresh fruit and vegetables under running water to remove dirt and bacteria clinging to the surface, using a vegetable brush if the skin is to be eaten. People have become ill from *Salmonella* introduced while cutting melons that were contaminated with surface bacteria. The bacteria were on the outside of the melons.
- Completely remove moldy portions of food, or do not eat the food. If a food is covered in mold, discard the food. Mold growth is prevented by properly storing food at cold temperatures and

cross-contamination Process by which bacteria or other microorganisms are unintentionally transferred from one substance or object to another, with harmful effect.

- Follow food recalls online at https://www.fsis.usda.gov/recalls. Note that a Class I recall means that there is a *reasonable probability* that consuming the food will cause serious health consequences or death.

Cook

- When thawing foods, do so in the refrigerator, under cold potable running water, or in a microwave oven. Also, cook foods immediately after thawing under cold water or in the microwave. Never let frozen foods thaw unrefrigerated all day or night. Also, marinate food in the refrigerator.
- During microwave cooking, cover food with glass or ceramic to decrease evaporation. Stir and rotate food at least once or twice for even cooking. Then, allow microwaved food to stand, covered, after heating is completed to help cook the exterior and equalize the temperature throughout. Use the oven temperature probe or a meat thermometer to check that food is done in several spots.
- If thawing meat in the microwave, use the oven's defrost setting. Ice crystals in frozen foods are not heated well by the microwave oven and can create cold spots, which later cook more slowly.
- Cook food thoroughly and use a bimetallic thermometer to check for doneness, especially for fresh beef and fish (145°F [63°C]), pork (145°F [63°C]), and poultry (165°F [74°C]). Minimal internal temperatures for doneness are shown in Figure 12-15. Eggs should be cooked until the yolk and white are hard. The FDA does not recommend that eggs be prepared sunny-side up. Alfalfa sprouts and other types of sprouts should be cooked until they are steaming. Cooking is by far the most reliable way to destroy foodborne viruses and bacteria, such as norovirus and toxic strains of *E. coli*. Freezing only temporarily halts viral and bacterial growth.
- A general precaution is to not eat raw animal products. As noted, many restaurants now include an advisory on menus stating that

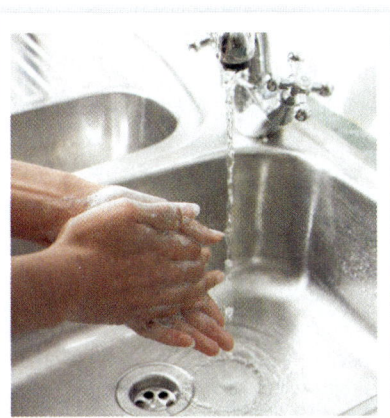

Washing hands thoroughly (for at least 20 to 30 seconds) with warm water and soap should be the first step in food preparation. **What are the *four F's* of food contamination?** Dave & Les Jacobs/Blend Images/Getty Images

using the food promptly. Also discard soft foods with high moisture content such as bread, yogurt, soft cheeses, and deli meats if there are spots of mold on them. It is safe to trim off any moldy spots of dense foods such as hard cheeses or firm fruits and vegetables.
- Avoid coughing or sneezing over foods, even when you are healthy. Cover cuts on hands with a sterile bandage. This helps stop *Staphylococcus* bacteria from contaminating food.
- Ignore the *5-second rule*. Food that has fallen on the floor picks up bacteria immediately upon contact.

Separate

- When shopping, select frozen foods and perishable foods such as meat, poultry, or fish last. Always place fresh meat, poultry, and fish in separate plastic bags so that drippings do not contaminate other foods in the shopping cart. Do not let groceries sit in a warm car; this allows bacteria to grow. Also consider using recyclable insulated grocery bags to transport your cold items. Get the perishable foods such as meat, eggs, and dairy products home quickly and promptly refrigerate or freeze them.
- Do not buy or use food from damaged containers that leak, bulge, or are severely dented, or from jars that are cracked or have loose or bulging lids. Do not taste or use food that has a foul odor or spurts liquid when the can is opened; the deadly *Clostridium botulinum* toxin may be present.
- Purchase only pasteurized milk and cheese (check the label). This is especially important for females who are pregnant because highly toxic bacteria and viruses that can harm the fetus thrive in unpasteurized milk.
- Purchase only the amount of produce needed for a week's time. The longer you keep fruits and vegetables, the more time is available for bacteria to grow.
- When purchasing precut produce or bagged salad greens, avoid those that look slimy, discolored, or dry; these are signs of improper holding temperatures.
- Observe sell-by and expiration dates on food labels, and do not buy products that are near or past these dates.

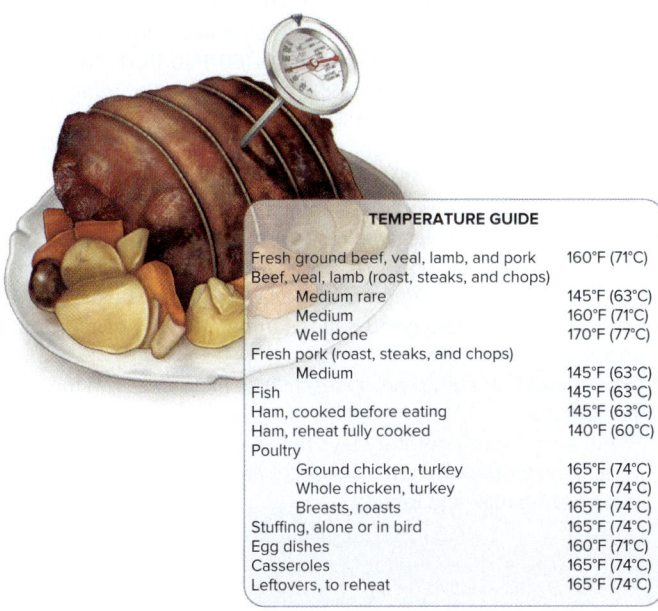

TEMPERATURE GUIDE	
Fresh ground beef, veal, lamb, and pork	160°F (71°C)
Beef, veal, lamb (roast, steaks, and chops)	
Medium rare	145°F (63°C)
Medium	160°F (71°C)
Well done	170°F (77°C)
Fresh pork (roast, steaks, and chops)	
Medium	145°F (63°C)
Fish	145°F (63°C)
Ham, cooked before eating	145°F (63°C)
Ham, reheat fully cooked	140°F (60°C)
Poultry	
Ground chicken, turkey	165°F (74°C)
Whole chicken, turkey	165°F (74°C)
Breasts, roasts	165°F (74°C)
Stuffing, alone or in bird	165°F (74°C)
Egg dishes	160°F (71°C)
Casseroles	165°F (74°C)
Leftovers, to reheat	165°F (74°C)

FIGURE 12-15 Minimum internal temperatures when cooking or reheating foods.

Source: USDA Food Safety and Inspection Service, Safe Minimum Internal Temperature Chart, www.fsis.usda.gov

an increased risk of foodborne illness is associated with eating undercooked eggs. As long as restaurants provide this warning on their menus, however, they are allowed to cook eggs to any temperature requested by the consumer. The FDA warns us not to consume homemade ice cream, eggnog, and mayonnaise if made with unpasteurized, raw eggs because of the risk of *Salmonella* foodborne illness. The pasteurization of eggs or egg products kills *Salmonella* bacteria. Consuming raw seafood, especially oysters, also poses a risk of foodborne illness. Properly cooked seafood should flake easily and/or be opaque or dull and firm. If it is translucent or shiny, it is not done.

- Cook stuffing separately from poultry (or stuff immediately before cooking, and then transfer the stuffing to a clean bowl immediately after cooking). Make sure the stuffing reaches 165°F (74°C). *Salmonella* is the major concern with poultry.
- For outdoor cooking, cook food completely at the picnic site, with no partial cooking in advance.
- Serve meat, poultry, and fish on a clean plate—never the same plate used to hold the raw product. For example, when grilling hamburgers, do not put cooked items on the same plate used to carry the raw product out to the grill.
- Once a food is cooked, consume it right away, or cool it to 70°F (21°C) within 2 hours, and then make sure any leftovers are cooled to 40°F (4.4°C) within 4 hours. If it is not to be eaten immediately, in hot weather (80°F and above) make sure that this cooling is done within 1 hour. Do this by separating the food into as many shallow pans as needed to provide a large surface area for cooling. Be careful not to recontaminate cooked food by contact with raw meat or juices from hands, cutting boards, or other dirty utensils.

Chill

- Keep foods out of the *danger zone* (see Fig. 12-10) by keeping hot foods hot and cold foods cold. Hold food below 40°F (4.4°C) or above 140°F (60°C). Foodborne microorganisms thrive in more moderate temperatures (60°F to 110°F [16°C to 43°C]). Some microorganisms can even grow in the refrigerator. Store dry food at 60°F to 70°F (16°C to 21°C).
- Keep leftovers in the refrigerator only for the recommended length of time (Fig. 12-16).
- Use refrigerated ground meat and patties in 1 to 2 days and frozen meat and patties within 3 to 4 months.
- Reheat leftovers to 165°F (74°C); reheat gravy to a rolling boil to kill *Clostridium perfringens* bacteria, which may be present. Merely reheating to a good eating temperature is not sufficient to kill harmful bacteria.
- Store peeled or cut-up produce, such as melon balls, in the refrigerator.
- Make sure the refrigerator stays below 40°F (4.4°C). Either use a refrigerator thermometer or keep it as cold as possible without freezing milk and lettuce.

The FoodKeeper app (https://www.foodsafety.gov/keep-food-safe/foodkeeper-app) will guide you on appropriate storage of foods. Developed by the Food Safety and Inspection Service, this resource is also available as a mobile app.

When in doubt, throw it out!

Food	Refrigerator Storage at 40°F (4.4°C) Time (days)
Meats	
Cooked beef, bison, lamb	3–4
Cooked ground beef/turkey	3–4
Cooked pork	3–4
Cooked poultry	3–4
Deli meat	3–5
Seafood	
Cooked	3–4
Raw (e.g. sushi/sashimi)	Consume on day of purchase
Other Entrees	
Casserole	3–4
Pasta	3–5
Pizza	3–4
Rice	4–6
Soups and Chili	
Chili	3–4
Soup/stew	3–4
Side Dishes	
Cooked vegetables	3–4
Deviled egg	3–4
Fresh salad	1–4
Fresh vegetables	1–6
Hard-boiled egg	7
Pasta or potato salad	3–5
Potato (any style)	3–4
Dessert	
Cake	7–10
Cheesecake	7–10
Cream pie	3–4
Fruit pie	2–7
Pastries	7

FIGURE 12-16 Length of time to keep leftovers safely in the refrigerator.
Source: www.foodsafety.gov

- When the power goes out, keep the freezer and refrigerator doors closed as much as possible. Food can stay cold in an unopened refrigerator for about 4 hours; after 4 hours without power, discard perishable foods such as milk, meat, leftovers, and deli meats. Unopened freezers will keep food frozen for 2 days if full and 1 day if half full. Meat, poultry, and seafood can be refrozen if the freezer has not risen above 40°F (4.4°C).

- Cross-contamination is not only a threat during food preparation; it can also become a problem during food storage. Make sure all foods, including leftovers, are contained and covered in the refrigerator to prevent drippings from uncooked and potentially hazardous foods from tainting other foods. It is a good idea to store foods likely to pose risk of foodborne illness on lower shelves of the refrigerator, beneath other foods to be eaten raw.
- Raw fish dishes, such as sushi, can be safe for most people to eat if they are made with very fresh fish that has been commercially frozen and then thawed. The freezing is important to eliminate potential health risks from parasites. The FDA recommends that the fish be frozen to an internal temperature of −10°F (−23°C) for 7 days. If you choose to eat uncooked fish, purchase the fish from reputable establishments that have high standards for quality and sanitation. If you are at high risk for foodborne illness, it is wise to avoid raw fish products.
- Keep your hands, surfaces, and utensils clean. Separate raw foods from cooked and ready-to-eat foods at all stages of food preparation, cooking, and storage to prevent cross-contamination. Use a food thermometer to ensure that you have cooked foods to the proper temperatures to kill harmful pathogens. Finally, chill the leftovers promptly, being sure that foods are not kept in the danger zone for more than 2 hours. These simple strategies will help to keep you safe from foodborne illness.

> **World Health Organization's Golden Rules for Safe Food Preparation:**
> 1. Choose foods processed for safety.
> 2. Cook food thoroughly.
> 3. Eat cooked foods immediately.
> 4. Store cooked foods carefully.
> 5. Reheat cooked foods thoroughly.
> 6. Avoid contact between raw and cooked foods.
> 7. Wash hands repeatedly.
> 8. Keep all kitchen surfaces meticulously clean.
> 9. Protect foods from insects, rodents, and other animals.
> 10. Use pure water.
>
> Source: WHO "Golden Rules" for Safe Food Preparation. https://www.paho.org/en/health-emergencies/who-golden-rules-safe-food-preparation

CASE STUDY: Preventing Foodborne Illness at Gatherings

Nicole attended a gathering of her coworkers on a warm Saturday in July. The theme of the party was international dining. Nicole and her husband brought an Argentinian dish: potato and beef empanadas. They followed the recipe and cooking time carefully, removing the dish from the oven at 1:00 P.M. and keeping it warm by wrapping the pan in a towel. They traveled in their car to the party and set the dish out on the buffet table at 3:00 P.M. Dinner was to be served at 4:00 P.M. However, the guests were enjoying themselves so much that no one began to eat until 6:00 P.M. Nicole made sure she sampled the empanadas that she and her husband made, but her husband did not. She also had some salad, garlic bread, and a sweet dessert made with coconut.

The couple returned home at 11:00 P.M. and went to bed. At about 2:00 A.M., Nicole knew something was wrong. She had severe abdominal pain and had to make a dash to the bathroom. She spent most of the next 3 hours in the bathroom with severe diarrhea. By dawn, the diarrhea subsided and she started to feel better. After a few cups of tea and a light breakfast, she was feeling like herself by noon. On Monday at work, she discovered that several of her coworkers also had diarrhea on Saturday night.

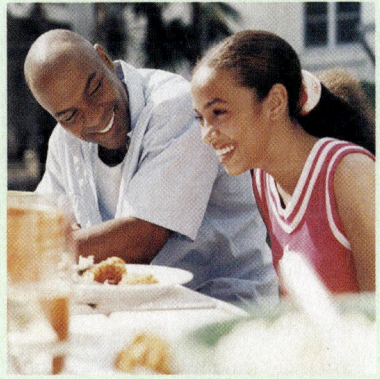

Nicole and her husband enjoying the international dining summer celebration with her coworkers. Digital Vision/Getty Images

1. Based on her symptoms, what type of foodborne illness did Nicole likely contract?
2. Why is consuming food at large gatherings risky?
3. What precautions for avoiding foodborne illness were ignored by Nicole and the rest of the people at the party?
4. How could this scenario be rewritten to substantially reduce the risk of foodborne illness?

Complete the Case Study. Responses to these questions can be provided by your instructor.

✓ CONCEPT CHECK 12.6

1. What are the four actionable items recommended by government agencies to prevent foodborne illnesses?
2. What is *cross-contamination,* and how can you avoid it?
3. What are some safe food-handling practices to implement during a power outage?

Summary (Numbers refer to numbered sections in the chapter)

12.1 Conventional agriculture emphasizes large yields and low costs, but the more recent trend toward sustainability considers the long-term environmental impact of agricultural practices. Consumers are driving up demand for organic, locally grown, and sustainable products. Food biotechnology is also on the rise to meet global demands and consumer trends. Sadly, food waste and losses are also increasing.

12.2 A variety of environmental contaminants and pesticide residues can be found in foods. It is helpful to know which foods pose the greatest risks and act accordingly to reduce exposure, such as washing fruits and vegetables before use.

12.3 Infants, children, older adults, patients post-surgery, individuals who are immunosuppressed, and females who are pregnant are most susceptible to foodborne illness. The risk of foodborne illness has increased as more of our foods are prepared outside of the home. In the past, salt, sugar, smoke, fermentation, and drying were used to protect against foodborne illness. Today, careful cooking, pasteurization, irradiation, attention to food temperature, and thorough handwashing provide additional insurance.

12.4 Viruses, bacteria, and other microorganisms in food pose the greatest risk for foodborne illness. Major causes of foodborne illness are norovirus and the bacteria *Campylobacter jejuni, Salmonella, Staphylococcus aureus,* and *Clostridium perfringens.* In addition, such bacteria as *Clostridium botulinum, Listeria monocytogenes,* and *Escherichia coli* have been found to cause illness.

12.5 Food additives are used primarily to extend shelf life by preventing microbial growth and the destruction of food components by oxygen, metals, and other substances. Food additives are classified as those directly (intentionally) added to foods and those that indirectly (incidentally) appear in foods. Under its jurisdiction in the United States, the Delaney Clause allows the FDA to ban the use of any direct food additive that increases cancer risk. Toxic substances occur naturally in a variety of foods, such as green potatoes, raw fish, mushrooms, and raw egg whites. Cooking foods limits their toxic effects in some cases; others are best to avoid altogether, such as toxic mushroom species and the green parts of potatoes.

12.6 Safe food handling can be summed up in four easy steps: (1) *clean* hands and surfaces often; (2) *separate* raw and ready-to-eat foods to prevent cross-contamination; (3) *cook* (and reheat) potentially hazardous foods thoroughly, measuring temperature with a food thermometer; and (4) *chill* foods by refrigerating promptly after eating. Two of these practices focus on food temperature; foods should not be held in the *danger zone* (40°F to 140°F; 4.4°C to 60°C) for more than 2 hours.

Check Your Knowledge (Answers are available at the end of this question set)

1. Nitrite prevents the growth of
   a. *Clostridium botulinum.*
   b. *Escherichia coli.*
   c. *Staphylococcus aureus.*
   d. yeasts.

2. Substances used to preserve foods by lowering the pH are
   a. smoke and irradiation.
   b. baking powder and baking soda.
   c. salt and sugar.
   d. vinegar and citric acid.

3. Food additives widely used for many years without apparent ill effects are on the _____ list.
   a. FDA
   b. GRAS
   c. USDA
   d. Delaney

4. The four actions that are part of the USDA food-safety program are clean, _____, cook, and chill.
   a. sterilize
   b. separate
   c. pasteurize
   d. freeze

5. *Salmonella* bacteria are usually spread via
   a. raw meats, poultry, and eggs.
   b. pickled vegetables.
   c. home-canned vegetables.
   d. raw vegetables.

6. It is unwise to thaw meats or poultry
   a. in a microwave oven.
   b. in the refrigerator.
   c. under cool running water.
   d. at room temperature.

7. Milk that can remain on supermarket shelves, free of microbial growth, for many years has been processed by which of the following methods?
   a. Use of humectants
   b. Using antibiotics in animal feed
   c. Use of sequestrants
   d. Aseptic processing

8. Those at greatest risk for foodborne illness include
   a. females who are pregnant.
   b. infants and children.
   c. immunosuppressed individuals.
   d. all of these individuals.

9. Pasteurization involves the
   a. exposure of food to high temperatures for short periods to destroy harmful microorganisms.
   b. exposure of food to heat to inactivate enzymes that cause undesirable effects in foods during storage.
   c. fortification of foods with vitamins A and D.
   d. use of irradiation to destroy certain pathogens in foods.

10. Food can be kept for long periods by adding salt or sugar because these substances
    a. make the food too acidic for spoilage to occur.
    b. bind to water, thereby making it unavailable to the microorganisms.
    c. effectively kill microorganisms.
    d. dissolve the cell walls in plant foods.

Answer Key: 1. a (LO 12.5), 2. d (LO 12.3), 3. b (LO 12.5), 4. b (LO 12.6), 5. a (LO 12.3), 6. d (LO 12.6), 7. d (LO 12.3), 8. d (LO 12.4), 9. a (LO 12.3), 10. b (LO 12.5)

Study Questions (Numbers refer to Learning Outcomes)

1. Describe some of the advances in agricultural science that are positively affecting our food supply. **(LO 12.1)**
2. Describe four recommendations for reducing the risk of ill effects from environmental contaminants. **(LO 12.2)**
3. What three trends in food purchasing and production have led to a greater number of cases of foodborne illness? **(LO 12.3)**
4. Which types of foods are most likely to be involved in foodborne illness? Why are they prone to contamination? **(LO 12.3)**
5. Identify three major classes of microorganisms responsible for foodborne illness. **(LO 12.4)**
6. Define the term *food additive*, and give examples of four direct or intentional food additives. What are their specific functions in foods? What is their relationship to the GRAS list? **(LO 12.5)**
7. Describe the federal process that governs the use of food additives, including the Delaney Clause. **(LO 12.5)**
8. Put into perspective the benefits and risks of using additives in food. Point out an easy way to reduce the consumption of food additives. Do you think this is worth the effort in terms of maintaining health? Why or why not? **(LO 12.5)**
9. Name some substances that occur naturally in foods but may cause illness. **(LO 12.5)**
10. List four techniques other than thorough cooking that are important in preventing foodborne illness. **(LO 12.6)**

References

1. U.S. agriculture—statistics & facts. Statista Research Department. Accessed November 10, 2023. https://www.statista.com/topics/1126/us-agriculture
2. Cassidy E, Snyder A. Map of the month: how many people work in agriculture. ResourceWatch. Accessed November 12, 2023. https://blog.resourcewatch.org/2019/05/30/map-of-the-month-how-many-people-work-in-agriculture/
3. Global Forum on Food Security and Nutrition. Food and Agriculture Organization of the United Nations. Accessed January 22, 2022. https://www.fao.org/fsnforum/
4. Organic market summary and trends. U.S. Department of Agriculture, Economic Research Service. Accessed November 10, 2023. https://www.ers.usda.gov/topics/natural-resources-environment/organic-agriculture/organic-market-overview.aspx
5. COVID-19 will shape organic industry in 2020 after banner year in 2019. News release. Organic Trade Association. Accessed November 12, 2023. https://ota.com/news/press-releases/21328
6. Worldwide sales of organic food from 1999 to 2019. Statista. Accessed November 12, 2023. https://www.statista.com/statistics/273090/worldwide-sales-of-organic-foods-since-1999/
7. Organic standards. U.S. Department of Agriculture, Agricultural Marketing Service. Accessed November 18, 2023. https://www.ams.usda.gov/grades-standards/organic-standards
8. Organic regulations. U.S. Department of Agriculture, Agricultural Marketing Service. Accessed November 12, 2023. https://www.ams.usda.gov/rules-regulations/organic
9. Smith-Spangler C, Brandeau MI, Hunter GE, et al. Are organic foods safer or healthier than conventional alternatives? a systematic review. *Ann Intern Med.* 2012 Sep 4;157(5):348-366. doi: 10.7326/0003-4819-157-5-201209040-00007
10. National Academies of Sciences, Engineering, and Medicine, Board on Agriculture and Natural Resources. *Report in Brief: Genetically Engineered Crops: Experiences and Prospects.* Accessed November 10, 2023. https://www.nap.edu/resource/23395/GE-crops-report-brief.pdf
11. BE disclosure. U.S. Department of Agriculture, Agricultural Marketing Service. Accessed November 28, 2023. https://www.ams.usda.gov/rules-regulations/be
12. GMO FAQs: what are CRISPR and other new breeding techniques (NBTs)? Genetic Literacy Project. Accessed November 18, 2023. https://gmo.geneticliteracyproject.org/FAQ/what-is-crisprcas9-and-other-new-breeding-technologies-nbts
13. Biotechnology. Center for Science in the Public Interest. Accessed November 10, 2023. https://cspinet.org/protecting-our-health/biotechnology
14. Klümper W, Qaim M. A meta-analysis of the impacts of genetically modified crops. *PLoS One.* 2014 Nov 3;9(11):e111629. doi: 10.1371/journal.pone.0111629
15. Vogliano C, Brown K. The state of America's wasted food and opportunities to make a difference. *J Acad Nutr Diet.* 2016 Jul;116(7):1199-1207. doi: 10.1016/j.jand.2016.01.022
16. Gunders D; National Resource Defense Fund. *Wasted: How America Is Losing Up to 40 Percent of Its Food from Farm to Fork to Landfills.* Second edition of NRDC's original 2012 report. Accessed November 13, 2023. https://www.nrdc.org/sites/default/files/wasted-2017-report.pdf

17. Papargyropoulou E, Lozano R, Steinberger JK, Wright N, bin Ujang Z. The food waste hierarchy as a framework for the management of food surplus and food waste. *J Clean Prod.* 2014 Aug 1;76:106-115. doi: 10.1016/j.jclepro.2014.04.020

18. New record: number of overfished stocks in the U.S. reaches all time low. U.S. Department of Commerce, National Oceanic and Atmospheric Administration (NOAA). Accessed November 13, 2023. https://www.noaa.gov/media-release/new-record-number-of-overfished-stocks-in-us-reaches-all-time-low

19. Fisheries of the United States, 2019. U.S. Department of Commerce, National Oceanic and Atmospheric Administration (NOAA), National Marine Fisheries Service. Accessed November 17, 2023. https://media.fisheries.noaa.gov/2021-05/fus-2019-fact-sheet-v4.2-webready.pdf?null

20. Kearns M. NFI releases new list detailing the top 10 seafood species Americans consume most. Seafood Source. Accessed November 17, 2023. https://www.seafoodsource.com/news/foodservice-retail/nfi-releases-new-top-10-list-detailing-the-seafood-species-americans-consume-most

21. Berge A. US consumption can be doubled. Salmon Business. Accessed November 17, 2023. https://salmonbusiness.com/us-consumption-can-be-doubled/

22. Pelletier JE, Laska MN, Neumark-Sztainer D, Story M. Positive attitudes toward organic, local, and sustainable foods are associated with higher dietary quality among young adults. *J Acad Nutr Diet.* 2013 Jan;113(1):127-132. doi: 10.1016/j.jand.2012.08.021

23. About farm to school. National Farm to School Network. Accessed November 17, 2023. https://www.farmtoschool.org/about/what-is-farm-to-school

24. Popp J, Pető K, Nagy J. Pesticide productivity and food security. A review. *Agron. Sustain. Dev.* 2013 Jan;33:243-255. doi: 10.1007/s13593-012-0105-x

25. Henley SJ, Anderson RN, Thomas CC, Massetti GM, Peaker B, Richardson LC. Invasive cancer incidence, 2004–2013, and deaths, 2006–2015, in nonmetropolitan and metropolitan counties—United States. *MMWR Surveill Summ.* 2014 Jul 7;66(14):1-13. doi: 10.15585/mmwr.ss6614a1

26. Glyphosate. U.S. Environmental Protection Agency. Accessed November 18, 2023. https://www.epa.gov/ingredients-used-pesticide-products/glyphosate

27. Curl CL, Beresford SAA, Fenske RA, et al. Estimating pesticide exposure from dietary intake and organic food choices: the Multi-Ethnic Study of Atherosclerosis (MESA). *Environ Health Perspect.* 2015 May;123(5):475-483. doi: 10.1289/ehp.1408197

28. Advice about eating fish. U.S. Food & Drug Administration. Accessed November 18, 2023. https://www.fda.gov/food/consumers/advice-about-eating-fish

29. Kantor L. Americans' seafood consumption below recommendations. U.S. Department of Agriculture, Economic Research Service. Accessed November 17, 2023. https://www.ers.usda.gov/amber-waves/2016/october/americans-seafood-consumption-below-recommendations/

30. Mohan D, Mente A, Dehghan M, et al. Associations of fish consumption with risk of cardiovascular disease and mortality among individuals with or without vascular disease from 58 countries. *JAMA Intern Med.* 2021 May 1;181(5):631-649. doi: 10.1001/jamainternmed.2021.0036

31. U.S. Department of Agriculture, Office of Inspector General. *USDA Agency Activities for Agroterrorism Prevention, Detection, and Response. Audit Report 50701-0001-21.* Accessed November 22, 2023. https://www.usda.gov/sites/default/files/50701-0001-21.pdf

32. Pal S. Incidence of foodborne illness. *US Pharm.* 2017 Dec 15;42(12):14.

33. Painter JA, Hoekstra RM, Ayers T, et al. Attribution of foodborne illnesses, hospitalizations, and deaths to food commodities by using outbreak data, United States, 1998–2008. *Emerg Infect Dis.* 2013 Mar;19(3):407-415. doi: 10.3201/eid1903.111866

34. Estimates of foodborne illness in the United States. Centers for Disease Control and Prevention. Accessed November 18, 2023. https://www.cdc.gov/foodborneburden

35. Cleanliness helps prevent foodborne illness. U.S. Department of Agriculture, Food Safety and Inspection Service. Accessed November 18, 2023. https://www.fsis.usda.gov/wps/portal/fsis/topics/food-safety-education/get-answers/food-safety-fact-sheets/safe-food-handling/cleanliness-helps-prevent-foodborne-illness/CT_Index

36. Carothers M. Are you and your food prepared for a power outage? *USDA Blog.* Accessed November 19, 2023. https://www.usda.gov/media/blog/2016/09/26/are-you-and-your-food-prepared-power-outage

37. Thatte D. The Food Safety Modernization Act in a nutshell. *National Institute of Standards and Technology Blog.* Accessed November 14, 2023. https://www.nist.gov/blogs/manufacturing-innovation-blog/food-safety-modernization-act-nutshell

38. Dall C. FDA reports major drop in antibiotics for food animals. *Center for Infectious Disease Research and Policy News.* Accessed November 16, 2023. http://www.cidrap.umn.edu/news-perspective/2018/12/fda-reports-major-drop-antibiotics-food-animals

39. Atreya CD. Major foodborne illness causing viruses and current status of vaccines against the diseases. *Foodborne Pathog Dis.* Summer 2004;1(2):89-96. doi: 10.1089/153531404323143602

40. Burden of norovirus illness in the U.S. Centers for Disease Control and Prevention. Accessed November 18, 2023. Available at https://www.cdc.gov/norovirus/trends-outbreaks/burden-US.html

41. Inventory of food contact substances listed in 21 CFR. U.S. Food & Drug Administration. Accessed November 18, 2023. Available at https://www.fda.gov/food/packaging-food-contact-substances-fcs/inventory-food-contact-substances-listed-21-cfr

42. AskUSDA. U.S. Department of Agriculture. Accessed November 18, 2023. https://ask.usda.gov/s/article/What-are-the-most-widely-used-food-additives

43. FDA issues final rule on food ingredients that may be "generally recognized as safe." U.S. Department of Agriculture, U.S. Food & Drug Administration. Accessed November 20, 2023. https://www.fda.gov/food/newsevents/constituentupdates/ucm516332.htm

44. McCann D, Barrett A, Cooper A, et al. Food additives and hyperactive behaviour in 3-year-old and 8/9-year-old children in the community: a randomised, double-blinded, placebo-controlled trial. *Lancet.* 2007 Nov 3;370(9598):1560-1567. doi: 10.1016/S0140-6736(07)61306-3

45. Kennedy OJ, Roderick P, Buchanan R, Fallowfield JA, Hayes PC, Parkes J. Coffee, including caffeinated and decaffeinated coffee, and the risk of hepatocellular carcinoma: a systematic review and dose–response meta-analysis. *BMJ Open.* 2017 May 9;7(5):e013739. doi: 10.1136/bmjopen-2016-013739

46. American College of Obstetricians and Gynecologists. ACOG Committee Opinion No. 462: moderate caffeine consumption during pregnancy. *Obst Gynecol.* 2010 Aug;116(2 Pt 1):467-468. doi: 10.1097/AOG.0b013e3181eeb2a1

47. American College of Obstetricians and Gynecologists. How much coffee can I drink while I'm pregnant? *Ask ACOG.* Accessed November 18, 2023. https://www.acog.org/womens-health/experts-and-stories/ask-acog/how-much-coffee-can-i-drink-while-pregnant

48. Reis CEG, Dórea JG, da Costa THM. Effects of coffee consumption on glucose metabolism: a systematic review of clinical trials. *J Tradit Complement Med.* 2018 May 3;9(3):184-191. doi: 10.1016/j.jtcme.2018.01.001

Design Element Credits: Fact Check/magnifying glass icon: McGraw Hill; Magnificent Microbiome background image: Alena Ohneva/Shutterstock; Sustainable Solutions icon: McGraw Hill; Roots icon: McGraw Hill; Medicine Cabinet icon: Peter Dazeley/Photographer's Choice/Getty Images

Chapter 13: Global Nutrition

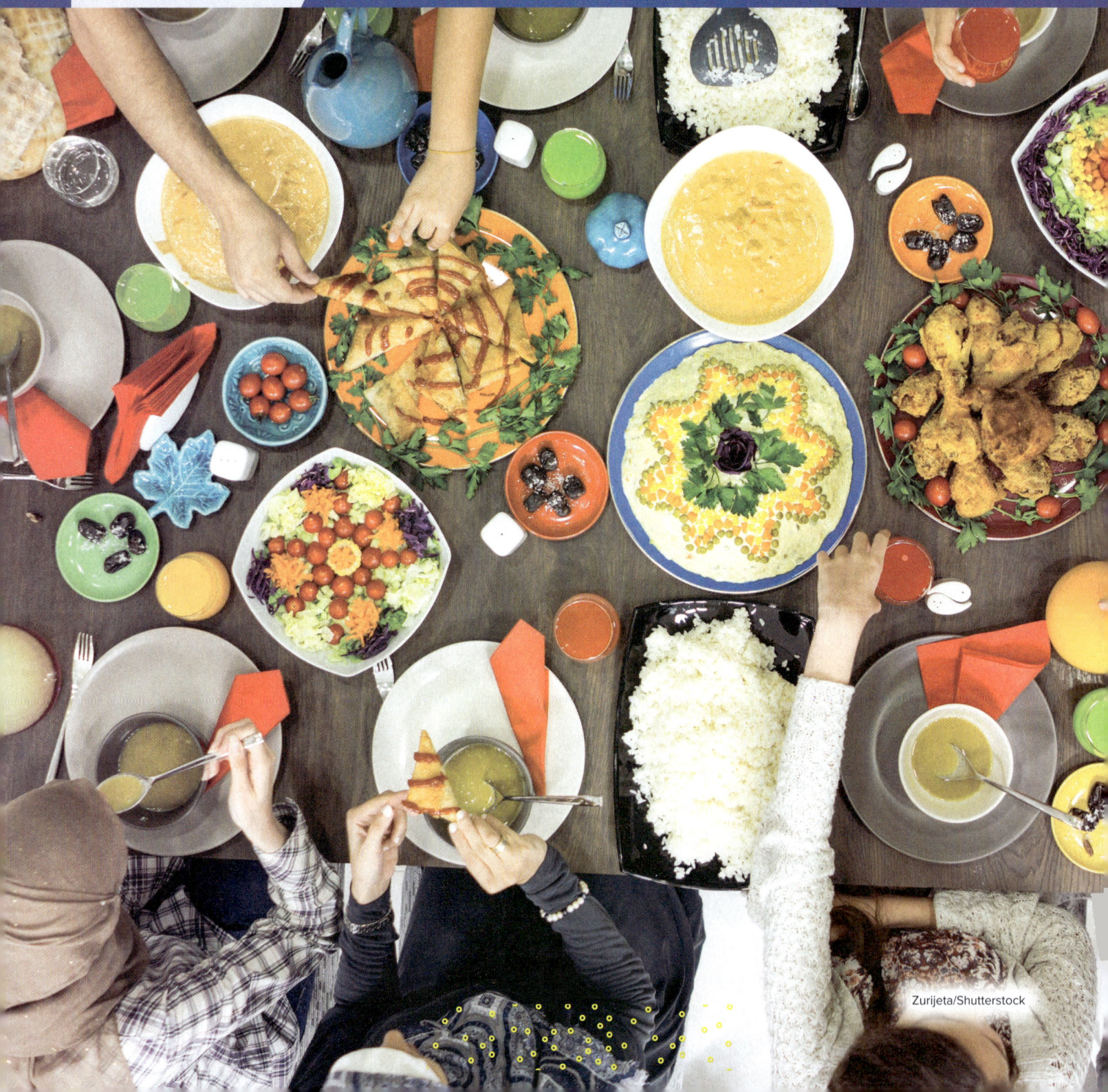

Zurijeta/Shutterstock

Student Learning Outcomes

Chapter 13 is designed to allow you to:

13.1 Define the state of global food and nutrition security.

13.2 Describe malnutrition in the United States and highlight efforts to combat suboptimal nutrition.

13.3 Examine global nutrition and evaluate the factors related to health outcomes.

13.4 Outline global strategies to combat malnutrition.

13.5 Evaluate the consequences of malnutrition during critical periods in a person's life.

FACT CHECK

Is there a difference between *malnutrition* and *hunger*?

We learned much of what we know about malnutrition in the 1940s when a group of researchers, led by Dr. Ansel Keys, examined the general effects of malnutrition on adults. In this study, healthy males were placed on a calorie-restricted diet for 6 months. During this time, they lost an average of 24% of their body weight and complained of fatigue, muscle soreness, irritability, intolerance to cold, and hunger. This was accompanied by a lack of ambition, self-discipline, and concentration and were often moody, apathetic, and depressed. Their heart rate and muscle tone decreased, and they developed edema. When the men were permitted to eat normally again, feelings of recurrent hunger and fatigue persisted, even after 12 weeks of rehabilitation. Full recovery required about 8 months. This landmark study helps us to better understand the general effects of adult malnutrition worldwide.

Plentiful food is a source of not only nourishment but also comfort and sustainability. This chapter examines global nutrition and focuses on the problem of malnutrition, contributing factors, and potential solutions. If we are to fully eradicate this issue, we have to understand the problem. We must begin to assume responsibility today, not tomorrow, to work on solutions to hunger and malnutrition both close to home and in faraway nations. The United Nations has led the charge to adopt and promote a set of goals to alleviate global poverty, protect the planet, and ensure prosperity for all. These 17 *Sustainable Development Goals* comprise the core of the global agenda. To coordinate and achieve this initiative, stakeholders, governments, the private sector, society, and individuals (just like you!) will be called on to support these sustainable goals. Visit Section 13.1 for more information describing the difference between hunger and malnutrition.

Source: Keys A. Will you starve that they be better fed? Brochure. May 27, 1944.

13.1 World Hunger

wasting Low weight for height (thinness) that typically indicates a recent and severe process of weight loss, often associated with acute starvation or severe disease.

stunting Low height (or length) for age, which indicates inadequate growth due to chronic undernutrition.

Our global food system currently faces simultanous challenges related to overnutrition (overweight and obesity), undernutrition (underweight, **wasting,** and **stunting**), and hidden hunger (micronutrient deficiencies). Expanding economic globalization has contributed to widespread access to lower cost, energy-dense foods that is widening the gap between lower- and higher-income countries. The result is the coexistence of overnutrition and undernutrition plaguing our poorest countries.[1]

Compounding these issues, the United Nation's State of Food Security and Nutrition in the World (SOFI) Report documents that over 122 million more people are now facing hunger across the globe secondary to persistent food waste and loss, the recent pandemic, climate extremes, political conflicts, economic crises, and growing inequality. As noted in Figure 13-1, the prevalence of hunger is the greatest in Africa and Asia.

HUNGER

To ensure optimal nutritional status, many nations provide key recommendations, like the U.S. *Dietary Guidelines,* encouraging adoption of healthy lifestyle behaviors across the life span. Yet for 2.4 billion (nearly 1 in 3) people around the world, uncertainty exists regarding the source of their next meal.[2] This situation is troubling, considering that agriculture worldwide produces more than enough food to meet the energy requirements of each of the planet's 8 billion people.[3] Even with this abundance, over 30% of people are still unable to access enough food to lead active, healthy lives.

food security A condition when all people, at all times, have physical and economic access to sufficient safe and nutritious food that meets their dietary needs and food preferences for an active and healthy life.

nutrition security Consistent access, availability, and affordability of foods and beverages that promote well-being, prevent disease, and, if needed, treat disease, particularly among racial/ethnic minority populations, lower income populations, and rural and remote populations.

Food availability, access, utilization, and stability are the pillars of **food security.** People who are food secure have physical, social, and economic access to sufficient, safe, and nutritious food to meet their dietary needs and food preferences for an active and healthy life (Fig. 13-2).[2]

Worldwide, the Food and Agriculture Organization (FAO) identifies five levels of food security (Fig. 13-3). The FAO's Integrated Food Security Phase Classifications (IPC) are based on global mortality, malnutrition, food and water access and availability, dietary diversity, coping strategies, and livelihood assets.[4] Yet food security is actually a component of a larger concept called **nutrition security.** The global definition of nutrition security encompasses secure access to an appropriately nutritious diet (i.e., protein,

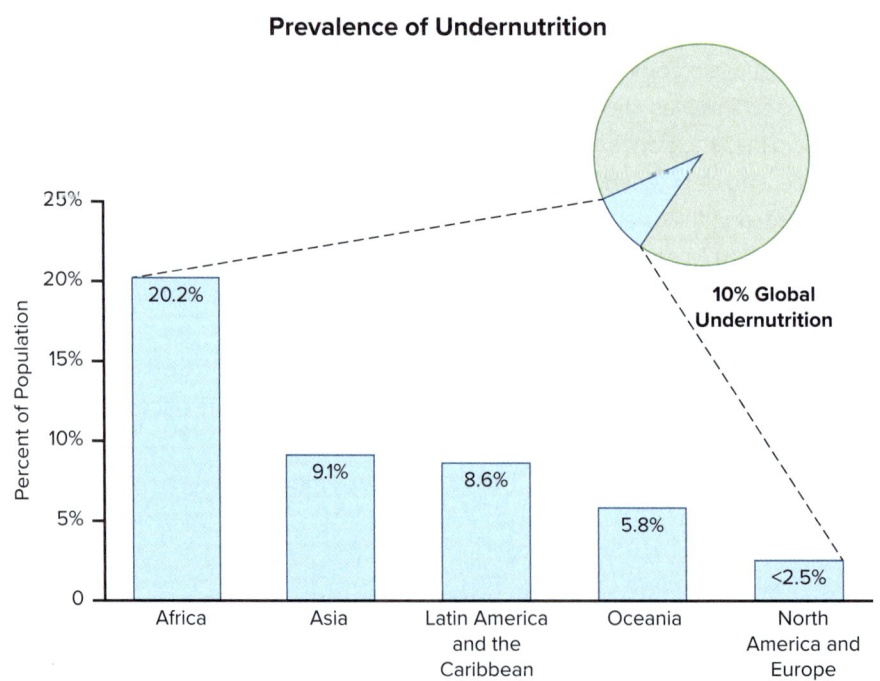

FIGURE 13-1 Prevalence and regions of hunger across the globe.

Source: FAO. 2023. FAOSTAT: Suite of Food Security Indicators. In: *FAO.* [Cited 12 July 2023].

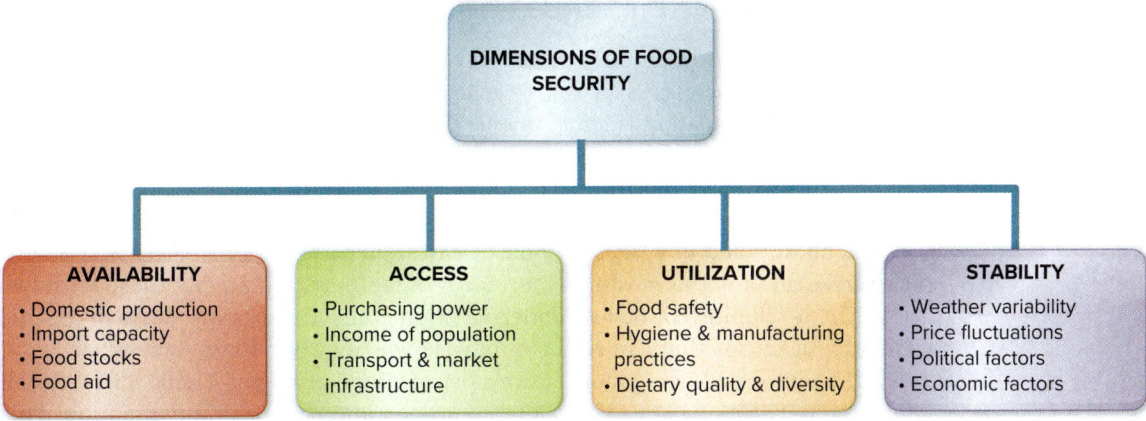

FIGURE 13-2 The four dimensions of food security.
Source: FAO, http://www.fao.org/docrep/013/al936e/al936e00.pdf

carbohydrate, fat, vitamins, minerals, and water), coupled with a sanitary environment and adequate health services and care, in order to ensure a healthy and active life for all household members.[5] The USDA has also adopted the terminology of nutrition security, which will be discussed in the next section.

CHRONIC MALNUTRITION

As you learned in this chapter's *Fact Check,* chronic malnutrition contributes to lowered resistance to disease, infection, and death. Recall that the physiological state that results when not enough food is eaten to meet energy needs is called *hunger.* This sensation is often described as an uneasiness, discomfort, weakness, or pain caused by a lack of food. Malnutrition can occur with or without hunger.

Malnutrition occurs when a dietary pattern is suboptimal and results over time in a diet that is lacking in nutrients. The increased demand and accessibility of affordable, convenient, pre-packaged, and quick meals have resulted in consumption of energy-dense foods rich in saturated fats, added sugars, and sodium—all contributing to malnutrition. Additionally, there is an inadequate supply of vegetables, fruits, and whole grains to meet daily nutritional needs for individuals.

The medical and societal costs of chronic malnutrition include high rates of preterm births, intellectual disabilities, inadequate or stunted growth and development, poor academic performance, decreased work output, chronic disease, and many other preventable issues. Malnutrition is not always a result of extreme poverty over a large segment of the population. Instead, there are often specific causes, such as disordered eating, alcohol use disorders, unavailable or inadequate caregiving, or homelessness that contribute to and compound this issue.[5]

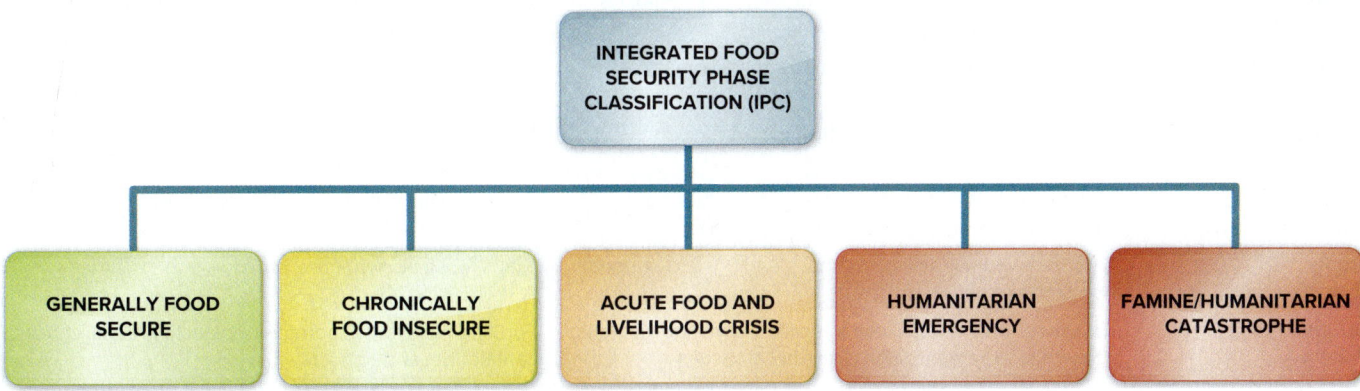

FIGURE 13-3 Integrated food security phase classifications.
Source: FAO, http://www.fao.org/docrep/013/al936e/al936e00.pdf

MALNUTRITION AND MICRONUTRIENT DEFICIENCIES

Malnutrition is a condition of impaired development or function caused by either a chronic deficiency or excess in calorie and/or nutrient intake. When food supplies are low and the population is large, undernutrition is common, leading to nutritional deficiency diseases, such as goiter (iodine deficiency), anemia (iron deficiency), and xerophthalmia (vitamin A deficiency). However, when the food supply is ample or overabundant, energy-dense food choices coupled with an excessive intake can lead to overnutrition, obesity, and its related chronic diseases, such as type 2 diabetes.

Undernutrition is the most common form of malnutrition among those with low incomes in developing countries. Undernutrition is also the primary cause of specific nutrient deficiencies that can result in muscle wasting, blindness, scurvy, pellagra, beriberi, anemia, rickets, goiter, and a host of other problems (Table 13-1). Recall that the term *hidden hunger* affects a large proportion of the world population. This refers to those with micronutrient (vitamin and mineral) deficiencies, often with no observable signs or symptoms. Protein-calorie malnutrition (PCM) is a form of undernutrition caused by an extremely deficient intake of calories or protein and is generally accompanied by worse outcomes of illness and functional impairments that are reversible with nutrition support. Kwashiorkor and marasmus are both forms of PCM.

The most critical micronutrients missing from diets worldwide are iron, vitamin A, iodine, zinc, and various B vitamins (e.g., folate), as well as selenium and vitamin C. Over 2 billion people, mostly in the developing world, are affected by iron and zinc deficiencies.[6] With poor iron status, cognitive development will likely be impaired, particularly if prolonged deficiency occurs during early infancy. The United Nations International Children's Emergency Fund (UNICEF) estimates that approximately 90% of people around the globe now consume iodized salt, representing a colossal large-scale food fortification achievement. Although severe vitamin A deficiency is on the decline, up to 500,000 preschool-age children are still blinded by it each year, with half of them likely to die within 12 months of losing their sight.[7] The lives of one in three children could be spared annually in the developing world

TABLE 13-1 ■ Nutrient-Deficiency Diseases That Commonly Accompany Undernutrition

Disease and Key Nutrient Involved*	Typical Effects of Deficiency	Sources of Nutrients Involved
Ariboflavinosis Riboflavin	Inflammation of oral cavity; nervous system disorders	Milk, mushrooms, spinach, liver, and enriched grains
Beriberi Thiamin	Nerve degeneration, altered muscle coordination, and cardiovascular problems	Sunflower seeds, pork, whole and enriched grains, and dried beans
Goiter Iodine	Enlarged thyroid gland in teenagers and adults, possible intellectual disabilities, and congenital hypothyroidism	Iodized salt and saltwater fish
Iron-deficiency anemia Iron	Reduced work output, delayed growth, and increased health risk in pregnancy	Meats, seafood, broccoli, peas, bran, whole grains, and enriched products
Macrocytic anemia Folate	Enlarged red blood cells, fatigue, and weakness	Green leafy vegetables, legumes, oranges, and liver
Pellagra Niacin	Diarrhea, dermatitis, dementia, and death	Mushrooms, bran, tuna, chicken, beef, peanuts, and whole and enriched grains
Rickets Vitamin D	Poorly calcified bones, bowed legs, and other bone deformities	Fortified milk, fish oils, and sun exposure
Scurvy Vitamin C	Delayed wound healing, internal bleeding, and abnormal formation of bones and teeth	Citrus fruits, strawberries, broccoli, and tomatoes
Xerophthalmia Vitamin A	Blindness from chronic eye infections, dryness, restricted growth, and keratinization of epithelial tissues	Fortified milk, sweet potatoes, spinach, greens, carrots, cantaloupe, and apricots

*Although the nutrients are listed separately to illustrate the important role of each one, often two or more nutrition-deficiency diseases are simultaneously found in an undernourished person in the developing world.

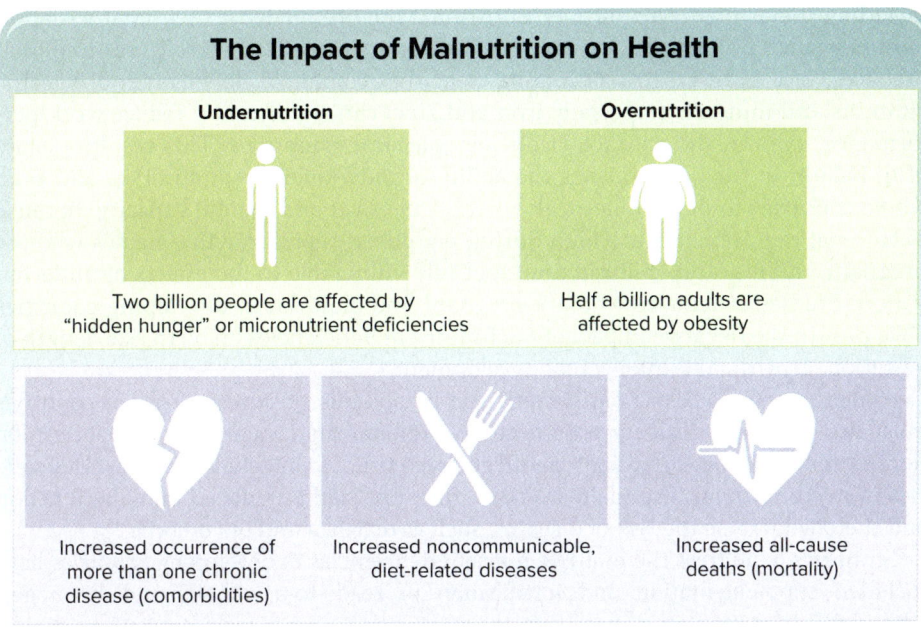

FIGURE 13-4 Malnutrition includes both undernutrition and overnutrition and occurs when a person's diet contains too few or too many nutrients.

Source: FAO of the United Nations.

if vitamin A supplements were provided a few times each year—with an annual cost of approximately 4 cents per child. In the 1990s, UNICEF created micronutrient powders (MNP) designed to address micronutrient deficiencies by improving the diet quality of children to prevent vitamin and mineral deficiencies where access to diverse nutritious foods is limited.[8]

In developed countries, undernutrition is a much more subtle problem than in developing countries. To the untrained eye, children who are undernourished may just seem lean, when, in fact, their growth is being stunted by insufficient nutrients. More likely, though, children from nutrition-insecure households are prone to be overweight. The coexistence of undernutrition with overweight or obesity is referred to as the *double burden of malnutrition*. This form of malnutrition may be the result of considerable reliance on highly processed convenience foods that provide excessive calories, saturated fat, and added sugars. The availability of cooking facilities also affects nutrient intake among those with low incomes. Without adequate cooking facilities, people may buy expensive convenience foods that require little to no preparation. These are typically highly processed foods that provide calories but are often lacking in nutrients. Malnutrition in either form (underweight or overweight) leads to significant health issues and greater mortality (Fig. 13-4).

EFFECTS OF SEMISTARVATION

In the initial stages, the results of undernutrition from semistarvation are often so mild that observable physical symptoms are absent and blood tests do not usually detect these slight metabolic changes. Even in the absence of detectable symptoms, however, undernourishment may affect the ability to work, learn, reproduce, and recover from illnesses or injuries. Recall that as tissues continue to be depleted of nutrients, blood tests eventually detect biochemical changes, such as a drop in blood hemoglobin concentration. Physical symptoms, such as body weakness or fatigue, tend to follow with further depletion. Finally, the full-blown symptoms of the deficiency are recognizable, such as stunting or blindness (vitamin A deficiency).

When a few people in a population develop a severe deficiency, this may represent only the tip of the iceberg. Typically, a much greater number of individuals in that area may be experiencing milder degrees of undernutrition. These deficiencies should not, therefore, be dismissed as trivial, especially in the developing world. In many low- and middle-income countries, it is typical for a combination of micronutrient deficiencies to occur together. These are caused by any number of factors, including dietary patterns of poor nutritional quality related to seasonal variation in food availability, low bioavailability of nutrients from plant sources, cultural food practices, and poverty. It is becoming clear that combined deficiencies of specific vitamins and minerals (especially iron and zinc) can significantly reduce work performance, even in the absence of obvious physical symptoms. This resulting state of ill health, in turn, diminishes the ability of individuals, communities, and even whole countries to perform at peak levels of physical and mental capacity. Because nutritional requirements are high during periods of rapid growth, females who are pregnant, infants, and children are especially vulnerable to the effects of undernutrition. Studies of females who are pregnant and children in developing countries have proven the negative impact of micronutrient deficiencies on birth size, length of gestation, growth, and intellectual development.

Added to their lack of nourishment, the inhabitants of poverty-stricken countries must also contend with recurrent infections, contaminated water sources, poor sanitation, extreme weather conditions, and regular exposure to infectious diseases. Deficiencies of micronutrients, especially iron and zinc, can lead to reduced immune function and thereby increase the risk of diseases, such as diarrhea and pneumonia.

Strategies to address the multiple nutrient deficiencies in developing countries have included supplementation and fortification of ready-to-use foods and beverages. Although supplementation has been the most widely practiced intervention, public health experts believe that fortification of a commonly consumed food could be a single, cost-effective intervention strategy to target a larger population. Studies of micronutrient supplementation during pregnancy have shown an increase in birth weight and a reduction in **low birth weights** but no impact on preterm births or perinatal mortality. In children, micronutrient supplementation with three or more nutrients has resulted in increases in height and weight.[9]

low birth weight (LBW) Referring to any infant weighing less than 2.5 kilograms (5.5 pounds) at birth; most commonly results from preterm birth.

✓ CONCEPT CHECK 13.1

1. What are the most critical micronutrients missing from diets worldwide?
2. What is the *double burden of malnutrition?*
3. List three health consequences of chronic malnutrition.
4. At which stages of the life cycle is undernutrition especially damaging?

13.2 Malnutrition in the United States

Roughly 38 million (12%) people in the United States are living at or below the poverty level.[10] Of these, approximately 57% of households report having to choose between purchasing food and housing costs, 69% between food and utilities, 66% between food and medicine, and 67% between food and access to transportation.[11] While housing and utility costs, medical care, and transportation fares are nonnegotiable, a person may choose to eat less. Food is one of the few optional items in a household budget. The short-term consequences of eating less may be less dramatic than getting evicted, but the long-term cumulative effects are significant. A healthy eating pattern will only be achieved when adequate resources and supports exist in places where individuals live, work, and gather.

NUTRITION SECURITY

Nutrition security is an emerging concept that complements efforts to improve food security while acknowledging health inequities. This expanded food and nutrition security approach is critical in recognizing that structural inequities pose significant barriers for many individuals to eat healthy dietary patterns and remain physically active (Fig. 13-5).

emergency departments and inpatient beds, detox programs, jails, prisons, and psychiatric institutions, all at high public expense.

Inadequate Healthy Food Access. Access to affordable and nutritious foods from supermarkets, grocery stores, or other retailers is a challenge for many Americans, making it harder for them to follow a balanced, nutrient-dense dietary pattern. Low-income, low-access areas with inadequate availability of nutritious foods were originally called **food deserts** and more recently are termed *healthy food priority areas.* USDA's online *Food Access Research Atlas* presents a spatial overview of food access indicators for low-income and other neighborhoods.[22] Measures include accessibility to sources of healthy food, as measured by distance to a store or by the number of stores in an area; individual-level resources that may affect accessibility, such as family income or vehicle availability; and neighborhood-level indicators of resources, such as the average income of the neighborhood and the availability of public transportation.[22]

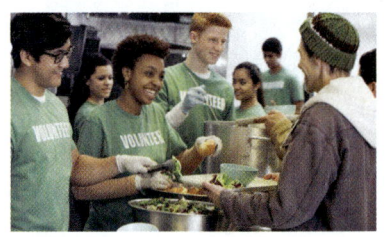

Food pantries and soup kitchens are important sources of nutrients for a growing number of people in the United States. **Do you know how to locate your local food pantry?** Ariel Skelley/Blend Images/Getty Images

food deserts Urban neighborhoods and rural towns without ready access to fresh, healthy, and affordable food. Also referred to as *low-income, low-access areas (LILA).*

The federal Healthy Food Financing Initiative (HFFI) provides government financing for developing and equipping grocery stores, small retailers, corner stores, and farmers' markets selling healthy food in low-income communities. In addition, this initiative provides employment and business opportunities in underserved areas. Farmers' markets are gaining attention as a simple and local approach in impacting hunger and health. Many farmers' markets now participate in programs for older adults, WIC, SNAP, and the SNAP Double Dollar program, where shoppers using their SNAP EBT card will receive matching funds that can be redeemed for produce at that market.

For many years, government-funded food assistance programs have helped to alleviate undernutrition in the United States.[23] Obtaining adequate food to not only survive, but thrive, is a tremendous challenge, especially when people experiencing homelessness are forced to live outside. Although many people assume that food pantries and soup kitchens are abundant and accessible for those in need, there are many barriers to accessing these resources. The majority of food pantries are staffed by volunteers and dependent upon food donations. They often have limited hours of operation, require appointments well in advance, often require proof of residence, and limit the amount of food that patrons can take home per month. Individuals who are homeless often lack proper identification and proof of residence, do not have cooking facilities and equipment needed for food preparation, and do not have adequate storage to prevent foodborne illnesses and practice safe food-handling procedures. Food availability through soup kitchens is limited in most cities and absent in most rural areas.

An additional challenge is that a growing number of cities have taken strides to restrict or ban the act of sharing food with the homeless. These laws are concerning, considering that most cities do not have adequate food resources to meet the needs of their poor and homeless. Advocates and food providers are eager to work with cities and other government agencies to help address the problems of hunger and homelessness by improving access to federal food benefits and other food resources. State governments have also begun moving to protect the right of individuals and groups to share excess food with others.

Cultural Traditions, Personal Preferences, and Budget. Exposure to a variety of foods and beverages early in life promotes a child's willingness to consume and enjoy a variety of foods throughout each life stage. Establishing and maintaining a healthy dietary pattern that aligns with individual and cultural preferences should be a priority. *Cultural foodways* refers to the intersection of food in culture, traditions, and history. Indeed, culture has a significant influence on both individual and family food and beverage choices. The *Dietary Guidelines* highlights that nutrient-dense and culturally relevant foods are part of all the food groups. For instance, spices and herbs can improve food flavor while reducing added sugars, saturated fat,

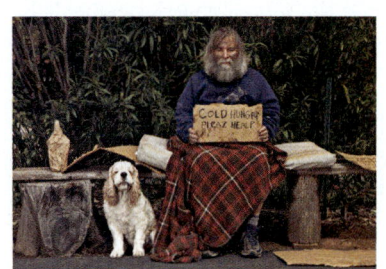

This man is hoping to find work to fill his basic need of food. **What may be feasible for you to help this person find employment, food, and/or shelter?** DebbiSmirnoff/Vetta/Getty Images

ASK THE RDN: College Food and Nutrition Security

Dear RDN: *I'm learning about the importance of food and its nutrients. What do I do if I, or a friend of mine, cannot afford healthy food to eat?*

We know that a nutritionally adequate dietary pattern can help you meet the demands of your busy lifestyle as a college student. Optimal nutrition supports both physical and mental wellness, which is necessary to reach your goals. Unfortunately, far too many college students face food and nutrition insecurity.

The *#RealCollege Survey* is the nation's largest annual assessment of college students' basic needs. The results showed that about one out of three college students reported recent food insecurity. These students must regularly meet the rigors of their academic schedules without the nutrition that is required to properly fuel their bodies and brains.

If you are struggling with food and nutrition insecurity, what can you do? First, you must understand that there is no shame in needing assistance. All college students deserve to be well nourished. Next, reach out to a trusted faculty person, counselor, or advisor. Your nutrition instructor is very aware of the ramifications of food and nutriton insecurity and will also be familiar with resources both on and off campus. Colleges and universities are providing food to students through food pantries, gardens, and cafeteria vouchers. Many universities also have an office (e.g., Single Stop, https://singlestop.org) where staff screen students for eligibility for benefits including SNAP and emergency funds. Most localities have food pantries for the community as well as nonprofit groups that connect students to benefits. Encourage your friends to use the resources they need when they need them.

All members of college communities must step up to advocate for those in need. The *#RealCollege Survey* also found that on-campus resources are underutilized by those who need them. If your college has not yet addressed food and nutrition insecurity, form a student group to begin the movement. If they have established resources, volunteer to raise awareness and gather donations. Let's normalize the provision of healthy food to all students who need it!

You can also harness the power of knowledge gained as a nutrition student to encourage budget-smart and nutritious choices for those in your social network. Make a large pot of homemade soup and pack it up to share. Form a dinner club that rotates meal duties between your friends. Have a meal prep party where everyone brings the ingredients for one dish, ingredients are prepped, and recipes shared. Share coupons and information on budget-friendly markets with your classmates and friends. As you learn more about food and its nutrients, you can talk to others about building a healthy dietary pattern within a strict budget.

Finally, it is important to work at all levels to solve this problem. You can join the student-led campaign to FUELHIgherEd at https://www.campushunger.org/. Write to your lawmakers at the state and federal levels to show your support of legislation that would address hunger on college campuses. States can expand benefits eligibility to allow more college students to have access to SNAP and other forms of aid. Some examples of bills that have been proposed are the Emergency Grant Aid for College Students Act, which would establish permanent emergency aid for students, and the Food for Thought Act, which would expand the National School Lunch Program to eligible community college students. This problem has solutions. Let's work to put those solutions into action!

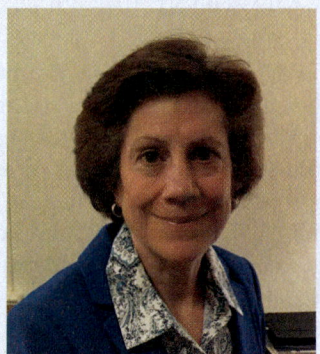

Laura Davidson/Andrew Davidson

Make a difference,

Laura Davidson, MS, RDN, LDN
Associate Professor of Nutrition and Allied Health, Community College of Philadelphia

and sodium. A healthy dietary pattern can be affordable and fit within budgetary constraints. Strategies for success require some advanced planning; consideration of regional and seasonal food availability; and incorporation of a variety of fresh, frozen, dried, and canned options as low-cost options to meet nutrient needs within a budget.

✓ CONCEPT CHECK 13.2

1. Name two food assistance programs in the United States.
2. What factors influence the presence of poverty, hunger, and malnutrition in the United States?
3. What is the difference between *situational* and *generational poverty*?

13.3 Global Malnutrition

Malnutrition in the developing world is also tied to poverty, and any sustainable solution must address this issue. However, such countries have a multitude of problems so complex and interrelated that they cannot be treated separately. The major obstacles challenging those seeking a solution are illustrated in Figure 13-8 and described in the next few sections.

FAMINE

Famine can also lead to chronic hunger. Periods of famine are characterized by large-scale loss of life, climate change, social disruption, economic chaos, and political conflicts. As a result of these extreme events, the affected community may experience the following: a downward spiral characterized by human distress; sales of land, livestock, and other farm assets; mass migration; division and impoverishment of the poorest families; crime; and humanitarian crises. The most at-risk countries for humanitarian catastrophes are ranked by the International Rescue Committee (IRC). The top 20 countries account for about 80% of internally displaced individuals and are experiencing the worst humanitarian crises in the world.[24] Focused and global efforts are needed to eradicate the fundamental causes of famine. These causes vary by region and decade, but the most common cause of famine is crop failure. The most obvious reasons are extreme weather conditions such as floods or drought, war, and civil strife.

FOOD-TO-POPULATION RATIO

The world has more than 8 billion inhabitants and this number is projected to increase by 2 billion by 2050. Population growth exceeds economic growth in much of the developing world, and as a result, poverty is on the rise globally. This disrupts the balance in the food-to-population ratio, tipping it toward food shortages. To ensure a decent life for a widening segment of humanity, many experts suggest that the growth in the earth's most vulnerable populations should slow.

According to the FAO, there are 735 million individuals affected by hunger in the world, and 98% reside in developing countries.[2] More than 90% of these people live in rural areas of Africa and Asia and remain totally dependent on local agriculture for all of their nutritional needs. Unfortunately, major food and health disparities continue to exist between developed and developing countries, among those with high and low incomes, and even within the family unit (e.g., males may be fed before females).

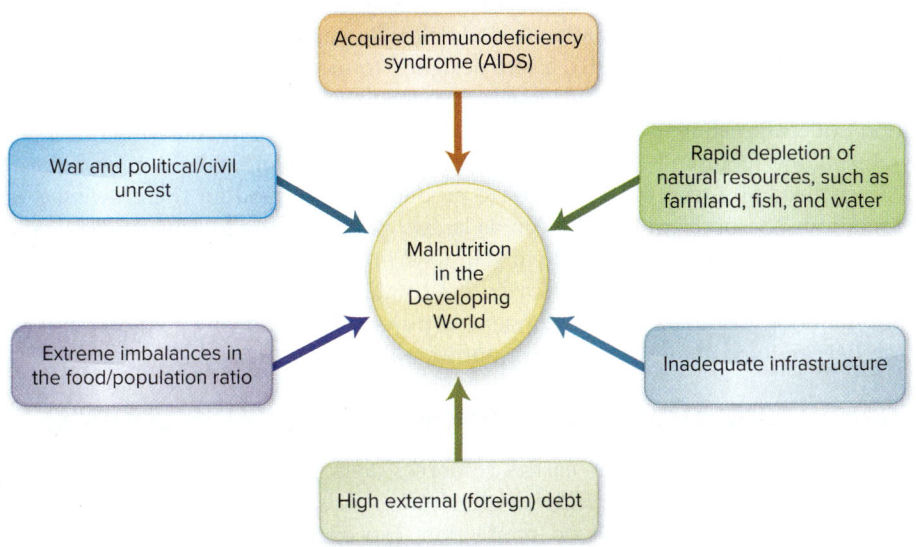

FIGURE 13-8 Many factors contribute to malnutrition in the developing world. Any solutions to the problem must take these multifaceted factors into consideration.

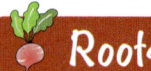

Roots

Insect Farming

Historical records and artifacts dating back over 1.5 million years in South Africa provide evidence that humans have farmed and consumed insects. This practice is known as *entomophagy* and is seen as a delicacy in some cultures. As a high-protein food source, insect farming is a form of sustainable agriculture requiring minimal inputs compared to other high-protein food sources. In addition to protein, insects are high in iron, calcium, and B vitamins and low in both carbohydrates and fat.

Top 10 Countries at Risk for a Humanitarian Crisis

1. Yemen
2. Afghanistan
3. Syria
4. Democratic Republic of Congo
5. Ethiopia
6. Burkina Faso
7. South Sudan
8. Nigeria
9. Venezuela
10. Mozambique

Source: International Rescue Committee.

Global Hunger Index (GHI) A tool that tracks the state of hunger worldwide and calls attention to locations where immediate hunger relief is urgently needed.

Economists estimate that world food production will continue to increase more rapidly than the world population. This will come at a high cost in terms of the water, fertilizer, and chemicals (pesticides, fungicides) needed to allow for adequate food production. In the short term, the primary problem is not related to production but rather to the supply chain—both distribution and use. This reality is even more dire in poverty-stricken areas of developing nations. Unfortunately, many people who are vulnerable do not have the income to purchase their own farmland or to have access to nonlocal sources.

Most viable farmland in the world is already in use, and because of inadequate farming practices or competing land-use demands, the number of farmable acres is decreasing annually. For these reasons, the world's *sustainable* food output—an amount that does not deplete the earth's resources—is now running well behind food consumption. This discrepancy suggests that food production in less-developed countries will not keep up with population growth and will soon lag behind.

Increasing per capita income, improving the standard of living, and improving education, especially for females in developing nations, can contribute to successful long-term solutions to excessive population growth. Yet the major concern remains whether there are enough resources worldwide to raise per capita income and provide enough education to slow total global population growth.

WAR AND POLITICAL/CIVIL UNREST

Global military spending hovers at almost $2 trillion.[25] Aside from the economic impact of military spending, civil disruptions and wars continue to set back the progress of addressing poverty and contribute to massive undernutrition. Globally, 1 in every 95 humans is now either a refugee, internally displaced, or seeking political or religious asylum. The UN Refugee Agency reports that worldwide, over 108 million people have been forcibly displaced.[26] Specifically, the Afghan refugee crisis is one of the longest and most protracted in the world, with nearly 6 million Afghans driven from their homes and their country by conflict, violence, and persecution. At least 80% of all recently displaced Afghans are females with children. As war rages on, health, education, and public services continue to decline for affected populations. All the while, poverty and malnutrition increase.

Sadly, food has become a weapon in many wars. At the local level, fields are often mined and water wells intentionally contaminated. Even when food is readily available and accessible, political divisions may impede its distribution to the point that undernutrition will plague countries for years. Especially during emergencies, programs designed to aid the hungry have been undermined by unstable administrations, corruption, and political influence. During this chaos, relief agencies may be caught between warring factions and those attempting to alleviate suffering.

To assess hunger, the International Food Policy Research Institute annually calculates the **Global Hunger Index (GHI),** a tool designed to measure and track hunger worldwide. The GHI uses a multidimensional approach to assess hunger that includes population undernourishment, child wasting, child stunting, and child mortality.[27]

During the 1960s and 1970s, the problem of undernutrition in developing countries was perceived as a technical one: how to produce enough food for the growing world population. The problem is now seen as largely political: how to achieve cooperation among and within nations so that gains in food production and infrastructure are not weapons of war. The best answer may lie in a combination of approaches: finding technical solutions to address chronic hunger and poverty, and resolving political crises that push developing nations into a state of nutrition despair and chaos.

AGRICULTURE AND THE DEPLETION OF NATURAL RESOURCES

As we continue to deplete the earth's resources, agriculture production is approaching its limits in many areas worldwide. Environmentally unsustainable farming methods have been undermining food production, especially in developing countries. In addition, climate change is increasingly linked to hunger and poverty. Climate change patterns, characterized by drought, flooding, and severe storms, require significant alterations in farming practices.

The **green revolution** was a phenomenon that began in the 1960s that resulted in a dramatic rise in crop yields in some countries, such as the Philippines, India, and Mexico. The increased use of fertilizers and irrigation, and the development of superior crops through careful plant breeding, made this boost in agricultural production possible. The more recent movement toward **sustainable agriculture** practices and the development of new crops through food biotechnology have begun to improve crop yields on the shrinking amount of farmable land. Crops that are pest or chemical resistant or biofortified have been produced as a result of biotechnology. Ongoing research is warranted to assess the effects of these crops on human health and the environment.

Today, many areas of the world are uncultivated or ungrazed and cannot sustain farming because they are too rocky, steep, infertile, dry, wet, or inaccessible. Fertile farmland is threatened by increased land and soil degradation and depletion of freshwater resources. China is experiencing a growing scarcity of fresh water that may impact the globe. Currently, China produces approximately 25% of the world's grain and feeds about 20% of the world's population—with less than 10% of the world's arable land.[28]

The impact of globalization can affect the dietary patterns and subsequent health of countries that depend on fish for their protein and overall nutritional needs. Globally, the amount of fish caught has leveled off as fish consumption has increased to about 17% of animal consumption. Fish are quickly becoming depleted in our oceans, and fish farming simply cannot compensate for the decline in wild fish populations.

If the world population continues to expand at its current rate, we face the potential threats of serious famine, disease, and death. A profound change is needed if we are to nourish an estimated 10 billion inhabitants of planet Earth by 2050. The FAO calls for global sustainability support and practices. Food systems should sustain the environment while providing adequate, healthy food. If food production is to keep up with the expanding population, immediate action is needed to protect the earth's already deteriorated environment from further destruction.[2]

green revolution Refers to increases in crop yields that accompanied the introduction of new agricultural technologies in less-developed countries. The key technologies were high-yielding, disease-resistant strains of rice, wheat, and corn; greater use of fertilizer and water; and improved cultivation practices.

sustainable agriculture Agricultural system that provides a secure living for farm families; maintains the natural environment and resources; supports the rural community; and offers respect and fair treatment to all involved, from farm workers to consumers to the animals raised for food.

INADEQUATE SHELTER AND SANITATION

When people die from undernutrition, other factors, such as inadequate shelter and sanitation, almost always contribute. No one can survive without clean water, nor can we stay healthy for any length of time without proper sanitation and shelter. Many more people experience the effects of poor sanitation and an unreliable water supply in developing countries than are affected by war and political/civil unrest. Without water, sanitation, and hygiene, sustainable development remains impossible.

Fortunately, organizations such as UNICEF are working in more than 100 countries across the globe to improve water supplies and sanitation facilities in schools and communities and to promote safe hygiene practices. The UNICEF *WASH* (water, sanitation, and hygiene) programs are designed to support the Sustainable Development Goal (discussed in next section) for clean water and sanitation to achieve universal and equitable access to safe and affordable drinking water for all by 2030. This goal can't come soon enough as about 2.2 billion people still lack access to safe water (Fig. 13-9).[29]

The tremendous movement of individuals to urban settings has caused a population redistribution that has challenged the capacity for shelter and sanitation. In 1950, 30% of the world's population resided in urban areas, but by 2050, over 68% of the world's population is projected to be urban. It is expected that in the next 30 years, most urban population growth will be in cities of developing countries, reaching almost 5.2 billion in 2050. People go to the cities to find employment and resources the countryside can no longer provide. In developing countries, low-income individuals make up most of the urban population, and their needs for housing and community services often exceed available governmental resources. About 25% of current urban dwellers live in slum-like conditions worldwide.[30]

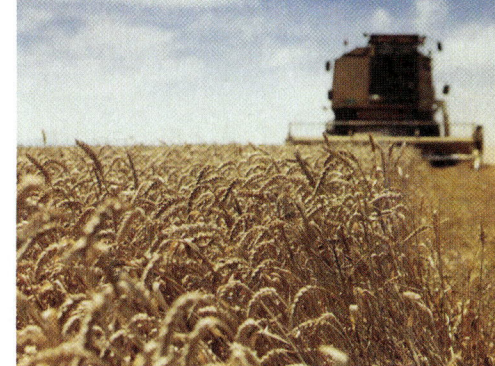
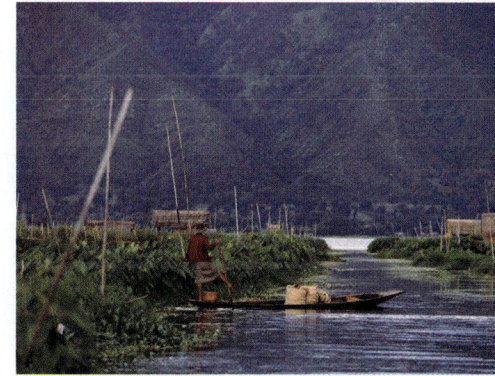

Rich agricultural resources as seen in these wheat fields (top) contrast with gardens being tended by a farmer on a floating island in Myanmar (bottom).
top: Aleksandar Dickov/Shutterstock; bottom: Kevin RMorris/Photodisc/Getty Images

FIGURE 13-9 Water quality and safety are paramount to optimal human development and well-being. Access to safe water is one of the most effective ways to promote health and reduce poverty.

Source: World Health Organization (WHO).

Water Access and Safety

2 billion do not have access to safe water services

122 million obtain water from streams or lakes

282 million travel over 30 minutes per trip to obtain water

Most urban residents who are impoverished live in overcrowded, self-made shelters, which lack a safe and adequate water supply and are only partially served by public utilities. The WHO/UNICEF Joint Monitoring Program for Water Supply and Sanitation has estimated that more than half of the global population lack access to safely managed sanitation, and over 2 billion lack safe and readily available water at home.[31] The shantytowns and ghettos of the developing world are often worse than the rural areas left behind. Urban individuals who are poor also need resources to purchase food, so they often subsist on food even more meager than the homegrown rural fare. Making matters worse, haphazard shelters often lack facilities to protect food from spoilage or damage by insects and rodents. This inability to protect food supplies in some developing countries leads to the loss of as much as 40% of all perishable foods.[2]

The shift from rural to urban life takes its greatest toll on infants and children. WHO/UNICEF reports that inadequate access to safe water and sanitation services, combined with poor hygiene practices, kills 395,000 children under age 5 annually.[32] Contributing to this issue is the fact that infants are often weaned early from breast milk to infant formula, partly because the mother must find employment. Mothers may also be influenced by advertisements depicting images of sophisticated, formula-feeding females. Unfortunately, because infant formulas are expensive, food-insecure parents may try to conserve the formula by either overdiluting the mixture or reducing the feeding volume. In addition, the water supply may not be safe, so the prepared formula is also likely to be contaminated with pathogens or contaminants. Human milk, in contrast, is much more economical, hygienic, readily available, and nutritious. It also provides infants with immunity to some ailments. In most situations, breastfeeding should be promoted as the safest and most nutritious choice for infant feeding.

Poor sanitation also creates a critical public health problem and, along with undernutrition, particularly raises the risk of infection. Inadequate sanitation is another example of the inferior infrastructure in the developing world. Human urine and feces are two of the most dangerous substances encountered in overcrowded urban areas. In addition, rotting garbage and associated insect and rodent infestations are potent sources of disease-causing organisms commonly seen in urban areas of the developing world. The inability to dispose of the massive numbers of deceased people (and animals) resulting from disease and wars causes additional sanitation problems. In some developing countries, diarrheal diseases account for almost 9% of all deaths in children younger than 5 years of age.[33] Additional repercussions of poor sanitation are that children are denied access to education because their schools lack private and decent sanitation facilities.

THE IMPACT OF HIV/AIDS WORLDWIDE

Nutrition security is impacted greatly in developing countries by the high prevalence of human immunodeficiency virus (HIV) and **acquired immunodeficiency syndrome (AIDS)**. HIV/AIDS impairs absorption of nutrients, increases nutrient requirements, and decreases the capacity to work. About 39 million people around the world are

acquired immunodeficiency syndrome (AIDS) Late stage HIV when the body's immune system is badly damaged because of the virus.

infected with HIV/AIDS. Cases in sub-Saharan Africa account for almost 65% of the global total of new HIV/AIDS infections.[34]

An individual can be infected with HIV through contact with bodily fluids including blood, semen, vaginal secretions, and human milk. Thus, the virus can be transmitted through sexual contact, through blood-to-blood contact, and from mother to child during pregnancy, delivery, or breastfeeding. The virus has a very limited ability to exist outside the body. Once infected with HIV, the individual is said to be *HIV positive*. If untreated, the viral disease progresses over the next few years, and the individual develops opportunistic infections with symptoms such as diarrhea, lung disease, weight loss, and a form of cancer. Once the individual has developed these symptoms, that person is said to have AIDS. Without treatment, an individual will likely die from AIDS in about 3 years.[35]

Universal Treatment for HIV/AIDS. Until a vaccine is available to prevent AIDS, the latest antiretroviral therapy (ART) can significantly slow the progression of the disease. Providing AIDS drugs to females who are pregnant is also an effective preventive measure. The goal of therapy for females who are pregnant is to maximize viral suppression to reduce the transmission of HIV to the fetus and newborn.

Although ART is effective, it is very costly. Currently, ART reaches only 76% of those who need it, meaning millions of people are still waiting to be treated. Progress toward the goal of ensuring access to HIV treatment has been slower for children than for adults. Sadly, just 57% of HIV-infected children had access to antiretroviral therapy.[36]

Nutrition and HIV/AIDS. Although adequate nutrition cannot prevent or cure HIV infection or AIDS, nutritional status can affect the progression of the disease. A focus on eliminating or reducing malnutrition can significantly slow disease progression and severity and can improve longevity. A dietary pattern adequate in energy, protein, and micronutrients can lessen the impact of infections associated with AIDS. Low levels of vitamins A and E can contribute to a more rapid onset of symptoms, including body wasting and fever. Maintenance of an optimal nutritional status should be an integral focus of the treatment for AIDS. Daily use of a balanced vitamin and mineral supplement has also been shown to slow health declines in people with HIV/AIDS. Nutritional counseling by a registered dietitian nutritionist (RDN) is paramount in assessing nutritional status, providing personalized education and recommendations, and monitoring outcomes. The main goals of nutritional treatment are to achieve and maintain a healthy body weight, body composition, and optimal nutritional status; minimize nutrition-related side effects and complications; improve quality of life; and expand access to nutrition services.[37]

 Sustainable Solutions

Offal

Does consuming offal sound awful? Offal refers to the entrails and organs, sometimes called *variety meats* or the *odd bits* of animals. Compared to other regions of the world, the United States is one of the lowest consumers of offal. In fact, nearly 60% of U.S. variety meats are exported to Asia. However, if you choose to consume animal products, including offal in your dietary pattern is a sustainable choice. From an agricultural standpoint, consuming everything *from nose to tail* is an efficient use of agricultural resources and cuts down on food waste. From environmental and economic perspectives, consuming these products locally helps to decrease the costs of exporting variety meats to other countries. Furthermore, organ meats are nutrient dense—especially for blood health! They are rich in high-quality protein and provide more iron, zinc, vitamin B-6, and vitamin B-12 than lean muscle meat.

Source: Ratliff E. Offal—health benefits of organ meat. *Today's Dietitian*. 2020 May;22(5):44.

> ✓ **CONCEPT CHECK 13.3**
>
> 1. Why does malnutrition continue despite an adequate food supply in many areas?
> 2. How have war and declines in natural resources contributed to malnutrition in developing countries?
> 3. What role does nutrition play in combating HIV/AIDS?

13.4 Global Malnutrition Strategies

Reducing malnutrition in the developing world is quite a complex goal and takes considerable time to accomplish. It has been a common practice for affluent nations to supply famine-stricken areas with direct food aid; however, this is not a long-term solution. Although it reduces the number of deaths from famine, it can also reduce incentives for local production by driving down food prices. In addition, the affected countries may have little or no means of transporting the food to those who need it most, and the donated foods may not be culturally acceptable or nutrient dense. In the short run or during a crisis, there is no choice: aid must be provided because people are starving.[38] Still, improving the infrastructure for people who are poor, especially those living in rural areas, must be the long-term focus.

With the adoption of the *Sustainable Development Goals (SDGs)* by all United Nations member states, world leaders committed to address the many dimensions of extreme poverty and create a better life for those in need by 2030 (Fig. 13-10). Pertinent hunger-related goals include reducing by half the proportion of males, females, and children of all ages living in poverty; eradicating extreme poverty for all, currently measured as people living on less than $2.15 a day; and ensuring that the most vulnerable have equal rights to economic resources, as well as access to basic services, ownership and control

SUSTAINABLE DEVELOPMENT GOALS

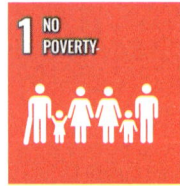 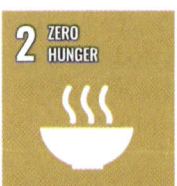 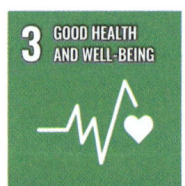 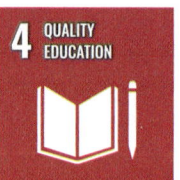 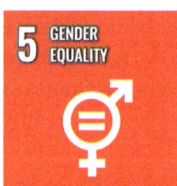 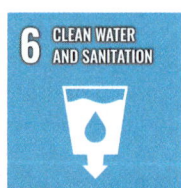
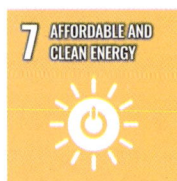 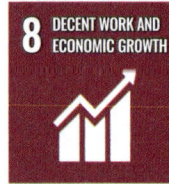 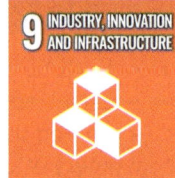 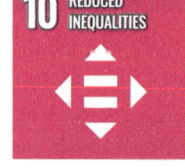 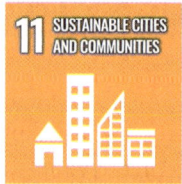 
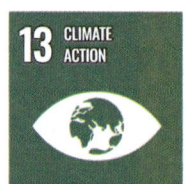  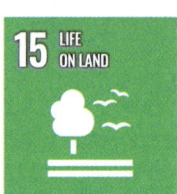 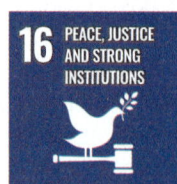 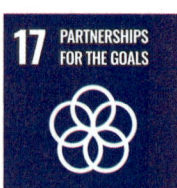 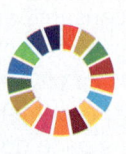

FIGURE 13-10 Achieving these targets will contribute to achievement of the United Nations Sustainable Development Goals (SDGs). Goals 2 and 3 aim to end hunger, achieve food security, improve nutrition, address all forms of malnutrition for all age groups, and ensure health and well-being for all at every stage of life. Used with permission of the United Nations, www.un.org/sustainabledevelopment/. The content of this publication has not been approved by the United Nations and does not reflect the views of the United Nations or its officials or Members States.

over land and other forms of property, inheritance, natural resources, appropriate new technology, and financial services.

Twelve of the seventeen SDGs contain nutrition-related metrics. Without substantial and sustained investments in adequate nutrition, the SDGs will certainly fail. As the SDGs emphasize, malnutrition results not only from a lack of nutritious and safe food but also from an intertwined and complex series of factors including health care, sociodemographics, education, water, sanitation, hygiene, food access, available resources, human empowerment, and more.

DEVELOPMENT TAILORED TO LOCAL CONDITIONS

Although world food supplies have grown in recent years, an increase in malnutrition has resulted from inadequate food distribution and access. In addition, millions of farmers are losing access to resources they need to be self-reliant. There is a growing realization that unless economic opportunities can be created as part of a plan for sustainable development, residents who live in rural areas and do not own land will flock to the overcrowded cities.

For the most part, the sustainable solutions lie in helping people meet their own needs and directing them to resources and employment opportunities. History has shown that the provision of credit—along with education and training, food storage facilities, and marketing support—allows people who live in rural areas to actively participate in their success, which benefits their families and communities. Understanding and appreciating the local conditions, including crop rotation, utilization of varieties of plants, and crop diversification, are essential to understanding barriers to success. Agroforestry initiatives and promotion of local and culturally sensitive foods are needed. Communities that have significant land and water limitations may require the intervention and assistance of local authorities.

One U.S. program, the Peace Corps, has helped to improve conditions in developing nations for over 50 years by providing education, distributing food and medical supplies, and building structures for local use. The aim of the Peace Corps is to help create independent, self-sustaining economies around the world. Becoming a Peace Corps volunteer is a meaningful way to make a difference around the world. Learn more about this program at www.peacecorps.gov.

Suitable technologies for processing, preserving, marketing, and distributing nutritious local staples also should be fostered so that small farmers can flourish. Education and training on how to use whole foods to create healthful eating plans adds further benefit. Pineapples, discussed in the *Farm to Fork* feature in this section, are an example of a local food source that provides economic benefits to developing nations. Supplementing indigenous foods with nutrients that are in short supply, such as iron, various B vitamins, zinc, and iodine, also deserves consideration. One such program involves enriching rice with vitamin A in various parts of the world. Later in this section, we examine the role of biotechnology in improving nutrient quality and other characteristics of plants and animals, another positive step in reducing malnutrition. In addition, advances in water purification must be employed.

Another SDG aims to ensure environmental sustainability, which may include promoting extensive land ownership and thus increasing the availability of food. If food resources are concentrated among a minority of people, as often happens with unequal land ownership, food is unlikely to be equally distributed unless efficient transportation systems are in place. Small-scale industrial development is another way to create meaningful employment and purchasing power for vast numbers of individuals who are poor and live in rural areas.

Raising the economic status of people living in poverty by employing them is as important as expanding the food supply. If an increase in food supply is achieved without an accompanying rise in employment, there may be no long-term change in the number of people who are undernourished. Although food prices may fall with increased mechanization, use of fertilizers, and other modern farming technologies, these advances can also displace people from jobs, a result that may harm, rather than help, the population.

Sustainable Development Goal Report Card

The SDG Report highlights progress had been made in some key areas including maternal and child health, increasing global access to electricity, and expanding representation of females in government.

Unfortunately, these gains were offset by increasing food insecurity, continued environmental deterioration, and persistent inequalities. The impact of COVID-19 caused further disruption to SDG progress, especially for our poorest and most vulnerable populations. Among the key findings:

- Over 70 million people are expected to be pushed back into extreme poverty, the first rise in global poverty since 1998.
- Underemployment and unemployment impacted half the global workforce with incomes reduced by approximately 60%.
- More than 1 billion people experienced inadequate housing, overcrowded public transport, and inadequate access to health care.
- Females and children experienced disruptions to health and vaccination services and limited access to nutrition services. A surge in domestic violence had been documented against females and children.
- Mandatory school closures affecting 90% of children worldwide caused over 370 million children to miss school breakfasts and lunches that they depend on.

For more details, visit https://sdgs.un.org/goals.

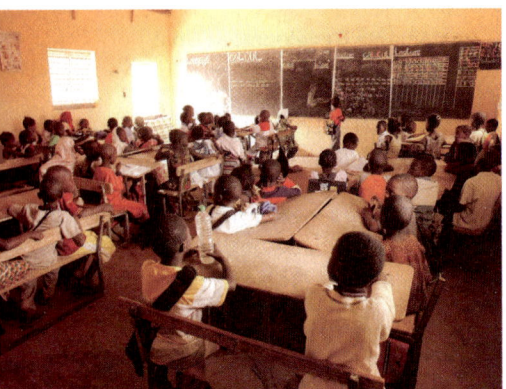

This school teacher and her students are in a classroom in a village in Senegal, Africa. Eliminating disparity is a goal of the Sustainable Development Goals. See https://www.nutritionintl.org for more on this issue. Andia/UIG/Getty Images

sustainable development Economic growth that will simultaneously reduce poverty, protect the environment, and preserve natural capital.

IMPROVING EQUALITY

Females living in poverty are a special concern. In addition to working longer hours than males, they grow most of the food for family consumption and account for 39% of the labor force in the informal sector of the economy and an increasing proportion in the formal sector.[30] Of the 700 million people in the world living on less than $2.15 a day, the majority are females. Clearly, economic opportunities for females and education regarding family planning must be augmented. Empowerment of females is critical to improve the level of food and nutrition security, increase the production and distribution of food and other agricultural products, and enhance living conditions in general (see *Newsworthy Nutrition*).

Goal 5 of the SDGs aims to achieve gender equality and empower all females. Increasing females' access to education, information and communication technologies, economic resources, and governance reduces poverty, promotes development, achieves equality, protects females' human rights, and eliminates violence against females. Although the proportion of females who are paid to work in jobs outside of agriculture is increasing, females continue to experience significant gaps in terms of poverty, labor market and wages, and participation in private and public decision making. There is still plenty of room for improvement.

SUSTAINABLE AGRICULTURE

Over the years, changes in agricultural practices have positively impacted the availability of food around the world. This chapter's *Farm to Fork* feature highlights pineapples, an economic tropical fruit. Along with the positive effects on farming, however, negative results have occurred. Most significant among these are the depletion of topsoil, contamination of groundwater, decline of family farms, neglect of living and working conditions for farm laborers, increasing costs of production, and lack of integration of economic and social conditions in rural communities.

The concept of **sustainable development** has been embraced as a means of economic growth that will reduce poverty while protecting the environment and preserving

Newsworthy Nutrition

Maternal depression and child severe acute malnutrition

INTRODUCTION: Maternal depression is the leading cause of disability and adversely affects the health of mothers and growth of their infants. **OBJECTIVE:** The aim of this *case-control study* was to assess maternal depression and its impact on malnutrition in Kenyan children ages 6 to 60 months. **METHODS:** A matched case-control study design was conducted with children admitted to a Kenyan hospital with severe acute malnutrition. The controls were normal-weight children who were age, acute diagnosis, and sex matched. Mothers of both groups were assessed for depression using the PHQ-9 questionnaire. Logistic regression was used to compare the odds of maternal depression in cases and controls, controlling for other factors associated with youth malnutrition. **RESULTS:** The prevalence of moderate to severe maternal depression of malnourished children was high (64%) compared to mothers of normal-weight children (5%). In multivariate analyses, the odds of maternal depression were higher in cases than in controls (adjusted OR = 53.5, 95% CI = 8.5–338.3), as were the odds of having very low income (adjusted OR = 77.6 95% CI = 5.8–1033.2). **CONCLUSION:** Kenyan mothers whose children were diagnosed with malnutrition carry a significant mental health burden. The authors recommend implementation of interventions that offer social support, mental health counseling, strategies to address food insecurity, and economic wellness training for mothers of malnourished children.

Source: Haithar S, Kuria MW, Sheikh A, Kumar M, Vander Stoep A. Maternal depression and child severe acute malnutrition: a case-control study from Kenya. *BMC Pediatr.* 2018 Sep 3;18(1):289. doi: 10.1186/s12887-018-1261-1

natural capital. The UN cites economic development, social development, and environmental protection as the *reinforcing pillars* of sustainable development. The role of the agriculture industry in promoting practices that contribute to environmental and social issues has been at the center of discussions of **sustainable intensification** in agriculture (Fig. 13-11).[39] As a result, interest in alternative farming practices has grown and reinforced a movement toward sustainable agriculture. Sustainable agriculture flows directly from the SDGs to ensure sustainable consumption and production patterns globally. Meeting these targets depends on integration of several goals, including environmental health, economic profitability, and social and economic equity. Sustainable agriculture addresses many environmental and social concerns and offers innovative and economically viable opportunities for many in the food system, including growers, laborers, consumers, and policy makers. It is gaining support and acceptance from conventional farmers in many countries.

Sustainable agriculture involves maintaining or enhancing the land and natural resources for use long into the future. It also requires consideration for human resources, including working and living conditions of laborers, the needs of rural communities, and consumer health and safety. The potential of sustainability is best understood when the consequences of farming practices on both human communities and the environment are considered. Many farmers around the globe are transitioning to sustainable agriculture by taking small, realistic steps based on their personal goals and family economics. Reaching the goal of worldwide sustainable agriculture requires participation by all stakeholders, including farmers, laborers, retailers, consumers, researchers, and policy makers.

Regenerative agriculture is a system of farming that focuses on restoring degraded soils, increasing biodiversity, improving watersheds, and enhancing the ecosystem. The principles and practices strive to capture carbon in the soil and above ground to counter atmospheric carbon accumulation. Critics of regenerative agriculture claim that it is a watered-down version of organic farming promoted by industry to appease environmentally conscious consumers. Ultimately, more rigorous research is needed to fully assess the long-term impact of various farming practices on the health of plants and the planet.

A novel area of agricultural technology that is gaining momentum is hydroponics. Implemented correctly, this soilless method of plant production can grow plants 25% faster and produce up to 30% greater yield as compared to traditional soil-grown plants. These significant benefits are possible through

sustainable intensification Agricultural practices that consider whole landscapes, territories, and ecosystems to optimize resource utilization and management.

regenerative agriculture A system of farming and grazing practices that aims to reverse climate change by rebuilding soil organic matter and restoring degraded soil biodiversity, resulting in both carbon drawdown and improving the water cycle.

FARM to FORK Pineapples

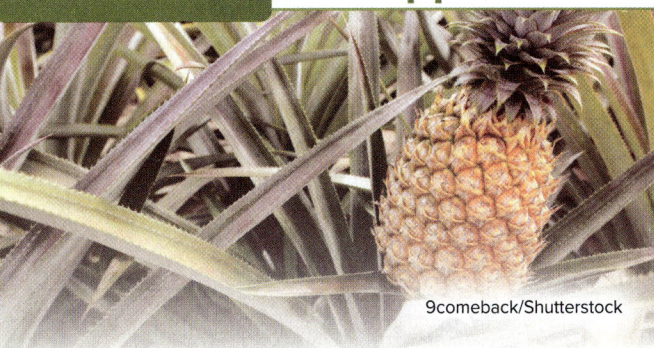
9comeback/Shutterstock

Luscious tropical fruits, like pineapples, not only provide key nutrients but also an economic advantage for developing countries. After bananas, pineapples are the most consumed tropical fruit in the U.S. Typically imported from Costa Rica and Hawaii, pineapples have a long history of being bred for certain traits, resulting in the sweet and low-acidic varieties available today. James Dole, the most famous pineapple industrialist, moved to Hawaii in 1899 and started the first pineapple plantation.

Grow
- To plant a pineapple at home, slice off the pineapple crown (top) from a fresh pineapple. Remove all fresh fruit to avoid rot. Make thin slices in the stalk, displaying a ring of brown root dots. Remove the lower leaves on the stalk to expose approximately 1" of bare stalk.
- Allow the stalk to dry well for a few days. Plant the pineapple 1" deep in a pot with fast-draining potting mix.
- Water lightly and place in a sunny location. The pineapple should root in 1 to 3 months.
- Repot as needed to encourage growth.

Shop
- When purchasing tropical fruits, look for *fair trade* fruits, signifying that the fruit was grown under environmentally friendly conditions with attention to small-scale producers.
- When shopping for pineapple, select the golden sweet varieties. Although sweet pineapples have 25% more sugar, they have 135% more beta-carotene and 350% more vitamin C than traditional Cayenne pineapples.
- To select the freshest pineapple, look for dark green crown leaves that are difficult to pluck and free of browning or fading.

Store
- Pineapples are harvested ripe and do not continue to ripen, so they should be kept refrigerated and eaten within 4 days.

Prep
- Pineapple juice and flesh are used in cuisines around the globe.
- Pineapple slices or chunks are used in desserts, fruit salads, and savory dishes such as pizza toppings or grilled with a hamburger.
- Crushed pineapple is often added to yogurt, jams, and ice cream.
- Pineapple juice is often consumed straight, added to smoothies, or used as a main ingredient in piña coladas. Pineapple juice can also serve as a meat marinade and tenderizer.

Source: Robinson J. Tropical fruits: make the most of eating globally. In: *Eating on the Wild Side: The Missing Link in Optimum Health.* New York: Little, Brown 7 Co.; 2013.

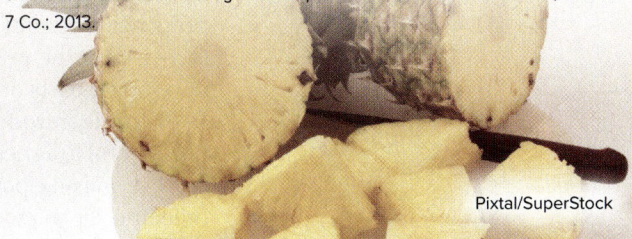
Pixtal/SuperStock

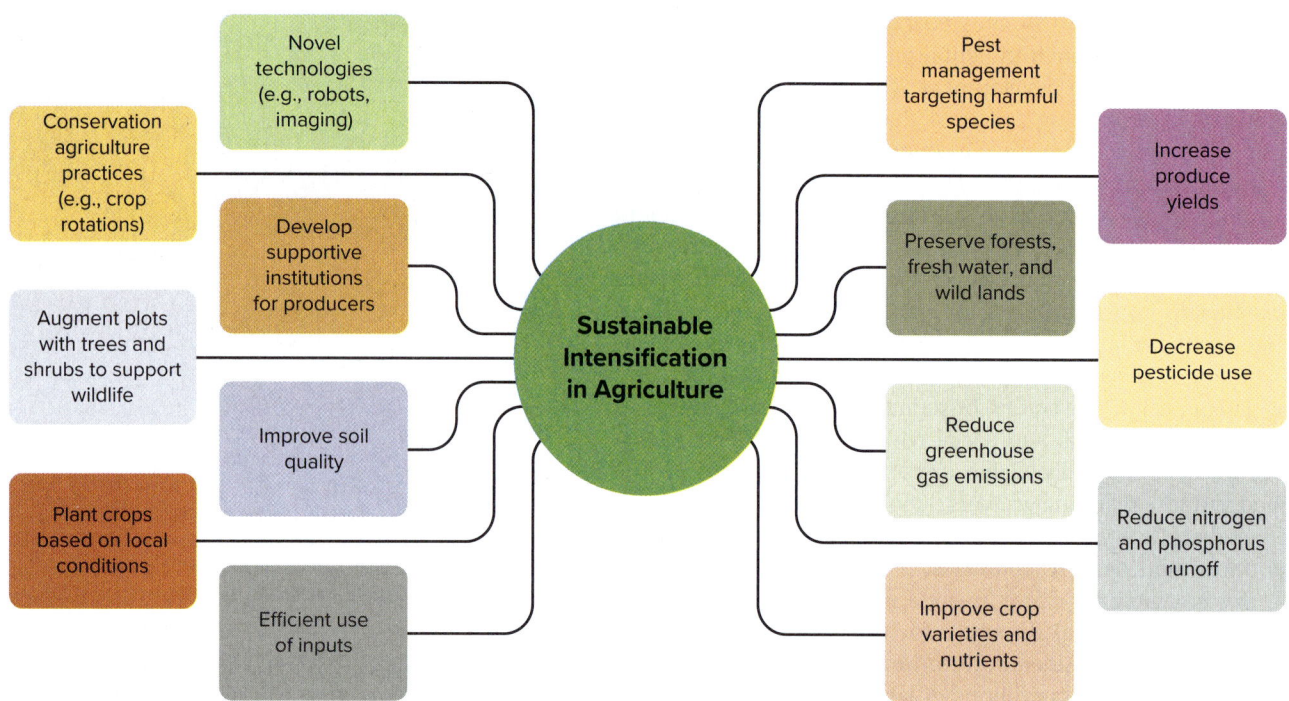

FIGURE 13-11 Goals of sustainable intensification of agriculture needed to efficiently produce enough food for the world's population using environmentally friendly techniques.
Source: Adapted from FAO.

intense control of the nutrient solution, water, and pH levels. In addition, hydroponics is environmentally friendly and reduces the waste and pollution often associated with soil runoff. Yet despite these positives, there remain limitations to hydroponics as well. Initially, system start-ups require extensive training, time, space, and money. Starting small is a wise choice for novice growers.

ADVANCES IN BIOTECHNOLOGY

Each year, up to 17 million farmers in 26 countries have planted over 190 million hectares of biotech crops. The top four GMOs include maize, soybean, canola, and cotton. The 72 million U.S. biotech hectares include maize, soybeans, cotton, canola, sugar beets, alfalfa, papaya, squash, potatoes, and apples. These crops help to alleviate poverty by improving the economic situation of over 16 million small farmers.[40]

Whether applications of genetic engineering will help to significantly reduce malnutrition in the developing world remains to be seen. Unless price cuts accompany the increased production, only landowners and suppliers of biotechnology will enjoy the benefits. Small farmers may benefit if they can afford to purchase the genetically modified seeds. This point deserves emphasis: the person who cannot afford to buy enough food today will still face that same predicament in the future. As with most innovations, the more successful farmers—often those with larger farms—will adopt new biotechnology first. Because of this, the present trend toward fewer and larger farms will continue in the developing world, a movement that undermines the solution to one of the most pressing undernutrition issues. Furthermore, biotechnology does not promise dramatic increases in the production of most grains and cassava, the primary food resources in developing parts of the world.

With the introduction of more drought- and pest-resistant crops, as well as self-fertilizing crops, agricultural biotechnology may help to reduce world hunger. Perhaps the most promising potential of genetically modified foods lies within the realm of plant breeding for micronutrients. If they have access to farming resources to increase the micronutrient composition of crops, developing countries will have a tool to treat and prevent nutrient deficiencies. In addition, greater yields for indigenous plants, such as tomatoes that tolerate high soil salinity, are another hopeful outcome. Biotechnology will likely be a useful tool against the complex scourge of world undernutrition. Improved crops produced by this technology, together with political and other efforts, can contribute to success in the battle against worldwide malnutrition.

Another exciting bioengineering technique includes biofortification. This process can improve the nutritional quality of crops while the plants are growing rather than through conventional fortification during food processing. Examples of successful biofortification of crops with nutrients include iron (rice, beans, sweet potatoes, cassava, and legumes), zinc (wheat, rice, beans, sweet potatoes, and maize), provitamin A carotenoid (sweet potatoes, maize, and cassava), and amino acid and protein (sorghum and cassava). UNICEF estimates that biofortification could impact over 5 million children under age 5 affected by iron deficiency.[41]

Any technology comes with risks. The public has long been opposed to *unnatural* products or processes perceived as harmful to the environment. Concern exists regarding potential cumulative effects of biotechnology over time. With these concerns in mind, the FDA carefully examines all products developed using this technology and will enforce labeling of potential allergens that may be newly present in food altered by biotechnology.

Magnificent microbiome

Soil Microbiome
Like humans, soil also has a vast and dynamic microbiome. This vibrant living community has a profound effect on the life and death of plants. The soil microbiome is a rich reservoir of biodiversity that has enormous functional potential in health care, agriculture, food production, and climate regulation.

Source: Plant Soil Microbial Community Consortium, NC State.

CONCLUDING THOUGHTS

The economic loss from malnutrition is staggering, and the amount of human pain and suffering it causes is incalculable. With all the international relief efforts and assistance from governments and private organizations combined, the battle is far from over. Read more about the progress toward the Sustainable Development Goals and the ongoing challenges of hunger in several regions of the world, even as poverty has decreased, at https://sdgs.un.org.[30]

Ultimately, the rapid depletion of world resources, massive debt incurred by poorer countries, threat of danger to more prosperous countries nearby, and toll of war and famine all affect the population's physical and economic well-being. Planet Earth has enough food and the technical expertise to alleviate hunger. With world leaders affirming the UN Sustainable Development Goals and working to achieve its targets by 2030, we have a promising coordinated political effort that is making progress toward lasting reductions in hunger and optimal health for all.

✓ CONCEPT CHECK 13.4

1. Why is development tailored to local conditions important in combating global hunger?
2. List three benefits of regenerative agriculture.
3. Describe one way biotechnology could help to relieve global malnutrition.

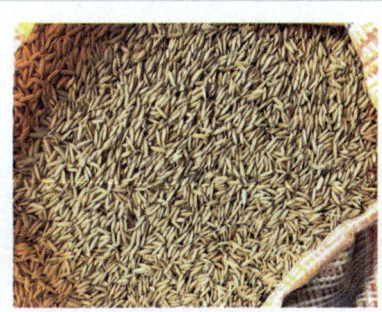

Fortification refers to adding nutrients to foods during processing. In contrast, biofortification uses plant breeding or biotechnology to grow plants with increased levels of certain nutrients. **What advantages does biofortification offer compared to other public health efforts to correct undernutrition?** ratharath nimhattha/Shutterstock

13.5 Nutrition and Your Health: Malnutrition at Critical Life Stages

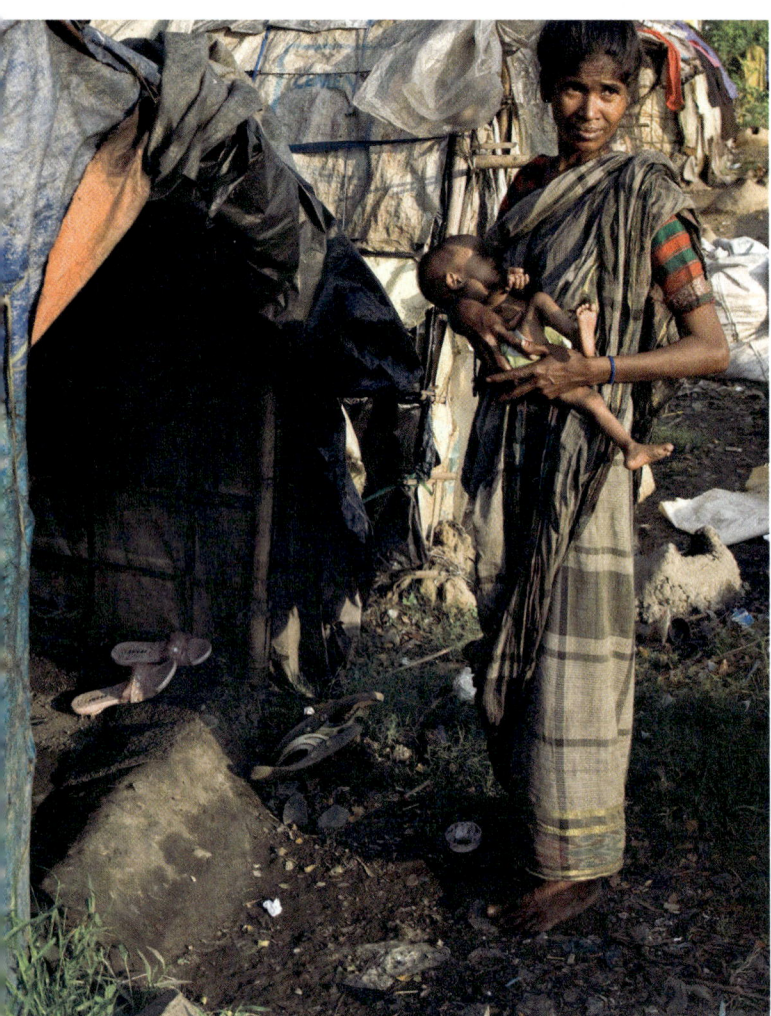

Andrew Holbrooke/Corbis/Getty Images

Pregnancy

Undernutrition poses the greatest health risk during pregnancy. Every day, approximately 800 females die from preventable causes, with 95% occurring in low- and middle-income countries.[42] A female who is pregnant needs extra nutrients to meet both her own needs and those of her developing offspring. Nourishing the fetus may deplete maternal stores of nutrients. Maternal iron-deficiency anemia is one possible consequence of malnutrition during pregnancy.

Birth rates in Africa are the highest in the world. In Niger, for example, a female gives birth to an average of nearly seven children. Coupled with chronic malnutrition, a female's risk of dying increases with every pregnancy and birth. This results in a strong connection between a high fertility rate and high maternal mortality rates. Although most of us consider pregnancy and childbirth as natural parts of life, for females living in developing countries and without adequate access to health care, pregnancy and childbirth complications are among the leading causes of death. The cumulative effect of successive pregnancies does not allow the mother to recover key nutrients, such as iron and folate, lost during pregnancy and breastfeeding. In South Asia, the maternal mortality ratio has declined by 67%, and in sub-Saharan Africa it has fallen by

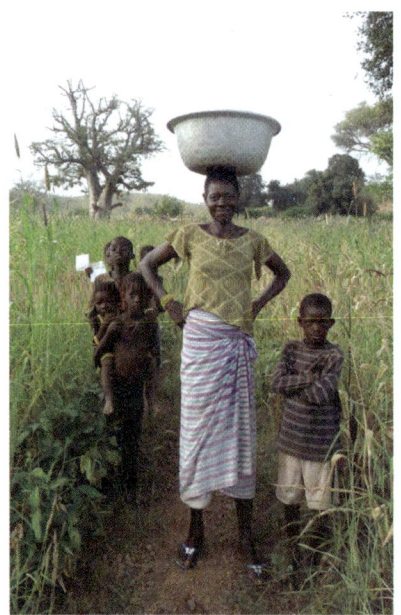

This Lobi tribeswoman, standing with her six children in a grassy field in Burkina Faso, Africa, is an illustration of the typical birth rate in this region. **Why do successive pregnancies and breastfeeding put this mother at nutritional risk?** Lissa Harrison

Prolonged malnutrition is detrimental to many aspects of human health, resulting in increased maternal, infant, and child mortality; loss of parents (especially linked to AIDS); exploitation of females reduced work capacity; reduced intellectual and social development; and overall human suffering, especially during a famine. It is particularly damaging during periods of growth and old age. A conceptual framework of malnutrition lists the immediate causes as inadequate dietary intake and unsatisfactory health. These underlying causes relate to families and include lack of access to food, inadequate care for females and children, and inadequate health services. Effective strategies to combat malnutrition should embrace a life cycle approach. Public health programs should be complementary and comprehensive across vulnerable periods of the whole reproductive cycle.

almost 33%.[42] The SDG is to reduce the global maternal mortality ratio to less than 70 per 100,000 live births by 2030.

Fetal Development and Infant Stages

An unborn baby faces major health risks from malnutrition during gestation. To support growth and development of the brain and other body tissues, a growing fetus requires a rich supply of protein, lipids, vitamins, and minerals. When these nutrient needs are not met, it is more likely that the infant will be born before 37 weeks of gestation, well before the ideal 40 weeks. Preterm birth and low birth weight (5.5 pounds or less) contribute to 60% to 80% of all neonatal deaths.[43] If the infant survives, abnormal growth and development can result. In extreme cases, low-birth-weight infants face exponentially greater risk of dying before their first birthday, primarily due to complications of reduced lung development. When low birth weight is accompanied by other physical abnormalities, medical costs may exceed hundreds of thousands of dollars.

Childhood

Early childhood, when growth is rapid, is another period when malnutrition is extremely risky. The greatest impact of undernutrition occurs in the first 1000 days of life: from conception to a child's second birthday. Irreversible damage is the result if optimal nutrition is not available at critical times in development. The central nervous system—including the brain—is highly vulnerable because of rapid growth through early childhood. After the preschool years, brain growth and development slow dramatically. Nutritional deprivation, especially in early infancy, can lead to permanent brain impairment. Without an effective intervention, it is projected that ongoing undernutrition could leave more than 1 billion children with mental impairments by 2020.[44]

In general, children living in poverty are at the greatest risk for nutrient deficiencies and their subsequent consequences. The WHO reports that nearly 150 million experience *stunted growth*. Iron-deficiency anemia is also more common among low-income children. This deficiency can lead to fatigue, reduced stamina, stunted growth, impaired motor development, and learning problems. Undernutrition in childhood can also weaken immune function and increase the risk of infection when nutrients such as protein, vitamin A, and zinc are low in a dietary pattern. Clearly, malnutrition and illness have a cyclical relationship. Not only does undernutrition lead to illness, but diarrheal and other infectious diseases increase malnutrition. For this reason, millions of children in developing countries are dying from the combination of malnutrition and infection. Conversely, when missing nutrients, such as vitamin A and iron, are restored to a child's diet, improvements in health are evident.

CASE STUDY: Undernutrition During Childhood

Jamal traveled to the Philippines with his church group last summer. During their stay, the group helped build shelters in a village where, a few weeks before, a storm had destroyed several houses. Jamal noticed that many of the children were very short, much shorter than the children in his neighborhood in the United States. His group worked in a remote, low-elevation area where the storm and subsequent flooding had caused the most damage. On several occasions, he noticed young mothers crouched on curbs or in doorways, holding their children. These children rarely moved; they appeared pale and listless. In contrast to the children Jamal's group had met at a church in the capital city, most of the children in this village were not active and lively. One evening, a nurse from the local clinic came to speak to Jamal's group. She said that many children in this area do not get enough to eat and that malnutrition was rampant. She considered the recent storm a blessing in disguise, hoping it would spur the Philippine government to send supplies to the village, particularly food and medicines. Jamal was shocked by such a degree of suffering. He wonders why children in the Philippines can be starving to death while so many children in his hometown in the United States have more food than they need.

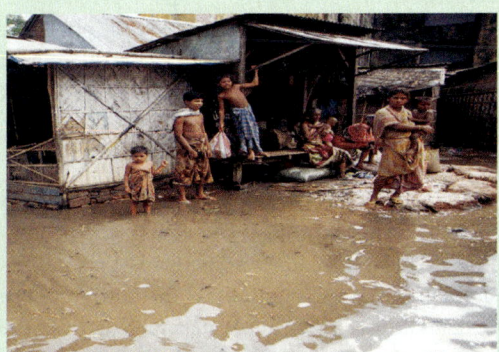

Family members from a small village in the Philippines are coping with recent flood waters encroaching on their living space. What are some potential health issues associated with living in these conditions? Digital Vision/Getty Images

1. Which nutrients are likely to be deficient in the diets of these children?
2. Which nutrient deficiencies contribute to *stunted* growth?
3. Which nutrient deficiencies may be reducing immune defenses?
4. Are these children likely to be consuming adequate calories? What effect does inadequate consumption of calories have on growth?
5. How might the recent flooding impact the health of the children in the village?

Complete the Case Study. Responses to these questions can be provided by your instructor.

Reducing wasting in children under 5 years of age and addressing the nutritional needs of adolescent girls are SDGs. Death rates for children under 5 years of age have been reduced to 1 in 26 children in 2018 compared to 1 in 11 in 1990. Despite this progress, over 5 million children under 5 years of age still died in 2019.[45] These statistics indicate that undernutrition is one of the most important challenges to overcome because it is estimated to be an underlying cause in as many as 50% of the preventable deaths among children under age 5.[43]

Later Years

The WHO predicts a significant increase in the number of people age 65 years or older, from an estimate of 524 million in 2010 to almost 1.4 billion in 2050.[46] Most of this increase in global aging will be in developing countries. Older adults, especially older females living alone in poverty, are at risk for undernutrition. All older adults require nutrient-dense foods in amounts dependent on their current health and degree of physical activity. Many older adults have fixed incomes and incur significant medical costs over time, so food often becomes a low-priority item. In addition, depression, social isolation, and declining physical and mental health can compound the problem of undernutrition in older adults.

✓ CONCEPT CHECK 13.5

1. What are some underlying causes of malnutrition?
2. What two factors contribute to neonatal deaths?
3. During childhood, when is the period when undernutrition is most impactful?

Summary (Numbers refer to numbered sections in the chapter)

13.1 Malnutrition includes undernutrition, overnutrition, and hidden hunger—resulting in poor physical and mental health and diet-related chronic disease. In poor countries, this is worsened by recurrent infections, unsanitary conditions, extreme weather, inadequate shelter, and exposure to pathogens and diseases.

Food security exists when people have physical, social, and economic access to sufficient, safe, and nutritious food to meet their dietary needs and food preferences for an active and healthy life. Nutrition security builds upon this while acknowleging global health inequities.

13.2 Many in the U.S. live at or below the federal poverty level and are impacted by hunger and malnutrition. Meals on Wheels, SNAP benefits, school lunch and breakfast programs, WIC, and other programs focus on improving the nutritional health of individuals at risk. When adequately funded, these programs have proved effective in reducing malnutrition and improving food and nutrition security.

13.3 Multiple factors contribute to the problem of global malnutrition. In densely populated countries, food resources, as well as the means for distributing food, may be inadequate. Environmentally unsustainable farming methods hamper future efforts to grow food. Limited water availability hinders food production. Natural disasters, urbanization, war, and disease all contribute to the major problem of undernutrition.

13.4 Proposed solutions to global malnutrition must consider multiple interacting factors, many thoroughly embedded in cultural traditions. Through education and training, efforts should be made to upgrade farming methods, improve crops, encourage breastfeeding, and improve sanitation and hygiene.

Direct food aid is a short-term solution. Many experts recommend more subsistence-level sustainable farming. Small-scale industrial development is another way to create meaningful employment and purchasing power for vast numbers of residents that live in rural areas and are poor. Various biotechnology applications may also prove beneficial. The UN's 17 *Sustainable Development Goals* focus on global solutions.

13.5 The greatest risk of malnutrition occurs during critical periods of growth and development: pregnancy, infancy, and childhood. People in their senior years are also at great risk.

Check Your Knowledge (Answers are available at the end of this question set)

1. The complex characteristics of include decreased or impaired concentration, immunity, productivity, infant birth weights, and mental health.
    a. stunting
    b. malnutrition
    c. wasting
    d. food deserts

2. The number-one killer of children in developing countries is
    a. xerophthalmia.
    b. iron-deficiency anemia.
    c. iodine deficiency.
    d. diarrhea.

3. A human is particularly susceptible to the effects of undernutrition during
   a. pregnancy.
   b. infancy.
   c. childhood.
   d. all of these stages.

4. Which is a barrier to solving undernutrition in the developing world?
   a. Ill-defined solutions
   b. Poor infrastructure
   c. A lack of manpower
   d. A lack of interest

5. Many of the child deaths each year in developing countries could be prevented if
   a. technology were improved.
   b. doctors were more specialized.
   c. mothers could learn more about nutrition.
   d. sanitation and hygiene were improved.

6. The Supplemental Nutrition Assistance Program (SNAP) allows
   a. families with low income to buy surplus food at government stores with government-issued electronic benefit transfer cards.
   b. individuals with low income to purchase food, cleaning supplies, alcoholic beverages, and anything else sold in supermarkets with electronic benefit transfer cards.
   c. individuals with low income to turn in government-issued electronic benefit transfer cards for cash to buy food.
   d. individuals with low income to purchase food and seeds with government-issued electronic benefit transfer cards.

7. A long-term solution to world hunger is
   a. the green revolution.
   b. cash crops.
   c. jobs and self-sufficiency.
   d. government and private aid.

8. How many of the Sustainable Development Goals are focused on nutrition-related metrics?
   a. 0
   b. 2
   c. 12
   d. 17

9. A system of farming that focuses on restoring degraded soils, increasing biodiversity, improving watersheds, and enhancing the ecosystem is called
   a. sustainable agriculture.
   b. biofortification.
   c. hydroponics.
   d. regenerative agriculture.

10. The WHO predicts a significant increase in the number of people in which category?
    a. Adults over 65 years of age
    b. Children born to teen mothers
    c. Adults who are nutrition secure
    d. Infants born with HIV/AIDS

Answer Key: 1. b (LO 13.1), 2. d (LO 13.3), 3. d (LO 13.5), 4. b (LO 13.3), 5. d (LO 13.3), 6. d (LO 13.2), 7. c (LO 13.2), 8. c (LO 13.4), 9. d (LO 13.4), 10. a (LO 13.4)

Study Questions (Numbers refer to Learning Outcomes)

1. Describe the difference between malnutrition, overnutrition, and undernutrition. **(LO 13.1)**
2. Name three nutrients often lacking in the diets of people who lack access to an adequate, safe food supply. What effects can be expected with each deficiency? **(LO 13.1)**
3. What are the major factors contributing to malnutrition in affluent nations, such as the United States? **(LO 13.2)**
4. What federal programs are available to address the problem of malnutrition in the United States? **(LO 13.2)**
5. Outline how war and civil unrest in developing countries have worsened issues of chronic hunger over the past few years. **(LO 13.3)**
6. How important is population control in addressing the problem of world hunger now and in the future? **(LO 13.3)**
7. Why is solving the problem of malnutrition a key factor in the ability of developing countries to reach their full potential? **(LO 13.3)**
8. Describe how sustainable agriculture and biotechnology can improve food availability worldwide. **(LO 13.4)**
9. List three long-term consequences of malnutrition during fetal development or infancy. **(LO 13.5)**
10. Related to nutrition, what are the critical stages of life when individuals are most vulnerable? **(LO 13.5)**

References

1. Seferidi P, Hone T, Duran AC, Bernabe-Ortiz A, Millett C. Global inequalities in the double burden of malnutrition and associations with globalisation: a multilevel analysis of demographic and health surveys from 55 low-income and middle-income countries, 1992–2018 [published correction appears in *Lancet Glob Health*. 2022 Apr;10(4):e481]. *Lancet Glob Health*. 2022 Apr;10(4):e482-e490. doi: 10.1016/S2214-109X(21)00594-5

2. FAO, IFAD, UNICEF, WFP, WHO. *The State of Food Security and Nutrition in the World 2023. Transforming Food Systems for Food Security, Improved Nutrition and Affordable Healthy Diets for All*. Available at https://www.fao.org/documents/card/en/c/cb4474en

3. World population. United States Census Bureau. Accessed November 26, 2023. https://www.census.gov/library/stories/2023/11/world-population-estimated-eight-billion.html.

4. FAO, IFAD, UNICEF, WFP, WHO. *The State of Food Security and Nutrition in the World 2019*. Available at https://www.unicef.org/media/55921/file/SOFI-2019-full-report.pdf. Accessed November 24, 2023.

5. Nordin SM, Boyle M, Kemmer TM; Academy of Nutrition and Dietetics. Position of the Academy of Nutrition and Dietetics: nutrition security in developing nations: sustainable food, water, and health [published correction appears in *J Acad Nutr Diet.* 2013 Dec;113(12):1759]. *J Acad Nutr Diet.* 2013;113(4):581-595. doi:10.1016/j.jand.2013.01.025

6. Addressing iron and zinc deficiency across the globe. U.S. Department of Agriculture, Agricultural Research Service. Accessed November 26, 2023. https://www.ars.usda.gov/oc/utm/addressing-iron-and-zinc-deficiency-across-the-globe/

7. Vitamin A deficiency. World Health Organization, Nutrition Landscape Information System. Accessed November 26, 2023. https://www.who.int/data/nutrition/nlis/info/vitamin-a-deficiency

8. UNICEF. *Multiple Micronutrient Powder (MNP): Supply and Market Outlook.* July 2021. Accessed November 26, 2023. https://www.unicef.org/supply/reports/multiple-micronutrient-powder-mnp-supply-and-market-outlook

9. Micronutrient facts. Centers for Disease Control and Prevention. Accessed November 15, 2023. https://www.cdc.gov/nutrition/micronutrient-malnutrition/micronutrients/index.html

10. Poverty in the U.S. U.S. Census Bureau. Accessed November 15, 2023. http://www.census.gov/topics/income-poverty/poverty.html

11. Hunger in America. Feeding America. Accessed November 22, 2023. https://www.feedingamerica.org/hunger-in-america/impact-of-hunger

12. U.S. Department of Agriculture. *FY 2022 Budget Summary.* Accessed November 31, 2023. https://www.usda.gov/sites/default/files/documents/2022-budget-summary.pdf

13. Foods typically purchased by Supplemental Nutrition Assistance Program (SNAP) households. U.S. Department of Agriculture, Food and Nutrition Service. Accessed Novermber 15, 2023. https://www.fns.usda.gov/snap/foods-typically-purchased-supplemental-nutrition-assistance-program-snap-households

14. USDA food plans: cost of food. U.S. Department of Agriculture. Accessed November 20, 2023. https://www.fns.usda.gov/cnpp/usda-food-plans-cost-food-reports

15. U.S. Department of Agriculture, Food and Nutrition Service. *Program Information Report: U.S. Summary FY 2018–FY 2019.* In: Hayes TO, Williams A. The School Breakfast Program and National School Lunch Program: a primer. American Action Forum. Accessed November 20, 2023. https://www.americanactionforum.org/research/primer-school_breakfast_program_national_lunch_program/

16. Older Americans Act for advocates. National Council on Aging. Accessed November 20, 2023. https://www.ncoa.org/advocates/public-policy/issues/aging-services/older-americans-act

17. Feeding America. *The Impact of the Coronavirus on Food Insecurity in 2020 & 2021.* Accessed November 26, 2023. https://www.feedingamerica.org/sites/default/files/2021-03/National%20Projections%20Brief_3.9.2021_0.pdf

18. Poverty in the United States: 2022. U.S. Census Bureau. Accessed December 7, 2023. Available at https://www.census.gov/data/tables/2023/demo/income-poverty/p60-280.html

19. Poverty guidelines. Office of the Assistant Secretary for Planning and Evaluation. Accessed December 7, 2024. Available at https://aspe.hhs.gov/topics/poverty-economic-mobility/poverty-guidelines.

20. U.S. Department of Housing and Urban Development, Office of Community Planning and Development. *The 2020 Annual Homeless Assessment Report (AHAR) to Congress.* Accessed November 26, 2023. https://www.huduser.gov/portal/sites/default/files/pdf/2020-AHAR-Part-1.pdf

21. U.S. Department of Housing and Urban Development Office of Community Planning and Development. *The 2022 Annual Homelessness Assessment Report (AHAR) to Congress.* Accessed December 7, 2023. Available at Annual Homelessness Assessment Report (AHAR) to Congress.

22. Food Access Research Atlas. U.S. Department of Agriculture, Economic Research Service. Accessed November 15, 2023. http://www.ers.usda.gov/data-products/food-access-research-atlas.aspx

23. Holben DH, Marshall MB. Position of the Academy of Nutrition and Dietetics: food insecurity in the United States. *J Acad Nutr Diet.* 2017 Dec;117(12):1991-2002. doi: 10.1016/j.jand.2017.09.027

24. International Rescue Committee. *Watchlist 2021.* Accessed November 26, 2023. https://www.rescue.org/sites/default/files/document/5481/2021emergencywatchlistirc.pdf

25. World military expenditure grows to $1.8 trillion in 2018. News release. Stockholm International Peace Research Institute (SIPRI). Accessed November 29, 2023. https://www.sipri.org/media/press-release/2019/world-military-expenditure-grows-18-trillion-2018

26. Figures at a glance. UN Refugee Agency. Accessed November 26, 2023. https://www.unhcr.org/en-us/figures-at-a-glance.html

27. Global Hunger Index scores by 2021 GHI rank. Global Hunger Index. Accessed November 10, 2023. https://www.globalhungerindex.org/results.html

28. FAO in China: China at a glance. Food and Agriculture Organization of the United Nations. Accessed November 19, 2023. http://www.fao.org/china/fao-in-china/china-at-a-glance/en

29. Drinking-water. World Health Organization (WHO). Accessed November 22, 2023. https://www.who.int/news-room/fact-sheets/detail/drinking-water

30. 17 goals to transform our world. United Nations, Sustainable Development Goals. Accessed November 15, 2023. http://www.un.org/sustainabledevelopment

31. Water, Sanitation and Hygiene (WASH). UNICEF. Accessed November 29, 2023. https://www.unicef.org/wash

32. Sanitation. World Health Organization (WHO). Accessed November 28, 2023. https://www.who.int/news-room/fact-sheets/detail/sanitation

33. Diarrhoea. UNICEF. April 2021. Accessed November 12, 2023. https://data.unicef.org/topic/child-health/diarrhoeal-disease

34. The Global Health Observatory data: HIV/AIDS. World Health Organization (WHO). Accessed November 4, 2023. https://www.who.int/gho/hiv/en

35. About HIV. Centers for Disease Control and Prevention. Accessed November 31, 2023. https://www.cdc.gov/hiv/basics/whatishiv.html

36. U.S. statistics: fast facts. HIV.gov. Accessed November 12, 2023. https://www.hiv.gov/hiv-basics/overview/data-and-trends/statistics

37. Willig A, Wright L, Galvin TA. Practice paper of the Academy of Nutrition and Dietetics: nutrition intervention and human immunodeficiency virus infection. *J Acad Nutr Diet.* 2018 Mar;118(3):486-498. doi: 10.1016/j.jand.2017.12.007

38. Food security in the U.S.: survey tools. U.S. Department of Agriculture, Economic Research Service. Accessed November 25, 2023. https://www.ers.usda.gov/topics/food-nutrition-assistance/food-security-in-the-us/survey-tools

39. Sustainable crop production intensification (SCPI) in FAO. Food and Agriculture Organization of the United Nations. Accessed November 22, 2023. https://www.fao.org/agriculture/crops/thematic-sitemap/theme/spi/scpi-home/framework/sustainable-intensification-in-fao/en/

40. Pocket K No. 16: biotech crop highlights in 2019. International Service for the Acquisition of Agri-biotech Applications (ISAAA). Accessed November 15, 2023. https://www.isaaa.org/resources/publications/pocketk/16

41. UNICEF. *The State of the World's Children 2019: Children, Food and Nutrition: Growing Well in a Changing World.* October 2019. Accessed November 10, 2023. https://www.unicef.org/media/60806/file/SOWC-2019.pdf

42. Maternal mortality. World Health Organization (WHO). Accessed November 11, 2023. https://www.who.int/news-room/fact-sheets/detail/maternal-mortality
43. Maternal, newborn, child and adolescent health and ageing. World Health Organization (WHO). Accessed November 15, 2023. https://www.who.int/teams/maternal-newborn-child-adolescent-health-and-ageing
44. The state of the world's children 2019: children, food and nutrition. UNICEF. Accessed November 17, 2023. https://data.unicef.org/resources/state-of-the-worlds-children-2019
45. Under-five mortality. UNICEF. Accessed November 25, 2023. https://data.unicef.org/topic/child-survival/under-five-mortality
46. Ageing and health. World Health Organization (WHO). Accessed November 31, 2023. https://www.who.int/news-room/fact-sheets/detail/ageing-and-health

Design Element Credits: Fact Check/magnifying glass icon: McGraw Hill; Magnificent Microbiome background image: Alena Ohneva/Shutterstock; Sustainable Solutions icon: McGraw Hill; Roots icon: McGraw Hill; Medicine Cabinet icon: Peter Dazeley/Photographer's Choice/Getty Images

Chapter 14

Nutrition During Pregnancy and Breastfeeding

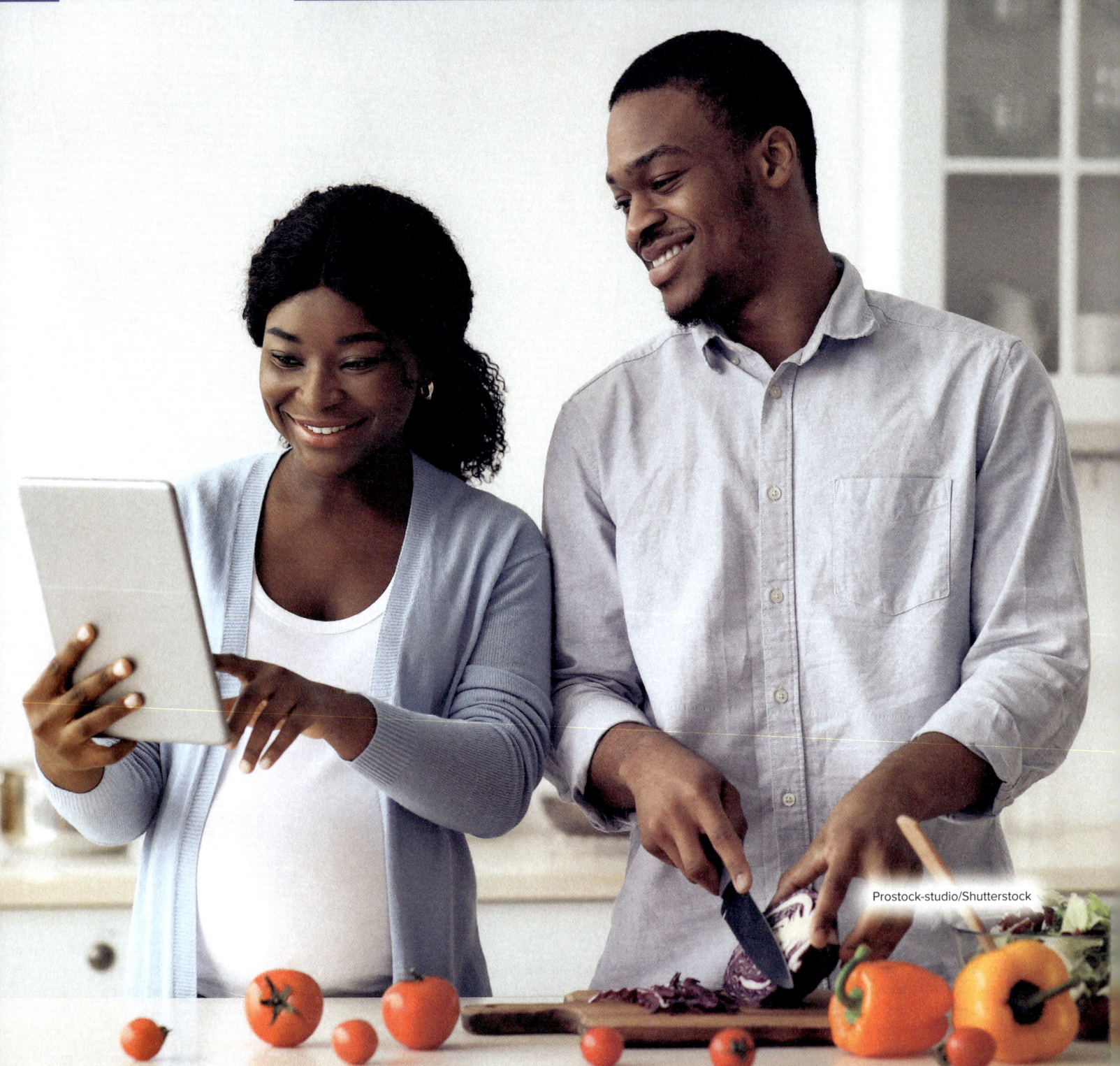

Prostock-studio/Shutterstock

Student Learning Outcomes

Chapter 14 is designed to allow you to:

14.1 Describe how nutrition affects fertility.

14.2 Summarize the physiological changes of pregnancy and how these changes affect key nutrient requirements.

14.3 Define *success* in terms of positive health outcomes during pregnancy and identify lifestyle factors that promote a successful pregnancy for both the mother and the infant.

14.4 Specify optimal ranges of gestational weight gain for individuals with low, healthy, or high prepregnancy BMI.

14.5 Outline guidelines for physical activity during pregnancy.

14.6 Describe how dietary changes can prevent or alleviate some discomforts and complications of pregnancy.

14.7 Summarize the physiological processes involved in breastfeeding and how breastfeeding affects maternal nutritional requirements.

14.8 Design an adequate, balanced meal plan for a female who is pregnant or breastfeeding based on MyPlate.

14.9 List several advantages of breastfeeding for both the mother and the infant.

14.10 Relate the nutritional status of the parents to the risk of birth defects in the child.

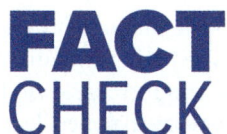

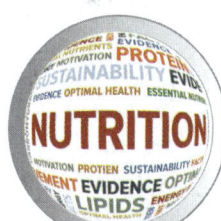

Is it necessary to avoid potential food allergens during pregnancy and breastfeeding to reduce the risk for food allergies in the infant?

There is no evidence that maternal dietary restrictions (e.g., peanuts, eggs, and fish) during pregnancy or breastfeeding prevent food allergies in infants. Read more about the impact of breastfeeding on the development of the infant's immune system in Section 14.7.

Source: Greer FR, Sicherer SH, Burks AW; Committee on Nutrition; Section on Allergy and Immunology. The effects of early nutritional interventions on the development of atopic disease in infants and children: the role of maternal dietary restriction, breastfeeding, hydrolyzed formulas, and timing of introduction of allergenic complementary foods. *Pediatrics*. 2019 Apr;143(4):e20190281. doi: 10.1542/peds.2019-0281

14.1 Nutrition and Fertility

"Surprise, we're pregnant!" Considering the fact that only about half of all pregnancies are planned, a positive pregnancy test can be shocking news. Even when planned, females often do not suspect they are pregnant during the first few weeks after conception. They may not seek medical attention until 2 to 3 months after conception. Without fanfare, though, the **embryo** grows and develops daily. As you will learn in this chapter, the mother's nutritional status will affect the health of the baby before and long after birth. For that reason, the health and nutrition habits of a female who is trying to become pregnant—or has the potential to become pregnant—are vitally important.

For up to 19% of couples who are planning for pregnancy, however, that pregnancy test shows a negative result month after month.[1] **Infertility** refers to the inability of a couple to conceive after 1 year of unprotected intercourse. There are numerous causes for male and female infertility, many of which are outside the couple's control. In some cases, however, modifying nutrition and other lifestyle behaviors can improve a couple's chances of conceiving a child.

The nutritional status of both the mother- and the father-to-be can affect the likelihood of conception.[2] Some of the nutritional factors discussed in this section affect the hormone levels involved in reproduction. Others directly affect the viability of the egg or the sperm. Thus far, research clearly supports a link between body fat and fertility, and some evidence points to roles of certain nutrients, such as dietary fats, carbohydrates, antioxidant nutrients, B vitamins, zinc, and iron. Overall dietary patterns, such as a Mediterranean dietary pattern, may also influence fertility.

ENERGY BALANCE

Recall from Section 7.1 that energy balance refers to matching calorie intake to energy expenditure. Positive energy balance describes a situation in which the amount of calories consumed exceeds the amount of calories required to support basic body processes and physical activity. Sustained over time, positive energy balance leads to gains in both lean mass and adipose tissue. Negative energy balance occurs when calorie intake falls short of calorie needs. Prolonged negative energy balance leads to the loss of both lean and adipose tissue. At either extreme, prolonged energy imbalance can impair fertility.

It is important to note that adipose tissue serves as more than just a storage depot for energy; it also produces estrogen and other hormones and cellular signaling molecules with widespread effects. For example, leptin, a hormone produced primarily by adipose tissue, affects appetite, metabolic rate, immune function, growth, and reproduction.

In terms of energy, reproductive function is costly! Synthesis of reproductive hormones, maintenance of normal menstrual cycles, pregnancy, and breastfeeding require calories. With negative energy balance, little energy is available to maintain normal reproductive function. Consequently, many females with underweight BMI experience **amenorrhea**, a sign of impaired ovulation. Some causes of low energy availability include undernutrition that stems from low food security, eating disorders, or high levels of athletic training. During World War II, for example, a famine in Holland drastically cut the calorie intake of females to about 1000 kcal per day. Many females became amenorrheic, and birth rates declined by about 50% during that time period. Studies in female athletes indicate that energy intake of at least 30 kcal per kilogram of lean mass is needed for normal female reproductive function. For males, as well, low body fat can decrease sex drive and sperm count.

On the opposite end of the spectrum, prolonged positive energy balance also decreases fertility. Excess adipose tissue affects the availability of reproductive hormones and induces insulin resistance. These endocrine changes impair the success of ovulation and implantation. In fact, females with a BMI of 27 kg/m² or higher are about

---

embryo In humans, the developing offspring in utero from about the beginning of the third week to the end of the eighth week after conception.

infertility Inability of a couple to conceive after 1 year of unprotected intercourse.

amenorrhea Absence of menstrual periods in a female of reproductive age.

three times more likely to experience infertility than those with a healthy BMI.[3] Among males, excess body fat increases estrogen levels and decreases testosterone. Also, extra fat tissue increases the temperature of the testicular area. The changes in hormones and temperature result in lower sperm production. Obesity is also associated with increased oxidative stress, which damages DNA in both the egg and the sperm. For adults who are overweight or obese, losing just 5% to 10% of body weight can increase the chances of conception.

HORMONAL BALANCE

As we discuss the ways energy imbalances influence fertility, it is important to mention **polycystic ovary syndrome (PCOS)**. Females with PCOS have hormonal imbalances that may lead to problems with ovulation, unusually high levels of androgen hormones (e.g., testosterone), and the presence of many tiny cysts that surround the ovaries like a strand of pearls. All females secrete some testosterone, but those with PCOS secrete more than normal. The high levels of male hormones lead to some of the signs and symptoms of PCOS: excess hair growth on the face, acne, and a tendency to deposit fat around the waist. Insulin resistance is another common feature of the syndrome. Thus, individuals with PCOS are at higher risk for diabetes, high blood pressure, and cardiovascular disease. Individuals with PCOS may experience irregular or absent periods, difficulty becoming pregnant, and higher-than-average rates of **spontaneous abortions.** Indeed, PCOS is the leading cause of female infertility.[4]

Several dietary and lifestyle interventions have been studied to see how they can alter the course of PCOS. To date, the evidence most clearly shows that modest weight loss may improve metabolic health and fertility issues among individuals who have PCOS and excess body fat. If a person with PCOS who is overweight or obese loses just 5% of initial body weight, the chances of conception improve.[5] Daily physical activity, known to improve insulin sensitivity, is a key component of any weight-management strategy.

At this time, there is no clear evidence to recommend any particular dietary macronutrient composition over another (e.g., low-fat versus low-carbohydrate dietary pattern). Individuals should consume a variety of foods from all different food groups to meet their energy and essential nutrient needs, tailoring the specific composition of the diet to personal and cultural preferences. However, because PCOS often cooccurs with insulin resistance, the quality of carbohydrates may make a difference in improving metabolic health and fertility. Experts often recommend choosing carbohydrates with a lower glycemic load.[5] For example, individuals with PCOS are urged to choose whole grains instead of refined grains and whole fruits and vegetables rather than juices, and to steer clear of sugar-sweetened beverages. These dietary changes can help to maintain blood sugar within a healthy range. Beware of unproven advice to reduce carbohydrate intake below the RDA during pregnancy. Severely restricting carbohydrate choices could limit the intake of important nutrients, such as fiber and B vitamins.

KEY NUTRIENTS

Vitamins. A variety of micronutrients may contribute to fertility, but folic acid tops the list for both males and females.[2] Folate is involved in DNA synthesis and the metabolism of homocysteine. For no other cells is proper DNA synthesis so important as for the egg and sperm, which transmit genetic information from one generation to the next. Foods such as leafy green vegetables, strawberries, and orange juice are sources of natural folate. The synthetic form, folic acid, can be found in fortified foods (e.g., ready-to-eat breakfast cereals) and dietary supplements.

The chemical reactions of metabolism produce free radicals (molecules with unpaired electrons) that can damage cell membranes and DNA. The body has some antioxidant

polycystic ovary syndrome (PCOS) A condition of hormonal imbalance (e.g., elevated testosterone and insulin) in a female that can lead to infertility, weight gain in the abdominal region, excessive growth of body hair, and acne.

spontaneous abortion Cessation of pregnancy and expulsion of the embryo or nonviable fetus prior to 20 weeks of gestation. This is the result of natural causes, such as a genetic defect or developmental problem; also called *miscarriage*.

mechanisms that limit the activity of free radicals, but when the production of free radicals exceeds the antioxidant capacity of the body, oxidative damage to cells is likely. Free radicals can damage egg and (especially) sperm cells and can affect how well a fertilized egg implants and matures. Research studies show that dietary patterns rich in antioxidants—vitamin E, vitamin C, selenium, zinc, beta-carotene, and some other plant pigments—are linked to improved fertility for both males and females.

Routine intake of a daily multivitamin and mineral supplement has been associated with improved fertility in many studies, but food sources of nutrients appear to offer multiple benefits beyond their vitamin and mineral content.[6] Foods of plant origin—including brightly colored fruits and vegetables, whole grains, and plant oils—are rich sources of vitamins linked to improved fertility.

Minerals. Iron and zinc are two minerals that have been linked to fertility. Zinc appears to be especially important for male fertility. Not only is it involved as a cofactor in antioxidant reactions that could protect the sperm from oxidative damage, but zinc also is required for normal sexual maturation and the production of sperm and reproductive hormones. Males with poor zinc status may have poor sperm quality (e.g., low sperm production, impaired sperm motility, and/or damaged DNA). Studies have shown that zinc supplements can improve sperm quality in individuals who are deficient in zinc.[7] However, a recent trial showed that zinc supplementation (in combination with folic acid supplementation) in males did not improve rates of live births or markers of sperm quality.[8] Rather than relying on supplements, males should strive to adhere to a *dietary pattern* that meets the RDA for zinc.

For females, iron and zinc are needed for normal ovulation. Data from a large observational study of nurses showed that iron intake before conception was linked to improved ovulatory function and therefore better fertility. Interestingly, in this study, higher intakes of nonheme iron (i.e., iron from plant sources, such as legumes and leafy green vegetables) were specifically related to improved fertility.[9]

Dietary Fat. As recommended for the general population of healthy adults, those who are trying to conceive should try to limit sources of saturated fats (and *trans* fats, which were recently banned from use in food manufacturing in the United States). For females, a dietary pattern rich in saturated fat promotes insulin resistance and impairs ovulation. For males, high intakes of saturated fat are linked to poor sperm quality.[2] Instead of consuming the typical American fare of pizza and fast foods, emphasize plant oils and fish oils, which provide more unsaturated fats. Among males experiencing infertility, boosting intakes of omega-3 fatty acids, which are the type of polyunsaturated fatty acids found in fish oils and walnuts, can improve sperm quality.

ALCOHOL

To date, research does not demonstrate a clear relationship between alcohol consumption and fertility.[2] However, in Section 14.8, you will learn about the devastating effects of alcohol on the developing **fetus** in utero. Given the fact that many individuals do not realize they are pregnant until several weeks after conception, it seems prudent to avoid alcohol while trying to conceive.

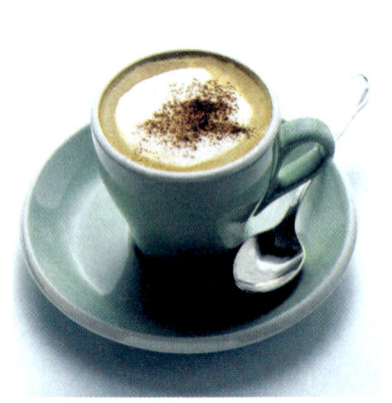

When trying to conceive, should you switch to decaf? The evidence is mixed. In some studies, intake of more than 4 cups of coffee (about 500 mg caffeine) has been linked to decreased fertility, but most studies show no clear link between moderate caffeine intake and fertility. Photo: Foodcollection

Text Source: Gaskins AJ, Chavarro JE. Diet and fertility: a review. *Am J Obstet Gynecol.* 2018 Apr;218(4):379-389. doi: 10.1016/j.ajog.2017.08.010

fetus The developing organism from about the beginning of the ninth week after conception until birth.

✓ CONCEPT CHECK 14.1

1. How is energy balance related to fertility?
2. What hormonal changes characterize polycystic ovary syndrome? List two dietary or lifestyle modifications that may help a person with PCOS to conceive.
3. Suggest one reason why a dietary pattern rich in fruits and vegetables is beneficial for fertility.

ASK THE RDN: Male Fertility

Dear RDN: My wife and I have been trying to conceive for the past 2 years. My wife has received so much advice about lifestyle changes to support fertility, but I know there must be some things I could be doing, as well. What are the best nutritional strategies to support male fertility?

Although it is not uncommon for the focus to be on the female when a couple is trying to conceive, 1/3 of all fertility challenges stem from male factors. (Another 1/3 of fertility challenges are due to female factors, and the remaining 1/3 are unexplained.) A male's lifestyle choices can impact his fertility, specifically via his dietary choices, whether he uses recreational drugs, which exercises he participates in, and whether he lives a stressful life.

When it comes to diet, here are some nutritional strategies that have been shown to support male fertility:

Maintain a healthy weight

Males who are considered obese are at higher risk of having fertility challenges. If you are not currently maintaining what is considered to be a healthy weight for your body, consider meeting with a registered dietitian to safely lose weight.

Follow a Mediterranean diet

From keto to paleo to everything in between, there are tons of "diets" that people can follow. But the one dietary pattern that has been linked to better male fertility outcomes is the Mediterranean diet.

Below are the basic principles of the Mediterranean diet:

- High consumption of fruits, vegetables, whole-grain bread and other cereals, beans, nuts, and seeds.
- Olive oil (a source of monounsaturated fatty acids) is the predominant source of fat.
- Fish and seafood are consumed at least two times a week.
- Dairy products and poultry are consumed in low to moderate amounts.
- Eggs are consumed zero to four times a week.
- Wine is consumed in low to moderate amounts.
- Red meat and sweets are rarely eaten.

Eat plenty of antioxidant-rich foods

Antioxidants protect cells from the damage caused by free radicals, which can come from sources like smoking or exposure to pollutants. Too many free radicals can cause oxidative stress, a condition that can negatively impact male fertility.

Focusing on antioxidant-rich foods by eating plenty of fruits, vegetables, beans, nuts, and whole grains may help support male fertility. Tomato intake has specifically been linked to supporting male fertility.

It is important to note that while dietary intakes of antioxidants have been consistently linked to improved male fertility parameters, the data on supplemental sources of antioxidants and male fertility parameters are mixed.

Include healthy fats in your dietary pattern

Oily fish like salmon are rich in omega-3 fatty acids, and higher fish intake is linked to improved male fertility. Eating a daily dose of walnuts, a plant-based source of omega-3 fatty acids, is linked to improved fertility parameters as well.

Limit intakes of alcohol and caffeine

While it doesn't appear that alcohol and caffeine need to be completely avoided when supporting male fertility, over-indulging may negatively affect fertility outcomes. Limiting caffeinated and alcoholic drinks when trying to conceive is a wise choice. Some data show that a maximum of one caffeinated drink and one alcoholic beverage a day won't have a large impact on male fertility parameters.

To future healthy babies,

Lauren Manaker, MS, RDN, LD, CLEC
Author of *Fueling Male Fertility*

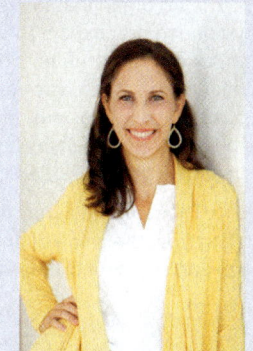
Erin Turner

Source: Turner KA, Rambhatla A, Schon S, et al. Male infertility is a women's health issue—research and clinical evaluation of male infertility is needed. *Cells*. 2020 Apr 16;9(4):990. doi: 10.3390/cells9040990

FIGURE 14-1 The fetus in relationship to the placenta. The placenta is the organ through which nourishment flows to the fetus.

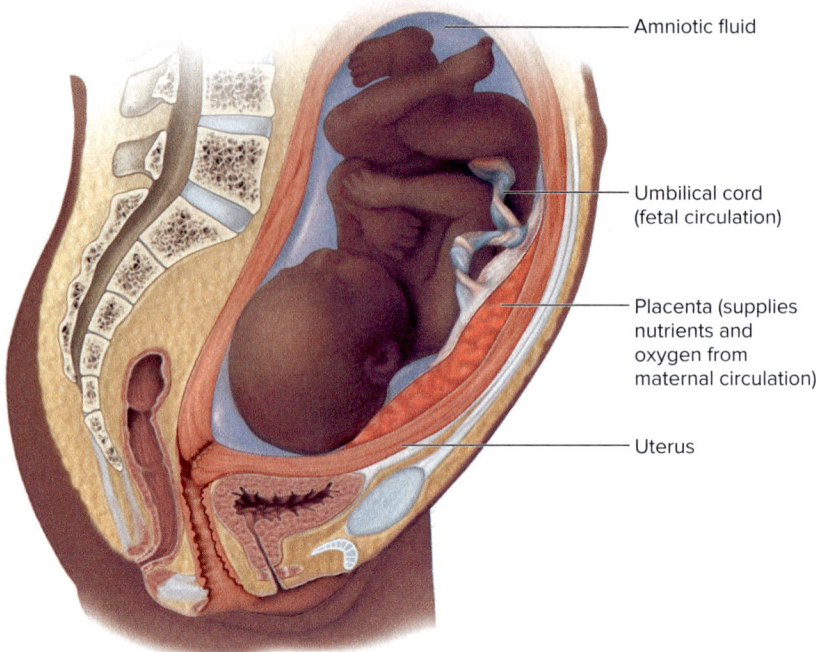

14.2 Prenatal Growth and Development

The length of a normal pregnancy is 38 to 42 weeks, measured from the first day of the last menstrual period. For purposes of discussion, the duration of pregnancy is commonly divided into three periods, called **trimesters.** For 8 weeks after conception, a human embryo develops from a fertilized **ovum** into a fetus.

Until birth, the mother nourishes the fetus via a **placenta,** an organ that forms in the uterus to accommodate the growth and development of the fetus (Fig. 14-1). The role of the placenta is to exchange nutrients, oxygen, and other gases between the mother and fetus and to eliminate waste products. This occurs through a network of capillaries that bring the fetal blood close to the maternal blood supply, but the two blood supplies do not mix.

EARLY GROWTH—THE FIRST TRIMESTER IS A CRITICAL TIME

In the formation of the human organism, the egg and sperm unite to produce a **zygote** (Fig. 14-2). From this point, the reproductive process occurs rapidly:

- Within 30 hours: the zygote divides in half to form two cells.
- Within 4 days: the cell number climbs to 128 cells.
- At 14 days: the group of cells is called an embryo.
- Within 35 days: the heart is beating, the embryo is 1/30 of an inch (8 millimeters) long, and the eyes and limb buds are clearly visible.
- At 8 weeks: the embryo is known as a fetus.
- At 13 weeks (end of first trimester): most organs are formed, and the fetus can move.

Growth begins within a day of conception with a rapid increase in cell number. This type of growth dominates embryonic and early fetal development. The newly formed cells then begin to grow larger. Further growth is a mix of increases in cell number and cell size. By the end of 13 weeks—the first trimester—most organs are formed and the fetus can move (Fig. 14-2).

As the offspring develops, nutritional deficiencies, toxicities, and other harmful environmental exposures have the potential to damage organ systems. For example, adverse reactions to medications, excessive intakes of vitamin A, exposure to radiation, or trauma can alter or arrest the current phase of fetal development, and the effects may last a lifetime (Fig. 14-2). The most critical time for these potential problems is

trimesters Three 13- to 14-week periods into which the normal pregnancy (on average, 40 weeks) is divided somewhat arbitrarily for purposes of discussion and analysis. Development of the offspring, however, is continuous throughout pregnancy, with no specific physiological markers demarcating the transition from one trimester to the next.

ovum The egg cell from which a fetus eventually develops if the egg is fertilized by a sperm cell.

placenta An organ that forms within the uterus during pregnancy. Through this organ, oxygen and nutrients from the mother's blood are transferred to the fetus, and fetal wastes are removed. The placenta also releases hormones that maintain the state of pregnancy.

zygote The fertilized ovum; the cell resulting from the union of an egg cell (ovum) and sperm until it divides.

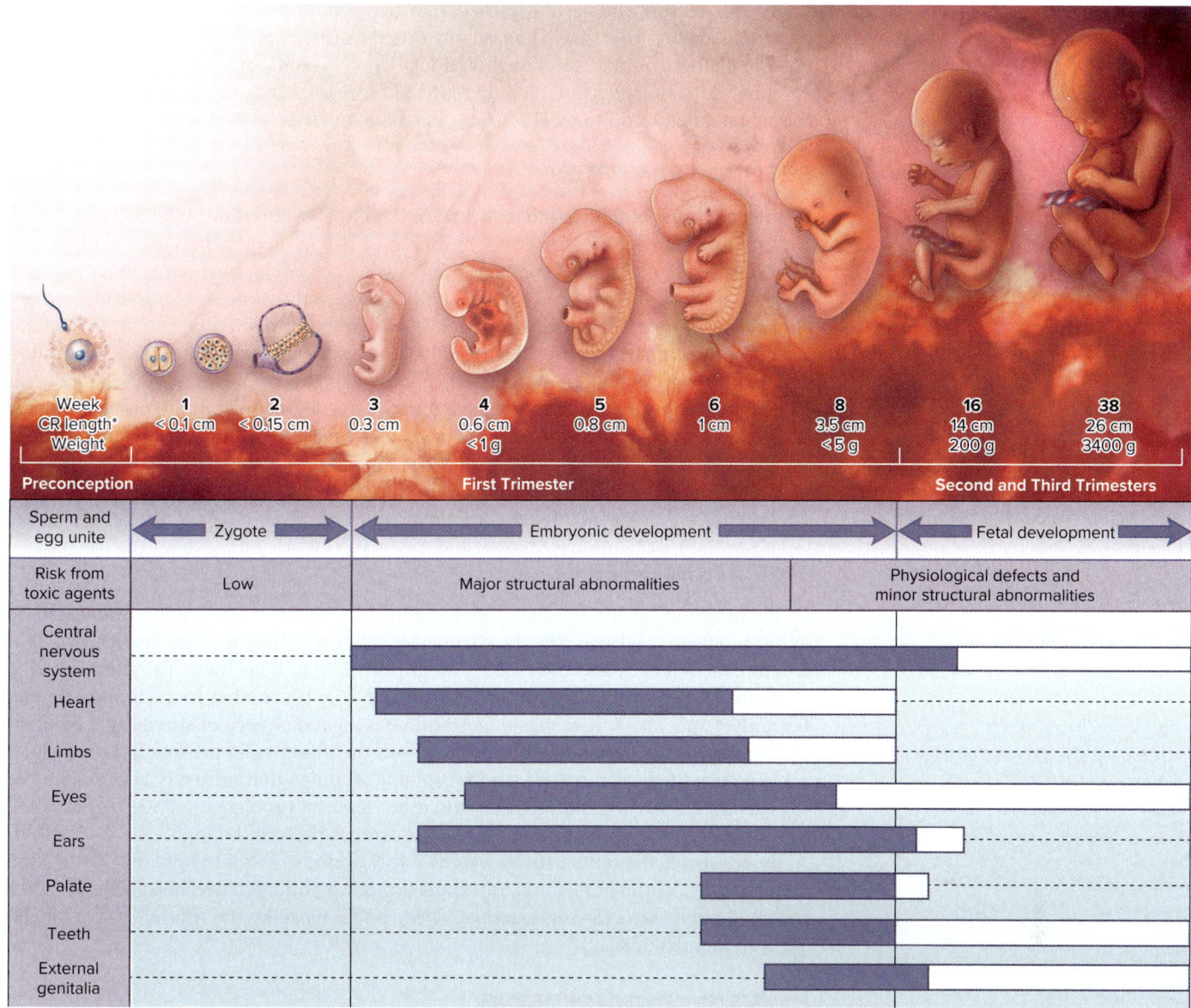

FIGURE 14-2 Harmful effects of toxic agents during pregnancy. Vulnerable periods of fetal development are indicated with purple bars. The purple shading indicates the time of greatest risk to the organ. The most serious damage to the fetus from exposure to toxins is likely to occur during the first 8 weeks after conception, two-thirds of the way through the first trimester. As the white bars in the chart show, however, damage to vital parts of the body—including the eyes, brain, and genitals—can also occur during the later months of pregnancy.
*CR length = measurement from the crown (top of the head) to the rump (lowest part of the buttocks)

during the first trimester. Most spontaneous abortions happen at this time. About 10% of clinically recognized pregnancies end in spontaneous abortion.[10] (Many additional cases of spontaneous abortion may go unrecognized, without awareness of the pregnancy.) Early spontaneous abortions usually result from a genetic defect or fatal error in fetal development. Smoking (any form of nicotine or marijuana), alcohol abuse, use of aspirin and NSAIDs, and illicit drug use raise the risk for spontaneous abortion.

Avoid substances that may harm the developing fetus, especially during the first trimester. This holds true, as well, for the time when a female is trying to become pregnant. As previously mentioned, it is common for pregnancy to go unrecognized in the early weeks. In addition, the fetus develops so rapidly during the first trimester that, if an essential nutrient is not available, the fetus may be affected even before evidence of the nutrient deficiency appears in the mother.

For this reason, the *quality*—rather than the *quantity*—of the eating pattern is most important during the first trimester. In other words, overall calorie intake does not need to change, but the mother should focus on choosing more nutrient-dense foods. Although some females lose their appetite and feel nauseated during the first trimester, they should be careful to meet nutrient needs as much as possible.

SECOND TRIMESTER

By the beginning of the second trimester (i.e., 13 weeks' **gestation**), a fetus weighs about 1 ounce and is about the size of a lemon. Arms, hands, fingers, legs, feet, and toes are fully formed. The fetus has ears and tooth sockets have begun to form in its jawbone. Organs continue to grow and mature, and, with a stethoscope or Doppler instrument, clinicians can detect the fetal heartbeat. Most bones are distinctly evident throughout the body. Eventually, the fetus begins to look more like an infant. It may suck its thumb and kick strongly enough to be felt by the mother. As shown in Figure 14-2, the fetus can still be affected by exposure to toxins, but not to the degree seen in the first trimester.

During the second trimester, the mother's breast weight typically increases by approximately 30% due to the development of milk-producing cells and the deposition of 2 to 4 pounds of fat for **lactation.** This stored fat serves as a reservoir for the extra energy that will be needed to produce breast milk.

THIRD TRIMESTER

By the beginning of the third trimester, a fetus weighs about 2 to 3 pounds and is about as big as a head of lettuce. The third trimester is a crucial time for fetal growth. The fetus will double in length and increase its weight by three to four times. The third trimester is the time when many nutrients are transferred from the mother to the fetus. An infant born after only about 26 weeks of gestation has a good chance of surviving if cared for in a nursery for high-risk newborns. However, the infant will have low stores of minerals (e.g., iron and calcium), fat, and fat-soluble vitamins that normally accumulate during the last month of gestation. This and other medical problems, such as a poor ability to suck and swallow, complicate nutritional care for **preterm** infants.

By 40 weeks, the fetus usually weighs 7 to 9 pounds (3 to 4 kilograms) and is about 20 inches (50 centimeters) long. Soft spots (fontanels) on top of the head indicate where the skull bones are growing together. These bones close by the time the baby reaches 12 to 18 months of age.

gestation The period of intrauterine development of offspring, from conception to birth; in humans, normal gestation is 38 to 42 weeks.

lactation The period of milk secretion following pregnancy; typically called *breastfeeding*.

preterm Referring to an infant born before 37 weeks of gestation; also referred to as *premature*.

✓ CONCEPT CHECK 14.2

1. What is the role of the placenta?
2. Describe how risks for fetal malformations vary throughout pregnancy.
3. During which trimester are most organs being formed?
4. During which trimester does fetal size increase the most?

14.3 Success in Pregnancy

The goal of pregnancy is to achieve optimal health for both the baby and the mother. For the mother, a successful pregnancy is one in which physical and emotional health are protected to facilitate an easy return to prepregnancy health status. For the infant, two widely accepted criteria are (1) a gestation period longer than 37 weeks and (2) a birth weight greater than 5.5 pounds (2.5 kilograms). Sufficient lung development, likely to have occurred by 37 weeks of gestation, is critical to the survival of a newborn. The longer the gestation (up to 42 weeks), the greater the ultimate birth weight and maturity of the organ systems, leading to fewer medical problems and a better quality of life for the infant.

As you read this chapter, you will notice frequent references to lifelong effects of maternal nutrition, physical activity, and other lifestyle practices on the child. This is called the *developmental origins of health and disease hypothesis* or, more simply, the **fetal origins hypothesis.** Emerging evidence links prenatal influences, such as famines, fasting, exposure to alcohol, environmental pollution, and even maternal stress, to the child's risks for disease later in life (see *Newsworthy Nutrition* in Section 14.4). As we learn more about how environmental factors modify the ways our genes are expressed, it becomes increasingly evident that many aspects of our physical and mental health are initially programmed while we are yet in utero. What's more, these epigenetic changes may be passed down from generation to generation.[11]

Overall, a successful pregnancy is the outcome of many complex gene–environment interactions. The decisions both parents make today can affect the health of their child for years to come. Although a mother's decisions, practices, and precautions before conception and during pregnancy contribute to the health of the fetus during all three trimesters, the parents cannot guarantee good health for their offspring because some genetic and environmental factors are beyond their control.

On average, a healthy newborn weighs about 7.5 pounds and is 20 inches long. **Low-birth-weight (LBW)** infants are those weighing less than 5.5 pounds (2.5 kilograms) at birth. In the United States, 1 in 12 infants is born LBW.[12] Most commonly, LBW is associated with preterm birth. Medical costs for preterm and LBW infants are much higher than those for normal-weight infants. In a recent study of health care expenditures in the United States, the average medical costs during the first 6 months of life were approximately $76,000 for an infant born preterm or approximately $114,000 for an infant with LBW. For comparison, average medical costs during the first 6 months of life for a **term** infant at a healthy birth weight are around $6500.[13]

Term and preterm infants who weigh less than the expected weight for their duration of gestation as a result of insufficient growth are described as **small for gestational age (SGA).** Thus, a full-term infant weighing less than 5.5 pounds at birth is SGA but not preterm, whereas a preterm infant born at 30 weeks of gestation is probably LBW without being SGA. Infants who are SGA are more likely than normal-weight infants to have medical complications, including problems with feeding, blood glucose control, temperature regulation, growth, and development in the weeks after birth.

PRENATAL CARE AND COUNSELING

Despite the availability of state-of-the-art health care, the infant mortality rate in the United States is higher than that of many other industrialized nations: about 5 of every 1000 infants per year die before their first birthday.[14] Adequate prenatal care helps to promote success in pregnancy. Ideally, families should seek examinations and counseling *before* becoming pregnant and should continue regular prenatal care throughout pregnancy. However, about 25% of those who are pregnant in the United States receive inadequate prenatal care.[15] If prenatal care is inadequate, delayed, or absent, untreated maternal nutritional deficiencies can deprive a developing fetus of needed nutrients. In addition, untreated health conditions, such as infections, anemia, hypertension, diabetes, or depression, must be carefully addressed to minimize complications during pregnancy. Without prenatal care, a female is three times more likely to deliver an LBW baby—one who will be 40 times more likely to die during the first 4 weeks of life than a normal-birth-weight infant.

Eating patterns cannot be predicted from income, education, or lifestyle. Although some individuals already have healthy dietary patterns, most can benefit from nutritional advice. All should be reminded of behaviors that may harm the growing fetus, such as extreme calorie restriction or fasting. By focusing on appropriate prenatal care, nutrient intake, and healthy behaviors, parents give their fetus—and, later, their infant—the best chance of thriving. Overall, the chances of having a healthy baby are maximized with education, an adequate eating pattern, and early and consistent prenatal medical care.

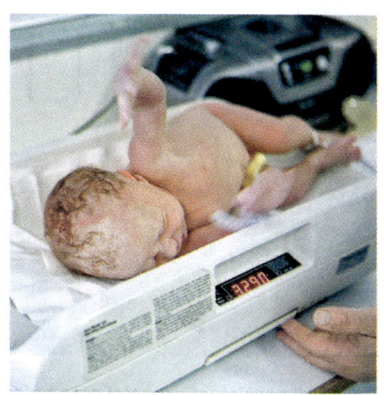

This newborn weighs 3290 grams (about 7 pounds, 3 ounces). **Is this a healthy birth weight?** Don Bayley/E+/Getty Images

fetal origins hypothesis A theory that links nutritional and other environmental factors during gestation to the future health of the offspring.

low birth weight (LBW) Referring to any infant weighing less than 2.5 kilograms (5.5 pounds) at birth; most commonly results from preterm birth.

term Referring to an infant born after a gestational period of 37 weeks up to 42 weeks, counting from the date of the mother's last menstrual period. The American College of Obstetrics and Gynecology further subdivides term pregnancy into *early term* (37 weeks up to 39 weeks), *full term* (39 weeks up to 41 weeks), and *late term* (41 weeks up to 42 weeks).

small for gestational age (SGA) Referring to infants who weigh less than the expected weight for their length of gestation. This corresponds to less than 2.5 kilograms (5.5 pounds) in a full-term newborn.

those with a healthy BMI, which could negatively affect fetal growth and development. A female who is underweight can improve nutrient stores and pregnancy outcomes by gaining weight before pregnancy (preferable) or gaining extra weight during pregnancy.

NUTRITIONAL STATUS

Is attention to good nutrition worth the effort? Yes! Extensive research suggests that an adequate vitamin and mineral intake at least 8 weeks before conception and throughout pregnancy can improve the outcomes of pregnancy.[18] Extra nutrients and calories support fetal growth and development, of course, but also undergird the synthesis of maternal tissues. The uterus and breasts grow, the placenta develops, total blood volume increases, the heart and kidneys work harder, and stores of body fat increase. In particular, meeting folate needs (400 micrograms of synthetic folic acid per day) helps to prevent birth defects such as **neural tube defects** (see Section 14.8) and decrease the risk of preterm delivery. Low intakes of calcium and iron or excessive intakes of vitamin A also are causes for concern during pregnancy.

Although it is difficult to predict the degree to which poor nutrition will affect each pregnancy, a daily eating pattern containing only 1000 kcal has been shown to greatly restrict fetal growth and development. Increased maternal and infant death rates seen in famine-stricken areas of Africa provide further evidence.

Genetic background can explain little of the observed differences in birth weight between developed and developing countries. Environmental factors, including nutritional factors, are important. The worse the nutritional status of the mother at the beginning of pregnancy, the more valuable a healthy prenatal dietary pattern and/or use of prenatal supplements are in improving the course and outcome of pregnancy.

NUTRITION ASSISTANCE FOR FAMILIES AFFECTED BY FOOD INSECURITY

Poverty impacts pregnancy in many ways. Families with low socioeconomic status tend to receive inadequate health care. A lack of education, limited access to health care, or scant financial resources may contribute to poor health practices, such as dietary patterns that fail to meet the mother's increased nutrient requirements.

Several U.S. government programs provide high-quality health care and foods to reduce infant mortality and improve the nutritional status of individuals who are pregnant (and their children). These government-subsidized programs are designed to alleviate the negative impact of poverty, insufficient education, and inadequate nutrient intake on pregnancy outcomes. An example of such a program is the Special Supplemental Nutrition Program for Women, Infants, and Children (WIC), described in Section 13.2. This program offers health assessments, education, and electronic benefit transfer (EBT) cards to purchase foods that supply high-quality protein, calcium, iron, and vitamins A and C to females who are pregnant or breastfeeding, infants, and children (up to 5 years of age) from eligible populations. The WIC program is available in all areas of the United States and has a staff trained to promote healthy behaviors during pregnancy. Participation in WIC has been shown to improve the nutrient intakes of mothers, infants, and children.[27] More than 6 million adult females, infants, and young children benefit from this program each month,[28] yet many eligible individuals are not participating.

neural tube defect A defect in the formation of the neural tube occurring during early fetal development. This type of defect results in various nervous system disorders, such as spina bifida. Maternal folate deficiency during pregnancy increases the risk that the fetus will develop this disorder.

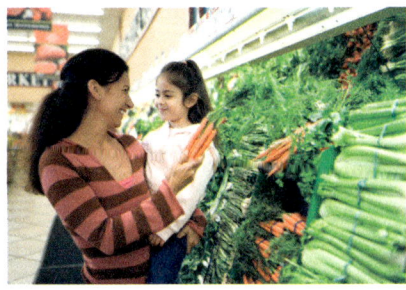

In the United States, individuals with low income can benefit from federal nutrition assistance programs:

Special Supplemental Nutrition Program for Women, Infants, and Children (WIC)
www.fns.usda.gov/wic

Supplemental Nutrition Assistance Program (SNAP)
www.fns.usda.gov/snap
/supplemental-nutrition
-assistance-program

Food Distribution Program on Indian Reservations (FDPIR)
www.fns.usda.gov/fdpir/food
-distribution-program-indian
-reservations

UpperCut Images/Getty Images

✓ CONCEPT CHECK 14.3

1. In one or two sentences, how would you define success in pregnancy?
2. Define the terms *preterm, low birth weight,* and *small for gestational age* and describe how these terms are related.
3. How is maternal age related to the outcome of pregnancy?
4. Is attention to good nutrition during pregnancy worth the effort? Why or why not?

14.4 Increased Nutrient Needs to Support Pregnancy

Pregnancy is a time of increased nutrient requirements. This section provides some generalized nutrition recommendations to meet the increased nutrient demands of pregnancy. However, recognize that each person will benefit from individualized counseling tailored to their unique physical needs and personal preferences.

CALORIE NEEDS

To support the growth and development of the fetus, females who are pregnant need adequate calories. Calorie needs during the first trimester are essentially the same as for females who are not pregnant. However, during the second and third trimesters, it is necessary to consume approximately 350 to 450 kcal more per day above prepregnancy needs. Energy needs can be estimated using Estimated Energy Requirement (EER) equations, which take into account the individual's age, current weight, height, physical activity level, weeks of gestation, and prepregnancy weight status (based on prepregnancy BMI).[29] The latest EER equations include additional calories to support healthy weight gain throughout gestation. They also factor in some adjustments for those who begin pregnancy above or below a healthy BMI. These adjustments allow for slightly higher weight gain for individuals who begin pregnancy at a low (underweight) BMI or slightly lower weight gain for individuals who begin pregnancy with a high (overweight or obese) BMI. The sample calculations that follow show the estimated energy needs of a 25-year-old female who begins pregnancy at a healthy BMI. See Appendix F for a complete set of EER equations for individuals at various stages of the life cycle.

Selena is a 25-year-old female. She is 5 feet, 7 inches (170 cm) tall and weighed 136 pounds (62 kg) before pregnancy. Her physical activity level before and during pregnancy is *low active*.

FIRST TRIMESTER (same as prepregnancy EER)

$575.77 - (7.01 \times \text{age}) + (6.6 \times \text{height}) + (12.14 \times \text{weight})$

$575.77 - (7.01 \times 25 \text{ y}) + (6.6 \times 170 \text{ cm}) + (12.14 \times 62 \text{ kg}) = 2275 \text{ kcal}$

SECOND TRIMESTER (20 weeks, weight has increased to 148 pounds)

$693.35 - (2.04 \times \text{age}) + (5.73 \times \text{height}) + (10.2 \times \text{weight}) + (9.16 \times \text{gestation}) + \text{energy deposition}$

$693.35 - (2.04 \times 25 \text{ y}) + (5.73 \times 170 \text{ cm}) + (10.2 \times 67 \text{ kg}) + (9.16 \times 20 \text{ weeks}) + 200 = 2683 \text{ kcal}$

THIRD TRIMESTER (32 weeks, weight has increased to 158 pounds)

$693.35 - (2.04 \times \text{age}) + (5.73 \times \text{height}) + (10.2 \times \text{weight}) + (9.16 \times \text{gestation}) + \text{energy deposition}$

$693.35 - (2.04 \times 25 \text{ y}) + (5.73 \times 170 \text{ cm}) + (10.2 \times 72 \text{ kg}) + (9.16 \times 32 \text{ weeks}) + 200 = 2844 \text{ kcal}$

Rather than seeing this as an opportunity to fill up on sugary desserts or fat-filled snacks, expectant mothers should consume these extra calories in the form of nutrient-dense foods. For example, throughout the day, about six whole wheat crackers, 1 tablespoon of peanut butter, 1 cup of grapes, and 1 cup of fat-free milk would supply the extra calories (and also some calcium). Although the mother "eats for two," a female who is pregnant must not double her normal calorie intake. Energy needs only increase by about 20% to 25% (and only during the second and third trimesters).

Keep in mind that any time you use an equation to estimate energy needs, the calculation is just a starting point. Individual variations in metabolic rate, prepregnancy weight status, body composition, and physical activity level may influence energy needs during pregnancy. The EER equations are established for singleton pregnancies; females who are pregnant with multiple fetuses may need even more calories. Changes in weight over time (i.e., gaining weight within the recommended ranges) are the best way to evaluate the adequacy of energy intake during pregnancy.

STAYING ACTIVE DURING PREGNANCY

Pregnancy is not the time to begin an intense fitness regimen, but females can generally take part in most low- or moderate-intensity activities during pregnancy. In fact, the *Physical Activity Guidelines* and current advice from the American College of Obstetrics and Gynecology recommend at least 30 minutes per day of moderate-intensity physical activity during pregnancy. Walking, cycling, swimming, or light aerobics for at least 150 minutes per week is generally advised. Such activity may prevent pregnancy complications and promote an easier delivery.[30,31,32] Some research indicates that regular physical activity during pregnancy lowers the risk of developing gestational diabetes by up to 60% and gestational hypertension by nearly 40%.[33] These disorders of pregnancy are discussed further in Section 14.6. Figure 14-4 illustrates the broad range of benefits of exercise during pregnancy for both the mother and the baby.

Individuals who were highly active prior to pregnancy can maintain their activities as long as they remain healthy and review plans with their health care providers. Adequate fluid intake before, during, and after physical activity is of heightened importance to regulate body temperature because heat stress can be harmful to the developing fetus. Activities with inherent risk of falls or abdominal trauma—downhill skiing, horseback riding, and contact sports (e.g., soccer and basketball)—can potentially harm the fetus and should be avoided. In addition, females who are pregnant should avoid activities that require excess straining (e.g., heavy weightlifting) or exposure to extremes in air pressure (e.g., SCUBA diving).

Females with high-risk pregnancies, such as those experiencing premature labor contractions, may need to restrict physical activity. To ensure optimal health for both themselves and their infants, expectant mothers should consult a primary care provider about physical activity and possible limitations during pregnancy.

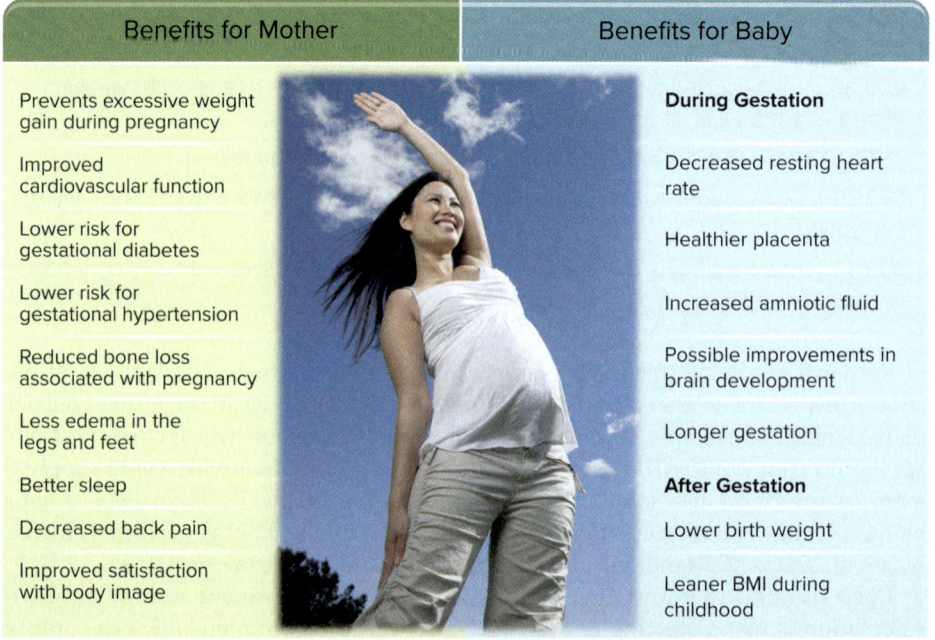

FIGURE 14-4 Benefits of physical activity during pregnancy for the mother and baby. Tanya Constantine/Blend Images LLC

Benefits of Physical Activity During Pregnancy

Benefits for Mother	Benefits for Baby
Prevents excessive weight gain during pregnancy	**During Gestation**
Improved cardiovascular function	Decreased resting heart rate
Lower risk for gestational diabetes	Healthier placenta
Lower risk for gestational hypertension	Increased amniotic fluid
Reduced bone loss associated with pregnancy	Possible improvements in brain development
Less edema in the legs and feet	Longer gestation
Better sleep	**After Gestation**
Decreased back pain	Lower birth weight
Improved satisfaction with body image	Leaner BMI during childhood

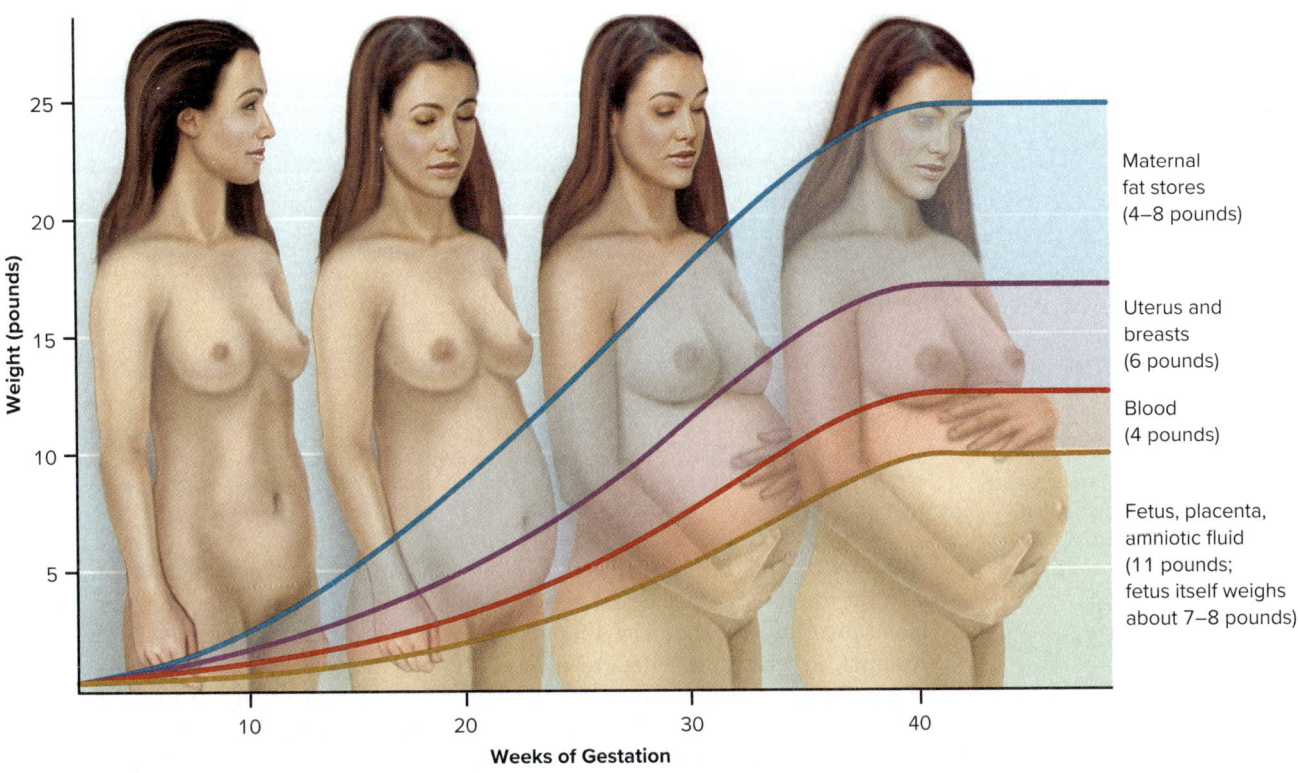

FIGURE 14-5 The components of weight gain in pregnancy. A total weight gain of 25 to 35 pounds throughout the whole pregnancy is recommended for most females. The various components shown in this figure total about 25 pounds.

OPTIMAL WEIGHT GAIN

Healthy prepregnancy weight and appropriate weight gain during pregnancy are excellent predictors of pregnancy outcome.[34,35] The mother's dietary pattern should allow for approximately 2 to 4 pounds (0.9 to 1.8 kilograms) of weight gain during the first trimester and then a subsequent weight gain of 0.8 to 1 pound (0.4 to 0.5 kilogram) weekly during the second and third trimesters (Fig. 14-5). A healthy goal for total weight gain for a female of normal weight (based on prepregnancy BMI; Table 14-1) averages about 25 to 35 pounds (11.5 to 16 kilograms).

For females who begin pregnancy with a low BMI, the goal for total weight gain increases to 28 to 40 pounds (12.5 to 18 kilograms). The goal decreases to a total of 15 to 25 pounds (7 to 11.5 kilograms) for females who are overweight at conception. Target weight gain for females who are obese at conception is a total of 11 to 20 pounds (5 to 9 kilograms). Figure 14-5 shows why the typical recommendation begins at 25 pounds.

A total weight gain of between 25 and 35 pounds for an individual starting pregnancy at a normal BMI has repeatedly been shown to yield optimal health for both mother and fetus if gestation lasts at least 38 weeks. The weight gain should yield a birth weight of about 7.5 pounds (3.5 kilograms). Although some extra weight gain during pregnancy is usually not harmful (about 5 to 10 pounds), it can set the stage for a pattern of excess weight gain during the childbearing years.

Mothers who are carrying more than one fetus need to gain additional weight to support fetal growth and development. There are provisional guidelines for females carrying multiple fetuses. Females of normal prepregnancy BMI carrying twins should aim to gain within the range of 37 to 54 pounds, whereas females who are overweight or obese and carrying twins should gain less (a total of 31 to 50 pounds or a total of 25 to 42 pounds, respectively).

Overweight and obesity contribute to complications during pregnancy. Excess maternal body fat increases risk for diabetes, hypertension, blood clots, and spontaneous

Check out the pregnancy weight-gain trackers at https://www.cdc.gov/reproductivehealth/maternalinfanthealth/pregnancy-weight-gain.htm/

TABLE 14-1 ■ Recommended Weight Gain in Pregnancy Based on Prepregnancy Body Mass Index (BMI)

Prepregnancy BMI Category	Total Weight Gain*	
	pounds	kilograms
Low (BMI less than 18.5)	28 to 40	12.5 to 18
Normal (BMI 18.5 to 24.9)	25 to 35	11.5 to 16
High (BMI 25.0 to 29.9)	15 to 25	7 to 11.5
Obese (BMI greater than 30.0)	11 to 20	5 to 9

*The listed values are for pregnancies with one fetus. For females of normal prepregnancy BMI carrying twins, the range is 37 to 54 pounds (17 to 24.5 kilograms), or less for heavier females.

Source: Data from Weight Gain During Pregnancy: Reexamining the Guidelines, Copyright 2009 by the Institute of Medicine and National Research Council of the National Academies. National Academies Press, Washington, DC.

fetal macrosomia A condition in which an infant grows excessively large (e.g., birth weight > 4000 grams) in utero, usually as a consequence of maternal hyperglycemia.

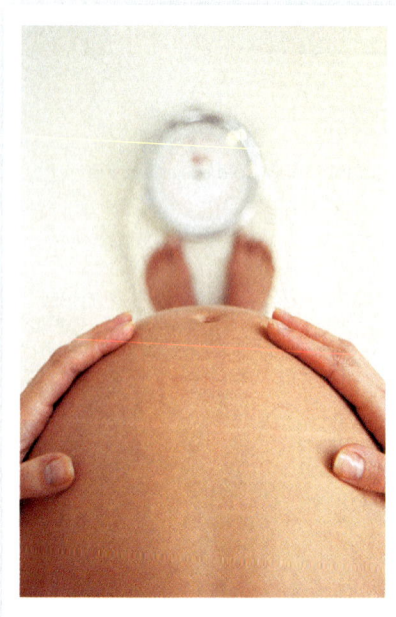

Health care providers must be on the lookout for individuals who exhibit disordered eating behaviors during pregnancy. Although it is not yet recognized as a distinct diagnosis, *pregorexia* is gaining attention among practitioners who work with expectant moms. Some individuals are exceptionally concerned about weight gain and may restrict food intake, exercise excessively, or engage in other methods of purging excess calories to prevent weight gain. **What are the risks of inadequate weight gain during pregnancy?** Photo: John Slater/Getty Images

Text Source: Getz L. Starving for two. *Today's Dietitian*. 2015 Jan;17(1):14.

abortions during pregnancy. After childbirth, lasting effects of excess gestational weight gain for the mother include increased BMI, central body fat distribution, and elevated blood pressure. For the baby, there is a greater chance of birth defects and **fetal macrosomia,** in which the fetus grows larger than average in utero. Compared to infants of normal birth weight, larger infants require surgical delivery (i.e., Cesarean sections) more often. Over the long term, excessive maternal weight gain during pregnancy has been linked to increased risk for obesity and metabolic syndrome in the child.

Gestational weight gain is a key issue in prenatal care and a concern of many mothers-to-be. Even after the 2009 release of the weight-gain guidelines summarized in Table 14-1, many females report receiving *no* guidance regarding weight gain from health care providers before or during pregnancy. Considering the extensive consequences of either inadequate or excessive weight gain during gestation, health professionals should take a more active role in educating clients about what weight changes to expect, the consequences of too little or too much weight gain during pregnancy, and how to make adjustments if the weight-gain trajectory veers off course.[36,37,38] Weight gain during pregnancy should generally follow the pattern in Figure 14-5. Weekly monitoring of weight changes during pregnancy, especially on a chart that shows expected weight gains, can help an expectant mom to assess and adjust food intake and physical activity.

Realistic information about increased calorie requirements should be provided. "Eating for two" is more about increasing the *quality* of the dietary pattern (i.e., choosing nutrient-dense foods) rather than the *quantity* of foods consumed. Furthermore, successful weight-management strategies involve a behavioral component; some individuals need to learn skills, such as self-monitoring of weight, dietary intake, and physical activity. Online tools and smartphone apps (e.g., Sprout Pregnancy) offer specialized tools to make self-monitoring tasks simple and social.

Recognize that weight loss during pregnancy is never advised. Even if an expectant mother gains 35 pounds in the first 7 months of pregnancy, it is still important to gain weight during the last 2 months. The mother should, however, slow the increase in weight to parallel the rise on the prenatal weight-gain chart. In other words, the sources of the unnecessary calories should be found and minimized. On the other hand, if an expectant mother has not gained the desired amount of weight by a given point in pregnancy, the recommendation is to slowly gain a little more weight than the typical pattern to meet the goal by the end of the pregnancy. When adjustments are needed, an RDN can make appropriate recommendations to help the individual meet their goals.

PROTEIN NEEDS

The RDA for protein increases to 1.1 grams per kilogram per day, which equates to an additional 25 grams per day during pregnancy[39] (Fig. 14-6). All females who are pregnant should check to make sure they are eating enough protein as well as enough calories (so that protein can be spared for synthesis of new tissue). However, many individuals already consume this much extra protein and therefore do not need to focus specifically on increasing protein intake. Small changes are usually all that is necessary. For example, simply adding a cup of fat-free milk to the daily menu adds 90 nutrient-dense kcal and 8 grams of protein.

CARBOHYDRATE NEEDS

The RDA for carbohydrate increases to 175 grams daily, primarily to prevent ketosis.[39] Ketone bodies, a by-product of metabolism of fat for energy, are poorly used by the fetal brain and may impair fetal brain development. The carbohydrate intakes of most females, pregnant or not, already fulfill this requirement (Fig. 14-6).

LIPID NEEDS

Fat intake should increase proportionally with calorie intake during pregnancy to yield around 20% to 35% of total calories from fat.[39] Pregnancy is not a time for a low-fat diet; individuals need some extra calories and essential fatty acids during pregnancy. Recommendations for the types of lipids needed during pregnancy are generally the same as for females who are not pregnant: saturated fat should contribute no more than 10% of total calories and *trans* fat should be avoided.

During pregnancy, it is particularly important to make sure to consume adequate essential fatty acids: linoleic acid (omega-6) and alpha-linolenic acid (omega-3). Essential fatty acids cannot be synthesized in the body and must be consumed as part of the dietary pattern. For the developing fetus, essential fatty acids are required for growth, brain development, and eye development. Children whose mothers consumed sources of omega-3 fatty acids during pregnancy tend to have better sleep patterns, better speech development, higher intelligence, and fewer behavioral problems as they grow and develop.[40] For mothers, a healthy dietary pattern that provides adequate omega-3 fatty acids during pregnancy may help to reduce postpartum depression.[41]

Recommendations are slightly increased during pregnancy to 13 grams per day of linoleic acid and 1.4 grams per day of alpha-linolenic acid. These needs can be met by consuming 2 to 4 tablespoons per day of plant oils. However, usual intakes of omega-3 fatty acids among females—pregnant or not—fall short of recommendations.[42] Consumption of two to three servings (8 to 12 ounces) per week of fish is recommended for meeting needs for essential fatty acids.[43] Those who choose not to eat fish can also obtain the same omega-3 fatty acids found in fish from specially raised eggs (it's in the chicken feed!) or fish oil supplements. For supplements, consumers should choose brands that have been purified to remove environmental contaminants. (See Section 14.8 for a discussion of mercury in fish.)

FLUID NEEDS

During pregnancy, extra water is needed to support increased plasma volume, heart function, and kidney function and to ensure an adequate amount of **amniotic fluid,** which surrounds and protects the growing fetus. Inadequate fluid intake contributes to constipation, a common complaint during pregnancy. More severe dehydration during pregnancy can cause electrolyte imbalances and restrict the transfer of oxygen, nutrients, and wastes between the mother and fetus. The Adequate Intake for total water increases by 0.3 liter (1¼ cups) above prepregnancy needs to 3 liters (about 12½ cups) per day.[39] Remember that total water includes water from foods and beverages. Increasing fluid (i.e., beverage) intake to about 10 cups per day is sufficient for most females during pregnancy. More fluid may be needed by individuals with high levels of physical activity and those who live in hot or dry climates. Thus, fluid intake goals should be individualized. An easy way to monitor hydration status is to check the color of the urine: pale yellow or straw-colored urine indicates adequate hydration.[44]

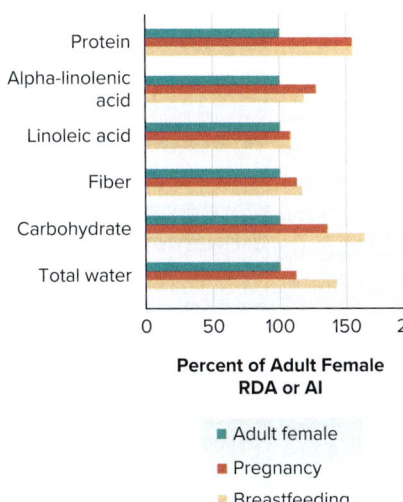

FIGURE 14-6 Relative macronutrient and water requirements for pregnancy and breastfeeding. Note that there is no RDA or AI for total fat; needs are based on 20% to 35% of overall energy intake.

amniotic fluid The water-based fluid that surrounds the developing fetus within the amniotic sac during gestation. It cushions the developing fetus, allows for fetal movement, maintains the fetal temperature, and facilitates the development of the lungs and digestive system.

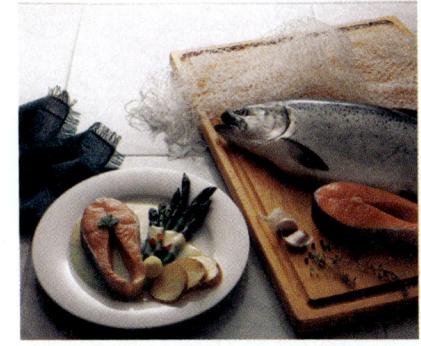

Use the *SMASH* acronym to remember the safest sources of fish:
- Salmon
- Mackerel
- Achovies
- Sardines
- Herring

These types of fish are high in omega-3 fatty acids but are less likely to be contaminated with heavy metals and other environmental pollutants. David Papazian/Corbis/Getty Images

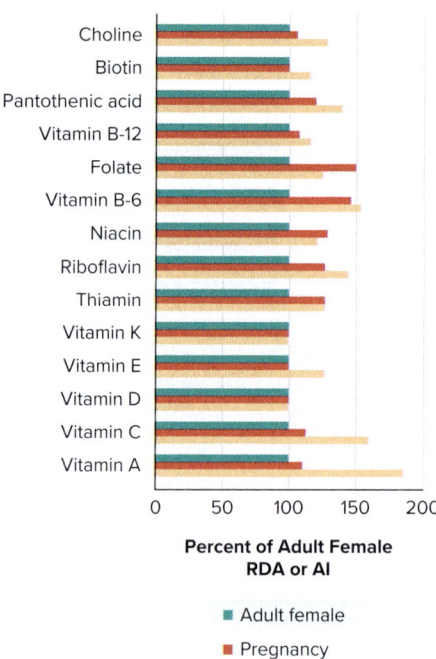

FIGURE 14-7 Relative vitamin requirements for pregnancy and breastfeeding.

Water is the best choice for hydration, but some nutrient-dense beverages may also be included. Low-fat or fat-free milk would help to ensure adequate calcium and vitamin D intake. Although it can also be a source of added sugars, 100% fruit juice does provide some vitamins and minerals. (In general, it is better to choose whole fruit instead of fruit juice.) Unsweetened coffee and tea can also contribute to meeting fluid needs, but most authorities recommend that females limit caffeine intake to 200 milligrams per day (equivalent to about 2 cups of coffee) during pregnancy.

Even though individuals who are pregnant do have room for some extra calories, they should not fill up on sugary beverages. High intakes of sugar-sweetened beverages promote excessive weight gain and may complicate blood sugar control. There is evidence, as well, that intake of sugar-sweetened beverages may have effects on body weight and disease risk later in life for the offspring.[45,46]

VITAMIN NEEDS

Vitamin needs increase from prepregnancy RDAs/AIs by up to 30% for most of the B vitamins, by 45% for vitamin B-6, and by 50% for folate (Fig. 14-7). Vitamin A needs only increase by 10%, so a specific focus on this vitamin is not needed.[39] Recall that excess amounts of vitamin A can be harmful to the developing fetus.

Folate. The extra amounts of vitamin B-6 and other B vitamins (except folate) needed in the dietary pattern are easily met via nutrient-dense food choices, such as a serving of a typical ready-to-eat breakfast cereal and some lean animal protein sources. Folate needs, however, often merit strategic menu planning and possible vitamin supplementation.[11]

Ultimately, both fetal and maternal health depend on an ample supply of folate. The synthesis of DNA, and therefore cell division, requires folate, so this nutrient is especially crucial for early fetal development. A lack of folate during early gestation could result in birth defects, such as neural tube defects, which are discussed in further detail in Section 14.8. Maternal red blood cell formation, which requires folate, increases during pregnancy. Serious folate-related anemia therefore can result if folate intake is inadequate. For these reasons, the RDA for folate increases during pregnancy to 600 micrograms DFE per day (review Section 8.14 for calculation of DFE).

Increasing folate intakes to meet 600 micrograms DFE per day during pregnancy can be achieved through dietary sources (see *Farm to Fork* in this section), a supplemental source of folic acid, or a combination of both. Choosing foods that are rich in synthetic folic acid, such as fortified, ready-to-eat breakfast cereals (look for approximately 50% to 100% of the Daily Value), is especially helpful in meeting folate needs. Recall that synthetic folic acid is much more easily absorbed than the forms of folate found naturally in foods.[47]

Vitamin D. Low maternal levels of vitamin D during pregnancy may affect multiple health parameters in the mother and the offspring. About 54% of Black females and 42% of white females have insufficient blood levels of the active form of vitamin D, even though many take a daily supplement containing 10 micrograms of vitamin D. Aside from its well-known role in bone health, vitamin D is also involved in cell differentiation, immune function, and regulation of blood glucose and blood pressure.

Because of the ability of vitamin D to modulate gene expression, vitamin D status is critically important during early fetal development through infancy. Poor vitamin D status has been implicated in several serious complications of pregnancy, including fetal growth restriction and the development of diabetes and hypertension.[48] Vitamin D's role in immune regulation is evidenced by higher rates of respiratory infections and mother-to-child transmission of HIV when vitamin D is deficient. Diseases that develop later in childhood or adulthood, such as type 1 diabetes, multiple sclerosis, allergies, asthma, schizophrenia, and certain types of cancer, are associated with low vitamin D status during gestation.

The RDA during pregnancy is 15 micrograms of vitamin D daily (the same as for adult females who are not pregnant). Including three servings per day of dairy products and 8 to 12 ounces of seafood per week, as recommended by the *Dietary Guidelines*,

Newsworthy Nutrition

Prenatal folic acid supplementation improves cognitive outcomes in offspring

INTRODUCTION: The benefits of folic acid supplementation during the periconceptional period for prevention of neural tube defects are well established. Given that the folate-dependent processes of myelination of the nervous system, neurotransmitter synthesis, and methylation of DNA occur throughout gestation, continued folate supplementation past the first trimester may be beneficial for neurocognitive development of the offspring. However, the effects of continued folic acid supplementation during the second and third trimesters on long-term cognitive outcomes of offspring have not been adequately studied. **OBJECTIVES:** In this follow-up investigation of a *randomized, placebo-controlled trial,* the researchers aimed to evaluate the effects of maternal folic acid supplementation during the second and third trimesters on the cognitive performance and brain function of the offspring at 11 years of age. **METHODS:** In the original Folic Acid Supplementation in the Second and Third Trimesters (FASSTT) trial, 119 females who were pregnant and had taken folic acid supplements during the first trimester were randomized to receive either continued folic acid supplementation (400 micrograms per day) or placebo during the second and third trimesters. This follow-up investigation included 68 of the offspring from the original cohort. Cognitive performance of the 11-year-old offspring was assessed using the Wechsler Intelligence Scale for Children 4th UK Edition (WISC-IV), which provides scores on several cognitive domains: verbal comprehension, perceptual reasoning, working memory, and processing speed. In addition, in a subset of the children (n = 33), brain functioning during a language processing test was measured using magnetoencephalography (i.e., brain imaging). **RESULTS:** At 11 years of age, the offspring of mothers who received folic acid supplementation during the second and third trimesters scored significantly higher on tests of processing speed (male and female offspring) and verbal comprehension (female offspring only) compared to the offspring of mothers in the control group. Brain imaging studies revealed increased neuronal activity indicative of more efficient language processing among offspring of mothers who received folic acid supplementation during the second and third trimesters. **CONCLUSION:** Continued folic acid supplementation during the second and third trimesters of pregnancy improves cognitive performance and brain function of the offspring during childhood up to 11 years of age.

Source: Caffrey A, McNulty H, Rollins M, et al. Effects of maternal folic acid supplementation during the second and third trimesters of pregnancy on neurocognitive development in the child: an 11-year follow-up from a randomised controlled trial. *BMC Med.* 2021 Mar 10;19(1):73. doi: 10.1186/s12916-021-01914-9

would go a long way toward meeting the RDA for vitamin D. On average, females who are pregnant consume about half of the recommended servings of dairy foods and seafood.[49] Currently, there is no recommendation for universal vitamin D screening or supplementation, but the American College of Obstetricians and Gynecologists advises 25 to 50 micrograms per day for individuals with vitamin D deficiency is a safe level of supplemental vitamin D during pregnancy.[50]

MINERAL NEEDS

Mineral needs generally increase during pregnancy, especially the requirements for iodine, iron, and zinc (Fig. 14-8).[11,51] Calcium needs do not increase but still deserve special attention because many females find it difficult to meet their calcium needs.

Iodine. Females who are pregnant need to consume extra iodine (RDA of 220 micrograms per day) to support thyroid hormone synthesis (for the mother and the developing fetus) and fetal brain development.[39] A mother who is deficient in iodine during pregnancy may develop a goiter (see Section 9.12), and the child may be born

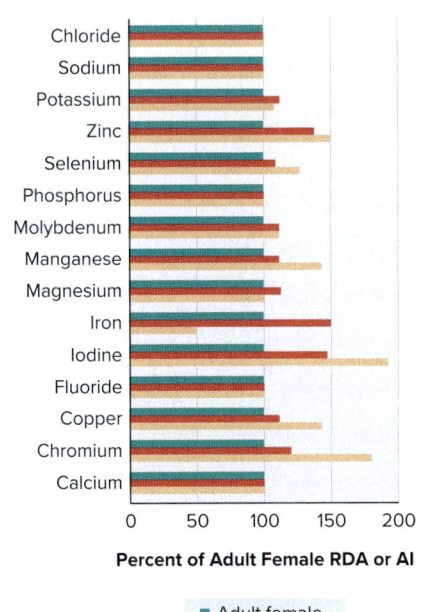

FIGURE 14-8 Relative mineral requirements for pregnancy and breastfeeding.

with congenital hypothyroidism, a devastating birth defect. Section 14.8 provides further information on this and other nutrition-related birth defects. In countries where salt is commonly fortified with iodine, use of iodized salt ensures a plentiful intake of this mineral throughout the life span.

Iron. Extra iron (RDA of 27 milligrams per day) is needed to synthesize a greater amount of hemoglobin during pregnancy and to establish iron stores for the fetus.[39] Less than 5% of females begin pregnancy with clinically diagnosed iron-deficiency anemia, but an estimated one-third of females have poor iron stores during pregnancy, which means the heavy demands for iron during pregnancy cannot be met.[52] The consequences of iron-deficiency anemia—especially during the first trimester—can be severe. Negative outcomes include preterm delivery, LBW infants, and increased risk for fetal death in the first weeks after birth.

To meet the increased RDA during pregnancy, females often need a supplemental source of iron, especially if they do not consume iron-fortified foods, such as highly fortified breakfast cereals containing close to 100% of the Daily Value for iron (18 milligrams). The American College of Obstetricians and Gynecologists recommends screening for iron deficiency for all females who are pregnant and provision of iron supplements for those with iron deficiency. Most prenatal supplements contain iron. A potential pitfall is that iron supplements can decrease appetite and can cause nausea and constipation. To alleviate these problems, it may be helpful to take these supplements between meals or just before going to bed. Milk, coffee, or tea should not be consumed with an iron supplement because these beverages contain compounds that interfere with iron absorption. On the other hand, eating foods rich in vitamin C helps increase iron absorption. Females who are not anemic may wait until the second trimester, when pregnancy-related nausea generally lessens, to start prenatal supplements if gastrointestinal side effects are a problem.

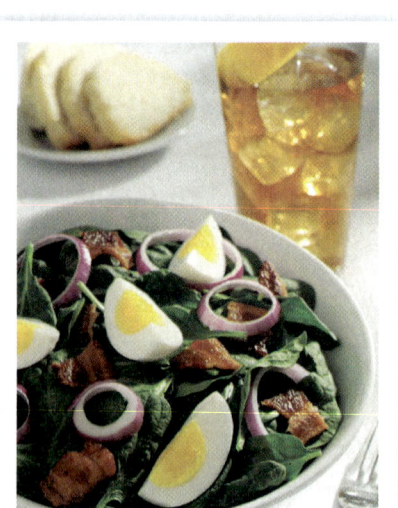

This lunch of spinach salad and sliced French bread has several sources of nonheme iron. **Is iced tea a good beverage choice to accompany this meal? Why or why not?** TheCrimsonMonkey/Getty Images

Zinc. The RDA for zinc increases from 8 to 11 milligrams per day during pregnancy.[39] Zinc is involved in protein synthesis and the function of many enzymes. Zinc deficiency during pregnancy has been linked to preterm and LBW births. In the United States, zinc intakes during pregnancy are generally adequate, but females with low income and those who follow vegan or vegetarian dietary patterns are more susceptible to low zinc status. Also, because iron and zinc compete for absorption, high levels of iron supplementation during pregnancy may impair zinc absorption. Incorporating lean animal proteins or a fortified, ready-to-eat breakfast cereal in the dietary pattern is a good way to obtain enough extra zinc during pregnancy.

USE OF PRENATAL VITAMIN AND MINERAL SUPPLEMENTS

With the exceptions of folate, iron, and vitamin D, the vitamin and mineral intakes of females during pregnancy in developed countries are generally adequate.[53] Research evidence supports routine supplementation with folic acid for the prevention of neural tube defects during pregnancy. Supplementation with iron is beneficial, specifically for those at risk of iron-deficiency anemia.[54] Beyond these nutrients, some studies indicate that the use of a multivitamin and mineral supplement is advantageous for reducing the number of LBW and SGA births.[55] More research is needed to know if prenatal supplements are effective for reducing many other pregnancy complications.[56] To date, there is not enough evidence to recommend prenatal multivitamin and mineral supplements for all females during pregnancy, but they are prescribed routinely by most health care providers. Some supplements formulated for pregnancy are sold over the counter, while others are dispensed by prescription because of their high synthetic folic acid content (1000 micrograms), which could pose problems for others, such as people who are older. These supplements are high in iron (27 milligrams per pill). There is no evidence that the use of such supplements causes significant health problems in pregnancy, with the possible exception of combined amounts of supplemental and dietary vitamin A (see Section 14.8).

Prenatal supplements may especially contribute to successful pregnancy outcomes for females living in poverty, teenagers, females with an inadequate dietary pattern, those pregnant with multiple fetuses, those who smoke or use alcohol or illegal drugs, and those who follow a vegan dietary pattern. In other cases, healthy eating patterns can provide the needed nutrients.

When choosing a multivitamin, discuss options with a primary care provider and rely on brands that display the USP symbol on their label, signifying that the supplement meets the content, quality, purity, and safety standards of the U.S. Pharmacopeial Convention (see Section 8.18). Of course, avoid megadoses of any nutrient. Skip supplements containing herbs, enzymes, and amino acids. Many of these ingredients have not been evaluated for safety during pregnancy or breastfeeding and may be toxic to the fetus. Furthermore, discard supplements that are past the expiration date, as some ingredients lose potency over time.

✓ CONCEPT CHECK 14.4

1. Danica is a 28-year-old female who needed about 2450 kcal per day before conception. By 24 weeks' gestation, she has gained 15 pounds, and her activity level has declined a bit. Her EER is now about 2800 kcal per day. Suggest a few nutrient-dense foods Danica could incorporate into her dietary pattern to supply these extra 350 kcal per day.
2. What is the optimal range of weight gain during pregnancy for a female who begins pregnancy at a healthy BMI? How does this differ for a female who begins pregnancy underweight? Overweight? Obese?
3. List two nutrients that may need to be supplemented in the dietary pattern of a female who is pregnant and explain the reason for each.

14.5 Eating Patterns for Females During Pregnancy

One dietary approach to support a successful pregnancy is based on MyPlate. For a 24-year-old female with a low level of physical activity, about 2200 kcal is recommended during the first trimester (the same as recommended for such a female when not pregnant). Her MyPlate plan should include 7 ounce equivalents from the grains group, 6 ounce equivalents from the protein foods group, 3 cups from the dairy group (or dairy alternatives), 3 cups of vegetables, and 2 cups of fruit. In addition, about 6 teaspoons per day of plant oil, used in cooking or as salad dressing, will supply essential fatty acids. Figure 14-9 shows a balanced dietary pattern, based on MyPlate, for a female in the first trimester. By selecting nutrient-dense foods from the food groups, the dietary pattern should be moderate in sodium (no more than 2300 milligrams per day), saturated fat (limit to 10% of total calories), and added sugars (limit to 10% of total calories).

FARM to FORK Greens

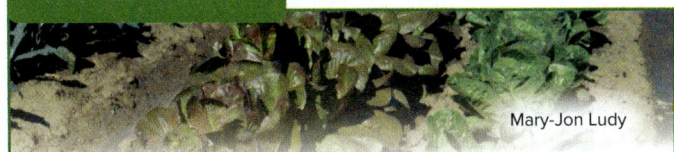

Mary-Jon Ludy

Leafy green vegetables are good sources of folate, a vital nutrient for the prevention of neural tube defects.

Grow
- Even if you don't have space for gardening, it's easy to grow lettuce and other greens in containers on your patio or balcony. Garden-fresh greens will be ready to eat in 30 to 60 days.
- Seed catalogs offer a much wider variety of greens than you can find in the grocery store. Find greens that will grow where you live, and try something new and nutritious!

Shop
- To identify greens that are highest in phytochemicals and nutrients, look for the deepest colors. Dark green, red, purple, and reddish-brown leaves have the most disease-fighting phytochemicals and the highest levels of micronutrients, including folate.
- Choose lettuces with leaves that are loose and open. These lettuce leaves produce more phytochemicals to protect themselves from the sun. Lettuces such as iceberg, with tightly wrapped leaves, provide only a fraction of the nutrients found in more colorful, loosely packed leaves.
- Fresh heads of lettuce or bunches of spinach tend to last longer than precut, prewashed greens sold in bags and plastic containers.

Store
- Greens need just the right amount of humidity and oxygen to stay fresh. After you bring home fresh greens, pull the lettuce apart, soak it in cold water for about 10 minutes, and spin it dry before storing. This increases the moisture content within the leaves but keeps the outside of the leaves dry, delaying spoilage.
- Use a pin to prick 10 to 20 holes in a gallon-size plastic bag. Store your greens in the perforated bag in the crisper drawer of your refrigerator to maintain optimal freshness. The bag helps the greens to retain their moisture. The tiny holes allow for some exchange of gases.

Prep
- Even though plants with the darkest colors have the most nutritional value, some people do not tolerate their somewhat bitter or peppery flavors. Harvesting the leaves early (i.e., baby lettuce greens) will yield a milder salad. Try mixing some bitter greens, such as arugula, with milder varieties, such as romaine or Bibb lettuce. Add sweet flavors, such as chopped fruit or a touch of honey in your salad dressing, to balance the stronger flavors.
- Don't skimp on the dressing! Many of the healthy compounds in these plants are fat-soluble. You will absorb more of the vitamin E and phytochemicals if you consume some fat as part of your meal. Olive oil is an excellent choice for homemade salad dressing.
- Boiling causes more than half of the nutrients to leach out of the vegetables and into the cooking water. If you cook your greens, sauté, steam, or microwave them.

Source: Robinson J. From wild greens to iceberg lettuce: breeding out the medicine. In: *Eating on the Wild Side: The Missing Link to Optimum Health*. New York: Little, Brown & Co.; 2013.

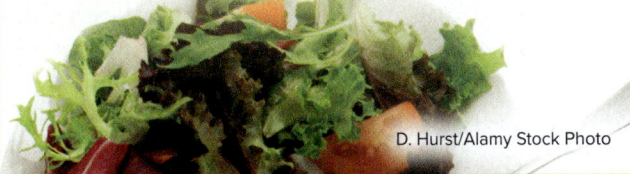

D. Hurst/Alamy Stock Photo

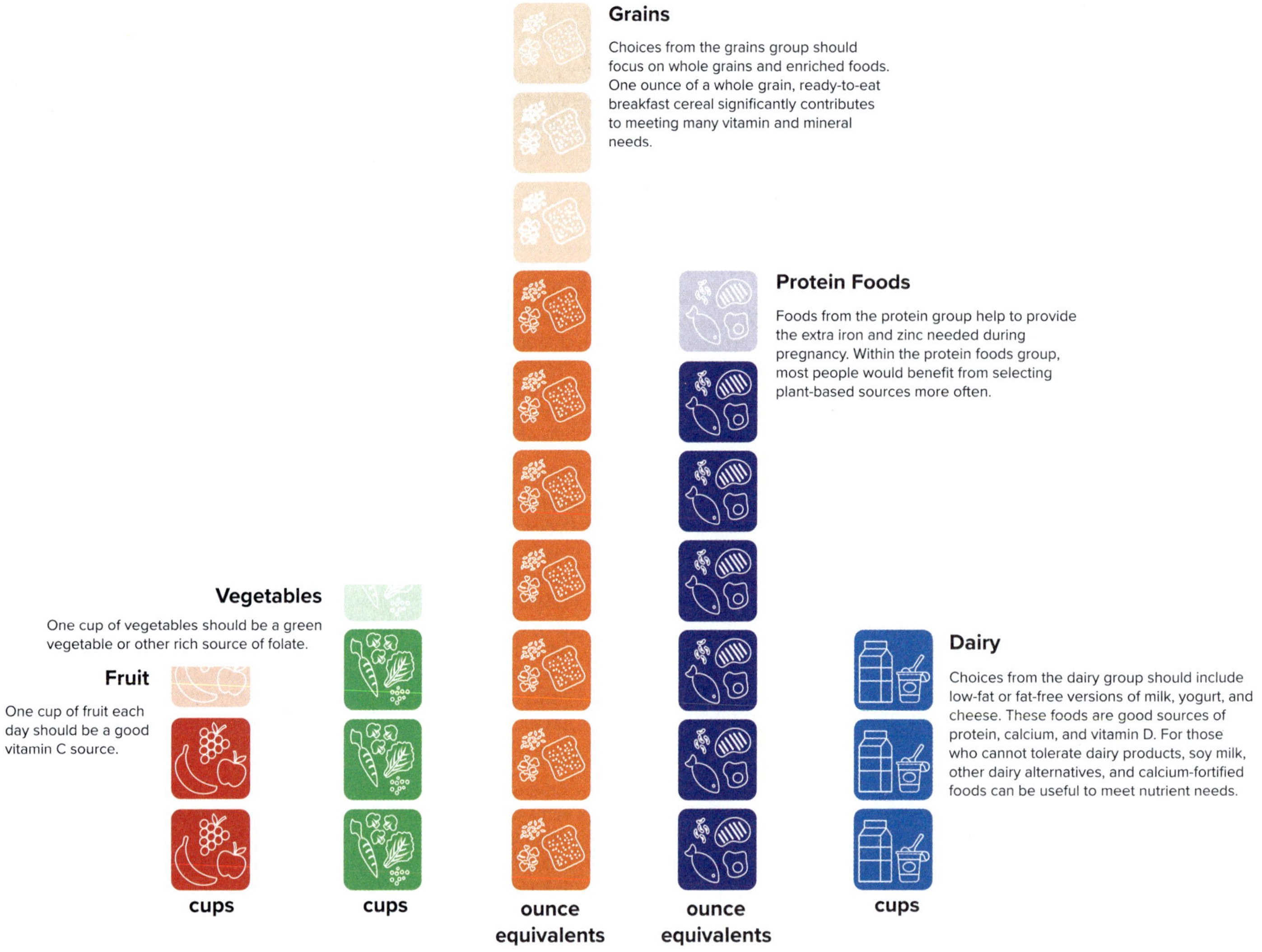

Fruit
One cup of fruit each day should be a good vitamin C source.

Vegetables
One cup of vegetables should be a green vegetable or other rich source of folate.

Grains
Choices from the grains group should focus on whole grains and enriched foods. One ounce of a whole grain, ready-to-eat breakfast cereal significantly contributes to meeting many vitamin and mineral needs.

Protein Foods
Foods from the protein group help to provide the extra iron and zinc needed during pregnancy. Within the protein foods group, most people would benefit from selecting plant-based sources more often.

Dairy
Choices from the dairy group should include low-fat or fat-free versions of milk, yogurt, and cheese. These foods are good sources of protein, calcium, and vitamin D. For those who cannot tolerate dairy products, soy milk, other dairy alternatives, and calcium-fortified foods can be useful to meet nutrient needs.

FIGURE 14-9 Daily meal plan for a female during pregnancy based on MyPlate. Servings per day for the first trimester (2200 kcal per day) are shown in dark colors. Additional servings per day for the second and third trimesters (2800 kcal per day) are shown in lighter colors.
Source: United States Department of Agriculture, Find your Healthy Eating Style, retrieved from https://choosemyplate-prod.azureedge.net/sites/default/files/myplate/checklists/MyPlateDailyChecklist_2200cals_Age14plus.pdf

In the second trimester, about 2600 kcal is recommended for this person. In the third trimester, the EER goes up to about 2800 kcal per day. By the third trimester, the plan may include up to 3 additional ounce equivalents from the grains group, an extra ounce equivalent from the protein group, an additional ½ cup from the vegetables group, an additional ½ cup from the fruit group, and 1 to 2 additional teaspoons of plant oil throughout the day. These additional servings are shown in lighter color in Figure 14-9.

Table 14-2 illustrates a sample menu based on the 2600 kcal plan for pregnancy for females in the second trimester. This menu meets the extra nutrient needs associated with pregnancy. Individuals who need to consume more than this—and some do for various reasons—should incorporate additional fruits, vegetables, and whole grain breads and cereals, not nutrient-poor snacks and sugar-sweetened beverages.

Do food cravings during pregnancy serve a purpose? Food cravings during pregnancy may be related to hormonal changes or may simply stem from family or cultural traditions. It is okay to give in to pregnancy cravings in moderation. In fact, some researchers think this may be a subtle way individuals cope with stress and anxiety during pregnancy.[57] However, there is no evidence that consuming the foods craved during pregnancy will correct nutrient deficiencies. Following the nutrition advice of respected health professionals, such as registered dietitian nutritionists, is much more

TABLE 14-2 ■ Sample 2600 kcal Daily Menu*

	Vitamin B-6	Folate	Iron	Zinc	Calcium
Breakfast					
1 cup multigrain cereal	✓	✓	✓	✓	✓
1 cup orange juice	✓	✓			
1 cup fat-free milk					✓
Snack					
2 tbsp peanut butter					
1 slice whole wheat toast					
1 cup plain low-fat yogurt				✓	✓
1 cup strawberries					
Lunch					
2 cups spinach and berry salad with	✓	✓	✓	✓	✓
2 tbsp oil and vinegar dressing					
4 ounces roasted chicken breast	✓			✓	
2 slices whole wheat toast					
Snack					
6 whole wheat crackers					
1½ ounces provolone cheese				✓	✓
1 cup grape juice					
Dinner					
1 bean and cheese burrito	✓	✓	✓	✓	✓
1 cup cooked broccoli	✓	✓			
1 ear of corn					
1 tbsp soft margarine					
1 cup unsweetened iced tea					
Snack					
2 oatmeal raisin cookies					
1 medium banana	✓				

*This dietary plan meets nutrient needs for pregnancy and breastfeeding. Check marks indicate that the menu item is a good source of the nutrient, whereas the lack of a check indicates a poor source of the nutrient. The vitamin- and mineral-fortified breakfast cereal used in this example makes an important contribution to meeting nutrient needs. Fluids can be added as desired. Total intake of fluids, such as water, should be 10 cups per day for females who are pregnant or about 13 cups per day for females who are breastfeeding.

reliable than trusting cravings to meet nutrient needs. See *Roots* in this section to learn about cravings for nonfood items during pregnancy.

VEGETARIAN DIETARY PATTERNS DURING PREGNANCY

Individuals who follow lactoovovegetarian or lactovegetarian dietary patterns generally do not face special difficulties in meeting their nutritional needs during pregnancy. Although many people assume that vegetarian dietary patterns are deficient in protein, as long as overall energy needs are met, protein intake is usually adequate. Females who follow a vegetarian dietary pattern during pregnancy should plan to consume a variety of plant sources of protein to get all of the essential amino acids.

pica A disorder characterized by eating nonfood items, such as dirt, laundry starch, or clay.

> ### 🥕 Roots
>
> #### Cultural Pica
>
> In the United States, an estimated 25% of females who are pregnant report consuming nonfood items, such as clay, dirt, or chalk. As you learned in Chapter 11, the persistent practice of eating nonfood items is classified as a mental disorder known as **pica.** Various forms of pica exist: *geophagia* (clay, dirt, chalk, or metal), *amylophagia* (laundry starch), and *pagophagia* (ice, freezer frost). However, the definition of pica specifies that the practice is not performed as part of a culturally supported or socially normative practice. Many cases of consuming nonfood items during pregnancy are rooted in family or cultural traditions. Researchers have termed this behavior *cultural pica.*
>
> The practice varies by region. In some African countries, where consuming dirt or clay is believed to reduce nausea and vomiting, reduce infectious diseases during pregnancy, or provide minerals that are lacking in the body, more than 90% of females who are pregnant engage in geophagia. In the United States, cultural pica is especially prevalent in African American communities, particularly those living in rural areas in southeastern states.
>
> Geophagia poses some risks: rather than correcting nutrient deficiencies, substances in clay or dirt may actually bind to minerals and make them less available for absorption. Several studies have linked poor iron status to cravings for nonfood items, but it is unclear whether it is a cause or a consequence of nutritional problems. Other risks may include intestinal blockages, parasitic infections, or exposure to lead or other toxins. Given these potentially serious health risks, health care professionals who work with females who are pregnant must ask about the consumption of nonfood items and educate their patients about safe food sources of nutrients.
>
> Source: Fawcett EJ, Fawcett JM, Mazmanian D. A meta-analysis of the worldwide prevalence of pica during pregnancy and the postpartum period. *Int J Gynaecol Obstet.* 2016 Jun;133(3):277-283. doi: 10.1016/j.ijgo.2015.10.012

On the other hand, for a female who follows a vegan dietary pattern during pregnancy, careful meal planning during preconception and pregnancy is crucial to ensure sufficient iron, zinc, calcium, vitamin D, vitamin B-12, and omega-3 fatty acids, in addition to protein.[58] The basic vegan dietary pattern described in Section 6.4 should be modified to include more whole grains, beans, nuts, and seeds to supply the necessary extra amounts of some of these nutrients. As mentioned, use of a prenatal multivitamin and mineral supplement also is generally advocated to help fill micronutrient gaps. However, although these are high in iron, this is not true for calcium (200 milligrams per pill). If iron and calcium supplements are used, they should not be taken together to avoid possible competition for absorption.

✓ CONCEPT CHECK 14.5

1. In Chapter 5, review the Mediterranean diet and how it compares to MyPlate. Is the Mediterranean diet suitable to meet the nutrient needs of a female during pregnancy?
2. Modify the sample 2600 kcal daily menu in Table 14-2 so that it would be suitable for a female who follows a vegan dietary pattern during pregnancy.
3. Michaela tells you about her pregnancy craving for ice cream. She says she has been eating one or two ice cream bars after lunch every day and usually stops for a milkshake at a fast-food restaurant on her way home from work. What nutrition information would you share with her?

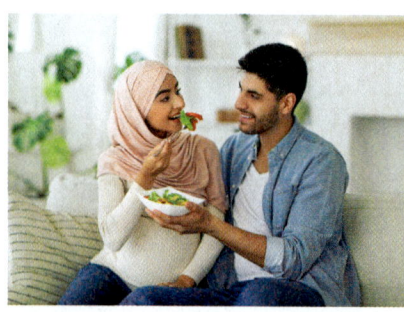

Dietary advice should be tailored to fit the individual's personal preferences, cultural traditions, and budget. Moms-to-be can personalize MyPlate for each trimester at www.myplate.gov/myplate-plan. milkos/123RF

CASE STUDY: Eating for Two

Lily and her husband have just found out that Lily is pregnant with their first child. She is 25 years old, weighs 135 pounds, and is 67 inches tall. Lily has been reading everything she can find on pregnancy because she knows that her health is important to the success of her pregnancy.

Lily knows she should avoid alcohol, especially because alcohol is potentially toxic to the growing fetus. Lily is not a smoker, does not take any medications, and limits her coffee intake to 4 cups a day and soft drink intake to 3 colas per day. Based on her reading, she has decided to breastfeed her infant and has already inquired about childbirth classes. She has modified her dietary pattern to include some extra protein, along with more fruits and vegetables. She has also started taking an over-the-counter vitamin and mineral supplement. Lily has always kept in good shape, and she is admittedly worried about gaining too much weight during pregnancy. Recently, she started a running program 5 days a week, and she plans to continue running throughout her pregnancy.

1. What recommendations do you have regarding Lily's use of dietary supplements?
2. What is Lily doing to prevent neural tube defects? What else could she do?
3. What recommendations would you make regarding Lily's caffeine consumption?
4. Should Lily include fish as a source of protein in her meals? Why or why not?
5. Constipation is a common complaint during pregnancy. What suggestions do you have to help Lily avoid this health concern?
6. What information would you share with Lily about appropriate weight gain during pregnancy?

Complete the Case Study. Responses to these questions can be provided by your instructor.

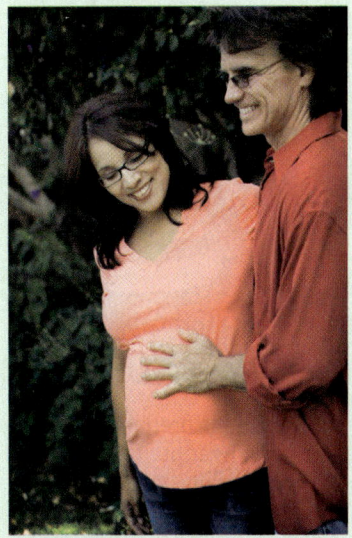

Lily and her husband want to do everything they can to ensure a healthy pregnancy. Hill Street Studios/Blend Images LLC

14.6 Nutrition-Related Concerns During Pregnancy

During pregnancy, fetal needs for oxygen and nutrients as well as excretion of waste products increase the workload for the mother's lungs, heart, and kidneys. Although a mother's organ systems work efficiently, some discomfort may accompany the changes her body undergoes to accommodate the fetus.

HEARTBURN

Hormones (such as progesterone) produced by the placenta relax smooth muscles in the uterus and the gastrointestinal tract. This often causes heartburn as the lower esophageal sphincter relaxes, allowing stomach acid to reflux into the esophagus (review Section 3.11). To prevent or reduce heartburn, avoid lying down for at least 3 hours after eating, choose meals that are lower in fat so that foods pass more quickly from the stomach into the small intestine, and avoid spicy foods, which can worsen symptoms. Also, consume most liquids between (rather than with) meals to limit the volume of stomach contents; this helps to decrease some of the pressure inside the stomach that encourages reflux. Individuals with more severe cases should consult a primary care provider about using antacids or related medications.[59]

CONSTIPATION AND HEMORRHOIDS

The hormone-induced relaxation of muscles in the GI tract may also lead to constipation. This is especially likely to develop late in pregnancy, when the fetus competes with the GI tract for space in the abdominal cavity. To alleviate constipation, focus on

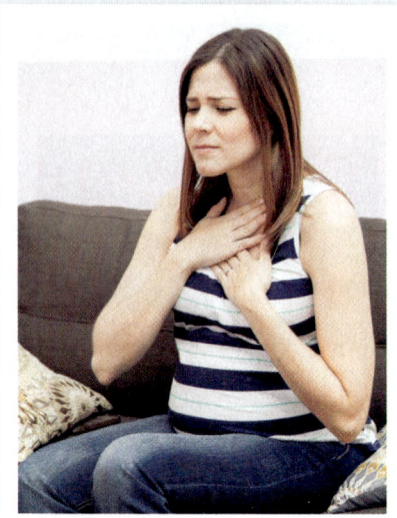

Sandy, 5 months pregnant, has been having heartburn and difficult bowel movements. As a student of nutrition, you understand the digestive system and the role of nutrition in health. **What dietary and lifestyle strategies could you suggest to Sandy to relieve her digestive complaints?** antoniodiaz/123RF

consuming adequate fluid and fiber and perform regular physical activity. The AI for fiber in pregnancy is 28 grams, slightly more than the AI for females who are not pregnant. Fluid needs are 10 cups per day. The extra iron in prenatal supplements may also contribute to constipation. If this is the case, a clinician can reevaluate the individual needs for supplemental iron. Alleviating constipation can also help to prevent hemorrhoids, which affect about one-third of females during pregnancy.

EDEMA

Placental hormones cause various body tissues to retain fluid during pregnancy. Blood volume also greatly expands during pregnancy. The extra fluid may cause some swelling (edema), especially in the extremities. However, there is no reason to restrict salt severely or use diuretics to limit mild edema. Mild edema during pregnancy simply reflects normal and expected changes in plasma volume and kidney function. Edema may limit physical activity late in pregnancy and occasionally requires an expectant mother to elevate her feet or wear compression stockings to control the symptoms. Overall, edema is only a mild nuisance unless it is accompanied by hypertension and evidence of organ dysfunction, such as the appearance of protein in the urine (see "Hypertensive Disorders of Pregnancy" later in this section).

NAUSEA AND VOMITING OF PREGNANCY

About 85% of females experience nausea during the early stages of pregnancy, but it usually resolves by the end of the first trimester.[60] Nausea and vomiting of pregnancy are probably related to changes in GI motility induced by pregnancy-related hormones. Although commonly called *morning sickness,* pregnancy-related nausea may occur at any time and may persist all day. It is often the first indication of pregnancy.

To help control mild nausea during pregnancy, try the following: avoid foods that are likely to trigger nausea (e.g., greasy, spicy, or acidic foods); cook foods in an environment with good ventilation to dissipate nauseating smells; eat saltine crackers or dry cereal before getting out of bed; avoid large fluid intake early in the morning; and eat smaller, more frequent meals instead of two or three large meals per day. The iron in prenatal supplements triggers nausea in some individuals, so changing the type of supplement or postponing use until the second trimester may provide relief in some cases. If the nausea seems to be exacerbated by the prenatal supplement, the primary care provider may consider modifying the prescription.

In persistent cases of nausea and vomiting, a physician may prescribe a dietary supplement of vitamin B-6, taken alone or in combination with doxylamine (a sleep aid). The dose of vitamin B-6 used to treat nausea and vomiting of pregnancy is typically 10 to 25 milligrams per day, which is quite a bit higher than the RDA (1.9 milligrams per day during pregnancy), but not high enough to exceed the UL (100 milligrams).[60,61] To avoid toxicity, which can cause neurological damage, use of vitamin B-6 for treatment of nausea and vomiting of pregnancy should be monitored by a physician.

Usually, nausea is mild and stops after the first trimester. However, in up to 3% of pregnancies, nausea and vomiting are prolonged and severe enough to cause weight loss, dehydration, and dangerous electrolyte imbalances.[62] In these cases, the preceding practices offer little relief; medical attention is needed to protect the health of the mother and the growing baby.

ANEMIA

To supply the fetus with nutrients and oxygen, the mother's blood volume expands by approximately 50%. The number of red blood cells, however, increases by only 20% to 30%, and this occurs more gradually. As a result, a female has a lower ratio of red blood cells to total blood volume during pregnancy. This hemodilution is known as

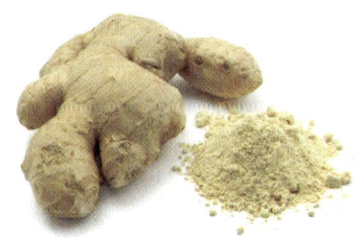

Some studies show a potential benefit of foods or dietary supplements made with ginger to alleviate nausea and vomiting of pregnancy for some individuals. **However, why is it important to consult your primary care provider before taking dietary supplements?** Toltek/iStock/Getty Images

physiological anemia. It is a normal response to pregnancy rather than the result of inadequate nutrient intake.

However, if iron stores and/or dietary iron intake are not sufficient to meet the increased needs of pregnancy, the individual may develop iron-deficiency anemia. The *Dietary Guidelines* identifies iron as a nutrient of public health concern because several population groups, including those who are pregnant, are likely to have low intakes of this nutrient. Iron-deficiency anemia requires medical attention at any stage of the life cycle, but consequences for the fetus are especially severe (see Section 14.4).[63] Maternal anemia is associated with LBW, preterm birth, and infant mortality. To identify problems with iron status during pregnancy, all females should be screened for iron deficiency at least once per trimester. Lean meats, beans, and fortified grains are nutrient-dense sources of iron that should be emphasized to prevent anemia during pregnancy. Importantly, once anemia has developed, *dietary supplements will be needed to replenish iron status;* dietary changes alone are not sufficient to correct iron deficiency.

GESTATIONAL DIABETES

Hormones synthesized by the placenta decrease the efficiency of insulin. This leads to a mild increase in blood glucose, which is normal and helps supply calories to the fetus. If the rise in blood glucose becomes excessive, this leads to **gestational diabetes,** often beginning between weeks 20 and 28, particularly among those with a family history of diabetes or who had a prepregnancy BMI in the obese range. Other risk factors include maternal age over 35 and gestational diabetes in a prior pregnancy.

In the United States, gestational diabetes develops in as many as 10% of pregnancies (estimates vary based on the diagnostic criteria used).[64] Individuals with risk factors for type 2 diabetes (e.g., obesity, family history) should be screened for undiagnosed type 2 diabetes at the first prenatal visit. Females who are pregnant who do not have type 2 diabetes should be screened for gestational diabetes between 24 and 28 weeks. Various testing methods are used but typically involve being given an oral dose of glucose, then testing blood glucose levels one, two, or three hours later.[65] If gestational diabetes is detected, a special dietary pattern that distributes carbohydrates throughout the day must be implemented. Carbohydrate choices should be mostly whole, unprocessed grains, vegetables, fruits, and beans, which have a lower impact on blood glucose than refined grains or foods with lots of added sugars. Sometimes insulin injections or oral medications are also needed. Regular physical activity also helps to control blood glucose.

The primary risk of uncontrolled diabetes during pregnancy is fetal macrosomia, which means that the fetus grows to a large size in utero. This is a result of the oversupply of glucose from maternal circulation coupled with an increased production of insulin by the fetus, which allows fetal tissues to take up an increased amount of building materials for growth. The mother may require a Cesarean section if the fetus is too large for a vaginal delivery. Another threat is that the infant may have low blood glucose at birth because of the tendency to produce extra insulin that began during gestation. Other concerns are the potential for early delivery, low iron stores, hyperbilirubinemia, and increased risk of birth trauma and malformations.

Although gestational diabetes usually resolves after the infant's birth, it increases the mother's risk of developing diabetes later in life, especially if the mother's BMI is in the overweight or obese range. About half of those who have gestational diabetes will later develop type 2 diabetes.[64] Hyperglycemia during gestation may have some long-term repercussions for the child as well. Studies show that infants of mothers with gestational diabetes may also have higher risks of developing obesity, metabolic syndrome, and type 2 diabetes as they grow to adulthood. For all these reasons, proper control of blood glucose during pregnancy is extremely important.

Researchers are working to understand how breastfeeding may be helpful for females who had gestational diabetes. Some studies indicate that breastfeeding may

physiological anemia The normal decrease in red blood cell concentration in the blood due to increased blood volume during pregnancy; also called *hemodilution*.

gestational diabetes A high blood glucose concentration that develops during pregnancy and returns to normal after birth; one cause is the placental production of hormones that antagonize the regulation of blood glucose by insulin.

lower the risk of developing type 2 diabetes later in life.[66] Breastfeeding may also help to protect the offspring from obesity, diabetes, and cardiovascular disease later in life.[67,68]

HYPERTENSIVE DISORDERS OF PREGNANCY

Hypertension occurs in about 6% to 8% of pregnancies in the United States.[69] Sometimes, females enter pregnancy with chronic hypertension. However, when hypertension first appears after 20 weeks of gestation, it is termed **gestational hypertension** (formerly called *pregnancy-induced hypertension*).

Up to 46% of individuals with gestational hypertension eventually develop **preeclampsia** (mild form) or **eclampsia** (severe form).[70] Early symptoms include a rise in blood pressure, excess protein in the urine, edema, changes in blood clotting, headache, and visual disturbances. Very severe effects, including convulsions, can occur in the second and third trimesters. If not controlled, eclampsia could restrict fetal growth, trigger preterm birth, or cause maternal or fetal death.

The causes of hypertensive disorders of pregnancy are not well understood but likely involve interactions among genetics, certain environmental or lifestyle influences, and abnormal function of the placenta. The populations most at risk for these disorders are females under age 17 or over age 35, females who have a BMI in the overweight or obese range, and those who have had multiple-birth pregnancies. A family history of gestational hypertension in the mother's or father's side of the family, diabetes, African-American race, and a first pregnancy also raise risk.

Gestational hypertension usually resolves once the pregnancy ends, making delivery the most reliable treatment for the mother. However, if eclampsia develops before the fetus is ready to be born, medical intervention is necessary. Bed rest and administration of magnesium sulfate are the most effective treatment methods. Magnesium likely acts to relax blood vessels and so leads to a reduction in blood pressure. There is good evidence that adequate intakes of calcium and vitamin D are involved in reducing the incidence of hypertensive disorders of pregnancy. There is interest in the use of antioxidants to prevent or treat hypertensive disorders of pregnancy, but current evidence does not support the use of antioxidant supplements for preventing these disorders.[71,72]

Although public health advice urges all Americans to keep sodium intake under 2300 milligrams per day, there is no evidence that extreme sodium restrictions (i.e., less than the AI of 1500 milligrams per day) influence the development or progression of preeclampsia or eclampsia. In fact, severe sodium restrictions could restrict fetal growth, impair nervous system development, and contribute to cardiovascular risks for the offspring later in life.[73,74] Current guidelines for those who are pregnant encourage sodium intake that meets the AI but does not exceed the CDRR.[39] Several other treatments are under study. In the meantime, the best advice is to comply with the key recommendations of the *Dietary Guidelines*, aiming to meet nutrient needs with a variety of foods.

gestational hypertension Blood pressure of 140/90 mmHg or higher that is first diagnosed after 20 weeks of gestation. This may evolve into preeclampsia or eclampsia.

preeclampsia A form of gestational hypertension characterized by signs of organ dysfunction, such as liver or kidney damage and/or blood clotting abnormalities.

eclampsia A severe form of gestational hypertension accompanied by signs of organ dysfunction and seizures; formerly called *toxemia*.

lactation consultant Health care professional (often a registered nurse or RDN) with special training to provide education and support for mothers who are breastfeeding and their infants.

alveoli (singular: alveolus). Small, saclike structures. Milk is produced in the alveoli of the breast.

✓ CONCEPT CHECK 14.6

1. What dietary and lifestyle strategies would you suggest for someone who complains of morning sickness during pregnancy?
2. Define *gestational diabetes*. What are the potential consequences of this disorder for the mother and baby?
3. Differentiate between chronic hypertension and gestational hypertension. Have any dietary supplements been shown to reliably prevent or treat hypertensive disorders of pregnancy?

14.7 Breastfeeding

Breastfeeding provides the newborn optimal nutrition from the start of life. The *Dietary Guidelines,* the Academy of Nutrition and Dietetics (AND), and the American Academy of Pediatrics (AAP) recommend breastfeeding *exclusively* (i.e., with no other foods or beverages) for the first 6 months, followed by the combination of breastfeeding and infant foods until 1 year.[75,76] The World Health Organization goes beyond that to recommend breastfeeding (along with age-appropriate solid foods; see Section 15.3) for at least 2 years.[77] In the United States, surveys show that about 83% of mothers breastfeed their infants in the hospital. By 6 months, about 56% of mothers are still breastfeeding their infants, but only about 25% are *exclusively* breastfeeding. At 1 year of age, about 36% of mothers are still breastfeeding (in addition to providing solid foods).[78]

Individuals who choose to breastfeed usually find it an enjoyable, special time in their lives that strengthens the bond with their new infant. Although bottle feeding with an infant formula is also safe for infants, it cannot replicate all of the benefits derived from breastfeeding. If a female does not breastfeed her newborn, milk production ceases within a few days after birth.

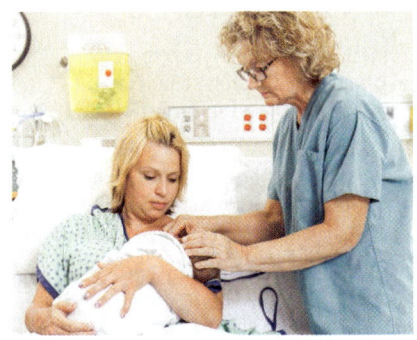

The Baby-Friendly Hospital Initiative promotes and supports breastfeeding. Guidelines include training hospital personnel to assist mothers with lactation, initiating breastfeeding within 30 minutes of birth, allowing infants to "room in" with mothers, not offering formula or pacifiers to newborn babies, and having a plan to support moms who are breastfeeding after they leave the hospital. Simplefoto, Tyler Olson/leaf/123RF

PLANNING TO BREASTFEED

Almost all females are physically capable of breastfeeding their children (see the later section "Medical Conditions Precluding Breastfeeding" for exceptions). In most cases, problems encountered in breastfeeding are due to a lack of knowledge or support. Anatomical problems in breasts, such as inverted nipples, can be corrected during pregnancy. Breast size generally increases during pregnancy and is no indication of success in breastfeeding. Most females notice a dramatic increase in the size and weight of their breasts by the third or fourth day of breastfeeding. If these changes do not occur, a new mother needs to seek advice from her primary care provider or a **lactation consultant.**

Infants who are breastfed must be monitored closely by caregivers over the first few days of life to ensure that feeding and weight gain are proceeding normally. Monitoring is especially important with a mother's first child because the mother will be inexperienced with the technique of breastfeeding. The infant is at risk of undernutrition and dehydration if feeding does not proceed smoothly.

Although it is the most natural way to feed a newborn child, the *technique* does not always come naturally. Gathering information on breastfeeding, what obstacles to anticipate, and how to respond to such obstacles will help new mothers and their babies to succeed with breastfeeding. It also helps to have an experienced friend, family member, or a professional lactation consultant to call for advice when questions arise.

lobule A cluster of alveoli in the human breast.

lobe A group of several lobules within the human breast; also called a *mammary gland.*

HUMAN MILK PRODUCTION

During pregnancy, breast weight increases by 1 to 2 pounds due to the action of placental hormones that stimulate the formation of milk-producing cells. Milk will be produced in small, saclike structures called **alveoli.** A cluster of alveoli makes up a **lobule;** a group of several lobules is called a **lobe.** Each breast houses 12 to 20 lobes (Fig. 14-10). Ducts lead from each lobe to the nipple, where milk is ejected from the breast.

Most of the protein found in human milk is synthesized by breast tissue. Some proteins also enter the milk directly from the mother's bloodstream. These proteins include immune factors (e.g., antibodies) and enzymes. Some of the fats in human milk

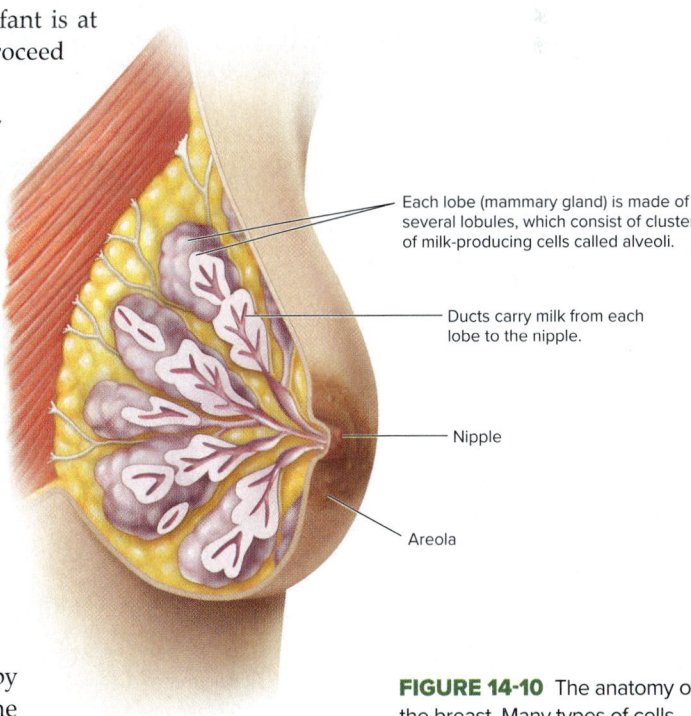

Each lobe (mammary gland) is made of several lobules, which consist of clusters of milk-producing cells called alveoli.

Ducts carry milk from each lobe to the nipple.

Nipple

Areola

FIGURE 14-10 The anatomy of the breast. Many types of cells form a coordinated network to produce and secrete human milk.

come from what the mother has eaten; other fats are synthesized by breast tissue. The sugar galactose is synthesized in the breast, whereas glucose enters from the mother's bloodstream. Together, these sugars form lactose, the main carbohydrate in human milk.

Lactation is regulated by two hormones: prolactin and oxytocin. **Prolactin** is the hormone that stimulates milk production in the lobules of the breast. As milk is produced between feedings, it is stored in the lobules. An important brain–breast connection—commonly called the **let-down reflex**—is necessary to release the milk stored in the lobules. This reflex occurs in response to the infant suckling at the breast. Stimulation of the nerves in the nipple area signals the pituitary gland to release **oxytocin,** which allows the lobules to contract and let down (release) stored milk (Fig. 14-11). The milk then travels via ducts to the nipple. The mother may feel a tingling sensation shortly before milk flow begins. Throughout the feeding, the suckling of the infant further stimulates prolactin release from the pituitary gland, so milk synthesis within the lobules continues. The more the infant suckles, the more milk is produced. As the quantity of milk production increases, the quality does not change. Because of this, even twins (and triplets) can be breastfed adequately.

If the let-down reflex does not operate properly, the infant will not receive enough milk. The infant gets frustrated, which then frustrates the mother. The let-down reflex is easily inhibited by nervous tension, a lack of confidence, and fatigue. Mothers should be especially aware of the link between tension and a weak let-down reflex. They need to find a relaxed environment where they can breastfeed.

After a few weeks, the mother's let-down reflex becomes automatic. Milk ejection can be triggered just by thinking about the infant or seeing or hearing another one cry. At first, however, the process can be a bit bewildering. Because they cannot directly measure the amount of milk the infant takes in, many new moms worry about underfeeding the infant.

As a general rule, a well-nourished breastfed infant should (1) have three to five wet diapers per day by 3 to 5 days of age and four to six wet diapers per day thereafter,

prolactin A hormone secreted by the pituitary gland that stimulates the synthesis of milk in the breast.

let-down reflex A reflex stimulated by infant suckling that causes the release (ejection) of milk from milk ducts in the mother's breasts; also called *milk ejection reflex.*

oxytocin A hormone secreted by the pituitary gland. It causes contraction of the musclelike cells surrounding the ducts of the breasts and the smooth muscle of the uterus.

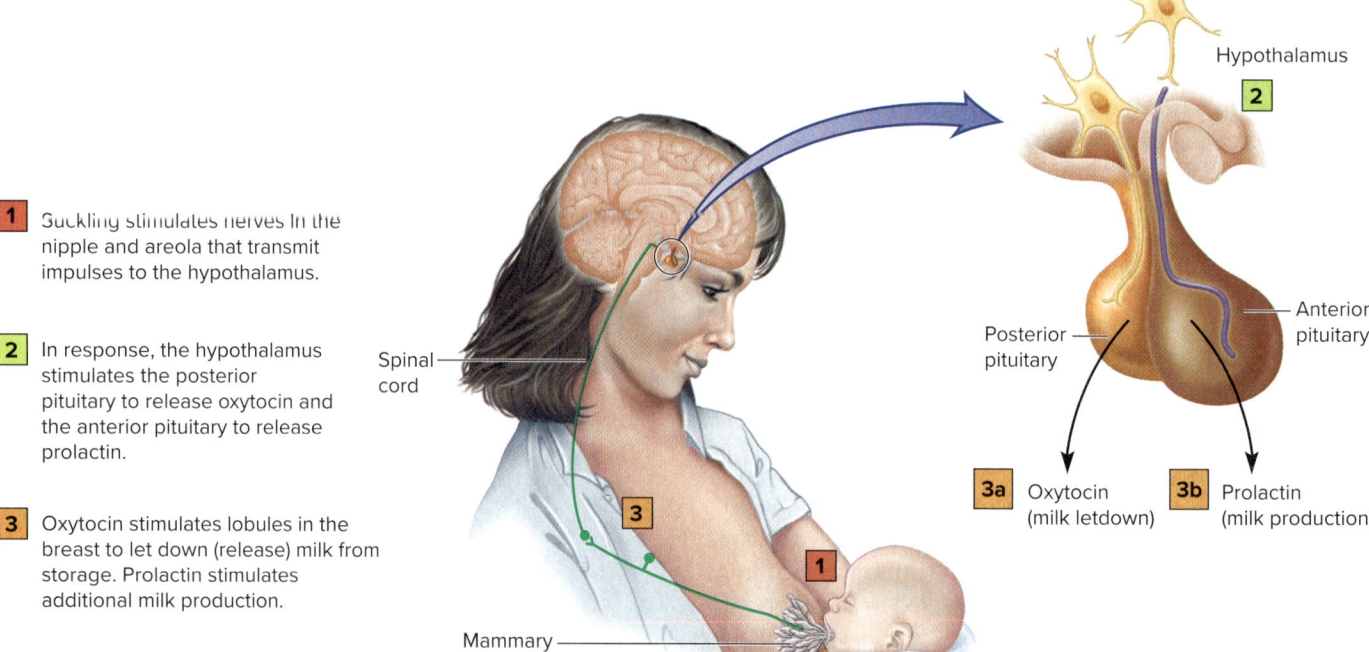

1. Suckling stimulates nerves in the nipple and areola that transmit impulses to the hypothalamus.

2. In response, the hypothalamus stimulates the posterior pituitary to release oxytocin and the anterior pituitary to release prolactin.

3. Oxytocin stimulates lobules in the breast to let down (release) milk from storage. Prolactin stimulates additional milk production.

FIGURE 14-11 Let-down reflex. Suckling sets into motion the sequence of events that lead to milk let-down, the flow of milk into ducts of the breast. Both milk production and let-down are regulated by hormones produced by the pituitary gland.

(2) show a normal pattern of weight gain, and (3) pass at least one or two stools per day that look like lumpy mustard. In addition, softening of the breast during the feeding indicates that milk is being removed from the breast. Parents who sense their infant is not consuming enough milk should consult their primary care provider immediately because dehydration can develop rapidly. It is normal for newborn infants to lose some weight (up to 10% of birth weight) in the first few days after birth. However, losing more than 10% of birth weight indicates a feeding problem that requires intervention.[79]

It generally takes 2 to 3 weeks to fully establish the feeding routine: infant and mother begin to feel comfortable, the milk supply meets infant demand, and initial nipple soreness disappears. Establishing the breastfeeding routine requires patience, but the rewards are numerous. The adjustments are easier if supplemental formula feedings are not introduced until breastfeeding is well established, after at least 3 to 4 weeks. Then it is fine if a supplemental bottle or two of infant formula per day is needed, but supplemental feedings will decrease the infant's demand for the breast, and thereby decrease milk production.

NUTRITIONAL QUALITIES OF HUMAN MILK

Human milk is different in composition from cow's milk. Unless altered (i.e., to make infant formula), cow's milk is not a suitable replacement for human milk until the infant is at least 12 months old. Unaltered cow's milk is too high in minerals and protein and does not contain enough carbohydrate to meet an infant's nutritional needs. In addition, the major protein in cow's milk is harder for an infant to digest than the major proteins in human milk. The proteins in cow's milk may also spur allergies in some infants.

Colostrum. At the end of pregnancy, the first fluid made by the human breast is **colostrum**. This thick, yellowish fluid may leak from the breast during late pregnancy and is produced in earnest for a few days after birth. Colostrum differs from mature human milk in that it contains a higher concentration of antibodies, immune system cells, and growth factors, some of which pass intact through the lining of the infant's immature GI tract into the bloodstream. The first few months of life are the only time when we can readily absorb whole proteins, such as immune factors, across the GI tract. These immune factors and cells protect the infant from some GI tract diseases and other infectious disorders, compensating for the infant's immature immune system during the first few months of life. These protective qualities of colostrum are an important reason for mothers to breastfeed their infants, even if for just the first few weeks after birth.

Colostrum is particularly rich in **human milk oligosaccharides.** These small carbohydrates cannot be digested by human enzymes, but they help to establish a healthy gut microbiota by promoting the growth of beneficial bacteria, including *Lactobacillus bifidus*. These beneficial bacteria limit the growth of potentially toxic bacteria in the intestine. Human milk oligosaccharides are thought to promote the health of the infant's gut and stimulate normal immune function. This is one way breastfeeding supports the infant's digestive health.[80] Beyond gut health, human milk oligosaccharides may have effects on infant growth, immune function, and neurological development.[81,82,83]

Mature Milk. Human milk composition gradually changes from colostrum to mature milk several days after delivery. Human milk looks very different from cow's milk. (Table 15-2 provides a direct comparison.) Human milk is thin and almost watery in appearance and often has a slightly bluish tinge. Its nutritional qualities, however, are impressive!

Human milk's proteins form a soft, light curd in the infant's stomach and are easy to digest. Some human milk proteins offer immune protection. Still others bind iron, reducing the growth of some bacteria that can cause diarrhea.

The lipids in human breast milk are high in linoleic acid and cholesterol, which are needed for brain development. Breast milk also contains long-chain omega-3 fatty acids, such as docosahexaenoic acid. This polyunsaturated fatty acid is used for the

colostrum The first fluid secreted by the breast during late pregnancy and the first few days after birth. This thick fluid is rich in immune factors and protein.

human milk oligosaccharides Small, indigestible carbohydrates made in the human breast from lactose and other simple sugars.

magnificent

Colonizing the Infant's GI Tract
Did you know that human breast milk is not sterile? Along with human milk oligosaccharides, the unique collection of microorganisms from the mother's breast helps to colonize the infant's GI tract.

microbiome

synthesis of tissues in the central nervous system, especially in the brain and the retina of the eye.

The fat composition of human milk changes during each feeding. The consistency of milk released at the start of a feeding (*fore milk*) resembles that of skim milk. The milk released after 10 to 20 minutes of feeding (*hind milk*) is much higher in fat, similar to cream. Babies need to nurse long enough (e.g., a total of 20 or more minutes) to get the calories in the rich hind milk to be satisfied between feedings and to grow well. The overall calorie content of infant formulas has been based on that of human milk (on average, 67 kcal per 100 milliliters).

Human milk composition also allows for adequate fluid status of the infant, provided the baby is exclusively breastfed. Caregivers often wonder if the infant needs additional water if stressed by hot weather, diarrhea, vomiting, or fever. The AAP advises against supplemental water or juice during the first 6 months of life. The practice may unnecessarily introduce pathogens or allergens. Excessive water can lead to brain disorders, low blood sodium, and other problems. Thus, before 6 months of age, supplemental fluids should be given only with a clinician's guidance.

Human Milk for Preterm Infants. Can a mother breastfeed a preterm infant? In some cases, human milk is the most desirable form of nourishment, depending on infant weight and length of gestation. Feeding of human milk to preterm infants has been linked to lower infant mortality, decreased risk of infections, reduced stays in the neonatal intensive care unit, fewer hospital readmissions, better growth, and improved brain development.[76]

Breastfeeding a preterm infant, however, demands a high level of dedication from caregivers. Preterm infants sometimes have a weak or uncoordinated suck-and-swallow reflex, so the mother may need to express milk from the breast and feed that milk to the infant through a tube until the infant's feeding ability improves. Fortification of the milk with calcium, phosphorus, sodium, and protein is often necessary to meet the needs of a rapidly growing preterm infant. In some cases, special feeding problems may prevent the use of human milk or necessitate supplementing it with specialized formula. For some preterm infants with gastrointestinal malformations or severe infections, intravenous feeding is the only option. Working as a team, the pediatrician, neonatal nurses, and RDN will guide the parents in this decision.

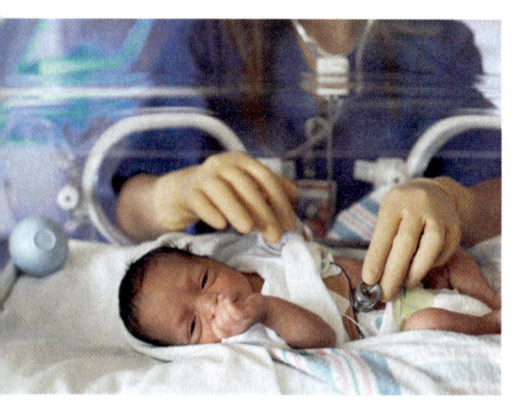

If human milk is used to feed the preterm infant, fortification of the milk with certain nutrients is often needed. ERproductions Ltd./Blend Images LLC

EATING PATTERN FOR FEMALES WHO BREASTFEED

The nutrient needs for a female who breastfeeds are somewhat different from those of the female in the second and third trimesters of pregnancy (review Fig. 14-7 and Fig. 14-8 and see the DRI summary tables in Appendix F). The DRIs for folate and iron decrease while the DRIs for calories; vitamins A, E, and C; riboflavin; copper; chromium; iodine; manganese; selenium; and zinc increase. Still, the increased dietary demands of breastfeeding will be met by the general dietary plan proposed for a female in the latter stages of pregnancy:

- 3 cups from the dairy group (which includes fortified soy beverages), or use of calcium-fortified foods to make up for any gap between calcium intake and need
- 6½ to 7 ounce equivalents from the protein group
- 3½ cups from the vegetables group
- 2 to 2½ cups from the fruits group
- 9 to 10 ounce equivalents from the grains group
- 8 teaspoons of plant oils

Table 14-2 provides a sample menu. As in pregnancy, a serving of fortified ready-to-eat breakfast cereal (or use of a balanced multivitamin and mineral supplement) is helpful to meet extra nutrient needs. As during pregnancy, individuals who are breastfeeding should consume 8 to 12 ounces of low-mercury fish per week (or 1 gram per day of omega-3 fatty acids from a fish oil supplement) because the omega-3 fatty acids present in fish are secreted into breast milk and are likely to be important for development of the infant's nervous system.[43]

Depending on the infant's demand for milk (which varies over time as the infant grows and begins to consume solid foods), milk production may require 500 kcal (or more) every day. The EER for lactation includes an extra 380 to 400 kcal per day above prepregnancy recommendations (see the sample equations that follow).[29] The equations to calculate energy needs during lactation take into account the individual's age, height, weight, physical activity level, plus the energy needed for milk production. The equations for 0 to 6 months postpartum also include a small energy deficit, which allows for a gradual loss of the extra body fat accumulated during pregnancy.

> Selena is a 26-year-old female. She gave birth to a healthy, term infant 3 months ago and she is exclusively breastfeeding the infant. She is 5 feet, 7 inches (170 cm) tall and now weighs 145 pounds (66 kg). Her physical activity level is *low active*.
>
> **EXCLUSIVELY BREASTFEEDING, 0 TO 6 MONTHS POSTPARTUM**
>
> 575.77 − (7.01 × age) + (6.6 × height) + (12.14 × weight) + energy cost of milk production − energy mobilization
>
> 575.77 − (7.01 × 26 y) + (6.6 × 170 cm) + (12.14 × 66 kg) + 540 kcal − 140 kcal = 2717 kcal
>
> Selena is a 26-year-old female. She gave birth to a healthy, term infant 9 months ago and she is still partially breastfeeding the infant, even as the infant is beginning to consume complementary foods. She is 5 feet, 7 inches (170 cm) tall and now weighs 132 pounds (60 kg). Her physical activity level is *low active*.
>
> **PARTIALLY BREASTFEEDING, 7 TO 12 MONTHS POSTPARTUM**
>
> 575.77 − (7.01 × age) + (6.6 × height) + (12.14 × weight) + energy cost of milk production
>
> 575.77 − (7.01 × 26 y) + (6.6 × 170 cm) + (12.14 × 60 kg) + 380 kcal = 2624 kcal

After giving birth, new mothers are often eager to shed the excess "baby fat." Breastfeeding, however, is no time for crash diets. A gradual weight loss of 1 to 4 pounds per month by a mother who is breastfeeding is appropriate. At significantly greater rates of weight loss—when calories are restricted to less than about 1500 kcal per day—milk output decreases. A reasonable approach for a mother who is breastfeeding is to follow a dietary plan that supplies at least 1800 kcal per day, has moderate fat content, and includes a variety of nutrient-dense foods from all food groups.

Hydration is especially important during breastfeeding; the mother should drink fluids every time the infant nurses. Drinking about 13 cups of fluids per day encourages ample milk production. Detrimental habits, such as smoking cigarettes or drinking more than two alcoholic beverages a day, can decrease milk output. (Even very small amounts of alcohol can have a deleterious effect on milk output for some individuals.)

EXPRESSING AND STORING HUMAN MILK

There are many reasons why lactating females may wish to express their milk and store it for later use. Infants who are born preterm or who have certain medical conditions may have difficulty latching on to the breast for effective feedings. In these cases, expressed breast milk can be fed to the infant by bottle or tube to provide nutritional and immunological benefits beyond what infant formula can provide. For mothers with low milk supply, pumping can stimulate the breast to increase milk production. Even for healthy mother/infant dyads, the ability to let another caregiver feed the infant allows the mother some freedom to spend a few hours away from home, return to work outside the home, or simply get a full night's sleep! Some mothers also donate milk to milk banks for use by infants whose mothers cannot breastfeed.

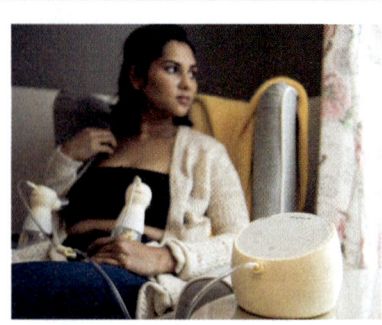

Breast milk can be expressed by the mother using a manual, battery-operated, or electric (shown) breast pump. In 2010, an amendment to the Fair Labor Standards Act mandated that most U.S. employers allow break time and a private setting for moms who are breastfeeding to express milk. **Why would it be advantageous for employers to support families in their efforts to breastfeed their children?** Medela 2019

Breast milk can be expressed by hand (i.e., manual expression) into a sterile plastic bottle or nursing bag. Several styles of breast pumps are also available: manually operated or electric, single or double. For a mother who wishes to return to work while continuing to breastfeed the infant, an electric double pump is a worthwhile investment. The cost for these supplies may be covered by insurance or may be tax-deductible.

Expressing and storing human milk requires careful sanitation and rapid chilling to ensure safety for the infant. Hands, surfaces, and all pumping equipment should be thoroughly washed before expressing milk. Pumps should not be shared with others. Any parts (e.g., tubing) that appear contaminated with mold should be replaced immediately. Freshly expressed human milk is safe at room temperature for up to 4 hours or can be kept in the refrigerator for up to 4 days. For longer-term storage, human milk will maintain its highest quality in the freezer for up to 6 months but can be kept up to a year. Sterile nursing bags are a practical, space-saving option for mothers who plan to keep a sizable supply of milk in the freezer. Thawed milk should be used within 24 hours. Any milk left over after a feeding should be used within 2 hours or discarded because bacteria and enzymes from the infant's saliva may make the milk unsafe.[84] See Chapter 15 for more information on infant feeding techniques.

Expressing milk may seem awkward at first; it takes some practice! The breastfed infant may need some time to adapt to drinking human milk from a bottle, as well. After 1 month or so, the breastfeeding routine should be well established, and the infant can easily transition between breast and bottle feedings. It is worth the effort to be able to provide optimal nutrition for the infant even when the mother cannot be present.

Advantages of Breastfeeding. With appropriate training and support, the vast majority of females are capable of breastfeeding, and their infants would benefit from it (see Table 14-3).[76] Nonetheless, individual circumstances may make breastfeeding impractical or undesirable. Mothers who do not want to breastfeed their infants should not feel pressured to do so. Breastfeeding provides advantages, but none so great that a mother who decides to feed the infant an infant formula should feel anxious about the infant's well-being.

Human milk is tailored to meet infant nutrient needs for the first 4 to 6 months of life. Beyond meeting nutritional needs, there are many other benefits of breastfeeding.

TABLE 14-3 ■ Advantages of Breastfeeding

For Infant
Bacteriologically safe
Always fresh and ready to go
Provides antibodies and other substances that contribute to the maturation of the immune system
Helps to establish a healthy gut microbiota and contributes to the maturation of the gastrointestinal tract
Decreases the risk of infections, such as diarrhea, respiratory disease, and ear infections
Reduces the risk of atopic diseases, such as eczema and asthma
Reduces the risk of celiac disease and inflammatory bowel diseases
Establishes the habit of eating in moderation, which is linked to 15% to 30% lower risk of obesity and 40% lower risk of type 2 diabetes later in life
Contributes to the proper development of jaws and teeth for better speech development
May enhance nervous system development and eventual learning ability
Decreases the risk of childhood leukemia and lymphoma
For Mother
Contributes to earlier recovery from pregnancy due to the action of hormones that promote a quicker return of the uterus to its prepregnancy state
Decreases the risk of several chronic diseases later in life, including hypertension, cardiovascular disease, and diabetes
Decreases the risk of ovarian and premenopausal breast cancer
Potential for a quicker return to prepregnancy weight
Potential for delayed ovulation, thus reducing the chances of pregnancy in the short term

Source: American Academy of Pediatrics. Policy Statement: breastfeeding and the use of human milk. *Pediatrics* 129:e827, 2012. DOI:10.1089/bfm.2012.0067.

Fewer Infections. Breastfeeding reduces the infant's overall risk of developing infections. This may be due to the antibodies passed from the mother to the infant through colostrum or perhaps due to positive effects on the infant's microbiome, which influences the development of the infant's immune system.[85] Studies demonstrate a lower risk of respiratory tract infections and gastrointestinal infections. Infants who are breastfed also have fewer ear infections (otitis media) because they do not sleep with a bottle in their mouth. Experts strongly discourage allowing an infant to sleep with a bottle in the mouth; milk can pool in the mouth, throat, and inner ear, creating a growth medium for bacteria, which can lead to ear infections and dental caries. By reducing these common ailments, parents can decrease discomfort for the infant, reduce the number of visits to the doctor's office, and prevent possible hearing loss.

Lower Risk for Noncommunicable Diseases. Research now links breastfeeding with reduced risks for many obesity-related, chronic diseases. Infants who are breastfed may learn to self-regulate food intake and avoid overeating, which may explain the connection to a lowered risk for obesity and type 2 diabetes among adults who were breastfed as infants. The immunologic benefits of breastfeeding seem to be involved in lowered rates of type 1 diabetes, **celiac disease,** and inflammatory bowel diseases. Reductions in risks of childhood leukemia and lymphoma have also been observed.

 Lower Risk for Atopic Diseases. Breastfeeding also reduces the chances of some **atopic diseases** (see Section 15.7). Currently, there is not enough evidence to draw conclusions about the duration of breastfeeding and the risk for food allergies. However, breastfeeding for at least 3 to 4 months lowers the risk for eczema and asthma.[86] Infants are also better able to tolerate human milk than formulas. Formulas sometimes must be switched several times until caregivers find the best one for the infant.

Convenience and Cost. Breastfeeding frees the mother from the time and expense involved in buying and preparing formula and washing bottles. Human milk is ready to go and safe to consume. This allows the mother to spend more time with the baby.

POSSIBLE BARRIERS TO BREASTFEEDING

Widespread misinformation, the mother's need to return to a job, and social reticence are some possible barriers to breastfeeding.

celiac disease Chronic, immune-mediated disease precipitated by exposure to dietary gluten in genetically predisposed people.

atopic disease A condition involving an inappropriate immune response to environmental allergens; examples include asthma, eczema, and seasonal allergies.

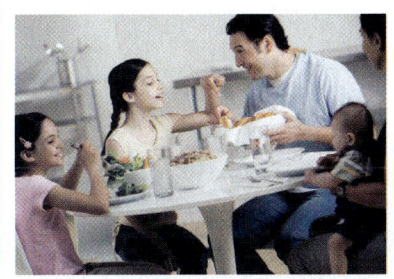

Some researchers propose that the passage of flavors from the mother's eating pattern into breast milk affords an opportunity for the infant to learn about the flavor of the foods of its family long before solids are introduced. **What are the favorite flavors at your family meals?** Andersen Ross/Blend Images/SuperStock

> ### 🌱 Sustainable Solutions
>
> #### Feeding the Next Generation
> Sustainability aims to ensure vitality for generations to come. One way to ensure the well-being of future generations is to promote breastfeeding as optimal nutrition for infants and a positive health behavior for mothers. What if more mothers chose to breastfeed their infants? A recent analysis estimated the potential public health impact of near universal breastfeeding. By reducing the risk of a multitude of health problems, such as gastrointestinal and respiratory infections, researchers projected that 823,000 infant deaths and 20,000 cases of breast cancer could be prevented per year. In fact, increasing the number of mothers who choose to breastfeed their infants would help to meet several of the United Nations' Sustainable Development Goals, including those focused on physical health, economic growth, education, and protecting the environment.
>
> Sources: Victora CG, Bahl R, Barros AJ, et al.; Lancet Breastfeeding Series Group. Breastfeeding in the 21st century: epidemiology, mechanisms, and lifelong effect. *Lancet.* 2016 Jan 30;387(10017):475-490. doi: 10.1016/S0140-6736(15)01024-7
>
> World Alliance for Breastfeeding Action. World Breastfeeding Week: Breastfeeding: a key to sustainable development. 2016. Accessed December 8, 2023. https://worldbreastfeedingweek.org/2016/images/wbw2016-af-i.jpg

Misinformation. The major barriers to breastfeeding stem from misinformation, such as the idea that one's breasts are too small to adequately nourish an infant, and the lack of role models. One positive note has been the widespread increase in the availability of lactation consultants over the past several years. First-time mothers who are interested in breastfeeding can find invaluable support from lactation consultants or by talking to others who have experienced breastfeeding successfully. In almost every community, a group called La Leche League offers classes in breastfeeding and advises mothers who are facing challenges with breastfeeding (800-LALECHE or www.lalecheleague.org).

Return to an Outside Job. Certainly, continuing to breastfeed after the mother returns to work is beneficial for the infant and the mother. It is also in the employer's best interest to support continued breastfeeding because infants who are breastfed are usually sick less often, which will reduce absenteeism and medical costs.[87] However, working outside the home can complicate plans to breastfeed.

Employers can support individuals who breastfeed with flexible work hours or remote working arrangements. If the job necessitates on-site hours, the employer should provide appropriate time and space to express milk. In fact, companies with 50 employees or more are required by federal law to provide reasonable breaks and a private space (other than a bathroom) for moms who breastfeed to pump milk. (See the earlier section on "Expressing and Storing Human Milk.") State laws may provide additional accommodations.

Some individuals can juggle both a job and breastfeeding, but demanding schedules, lack of appropriate equipment or facilities, and unsupportive coworkers can make it difficult to keep up with breastfeeding. A compromise—balancing some feedings of human milk (e.g., early morning and bedtime), with infant formula feedings during the day—is possible. The use of supplemental feedings will decrease milk production, but some breast milk is better than no breast milk!

Social Concerns. Another possible barrier is embarrassment about nursing a child in public. Historically, social mores in the U.S. have stressed modesty and discouraged public displays of breasts—even for as good a cause as nourishing babies. In the United States, no state or territory has a law prohibiting breastfeeding. However, indecent exposure (including the exposure of female breasts) has long been a common law or statutory offense. Now, all 50 states, the District of Columbia, and the Virgin Islands have specific laws that protect the right to breastfeed in any location. Those who feel reluctant should be reassured that they do have social support and that breastfeeding can be done discreetly.

Medical Conditions Precluding Breastfeeding. Breastfeeding may be ruled out by certain medical conditions in either the infant or the mother. For example, breastfeeding is contraindicated for infants with **galactosemia**, an inherited disorder in which the body cannot break down galactose. Lactose, the main carbohydrate in human breast milk, is made of glucose and galactose. When galactose is not broken down properly, its by-products can damage body organs. Infants with galactosemia cannot tolerate breast milk or cow's milk; they require lactose-free infant formula.

Certain medications can pass into the milk and adversely affect the infant. A mother should discuss all medications (prescription and over-the-counter) with a health care provider to make sure they are compatible with breastfeeding. In addition, a mother in the United States or other developed region of the world who has a transmissible disease (such as tuberculosis or HIV) or who is being treated with chemotherapy medications should not breastfeed.

Cosmetic Alterations to the Breast. Nipple piercings should have no impact on the ability to breastfeed, but the jewelry should be removed before each feeding. Repeated removal and reinsertion of the jewelry may be inconvenient and irritating, so it may be best to leave the jewelry out for the entire period of breastfeeding. Breast tattoos will

galactosemia Inborn error of metabolism in which the enzyme that converts galactose into glucose is missing or deficient.

not impair breastfeeding, either. However, getting a new nipple piercing or breast tattoo while breastfeeding is not advised due to the pain of healing and possibility of infection. Past breast augmentation or reduction surgeries may impair a person's ability to breastfeed if milk-producing tissue was damaged during the surgery.

Environmental Contaminants in Human Milk. There is some legitimate concern over the levels of various environmental contaminants in human milk. However, the benefits of human milk are well established, and the risks from environmental contaminants are still largely theoretical. A few measures a mother could take to counteract some known contaminants are to (1) consume a variety of foods within each food group, (2) avoid freshwater fish from polluted waters, (3) carefully wash and peel fruits and vegetables (or choose organically raised produce, which has lower levels of pesticides than conventional produce), and (4) remove the fatty edges of meat, as pesticides can become concentrated in fat tissue. In addition, new mothers should not try to lose weight rapidly while nursing (more than 0.75 to 1 pound per week) because contaminants stored in the fat tissue might be released into her bloodstream and then appear in breast milk. If there are concerns about the safety of breast milk, especially if the mother has lived in an area known to have a high concentration of toxic wastes or environmental pollutants, consult the local health department.

DIETARY SUPPLEMENTS FOR BREASTFED INFANTS

There are some cases in which infant dietary supplements, used under a pediatrician's guidance, are recommended.

- The AAP recommends *all* infants, including exclusively breastfed infants, be given 10 micrograms of vitamin D per day, beginning shortly after birth and continuing until the infant consumes that much from food (see Section 15.2 for more information about vitamin D supplements for infants).[88] Alternatively, under physician supervision, the mother can take high-dose vitamin D supplements (160 micrograms per day) to boost the vitamin D content of breast milk to levels sufficient to meet the infant's needs.[89] Some sun exposure also helps in meeting vitamin D requirements.
- Term infants are usually born with adequate iron stores to last for the first 4 to 6 months of life. However, to prevent anemia, the AAP recommends iron supplements for exclusively breastfed infants starting at 4 months of age. More aggressive iron supplementation may be needed for infants born preterm or LBW or to mothers with iron deficiency.[90]
- The AAP does not advise fluoride supplements before 6 months of age. After 6 months, the pediatrician or dentist may recommend supplemental fluoride if the infant's exposure to fluoride from drinking water, foods, and oral hygiene products is insufficient.[91]
- Vitamin B-12 supplements are recommended for infants who are breastfed by mothers who follow a vegetarian dietary pattern.[92]

For more information on successful breastfeeding, see *Your Guide to Breastfeeding* from the Office on Women's Health, available at https://www.womenshealth.gov/your-guide-to-breastfeeding

✓ CONCEPT CHECK 14.7

1. What do AND and AAP recommend for the duration of breastfeeding?
2. Describe the physiological processes of milk production and let-down. Be sure to mention the hormones involved in these processes.
3. List three advantages of breastfeeding for the mother and three advantages for the infant.
4. Describe three potential barriers to breastfeeding, and suggest ways to overcome them.
5. Identify three micronutrients that may need to be supplemented in the dietary patterns of infants who are breastfed, and give the rationale for each.

14.8 Nutrition and Your Health: Reducing the Risk of Birth Defects

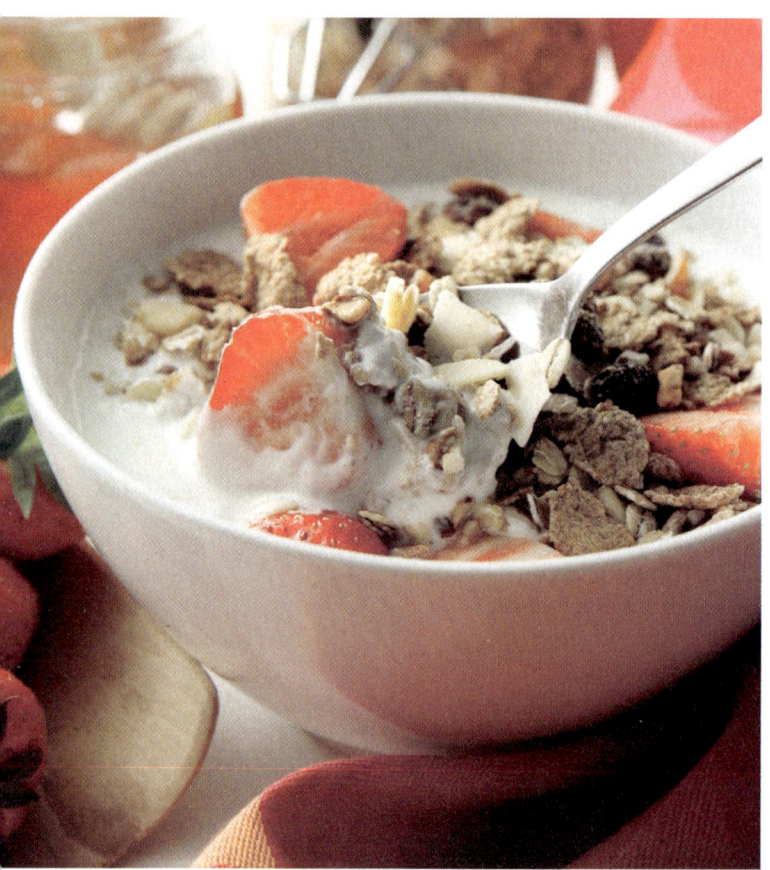

Floortje/Vetta/Getty Images

Eating well for a healthy pregnancy not only supplies materials for fetal growth and development but also helps to direct the amazing process of building a new life. Considering the complexity of the human body and its more than 20,000 genes, it is not surprising that abnormalities of structure, function, or metabolism are sometimes present at birth. Birth defects impact 1 in every 33 babies born in the United States.[93] In some cases, they are so severe that a baby cannot survive or thrive. Defects in embryonic or fetal development are the presumed cause of many spontaneous abortions and are at the root of about 20% of infant deaths before 1 year of age. However, many babies with birth defects can go on to live healthy and productive lives.

A wide range of physical or mental disabilities result from birth defects. Heart defects are present in approximately 1 in every 100 to 200 newborn babies, accounting for a large proportion of infant deaths. Cleft lip and/or cleft palate are malformations of the lip or roof of the mouth and occur in approximately 1 in 700 to 1000 births. Neural tube defects are malformations of the brain or spinal cord that occur during embryonic development. Examples include **spina bifida,** in which all or part of the spinal cord is exposed, and **anencephaly,** in which some or all of the brain is missing (Fig. 14-12). Babies born with spina bifida can survive to adulthood but in many cases have disabilities, such as paralysis, incontinence, and cognitive disorders. Babies born with anencephaly die soon after birth. Neural tube defects occur in 1 in 1000 births. Down syndrome, a condition in which an extra chromosome leads to intellectual disability and other physical alterations, occurs in about 1 in 800 births. Other common birth defects include musculoskeletal defects, gastrointestinal defects, and metabolic disorders.

What causes a birth defect? About 15% to 25% of birth defects are known to be genetic (i.e., inherited or spontaneous mutations of the genetic code). Another 10% are due to environmental influences (e.g., exposure to **teratogens**). The specific cause of the remaining 65% to 75% of birth defects is unknown. Although the etiology of birth defects is multifactorial and many elements are beyond human control, good nutrition practices can positively influence the outcome of pregnancy.

Folic Acid

During the 1980s, researchers in the United Kingdom noticed a relationship between poor dietary habits and a high rate of neural tube defects among children of families living in poverty. Subsequent intervention studies demonstrated that administration of a multivitamin supplement to the mother during the periconceptional period—the months before conception and during early pregnancy—reduced the recurrence of these birth defects. The specific link between dietary folic acid and neural tube defects was tested and confirmed in several follow-up studies. Folate plays a leading role in the synthesis of DNA and the metabolism of amino acids. The rapid cell growth of pregnancy increases needs for folate during pregnancy to 600 micrograms DFE per day. Some females, for genetic reasons, may have an even higher requirement. Adequate folic acid in the periconceptional period decreases the risk of neural tube defects by about 70% and has also been associated with decreased risk of cleft lip/palate, heart defects, and Down syndrome.

spina bifida Birth defect resulting from improper closure of the neural tube during embryonic development. The spinal cord or fluid may bulge outside the spinal column.

anencephaly Birth defect characterized by the absence of some or all of the brain and skull.

teratogen A compound (natural or synthetic) that may cause or increase the risk of a birth defect. Exposure to a teratogen does not always lead to a birth defect; its effects on the fetus depend on the dose, timing, and duration of exposure. Examples: alcohol, some drugs, some industrial or household chemicals, certain infections, and extreme heat.

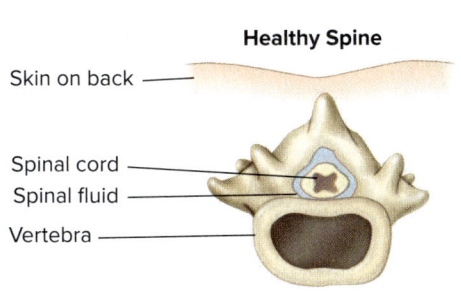
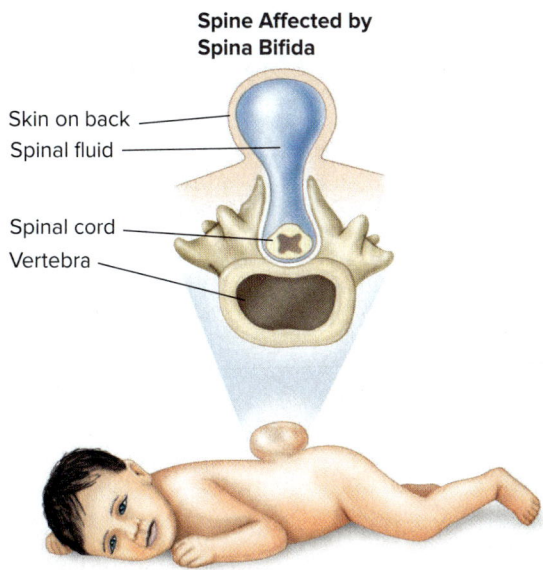

FIGURE 14-12 Spina bifida is one type of neural tube defect. Very early in fetal development, a ridge of neural-like tissue forms along the back of the embryo. As the fetus develops, this ridge develops into both the spinal cord and nerves at the lower end and the brain at the upper end. At the same time, the bones that make up the back gradually surround the spinal cord on all sides. In spina bifida, the backbones do not form a complete ring to protect the spinal cord. Deficient folate status in the mother during the beginning of pregnancy, especially in combination with a genetic abnormality in folate metabolism, greatly increases the risk of neural tube defects.

In 1998, the U.S. Food and Drug Administration (FDA) mandated fortification of grain products to provide 140 micrograms of folic acid per 100 grams of grain consumed. In Canada, the level of fortification is 150 micrograms of folate per 100 grams of grain consumed. In general, this fortification program increases the average consumption of dietary folic acid by 100 micrograms per day.

Adequate folate status is crucial for all females of childbearing age because the neural tube closes within the first 28 days of pregnancy, a time when many individuals are unaware they are pregnant. A well-planned dietary pattern can meet the RDA for folate, but the U.S. Public Health Service, March of Dimes, and *Dietary Guidelines* recommend that all females of childbearing age take a daily multivitamin and mineral supplement that contains 400 micrograms of folic acid. Females who have already had a child with a neural tube defect are advised to consume megadoses of folic acid—4000 micrograms per day. They are to begin supplementation at least 1 month before any future pregnancy. This must be done under the supervision of a primary care provider.[94]

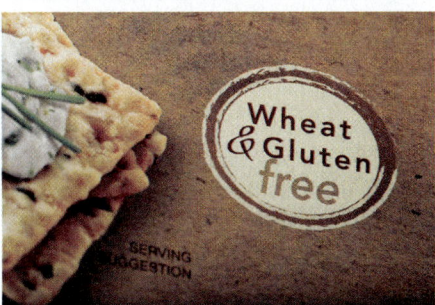

A surge in the popularity of low-carb diets may be undermining recent progress toward reducing rates of neural tube defects. By cutting out fortified grains (e.g., cereal, pasta, and bread), females who follow low-carb diets during pregnancy may miss out on important sources of folic acid. Photo: Mark Steinmetz

Text Source: Desrosiers TA, Siega-Riz AM, Mosley BS, Meyer RE; National Birth Defects Prevention Study. Low carbohydrate diets may increase risk of neural tube defects. *Birth Defects Res.* 2018 July 3;110(11):901-909. doi: 10.1002/bdr2.1198

Iodine

Low iodine status during the first trimester of pregnancy—a critical period of brain development—may lead to congenital hypothyroidism (formerly called *cretinism*).[95] If left untreated, consequences (which may vary in severity) include intellectual disability, stunting of growth, impaired hearing and speech, and infertility. Some other physical features are evident in Figure 14-13. When the defect is identified early (by newborn screening tests), these harmful effects can be prevented by treatment with thyroid hormones. Please note that iodine deficiency is just one possible cause of congenital hypothyroidism. The condition may also arise due to genetic abnormalities, autoimmune disorders, or exposure to some medications during pregnancy. Congenital hypothyroidism due to iodine deficiency is most common in developing nations without food fortification programs. With the use of iodized salt, however, congenital hypothyroidism due to iodine deficiency is rare in developed nations.

Antioxidants

A case can be made for antioxidants in the prevention of birth defects as well. Free radicals are constantly generated within the body as a result of normal metabolic processes. An abundance of free radicals results in damage of cells and their DNA, which can lead to gene mutations or tissue malformations. Some research points to free radicals as a source of damage during embryonic development, when organs are first being formed. Antioxidant systems within the body act to minimize the damage caused by free radicals, and researchers hypothesize that dietary sources of antioxidants may aid in the prevention of birth defects. At this time, there is insufficient evidence to support supplementation of individual nutrients that participate in antioxidant systems—vitamin E, vitamin C, selenium, zinc, and copper—for the prevention of birth defects. However, use of a balanced multivitamin and mineral supplement while consuming meals rich in whole grains, legumes, and a variety of fruits and vegetables will provide enough of these nutrients to meet current recommendations.

In the United States, typical dietary patterns supply adequate vitamin A from foods, so supplemental use is not generally necessary. During pregnancy, supplemental preformed vitamin A should not exceed 3000 micrograms RAE per day. Most multivitamins and prenatal vitamins supply less than 1500 micrograms RAE per day. A balanced eating plan and prudent use of dietary supplements are actions that can sidestep potential problems with vitamin A toxicity.

Caffeine

Caffeine has been scrutinized for its safety during pregnancy, especially for any link with the rate of birth defects. Caffeine decreases the mother's absorption of iron and may reduce blood flow through the placenta. In addition, the fetus is unable to detoxify caffeine. Research shows that as caffeine intake increases, so does the risk of miscarriage or delivering an LBW infant. Heavy caffeine use during pregnancy may also lead to caffeine withdrawal symptoms in the newborn. These risks are reported with caffeine intakes in excess of 500 milligrams, or the equivalent of about 5 cups of coffee per day. Moderate use of caffeine (up to 200 milligrams of caffeine, or the equivalent of about 2 cups of regular coffee per day), however, is not associated with risk for birth defects.[39] Accounting for caffeine intake from tea, over-the-counter medicines containing caffeine, and chocolate is also important.

Aspartame

Phenylalanine, a component of the alternative sweetener aspartame (NutraSweet® and Equal®), is a cause for concern for some individuals during pregnancy. High amounts of phenylalanine in maternal blood disrupt fetal brain development if the mother has a disease known as *phenylketonuria* (see "Obesity and Chronic Health Conditions" in this section). If the mother does not have this condition, however, it is unlikely that the baby will be affected by moderate aspartame use.

For most adults, diet soft drinks are the primary source of alternative sweeteners. Of greater concern than the safety of sweeteners during pregnancy is the quality of foods and beverages consumed. A high intake of diet soft drinks may crowd out healthier beverages, such as water and low-fat milk.

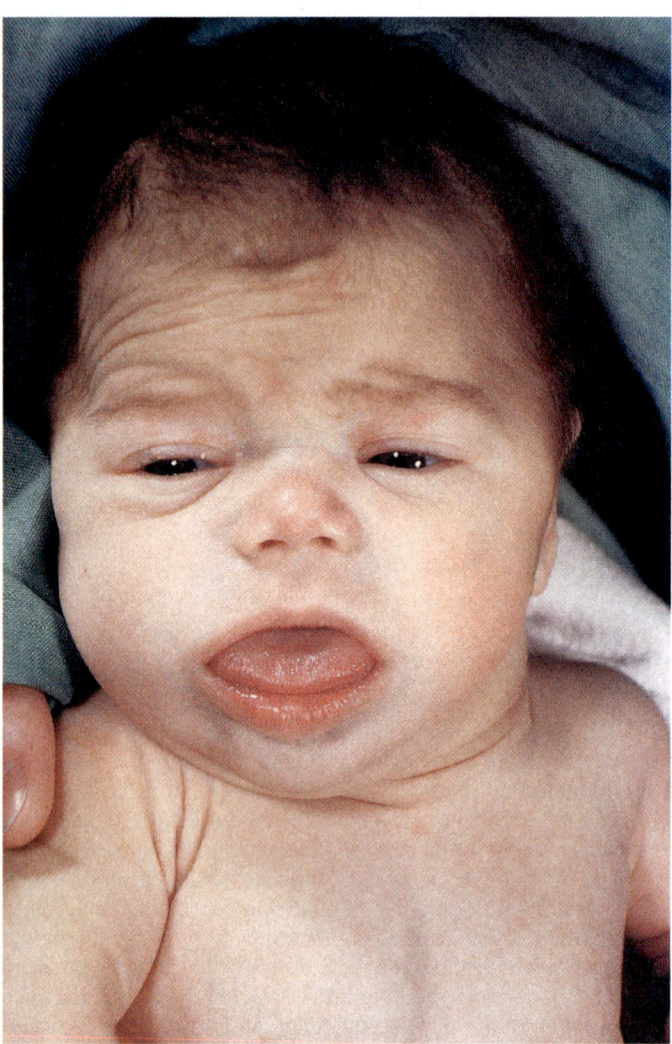

FIGURE 14-13 Child with congenital hypothyroidism due to maternal iodine deficiency. This birth defect leads to intellectual disability, stunting of growth, and other physical defects, such as goiter, large tongue, enlarged head, and puffy eyes. Mediscan/Alamy Stock Photo

Vitamin A

Although the requirements for most vitamins and minerals increase by about 30% during pregnancy, the RDA for vitamin A increases by only 10%. Studies have shown the teratogenic potential of vitamin A in doses as low as approximately 3000 micrograms RAE per day. This is just over three times the RDA of 770 micrograms RAE per day for adult females during pregnancy.

Fetal abnormalities resulting from vitamin A toxicity primarily include facial and cardiac defects, but a wide range of defects have been reported. It is rare that food sources of vitamin A would lead to toxicity. Preformed vitamin A is found in liver, fish, fish oils, fortified milk and yogurt, and eggs. Carotenoids, found in fruits and vegetables, are precursors of vitamin A that are converted into vitamin A in the small intestine, liver, and kidneys. However, the efficiency of absorption of carotenoids decreases as intake increases. Vitamin A excesses typically arise from high-dose dietary supplements rather than food sources.

Obesity and Chronic Health Conditions

Even before becoming pregnant, females of childbearing age should have regular medical checkups to keep an eye on any health conditions that already exist or to identify any developing health problems. In some cases, the condition itself increases risk for birth defects. Obesity, high blood pressure, and uncontrolled diabetes are common health problems known to increase the risk for birth defects, including neural tube defects. In other cases, medications used to control illnesses may pose a risk to the developing fetus. Other health issues, such as seizure disorders and metabolic disorders, could also affect fetal development. A preconception visit with a health professional can help to identify and make plans to minimize such risks. Once a female has become pregnant, early and regular prenatal care promote the success of a pregnancy.

Females with diabetes are more likely to give birth to a baby with birth defects compared to those with normal glucose metabolism.[96] Examples of birth defects common in this group include malformations of the spine, legs, and blood vessels of the heart. Some experts speculate that the mechanism by which diabetes increases birth defects is via excessive free radicals, which lead to oxidative damage of DNA during early gestation. Careful control of blood glucose drastically lowers the risk for birth defects for infants of females with diabetes. Optimal blood glucose control can be achieved through a combination of dietary modifications and medications. Given that diabetes is on the rise among females of childbearing age, this elevated rate of birth defects has become an area of heightened concern.

Another health condition for which maternal nutritional control is of utmost importance is PKU. Recall from Section 6.8 that PKU is an error of metabolism in which the liver lacks the ability to process phenylalanine, leading to an accumulation of this amino acid and its metabolites in body tissues. Babies born to mothers who have phenylketonuria that is not controlled by a PKU diet are at heightened risk for brain defects, such as microcephaly and intellectual disability.[97]

Alcohol

Conclusive evidence shows that repeated consumption of four or more alcoholic drinks at one sitting harms the fetus.[98] Such binge drinking is especially perilous during the first 12 weeks of pregnancy, as this is when critical early developmental events take place in utero. Experts have not determined a safe level of alcohol intake during pregnancy. Until a safe level can be established, females are advised not to drink any alcohol—from beverages, foods, or medications (check the label)—during pregnancy or when there is a chance of conception. The embryo (and, at later stages, the fetus) has no means of detoxifying alcohol.

Females with alcohol use disorders give birth to children with a variety of physical and intellectual problems collectively called **fetal alcohol spectrum disorders (FASDs)**. The most severe of these disorders is **fetal alcohol syndrome (FAS)**. A diagnosis of FAS is based mainly on inadequate fetal and infant growth, physical deformities (especially of facial features), and intellectual disability (Fig. 14-14). Irritability, hyperactivity, short attention span, and limited hand–eye coordination are other symptoms of FAS. Defects in vision, hearing, and mental processing may also develop over time. Other FASDs consist of some but not all of the defects of FAS. **Alcohol-related neurodevelopmental disorders (ARNDs)** include behavior and learning problems resulting

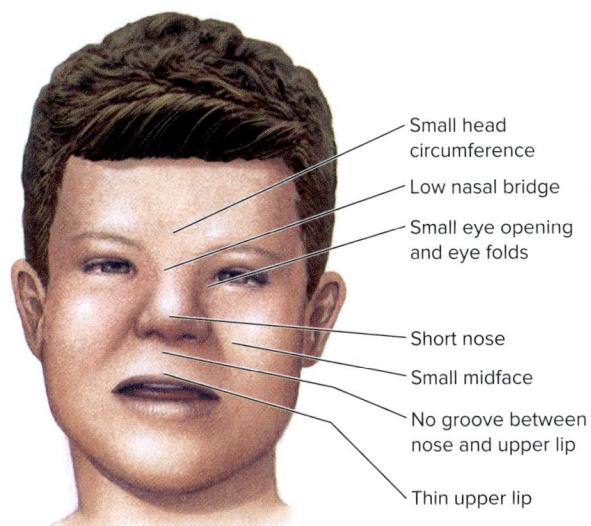

FIGURE 14-14 Fetal alcohol syndrome. The facial features shown are typical of affected children. Additional abnormalities in the brain and other internal organs accompany fetal alcohol syndrome but are not immediately apparent from simply looking at the child. Milder forms of alcohol-induced changes from a lower alcohol exposure to the fetus are known as alcohol-related neurodevelopmental disorders (ARNDs) and alcohol-related birth defects (ARBDs).

from exposure to alcohol in utero. **Alcohol-related birth defects (ARBDs)** typically include malformations of the heart, kidneys, bones, and/or ears.

Exactly how alcohol causes these defects is not known. One line of research suggests that alcohol, or products of the metabolism of alcohol (e.g., acetaldehyde), cause faulty movement of cells in the brain during the early stages of nerve cell development or block the action of certain neurotransmitters. In addition, inadequate nutrient intake, reduced nutrient and oxygen transfer across the placenta, concomitant tobacco and illicit drug use, and possibly other factors contribute to the overall result.

All major health authorities recommend that alcoholic beverages not be consumed by females during pregnancy. For more information about the effects of maternal alcohol use during pregnancy, visit the website www.cdc.gov/ncbddd/fasd.

Environmental Contaminants

There is insufficient evidence to link birth defects with the amounts of pesticides, herbicides, or other contaminants in foods or public water supplies. However, evaluating such a link can be difficult, and many would argue that regulations concerning contaminants in the food and water supply are too permissive. Thus, it seems prudent to take measures to decrease intake of pesticides and other contaminants wherever possible. For fruits and

---

fetal alcohol spectrum disorders (FASDs) A group of irreversible physical and mental abnormalities in the infant that result from the mother's consumption of alcohol during pregnancy.

fetal alcohol syndrome (FAS) Severe form of FASD that involves abnormal facial features and problems with development of the nervous system and overall growth as a result of maternal alcohol consumption during pregnancy.

alcohol-related neurodevelopmental disorders (ARNDs) One or more abnormalities of the central nervous system (e.g., small head size, impaired motor skills, hearing loss, or poor hand–eye coordination) related to confirmed alcohol exposure during gestation.

alcohol-related birth defects (ARBDs) One or more birth defects (e.g., malformations of the heart, bones, kidneys, eyes, or ears) related to confirmed alcohol exposure during gestation.

vegetables, peeling, removing outer leaves, and/or thoroughly rinsing and scrubbing with a brush under running water will remove the majority of contaminants. In animal products, toxins are most likely to accumulate in fatty tissues. Therefore, removing skin, discarding drippings, and trimming visible fat will decrease exposure from meat, poultry, and fish.

For fish, mercury is of particular concern because it can harm the nervous system of the fetus. Although females who are pregnant should consume 8 to 12 ounces per week of seafood to obtain omega-3 fatty acids, they should steer clear of a few types of fish that tend to have higher levels of mercury and other contaminants (e.g., swordfish, shark, king mackerel, and tilefish). When it comes to canned tuna, albacore tuna is a potential mercury source, so it should not be consumed in amounts exceeding 6 ounces per week.[43] Most experts agree that the benefits of consuming fish far outweigh the potential risks of environmental contaminants. As a rule of thumb, consuming a *variety* of foods minimizes risk of exposure to any one contaminant from the food supply.

In Summary

Although many risk factors for birth defects are beyond our control, parents-to-be can make some wise nutrition choices to improve the chances of having a healthy baby without birth defects. A varied and balanced dietary pattern, such as the food plan for pregnancy described in this chapter, along with a daily multivitamin and mineral supplement with 400 micrograms of folic acid, will ensure adequate nutrient status. It is estimated that daily use of a multivitamin and mineral supplement containing folic acid will decrease the rate of all birth defects by 50%.

Discuss the use of any other dietary supplements with a primary care provider or RDN to be sure that the fetus will not be exposed to toxic levels of vitamin A or other dangerous food components. Early and consistent prenatal care can help control obesity and any chronic health conditions that may complicate a pregnancy. Also, avoiding alcohol during pregnancy will eliminate any risk for fetal alcohol spectrum disorders.

Although it seems that advice for a healthy pregnancy is always directed at the mother, fathers-to-be are not off the hook! Health is a family affair, so encouraging healthy eating habits and avoiding smoking and alcohol are important for fathers, too. As you read in the beginning of this chapter, the genetics of the baby are certainly an outcome of both parents. Indeed, inadequate supplies of zinc, folate, antioxidants, and omega-3 fatty acids affect the quality of sperm. Overall, the periconceptional period is a time for good nutrition and careful lifestyle practices for mothers- and fathers-to-be.

✓ CONCEPT CHECK 14.8

1. Why are females of childbearing age encouraged to obtain 400 micrograms per day of folic acid from supplements or fortified foods?
2. What is the recommendation for seafood intake during pregnancy? How can you balance the health benefits of regular seafood consumption with concerns about environmental contaminants in fish?

Summary (Numbers refer to numbered sections in the chapter)

14.1 Energy imbalances can adversely affect fertility by altering hormone levels and promoting oxidative damage. Polycystic ovary syndrome, which tends to co-occur with upper-body obesity, is a condition of hormonal imbalance that causes infertility. Other than managing body weight, nutritional factors that may improve male and/or female fertility include adequate intakes of unsaturated fats, antioxidants, folate, iron, and zinc.

14.2 Pregnancy is arbitrarily divided into three trimesters of 13 to 14 weeks each. The first trimester is characterized by a rapid increase in cell number as the zygote grows to be an embryo, then a fetus. During the first trimester, the growing organism is most susceptible to damage from exposure to toxic agents or nutrient deficiencies. By the start of the second trimester, the organs and limbs have formed and will continue to grow and develop. The third trimester is marked by rapid fetal growth and storage of nutrients in preparation for life outside the womb.

14.3 A successful pregnancy results in optimal health for both the infant and the mother. Pregnancy success is defined as (1) gestation longer than 37 weeks and (2) birth weight greater than 5.5 pounds (2.5 kilograms). Factors that predict pregnancy success include early and regular prenatal care, maternal age within the range of 20 to 35 years, interpregnancy interval of at least 18 months, and adequate nutrient intake. Factors that contribute to poor pregnancy outcome include inadequate prenatal care, obesity, underweight, young age (<20 years), smoking, alcohol consumption, use of certain prescription medications and all illicit drugs, inadequate nutrient intake, heavy caffeine use, and various infections, such as listeriosis.

14.4 For females with a healthy prepregnancy BMI (18.5 to 24.9), total weight gain should be within the range of 25 to 35 pounds. Females who are underweight at conception and those carrying multiple fetuses should gain more; females who are overweight or obese at conception should gain less. During the first trimester, although they need not increase the quantity of food consumed, females should focus on the quality of the dietary pattern to meet increased requirements for protein, carbohydrate, essential fatty acids, fiber, water, and many vitamins and minerals. A female typically needs an additional 350 to 450 kcal per day during the second and third trimesters.

14.5 Following a plan based on the *Dietary Guidelines* as exemplified by MyPlate is recommended during pregnancy and breastfeeding. The mother-to-be should especially emphasize good sources of vitamin B-6, folate, vitamin D, iron, zinc, and calcium. Vegetarian dietary patterns are safe during pregnancy, but mothers following a vegan dietary plan should specifically seek out good sources of iron, zinc, calcium, vitamin D, vitamin B-12, and omega-3 fatty acids. Prenatal multivitamin and mineral supplements are useful for meeting increased nutrient requirements during pregnancy.

14.6 Gestational hypertension, gestational diabetes, heartburn, constipation, nausea, vomiting, edema, and anemia are all possible discomforts and complications of pregnancy. Nutrition therapy can help minimize some of these problems.

14.7 Almost all females are physically able to breastfeed their infants. For the infant, the advantages of breastfeeding (compared to formula feeding) are numerous, including fewer infections, reduced risk of atopic diseases, and lower rates of obesity and type 2 diabetes throughout life. Benefits for the mother include reduced risk of certain cancers, earlier recovery from pregnancy, and faster return to prepregnancy weight. When medical conditions of the mother (e.g., AIDS) or infant (e.g., galactosemia) preclude breastfeeding or if the mother chooses not to breastfeed, infants can be adequately nourished with formula.

14.8 During pregnancy, females can take several steps to reduce the risk of birth defects. They should achieve a healthy body weight before pregnancy. Adequate intakes of folic acid, iodine, and antioxidant nutrients are essential for prevention of many types of birth defects. Excesses of vitamin A and caffeine should be avoided. There is no safe level of alcohol intake known during pregnancy. Dietary control of diseases (e.g., diabetes and PKU) will also protect the fetus.

Check Your Knowledge (Answers are available at the end of this question set)

1. Which of the following nutrition interventions is most likely to improve fertility?
    a. Taking a vitamin E supplement
    b. Losing excess body fat
    c. Consuming a low-carbohydrate diet
    d. Taking an iron supplement

2. Increased carbohydrate needs during pregnancy are set to
    a. prevent ketosis.
    b. alleviate nausea.
    c. prevent gestational hypertension.
    d. supply adequate folate.

3. An infant born at 38 weeks' gestation weighing 5 pounds can be described as
    a. preterm.   c. SGA.
    b. LBW.   d. LBW and SGA.

4. Brianna is 5 feet 2 inches tall and weighs 150 pounds before becoming pregnant. How much weight should she gain during pregnancy?
    a. 28 to 40 pounds (12.5 to 18 kilograms)
    b. 25 to 35 pounds (11.5 to 16 kilograms)
    c. 15 to 25 pounds (7 to 11.5 kilograms)
    d. As little as possible

5. Benefits of physical activity during pregnancy include
    a. preventing excessive gestational weight gain.
    b. improved sleep.
    c. lower risk for gestational diabetes.
    d. all of these.

6. Which of the following may help to alleviate nausea during pregnancy?
    a. Postponing meals until the afternoon
    b. Drinking large amounts of water
    c. Postponing use of iron supplements until the second trimester
    d. All of these

7. Silvia breastfeeds her 8-month-old infant. She should consume approximately _____ extra kcal per day above her prepregnancy energy requirements.
    a. 200
    b. 400
    c. 700
    d. 1000

8. An eating pattern for a female in the third trimester of pregnancy differs from the prepregnancy dietary plan in that
    a. fluid needs are higher.
    b. protein requirements are higher.
    c. there are more servings from the grains group.
    d. all of these apply.

9. Advantages of breastfeeding include
    a. decreased ear infections in the infant.
    b. decreased diarrheal diseases in the infant.
    c. decreased risk of breast cancer for the mother.
    d. all of these.

10. Consuming a single cup of coffee per day is associated with
    a. spontaneous abortion.
    b. LBW.
    c. birth defects.
    d. none of these.

Answer Key: 1. b (LO 14.1), 2. a (LO 14.2), 3. d (LO 14.3), 4. c (LO 14.4), 5. d (LO 14.5), 6. c (LO 14.6), 7. b (LO 14.7), 8. d (LO 14.8), 9. d (LO 14.9), 10. d (LO 14.10)

Study Questions (Numbers refer to Learning Outcomes)

1. Provide three key pieces of nutrition advice for a couple seeking to maximize their chances of conceiving. Why did you identify those specific factors? **(LO 14.1)**
2. Identify four key nutrients for which intake should be significantly increased during pregnancy. **(LO 14.2)**
3. Describe some nutritional concerns related to teenage pregnancy. **(LO 14.3)**
4. Outline current weight-gain recommendations for pregnancy. What is the basis for these recommendations? **(LO 14.4)**
5. Suggest several safe exercises for an individual who is pregnant. **(LO 14.5)**
6. What nutrition advice would you give to a friend who experiences nausea during pregnancy? **(LO 14.6)**
7. Describe the physiological mechanisms that stimulate human milk production and release. How can knowing about these help mothers breastfeed successfully? **(LO 14.7)**
8. Starting in the second trimester of pregnancy, a female typically needs 350 to 450 kcal in excess of usual needs. Suggest a combination of nutrient-dense foods that would supply these extra calories. **(LO 14.8)**
9. Provide three reasons a new mother should give serious consideration to breastfeeding the infant. **(LO 14.9)**
10. Describe the importance of consuming adequate folic acid before and during pregnancy. **(LO 14.10)**

References

1. Infertility. Division of Reproductive Health, National Center for Chronic Disease Prevention and Health Promotion. Updated April 26, 2023. Accessed November 29, 2023. https://www.cdc.gov/reproductivehealth/infertility/index.htm
2. Gaskins AJ, Chavarro JE. Diet and fertility: a review. *Am J Obstet Gynecol.* 2018 Apr;218(4):379-389. doi: 10.1016/j.ajog.2017.08.010
3. Practice Committee of the American Society for Reproductive Medicine. Obesity and reproduction: a committee opinion. *Fertil Steril.* 2021 Nov;116(5):1266-1285. doi: 10.1016/j.fertnstert.2021.08.018
4. Polycystic ovary syndrome. Office on Women's Health. Updated February 22, 2021. Accessed November 29, 2023. https://www.womenshealth.gov/a-z-topics/polycystic-ovary-syndrome
5. Teede H, Tay CT, Laven J, et al. *International Evidence-Based Guideline for Assessment and Management of Polycystic Ovary Syndrome.* Melbourne, Australia: Monash University; 2023. https://www.monash.edu/__data/assets/pdf_file/0003/3379521/Evidence-Based-Guidelines-2023.pdf
6. Salas-Huetos A, Bulló M, Salas-Salvadó J. Dietary patterns, foods and nutrients in male fertility parameters and fecundability: a systematic review of observational studies. *Hum Reprod Update.* 2017 Jul 1;23(4):371-389. doi: 10.1093/humupd/dmx006
7. Fallah A, Mohammad-Hasani, Colagar AH. Zinc is an essential element for male fertility: a review of Zn roles in men's health, germination, sperm quality, and fertilization. *J Reprod Infertil.* Apr-Jun 2018;19(2):69-81. PMID: 30009140
8. Schisterman EF, Sjaarda LA, Clemons T, et al. Effect of folic acid and zinc supplementation in men on semen quality and live birth among couples undergoing fertility treatment: a randomized clinical trial. *JAMA.* 2020 Jan 7;323(1):35-48. doi: 10.1001/jama.2019.18714
9. Chavarro JE, Rich-Edwards JW, Rosner BA, Willett WC. Diet and lifestyle in the prevention of ovulatory disorder infertility. *Obstet Gynecol.* 2007 Nov;110(5):1050-1058. doi: 10.1097/01.AOG.0000287293.25465.e1
10. American College of Obstetricians and Gynecologists' Committee on Practice Bulletins—Gynecology. ACOG Practice Bulletin No. 200: early pregnancy loss. *Obstet Gynecol.* 2018 Nov;132(5):e197-e207. doi: 10.1097/AOG.0000000000002899
11. Koletzko B, Godfrey KM, Poston L, et al.; Early Nutrition Project Systematic Review Group. Nutrition during pregnancy, lactation and early childhood and its implications for maternal and long-term child health: The Early Nutrition Project recommendations. *Ann Nutr Metab.* 2019;74(2):93-106. doi: 10.1159/000496471
12. Low birth weight. March of Dimes. Updated June 2021. Accessed November 30, 2023. https://www.marchofdimes.org/complications/low-birthweight.aspx
13. Beam AL, Fried I, Palmer N, et al. Estimates of healthcare spending for preterm and low-birthweight infants in a commercially insured population: 2008-2016. *J Perinatol.* 2020 Jul;40(7):1091-1099. doi: 10.1038/s41372-020-0635-z
14. Mortality rate, infant (per 1,000 live births). World Bank. Accessed November 30, 2023. https://data.worldbank.org/indicator/SP.DYN.IMRT.IN
15. Increase the proportion of pregnant women who receive early and adequate prenatal care - MICH-08. Office of Disease Prevention and Health Promotion. 2021. Accessed December 1, 2023. https://health.gov/healthypeople/objectives-and-data/browse-objectives/pregnancy-and-childbirth/increase-proportion-pregnant-women-who-receive-early-and-adequate-prenatal-care-mich-08/data
16. Trends in teen pregnancy and childbearing. U.S. Department of Health & Human Services, Office of Population Affairs. Accessed December 1, 2023. https://opa.hhs.gov/adolescent-health/reproductive-health-and-teen-pregnancy/trends-teen-pregnancy-and-childbearing
17. Leftwich HK, Alves MVO. Adolescent pregnancy. *Pediatr Clin North Am.* 2017 Apr;64(2):381-388. doi: 10.1016/j.pcl.2016.11.007
18. Marshall NE, Abrams B, Barbour LA, et al. The importance of nutrition in pregnancy and lactation: lifelong consequences. *Am J Obstet Gynecol.* 2022;226(5):607-632. doi:10.1016/j.ajog.2021.12.035
19. Teenage pregnancy. March of Dimes. Updated July 2012. Accessed March 1, 2024. https://www.marchofdimes.org/glue/materials/teenage-pregnancy.pdf
20. Sauer MV. Reproduction at an advanced maternal age and maternal health. *Fertil Steril.* 2015 May;103(5):1136-1143. doi: 10.1016/j.fertnstert.2015.03.004
21. Pregnancy at age 35 years or older: ACOG Obstetric Care Consensus No. 11 *Obstet Gynecol.* 2022;140(2):348-366. doi:10.1097/AOG.0000000000004873
22. American College of Obstetricians and Gynecologists; Society for Maternal-Fetal Medicine. Obstetric Care Consensus No. 8: interpregnancy care. *Obstet Gynecol.* 2019 Jan;133(1):e51-e72. doi: 10.1097/AOG.0000000000003025

23. Medicine and pregnancy. Centers for Disease Control and Prevention. Updated April 10, 2023. Accessed December 1, 2023. https://www.cdc.gov/pregnancy/meds/treatingfortwo/

24. Listeria and pregnancy. American College of Obstetricians and Gynecologists. August 2022. Accessed December 1, 2023. https://www.acog.org/womens-health/faqs/listeria-and-pregnancy

25. Mohammadi M, Maroufizadeh S, Omani-Samani R, Almasi-Hashiani A, Amini P. The effect of prepregnancy body mass index on birth weight, preterm birth, cesarean section, and preeclampsia in pregnant women. *J Matern Fetal Neonatal Med.* 2019 Nov;32(22):3818-3823. doi: 10.1080/14767058.2018.1473366

26. Lisonkova S, Muraca GM, Potts J, et al. Association between prepregnancy body mass index and severe maternal morbidity. *JAMA.* 2017 Nov 14;318(18):1777-1786. doi: 10.1001/jama.2017.16191

27. Schultz DJ, Shanks CB, Houghtaling B. The impact of the 2009 Special Supplemental Nutrition Program for Women, Infants, and Children food package revisions on participants: a systematic review. *J Acad Nutr Diet.* 2015 Nov;115(11):1832-1846. doi: 10.1016/j.jand.2015.06.381

28. WIC program. U.S. Department of Agriculture, Economic Research Service. Updated July 19, 2023. Accessed December 2, 2023. https://www.ers.usda.gov/topics/food-nutrition-assistance/wic-program/

29. National Academies of Sciences, Engineering, and Medicine. *Dietary Reference Intakes for Energy.* Washington, DC: The National Academies Press. January 17, 2023. https://doi.org/10.17226/26818.

30. Physical activity and exercise during pregnancy and the postpartum period: ACOG Committee Opinion Summary, Number 804. *Obstet Gynecol.* 2020 Apr;135(4):991-993. doi: 10.1097/AOG.0000000000003773

31. Artal R. Exercise in pregnancy: guidelines. *Clin Obstet Gynecol.* 2016 Sep;59(3):639-644. doi: 10.1097/GRF.0000000000000223

32. U.S. Department of Health & Human Services. *Physical Activity Guidelines for Americans,* 2nd ed. 2018. Accessed January 31, 2020. https://health.gov/paguidelines/second-edition/pdf/Physical_Activity_Guidelines_2nd_edition.pdf

33. Ribeiro MM, Andrade A, Nunes I. Physical exercise in pregnancy: benefits, risks and prescription. *J Perinat Med.* 2021 Sep 6;50(1):4-17. doi: 10.1515/jpm-2021-0315

34. Rasmussen KM, Yaktine AL, eds.; Institute of Medicine; National Research Council. *Weight Gain During Pregnancy: Reexamining the Guidelines.* Washington, DC: National Academies Press; 2009.

35. Goldstein RF, Abell SK, Ranasinha S, et al. Association of gestational weight gain with maternal and infant outcomes: a systematic review and meta-analysis. *JAMA.* 2017 Jun 6;317(21):2207-2225. doi: 10.1001/jama.2017.3635

36. Stang J, Huffman LG. Position of the Academy of Nutrition and Dietetics: obesity, reproduction, and pregnancy outcomes. *J Acad Nutr Diet.* 2016 Apr;116(4):677-691. doi: 10.1016/j.jand.2016.01.008

37. Berenson AB, Pohlmeier AM, Laz TH, Rahman M, Saade G. Obesity risk knowledge, weight misperception, and diet and health-related attitudes among women intending to become pregnant. *J Acad Nutr Diet.* 2016 Apr;116(1):69-75. doi: 10.1016/j.jand.2015.04.023

38. Hamad R, Cohen AK, Rehkopf DH. Changing national guidelines is not enough: the impact of 1990 IOM recommendations on gestational weight gain among US women. *Int J Obes (Lond).* 2016 Oct;40(10):1529-1534. doi: 10.1038/ijo.2016.97

39. Kaiser LL, Campbell CG; Academy Positions Committee Workgroup. Practice paper of the Academy of Nutrition and Dietetics abstract: nutrition and lifestyle for a healthy pregnancy outcome. *J Acad Nutr Diet.* 2014 Sep;114(9):1447. doi: 10.1016/j.jand.2014.07.001

40. Emmett PM, Jones LR, Golding J. Pregnancy diet and associated outcomes in the Avon Longitudinal Study of Parents and Children. *Nutr Rev.* 2015 Oct;73(Suppl 3):154-174. doi: 10.1093/nutrit/nuv053

41. Firouzabadi FD, Shab-Bidar S, Jayedi A. The effects of omega-3 polyunsaturated fatty acids supplementation in pregnancy, lactation, and infancy: an umbrella review of meta-analyses of randomized trials. *Pharmacol Res.* 2022 Mar;177:106100. doi: 10.1016/j.phrs.2022.106100

42. Thompson M, Hein N, Hanson C, et al. Omega-3 fatty acid intake by age, gender, and pregnancy status in the United States: National Health and Nutrition Examination Survey 2003-2014. *Nutrients.* 2019 Jan 15;11(1):177. doi: 10.3390/nu11010177

43. Advice about eating fish: for those who might become or are pregnant or breastfeeding and children ages 1–11 years. U.S. Environmental Protection Agency; U.S. Food & Drug Administration. Revised October 2021. Accessed December 8, 2023. https://www.fda.gov/media/102331/download

44. McKenzie AL, Armstrong LE. Monitoring body water balance in pregnant and nursing women: the validity of urine color. *Ann Nutr Metab.* 2017;70(Suppl 1):18-22. doi: 10.1159/000462999

45. Gillman MW, Rifas-Shiman SL, Fernandez-Barres S, Kleinman K, Taveras EM, Oken E. Beverage intake during pregnancy and childhood adiposity. *Pediatrics.* 2017 Aug;140(2):e20170031. doi: 10.1542/peds.2017-0031

46. Jen V, Erler NS, Tielemans MJ, et al. Mothers' intake of sugar-containing beverages during pregnancy and body composition of their children during childhood: the Generation R Study. *Am J Clin Nutr.* 2017 Apr;105(4):834-841. doi: 10.3945/ajcn.116.147934

47. Procter SB, Campbell CG. Position of the Academy of Nutrition and Dietetics: nutrition and lifestyle for a healthy pregnancy outcome. *J Acad Nutr Diet.* 2014 Jul;114(7):1099-1103. doi: 10.1016/j.jand.2014.05.005

48. Pilz S, Zittermann A, Obeid R, et al. The role of vitamin D in fertility and during pregnancy and lactation: a review of clinical data. *Int J Environ Res Public Health.* 2018 Oct 12;15(10):2241. doi: 10.3390/ijerph15102241

49. U.S. Department of Agriculture; U.S. Department of Health & Human Services. *Dietary Guidelines for Americans, 2020–2025.* 9th ed. December 2020. http://DietaryGuidelines.gov

50. ACOG Committee Opinion No. 495: vitamin D: screening and supplementation during pregnancy. American College of Obstetricians and Gynecologists. July 2011. Reaffirmed 2021. Accessed March 19, 2022. https://www.acog.org/clinical/clinical-guidance/committee-opinion/articles/2011/07/vitamin-d-screening-and-supplementation-during-pregnancy

51. Grieger JA, Clifton VL. A review of the impact of dietary intakes in human pregnancy on infant birthweight. *Nutrients.* 2014 Dec;7(1):153-178. doi: 10.3390/nu7010153

52. Banjari I. Iron deficiency anemia and pregnancy. In: Khan J, ed. *Current Topics in Anemia.* Croatia: InTech; 2018. doi: 10.5772/intechopen.69114

53. Blumfield ML, Hure AJ, Macdonald-Wicks L, Smith R, Collins CE. A systematic review and meta-analysis of micronutrient intakes during pregnancy in developed countries. *Nutr Rev.* 2013 Feb;71(2):118-132. doi: 10.1111/nure.12003

54. Cantor AG, Bougatsos C, Dana T, Blazina I, McDonagh M. Routine iron supplementation and screening for iron deficiency anemia in pregnancy: a systematic review for the U.S. Preventive Services Task Force. *Ann Intern Med.* 2015 Apr 21;162(8):566-576. doi: 10.7326/M14-2932

55. Haider BA, Bhutta ZA. Multiple-micronutrient supplementation for women during pregnancy. *Cochrane Database Syst Rev.* 2017 Apr 13;4(4):CD004905. doi: 10.1002/14651858.CD004905.pub5

56. Lowensohn RI, Stadler DD, Naze C. Current concepts of maternal nutrition. *Obstet Gynecol Surv.* 2016 Aug;71(7):413-426. doi: 10.1097/OGX.0000000000000329

57. Blau LE, Lipsky LM, Dempster KW, et al. Women's experience and understanding of food cravings in pregnancy: a qualitative study in women receiving prenatal care at the University of North Carolina–Chapel Hill. *J Acad Nutr Diet.* 2020 May;120(5):815-824. doi: 10.1016/j.jand.2019.09.020

58. Melina V, Craig W, Levin S. Position of the Academy of Nutrition and Dietetics: vegetarian diets. *J Acad Nutr Diet.* 2016 Dec;116(12):1970-1980. doi: 10.1016/j.jand.2016.09.025

59. Altuwaijri M. Evidence-based treatment recommendations for gastroesophageal reflux disease during pregnancy: a review. *Medicine (Baltimore).* 2022;101(35):e30487. doi:10.1097/MD.0000000000030487

60. McParlin C, O'Donnell A, Robson SC, et al. Treatments for hyperemesis gravidarum and nausea and vomiting in pregnancy: a systematic review. *JAMA.* 2016 Oct 4;316(13):1392-1401. doi: 10.1001/jama.2016.14337

61. ACOG Practice Bulletin No. 189 summary: nausea and vomiting of pregnancy. *Obstet Gynecol.* 2018 Jan;131(1):190-193. doi: 10.1097/AOG.0000000000002450

62. London V, Grube S, Sherer DM, Abulafia O. Hyperemesis gravidarum: a review of recent literature. *Pharmacology.* 2017;100(3-4):161-171. doi: 10.1159/000477853

63. American College of Obstetrics and Gynecologists. ACOG Practice Bulletin No. 95: anemia in pregnancy. *Obstet Gynecol.* 2008 Jul;112(1):201-207. doi: 10.1097/AOG.0b013e3181809c0d

64. Gestational diabetes. Centers for Disease Control and Prevention. Updated December 30, 2022. Accessed December 6, 2023. https://www.cdc.gov/diabetes/basics/gestational.html

65. ElSayed NA, Aleppo G, Aroda VR, et al. 15. Management of Diabetes in Pregnancy: Standards of Care in Diabetes-2023. *Diabetes Care.* 2023;46(Suppl 1):S254-S266. doi:10.2337/dc23-S015

66. Ikoh Rph CL, Tang Tinong R. The incidence and management of type 2 diabetes mellitus after gestational diabetes mellitus. *Cureus.* 2023;15(8):e44468. Published 2023 Aug 31. doi:10.7759/cureus.44468

67. Doughty KN, Taylor SN. Barriers and benefits to breastfeeding with gestational diabetes. *Semin Perinatol.* 2021 Mar;45(2):151385. doi: 10.1016/j.semperi.2020.151385

68. Ong YY, Pang WW, Huang JY, et al. Breastfeeding may benefit cardiometabolic health of children exposed to increased gestational glycemia in utero. *Eur J Nutr.* 2022;61(5):2383-2395. doi: 10.1007/s00394-022-02800-7

69. High blood pressure during pregnancy. Centers for Disease Control and Prevention. Updated June 19, 2023. Accessed December 7, 2023. https://www.cdc.gov/bloodpressure/pregnancy.htm

70. Wilkerson RG, Ogunbodede AC. Hypertensive disorders of pregnancy. *Emerg Med Clin North Am.* 2019 May;37(2):301-316. doi: 10.1016/j.emc.2019.01.008

71. Achamrah N, Ditisheim A. Nutritional approach to preeclampsia prevention. *Curr Opin Clin Nutr Metab Care.* 2018 May;21(3):168-173. doi: 10.1097/MCO.0000000000000462

72. O'Callaghan KM, Kiely M. Systematic review of vitamin D and hypertensive disorders of pregnancy. *Nutrients.* 2018 Mar 1;10(3):294. doi: 10.3390/nu10030294

73. Asayama K, Imai Y. The impact of salt intake during and after pregnancy. *Hypertens Res.* 2018 Jan;41(1):1-5. doi: 10.1038/hr.2017.90

74. Sakuyama H, Katoh M, Wakabayashi H, Zulli A, Kruzliak P, Uehara Y. Influence of gestational salt restriction in fetal growth and in development of diseases in adulthood. *J Biomed Sci.* 2016 Jan 20;23:12. doi: 10.1186/s12929-016-0233-8

75. Lessen R, Kavanagh K. Position of the Academy of Nutrition and Dietetics: promoting and supporting breastfeeding. *J Acad Nutr Diet.* 2015 Mar;115(e):444-449. doi: 10.1016/j.jand.2014.12.014

76. Meek JY, Noble L. Technical report: breastfeeding and the use of human milk. *Pediatrics.* 2022 Jul;150(1):e2022057989. doi: 10.1542/peds.2022-057989

77. World Health Organization; UNICEF. *Global Strategy for Infant and Young Child Feeding.* 2003. Accessed December 7, 2023. https://apps.who.int/iris/rest/bitstreams/50491/retrieve

78. Breastfeeding report card. Centers for Disease Control and Prevention. 2022. Updated August 31, 2022. Accessed December 7, 2023. https://www.cdc.gov/breastfeeding/data/reportcard.htm

79. Holt K, Wooldridge N, Storuy M, Sofka D. *Bright Futures: Nutrition.* 3rd ed. Elk Grove Village, IL: American Academy of Pediatrics; 2011.

80. Okburan G, Kızıler S. Human milk oligosaccharides as prebiotics. *Pediatr Neonatol.* 2023;64(3):231-238. doi:10.1016/j.pedneo.2022.09.017

81. Brockway MM, Daniel AI, Reyes SM, et al. Human milk bioactive components and child growth and body composition in the first 2 years: a systematic review. *Adv Nutr.* 2024;15(1):100127. doi:10.1016/j.advnut.2023.09.015

82. Plaza-Diaz J, Fontana L, Gil A. Human milk oligosaccharides and immune system development. *Nutrients.* 2018 Aug;10(8):1038. doi: 10.3390/nu10081038

83. Berger PK, Ong ML, Bode L, Belfort MB. Human milk oligosaccharides and infant neurodevelopment: a narrative review. *Nutrients.* 2023;15(3):719. doi:10.3390/nu15030719

84. U.S. Department of Health and Human Services, Office on Women's Health. *Your Guide to Breastfeeding.* February 4, 2022. Accessed December 8, 2023. https://www.womenshealth.gov/your-guide-to-breastfeeding

85. Rosas-Salazar C, Shilts MH, Tang Z-Z, et al. Exclusive breast-feeding, the early-life microbiome and immune response, and common childhood respiratory illnesses. *J Allergy Clin Immunol.* 2022;150(3):612-621. doi: 10.1016/j.jaci.2022.02.023

86. Greer FR, Sicherer SH, Burks AW; Committee on Nutrition; Section on Allergy and Immunology. The effects of early nutritional interventions on the development of atopic disease in infants and children: the role of maternal dietary restriction, breastfeeding, hydrolyzed formulas, and timing of introduction of allergenic complementary foods. *Pediatrics.* 2019 Apr;143(4):e20190281. doi: 10.1542/peds.2019-0281

87. Abdulwudud OA, Snow ME. Interventions in the workplace to support breastfeeding for women in employment. *Cochrane Database Syst Rev.* 2012 Oct 17;10(10):CD006177. doi: 10.1002/14651858.CD006177.pub3

88. Wagner CL, Greer FR; American Academy of Pediatrics Section on Breastfeeding; American Academy of Pediatrics Committee on Nutrition. Prevention of rickets and vitamin D deficiency in infants, children, and adolescents. *Pediatrics.* 2008 Nov;122(5):1142-1152. doi: 10.1542/peds.2008-1862

89. Hollis BW, Wagner CL, Howard CR, et al. Maternal versus infant vitamin D supplementation during lactation: a randomized controlled trial [published correction appears in *Pediatrics.* 2019 Jul;144(1):e20191063]. *Pediatrics.* 2015 Oct;136(4):625-634. doi: 10.1542/peds.2015-1669

90. Baker RD, Greer FR; American Academy of Pediatrics, Committee on Nutrition. Diagnosis and prevention of iron deficiency and iron-deficiency anemia in infants and young children (0-3 years of age). *Pediatrics.* 2010 Nov;126(5):1040-1050. doi: 10.1542/peds.2010-2576

91. Lewis CW. Fluoride and dental caries prevention in children. *Pediatr Rev.* 2014 Jan;35(1):3-15. doi: 10.1542/pir.35-1-3

92. Baroni L, Goggi S, Battaglino R, et al. Vegan nutrition for mothers and children: practical tools for healthcare providers. *Nutrients.* 2018 Dec;11(1):5. doi: 10.3390/nu11010005

93. Data & statistics on birth defects. Centers for Disease Control and Prevention. Updated June 28, 2023. Accessed December 8, 2023. https://www.cdc.gov/ncbddd/birthdefects/data.html

94. van Gool JD, Hirche H, Lax H, De Schaepdrijver L. Folic acid and primary prevention of neural tube defects: a review. *Reprod Toxicol.* 2018 Sep;80:73-84. doi: 10.1016/j.reprotox.2018.05.004

95. Pearce EN, Lazarus JH, Moreno-Reyes R, Zimmermann MB. Consequences of iodine deficiency and excess in pregnant women: an overview of current knowns and unknowns. *Am J Clin Nutr.* 2016 Sep;104(Suppl 3):918S-923S. doi: 10.3945/ajcn.115.110429

96. Tinker SC, Gilboa SM, Moore CA, et al.; National Birth Defects Prevention Study. Specific birth defects in pregnancies of women with diabetes: National Birth Defects Prevention Study, 1997-2011. *Am J Obstet Gynecol.* 2020 Feb;222(2):176.e1-176.e11. doi: 10.1016/j.ajog.2019.08.028

97. Committee on Genetics. Policy Statement: maternal phenylketonuria. *Pediatrics.* 2008 Aug;122(2):445-449. Reaffirmed January 2013. doi: 10.1542/peds.2008-1485

98. Viteri OA, Soto EE, Bahado-Singh RO, Christensen CW, Chauhan SP, Sibai BM. Fetal anomalies and long-term effects associated with substance abuse in pregnancy: a literature review. *Am J Perinatol.* 2015 Apr;32(5):405-416. doi: 10.1055/s-0034-1393932

Design Element Credits: Fact Check/magnifying glass icon: McGraw Hill; Magnificent Microbiome background image: Alena Ohneva/Shutterstock; Sustainable Solutions icon: McGraw Hill; Roots icon: McGraw Hill; Medicine Cabinet icon: Peter Dazeley/Photographer's Choice/Getty Images

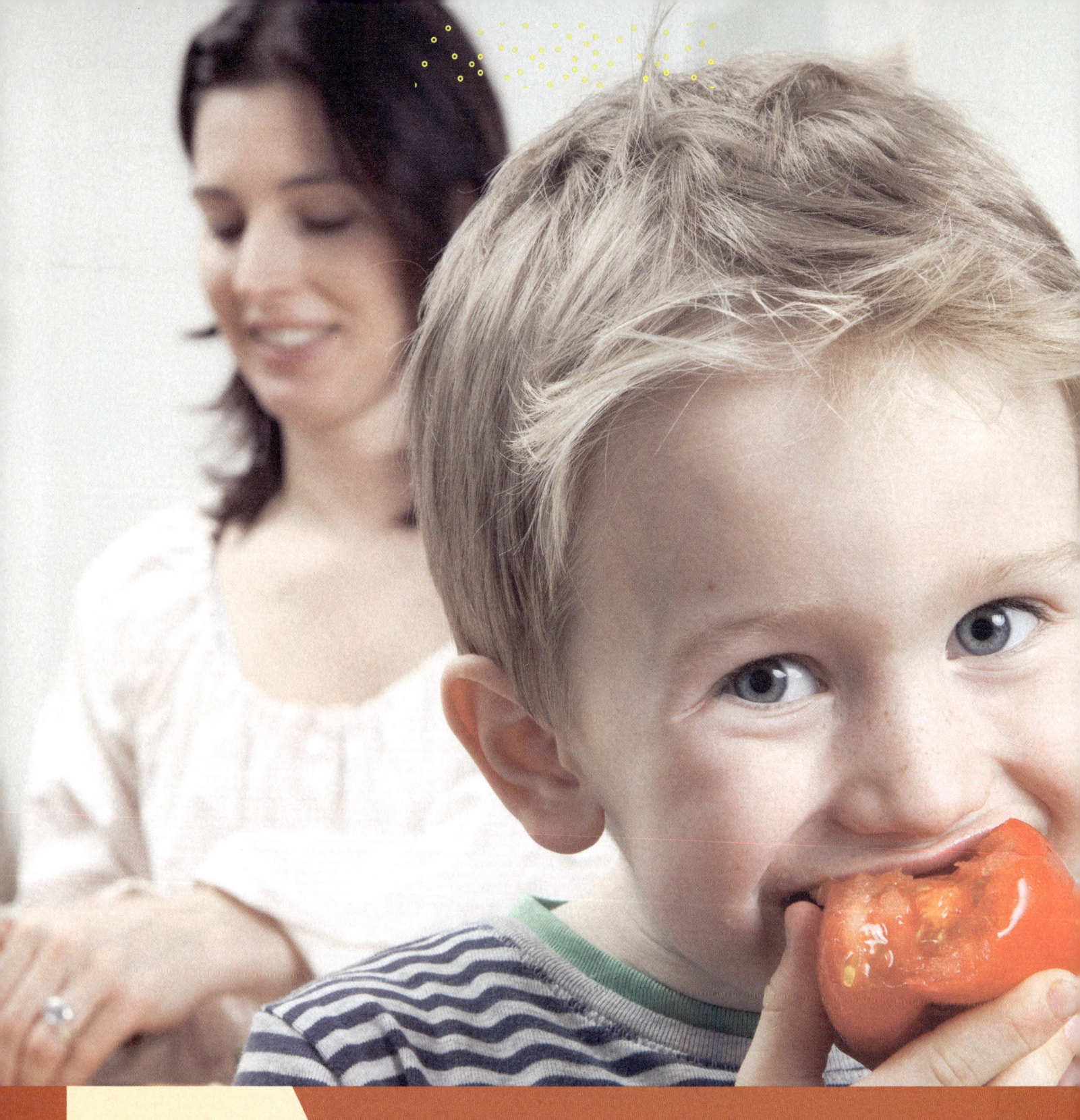

Chapter 15
Nutrition from Infancy Through Adolescence

Student Learning Outcomes

Chapter 15 is designed to allow you to:

15.1 Describe the impact of nutrition on growth and physiological development from infancy through adolescence.

15.2 List specific nutrients often found to be lacking in the dietary patterns of infants, toddlers, preschoolers, school-age children, and teenagers.

15.3 Identify appropriate dietary strategies to meet the nutritional needs for normal growth and development for infants.

15.4 Outline strategies to promote healthy eating behaviors during childhood and adolescence.

15.5 Describe the long-term effects of childhood obesity and suggest ways to prevent or treat the problem.

15.6 Identify common food allergens and suggest practices that may reduce the risk of food allergies.

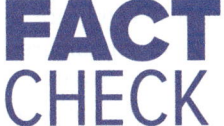

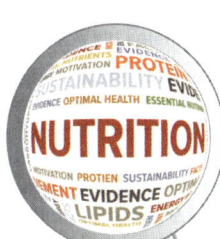

Do toddlers need special toddler drinks to meet nutrient needs?

Toddler drinks or "transition formulas," which are often packaged like infant formulas, may be perceived as a healthy step for child feeding after weaning from breast milk or infant formula. However, child nutrition experts do not advocate regular use of these products. Weaning is a critical time to expose children to a variety of tastes and textures. These sweet beverages may blunt the appetite and decrease the child's acceptance of foods at meals. Most provide added sugars and have less protein than cow's milk. Instead of relying on toddler drinks, offer water or milk to drink and provide a variety of nutrient-dense options at five or six meals or snacks each day. Let the child learn to rely on *whole foods* to meet nutrient needs! Read more about planning a healthy eating pattern for toddlers in Section 15.4.

Source: Lott M, Callahan E, Welker Duffy E, Story M, Daniels S. *Healthy Beverage Consumption in Early Childhood: Recommendations from Key National Health and Nutrition Organizations.* Technical Scientific Report. Durham, NC: Healthy Eating Research; 2019. http://healthyeatingresearch.org

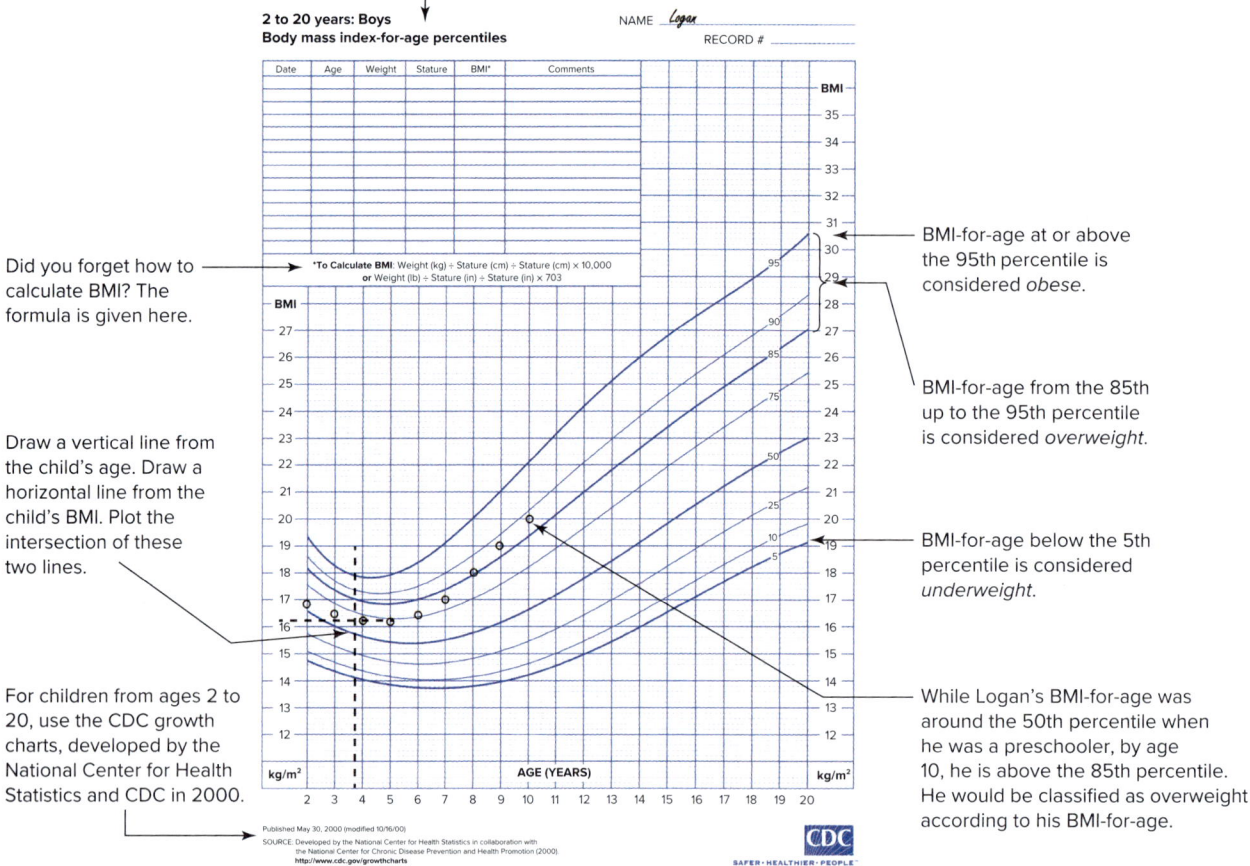

FIGURE 15-2 BMI-for-age plotted for a young male (Logan) up to age 10. See Table 15-1 for more information about interpreting BMI-for-age.
Centers for Disease Control and Prevention, based on WHO Child Growth Standards (2009)

PEDIATRIC MALNUTRITION (UNDERNUTRITION)

The human body needs a lot more food (per pound of body weight) to support growth and development than it does to merely maintain its size once growth ceases. Along with adequate energy, a few key nutrients are particularly important during these years: protein, calcium, iron, and zinc. When nutrients are missing at critical phases of this process, growth and development may slow or even stop.

Pediatric malnutrition is an imbalance between nutrient requirements and nutrient intake that leads to deficits of energy, protein, or micronutrients.[3] Depending on their severity, timing, and duration, such deficits may negatively affect growth, development, and long-term physical, mental, and socioeconomic outcomes. Please note, although malnutrition includes both undernutrition and overnutrition, the term *pediatric malnutrition* is usually used to describe undernutrition.

Pediatric malnutrition may be acute or chronic. A period of malnutrition lasting less than 3 months is considered acute. This may occur if a brief illness leads to low food intake, weight loss, and wasting. Chronic malnutrition lasts for 3 months or longer and may be evident as stunting, in which the child does not experience expected gains in stature.[4]

Sometimes, pediatric malnutrition is related to an *illness* that increases the needs for calories and nutrients and/or decreases the ability to ingest, digest, or absorb nutrients. For example, a child who needs a breathing tube for a lung disease may not be able to consume adequate nutrients by mouth. Even if a child consumes enough food and beverages, growth may still falter if there are digestive disorders, such as celiac disease,

pediatric malnutrition An imbalance between nutrient requirements and nutrient intake that results in cumulative deficits of energy, protein, or micronutrients and may negatively impact growth, development, and other physical and mental health outcomes; also called *pediatric undernutrition*.

which, if left untreated, can compromise nutrient absorption. Some medical conditions, such as heart or lung disorders, lead to greatly increased energy requirements. Other times, pediatric malnutrition is caused by *social or environmental conditions,* such as food insecurity, parental neglect, or eating disorders. For example, needing to stretch food dollars, caregivers may overdilute formula—a detrimental practice that fills the child's stomach without providing adequate calories.

Nutritional deficits at any stage of life can be detrimental to health, but children under 5 years of age are particularly vulnerable because this should be a stage of rapid growth and development. Globally, about one in five children under 5 years of age are short and underweight for their ages.[5] Pediatric malnutrition is at the root of an estimated 45% of child deaths around the world.[6] In developing nations, poverty and famine are major causes of pediatric malnutrition. In developed nations, it is most often related to a medical condition.[4]

As with the fetus in utero, nutritional problems in infancy and childhood may have enduring effects on health. An inadequate dietary pattern during a critical stage of infancy or childhood hinders the cell division that should occur at that stage. Mild zinc deficiencies, for example, have been linked to diminished growth and development during childhood.[7] Unfortunately, improving dietary patterns after a period of nutrient deficiency will not completely compensate for losses in physical or mental development because the hormonal and other conditions needed for growth will not likely be present. In addition, gains in height are no longer possible after the skeleton reaches full maturity. This happens as growth plates at the ends of the bones fuse, starting around 14 years of age in females and 15 years of age in males. This process is usually complete by age 19 in females and age 20 in males. Furthermore, muscles can increase in diameter later in life, but their linear growth is limited by the length of the bone.

For these reasons, a 15-year-old female who has experienced pediatric malnutrition and is only 4 feet 8 inches tall cannot attain the adult height of a typical American female simply by changing her dietary intake. Females experience their peak rate of growth right before the onset of menstrual periods. Once the time for growth ceases (for females, this is about 5 years after they start menstruating), adequate nutrient intake helps maintain health and weight but cannot make up for missed growth in height.

Whatever the cause—and there may be multiple causes—the consequences of pediatric malnutrition are serious and long-lasting. Possible outcomes include poor physical growth, impaired mental development, and behavioral problems. When health professionals encounter an infant or child with faltering growth, the true causes must be identified and then treated. If the problem stems from a lack of financial resources, appropriate referrals to social services should be made. Counseling about proper nutrition and the importance of healthy parent–child interactions can help to get a child's growth back on track.

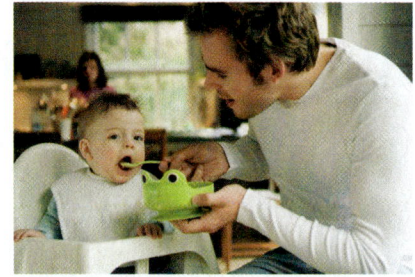

Having access to safe and nourishing food does not guarantee that a child will grow and thrive. Children also need a stimulating environment, a sense of security, and specific attention focused on them.
ONOKY-Photononstop/Alamy Stock Photo

OVERNUTRITION

When a child's BMI-for-age approaches the highest percentiles, caregivers should be concerned. A child from the 85th up to the 95th percentile for BMI-for-age is considered overweight. At or above the 95th percentile, a child is considered obese (Table 15-1).

Since 1970, researchers have speculated that overfeeding during infancy may increase the number of adipose tissue cells. Today, we know that the number of adipose cells can also increase with positive energy balance during adulthood. If energy intake is limited during infancy to minimize the number of adipose cells, the growth of other organ systems may also be severely restricted, especially brain and nervous system development. Furthermore, most infants who are overweight become normal-weight preschoolers without dietary restrictions. For these reasons, it is unwise for an infant's dietary pattern to be restrictive—especially related to fat intake. A healthy range of fat intake is 30% to 40% of total calories for ages 1 to 3 years and 25% to 35% of total calories for older children and teenagers.

TABLE 15-1 ■ Weight Status Classifications for Children, Ages 2 to 20

Weight Status Classifications	BMI-for-Age Percentile
Underweight	< 5th percentile
Healthy weight	5th up to 85th percentile
Overweight	85th up to 95th percentile
Obese	≥ 95th percentile

Source: Adapted from World Health Organization, 2018.

> ✓ **CONCEPT CHECK 15.1**
>
> 1. How do health care providers assess the growth of infants and children?
> 2. Define *pediatric malnutrition.* List two possible causes.
> 3. If a female adolescent is short for her age due to a brief period of undernutrition between ages 10 to 12, can she catch up in growth after proper nutrition is restored? Why or why not?
> 4. Define childhood overweight and obesity in terms of BMI-for-age.

15.2 Infant Nutritional Needs

Infants' nutritional needs vary as they grow. For the first 4 to 6 months of life, human milk or infant formula supplies all the required nutrients. Age-appropriate solid foods should be added to the infant's eating pattern around 6 months of age. (See the section "Expanding the Infant's Mealtime Choices" for additional guidance on the timing of introduction of solid foods.) Even after solid foods are added, the foundation of an infant's dietary pattern for the first year is still human milk or infant formula. Because of the critical importance of adequate nutrition in infancy and the difficulties encountered in feeding some infants, there is more discussion in this chapter on infancy than on the later periods of childhood.

ENERGY

Due to rapid growth and a high metabolic rate, the energy requirements per pound of body weight for an infant are the highest of any life stage. The sample calculations below show the estimated energy needs of a healthy male infant at 2, 6, and 12 months of age. See Appendix F for a complete set of EER equations for individuals at various stages of the life cycle.

Infants need a concentrated source of calories to meet these high demands. Exclusive feeding of either human milk or infant formula is ideal for the first 6 months of life; both are high in fat and supply about 640 kcal/quart (670 kcal/liter; Table 15-2). Beginning around 6 months of age, developmentally appropriate solid foods provide additional calories, nutrients, and variety for the developing infant.

> Gabriel is a male infant. Let's calculate his estimated energy needs as he grows.
>
> At 2 months, Gabriel was 22 inches (56 centimeters) long and weighed 12 pounds (5.4 kilograms).
>
> $$-716.45 - (1 \times age) + (17.82 \times height) + (15.06 \times weight) + \text{energy cost of growth}$$
>
> $$-716.45 - (1 \times 0.17) + (17.82 \times 56) + (15.06 \times 5.4) + 200 \text{ kcal} = 563 \text{ kcal}$$
>
> At 6 months, Gabriel was 26.5 inches (67.3 centimeters) long and weighed 18 pounds (8.2 kilograms).
>
> $$-716.45 - (1 \times age) + (17.82 \times height) + (15.06 \times weight) + \text{energy cost of growth}$$
>
> $$-716.45 - (1 \times 0.5) + (17.82 \times 67.3) + (15.06 \times 8.2) + 20 \text{ kcal} = 626 \text{ kcal}$$
>
> At 12 months, Gabriel was 30 inches (76.2 centimeters) long and weighed 22 pounds (10 kilograms).
>
> $$-716.45 - (1 \times age) + (17.82 \times height) + (15.06 \times weight) + \text{energy cost of growth}$$
>
> $$-716.45 - (1 \times 1) + (17.82 \times 76.2) + (15.06 \times 10) + 20 \text{ kcal} = 811 \text{ kcal}$$

TABLE 15-2 ■ Composition of Mature Human Milk, Cow's Milk, and Infant Formulas (per Liter)[a]

	Energy (kcal)	Protein (grams)	Fat (grams)	Carbohydrate (grams)	Minerals[b] (grams)
Milk					
Human milk	650–700[c]	9–12	32–36	67–78	2
Cow's milk, whole[d]	670	36	36	49	7
Cow's milk, fat-free[d]	360	36	1	51	7
Casein/Whey-Based Formulas					
Similac®	680	14	36	71	3
Enfamil®	670	15	37	69	3
Good Start®	670	16	34	73	3
Soybean Protein–Based Formulas					
ProSobee®	670	20	35	67	4
Isomil®	680	16	36	68	4

[a] At 3 months of age, infants typically consume 0.75 to 1 liter of human milk or formula per day.
[b] Calcium, phosphorus, and other minerals.
[c] Rough estimate; ranges from 650 to 700 kcal per liter.
[d] Not appropriate for infant feeding, based primarily on high protein and mineral content.

CARBOHYDRATES

Carbohydrate requirements in infancy are 60 grams per day from 0 to 6 months and 95 grams per day from 7 to 12 months. These needs are based on the typical intakes of human milk by breastfed infants and their eventual intake of solid foods. These carbohydrate goals are easily satisfied by a developmentally appropriate eating pattern.

Do infants need fiber? There is no set AI for fiber for infants younger than 1 year of age. For about the first 6 months of life, breast milk or formula, which contains no fiber, provides optimal nutrition. As solid foods are introduced, include some fruits, vegetables, and whole grains. Some experts recommend working up to about 5 grams of fiber per day by 1 year of age. Keep in mind that too much fiber can limit nutrient absorption because it binds to some minerals and speeds the passage of food through the GI tract. Let the child's bowel habits be your guide. If the child is constipated, try increasing fiber and fluid intakes. On the other hand, if the child is uncomfortably gassy or is having many soft bowel movements per day, decrease the amount of fiber in the dietary pattern.

PROTEIN

Daily protein needs in infancy are about 9 grams per day for younger infants and about 11 grams per day for older infants. These recommendations are based on the typical consumption of human milk by infants who are breastfed for 0 to 6 months and then on the increased protein needs for growth for older infants. About half of total protein intake should come from essential amino acids. As with carbohydrates, protein needs are easily satisfied by either human milk or infant formula. However, protein metabolism generates waste products that must be excreted by the kidneys. Dietary patterns that are excessive in protein may stress the infant's immature kidneys, so protein intake should not greatly exceed these recommendations.

In developed nations, protein deficiencies among infants are unlikely, except in cases of inappropriate formula preparation, such as when an infant's formula is excessively diluted with water. Protein deficiency may also be induced by elimination diets used to identify food allergies to certain foods. As foods are eliminated, infants may not be offered enough protein to compensate for that supplied by the suspected food allergen (see Section 15.7).

> **Quick Guide to Infant Macronutrient Needs**
>
> **Carbohydrates**
> - 0 to 6 months: 60 grams per day
> - 7 to 12 months: 95 grams per day
>
> **Protein**
> - 0 to 6 months: 9 grams per day
> - 7 to 12 months: 11 grams per day
>
> **Fat**
> - 0 to 6 months: 31 grams per day
> - 7 to 12 months: 30 grams per day

FAT

Fat makes up the largest proportion (about 50%) of an infant's overall energy intake during the first year of life. Infants need about 30 grams of fat per day. Essential fatty acids should make up about 15% of total fat intake (about 5 grams per day). Both recommendations are again based on the typical consumption of human milk by breastfed infants and the eventual intake of solid foods. Fats are an important part of the infant's dietary pattern because they are vital to the development of the nervous system. Also, fats are a concentrated source of energy (9 kcal per gram). The stomach capacity of an infant is limited, so a concentrated source of calories is necessary to meet overall energy requirements. Thus, restriction of fat intake is not advised for infants or children under age 2.

Arachidonic acid (ARA) and docosahexaenoic acid (DHA) are two fatty acids that have important roles in infant development. These fatty acids can be made in the body from the essential fatty acids or they can be supplied by foods. The nervous system, especially the brain and eyes, depends on these fatty acids for proper development. During the last trimester, DHA and ARA provided by the mother accumulate in the brain and retinas of the eyes in the fetus. Breastfed infants continue to acquire these fatty acids from human milk, especially if their mothers are regularly eating fish. Since 2002, infant formula manufacturers have been adding ARA and DHA to their products to match the average fatty acid composition of human milk. Such infant formulas are particularly useful for feeding preterm infants.[8]

VITAMINS OF SPECIAL INTEREST

All of the essential vitamins play important roles in infant growth and development, but three vitamins—K, D, and B-12—are of special interest for infants because stores of these nutrients tend to be low and the consequences of deficiency are dire.

Vitamin K. Newborn infants have low levels of vitamin K because (1) limited amounts of this vitamin are transferred from the mother to the fetus during gestation, (2) breast milk is not particularly high in vitamin K, and (3) newborn infants lack the intestinal bacteria that synthesize vitamin K. Infant vitamin K deficiency can lead to a rare but potentially fatal problem known as vitamin K deficiency bleeding. To prevent hemorrhage, vitamin K is routinely given by injection to all infants at birth.

Vitamin D. For bone health (to prevent rickets), immune function, and chronic disease prevention, the American Academy of Pediatrics (AAP) recommends that all infants and children consume 10 micrograms of vitamin D per day starting soon after birth. Supplemental vitamin D is necessary for all infants who are breastfed, as well as for formula-fed infants who consume less than 1 quart (approximately 1 liter) of formula per day.[9] However, no further benefits are seen beyond 10 micrograms per day, and toxicity is possible if intake exceeds 25 micrograms per day. Supplementation should continue until intake of vitamin D from other foods and beverages provides at least 10 micrograms per day.

Vitamin B-12. For infants who are breastfed by females who follow a vegan dietary pattern, ensuring adequate vitamin B-12 status is vitally important to prevent anemia and optimize growth and development (especially of the nervous system). Recall that vitamin B-12 is only found in foods of animal origin. Infant formula does contain vitamin B-12, but the breast milk of a mother who avoids all animal products may be deficient in vitamin B-12. A female who follows a vegan dietary pattern while breastfeeding should take care to obtain adequate vitamin B-12 from fortified foods or dietary supplements. If the mother's vitamin B-12 status is low, supplemental vitamin B-12 may be necessary for the infant.[10]

MINERALS OF SPECIAL INTEREST

Two minerals of special interest in the dietary patterns of infants are iron and fluoride. Infants also need adequate amounts of zinc and iodine to support growth. However, when human milk and infant formula are provided in quantities to meet energy needs, zinc and iodine requirements are generally met.

Iron. Infants are born with some internal stores of iron, transferred from the mother during the last few weeks of gestation. However, if food sources of iron are not part of the infant's dietary pattern, that stored iron will be depleted by about 6 months of age. If the mother was iron deficient during the pregnancy, the infant's iron stores will be exhausted even sooner. Iron-deficiency anemia can lead to poor cognitive development in infants. Several studies indicate that iron-deficiency anemia during infancy, even if corrected, has a lasting impact in terms of cognition, motor development, and behavior later in life.[11]

To maintain a desirable iron status, the AAP recommends that formula-fed infants should be fed an iron-fortified formula from birth.[12] In the past, low-iron formulas were sometimes recommended for infants with gastrointestinal distress, based upon the belief that iron is associated with constipation. However, current evidence shows that iron-free infant formulas do not improve GI symptoms in infants. In fact, use of low-iron infant formulas places an infant at risk for iron deficiency. Although they are still available, the use of low-iron infant formula is strongly discouraged.

Breast milk is lower in iron than fortified infant formulas, but the form of iron in breast milk is much more bioavailable than the form in infant formula. Even so, by about 6 months of age, breastfed infants need solid foods to supply extra iron. This need for iron is a major consideration in the decision to introduce **complementary foods**. To prevent iron deficiency, the AAP recommends that exclusively breastfed infants should receive iron supplements starting at 4 months of age and continuing until dietary sources of iron are introduced. Preterm and low-birth-weight infants, those with blood disorders, or infants born to mothers who have iron-deficiency anemia or diabetes may need higher levels of supplemental iron.[13]

complementary foods Solid or semi-solid foods that are introduced to an infant's dietary pattern to complement (not replace) breast milk or infant formula during the latter part of the first year of life. These foods provide energy and essential nutrients to meet the infant's requirements for growth and development.

Fluoride. Breast milk is a poor source of fluoride, and formula manufacturers use fluoride-free water in formula preparation, so intake of this mineral during the first 6 months of life is low. However, fluoride supplementation is not advised before 6 months of age. After 6 months, the pediatrician or dentist may recommend fluoride supplements to aid in tooth development if fluoride supplied by tap water, foods, and toothpaste is inadequate.[14]

The American Dental Association does not recommend fluoridated bottled water for use by infants because it heightens the risk for enamel fluorosis during early tooth development.

WATER

An infant needs about 3 cups (700 to 800 milliliters) of water per day to regulate body temperature and transport oxygen, nutrients, and wastes throughout the body. For the vast majority of infants, human milk or formula supplies enough water to keep the infant well hydrated.

In infants, dehydration can occur rapidly and have devastating consequences. In the first few days after birth, improper feeding techniques can leave an infant deprived of water and nutrients. In addition, protracted episodes of vomiting or diarrhea can quickly deplete an infant of fluid and electrolytes.

To identify dehydration, look for these signs:[15]

- More than 6 hours without a wet diaper
- Dark-yellow or strong-smelling urine
- Unusually tired and fussy
- Dry mouth and lips
- Absence of tears when crying
- Eyes and soft spot on the head appear sunken
- Cold and splotchy hands and feet

wet nursing The practice of breastfeeding (and caring for) another mother's child.

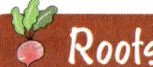

Roots

Milk from Another Mother

Within families and by contractual arrangements, females have been breastfeeding the infants of others for centuries. This practice, known as **wet nursing,** was documented in ancient Hebrew and Egyptian texts dating back to 2000 BC and was quite common until nutritionally adequate infant formulas were available. Wet nursing was merely a convenience for some mothers, but in cases when a mother died during childbirth or was unable to produce milk, wet nurses were a necessity for infant survival.

In many cultures and time periods, wet nursing was an honored profession. In the Islamic Mughal dynasty, for example, wet nurses tied families together. Two children from different families nursed by the same person were considered "milk siblings." As modern medicine evolved, physicians who worked in neonatal care units would often recruit wet nurses to live in the hospital or in the homes of families in need, where they could provide life-saving milk for infants who would otherwise die of malnutrition.

However, wet nurses were not always revered. There were many superstitions about the passage of physical and personality traits from the wet nurse to the infant. Sometimes, the fondness of an infant for the wet nurse provoked jealousy between mother and wet nurse. In the United States in the nineteenth and early twentieth centuries, those who served as wet nurses often came from uneducated and economically disadvantaged backgrounds. Out of dire financial straits, disadvantaged individuals would leave their own children at home with artificial milk to earn money as a wet nurse for a middle- or upper-class family, only to be mistreated and subject to firing at the whim of the employers. As wet nurses came to be regarded as poor, uncultured, and intellectually inferior, the hiring of a wet nurse was fraught with racial and class tensions.

In the mid-1900s, advances in electric breast pumps began to dissociate the wet nurse from her "product." Rather than infants and families interacting directly with wet nurses, females with abundant milk supplies could provide their extra milk to milk banks, where it could be stored, and later distributed to families in need. Today, the Human Milk Banking Association of North America coordinates a network of 31 milk banks in Canada and the United States, each of which is a sophisticated and regulated operation. Donors are screened, milk donations are tested for diseases, then milk is pooled, pasteurized, and safely stored for use by infants in need.

Wet nursing is still practiced around the world, both formally and informally. In their current guidelines for infant feeding, the World Health Organization recommends wet nursing when the mother is unable to breastfeed. Some individuals cross-nurse each other's infants to accommodate work schedules or social activities. There are also numerous informal networks of milk sharing within families, in lactation support groups, or via social media sites.

Sources: Stevens EE, Patrick, TE, Pickler R. A history of infant feeding. *J Perinat Educ.* 2009;18(2): 32-39. doi: 10.1624/105812409X426314

Wolf JH. "Mercenary hirelings" or "a great blessing"? Doctors' and mothers' conflicted perceptions of wet nurses and the ramifications for infant feeding in Chicago, 1871–1961. *J Soc History.* 1999; 33(1):97-120. https://www.jstor.org/stable/3789462

---

hydrolyzed protein formula Infant formula in which the proteins have been broken down into smaller peptides and amino acids to improve digestibility and reduce exposure to potential food allergens; sometimes called *predigested* or *hypoallergenic infant formula.*

Formulas generally contain lactose and/or sucrose for carbohydrate, heat-treated proteins from cow's milk, and plant oils for fat (review Table 15-2). Soy protein–based formulas are available for infants whose parents want the infant to begin a vegan dietary pattern or those who cannot tolerate lactose or the types of proteins found in cow's milk. Infants with milk protein allergies are often sensitive to soy as well, so the best choice for infants with allergies is a **hydrolyzed protein formula.** In this type of formula, the proteins have been broken down into small polypeptides and individual amino acids. A variety of other specialized formulas are also available for specific medical conditions. In any case, it is important to use an iron-fortified formula unless a pediatrician recommends otherwise.

Infant formula comes in several different forms. Some infant formulas come in ready-to-feed, liquid form. These can be simply poured into a clean bottle and fed to the infant without further preparation. Powdered and concentrated fluid formula preparations are also commonly used. Powdered or concentrated formulas should be combined with clean, cold water, precisely following the directions on the formula label. The formula is then warmed, if desired, and fed immediately to the infant.

The following are some tips for safe preparation and storage of infant formula:

- All containers and utensils used to prepare formula should be washed with hot, soapy water and thoroughly rinsed with clean water before use. Household dishwashers are a good way to clean bottles and utensils, too. Unless the infant's immune system is compromised, it is not necessary to boil the containers and utensils prior to use.
- Use cold water to prepare infant formula. Hot water that sits in a hot water heater or runs through pipes made with lead is more likely to accumulate contaminants than cold water (see Section 15.4). For homes with older plumbing systems, it is prudent to let cold tap water run for 1 to 2 minutes before filling a bottle or cup.
- If well water will be used to make infant formula, it should be tested regularly for contaminants, such as naturally occurring nitrates, which can lead to a severe form of anemia (especially among babies younger than 1 year).
- If microbial contamination of well water or municipal tap water is a concern, water should be brought to a rolling boil (for 1 minute) and then cooled to room temperature (for up to 30 minutes) before use in formula preparation. Caregivers should pay close attention to local water advisories. Some pediatricians recommend boiling (then cooling) the water to be used in formula preparation for infants up to 6 months of age, regardless of reports about water safety.
- The American Dental Association does not recommend that formula be mixed with bottled "nursery water," which can be found alongside infant formula in most supermarkets. These bottled water products may contain high levels of fluoride, which can lead to tooth discoloration.
- To warm a bottle of formula, run hot water over it or place it briefly in a pan of simmering water. Infant formulas should not be heated in a microwave oven because hot spots may develop, which can burn the infant's mouth and esophagus.
- Refrigerating prepared formula for 1 day is safe. However, formula left over from a feeding should be discarded if not used within 1 hour because it will be contaminated by microbes and enzymes from the infant's saliva.

Some transition formulas/beverages have been introduced for older infants and toddlers. A few of these products are intended for use after 6 months of age if the infant is consuming solid foods, but most are intended for use only by toddlers (i.e., age 12 months and older). These transition products are lower in fat than human milk or standard infant formulas; their iron content is higher than that of cow's milk; and their overall mineral content is generally more like that of human milk than cow's milk. According to the manufacturers, the advantages of these transition formulas/beverages over standard formulas for older infants and toddlers include reduced cost and better flavor. Recent recommendations from experts in pediatric medicine, nutrition, and dentistry advise caregivers to skip these transition formulas.[23] Instead, offer milk or water as beverage choices after 1 year of age.

Dentists and pediatricians warn caregivers to avoid putting infants to bed (or in infant seats) with a bottle. This advice aims to prevent **early childhood caries** (Fig. 15-3). When carbohydrate-rich fluid continuously bathes the teeth, this provides an ideal growth medium for oral bacteria. These bacteria feast on the carbohydrates and produce acids, which dissolve tooth enamel and lead to decay. It is okay to feed an infant at bedtime, but remove the bottle from the infant's mouth when she falls asleep or before putting her in her crib so that formula (or expressed breast milk) does not pool in the infant's mouth.

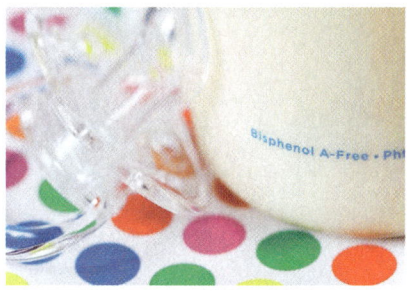

Bisphenol A (BPA) is a chemical used in the production of many plastics. It can leach into foods and liquids and has been detected in human tissues. The consensus among regulatory agencies in the United States and Canada is that current levels of BPA exposure are not harmful, even for infants. Nevertheless, in response to public concern, the U.S. Food and Drug Administration (FDA) has banned the use of BPA in the manufacture of baby bottles, sippy cups, and packaging for infant formulas. BSIP SA/Alamy Stock Photo

early childhood caries Tooth decay that results from formula or juice (and even human milk) bathing the teeth as the child sleeps with a bottle in the mouth. The upper teeth are mostly affected as the lower teeth are protected by the tongue; formerly called *nursing bottle syndrome* or *baby bottle tooth decay*.

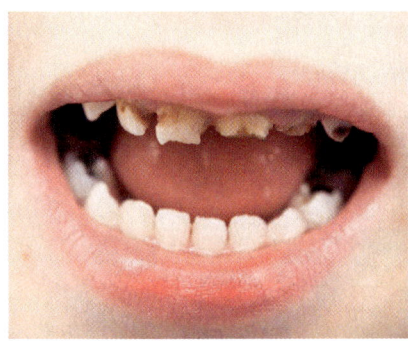

FIGURE 15-3 Early childhood caries. This type of tooth decay may have resulted from frequently putting the child to bed with a bottle. Some of the upper teeth have decayed almost all the way to the gum line. Zoonar GmbH/Alamy Stock Photo

responsive feeding A healthy feeding relationship between the caregiver and the child in which the caregiver pays attention to and respects the child's hunger and satiety.

FEEDING TECHNIQUE

Infants swallow a lot of air as they ingest either formula or human milk. To alleviate discomfort, it is important to burp an infant during feeding (every 1 to 2 ounces) and again at the end of the feeding. Spitting up a small amount of milk or formula is normal at this time.

Formula intake and feeding frequency may vary considerably from one infant to another and also from one day to the next. In general, a formula-fed infant should consume about 2½ fluid ounces (75 milliliters) of formula per pound of body weight each day (Table 15-3), up to about 32 fluid ounces (960 milliliters) in 1 day. In most cases, however, the infant's appetite is a better guide than any standardized recommendations. When the infant begins acting full, bottle feeding should be stopped, even if some milk is left in the bottle. Common signals that an infant has had enough include turning the head away, being inattentive, falling asleep, or becoming playful. Breastfeeding infants usually have had enough to eat after about 20 minutes. Although it is difficult to tell how much milk breastfed infants are getting, they also give recognizable signs when they are full.

By carefully observing and responding appropriately to the infant's cues during feeding, caregivers can (1) be assured that the infant's calorie needs are being met, (2) foster a climate of trust and responsiveness, and (3) help a child develop a habit of respecting internal cues of hunger and satiety.[24] This principle is called **responsive feeding** and should guide caregivers' feeding practices at all stages of infancy and childhood.

EXPANDING THE INFANT'S MEALTIME CHOICES

By about 6 months of age, the infant is ready to start eating complementary foods. Complementary foods are age-appropriate solid foods that *complement* (rather than *replace*) breast milk or infant formula, at least initially.

In the first attempts to introduce solid foods, just getting the food into the infant's mouth may be a challenge. By the end of the first year, though, the infant should be eating a variety of protein sources, vegetables, fruits, and grains so that the infant's daily menu begins to reflect a balanced pattern (Table 15-4). Throughout the process of expanding the infant's mealtime choices, the caregiver should continue to respond to the infant's cues of hunger or satiety. Feeding behaviors developed through early exposures to food will set the stage for healthy eating to last a lifetime.[25]

Determining the Infant's Readiness for Solid Foods. How does the caregiver know it is time to introduce solid foods? Infant size can serve as a rough indicator of readiness: Reaching a weight of at least 13 pounds (6 kilograms) is a preliminary sign of readiness for solid foods. Another physiological cue is volume or frequency of feeding, such as consuming more than 32 ounces (approximately 1 liter) of formula daily or breastfeeding more than 8 to 10 times within 24 hours. Underlying these noticeable signals are several important developmental factors:[2]

1. *Nutritional need.* Before the infant is 6 months old, nutritional needs can generally be met with human milk and/or formula. After 6 months of age, however, many

TABLE 15-3 ■ Typical Formula Intake of Infants

Age	Amount per Feeding	Frequency
< 1 month	2 to 3 fluid ounces (60 to 90 ml)	Every 3 to 4 hours
1 to 6 months	4 to 6 fluid ounces (120 to 180 ml)	Every 4 to 6 hours
6 to 12 months	6 to 8 fluid ounces (180 to 240 ml)*	Every 4 to 6 hours

Source: Data from American Academy of Pediatrics. *Caring for Your Baby and Young Child: Birth to Age 5.* 6th Ed. New York: Bantam Books; 2014.
*With introduction of age-appropriate solid foods.

TABLE 15-4 ■ Sample Daily Menu for a 1-Year-Old Child*

Breakfast	Snack
1 tbsp unsweetened applesauce	4 whole wheat crackers
¼ cup toasted oat cereal	½ cup water
½ cup whole milk	
Snack	**Dinner**
½ slice whole wheat toast	1 ounce roast beef (finely diced)
½ tsp smooth peanut butter	2 tbsp mashed potatoes
½ cup mandarin orange segments	2 tbsp cooked carrots (diced)
½ cup water	½ cup whole milk
Lunch	**Snack**
2 tbsp black beans	½ banana
2 tbsp rice with ½ tsp butter	1 oatmeal cookie (no raisins)
1 tbsp tomatoes	½ cup whole milk
½ cup whole milk	

Nutritional Analysis	
Total energy (kcal)	775
Approximate % energy from	
Carbohydrate	50%
Protein	20%
Fat	30%

*This menu is just a start. A 1-year-old may need more or less food. In those cases, serving sizes should be adjusted. The milk can be fed by cup; some can be put into a bottle if the child has not been fully weaned from the bottle.

infants need additional calories. In terms of individual nutrients, iron stores are exhausted by about 6 months of age. Developmentally appropriate, nutrient-dense foods will help to meet the infant's calorie and iron needs.

2. *Physiological capabilities.* Before about 3 months of age, an infant's digestive tract cannot readily digest starch. Also, kidney function is limited until about 4 to 6 weeks of age. Until then, waste products from excessive amounts of dietary protein or minerals are difficult to excrete. As the infant ages, the ability to digest and metabolize a wider range of food components improves.
3. *Physical ability.* Three observable markers indicate that a child is ready for solid foods: (1) the disappearance of the extrusion reflex (thrusting the tongue forward and pushing food out of the mouth), (2) head and neck control, and (3) the ability to sit up with support. These usually occur around 4 to 6 months of age, but they vary with each infant.
4. *Allergy prevention.* Because a newborn's digestive system is still immature, whole proteins can readily be absorbed from birth until 4 to 5 months of age. If the infant is exposed too early to some types of proteins, the infant may be predisposed to food allergies and autoimmune conditions (e.g., type 1 diabetes). However, there is no benefit to delaying introduction of solid foods beyond 6 months of age.

With these considerations in mind—nutritional need, physiological and physical readiness, and allergy prevention—the AAP and the *Dietary Guidelines* recommend introducing complementary foods to the infant's diet around 6 months of age.[26] Some infants may be developmentally ready for complementary foods earlier than 6 months of age, but caregivers are advised to wait until at least 4 months. Despite these recommendations, data from the National Health and Nutrition Examination Survey indicate that nearly 1 in 5 infants receives complementary foods before 4 months of age.[27]

One reason cited by caregivers for early introduction of solid foods is to satisfy infant hunger. Only occasionally does a rapidly growing infant need to add solid foods to meet calorie and nutrient needs before 6 months of age. In fact, most complementary foods are *less* energy dense than human milk or infant formula. Given the infant's small stomach capacity, providing complementary foods in place of human milk or infant formula before the infant is developmentally ready may actually lower the infant's energy and nutrient intake and hinder growth in the short term. Over the long term, some studies indicate that earlier introduction of solid foods is associated with overweight or obesity.[26]

Aside from hunger, many caregivers believe that early introduction of solid foods will help an infant sleep through the night (i.e., 6 to 8 hours of uninterrupted sleep). The age at which an infant begins to sleep through the night is of little consequence to the child's physical and mental outcomes,[28] yet sleep-deprived caregivers are eager for that blissful time of rest! Does early introduction of solid foods influence sleep duration? One recent analysis showed a modest but statistically significant relationship between early introduction of solid foods and longer sleep duration.[29] However, evidence has been mixed.[30] Overall, pediatric nutrition experts recommend waiting until *at least* 4 months—preferably closer to 6 months—before introducing complementary foods.

Foods to Match Needs and Developmental Abilities During the First Year. The primary goal of introducing complementary foods to the infant's dietary pattern is to meet nutrient needs, particularly for iron and zinc. Therefore, pediatric nutrition experts recommend iron-fortified infant cereals and lean ground (strained) meats as the first solid foods (Fig. 15-4).

When starting solid foods, begin with a teaspoon-size serving of a single-ingredient food item and increase the serving size gradually over the next few days. Once the new food has been fed for several days without adverse effects, another food can be added to the infant's eating pattern. There is no prescribed order for the introduction of specific types of foods or food groups, but food choices should be nutrient dense and developmentally appropriate.

Waiting about 3 to 5 days between the introduction of each new food is important because it can take that long for evidence of an allergy or intolerance to materialize. Also, it is best to avoid introducing mixed foods until each component of the combination dish has been given separately without an adverse reaction.[26] Signs of food allergies include diarrhea, vomiting, a rash, or wheezing. If one or more of these signs appears, the suspected problem food should be avoided for several weeks and then reintroduced in a small quantity. If the problem continues, consult a pediatrician. Fortunately, many babies outgrow food allergies later in childhood.

Until 2008, parents and caregivers were advised to avoid feeding children a wide range of potentially allergenic foods, including egg whites, chocolate, peanuts, tree nuts, fish, and other seafood. Now, pediatric nutrition experts acknowledge that there is no evidence that delaying introduction of solid foods—including these common food allergens—beyond 4 to 6 months of age is of any benefit for prevention of atopic diseases. Indeed, the most recent guidelines from the National Institute of Allergy and Infectious Diseases recommend early introduction of peanut protein—between 4 and 6 months of age—to infants at risk of food allergies.[31,32]

Many strained foods for infant feeding are available where groceries are sold. Single-food items are more desirable than mixed dinners and desserts, which are less nutrient dense. Most brands have no added salt, but some fruit desserts contain added sugar, which is not recommended for infant feeding.[33] Read food labels carefully to find the most nutrient-dense foods for infants.

As an alternative to store-bought baby foods, plain, unseasoned cooked foods—vegetables, fruits, and meats—can be ground up in an inexpensive baby food grinder at home. Another option is to purée a larger amount of food in a blender, freeze it in ice-cube portions, store in plastic bags, and defrost and warm as needed. Careful attention

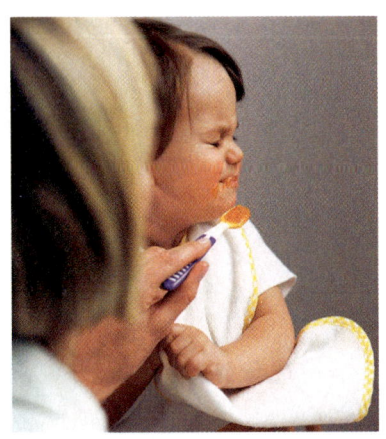

Infants and toddlers are often wary of trying new foods, so it is normal and expected for infants to refuse some foods. Repeated exposure fosters acceptance of new tastes and textures. **Should you force an infant to eat a new food?** Fuse/Corbis/Getty Images

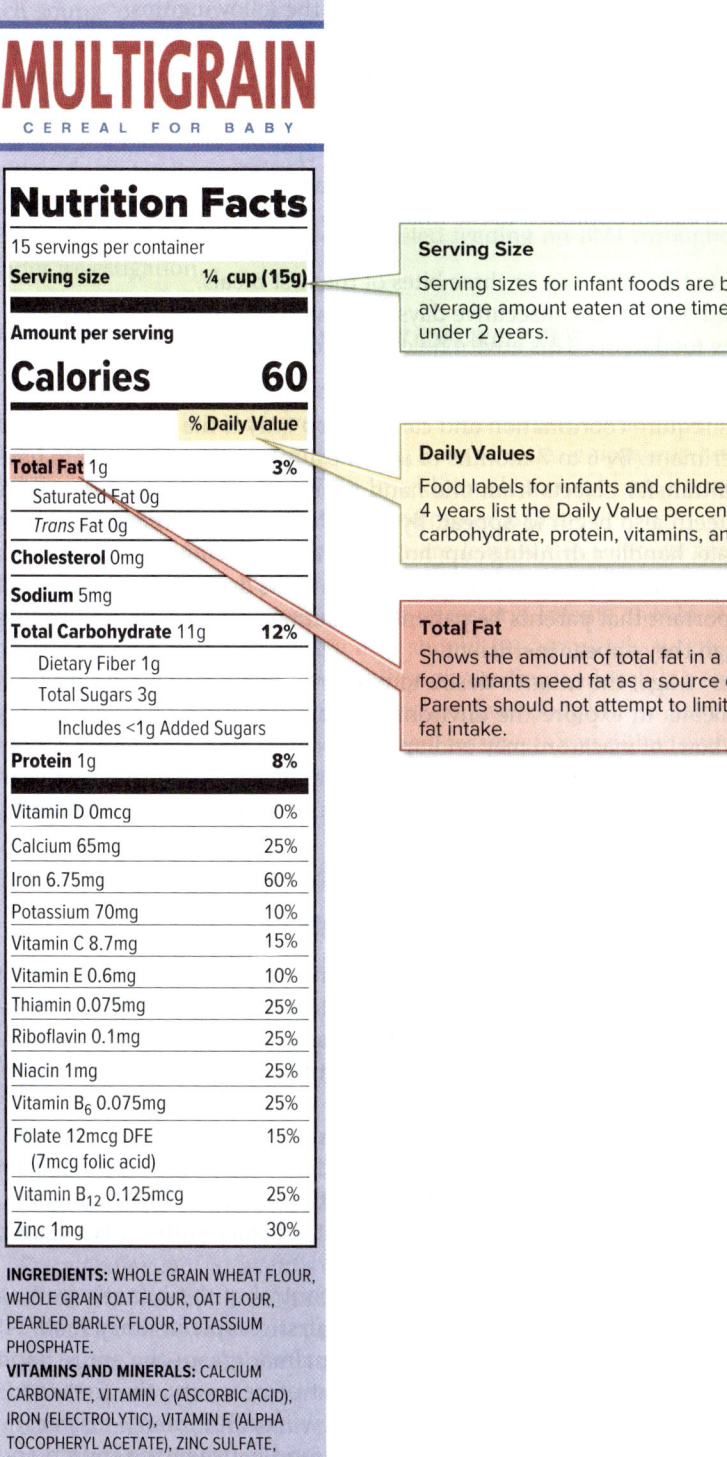

FIGURE 15-4 Infant foods, like adult foods, are required to have a Nutrition Facts label; however, the information provided on infant food labels differs from that on adult food labels (see Fig. 2-16). There are separate Daily Values set for infants through 12 months of age and children 1–3 years of age.

to food safety is necessary. Seasonings that may please the rest of the family should not be added to infant foods made at home. The infant does not notice the difference if salt, sugar, or spices are omitted. It is best to introduce infants to a variety of foods so that by the end of the first year, the infant is consuming many foods—human milk or formula, meats, fruits, vegetables, and grains.

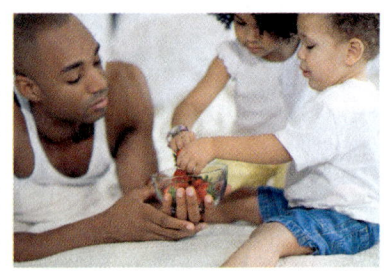

Can infants have alternative sweeteners? Although the FDA affirms the safety of all currently approved alternative sweeteners, foods that contain these additives (e.g., diet soft drinks, sugar-free candies) are typically not good sources of the nutrients infants need to support growth and development. Furthermore, alternative sweeteners given early in life may contribute to a preference for highly sweetened foods. A nutrient-dense snack with natural sugars, such as yogurt with fruit, would be a better option. Blend Images/123RF

- *Vary the veggies.* During the second half of the first year, infants have a big appetite and are relatively open to new flavors. This is a perfect opportunity to introduce a variety of vegetables, *especially* those with stronger flavors, such as beets, broccoli, and spinach. If infants learn to eat a variety of vegetables early in life, they will be more likely to continue to eat them throughout childhood. However, studies show that by 1 year of age, vegetable choices are dominated by white potatoes. Continuing to offer many colorful options during late infancy and the toddler years will enhance intakes of fiber, folate, vitamin A, vitamin C, vitamin E, magnesium, potassium, and phytochemicals.
- *Go for the grains.* Including both whole grains and enriched or fortified grain products will provide several nutrients of concern. Selecting a variety of different grains will help to reduce exposure to harmful environmental contaminants. Whole grains provide fiber to promote healthy digestion. Enriched or fortified grain products are good sources of iron. Iron-fortified infant cereals made of oats, barley, rice, or a mixture of grains should be among the first foods offered to infants. As motor skills develop, fortified dry breakfast cereals are desirable finger foods.

WHAT *NOT* TO FEED AN INFANT

The following are several foods and practices to avoid when feeding an infant:

- *Excessive infant formula or human milk.* After 6 months of age, solid foods should play an increasing role in satisfying an infant's growing appetite. Age-appropriate solid foods provide necessary calories and iron, plus they help the infant to develop motor skills. About 24 to 32 ounces (¾ to 1 liter) of human milk or formula daily is ideal after 6 months, with complementary foods supplying the rest of the infant's energy needs.
- *Foods that tend to cause choking.* Foods that are round or oval in shape, larger than ½ inch in diameter, or of a soft or sticky texture can easily get lodged in a child's throat. These foods include hot dogs, hard or gummy candies, whole nuts, grapes, coarsely cut meats, raw carrots, popcorn, and large portions of nut butters. Caregivers should not allow younger children to gobble snack foods during playtime and should supervise all meals.
- *Potential food allergens before 4 months of age.* The nine most common food allergens (in order of prevalence during childhood) include peanuts, milk, shellfish, tree nuts, eggs, fin fish, wheat, soy, and sesame. Until about 6 months of age, energy and nutrient needs of most infants can be met with exclusive breastfeeding or infant formula. If any solid foods are introduced before 4 months of age (not recommended), they should be iron-fortified infant cereals, puréed meats, vegetables, or fruits.
- *Cow's milk (as a replacement for human milk or infant formula).* Foods made with cow's milk, such as yogurt, can be safely introduced starting around 6 months of age. However, cow's milk is not recommended as a replacement for human milk or iron-fortified infant formula for infants until 1 year of age because it may displace good sources of iron in the infant's diet. In large amounts, cow's milk may also irritate the young infant's GI tract. In addition, the AAP strongly urges caregivers not to give reduced-fat or fat-free milk to children under age 2. Before age 2, the amount of reduced-fat or fat-free milk needed to meet energy needs would supply too many minerals, which could overwhelm the kidneys. Limiting fat intake at this age might also hinder nervous system development. After the second birthday, children can drink reduced-fat, 1%, or fat-free milk because by this age, they are consuming enough solid foods to meet calorie and fat requirements.

- *Other plant-based milk alternatives.* Plant-based milk alternatives (e.g., almond milk, rice milk) are not recommended for infants because of their low **energy density,** lower-quality protein, and lack of micronutrients that are critical for infant growth and development. Although many manufacturers do fortify plant-based milk alternatives with certain micronutrients (e.g., calcium and vitamin D), there is no federal mandate or standardization across the industry.
- *Goat's milk.* Although perceived by some to pose lower risk for food allergies, goat's milk is low in folate, iron, vitamin C, and vitamin D and should not be used as a source of nourishment for infants.
- *Do not overdo high-fiber foods.* The natural amounts of fiber in kid-size portions of fruits, vegetables, legumes, and grains are appropriate, but too much fiber can be harmful for infants. High-fiber dietary patterns are bulky and low in calories, so infants may feel full before calorie and nutrient needs are met. Furthermore, excessive fiber may limit the absorption of important minerals, such as iron, zinc, and calcium.
- *Skip the added sugars.* Natural sugars, such as those found in human milk, dairy products, and fruits, are excellent sources of energy for active, rapidly growing infants. However, the *Dietary Guidelines* states that added sugars should be avoided by infants and young children under age 2. Nutrient-dense foods are needed to support the infant's rapid growth and development. There is very little room in the infant's dietary pattern for sugar-sweetened beverages and sugary snacks—even those with "fruit" in their names. These choices supply calories without the benefits of fiber, vitamins, minerals, and phytochemicals.
- *Excessive fruit juice.* The fructose and sorbitol contained in some fruit juices, especially apple and pear juices, can lead to diarrhea because they are slowly absorbed. Also, if fruit juice or related drink products are displacing formula or milk in the dietary pattern, the infant may not be receiving adequate calories, calcium, or other nutrients essential for proper growth. Studies have shown a link between excessive amounts of fruit juice and pediatric malnutrition, GI tract complications, obesity, short stature, and poor dental health. Fruit juice (even 100% fruit juice) is not recommended at all for infants. See Sections 15.4 and 15.5 for age-specific recommendations.
- *Heavily seasoned and processed foods.* Sodium is an essential mineral found naturally in almost all foods. As part of a healthy dietary pattern, infants need sodium for their bodies to work properly. However, the average intakes of sodium among infants and toddlers are above the AI. Caregivers should refrain from offering heavily salted and highly processed foods.
- *Food safety hazards.* The immune system is still maturing during infancy and early childhood, so it is important to avoid potential sources of foodborne illness. For example, raw (unpasteurized) milk or soft cheeses (e.g., queso fresco) may be contaminated with bacteria or viruses. Meat, poultry, eggs, and seafood should be cooked to proper temperatures. In addition, honey may contain spores of *Clostridium botulinum,* which can lead to the potentially fatal foodborne illness known as *botulism.* Safe food handling starts with proper handwashing.
- *Excessive nutrient supplementation.* Supplemental vitamins or minerals that provide more than 100% of the RDA or AI for age can increase the risk for nutrient toxicities. Vitamin D supplementation is recommended for all infants until foods or beverages supply the RDA. For exclusively breastfed infants, iron supplements are recommended after 4 months of age until foods or beverages supply the RDA for iron. Except to correct a nutrient deficiency, other dietary supplements are not advised. Consult a pediatrician or RDN before giving dietary supplements to an infant.

energy density A comparison of the calorie (kcal) content of a food with the weight of the food. An energy-dense food is high in calories but weighs very little (e.g., potato chips), whereas a food low in energy density has few calories but weighs a lot (e.g., an orange).

Recommendations for Infant Feeding from the *Dietary Guidelines*

- **For about the first 6 months of life,** exclusively feed infants human milk. Continue to feed infants human milk through at least the first year of life, and longer if desired. Feed infants iron-fortified infant formula during the first year of life when human milk is unavailable.
- Provide infants with supplemental vitamin D beginning soon after birth.
- **At about 6 months,** introduce infants to nutrient-dense complementary foods.
- Introduce infants to potentially allergenic foods along with other complementary foods.
- Encourage infants and toddlers to consume a variety of foods from all food groups. Include foods rich in iron and zinc, particularly for infants fed human milk.
- Avoid foods and beverages with added sugars.
- Limit foods and beverages higher in sodium.
- As infants wean from human milk or infant formula, transition to a healthy dietary pattern.

CASE STUDY: Undernutrition During Infancy

Damon is a 7-month-old male who has been taken into a clinic for a routine checkup. On examination, he was found to be moderately underweight relative to his age and body length. His pediatrician scheduled a follow-up appointment in 3 months. At the 10-month visit, Damon appeared sluggish and was even more underweight for his age and length.

An RDN interviewed Damon's 16-year-old mother to collect information on Damon's dietary intake. His intake over the previous 24 hours consisted of two 8-ounce bottles of infant formula, three 8-ounce bottles of fruit punch, and a hot dog. Damon may have been fed some additional items on the nights that his mother left him with a neighbor so that she could go out with friends for a few hours. Thus, she was not aware of all that he ate.

1. Damon's mother did not specify what type of formula she gives to her child or how she prepares it. What questions would you ask about his formula?
2. Besides lagging growth, name three other potential consequences of inadequate calorie and nutrient intake during infancy.
3. What foods should Damon's caregivers offer that are appropriate for his age and nutritional needs?
4. What problems might arise from consumption of sugary drinks from a bottle?
5. Does Damon need any vitamin or mineral supplements?

Complete the Case Study. Responses to these questions can be provided by your instructor.

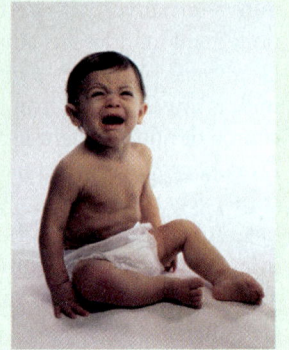

At his well-baby check-up, Damon is underweight compared to other infants his age. How can Damon's caregivers help him eat well to achieve optimal growth? Kwame Zikomo/Purestock/SuperStock

✓ CONCEPT CHECK 15.3

1. List three similarities between human milk and infant formula. List three differences.
2. Describe four ways to assess an infant's readiness for solid foods.
3. Excessive intake of added sugars is common in late infancy. Describe several ways to limit intake of added sugars in an infant's eating pattern.
4. List three foods that should *not* be fed to infants during the first year of life.

15.4 Toddlers and Preschool Children: Nutrition Concerns

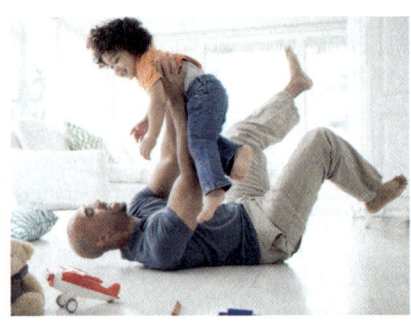

The *Physical Activity Guidelines for Americans* recommends that children should be physically active every day, starting as young as 3 years of age. Caregivers can encourage physical activity by setting aside time, providing a safe space, and engaging in active play with their children. Hero/Corbis/Fancy Photography/Glow Images

The rapid growth rate that characterizes infancy tapers off during the toddler and preschool years. The average annual weight gain is only 4.5 to 6.6 pounds (2 to 3 kilograms), and the average annual height gain is only 3 to 4 inches (7.5 to 10 centimeters) between the ages of 2 and 5. As the growth rate tapers off, energy needs decrease and eating behaviors change. For example, among toddlers, the decreased growth rate leads to a decreased appetite, which contributes to "picky eating."

Relative energy needs (i.e., kcal per kilogram of body weight) gradually decline from approximately 100 kcal per kilogram during infancy to about 80 or 90 kcal per kilogram for the preschooler. However, because body size is increasing, *absolute* calorie needs (i.e., kcal per day) gradually increase throughout childhood. For toddlers ages 12 to 23 months, typical energy needs are 700 to 1000 kcal per day (Table 15-5). From ages 2 through 5, energy requirements are 1000 to 1600 kcal per day (Table 15-6). Energy needs vary by age, biological sex, body size, physical activity level, and rate of growth. See Appendix F for a complete set of EER equations for individuals at various stages of the life cycle

Except in cases of poverty or homelessness, the dietary patterns of toddlers and preschoolers in the United States and Canada are adequate in calories and most nutrients. A few nutrients of particular concern among this age group are iron, calcium, and sodium.[38]

TABLE 15-5 ■ Healthy U.S.-Style Dietary Patterns for Toddlers Ages 12 Through 23 Months[a]

- Choose easy-to-chew whole **Fruits** rather than fruit juice. Choose options with little or no added sugars.
- Choose a variety of easy-to-chew (i.e., cooked) **Vegetables** from each subgroup. Choose options that are prepared with less added fat and salt.
- At least half of **Grain** choices should be whole grains.
- Incorporate a variety of lean, unprocessed meats, plant sources of **Protein**, and low-mercury seafood choices. Avoid choking hazards (e.g., large chunks of tough meat, nuts, and large spoonfuls of nut butters).
- Before age 2, choose whole milk. Strive to achieve the recommended daily amounts of **Dairy** foods to support bone health but remember that consuming too much milk can leave the dietary pattern short on iron.
- **Oils** refer to nontropical plant oils, such as canola, corn, olive, peanut, safflower, soybean, and sunflower oils.

Calorie Level	700	800	900	1000
Fruits (cups)	½	¾	1	1
Vegetables[b] (cups)	⅔	¾	1	1
Grains (oz-eq)	1¾	2¼	2½	3
Protein (oz-eq)	2	2	2	2
Dairy (cups)	1⅔	1¾	2	2
Oils (grams)	9	9	8	13

[a] These dietary patterns are for toddlers who are no longer receiving human milk or infant formula.
[b] Beans, peas, and lentils can count either as vegetables or protein foods.

Source: U.S. Department of Agriculture and U.S. Department of Health and Human Services. *Dietary Guidelines for Americans, 2020–2025*. 9th edition. December 2020. Available at DietaryGuidelines.gov.

Iron. Childhood iron-deficiency anemia is most likely to appear in children between the ages of 6 and 24 months—a time when iron stores from gestation become depleted but intake of iron from food sources may be inadequate. This can lead to decreases in both stamina and learning ability, as well as lowered resistance to disease. The targeted efforts of the Special Supplemental Nutrition Program for Women, Infants, and Children (WIC) have helped to decrease the occurrence of iron deficiency among children, but it still remains a problem for almost 15% of toddlers and about 4% of preschoolers.[39]

The RDA for iron is 7 milligrams per day for children ages 1 to 3 and 10 milligrams per day for children ages 4 to 8. The best way to prevent iron-deficiency anemia in children is to provide foods that are rich sources of iron. Even though some animal products are high in saturated fat and cholesterol, the high proportion of heme iron in many animal foods allows the iron to be more readily absorbed than is iron from plant foods. Focus on lean cuts of meat, such as ground sirloin. Fortified breakfast cereals also contribute to meeting iron (and other nutrient) needs. Consuming a source of vitamin C will aid absorption of the less readily absorbed form of iron in plants, fortified foods, and supplements. While dietary changes can be effective for preventing iron-deficiency anemia, supplementation will be required to correct existing.

Calcium. Childhood is a period of rapid bone growth and mineralization. The RDA for calcium for ages 1 to 3 is 700 milligrams per day. Between the ages of 4 and 8, calcium needs increase to 1000 milligrams per day. However, national surveys of food intake show that the dietary patterns of children—especially adolescent females—fall short of the RDA for this important nutrient.[40]

Milk and other dairy products are the primary source of calcium in the dietary patterns of children, but unfortunately milk consumption has declined as intake of sugar-sweetened beverages has increased. Consuming about two servings per day of milk or other foods from the dairy group will help toddlers and preschoolers meet their requirements for bone-building nutrients. Children up to 2 years of age should drink whole milk because they need the extra fat for energy, but after 2 years of age reduced-fat or fat-free milk are more nutrient-dense choices. For children who do not consume dairy products, whether due to choice or

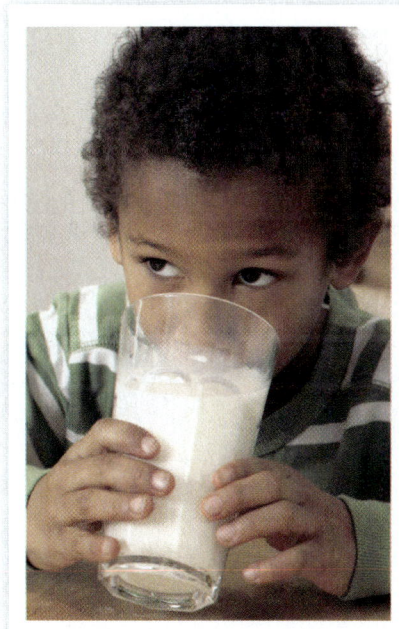

Cow's milk is a source of bioavailable calcium and vitamin D for toddlers and preschoolers, but overreliance on milk can crowd out other nutrient-dense foods. Children who drink more than 3 cups of milk per day are likely to consume inadequate amounts of iron and fiber. **What is the best way for toddlers and preschoolers to quench thirst?** Andrew Olney/OJO Images/age fotostock

TABLE 15-6 ■ **Healthy U.S.-Style Dietary Patterns for Children Ages 2 Through 18**

Choose whole **Fruit** rather than fruit juice. Choose options with little or no added sugars. Avoid choking hazards (e.g., large pieces of firm fruit, dried fruit) until molars emerge (around age 4).

Choose a variety of **Vegetables** from each subgroup. Choose options that are prepared with less added fat and salt. Avoid choking hazards (e.g., firm, raw vegetables) until molars emerge.

At least half of **Grain** choices should be whole grains.

Incorporate a variety of lean, unprocessed meats, plant sources of **Protein**, and low-mercury seafood choices. Avoid choking hazards (e.g., large chunks of tough meat, nuts, and large spoonfuls of nut butters) until molars emerge.

Choose unsweetened and reduced-fat or fat-free **Dairy** foods. Strive to achieve the recommended daily amounts of dairy foods to support bone health but remember that consuming too much milk can leave the dietary pattern short on iron.

Oils refer to nontropical plant oils, such as canola, corn, olive, peanut, safflower, soybean, and sunflower oils.

Calories for Other Uses include added sugars and rich sources of saturated fat, such as butter, shortening, lard, or tropical plant oils (e.g., coconut oil).

	Toddlers & Preschoolers (2 to 5 years)			School-Age Children (6 to 12 years)					Teenagers (13 to 18 years)		
Daily Amount of Food from Each Group Based on Calorie Level											
Calorie Level	1000	1200	1400	1600	1800	2000	2200	2400	2600	2800	3000	3200
Fruits (cups)	1	1	1½	1½	1½	2	2	2	2	2½	2½	2½
Vegetables[a] (cups)	1	1½	1½	2	2½	2½	3	3	3½	3½	4	4
Grains (oz-eq)	3	4	5	5	6	6	7	8	9	10	10	10
Protein (oz-eq)	2	3	4	5	5	5½	6	6½	6½	7	7	7
Dairy (cups)	2	2½	2½[b]	2½[b]	2½[b]	2½[b]	3	3	3	3	3	3
Oils (grams)	15	17	17	22	22[c]	24[c]	29	31	34	36	44	51
Limit on Calories for Other Uses												
Calories for Other Uses (kcal)	130	80	90[d]	150[d]	190[d]	280[d]	250	320	350	370	440	580

[a]Beans, peas, and lentils can count either as vegetables or protein foods.
[b]Older children at this Calorie level should have 3 cups per day from the Dairy group.
[c]Older children at this Calorie level need slightly more grams of Oils.
[d]Because they need more Dairy and Oils, older children at this Calorie level have a slightly lower allowance for Calories for Other Uses.

Source: U.S. Department of Agriculture and U.S. Department of Health and Human Services. *Dietary Guidelines for Americans, 2020–2025.* 9th Edition. December 2020. Available at DietaryGuidelines.gov

Quick Guide to Child Nutrition Needs

Carbohydrates
- 130 grams per day to supply energy for the central nervous system and prevent ketosis

Protein
- 13 to 19 grams per day (ages 1 to 3)
- 34 to 52 grams per day (older children)

Fat
- 30% to 40% of total kcal (ages 1 to 3)
- 25% to 35% of total kcal (older children)

food jag A period of time (usually a few days or weeks) during which a person will eat only a limited variety of foods.

necessity, there are alternative sources of calcium and other bone-building nutrients. Fortified beverages, such as soy milk, almond milk, or orange juice, can supply as much calcium per serving as cow's milk (check the label to be sure). Some legumes and vegetables are sources of calcium as well, but the mineral is not as bioavailable as it is from dairy products.

Sodium. While iron and calcium intakes fall short of needs in preschool children, excessive sodium intake is a concern.[41] For children 1 to 3 years of age, the CDRR for sodium is 1200 milligrams per day. For children 4 to 8 years of age, the CDRR is 1500 milligrams per day.[42] High intakes of fast foods and highly processed foods elevate sodium intakes to about 1000 milligrams per day *more* than preschoolers need. Caregivers can lower sodium intake by preparing meals at home instead of relying on fast foods or frozen meals, by limiting salt added during cooking and at the table, by cutting back on use of highly processed foods (e.g., luncheon meats and hot dogs), by rinsing canned beans and vegetables before cooking, and by encouraging consumption of fruits, vegetables, and whole grains in place of prepackaged snacks.

Feeding skills are an important part of physical and cognitive development. Young children explore their environment through the tastes and textures of foods, develop dexterity using utensils and drinking from a cup, and begin to express their autonomy by refusing certain foods. At this time in life, children are also testing boundaries to find out what is acceptable in their little corner of the world. Messy mealtimes, food refusals, and **food jags** can be sources of tension in families. Creating a more harmonious family atmosphere at mealtime is an important way to keep these behaviors from becoming serious feeding problems (see "Understanding Picky Eating" later in this section). Caregivers must understand that these are normal phases of child development but should also be consistent about setting limits for behavior at the dinner table.

Because of the preschool child's reduced appetite, planning a dietary pattern that meets nutrient needs poses a special challenge. Nutrient density is an important consideration for this age group. Overall, caregivers should focus on offering a variety of healthy choices, allowing the child to exert some autonomy over the specific type of food and the amount eaten.

Table 15-6 summarizes the healthy U.S.-style dietary patterns (from the *Dietary Guidelines*) at calorie levels appropriate for children ages 2 through 18. Keep in mind that Table 15-6 displays the quantity of food from each food group to be consumed throughout the course of a day. When it comes to planning individual meals, MyPlate is a useful, easy-to-understand tool for children. The *proportions* illustrated by MyPlate apply to all ages, even though the portions of foods at each meal will be smaller for children. Until a child is about 5 years of age, a good starting point for *portion* sizes in the vegetables group, fruits group, and protein group is about 1 tablespoon per year of life.

It is important to promote a healthy attitude about eating. While caregivers will want to focus on nutrient-dense foods, there is no reason to be overly restrictive about child food choices. In fact, when parents are extremely controlling about the family's food intake, children may be at risk for **body dissatisfaction** and **disordered eating.** There is room for occasional indulgences, a skipped meal or two, or once in a while "less than ideal" choices. It is eating and lifestyle patterns over the course of a month (and lifetime) that matter. Children develop healthy eating habits when adults set a good example, provide opportunities to learn, give support for exploration, and limit inappropriate behavior.

Next, we will consider some typical complaints and concerns of caregivers, explore the causes, and make suggestions for achieving optimal nutrition during the toddler and preschool years.

UNDERSTANDING PICKY EATING

Many parents are baffled by their toddler's erratic eating behaviors. Toddlers and preschoolers tend not to eat as much or as regularly as infants. One day, a young child may pick at his food and staunchly refuse to eat his green beans, but on the next day he might ask for a second helping. Parents often need reminding that toddlers and preschoolers cannot be expected to eat as voraciously as infants or to eat adult-size portions. Because the growth rate slows after infancy, a toddler's drive to eat is not so intense. In addition, children are sometimes more interested in playing and exploring than eating.

Youngsters also tend to be wary of new foods, a trait known as **neophobia.** One reason is that they have more taste buds, and their taste buds are more sensitive than those of adults. A general distrust of unfamiliar things is common in this age group. Thus, familiarity plays an important role in food acceptance. Adults can encourage young children to broaden their food repertoire with repeated exposures to new food choices. It may take 10 or more exposures to a new food before a child finds it acceptable, but if adults can be patient and persevere, children will build good food habits.[43]

Food preferences change rapidly in childhood and are influenced by food temperature, appearance, texture, and taste. The following are a few practical tips for improving acceptance of nutrient-dense foods.

- *Build on what they know and accept.* Pairing a new food item with a familiar one can help to foster acceptance of the new food.
- *Enlist the child's aid in food selection and preparation.* For example, let the child pick out the tomatoes and squash at the local farmers' market.
- *Serve meals on a sectioned plate.* Sometimes children object to having foods mixed, as in stews and casseroles, even if they normally like the ingredients separately.
- *Keep it crunchy.* Certain food characteristics, such as crisp textures and mild flavors, are appealing to children. Kids who reject mushy, cooked carrots may enjoy them raw or lightly steamed. (After about age 4, children can safely eat raw vegetables without fear of choking.)
- *Finger foods are fun.* Preschoolers eventually develop skill with spoons and forks and can even use dull knives, but it is still a good idea to serve some finger foods, especially with healthy dips such as yogurt sauce or hummus.
- *Save the best for last.* If a child is prone to leave their chicken on the plate untouched, serve the chicken first. Hunger is the best means of getting a child to eat!

Although picky eating is usually not cause for alarm, a child's sudden loss of appetite may be a sign of underlying illness, such as an infection or gastrointestinal problem. Be alert for signs of **eating disorders,** as well. Extreme, self-imposed dietary restrictions

---

Choking is a preventable hazard for young children. Some suggestions for caregivers include:

- Set a good example at the table by taking small bites and chewing foods thoroughly.
- During meals and snacks, limit distractions, such as television and electronic devices. Have children sit at the table, take their time, and focus on their food.
- Avoid giving children any foods that are round, firm, sticky, or cut into large chunks, especially before molars emerge (around age 4). For toddlers and preschoolers, some examples of foods to avoid are hot dogs, nuts, whole grapes, raisins, popcorn, peanut butter (unless it is thinly spread on another food), caramel, marshmallows, and hard pieces of raw fruits or vegetables.

body dissatisfaction Negative thoughts or attitudes about one's own body that may arise from a perceived gap between one's own physical appearance and one's ideal of attractiveness.

disordered eating Mild and short-term changes in eating patterns that occur in relation to a stressful event, an illness, or a desire to modify one's dietary pattern for a variety of health and personal appearance reasons.

neophobia Fear of new things, such as new foods.

eating disorder Severe alterations in eating patterns linked to physiological changes. The alterations are associated with food restriction, binge eating, inappropriate compensatory behaviors, and fluctuations in weight. They also involve a number of emotional and cognitive changes that affect the way a person perceives and experiences their body.

FARM to FORK: Blueberries

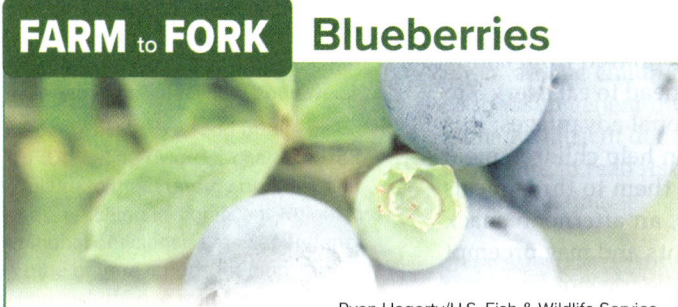

Ryan Hagerty/U.S. Fish & Wildlife Service

From a health standpoint, it's tough to beat these AMAZING berries! The antioxidant and phytochemical activities of berries are four times greater than those of most other fruits, 10 times greater than those of most vegetables, and 40 times higher than those of most cereal grains. Berries may play a role in prevention of diabetes, cancer, high blood pressure, cardiovascular disease, and dementia!

Grow
- Many urban landscapes are adding attractive berry patches as part of an edible environment. Although most blueberries thrive in cooler climates, some varieties do fine in warmer climates.
- Children love to pick berries! If you don't have your own berry patch, consider finding a local U-pick farm for building great family memories.

Shop
- When shopping, examine the berries carefully and look for plump, firm, and colorful fruit.
- The most nutrient-dense frozen berries are flash-frozen to preserve phytochemicals and vitamin C. Flash-frozen wild berries are the best choice.
- If purchasing juice, read the ingredients to be sure it is 100% pure berry juice. Most berry juices contain more juice from apples and white grapes than from berries.

Store
- Rinse fresh berries just prior to eating and eat them within several days to ensure the highest nutrient content.
- Before freezing your own berries, dust lightly with vitamin C powder or Fruit-Fresh® to retain nutrients.

Prep
- Berries may be enjoyed fresh, frozen, stewed, or dried. They can be used to sweeten any dish.
- Frozen berries thawed quickly in the microwave actually retain double the nutrient content as those thawed at room temperature or in the refrigerator.
- Heating increases the bioavailability of phytochemicals and nutrients in berries. Thus, cooked or canned berries are healthy choices.

Source: Robinson J. Blueberries and blackberries: extraordinarily nutritious. In: *Eating on the Wild Side: The Missing Link to Optimum Health.* New York: Little, Brown & Co.; 2013.

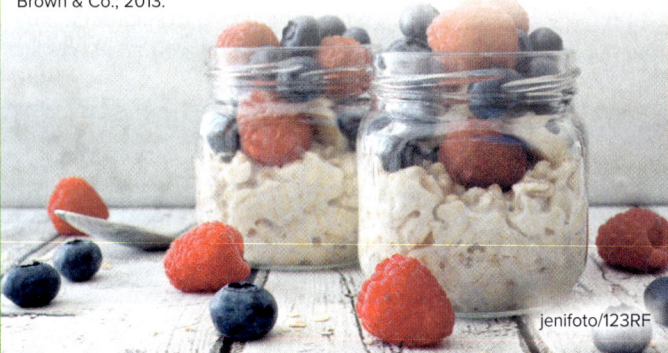

jenifoto/123RF

CHOOSE DIETARY SUPPLEMENTS CAREFULLY

Major scientific groups, such as the Academy of Nutrition and Dietetics and the American Society for Nutrition, state that multivitamin and mineral supplements are generally unnecessary for healthy children; it is better to emphasize whole foods. In fact, consuming fortified foods and supplements may lead to intakes above the UL for some nutrients, such as vitamin A and zinc. Supplements for children that are made to look like candy may result in accidental overdose, particularly of iron. Rather than relying on supplements, choose fortified, low-sugar, ready-to-eat breakfast cereals with milk to close any gaps between current micronutrient intake and needs, such as for folate, vitamin D, vitamin E, iron, or zinc.[26,47]

For a child who is ill, has a very poor appetite, is extremely selective about foods, or adheres to dietary restrictions (e.g., due to food allergies or metabolic disorders), a children's multivitamin and mineral supplement not exceeding 100% of Daily Values for any nutrient may be beneficial. Still, as mentioned many times in this book, dietary supplements cannot substitute for an otherwise healthy dietary pattern. If current childhood feeding practices are to become more healthful, the focus should be on whole grain breads and cereals, fruits, vegetables, lean sources of protein, and low-fat milk and milk products.

REDUCE LEAD POISONING

Humans may be exposed to lead from drinking contaminated water, consuming or inhaling lead dust (e.g., from cracked and peeling lead paint), contaminated dietary supplements (e.g., calcium supplements derived from bone meal), or foods stored or prepared in lead-containing vessels. In the United States, average blood lead levels have declined over the past 40 years due to the successes of public health programs aimed at reducing environmental lead exposure. Nevertheless, nearly all children have detectable levels of lead in their blood and, based on national data collected between 2011 and 2016, more than 250,000 children between the ages of 1 and 5 years had blood lead levels exceeding the reference value recommended by the CDC at the time of testing.[48] Young children are particularly vulnerable to lead poisoning because they are small, absorb lead quickly, spend a lot of time on the floor, and are apt to put objects in their mouths. Children in families with lower socioeconomic status are at highest risk for lead poisoning because they are more likely to live in older homes with lead-based paint. In the short term, symptoms of lead poisoning include gastrointestinal distress, lack of appetite, irritability, fatigue, and anemia. Over the long term, devastating effects include intellectual and behavioral impairments and increased risk for several chronic diseases in adulthood.

Although it does not address the source of exposure, proper nutrition can reduce the risks of lead poisoning for children. Consuming regular meals with moderate fat intake and ensuring adequate iron and calcium status are dietary practices known to reduce lead absorption. Adequate zinc, thiamin, and vitamin E intakes also reduce the harmful effects of absorbed lead. To minimize lead levels in drinking water, only use cold water for drinking and preparation of formula or food. Letting cold water run from the tap for 1 to 2 minutes after a long period of inactivity (e.g., overnight) will limit the amount of lead that has accumulated in tap water. If the public water supply contains a high concentration of lead, bottled water is a safer alternative, particularly for formula preparation. Overall, a balanced meal plan that offers a variety of whole grains, lean meats, and low-fat dairy products is especially useful for protecting children from lead poisoning.[49]

ALLEVIATE CONSTIPATION WITH LIFESTYLE CHANGES

Constipation, a common problem among children, can be defined as hard, dry stools that are difficult to pass. Typically, a 4-year-old child has one bowel movement per day, but normal bowel habits vary widely. Therefore, the frequency of bowel movements is not as important as the consistency of stools. Pediatricians diagnose constipation after 2 or more weeks of delayed or difficult bowel movements.[50] In rare situations, constipation can be a sign of a serious problem. If a child has a fever or vomiting along with constipation, if there is blood in the stool, or if the abdomen becomes swollen, caregivers should seek immediate medical attention.

What causes constipation? Although there could be a serious medical problem, most cases are related to lifestyle. Lack of physical activity contributes to constipation. Some cases may be due to inadequate fluid intake. Also, on average, children (and adults) in the United States barely obtain half of the AI for fiber. Altered bowel habits also may be a sign of a food allergy or intolerance to a food component such as cow's milk. Many times, constipation results from the child withholding bowel movements. For children, a painful bowel movement can be so traumatic that they try to resist subsequent bowel movements. The longer they hold their stools, the harder and drier they get, leading to another painful movement. This cycle disrupts regular bowel habits, leading to distress and, if not treated, **fecal impaction**.[51]

When presented with a constipated child, a primary care provider first has to rule out a medical cause, such as an intestinal blockage. Treatment of fecal impaction may require evacuation of the bowels (e.g., with an enema). Once bowels have been evacuated, lifestyle changes are necessary to prevent future problems. Although various types of laxatives may be prescribed by the primary care provider in the short term, dietary and lifestyle strategies are safest over the long term. First, regular bowel habits must be established. For example, caregivers should set aside time for the child to use the toilet, without rushing, after each meal. Rewards, such as stickers on a chart, may be used to reinforce good habits. Increasing physical activity while cutting back on sedentary activities (e.g., watching television or using electronic devices) can help to promote regular bowel movements. The primary dietary interventions to alleviate constipation include eating more fiber and drinking more fluids. In the initial stages of treatment, providing certain fruit juices (e.g., prune, grape, and apple) and trying soy milk instead of cow's milk may relieve constipation.[52]

Ultimately, whole fruits (e.g., plums, peaches, and apricots) are better choices than juices because whole fruits are less concentrated sources of calories. Pediatric nutrition authorities recommend limiting fruit juice to just 4 fluid ounces per day for toddlers (ages 1 to 3).[53] Other foods to emphasize for fiber include vegetables, whole grain breads and cereals, and beans. The daily fiber goals for children set by the Food and Nutrition Board vary by age (see box). Few children meet these goals. It is important to increase fluid consumption along with fiber to avoid another fecal impaction. Accompanying fluid recommendations are 4 cups (900 milliliters) per day for toddlers and about 5 cups (1200 milliliters) per day for older children.

Between 2014 and 2015, the water supply in the city of Flint, Michigan, became contaminated with dangerously high levels of lead. The problem was traced to the city's aging infrastructure. When the city switched its water supply from Lake Huron to the Flint River, corrosive compounds in the water caused lead to leach from aging pipes into the water. Contaminated water contributed to extremely high blood lead levels and a variety of serious health problems. Lead poisoning is problematic at any age, but it can cause neurological damage in infants and children. Infants born during this time had lower birth weights and affected families reported increased behavioral and physical health concerns. In the years since this crisis, the city of Flint has switched back to the Lake Huron water supply, replaced the outdated water infrastructure, increased blood lead screening and environmental testing, provided referrals and funds for health services, and enhanced efforts to educate the public about preventing lead exposure.

Source: Centers for Disease Control and Prevention. *Community Assessment for Public Health Emergency Response (CASPER): After the Flint Water Crisis: May 17–19, 2016*. July 2016. Accessed December 18, 2023. https://www.michigan.gov/documents/flintwater/CASPER_Report_540077_7.pdf

fecal impaction The presence of a mass of hard, dry feces that remains in the rectum as a result of chronic constipation.

Fiber Recommendations for Children

Young Children
1–3 years	19 grams/day
4–8 years	25 grams/day

Males
9–13 years	31 grams/day
14–18 years	38 grams/day

Females
9–13 years	26 grams/day
14–18 years	26 grams/day

Source: Food and Nutrition Board.

> The *Dietary Guidelines* provides a framework for healthy vegetarian dietary patterns for children, starting at 12 months of age. Notably, these patterns illustrate lactoovovegetarian eating patterns. Inclusion of dairy foods ensures nutrient-dense sources of protein, calcium, vitamin D, and vitamin B-12. See Appendix 3 of the *Dietary Guidelines* at DietaryGuidelines.gov.

> The **Healthy Drinks. Healthy Kids.** campaign highlights appropriate beverage choices for children from birth to 5 years of age. All children up to 5 years of age should avoid beverages with added sugars, such as flavored milks, toddler formulas, sweetened soft drinks, and plant-based/nondairy milks.
>
> **0 to 6 months**
> Only provide breast milk or infant formula.
>
> **6 to 12 months**
> Continue to provide breast milk or infant formula as complementary foods are added to the infant's dietary pattern.
> Introduce sips of plain water.
>
> **12 to 24 months**
> Introduce whole milk during weaning from breast milk or infant formula.
> Continue to offer plain water.
> If any fruit juice is offered, make sure it is 100% fruit juice.
>
> **2 to 5 years**
> Switch to low-fat or fat-free milk.
> Milk and water should be the primary beverages.
> If any fruit juice is offered, make sure it is 100% fruit juice.
>
> Sources: Academy of Nutrition and Dietetics, American Academy of Pediatric Dentistry, American Academy of Pediatrics, American Heart Association.

autism spectrum disorder (ASD)
A disorder of neurological development characterized by problems with social interaction, verbal and nonverbal communication, and/or unusual, repetitive, or limited activities and interests.

VEGETARIAN DIETARY PATTERNS FOR YOUNG CHILDREN

Appropriately planned vegetarian dietary patterns can meet the young child's needs for growth and development. However, caregivers should be aware of a few potential nutrition risks. These include the possibility of developing iron-deficiency anemia, a deficiency of vitamin B-12, and rickets from a vitamin D deficiency. During the first few years of life, children also may not consume enough calories when following a vegetarian eating pattern, which tends to consist of many foods with low energy density. These known pitfalls are easily avoided by informed meal planning (review Section 6.4). Dietary patterns for children who eat vegetarian fare should focus on the following:[54]

- A variety of plant sources of protein to provide a full complement of essential amino acids (e.g., beans, nuts, and grains)
- A synthetic source of vitamin B-12 (e.g., dietary supplement or fortified breakfast cereal)
- Plenty of plant sources of iron (e.g., beans, dried fruits, and fortified grain products)
- Good sources of zinc (e.g., whole grains, beans, nuts, and seeds)
- Foods that are fortified with vitamin D (e.g., fortified orange juice), along with regular sun exposure
- Rich plant sources of calcium (e.g., fortified milk or juice), almonds, some forms of tofu, and green, leafy vegetables

PROMOTE GOOD ORAL HEALTH

Approximately 23% of toddlers and preschoolers have dental caries in their primary teeth (i.e., baby teeth).[55] A healthy dietary pattern goes a long way toward reducing the risk for dental caries in young children. In addition to beginning oral hygiene when teeth start to appear and seeking early pediatric dental care, the following nutrition-related tips can help reduce dental problems in children:[14]

- Drink water (fluoridated, if available) as opposed to carbohydrate-rich or acidic beverages (e.g., fruit juice, soft drinks, sports drinks, and energy drinks). If sugary or acidic beverages are consumed, it is better to drink them *with* meals rather than *between* meals. Sipping juice continuously between meals (e.g., from a sippy cup) exposes teeth to caries-promoting sugars and acids, which, over time, can erode enamel.
- Use small amounts of fluoridated toothpaste twice daily. In areas without fluoridated water, discuss fluoride needs with a dentist or pediatrician.
- Snack in moderation. Again, constant exposure of teeth to sugars and acids throughout the day (i.e., grazing) tends to promote caries.
- Make wise snack choices. We automatically think of sticky, sugary snacks as promoters of dental caries, but foods such as pretzels and popcorn provide a source of carbohydrates for oral bacteria as well. In contrast, crunchy fruits and vegetables, such as apples or celery, can help to brush away sticky food particles. Snacking on dairy products, such as cheese, can actually buffer the acids that lead to tooth decay.

LINKS BETWEEN AUTISM AND NUTRITION

Autism spectrum disorder (ASD) is characterized by a range of problems with social interaction, verbal and nonverbal communication, and/or unusual, repetitive, or limited activities and interests. This disorder usually is diagnosed in early childhood and affects an estimated 1 in every 36 children, with higher prevalence in males than females.[56] The causes for ASD are not well understood, but there is a definite genetic component.

ASD can both affect and be affected by nutritional status.[57] In addition to developmental and behavioral abnormalities, many children with ASD experience GI disorders, such as constipation, diarrhea, or reflux disease. Such disorders may impair nutrient intake or absorption. Medications used to treat behavioral problems may alter appetite. Some children with ASD may have feeding problems related to developmental impairments. Also, selective eating behaviors may affect nutrient intake. Children with ASD can be very rigid with their food selections, rejecting foods or entire food groups based on sensory qualities such as texture, color, and temperature. Thus, careful attention to nutrient-dense food choices is of prime importance.

A new diagnosis of ASD can be bewildering, and the lack of treatment options leaves many families feeling helpless. A dietary intervention may seem like a reasonable, low-risk option. Thus, a variety of dietary restrictions and/or nutrient supplements are commonly employed by families affected by ASD.[58] Is there any evidence that nutritional interventions are effective?

A widely used nutritional intervention is the gluten-free, casein-free (GFCF) diet, which eliminates all wheat, barley, rye, and milk products. Proponents of the GFCF diet believe that some children have a "leaky gut," which allows food proteins to be absorbed intact from the GI tract, enter the bloodstream, and affect brain function. By eliminating the offending food proteins, could symptoms of autism be reduced? This sounds scientifically plausible, yet there is little science to support this theory. Certain proteins may cross the blood–brain barrier and exert druglike effects on the brain, but the levels of these druglike proteins in body fluids are no higher among children with ASD than among children without ASD.

As mentioned, many children with ASD display selective eating behaviors; they are more sensitive than other children to colors, tastes, temperatures, and textures. Also, children with ASD prefer consistent routines and may refuse new foods. There is a strong possibility that a restrictive diet may exacerbate problems with social and emotional functioning.

In addition, restricting food choices may further limit an already marginal nutrient intake, leading to deficiencies of iron, calcium, vitamin D, and several B vitamins. Eliminating gluten will entail cutting out many types of breads, pastas, bakery products, crackers, and snack foods. Removing casein will require avoidance of milk, yogurt, cheese, butter, and many frozen desserts. Indeed, studies have shown that the dietary patterns of children with ASD already may be deficient in key nutrients. Children who follow a casein-free diet may have low bone mass or delayed bone development related to inadequate intake of calcium and vitamin D. Children on a gluten-free diet have lower levels of folate and vitamin B-6. Nutrient shortfalls can have both short- and long-term implications for the child's health.

Clearly, the GFCF diet is not free of risks. But would the risks be acceptable if the eating plan helps to improve symptoms? Unfortunately, there is very little evidence to support either the safety or the efficacy of the GFCF diet. The few studies that do show a positive outcome are of poor quality, meaning they were of short duration and had small numbers of subjects, poor study designs, and a high risk of bias.[59,60]

Knowing that children with ASD are at risk for dietary inadequacies, the best dietary strategy is to offer a variety of nutrient-dense foods at each meal. A dietary restriction should only be used if there is evidence that a child has an allergy or intolerance to a food. Consulting with an RDN would be helpful to assess the child's dietary patterns and create a personalized plan to alleviate GI symptoms and ensure that nutritional needs are met. For a child with extremely limited dietary intake, multivitamin and mineral supplementation may be an option.

At this time, the AAP does not endorse any specific dietary plan or supplement as a treatment for ASD.[61] Despite the lack of evidence to support the efficacy of nutritional interventions for ASD, many parents will choose to try them anyway, hoping for positive results. There may, in fact, be a subset of children with ASD who do respond to dietary treatments. Because of the rising incidence of ASD and the lack of curative treatments, nutritional interventions for ASD will continue to be an active area of research.

Autism Spectrum Disorder
Researchers have observed differences between the gut microbiota of neurotypical children and those with autism spectrum disorder (ASD). Some researchers point to alterations in the gut microbiota as a causative factor for ASD. Perhaps some compounds produced by the microbiota are absorbed into the blood and can directly affect brain function. Scientists have seen that inoculating germ-free mice with the gut bacteria from a human with ASD led to ASD-like behaviors in the mice. Scientists are interested in learning about the potential for manipulating the microbiota (e.g., with prebiotics or probiotics) to alter the course of ASD.

Source: Sharon G, Cruz NJ, Kang D-W, et al. Human gut microbiota from autism spectrum disorder promote behavioral symptoms in mice. *Cell*. 2019 May 30;177(6):1600-1618.e17. doi: 10.1016/j.cell.2019.05.004

Helpful resources for planning nutritious, age-appropriate meals and snacks:
www.MyPlate.gov
www.fns.usda.gov/team-nutrition
brightfutures.aap.org

✓ CONCEPT CHECK 15.4

1. Why is picky eating common among preschoolers? Provide three or more suggestions to help a preschooler accept nutritious foods.
2. How often do preschoolers need to eat throughout the day? List three nutrient-dense snack ideas that would be appropriate for a 3-year-old child.
3. Should toddlers and preschoolers take a multivitamin and mineral supplement? Why or why not?
4. Explain the connections between nutrition and oral health. List three ways to reduce risk for dental caries with healthy eating habits.
5. What are some nutrition concerns of children with autism spectrum disorder?

15.5 School-Age Children: Nutrition Concerns

The dietary patterns of many school-age children can be improved, particularly with regard to fruit, vegetable, whole grain, and beverage choices. In recent years, whole fruit consumption has gone up and fruit juice consumption has gone down, but overall fruit intake among school-age children remains below the targets of the *Dietary Guidelines*. Similarly, vegetable intake is about half of the recommended servings per day for children.[62] White potatoes (including French fries) account for about 30% of vegetable intake.[63] Less than 1% of children meet the recommendation of the *Dietary Guidelines* to make half of grains whole.[64] Intakes of dairy foods, although they make a significant contribution to calcium, vitamin D, and potassium intakes among children, are below targets.[65] In general, the nutritional concerns and goals applicable to school-age children are the same as those discussed in relation to preschoolers. However, with the added pressures of peers, food advertisers, health messages from the media, and an increasing desire for independence, these goals may be harder to achieve as children grow older.

The healthy U.S.-style dietary patterns summarized in Table 15-6 are a good basis for meal planning. For school-age children from 6 to 12 years of age, daily calorie needs are usually within the range of 1200 to 2400 kcal per day, depending on age, biological sex, body size, activity level, and rate of growth. Families with school-age children should continue to use MyPlate (Fig. 15-5) as a guide for building healthy meals. Emphasize nutrient-dense sources of iron, zinc, calcium, and vitamin D while striving to limit intakes of saturated fat, added sugars, and sodium.

Now let us look at several nutritional issues of particular concern during the school-age years.

REVERSING TRENDS FOR OVERWEIGHT AND OBESITY

By far, the most troublesome nutritional problem facing children today is the rise in childhood obesity. The rate of obesity among children tripled from 1971 to 2017 but has stabilized within the past few years. Currently, about 35% of U.S. children are classified as overweight or obese. The rates of childhood obesity are highest among children from low-income families and minority populations.[66]

Childhood obesity can affect every body system (Fig. 15-6). The mechanical stress of excess weight impacts the development of bones, joints, and muscles. Changes in hormones affect growth and sexual maturation; puberty may begin earlier, resulting in an earlier adolescent growth spurt, but this may ultimately lead to short stature due to premature fusing of growth plates. Insulin resistance and increased inflammation contribute to the development of type 2 diabetes and cardiovascular disease. In addition to effects on physical health, childhood obesity is also associated with social concerns (e.g., bullying) and psychiatric disorders (e.g., depression, anxiety, and disordered eating behaviors). Compared to children at a healthy weight, children with obesity are

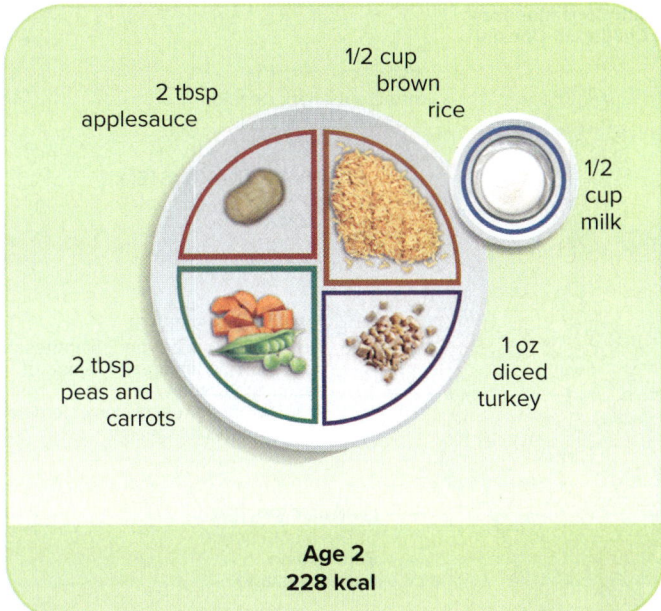
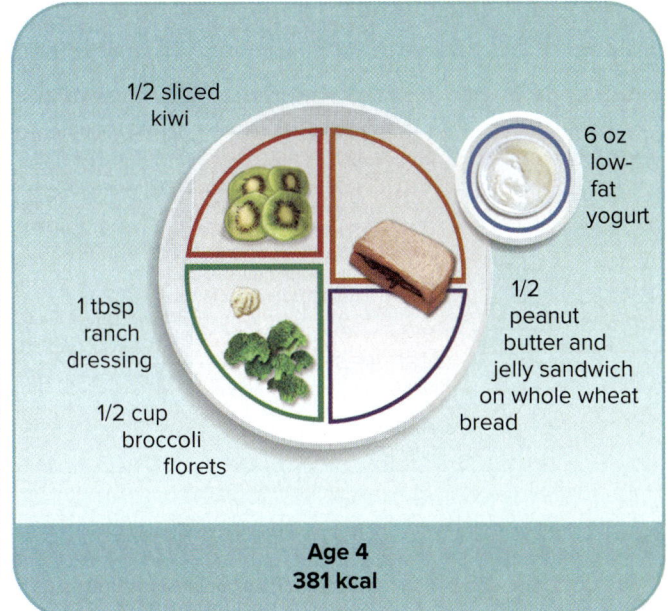
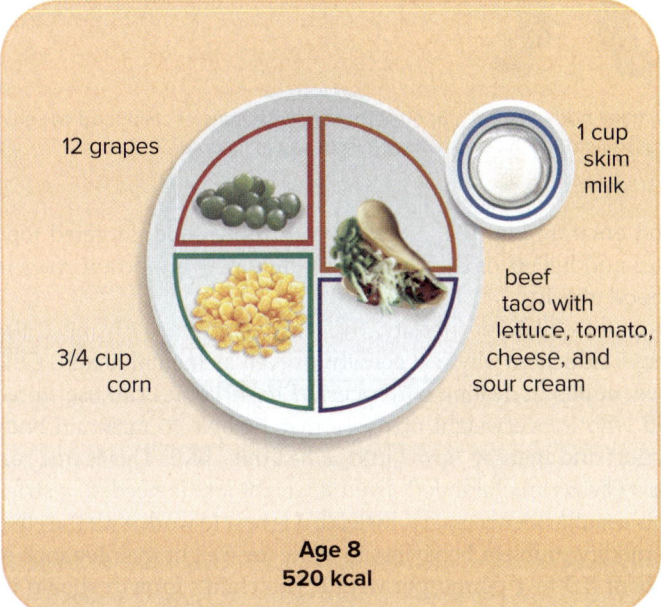
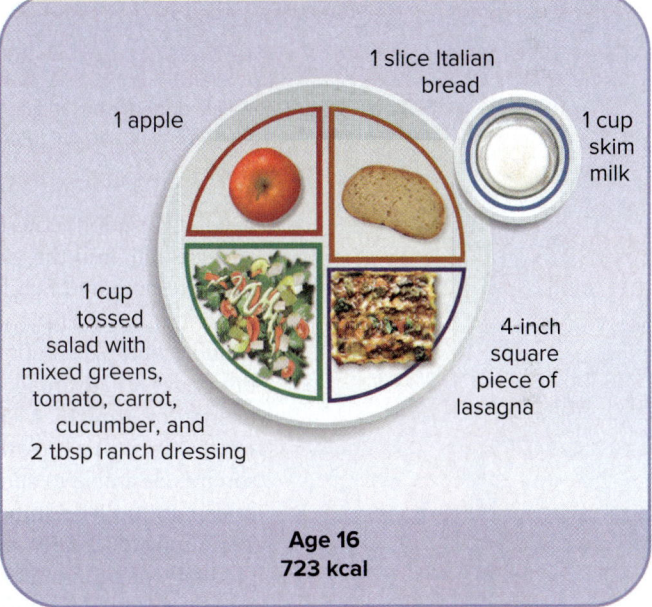

FIGURE 15-5 Using MyPlate to build a healthy meal for children. MyPlate is a useful tool for all Americans ages 2 and older. MyPlate proportions apply to children as well as adults, but portion sizes and food choices vary by age.

approximately five times more likely to have obesity during adulthood.[67] To identify cases and reverse these trends, the U.S. Preventive Services Task Force recommends screening children for obesity starting at 6 years of age.[68]

Research points to many potential causes of childhood obesity. When it comes to dietary patterns, excessive calories from sugar-sweetened beverages, unlimited snacking, oversized portions, and overreliance on fast foods all may contribute to excessive weight gain during childhood. Energy expenditure also tends to decline as children age. On average, children spend about 7.5 hours per day engaged in screen time, which includes time spent watching television, working at the computer, or using phones and other electronic devices.[69] As screen time goes up, "lean time" goes down; less than 30% of school-age children (ages 6 to 11) and less than 20% of adolescents (ages 12 to 17) are getting the recommended 60 minutes of physical activity per day.[70] Furthermore,

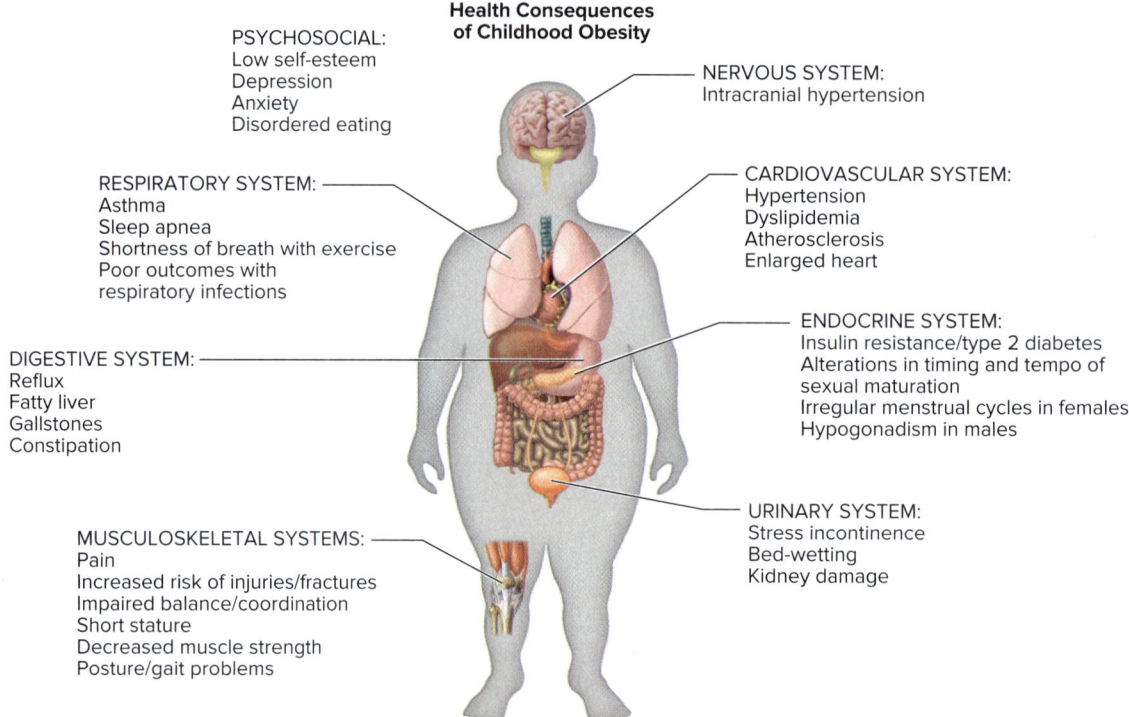

FIGURE 15-6 During childhood, obesity affects many body systems. Short-term consequences of childhood obesity are illustrated here. Long-term health outcomes associated with obesity were discussed in Chapter 7.

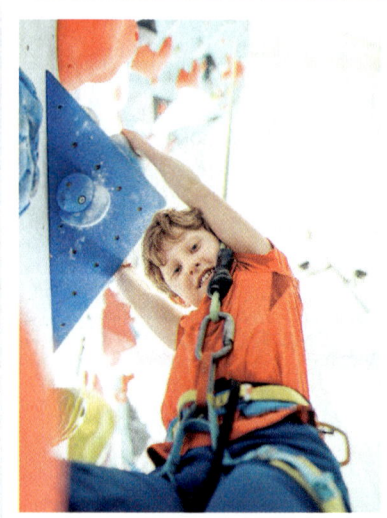

To get kids involved in physical activity, new physical education classes have been introduced in some schools. Classes on rock climbing, kayaking, and martial arts help to promote activity because they take the focus away from teams and competition, which often discourage and embarrass kids who lack athletic talent. **What are the recommendations of the *Physical Activity Guidelines* for children?** soloway/123RF

genetic variations, the food environment (i.e., access to nutritious food, targeted food advertising), and the values and beliefs of the child and family play important roles in the development of childhood obesity.[71]

Given the multiple causes of childhood obesity, the treatment approach must also include multiple components: nutrition, physical activity, as well as mental health. Children have an advantage over adults in dealing with obesity: Their bodies can use stored energy for growth. A child who is overweight or obese may be able to maintain body weight through a growth spurt and thereby "grow into" a healthier BMI. This is one reason it is desirable to address obesity in childhood. Even if weight loss is needed, a strict, calorie-controlled regimen is usually not necessary. Instead, it is best to work with the child and family to identify and modify problem behaviors to allow for weight maintenance or gradual weight loss (i.e., about 0.5 to 1 pound per week). The child's growth should be monitored closely; calorie intake should not be so low that gains in height diminish.

Modifying Physical Activity Habits. Typically, the initial approach in treating a child who is overweight or obese is to assess physical activity. The *Physical Activity Guidelines for Americans* recommends 60 minutes or more of moderate to vigorous physical activity per day for children and adolescents (Table 15-8). If a child spends too much time in sedentary activities, more physical activities should be encouraged. For school-age children, parents should set appropriate limits on screen time to facilitate increased physical activity.[72]

Younger children can engage in unstructured play to reap the benefits of several different forms of physical activity. For example, running, bicycling, and dancing are examples of aerobic activities, which help to build cardiorespiratory fitness. Some movements also naturally promote strengthening of muscles (e.g., climbing on playground equipment) and bones (e.g., the weight-bearing activity of jumping). As children grow and mature, they may become more interested in organized sports (e.g., soccer and basketball). Structured weight training with small weights can also be beneficial as long as children are properly supervised.[73]

TABLE 15-8 ■ Physical Activity Guidelines for Children

Guidelines for Preschool-Age Children (age 3–5 years)
Be physically active throughout the day to enhance growth and development.
Caregivers should encourage active play that includes a variety of types of activity.
Guidelines for Children and Adolescents
Provide opportunities and encouragement to participate in a variety of enjoyable, age-appropriate physical activities.
Engage in 60 minutes or more of moderate to vigorous physical activity daily, which should include:
Mostly moderate- or vigorous-intensity aerobic physical activity; include vigorous-intensity physical activity on at least 3 days per week.
Muscle-strengthening physical activity on at least 3 days per week.
Bone-strengthening physical activity on at least 3 days per week.

Source: *Physical Activity Guidelines for Americans*, 2nd ed., available from https://health.gov/paguidelines/secondedition/pdf/Physical_Activity_Guidelines_2nd_edition.pdf.

Making a habit of engaging in and enjoying regular physical activity will help children to maintain a healthy body weight throughout life. However, simply recommending an increase in physical activity will not make it happen; parents and other caregivers need to plan for and model these behaviors! For example, getting the family together for a brisk walk after dinner encourages healthy habits for all involved.[46]

Modifying Eating Habits. Many safe and effective dietary interventions are available to promote healthier body weight in the pediatric population, but there is not enough evidence to specifically recommend one intervention over another.[71] As discussed in Chapter 7 for the treatment of obesity in adults, dietary interventions must be tailored to the individual, taking into account medical needs, cultural traditions, personal and family preferences, and economic constraints. There are interventions that focus on building a healthy plate, particularly increasing fruit and vegetable intake. An emphasis on appropriate portion sizes may help youth learn to curb excessive food consumption. Some interventions teach families about the glycemic load of foods and encourage children to select foods with higher fiber and lower sugar content. Other interventions limit the frequency of meals consumed outside the home (i.e., fast foods). There are many tools in the toolbox, and it is up to the RDN, the child, and the family to figure out what tool (or combination of tools) will meet the child's needs and can be sustained long term. Given that children are still growing and developing, it is crucial to monitor growth over time and ensure that essential nutrient needs are being met.

Medical and Surgical Interventions. Approximately 8% of youth have severe obesity (i.e., BMI ≥ 35 kg/m² or ≥ 120% of the 95th percentile for BMI-for-age). Weight-loss medications may be prescribed by a primary care provider to complement lifestyle interventions. Currently, orlistat (Xenical) is the only weight-loss medication approved for the pediatric population (age 12 or older) by the FDA. On average, treatment with orlistat leads to about 3% reduction in BMI among youth with obesity.[74]

For children with severe obesity, particularly those with existing hypertension, cardiovascular disease, or type 2 diabetes, bariatric surgery is a safe and effective option for weight management.[75] The two most common forms of bariatric surgery performed on adolescents are Roux-en-Y gastric bypass and vertical sleeve gastrectomy. Outcomes of bariatric surgery in the pediatric population are good. On average, children lose more than 25% of body weight and experience significant improvements or resolution of comorbid health conditions. As discussed in Section 7.9, long-term follow-up is essential to monitor nutrition status, as deficiencies of vitamin B-12, iron, and folate are common.

The majority of children with obesity have experienced some degree of weight bias. Most often, they report weight bias from peers (at school or online), but some children also experience weight bias in the health care setting. Weight bias has been associated with poor health outcomes, including depression, low self-esteem, overeating, disordered eating, and avoidance of physical activity.[71]

When it comes to weight bias, health care professionals can either be part of the problem or part of the solution. Here are a few suggestions to reduce weight bias in childhood obesity management.

- Communicate with respect. Use people-first language (e.g., "person with obesity" rather than "obese person"). Ask the patient about their preferred words for describing body weight and body shape.
- Involve the child (and the child's family) in the treatment plan. Ask the patient if they want to engage in a plan for weight change. If weight change is a desired goal, engage the patient in setting realistic goals and making practical plans to reach those goals.
- Ensure that the clinical setting (e.g., furniture, scales, blood pressure cuffs, and hospital gowns) can accommodate patients with larger body sizes.
- Avoid blaming and shaming. Acknowledge the many genetic, medical, environmental, and social factors that influence body weight.

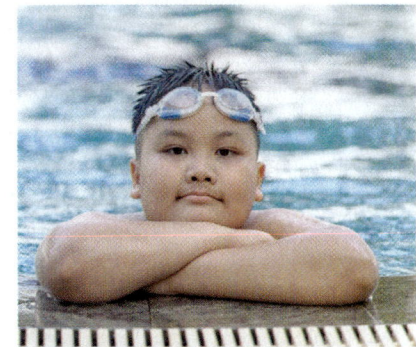

Some researchers have suggested that treatments for pediatric obesity may increase the risk for mental health disorders among children. However, there is currently no evidence that pediatric weight management interventions worsen depression or anxiety or increase the risk for disordered eating or eating disorders.[71] Kwanchai Chai-udom/123RF

Chronic Disease Risk Reduction Intake (CDRR) for Sodium for Children	
1 to 3 years	1200 milligrams per day
4 to 8 years	1500 milligrams per day
9 to 13 years	1800 milligrams per day
14 to 18 years	2300 milligrams per day

EARLY SIGNS OF CARDIOVASCULAR DISEASE

Parallel to the increase in childhood obesity, early signs of cardiovascular disease have become increasingly prevalent among children and adolescents. The CDC estimates that 7% of children have abnormal blood lipids.[76] Therefore, lifestyle modifications to delay the progression of the disease are important throughout the life span. The AAP recommends universal blood lipid screening for all children around the ages of 9 to 11. Even earlier screening is recommended for "at-risk" children who are overweight, have high blood pressure, smoke, or have diabetes; have a family history of cardiovascular disease; or whose family history is unknown.[77] For children whose cholesterol is elevated, lifestyle approaches such as weight management through dietary modification and increased physical activity are the first line of therapy.[78] An eating pattern that is consistent with the *Dietary Guidelines* would be appropriate for prevention of cardiovascular disease. To complement modifications to fat and sodium intakes, the American Heart Association recently released guidelines for children to limit added sugar intake to 25 grams per day.[33] This is quite a reduction from the average 80 grams of added sugars consumed by children and adolescents per day.

TYPE 2 DIABETES AMONG YOUTH

Type 2 diabetes was once regarded as an adult condition. However, an alarming increase in the frequency of the disease among children (and teenagers) has been documented.[79] This is primarily due to the rise in obesity in this age group. Up to 85% of children with the disease are overweight at diagnosis.[80] Infection with SARS-CoV-2, the virus that causes COVID-19, has also been linked to increased risk for developing type 1 and type 2 diabetes among children.[81]

Starting at age 10, children who are overweight or obese and who have risk factors for type 2 diabetes should be screened for type 2 diabetes every 3 years.[82] Besides obesity and a sedentary lifestyle, examples of risk factors include having a close relative with the disease or belonging to a nonwhite population. In 2013, the AAP released the first-ever guidelines for management of type 2 diabetes in children.[83] These guidelines provide recommendations for monitoring of blood glucose, use of medications, weight management, and physical activity. Dietary management strategies should be culturally appropriate and include a regular schedule of meals and snacks; education on appropriate portion sizes; limiting sugar-sweetened beverages, high-fat foods, snacks, and fast foods; and focusing on incorporating more fruits, vegetables, and low-fat or fat-free dairy products. For physical activity, experts advise children to engage in moderate- or vigorous-intensity physical activity for at least 60 minutes each day.

START THE DAY WITH BREAKFAST

You have heard it before: *breakfast is the most important meal of the day.* Yet, about 15% of school-age children skip breakfast. The problem gets worse as children reach the teenage years, when nearly 30% of adolescents skip breakfast on a given day.[84] Children who skip breakfast are missing out on important nutrients that fuel the brain and the body. A fortified, low-sugar, ready-to-eat breakfast cereal offers lots of nutrition in a tasty and convenient package; it is typically the greatest source of iron, vitamin A, and folic acid for children ages 2 to 18. Although there is disagreement over the true benefit of breakfast for cognitive ability, children who eat breakfast are more likely to meet their daily needs for vitamins and minerals compared to children not eating breakfast.[85] Also, a growing body of research shows that starting the day with breakfast reduces the risk for obesity.

Note that breakfast menus need not be limited to traditional fare. A little imagination can spark the interest of even the most reluctant eater. Instead of conventional breakfast foods, parents can offer leftovers from dinner, such as pizza, spaghetti, soups, yogurt topped with trail mix, chili with beans, or sandwiches. For lasting energy and satiety, combine traditional carbohydrate-rich breakfast foods with a source of protein, such as low-fat cheese, nuts, or eggs.

For kids who complain about waking up early to make time for breakfast, consider the convenience of healthy, grab-and-go options, such as leftover pancakes topped with peanut butter and bananas. **What quick and nutritious breakfast ideas would you recommend for a school-age child?** Alexis Joseph/McGraw Hill

CHOOSE HEALTHY FATS

Dietary patterns of school-age children should include a variety of foods from each major group, not necessarily excluding any specific food because of its fat content. Overemphasis on fat-reduced eating patterns during childhood has been linked to an increase in eating disorders and encourages an inappropriate "good food, bad food" attitude.

However, surveys of dietary intake among children show that they are consuming too much saturated fat, most of which comes from whole milk, other full-fat dairy products, and fatty meats.[65] Furthermore, few children (or adults) meet recommendations to include two servings of fish per week to ensure adequate intake of omega-3 fatty acids.[86] Emphasizing low-fat dairy products (from age 2 onward), offering broiled or baked fish, choosing leaner cuts of meat, trimming visible fat from meats, and removing the skin from poultry before serving foods will establish heart-healthy eating habits to last a lifetime. Snacks for children should emphasize fruits, vegetables, whole grains, and low-fat or fat-free dairy choices. Ideas for healthy snacks are found in Table 15-7.

SELECT APPROPRIATE BEVERAGES

Maintaining proper hydration is important for children. The fluid needs of school-age children range from approximately 1½ to 2½ liters per day, depending on age and sex. Instead of choosing water and milk, however, children often opt for sugar-sweetened beverages. Intake of sugar-sweetened beverages among children steadily increased from the 1970s, peaked around the turn of the century, and then decreased slightly over the past 20 years. Despite the recent decrease, intakes of sugar-sweetened beverages still contribute almost 100 empty kcal per day for school-age children.[87] Besides contributing to excess body weight, such high intakes of sugar-sweetened beverages are linked to increased levels of inflammation and worsened blood lipid profiles among children.[88]

Even 100% fruit juices, which are perceived by many to be an important source of vitamin C and potassium for children, may contribute to excessive weight gain among children.[89] Replacing 100% fruit juices with whole fruits would supply important nutrients in a lower-caloric package for children. Fruit juice should be limited to 6 fluid ounces per day for young children (ages 4 to 6) or 8 fluid ounces per day for older children (ages 7 to 18).[90] Overall, children should be given water and low-fat or fat-free milk as primary beverage choices.

PROMOTE SOUND NUTRITION IN SCHOOLS

Children spend the majority of their waking hours in school, so it is a great place to learn about and practice healthy eating behaviors.[91] A strong emphasis on nutrition education in schools can help children understand why healthy dietary patterns will make them feel more energetic, look healthier, and work more efficiently. The USDA's Team Nutrition initiative supports child nutrition programs with education materials that promote healthy food choices and physical activity.

Most schools have included nutrition education in their health or science curricula, but until recently these healthy nutrition messages were not consistently backed up by the food offerings in school cafeterias. In 2010, the Healthy, Hunger-Free Kids Act extended funding for the National School Lunch Program, School Breakfast Program, and several other federal nutrition programs. The law also authorized the USDA to make significant changes to the nutritional quality of foods provided in schools. Public school food-service programs now have to meet nutrition standards that stipulate the inclusion of fruits, vegetables, and whole grains, while limiting saturated fat and sodium content in meals.[92]

Breakfasts and lunches prepared by school cafeterias are not the only targets of school nutrition reforms. In 2014, standards for the quality of competitive foods sold on school campuses (e.g., from snack bars and vending machines) went into effect. These guidelines set calorie limits on snacks and restrict the levels of saturated fat, added sugars, and sodium in foods that can be sold to students.[93]

one in five children is deficient in vitamin D. Meanwhile, the adolescent growth spurt marks a critical time for bone development. About 50% of adult bone mass is accrued during adolescence. Calcium requirements for 14- to 18-year-old children are 1300 milligrams per day—higher than during any other time of life! Failure to maximize bone mineralization during childhood sets the stage for development of osteoporosis later in life.[26]

The *Dietary Guidelines* recommend three servings per day from the dairy group for all teenagers and young adults to meet calcium needs. If dairy products are not consumed, alternative calcium sources must be included. Nondairy sources of calcium include almonds, legumes, some green vegetables, and fortified foods (e.g., nondairy milks, fruit juices, cereal, and granola bars). However, it is important to note that these alternative sources of calcium may not provide other important nutrients supplied by dairy products, such as protein and vitamins A, D, and B-12.

Iron. About 10% of adolescent females have low iron stores or iron-deficiency anemia.[100] Iron-deficiency anemia is a highly undesirable condition for a teen. It can lead to fatigue and a decreased ability to concentrate and learn, such that academic and physical performance suffers. Iron-deficiency anemia sometimes appears in males during their growth spurt, but adolescent females are at risk of deficiency due to menstruation and poor dietary intake. It is important that teenagers choose good food sources of iron, such as lean meats and fortified grain products. Teenage females, in particular, need to eat good sources of iron. If dietary intake is insufficient to achieve optimal iron status, work with a primary care provider to determine whether dietary supplementation is necessary.

Many of the nutritional issues of adolescents—obesity, snacking, beverage choices, and skipping meals—have been adequately described with reference to younger children. Here, we present a few nutrition dilemmas that pertain especially to teenagers.

BREAK THE FAST-FOOD HABIT

It is convenient, casual, inexpensive, and their friends work there. These are reasons why, on any given day, about 40% of the nation's youth eat food from a fast-food restaurant. Unfortunately, the average trip to a fast-food establishment yields about 300 extra calories, 14 additional grams of fat, and 400 milligrams of sodium *in excess* of typical home-prepared meals for teenagers.[41,101]

With some small changes, teens can still enjoy dining out with friends without detriment to their health. When building a sandwich, opt for one layer of meat instead of double or triple patties, and select grilled instead of fried meat. For deli sandwiches, choose moderate portions of lean sources of protein, such as roasted turkey or chicken, rather than fatty slices of processed meats, such as bologna and salami. Skip the condiments or request them on the side; the mayonnaise on a typical fast food sandwich supplies about 100 fat-laden kcal. Each slice of cheese supplies another 80 to 100 kcal. When it comes to choosing a side dish, a small baked potato or a garden salad with reduced-fat dressing will provide fewer calories and more nutrients than the typical 500 kcal large serving of fries. Calories from regular soft drinks—especially when free refills are available—can quickly add up. Teens should choose reduced-fat or fat-free milk as a nutrient-dense alternative or opt for water. Order a pizza with veggie toppings, low-fat cheese, and whole grain crust.

When burgers are measured in pounds instead of ounces, portion control is an issue. Supersized meals, while they may seem economical, should be avoided unless they are to be divided and shared among friends. Choosing items from the kids' menu can lessen the impact of dining out on adolescent wallets and waistlines.

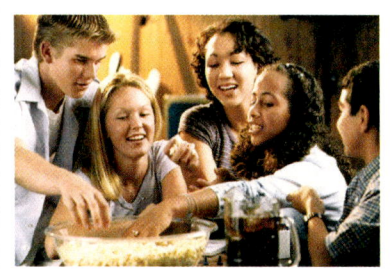

The teenage years are noted for snacking. **Suggest some snack choices to fill common nutrient gaps among teens.** SW Productions /Photodisc/Getty Images

CURB CAFFEINE INTAKE

The combined demands of school, work, extracurricular activities, social commitments, and late-night screen time leave many adolescents looking for a quick pick-me-up. Commonly, they are turning to caffeine, the most widely used stimulant on the planet. Soft drinks, a common choice among youth, provide about 25 milligrams

Newsworthy Nutrition

Glycemic load of food choices may influence acne

INTRODUCTION: About 80% to 90% of teens experience acne to some degree. Although it is popularly believed that nuts, chocolate, French fries, and pizza contribute to acne, scientific studies have failed to show a strong role for any of these dietary factors. Observational studies suggest a relationship between glycemic index or glycemic load of the dietary pattern and acne, but previous research has not adequately or accurately assessed dietary intake and biological factors relative to acne. **OBJECTIVES:** To examine differences in dietary intake (especially glycemic index and glycemic load of the dietary pattern) and biological markers of insulin resistance among young adults with or without acne. **METHODS:** In this *cross-sectional study*, 64 adults between the ages of 18 and 40 with BMI within the range of 18.5 to 30 kg/m^2 completed 5-day diet records. The researchers collected blood samples to assess biological markers of insulin resistance. Digital photos were taken and assessed by trained dermatologists who scored acne severity. **RESULTS:** Compared to the dietary patterns of subjects with no acne, the dietary patterns of subjects with moderate or severe acne were higher in total carbohydrates and glycemic load. In addition, the subjects with acne had higher insulin resistance than subjects without acne. **CONCLUSION:** Glycemic load of the dietary pattern is associated with acne among young adults. Insulin resistance appears to play a role in development of acne. Choosing whole, unprocessed grains, vegetables, and fruits instead of refined grains and foods with added sugars may assist efforts to reduce acne.

Source: Burris J, Rietkerk W, Shikany JM, Woolf K. Differences in dietary glycemic load and hormones in New York City adults with no and moderate/severe acne. *J Acad Nutr Diet.* 2017 Sep;117(9):1375-1383. doi: 10.1016/j.jand.2017.03.024

of caffeine per serving. On average, 40% of adolescents report consuming energy beverages, which typically contain between 100 and 200 milligrams of caffeine per serving.[102] Consumption of coffee and tea, which yield about 100 milligrams of caffeine per cup, is on the rise among teens. Various foods, including chocolate and some types of candies or sports nutrition products, contain caffeine as well. Average caffeine intake from all sources is just over 100 milligrams per day among teens. Many consumers are unaware of how much caffeine they are consuming; the exact amount of caffeine is not always listed on energy drink labels because (1) it is not currently required by food labeling laws and (2) some manufacturers (especially of energy drinks) consider it to be part of a "proprietary blend."

Considering diet quality, many caffeinated beverages are sources of added sugars. For children, added sugars contribute empty calories at a time of life when essential nutrients are in high demand to support growth and development. Caffeine itself may lead to sleep problems, shakiness, dizziness, feelings of anxiety, headaches, and gastrointestinal distress. For children, in particular, there is concern that excessive caffeine intake could affect normal neurological and cardiovascular development. Furthermore, disturbances in normal sleep patterns could affect growth and learning ability. Alarmingly, there have been thousands of reports of caffeine poisoning—and even some deaths—as a result of excessive intake of energy drinks.[103] For these reasons, caffeine is not recommended at all for children under age 12. For adolescents, caffeine intake should be limited to 100 milligrams per day, if it is used at all.[104]

VEGETARIAN DIETARY PATTERNS DURING ADOLESCENCE

Teenagers, who strive to forge an identity by adopting dietary patterns different from those of their families, may choose to follow a plant-based dietary pattern. Vegetarians enjoy many health benefits, including lower body weight and better control of blood glucose and cholesterol. Indeed, an increased focus on plant foods is needed

> The *Dietary Guidelines* outlines healthy vegetarian dietary patterns at various calorie levels for ages 2 and older. For additional information, see Appendix 3 at DietaryGuidelines.gov.

among adolescents, who often miss out on their recommended daily servings of fruits and vegetables. However, teens may not know enough about a vegetarian dietary pattern to keep from developing health problems, such as iron-deficiency anemia. The bulkiness of a plant-based eating pattern is not as much of a concern for teens as it is for younger children with smaller stomach capacity, but a strictly vegetarian eating pattern must be monitored for adequate energy, protein, iron, vitamin B-12, calcium, and vitamin D (the latter if sun exposure is not sufficient) at any age. These nutrients are particularly important in teenagers, as their dietary patterns are often already nutrient poor.

Teens often cite concern for the humane treatment of animals as their main reason for choosing vegetarian eating patterns, but be observant of teens who choose vegetarianism as a strategy to manage body weight. Vegetarian dietary patterns are sometimes used as a socially acceptable way to restrict food intake and, for some, can be an early sign of disordered eating.[105]

ALCOHOL ABUSE AMONG TEENS

In Section 15.5, we discussed how the beverage choices of school-age children are in need of improvement because they provide too much sugar and not enough micronutrients. The nutrient density of beverages continues to be a problem among teenagers, but a new problem arises: alcohol abuse. Developmentally, adolescents are prone to experimentation, rebellion, and risk taking, so use of this illegal and dangerous substance is common among teenagers. Results of the national Youth Risk Behavior Survey demonstrate that approximately 23% of high school students regularly use alcohol and about 10% of high school students engage in binge drinking.[106]

It is just harmless fun, right? Wrong! Alcohol use beginning in adolescence has severe consequences.[107] The adolescent's body and brain are still developing. Exposure to alcohol can decrease brain mass in the area of the brain involved in decision making, memory, and learning. This is evidenced by academic problems and poor decision making, which can lead to legal troubles, physical assault, and risky sexual behaviors. The most dangerous consequence of poor judgment is drinking and driving; about 1 in 20 teenagers admits to drinking and driving.[106] Alcohol also contributes to other causes of accidental injuries and deaths, such as drowning, falls, and burns.

Adolescent alcohol abuse exacts a toll on long-term physical health as well. Studies show that alcohol abuse beginning during adolescence is a strong predictor of alcohol abuse during adulthood. Nutritional status can be affected because alcohol abuse is often accompanied by nutrient-poor dietary patterns. Also, weight gain from empty calories increases the risk for obesity-related diseases, such as hypertension and cardiovascular disease. These physical consequences may not surface until later in life, but it is certain that the effects of alcohol on the liver, brain, and cardiovascular system can start early.

Alcohol use by teenagers should not be viewed as a normal part of growing up. On the contrary, the physical, emotional, and intellectual consequences of underage drinking can be long-standing and devastating. Parents and other caregivers should talk to their children about the consequences of alcohol abuse, set clear rules, monitor their children's behavior, and be positive role models.

✓ CONCEPT CHECK 15.6

1. Which two minerals are most likely to be deficient in the dietary patterns of teens? Name two rich food sources of each of these minerals.
2. Design a meal for a teen that resembles MyPlate and can be purchased from a fast-food restaurant.
3. Are energy drinks safe for consumption by children of any age? Why or why not?
4. List three consequences of alcohol abuse that are specific to adolescents.

15.7 Nutrition and Your Health: Food Allergies and Intolerances

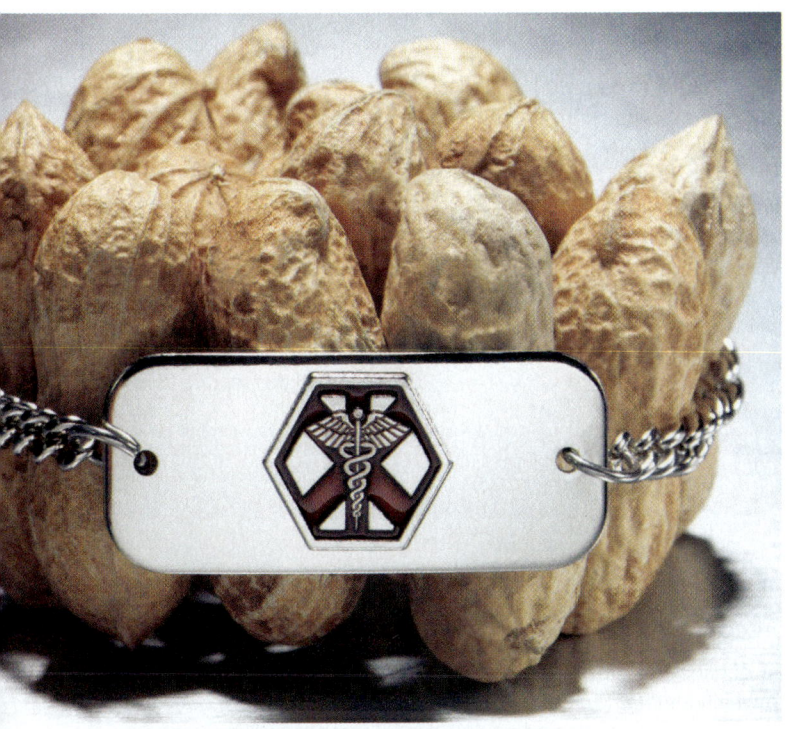

Peter Reali/Corbis Super RF/Alamy Stock Photo

Food allergies are on the rise. What used to be a rare medical incident is now the cause for 200,000 emergency department visits per year.[108] Accounting for direct medical costs, special foods, and time lost from work, food allergies cost Americans $25 billion per year. Today, food allergies affect about 8% (5.9 million) of children in the United States. About 40% of children with food allergies are allergic to more than one type of food. The most commonly reported food allergies among children are peanuts, milk, shellfish, and tree nuts (Fig. 15-7).[109]

Adverse reactions to foods—indicated by sneezing, coughing, nausea, vomiting, diarrhea, hives, and other rashes—are broadly classed as food allergies (also called *hypersensitivities*) or **food intolerances.** The term *food sensitivity* is ill defined but generally refers to any symptom that is perceived to be food related. In our discussion, we group adverse food reactions into two categories: those caused by an immune response are termed *food allergies,* and those not caused by an immune response are *food intolerances.*

Food Allergies: Symptoms and Mechanisms

Symptoms of food allergies may affect the following:

- *Skin:* itching, tingling,* redness, hives, and swelling
- *GI tract:* nausea, vomiting, diarrhea, intestinal gas, bloating, pain, constipation, and indigestion
- *Respiratory tract:* runny nose, wheezing, congestion, and difficulty breathing*
- *Cardiovascular system:* low blood pressure* and rapid heart rate*

These symptoms usually set in shortly after consuming the offending food protein and may last for a few seconds or a few days. The symptoms marked with an asterisk (*) are signs of a rapid and potentially fatal type of allergic response called **anaphylaxis.** This severe allergic response results in low blood pressure and respiratory distress. A person who is extremely sensitive to a food may not be able to touch the food or even be in the same room where it is being cooked without reacting to it. Although any food can trigger anaphylaxis, the most common culprits are peanuts (a legume, not a nut), tree nuts (e.g., walnuts, pecans), shellfish, milk (also beware of an ingredient called casein), eggs (look for

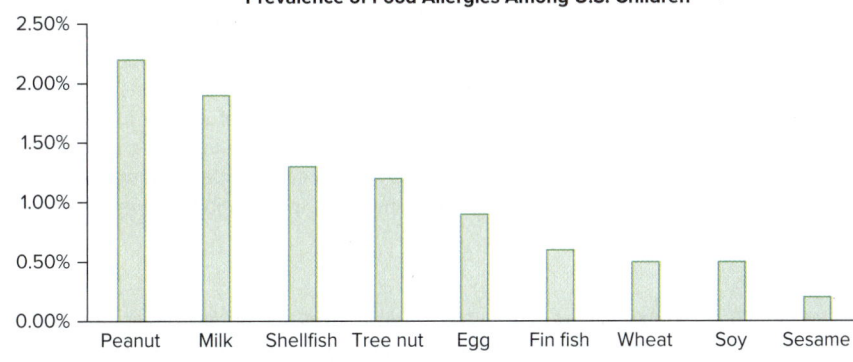

FIGURE 15-7 Prevalence of food allergies among U.S. children.
Source: Data from Gupta RS, Warren CM, Smith BM, et al. The public health impact of parent-reported childhood food allergies in the United States. *Pediatrics.* 2018; 142;e20181235.

food intolerance An adverse reaction to food that does not involve an immune response.

anaphylaxis A severe allergic response that results in lowered blood pressure and respiratory distress. This can be fatal.

the ingredient albumin), soybeans, wheat, fish, and sesame. Other foods frequently identified with adverse reactions include meat and meat products, fruits, and cheese. For a small number of people, avoiding foods such as peanuts or shellfish is a matter of life and death.

Basically, allergies are an inappropriate response of the immune system. When immune cells identify a harmful foreign protein (antigen), they destroy it and produce antibodies to it, so that the next response to the harmful substance will be swift and effective. Almost all food allergies are caused by proteins in foods that act as antigens (also called allergens). In these cases, the immune system mistakes the food protein for a harmful substance and mounts an immune response, leading to symptoms such as hives, runny nose, and GI disturbances.

No one is sure why the immune system sometimes overreacts to harmless proteins. The early introduction (e.g., before 4 months of age) of solid foods to infants may trigger food allergies. The reasoning is that the infant's GI tract is immature and "leaky," allowing some undigested proteins to be absorbed into the bloodstream. Gut permeability is beneficial for the absorption of immune proteins from breast milk; however, if some food proteins are introduced before the GI tract has matured, antigens may enter the bloodstream and stimulate an immune response.

The hygiene hypothesis offers another interesting explanation: in our "germophobic" society, with the protection of antibiotics, hand sanitizers, and antimicrobial soaps and cleaners, our immune systems are not vigorously challenged by antigens. As a result, the immune system may become sensitized to innocuous substances, such as food proteins. Current research supports the hygiene hypothesis. Children who grow up on farms or who have pets and are thereby exposed to many antigens have fewer allergies and a lower incidence of asthma than children who grow up in more sterile environments.

Researchers are currently interested in the connection between a healthy gut microbiota and the risk for food allergies. Also, researchers have proposed a link between low levels of vitamin D and food allergies. The relationship between vitamin D and food allergies may be mediated by the vitamin's role in immune function.

TESTING FOR A FOOD ALLERGY

The diagnosis of a food allergy can be a difficult task.[110] It requires the expertise of a skilled clinician. To determine whether a food allergy is present, the health professional will record a detailed history of symptoms, including the time from ingestion to onset of symptoms, duration of symptoms, most recent reaction, food suspected of causing a reaction, and quantity and nature of food needed to produce a reaction. A family history of allergic diseases can also help, as allergies tend to run in families. A physical examination may reveal evidence of an allergy, such as skin diseases and asthma. Various diagnostic tests can rule out other conditions (Table 15-9).

If the patient history and physical exam suggest a food allergy, the health professional then faces the task of identifying the source of the food allergy. The first step in diagnosing a food allergy is to eliminate from the eating pattern (for 1 to 2 weeks) all food

TABLE 15-9 ■ Diagnosing Food Allergies

History	Include description of symptoms, time between food ingestion and onset and severity of symptoms, duration of symptoms, most recent allergic episode, quantity of food required to produce reaction, suspected foods, and allergic diseases in other family members.
Physical examination	Look for signs of an allergic reaction (rash, itching, intestinal bloating, etc.).
Elimination diet	Remove the suspected food allergen for 1 to 2 weeks or until symptoms clear.
Food challenge	Add back small amounts of excluded foods, one at a time, as long as anaphylaxis is not a possible consequence.
Blood test	Determine the presence of antibodies in blood that bind to food antigens tested.
Skin test	Place a sample of the suspected allergen under the skin and watch for an inflammatory reaction.

components that appear to cause allergic symptoms. This is called an **elimination diet.** The person generally starts out eating foods to which almost no one reacts, such as rice, vegetables, noncitrus fruits, and fresh meats and poultry. If symptoms are still present, the person can more severely restrict the eating pattern or even use special formulas that are hypoallergenic.

Once a dietary pattern is found that causes no symptoms, foods can be added back one at a time. This type of food challenge is an option only when the culprit foods are known to pose no risk of anaphylaxis in the person. Doses of ½ to 1 teaspoon (2½ to 5 milliliters) are given at first. The amount is increased until the dose approximates usual intake. Any reintroduced food that causes significant symptoms to appear is identified as an allergen for the person.

Laboratory tests can also aid in diagnosis of food allergies. Skin testing involves pricking the skin with a small amount of purified food extract and observing any allergic response (e.g., a red eruption at the prick site). These types of tests are easy and safe, even for infants, but they may not clearly diagnose a food allergy. A positive skin-prick test merely indicates that a person has been sensitized to a food; it cannot clearly identify if that food is the cause for the symptoms in question. Newer types of

elimination diet A restrictive diet that systematically tests foods that may cause an allergic response by first eliminating them for 1 to 2 weeks and then adding them back, one at a time.

blood testing, however, have more diagnostic value. Blood tests estimate the blood concentration of antibodies that bind certain foodborne antigens.

LIVING WITH FOOD ALLERGIES

Once potential food allergens are identified, dietary modifications must be made.[111] In some cases, small amounts of the offending food can be consumed without an observable reaction. Also, some food allergens are destroyed by heating, so cooking may eliminate the allergic response. This is effective primarily for allergies to fruits or vegetables, not for the more common allergies to milk, peanuts, or seafood. For most cases, though, complete avoidance of allergy-causing food ingredients is the safest course of action. This makes careful reading of food labels essential.

In the United States, a few laws have been passed to ensure that manufacturers clearly identify the presence of major food allergens. Since 2006, to comply with the Food Allergen Labeling Consumer Protection Act (FALCPA), food manufacturers have been required to declare the presence of eight major food allergens (milk, eggs, fish, shellfish, peanuts, tree nuts, wheat, and soy) on food product labels.[112] Beginning in 2023, as a result of the Food Allergy Safety, Treatment, Education, and Research (FASTER) Act, sesame became the ninth major food allergen to be required on food labels.[113]

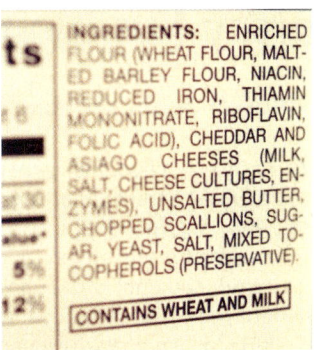

The Food Allergen Labeling and Consumer Protection Act of 2004 and the Food Allergy, Safety, Treatment, Education, and Research Act of 2021 are two laws to ensure that food manufacturers declare the presence of common food allergens in their products. FoodIngredients/Alamy Stock Photo

Nine Most Common Food Allergens:	
Peanuts	Tree nuts
Milk	Eggs
Fin fish	Shellfish
Wheat	Soy
Sesame	

A major challenge of managing a food allergy is to make sure that what remains in the dietary pattern can still provide essential nutrients. The small food intake of children permits less leeway in removing offending foods that may contain numerous nutrients. An RDN can help guide the diet-planning process to ensure that the remaining food choices still meet nutrient needs. Dietary supplements may be necessary.[111]

Studies show that about 25% of young children with food allergies outgrow them. Food allergies diagnosed after 3 years of age are more likely to be lifelong. It is common for children to outgrow allergies to milk, soy, or eggs, but allergies to peanuts, tree nuts, and shellfish are likely to endure. Periodic reintroduction of offending foods can be tried every 6 to 12 months or so to see whether the allergic reaction has decreased. If no symptoms appear, tolerance to the food has developed.[110]

Several strategies are being studied to ease the dietary restrictions imposed by food allergies. One possibility includes treatment with antibodies that will increase the threshold at which an allergic response occurs. For a person with an allergy to peanuts, for example, this would alleviate some anxiety about severe reactions to trace amounts of peanuts found in foods. Similarly, immunotherapy, which exposes individuals with allergies to very small but progressively larger amounts of food allergens, may help some people build up a tolerance to certain food components. In 2020, the FDA approved the first immunotherapy drug for peanut allergy.[114] It is important to recognize that immunotherapy does not cure food allergies; rather, immunotherapy promotes tolerance to prevent anaphylaxis in case of accidental exposure to food allergens. Vaccines are another area of research. Also, scientists are working on genetically engineered foods that do not contain common allergens.[115]

PREVENTING FOOD ALLERGIES

With the rising number of cases of food allergies, many new parents wonder when and how to introduce new foods during infancy and early childhood. Over the past 25 years, expert recommendations for the prevention of food allergies have undergone dramatic revisions. Out of an abundance of caution, experts once advised new parents to delay the introduction of potential food allergens—until after the third birthday for some foods. Females who were prone to allergies were advised to avoid highly allergenic foods during pregnancy and breastfeeding to limit the infant's exposure to allergens via the placenta or breast milk. Infants with a family history of food allergies were given extensively hydrolyzed infant formulas to limit their exposure to intact proteins. Based on observational studies comparing rates of food allergies among infants who were fed human milk versus infant formula, experts promoted exclusive breastfeeding as a tactic to prevent food allergies.[26]

Did any of these recommendations reduce the prevalence of food allergies? No! As it turns out, there is not enough evidence to support any of this past guidance. The best evidence we have at this time centers around *early*—not late—introduction of peanut protein to prevent food allergies.[32] This protocol may prove useful for other food allergens, but the data are not yet clear.

So, in 2019, the AAP released updated recommendations for food allergy prevention through diet:[116]

Newsworthy Nutrition

Early introduction of peanut protein reduces peanut allergy

INTRODUCTION: Based on a hypothesis that early introduction of food proteins to infants increased risk for food allergies, pediatricians once advised parents to delay introduction of potential food allergens (e.g., 2 years for eggs and 3 years for peanuts, tree nuts, and fish). However, in the 1990s, evidence started to accumulate that delaying introduction of a variety of foods provided no benefit for preventing food allergies. For instance, Jewish children raised in the United Kingdom, where peanuts were not introduced until after 1 year of age, were 10 times more likely to develop peanut allergies than Jewish children raised in Israel, where peanut-based foods are introduced within the first year of life. **OBJECTIVE:** The Learning Early About Peanut Allergy (LEAP) trial aimed to see if early introduction of peanut protein could prevent peanut allergies among at-risk children. **METHODS:** The *randomized, controlled trial* included 640 infants between 4 and 11 months of age who were at risk for food allergies (based on existing allergies, severe eczema, or both). Participants were divided into two groups based on previous sensitization to peanut protein (i.e., skin testing showed if the infants' immune systems had already reacted to peanut protein from dietary, skin, or respiratory exposure). Next, the infants were randomized to treatment or control groups. The treatment group received at least 6 grams of peanut protein per week in the form of a peanut-based snack food or smooth peanut butter, while the control group was advised to avoid dietary exposure to peanuts. **RESULTS:** At 5 years of age, the children were tested for peanut allergy using an oral food challenge. Among the children who were not sensitized to peanuts at baseline, peanut consumption reduced the risk of developing peanut allergy by 86.1% compared to controls. Among the children who were initially sensitized to peanut protein, treatment with peanut protein reduced the risk of developing peanut allergy by 70%. **CONCLUSION:** The researchers concluded that early (< 11 months), sustained peanut consumption reduced peanut allergy among children at risk of food allergies.

Source: Du Toit G, Roberts G, Sayre PH, et al.; LEAP Study Team. Randomized trial of peanut consumption in infants at risk for peanut allergy. *N Engl J Med.* 2015 Feb 26;372(9):803-813. doi: 10.1056/NEJMoa1414850

- There is *no evidence* to recommend maternal dietary restrictions of potential food allergens during pregnancy or breastfeeding.
- There is *no evidence* to recommend any specific duration of breastfeeding.
- There is *very limited evidence* to recommend partially or extensively hydrolyzed infant formula for high-risk infants.
- There is *no evidence* to delay the introduction of any potentially allergenic foods beyond 4 to 6 months of age.
- There is evidence that early introduction (between 4 and 6 months of age) of peanut protein reduces the risk for peanut allergies.

The AAP; the American Academy of Allergy, Asthma, and Immunology; and the latest edition of the *Dietary Guidelines* advise waiting to introduce solid foods until at least 4 months of age, but preferably around 6 months of age for the lowest risk of food allergies. Delaying introduction of solid foods beyond 6 months of age is not advised. Even highly allergenic foods, such as peanuts, egg whites, and milk, can be introduced in forms that are safe for infants to eat (e.g., mixing a small amount of peanut butter into infant cereal or yogurt) when the family chooses to offer complementary foods.[26]

FOOD INTOLERANCES

Food intolerances are adverse reactions to foods that do not involve immunologic mechanisms. Generally, larger amounts of an offending food are required to produce the symptoms of an intolerance than to trigger allergic symptoms. Common causes of food intolerances include the following:

- Constituents of certain foods (e.g., red wine, tomatoes, and pineapples) that have a drug-like activity, causing physiological effects such as changes in blood pressure
- Certain synthetic compounds added to foods, such as sulfites, food-coloring agents, and monosodium glutamate (MSG)
- Food contaminants, including antibiotics and other chemicals used in the production of livestock and crops, as well as insect parts not removed during processing
- Toxic contaminants, which may be ingested with improperly handled and prepared foods containing *Clostridium botulinum*, *Salmonella* bacteria, or other foodborne microorganisms
- Deficiencies in digestive enzymes, such as lactase

Almost everyone is sensitive to one or more of these causes of food intolerance, many of which produce GI tract symptoms. Sulfites, added to foods and beverages as antioxidants, cause flushing, spasms of the airway, and a loss of blood pressure in susceptible people. Wine, dehydrated potatoes, dried fruits, gravy, soup mixes, and restaurant salad greens commonly contain sulfites. A reaction to MSG may include an increase in blood pressure, numbness, sweating, vomiting, headache, and facial pressure. MSG is commonly found in restaurant food and many processed foods (e.g., soups). A reaction to tartrazine, a yellow food-coloring additive, includes spasm of the airway, itching, and reddening skin. Tyramine, a derivative of the amino acid tyrosine, is commonly found in "aged" foods such as cheeses and red wines. This natural food constituent can cause high blood pressure in people taking monoamine

ASK THE RDN: Alpha-Gal Syndrome

Dear RDN: *Can a person be allergic to red meat?*

Although it's not among the nine most common food allergens, some people do have allergies to red meat. Actually, over the past few years, the incidence of "red meat allergy," also known as **alpha-gal syndrome,** has been on the rise. First identified in 2009, alpha-gal syndrome is a type of food allergy that develops after a tick bite.

Alpha-gal is a nickname for a small carbohydrate molecule (galactose-α-1,3-galactose) that is produced by mammals, including deer, cows, pigs, sheep, and rabbits. However, alpha-gal is not produced by humans. A bite from a tick that has alpha-gal in its saliva (which was most likely acquired through a previous bite of another mammal) may transmit alpha-gal to the blood of a human host. For some people, exposure to this carbohydrate through a tick bite leads to the onset of an allergy to red meat.

In the United States, bites from the lone star tick are the most common presumed source of alpha-gal syndrome. The condition is common in the southern, central, and eastern United States, where the lone star tick typically lives, but cases have been found around the world. Also, bites from other ticks may initiate this allergic condition. Because it is relatively new, awareness of the condition is low, and a national reporting system is not yet in place, we don't have accurate numbers on the prevalence of alpha-gal syndrome. Some researchers estimate there may have been as many as 450,000 cases of alpha-gal syndrome since 2010, including many undiagnosed cases. Clinicians have witnessed a recent surge and spread in alpha-gal syndrome. This may be related to an increased number of ticks that carry alpha-gal, migration of the deer that carry the lone star tick, and/or an increased awareness of the condition.

After ingestion of red meat, a person with alpha-gal syndrome may experience hives, gastrointestinal distress, or anaphylactic shock. Alpha-gal syndrome is different from other food allergies in a few ways, however. It can take weeks or months from the initial tick bite to the onset of food allergy symptoms. Also, it may be several hours after ingestion of red meat before symptoms appear. These delayed reactions can make it difficult to identify the cause of the illness.

As with any food allergy, the only known treatment for alpha-gal syndrome is complete avoidance of the offending food(s), including beef, pork, lamb, and venison (deer meat). Up to one in five people with alpha-gal syndrome may even react to milk and other dairy products. Individuals with alpha-gal syndrome must be cautious about certain medical treatments, as they may react to medications, enzymes, or implants that are derived from animals. However, poultry, eggs, and seafood are still safe to eat.

For some people, alpha-gal syndrome subsides after a few years, but for others, the effects will last a lifetime. As awareness of this unusual food allergy increases, we will continue to learn about the progression of the disease, what makes some people susceptible to the condition, and what we can do to treat it. For now, the best prevention is to take precautions when you venture outdoors: avoid the woods or areas with long grasses, where ticks like to live; wear long sleeves and long pants; use tick repellents; shower and check your hair and skin for ticks after exploring outdoors; and remove any ticks with tweezers as soon as you find them.

Taking a bite out of food allergies,

Angela Collene, MS, RDN, LD

Senior Lecturer, The Ohio State University, Author of *Wardlaw's Contemporary Nutrition* and *Wardlaw's Contemporary Nutrition: A Functional Approach*

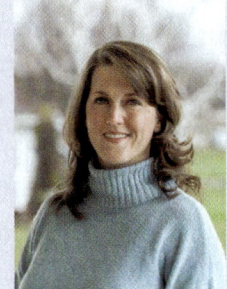
Tim Klontz

Sources: Alpha-gal syndrome. Centers for Disease Control and Prevention. Reviewed October 27, 2023. Accessed December 19, 2023. https://www.cdc.gov/ticks/alpha-gal/index.html

Mollah F, Zacharek MA, Benjamin MR. What is alpha-gal syndrome? *JAMA.* 2024;331(1):86. doi:10.1001/jama.2023.23097

---

oxidase (MAO) inhibitor medications, which may be prescribed for clinical depression.

The basic treatment for food intolerances is to avoid specific offending components. However, total elimination often is not required because people generally are not as sensitive to compounds causing food intolerances as they are to allergens.

alpha-gal syndrome A food allergy to galactose-α-1,3-galactose, an oligosaccharide found in mammalian meat and milk. Onset of the allergy occurs after a tick bite.

✓ CONCEPT CHECK 15.7

1. Name the nine common food allergens that must be listed on food labels in the United States.
2. What is the most common and most dangerous food allergen among children in the United States?
3. A new mom asks you how to prevent food allergies in her infant. What information can you provide?

Summary (Numbers refer to numbered sections in the chapter.)

15.1 Growth is rapid during infancy; birth weight doubles by 6 months of age, and length increases by 50% in the first year. An adequate dietary pattern, especially in terms of calories, protein, iron, and calcium, is essential to support normal growth. Growth charts can be used to assess changes in body weight, height (or length), head circumference, and body mass index over time.

15.2 Compared to other life stages, the relative energy needs of infants are high. Fat should make up about 50% of total energy intake. DHA and ARA are important fatty acids for nervous system development. Carbohydrate requirements range from 60 grams per day for younger infants to 95 grams per day for older infants. Protein requirements are 9 grams per day for younger infants and 11 grams per day for older infants. Supplementation with vitamin D, iron, and fluoride may be appropriate for some infants. During the first 6 months of life, exclusive feeding of breast milk or formula provides adequate calories, essential nutrients, and hydration.

15.3 Infant nutrient needs can usually be met by human milk or iron-fortified infant formula for the first 6 months of life. Introduction of solid foods should begin no earlier than 4 months of age, but preferably around 6 months of age, based on an infant's nutritional needs, physical abilities, and developmental readiness. Solid foods should be introduced one at a time, starting with iron-fortified infant cereals or ground meats (sources of iron). During the first year of life, avoid giving infants honey, unaltered cow's milk (especially fat-reduced varieties), foods with added salt or sugars, and foods that may cause choking.

15.4 A slower growth rate results in decreased relative energy needs and reduced appetite among toddlers and preschool children, which may lead to picky eating behaviors and inadequate intake of some nutrients, especially iron and calcium. It is crucial to offer several small meals and snacks with a variety of nutrient-dense foods. Follow the example set forth by MyPlate, but use smaller portions (e.g., 1 tablespoon of food per year of life). Other common nutrition-related concerns include constipation and dental caries. For autism spectrum disorders, although nutritional interventions are widely promoted in the media, none are endorsed by the AAP.

15.5 Among school-age children, excessive energy intakes coupled with low levels of physical activity have contributed to an alarming increase in overweight, obesity, type 2 diabetes, and cardiovascular disease. Parents can provide healthful food choices and encourage at least 60 minutes of physical activity per day. When addressed early through dietary and physical activity interventions, BMI-for-age may deflect downward as the child continues to grow in height. Other important nutrition strategies for school-age children include starting the day with breakfast and selecting low-fat or fat-free milk or water instead of sugar-sweetened beverages. Recent changes in meal offerings through schools are aimed at curtailing the rise in childhood obesity.

15.6 During the adolescent growth spurt, children have increased needs for iron, calcium, and overall calories. Inadequate calcium intake by female adolescents is a major concern because it can set the stage for the development of osteoporosis later in life. Adolescents need to limit their intakes of solid fats, added sugars, and sodium, and use caffeine in moderation (if at all). Alcohol abuse during adolescence has many severe consequences, including impaired brain development and increased risk for liver and cardiovascular diseases in adulthood.

15.7 The most common food allergies (in order of prevalence during childhood) are associated with peanuts, milk, shellfish, tree nuts, eggs, fin fish, wheat, soy, and sesame. Current treatment for food allergies involves complete avoidance of the food allergen. With the help of an RDN, the family can ensure adequate energy and nutrient intake of a child with food allergies, despite dietary restrictions.

Check Your Knowledge (Answers are available at the end of this question set)

1. Inadequate intake of which of the following results in poor growth?
   a. Calories
   b. Iron
   c. Zinc
   d. All of these

2. Cow's milk is a nutrient-dense source of all of the following except
   a. protein.
   b. iron.
   c. calcium.
   d. zinc.

3. To ensure adequate vitamin and mineral intake for a picky eater,
   a. provide a fortified breakfast cereal.
   b. promise dessert as a reward for eating meats and vegetables.
   c. use a multivitamin and mineral supplement.
   d. avoid sources of dietary fiber.

4. Should caregivers provide fruit juice in a bottle for infants?
   a. No. Continuous exposure of developing teeth to the carbohydrates in fruit juice could promote early childhood caries.
   b. Yes. Fruit juice is a rich source of several essential vitamins and minerals, including vitamin C and potassium.
   c. Yes. Regular intake of fruit juice helps to prevent constipation.
   d. Yes. Infants need a concentrated source of carbohydrates to provide energy for growth and development.

5. You are trying to introduce an apple and blueberry purée to a 7-month-old infant, but she rejects it. You should
   a. assume she doesn't like apples and blueberries.
   b. offer the food again on another day.
   c. force a spoonful into her mouth.
   d. do none of these.

6. Introduction of cow's milk should be delayed until 12 months of age because it
   a. contains too much fat.
   b. supplies too much lactose.
   c. contains too much protein.
   d. does all of these.

7. Which of the following is an outcome of consuming a fortified, ready-to-eat breakfast cereal instead of skipping breakfast?
   a. Increased intakes of saturated fat and cholesterol
   b. Improved intakes of iron and calcium
   c. Excessive weight gain
   d. All of these

8. Which of the following nutrition interventions is recommended by the AAP for treatment of autism spectrum disorder?
   a. Camel's milk
   b. Fish oil supplements
   c. Gluten-free, casein-free diet
   d. None of these

9. If moderate weight loss is needed, a school-age child should
   a. eat fewer meals.
   b. follow a low-carbohydrate eating plan.
   c. engage in physical activity for 60 minutes per day or more.
   d. avoid dairy products.

10. Your niece breaks out in hives and feels nauseous after eating a salad containing mango. She probably has a food
    a. sensitivity.
    b. allergy.
    c. intolerance.
    d. All of these are correct.

Answer Key: 1. d (LO 15.1), 2. b (LO 15.2), 3. a (LO 15.3), 4. a (LO 15.3), 5. b (LO 15.3), 6. c (LO 15.3), 7. b (LO 15.3), 8. d (LO 15.4), 9. c (LO 15.5), 10. b (LO 15.6)

Study Questions (Numbers refer to Learning Outcomes.)

1. List two factors that limit "catch-up" growth when a nutrient-deficient dietary pattern has been consumed throughout childhood. **(LO 15.1)**
2. What are two possible causes of pediatric malnutrition? **(LO 15.1)**
3. Which two nutrients are of particular concern in planning dietary patterns for teenagers? Why does each deserve special attention? **(LO 15.2)**
4. List three nutrients of concern for a child who is following a vegetarian lifestyle. **(LO 15.2)**
5. Outline three key factors that help to determine when to introduce solid foods into an infant's dietary pattern. **(LO 15.3)**
6. List three foods or beverages to avoid feeding infants. Explain why these items should be avoided. **(LO 15.3)**
7. Describe the pros and cons of snacking. What is the basic advice for healthful snacking from childhood through the teenage years? **(LO 15.4)**
8. List three reasons why preschoolers are noted for picky eating. **(LO 15.4)**
9. What three factors are likely to contribute to obesity in a typical 10-year-old child? **(LO 15.5)**
10. What is the difference between a food allergy and a food intolerance? **(LO 15.6)**

References

1. CDC extended BMI-for-age growth charts: what to know. Centers for Disease Control and Prevention. December 15, 2022. Accessed December 16, 2023. https://www.cdc.gov/growthcharts/extended-Healthcare-professionals.htm
2. Holt K, Wooldridge N, Storuy M, Sofka D. *Bright Futures: Nutrition.* 3rd ed. Elk Grove Village, IL: American Academy of Pediatrics; 2011.
3. Mehta NM, Corkins MR, Lyman B, et al.; American Society for Parenteral and Enteral Nutrition Board of Directors. Defining pediatric malnutrition: a paradigm shift toward etiology-related definitions. *JPEN J Parenter Enteral Nutr.* 2013 Jul;37(4):460-481. doi: 10.1177/0148607113479972
4. Becker PJ, Nieman Carney L, Corkins MR, et al. Consensus statement of the Academy of Nutrition and Dietetics/American Society for Parenteral and Enteral Nutrition: indicators recommended for the identification and documentation of pediatric malnutrition (undernutrition). *J Acad Nutr Diet.* 2014 Dec;114(12):1988-2000. doi: 10.1016/j.jand.2014.08.026
5. Malnutrition. UNICEF. May 2023. Accessed December 16, 2023. https://data.unicef.org/topic/nutrition/malnutrition/
6. Malnutrition. World Health Organization. June 9, 2021. Accessed December 16, 2023. https://www.who.int/news-room/fact-sheets/detail/malnutrition
7. Salgueiro MJ, Zubillaga MB, Lysionek AE, Caro RA, Weill R, Boccio JR. The role of zinc in the growth and development of children. *Nutrition.* 2002 Jun;18(6):510-519. doi: 10.1016/s0899-9007(01)00812-7
8. Delplanque D, Gibson R, Koletzko B, Lapillonne A, Strandvik B. Lipid quality in infant nutrition: current knowledge and future opportunities. *J Pediatr Gastroenterol Nutr.* 2015 Jul;61(1):8-17. doi: 10.1097/MPG.0000000000000818
9. Wagner CL, Greer FR; American Academy of Pediatrics Section on Breastfeeding; American Academy of Pediatrics Committee on Nutrition. Prevention of rickets and vitamin D deficiency in infants, children, and adolescents. *Pediatrics.* 2008 Nov;122(5):1142-1152. doi: 10.1542/peds.2008-1862
10. Baroni L, Goggi S, Battaglino R, et al. Vegan nutrition for mothers and children: practical tools for healthcare providers. *Nutrients.* 2018 Dec;11(1):5. doi: 10.3390/nu11010005

77. Richerson JE, Abularrage JJ, Almendarez YM, et al.; Committee on Practice and Ambulatory Medicine; Bright Futures Periodicity Schedule Workgroup. 2019 recommendations for preventive pediatric health care. *Pediatrics.* 2019 Mar;143(3):e201839971. doi: 10.1542/peds.2018-3971

78. Expert Panel on Integrated Guidelines for Cardiovascular Health and Risk Reduction in Children and Adolescents; National Heart, Lung, and Blood Institute. Expert panel on integrated guidelines for cardiovascular health and risk reduction in children and adolescents: summary report. *Pediatrics.* 2011 Dec;128(Suppl 5):S213-S256. doi: 10.1542/peds.2009-2107C

79. Lawrence JM, Divers J, Isom S, et al.; SEARCH for Diabetes in Youth Study Group. Trends in prevalence of type 1 and type 2 diabetes in children and adolescents in the US, 2001–2017 [published correction appears in JAMA. 2021 Oct 5;326(13):1331]. *JAMA.* 2021 Aug 24;326(8):717-727. doi: 10.1001/jama.2021.11165

80. Pulgaron ER, Delamater AM. Obesity and type 2 diabetes in children: epidemiology and treatment. *Curr Diab Rep.* 2014 Aug;14(8):508. doi: 10.1007/s11892-014-0508-y

81. Barrett CE, Koyama AK, Alvarez P, et al. Risk for newly diagnosed diabetes >30 days after SARS-CoV-2 infection among persons aged <18 years—United States, March 1, 2020–June 28, 2021. *MMWR Morb Mortal Wkly Rep.* 2022 Jan 14;71(2):59-65. doi: 10.15585/mmwr.mm7102e2

82. American Diabetes Association Professional Practice Committee. 2. Diagnosis and Classification of Diabetes: Standards of Care in Diabetes-2024. *Diabetes Care.* 2024;47(Suppl 1):S20-S42. doi:10.2337/dc24-S002

83. Copeland KC, Silverstein J, Moore KR, et al.; American Academy of Pediatrics. Management of newly diagnosed type 2 diabetes mellitus (T2DM) in children and adolescents. *Pediatrics.* 2013 Feb;131(2):364-382. doi: 10.1542/peds.2012-3494

84. Terry AL, Wambogo E, Ansai N, Ahluwalia N. Breakfast intake among children and adolescents: United States, 2015–2018. *NCHS Data Brief.* 2020 Oct;(386):1-8. PMID: 33054919

85. Gibney MJ, Barr SI, Bellisle F, et al. Breakfast in human nutrition: the International Breakfast Research Initiative. *Nutrients.* 2018 May 1;10(5):559. doi: 10.3390/nu10050559

86. Sheppard KW, Cheatham CL. Omega-6/omega-3 fatty acid intake of children and older adults in the U.S.: dietary intake in comparison to current dietary recommendations and the Healthy Eating Index. *Lipids Health Dis.* 2018 Mar 9;17(1):43. doi: 10.1186/s12944-018-0693-9

87. Marriott BP, Hunt KJ, Malek AM, Newman JC. Trends in intake of energy and total sugar from sugar-sweetened beverages in the United States among children and adults, NHANES 2003–2016. *Nutrients.* 2019;11(9):2004. doi:10.3390/nu11092004

88. Scharf RJ, DeBoer MD. Sugar-sweetened beverages and children's health. *Annu Rev Public Health.* 2016;37:273-293. doi: 10.1146/annurev-publhealth-032315-021528

89. Auerbach BJ, Wolf FM, Hikida A, et al. Fruit juice and change in BMI: a meta-analysis. *Pediatrics.* 2017 Apr;139(4):e20162454. doi: 10.1542/peds.2016-2454

90. Heyman MB, Abrams SA; Section on Gastroenterology, Hepatology, and Nutrition; Committee on Nutrition. Fruit juice in infants, children, and adolescents: current recommendations. *Pediatrics.* 2017 Jun;139(6):e20170967. doi: 10.1542/peds.2017-0967

91. Hayes D, Contento IR, Weekly C. Position of the Academy of Nutrition and Dietetics, Society for Nutrition Education and Behavior, and School Nutrition Association: comprehensive nutrition programs and services in schools. *J Acad Nutr Diet.* 2018 May;118(5):913-919. doi: 10.1016/j.jand.2018.03.005

92. National School Lunch Program. U.S. Department of Agriculture, Food and Nutrition Service. Accessed December 18, 2023. https://www.fns.usda.gov/nslp

93. Final rule: National School Lunch Program and School Breakfast Program: nutrition standards for all foods sold in school as required by the HHFKA of 2010. U.S. Department of Agriculture, Food and Nutrition Service. July 29, 2016. Accessed December 18, 2023. https://www.fns.usda.gov/cn/fr-072916d

94. Cullen KW, Dave JM. The new federal school nutrition standards and meal patterns: early evidence examining the influence on student dietary behavior and the school food environment. *J Acad Nutr Diet.* 2017 Feb;117(2):185-191. doi: 10.1016/j.jand.2016.10.031

95. Mozer L, Johnson DB, Podrabsky M, Rocha A. School lunch entrées before and after implementation of the Healthy, Hunger-Free Kids Act of 2010. *J Acad Nutr Diet.* 2019 Mar;119(3):490-499. doi: 10.1016/j.jand.2018.09.009

96. Perera T, Frei S, Frei B, Wong SS, Bobe G. Improving nutrition education in U.S. elementary schools: challenges and opportunities. *J Educ Pract.* 2015;6(30):41-20.

97. Das JK, Salam RA, Thornburg KL, et al. Nutrition in adolescents: physiology, metabolism, and nutritional needs. *Ann N Y Acad Sci.* 2017 Apr;1393(1) :21-33. doi: 10.1111/nyas.13330

98. Lange SJ, Moore LV, Harris DM, et al. Percentage of adolescents meeting federal fruit and vegetable intake recommendations—Youth Risk Behavior Surveillance System, United States, 2017. *MMWR Morb Mortal Wkly Rep.* 2021 Jan 22;70(3):69-74. doi: 10.15585/mmwr.mm7003a1

99. Childhood obesity facts. Centers for Disease Control and Prevention. Reviewed May 17, 2022. Accessed December 18, 2023. https://www.cdc.gov/obesity/data/childhood.html

100. Gupta PM, Hamner HC, Suchdev PS, Flores-Ayala R, Mei Z. Iron status of toddlers, nonpregnant females, and pregnant females in the United States. *Am J Clin Nutr.* 2017 Dec;106(Suppl 6):1640S-1646S. doi: 10.3945/ajcn.117.155978

101. Powell LM, Nguyen BT. Fast-food and full-service restaurant consumption among children and adolescents: effect on energy, beverage, and nutrient intake. *JAMA Pediatr.* 2013 Jan;167(1):14-20. doi: 10.1001/jamapediatrics.2013.417

102. Soós R, Gyebrovszki Á, Tóth Á, Jeges S, Wilhelm M. Effects of caffeine and caffeinated beverages in children, adolescents and young adults: short review. *Int J Environ Res Public Health.* 2021 Nov 25;18(23):12389. doi: 10.3390/ijerph182312389

103. Ruiz LD, Scherr RE. Risk of energy drink consumption to adolescent health. *Am J Lifestyle Med.* 2018 Sep 27;13(1):22-25. doi: 10.1177/1559827618803069

104. Caffeine and children. American Academy of Child and Adolescent Psychiatry. Updated July 2020. Accessed December 19, 2023. https://www.aacap.org/AACAP/Families_and_Youth/Facts_for_Families/FFF-Guide/Caffeine_and_Children-131.aspx

105. Bardone-Cone AM, Fitzsimmons-Craft EE, Harney MB, et al. The interrelationships between vegetarianism and eating disorders among females. *J Acad Nutr Diet.* 2012 Aug;112(8):1247-1252. doi: 10.1016/j.jand.2012.05.007

106. 1991-2021 High School Youth Risk Behavior Survey Data. Centers for Disease Control and Prevention (CDC). Accessed December 19, 2023. http://yrbs-explorer.services.cdc.gov/.

107. Substance Abuse and Mental Health Services Administration. *Underage Drinking: Myths versus Facts.* Revised May 2023. Accessed December 19, 2023. https://store.samhsa.gov/sites/default/files/pep23-03-10-004.pdf

108. Food Allergy Research and Education. *Food Allergy Facts and Statistics for the U.S.* Revised June 4, 2020. Accessed December 19, 2023. https://www.foodallergy.org/media/1012/download?attachment

109. Gupta RS, Warren CM, Smith BM, et al. The public health impact of parent-reported childhood food allergies in the United States. *Pediatrics.* 2018 Dec;142(6):e20181235. doi: 10.1542/peds.2018-1235

110. Oriel RC, Wang J. Diagnosis and management of food allergy. *Immunol Allergy Clin North Am.* 2021;41(4):571-585. doi:10.1016/j.iac.2021.07.012

111. Collins SC. Practice paper of the Academy of Nutrition and Dietetics: role of the registered dietitian nutritionist in the diagnosis and management of food allergies. *J Acad Nutr Diet.* 2016 Oct;116(10):1621-1631. doi: 10.1016/j.jand.2016.07.018

112. Food Allergen Labeling Consumer Protection Act of 2004 (FALCPA). U.S. Food & Drug Administration. Updated March 7, 2022. Accessed April 7, 2022. https://www.fda.gov/food/food-allergensgluten-free-guidance-documents-regulatory-information/food-allergen-labeling-and-consumer-protection-act-2004-falcpa

113. FASTER Act video for food industry and other stakeholders. U.S. Food & Drug Administration. Updated January 31, 2022. Accessed December 19, 2023. https://www.fda.gov/food/cfsan-constituent-updates/faster-act-video-food-industry-and-other-stakeholders

114. Pepper AN, Assa'ad A, Blaiss M, et al. Consensus report from the Food Allergy Research & Education (FARE) 2019 Oral Immunotherapy for Food Allergy Summit. *J Allergy Clin Immunol.* 2020 Aug;146(2):244-249. doi: 10.1016/j.jaci.2020.05.027

115. Collins SC. Food allergies/sensitivities: Will food allergies soon be eliminated? *Today's Dietitian.* 2019 Nov-Dec;21(11):12.

116. Greer FR, Sicherer SH, Wesley Burks A; Committee on Nutrition; Section on Allergy and Immunology. The effects of early nutritional interventions on the development of atopic disease in infants and children: the role of maternal dietary restriction, breastfeeding, hydrolyzed formulas, and timing of introduction of allergenic complementary foods. *Pediatrics.* 2019 Apr;143(4):e20190281. doi: 10.1542/peds.2019-0281

Design Element Credits: Fact Check/magnifying glass icon: McGraw Hill; Magnificent Microbiome background image: Alena Ohneva/Shutterstock; Sustainable Solutions icon: McGraw Hill; Roots icon: McGraw Hill; Medicine Cabinet icon: Peter Dazeley/Photographer's Choice/Getty Images

16.1 Healthy Aging

Due to advances in health care and sanitation, the demographics of developed countries are shifting so that, as a population, we are getting older. In the United States, the group constituting those aged 85+ years is the fastest-growing segment of the population. By 2040, the population aged 85+ years in the United States is expected to double its current size (Fig. 16-1).[1] Even more amazing is that 6 million or more people in the United States could be over 100 years old in 2050.

Although great news, the **aging** of adults poses some unique challenges. Individuals older than age 65 make up less than 17% of the U.S. population but account for more than 37% of all health care costs.[2] Among older adults, 80% or more have chronic conditions such as cardiovascular diseases, type 2 diabetes, hypertension, cancers, and osteoporosis.[3] Preventing or postponing the onset of chronic diseases for as long as possible can help control health care costs and improve quality of life.

Health and independence contribute quality—not just quantity—to life and lessen the load on an already overburdened health care system. Keep in mind that aging is not a disease. Furthermore, diseases that commonly accompany old age—obesity, osteoporosis, cancers, and atherosclerosis, for example—are not an inevitable part of aging. Many can be prevented or managed by adhering to positive lifestyle behaviors (Fig. 16-2).

CAUSES OF AGING

Adulthood, the longest stage of the normal life cycle, begins when an adolescent completes their physical growth. Unlike earlier stages of the life cycle, nutrients are used primarily to maintain the body rather than support physical growth. Recall that pregnancy is the only time during adulthood when substantial amounts of nutrients are used for growth. As adults get older, nutrient needs change. More on macro- and micronutrient recommendations for older adults will be discussed later in this chapter.

Aging is defined as the physical and physiological changes in body structure and function that occur throughout adulthood as humans mature and become older. There are two types of aging. *Intrinsic aging* refers to the genetically predetermined processes that occur naturally. This is estimated to account for about 25% of the aging process. *Extrinsic aging* refers to aging related to environmental factors including lifestyle patterns, stress levels, and surroundings.[4]

aging Time-dependent physical and physiological changes in body structure and function that occur normally and progressively throughout adulthood as humans mature and become older.

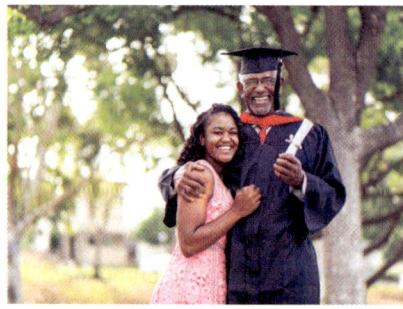

The World Health Organization (WHO) defines *healthy aging* as the process of developing and maintaining the functional ability that enables well-being in older age. Healthy aging enables individuals to be and do what they value, including a person's ability to:

- Meet their basic needs.
- Learn, grow, and make decisions.
- Be mobile.
- Build and maintain relationships.
- Contribute to society.

adamkaz/E+/Getty Images

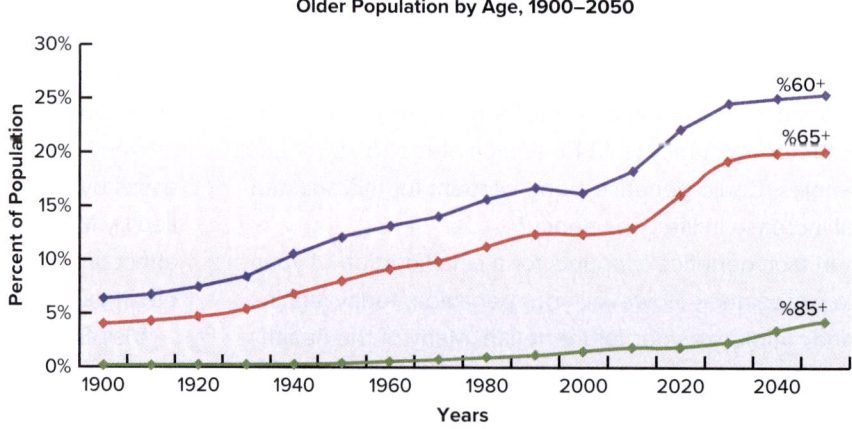

FIGURE 16-1 Growth of the U.S. population of older adults. This chart shows that the proportion of the total U.S. population composed of older adults has been steadily increasing over the past century and how these trends are expected to continue. The 85+ demographic group (green line), although still the smallest group in total numbers, is expected to experience the most rapid rate of growth. Conversely, most demographic groups under the age of 45 are shrinking as a percentage of overall population (not shown here). This means that fewer young people will be available to care for a growing population of older adults in years to come.

Source: U.S. Administration on Aging.

Genetics. Living to an old age tends to run in families. If your parents and grandparents lived a long life, you are more likely to live to an old age, too. Studies of twins indicate that about 20% to 30% of longevity can be attributed to genetics.[8] And there is not just one gene that predicts a long and healthy life. So far, a few genes have been identified, but there are likely many genes involved in regulating how long we can live, and we have no control over our DNA.

For humans, as well as most other species, females tend to live longer than males. Another genetic characteristic that may influence longevity is metabolic efficiency. Some researchers hypothesize that individuals with a thrifty metabolism require fewer calories for metabolic processes and are able to store body fat more easily than those with faster metabolic rates. Throughout history, it was the individuals with thrifty metabolism who tended to live the longest because they efficiently stored fat during times of plenty and thus had the energy stores needed to survive frequent periods of food scarcity. In today's environment of labor-saving devices and abundant, energy-dense foods, however, a thrifty metabolism may actually reduce longevity. Accumulation of excessive body fat increases the risk of developing health problems (e.g., heart disease, hypertension, and many cancers) that reduce life expectancy.

Is DNA your destiny? Although genetics remain largely unchangeable, the good news is we can exert some control over the environmental and lifestyle factors that determine how long we will live. Exposures to environmental toxins, our physical activity level, and—you guessed it—our food choices play significant roles in not only the amount of years in our lives but also the amount of life in our years! See the *Newsworthy Nutrition* in this section for more support that lifestyle matters!

Newsworthy Nutrition

Impact of nutrition on aging

INTRODUCTION: As life expectancy continues to rise, the later years of an individual's life often coincide with a decline in the overall quality of life. While biological changes inherent to the aging process remain beyond control, lifestyle-related risk factors offer an avenue for intervention. **OBJECTIVE:** The primary objective of this *systematic review* is to assess the modulatory effects of nutrition on aging by evaluating its efficiency, examining biomarkers associated with healthy aging, and exploring strategies to enhance longevity through nutritional interventions. **METHODS:** A total of 36 studies were chosen based on three key criteria: (1) the efficacy of nutrition in influencing aging, (2) the assessment of biomarkers contributing to healthy aging, and (3) methods to extend longevity through nutritional approaches. The selected studies underwent a rigorous quality assessment. **RESULTS:** The findings revealed that opting for low carbohydrate diets or those rich in vegetables, fruits, nuts, cereals, fish, and unsaturated fats—enriched with antioxidants, potassium, and omega-3—significantly reduced the risks of cardiovascular diseases and obesity. Furthermore, such dietary patterns demonstrated protective effects on the aging brain, mitigated the risk of telomere shortening, and contributed to an overall healthier life. **CONCLUSION:** In light of the inability to control the biological processes of aging, this study underscores the critical role of altering nutritional patterns. Choosing diets with specified characteristics is not only vital in preventing the onset and progression of diseases but also proves instrumental in promoting longevity. Above all, this dietary modification emerges as a key strategy to enhance overall quality of life and foster healthy aging.

Source: Leitão C, Mignano A, Estrela M, et al. The effect of nutrition on aging: a systematic review focusing on aging-related biomarkers. *Nutrients*. 2022 Jan 27;14(3):554. doi: 10.3390/nu14030554. PMID: 35276919; PMCID: PMC8838212.

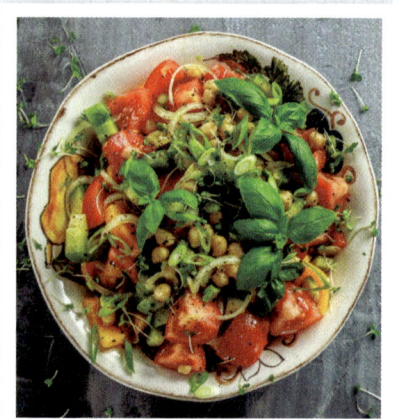

A plant-forward dietary pattern, exemplified by this bowl of chickpea salad with avocado and vegetables, is a common feature among populations who enjoy long, healthy, and productive lives. **What other lifestyle behaviors are associated with healthy aging?** DronG/iStock/Getty Images

Lifestyle. Lifestyle includes one's pattern of living; it includes food choices, physical activity, and substance use (e.g., alcohol, drugs, and tobacco). Lifestyle choices can have a major impact on health and longevity, partly by regulating gene expression. If individuals have a family history of premature heart disease, they would be wise to adjust their dietary and activity patterns and to avoid tobacco products to prevent the onset or slow the progression of the disease. The converse is true, too—that is, lifestyle choices (like consuming an unhealthy dietary pattern and not engaging in physical activity) can increase susceptibility to noncommunicable diseases that hasten the rate of aging, ultimately shortening life expectancy, even if a person does not have a genetic predisposition to disease.

Followers of the traditional Mediterranean diet also enjoy some of the lowest recorded rates of chronic disease in the world. Recall the Mediterranean diet features abundant daily intake of fruits, vegetables, whole grains, beans, nuts, and seeds. Olive oil, a source of heart-healthy monounsaturated fat, is the main dietary fat. Beans and fish are emphasized as sources of protein, whereas dairy products, eggs, poultry, and meats are consumed less frequently. Daily physical activity is a way of life. In addition, many Mediterraneans consume wine in moderation at mealtimes.

Environment. Income, education, health care, shelter, and other socioecological factors exert a powerful influence on the rate of aging. For instance, being able to access and purchase nutritious foods, obtain optimal health care, and reside in safe housing all decrease the rate of aging. Having the education to earn sufficient living wages, as well as the knowledge to make wise lifestyle choices, also can slow the aging process. In addition, the ability and willingness to seek health care promptly when it is needed, the health literacy to understand a health care provider, and the ability to accept responsibility for one's own health can slow the rate of aging. Likewise, safe shelter and neighborhoods that protect individuals from physical danger, environmental toxins, climate extremes, and sun exposure slow the aging process. Allowing people to make at least

Sustainable Solutions

Essential Oils

Growing in popularity, the use of essential oils and aromatherapy is expanding rapidly among claims of curbing appetite, promoting weight loss, reducing stress, alleviating pain, and other miraculous healing. In short, essential oils are highly concentrated plant extracts that are often promoted as "natural." Yet safety and environmental sustainability must be considered when using these products given many contain volatile and unregulated compounds that can cause more harm than good. For instance, some essential oils have been found to act as endocrine disruptors that interfere with normal hormone levels. Lavender oil has been linked to early breast development in young females and abnormal breast tissue growth in young males. Hives, dermatitis, and other skin irritations have been reported after essential oil use. Those with respiratory conditions, such as asthma or frequent bronchitis, should avoid using essential oil diffusers as they can irritate the lungs.

In terms of sustainability, a significant amount of plant matter is required to make essential oils. For instance, it takes approximately 625 pounds of rose petals to make 1 ounce of essential rose oil. Frankincense is a wildly popular essential oil derived from tree sap. Sadly, frankincense and sandalwood forests are now disappearing at alarming rates and are at risk of extinction due to growing manufacturing of these essential oils.

Before using essential oils, consider your living environment and the potential effects on youth, pets, females who are pregnant, seniors, and those living with comorbidities that may be harmed by essential oil exposure.

Source: Capritto A. The dangers of essential oils: natural isn't always safe. *CNET.* November 4, 2020. https://www.cnet.com/health/are-essential-oils-actually-safe/

some decisions for themselves and control their own activities, as well as providing psychosocial support and resources, promote successful aging and psychological well-being. In contrast, aging is likely to accelerate if any or all of the converse are true. Do you think you are aging in a healthy and successful manner?

✓ CONCEPT CHECK 16.1

1. Describe three causes of aging.
2. What is the difference between *usual* and *successful* aging?
3. Provide one example each to describe how genetics, lifestyle, and environment influence aging.

16.2 Nutrient Needs During Adulthood

The challenge of the adult years is to maintain the body, preserve optimal function, and avoid chronic disease—that is, to age successfully. A healthy dietary pattern can help achieve this goal. One blueprint for a healthy eating pattern comes from the *Dietary Guidelines.* The advice from those guidelines includes the following goals:

- Follow a healthy dietary pattern across the life span with special attention to potassium, calcium, vitamin D, vitamin B-12, vitamin C, and dietary fiber.
- Enjoy nutrient-dense foods and beverages that reflect personal preferences, cultural traditions, and budgetary considerations.
- Maintain a healthy weight and prevent additional weight gain by following a healthy dietary pattern and adopting an active lifestyle.
- Get ample protein to maintain muscle mass.
- Limit foods and beverages higher in added sugars, saturated fat, and sodium, and limit alcoholic beverages.

Meeting one's nutrient needs delays the onset of certain diseases; improves the management of existing diseases; speeds recovery from acute illnesses; and increases mental, physical, and social well-being.[9] As you will recall, overweight and obesity increase the risk of noncommunicable chronic diseases. Common dietary excesses are calories, saturated fat, sodium, and, for some, alcohol. Yet the dietary patterns of adult females tend to fall short of the recommended amounts of vitamins D and E, folate, magnesium, calcium, zinc, and fiber. The dietary patterns of adult males tend to be low in the same nutrients, except vitamin D, which becomes more problematic after age 50.[10]

MALNUTRITION RISK

People age 65 and older, particularly those in long-term care facilities and hospitals, are at heightened risk for malnutrition due to a number of factors (Fig. 16-5).[11] There are many nutrition screening tools to help pinpoint older adults who are at risk for malnutrition. One simplified tool, the *Malnutrition Screening Tool (MST),* relies on unintentional weight loss and appetite criteria to quickly identify individuals at nutritional risk.[12,13] Such screening tools are helpful because they are fast and noninvasive and require minimal training to administer. Once an individual is identified as *at risk,* a referral to a registered dietitian will help to ensure that the individual receives professional, personalized advice to optimize nutritional status. You will learn more about the factors that relate to the adequate or inadequate nutritional status of older adults in the next section.

DIETARY RECOMMENDATIONS

The DRIs for adults (Appendix F) are organized by sex and age. These changes in nutrient needs take into consideration aging-related physiological alterations in body composition, metabolism, and organ function.

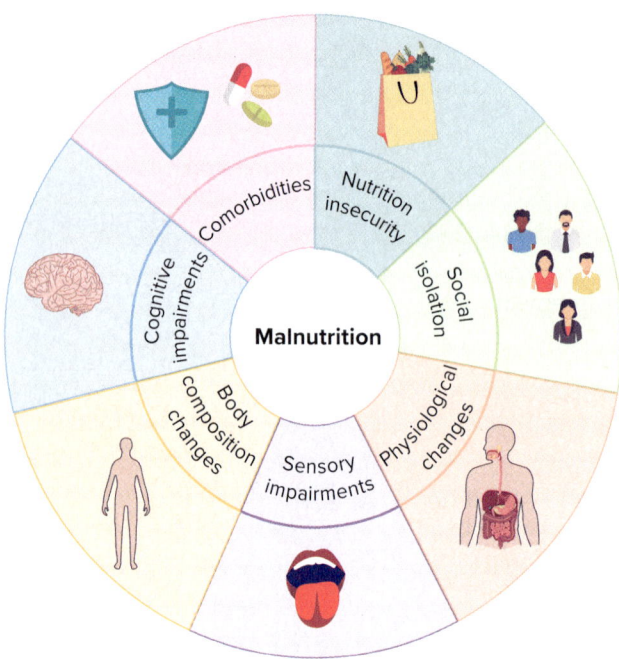

FIGURE 16-5 Factors impacting adult malnutrition risk.
Source: National Council on Aging.

Calories. In the past, many blamed increasing weight in adulthood on slowing metabolism after the age of 30. Yet recent research tells a different story. It appears metabolism peaks at age 1, then declines about 3% per year until age 20. Metabolism remains stable from age 20 to 60, then begins to decline again about 1% per year throughout older adulthood.[14]

Losses of lean body mass and decreases in physical activity also tend to accompany aging. To a considerable extent, adults can exert control over this reduction in calorie need by exercising. Physical activity can halt, slow, and even reverse reductions in lean body mass and subsequent declines in energy needs. Being able to consume more calories makes it much easier to meet micronutrient needs without dietary supplements.

Protein. The protein intake of younger adults typically exceeds the current RDA (0.8 gram per kilogram of body weight) and falls within the recommended range of 10% to 35% of total calories. Among older adults, however, several studies indicate that consuming protein in amounts slightly higher than the RDA (in the range of 1.0 to 1.2 grams per kilogram of body weight) may help preserve muscle and bone mass.[15] As with calorie needs, protein requirements should be determined in relation to routine physical activity. Furthermore, evenly distributing protein intake throughout the day (e.g., 25 to 30 grams of high-quality protein at each meal) appears to be best for preserving lean mass for aging adults.[16]

Protein recommendations are aimed at supporting immune function, improving wound healing, protecting bone health, and preventing malnutrition. Inclusion of some animal proteins can be helpful because these foods generally contain a higher proportion of the amino acid leucine, which plays a key role in stimulating muscle protein synthesis. Plant-based proteins, such as soy products (tofu, soy milk, and soy yogurt), lentils, beans, nuts, and seeds are excellent choices for vegetarians. Adults who have limited food budgets, have difficulty chewing meat, or are lactose intolerant may not get enough protein, especially animal protein. Keep in mind that any protein consumed in excess of that needed for the maintenance of body tissue will be broken down and used as energy or stored as fat. The waste products of metabolism of protein must be removed by the kidneys; excessive protein intake may accelerate kidney function decline in those with preexisting kidney issues.

Fat. The typical fat intake of adults of all ages is near the upper end of the 20% to 35% of total calories recommended by the Food and Nutrition Board. Looking specifically at saturated fat, usual intakes are slightly above the 10% of total calories limit suggested by the *Dietary Guidelines*.[17] It is a good idea for almost all adults to reduce their saturated fat intake because of the strong link between high saturated fat dietary patterns and obesity, heart disease, and certain cancers. A few strategies that would help most American adults to align with current recommendations for fat intake would be: (1) choose seafood, skinless poultry, lean meats, beans, peas, or lentils as protein sources for most meals; (2) prepare foods by steaming, grilling, broiling, or sautéing in a small amount of plant oil instead of deep-frying; and (3) choose skim or low-fat dairy products instead of full-fat varieties.

Carbohydrates. The AMDR for carbohydrates is 45% to 65% of total calories. Although total carbohydrate intake is typically adequate for older adults, fewer than 10% follow the advice to make *half your grains whole grains* (or consume 14 grams of dietary fiber per 1000 kcal) as recommended. Many adults need to shift their carbohydrate choices to emphasize complex carbohydrates and whole grains while minimizing the intake of added sugars and refined grains. Remember that the healthy eating pattern described in the *Dietary Guidelines* limits added sugars to 10% of calories per day and emphasizes the following carbohydrates:

- A variety of vegetables from all of the subgroups: dark green; red and orange; beans, peas, and lentils; starchy vegetables; and other vegetables
- Fruits, especially whole fruits
- Grains, at least half of which are whole grains
- Low-fat dairy, including milk, yogurt, cheese, and/or fortified soy beverages

A dietary pattern rich in complex carbohydrates helps us meet our nutrient needs without excess calories. Replacing sweets and refined grains with fiber-rich whole grains also improves blood glucose, cholesterol control, and bowel regularity. This is particularly helpful because inactivity and increasing body fatness that often accompany aging are connected to insulin resistance. Beyond these benefits, a dietary pattern rich in dietary fiber helps adults reduce their risk for heart disease and some forms of cancer. Indeed, adults could benefit from incorporating more whole grains into their dietary patterns.

Water. Many adults, especially as they approach their later years, fail to consume adequate quantities of water. In fact, many may be in a constant state of mild dehydration and at risk of electrolyte imbalances. Low fluid intakes in older adults may be caused by blunted thirst mechanisms, chronic diseases, and/or conscious reductions in fluid intake in order to reduce urination. Some may have alterations in fluid output due to certain medications (i.e., diuretics and laxatives) and/or experience an age-related decline in the kidneys' ability to concentrate urine. Dehydration is very dangerous and, among other symptoms, can cause disorientation and mental confusion, constipation, fecal impaction, and even death.

The AI for fluid is 13 cups per day for males and 9 cups per day for females. Initiatives to improve fluid intake, especially in older adults, should include assessments of barriers to drinking, hydration education, close intake monitoring, frequent prompting, offering a choice of healthy drinks, and addressing continence issues.

Minerals and Vitamins. Dietary requirements for many nutrients change throughout the adult years (Figs. 16-6 and 16-7). Most adults can get all the nutrients they need from foods. Adults who have impaired nutrient absorption, who have low overall food intake, or who are unable to follow a nutritious dietary pattern may benefit from mineral or vitamin supplements matched with their needs. For example, supplements or fortified foods can be especially helpful when it comes to meeting the RDAs for vitamin D and vitamin B-12. As always, it is best to discuss supplements with a doctor or an RDN. If older adults need to supplement their eating pattern, they should look for a supplement that supplies the needed nutrient(s) without other unnecessary ingredients. Megadoses of nutrients can be harmful.

In general, adults would benefit from lowering their intakes of sodium and consuming more food sources of calcium, vitamin D, potassium, iron, zinc, magnesium, vitamin B-6, folate, vitamin B-12, vitamin E, and carotenoids. Let's explore these dietary components in further detail in the next few pages.

Calcium and Vitamin D. These bone-building nutrients tend to be low in the dietary patterns of all adults. They become particularly problematic after age 50. Inadequate intake of these nutrients, combined with their decreased absorption, medication interactions, reduced synthesis of vitamin D in the skin (limited sun exposure), and the kidneys' decreased ability to convert vitamin D to its active form, greatly contributes to the development of osteoporosis. Getting enough of these nutrients is a challenge for many older adults because food sources of vitamin D are limited and the major sources—fatty fish and fortified milk—are not widely consumed by older adults. Plus, with increasing age, lactase production frequently decreases. As you will recall, one of the richest and most absorbable sources of these nutrients—milk—contains lactose.

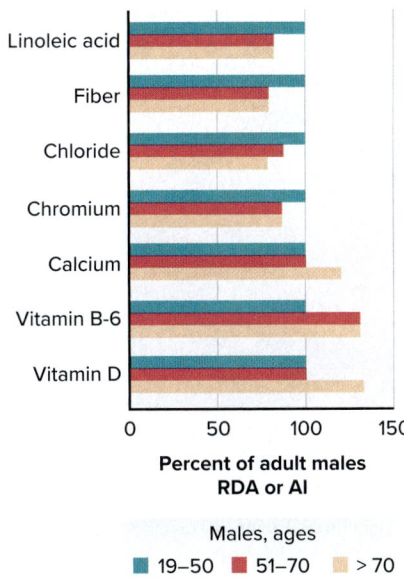

FIGURE 16-6 Relative nutrient requirements for aging adult males. Only nutrients that vary by age are shown.

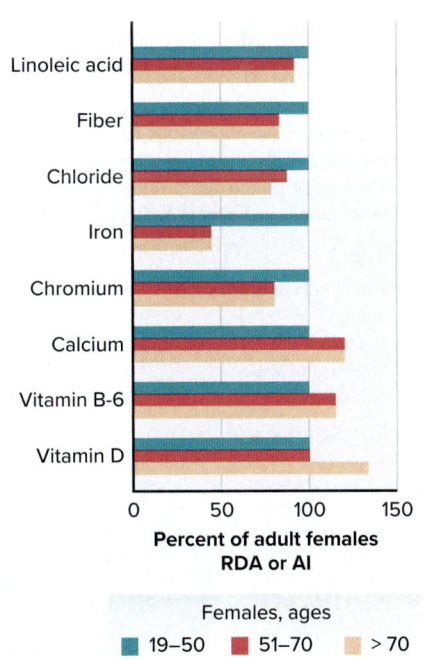

FIGURE 16-7 Relative nutrient requirements for aging adult females. Only nutrients that vary by age are shown.

FARM to FORK: Grapes and Raisins

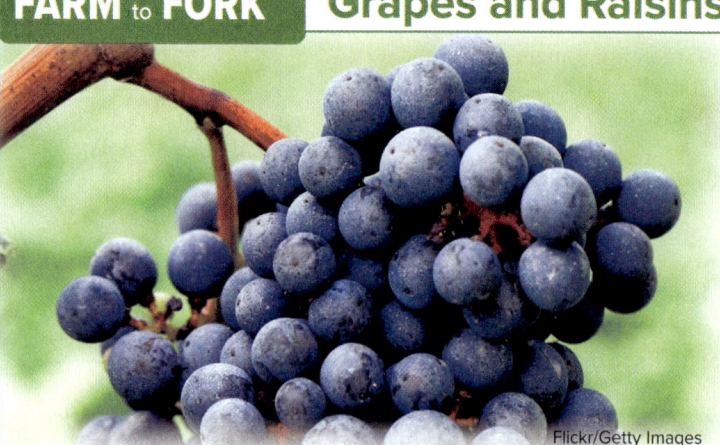

Flickr/Getty Images

Light green Thompson seedless grapes are the nation's most popular variety of grapes, outselling others by 1000 to 1. Yet the red, purple, and black varieties have 50% to 75% more phytochemicals than the pale Thompson. Sun-dried raisins, from Thompson grapes, are also the most popular dried fruit in the United States. Both are fantastic sources of nutrients and fiber for all ages.

Grow
- Home gardeners can successfully grow grapes if they select the correct site and cultivar, and an effective training and trellis system.
- Fertility and pest management programs are also necessary along with pruning the grapevines annually.
- A well-maintained grapevine can produce up to 20 pounds of grapes per year for over 50 years!

Shop
- As with many fruits, grapes are often harvested well before maximum ripeness to ensure stability during shipping.
- When shopping, look for vine-ripe grapes for maximum flavor and texture. Look for grapes that are firm and plump. Stems should be bright green and flexible, not dry and brittle.
- To check freshness, give the stem a gentle shake, and the grapes should remain on the vine.

Store
- Once harvested, cool grapes quickly in the coldest part of the refrigerator to extend shelf life and nutrient content.
- Store grapes in the plastic grape bag from the grocery store.
- Rinse grapes just prior to eating to reduce decay.

Prep
- The beauty of grapes is that they are a no-prep healthy snack for any time of the day!
- To add variety, try frozen grapes, add grapes or raisins to salads, or pair with low-fat cheeses.
- Home drying can be accomplished in a dehydrator or oven or by baking in the sun.

Source: Robinson J. Grapes and raisins: from muscadines to Thompson seedless. In: *Eating on the Wild Side: The Missing Link to Optimum Health.* New York: Little, Brown & Co.; 2013.

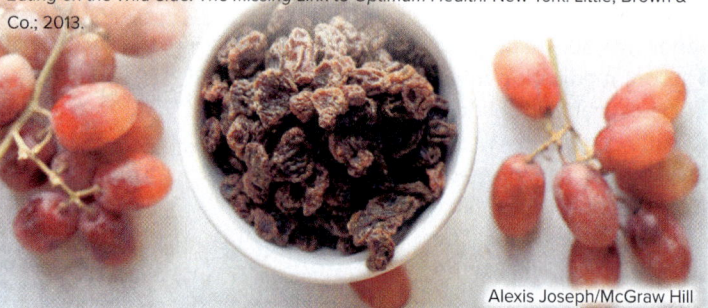

Alexis Joseph/McGraw Hill

After age 70, the RDA for vitamin D increases to 20 mcg/day (800 IU). To get the vitamin D and calcium they need, individuals with lactose intolerance may be able to consume small amounts of milk at mealtime with no ill effects. Calcium-fortified foods, cheese, yogurt, fish eaten with bones (e.g., canned sardines or salmon), and dark-green leafy vegetables can help those with lactose intolerance meet their calcium needs—but these sources often do not provide vitamin D. Just 10 to 15 minutes per day of sunlight can make a large difference in vitamin D status.

Potassium. Many older adults do not obtain adequate potassium although the AI remains constant in adulthood. This is an important mineral that plays a role in normal functioning of your heart, kidneys, nerves, and muscles. Inadequate potassium levels, often caused by inadequate intake and diuretic medication, can increase your blood pressure and kidney stone risk and even leach calcium out of your bones. Foods high in potassium include dried apricots, lentils, potatoes, and raisins. See this chapter's *Farm to Fork* for more on grapes and raisins.

Vitamin C. Vitamin C functions as an antioxidant and plays a role in immune function, wound healing, age-related macular degeneration, and cataracts in older individuals. Oxidative stress might contribute to the etiology of both conditions. Fruits and vegetables are some of the best sources of vitamin C. Citrus fruits, tomatoes, and potatoes can be a large source of vitamin C.

Iron. As females reach menopause (around age 50), the RDA for iron decreases to 8 mg/d (same as for males). Iron deficiency is the most common nutrient deficiency during all stages of the life cycle. Recall that iron deficiency can impair red blood cell synthesis, which leads to weakness, fatigue, shortness of breath, confusion, and disorientation. Common causes of iron deficiency in adults of all ages include digestive tract injuries that cause bleeding (i.e., bleeding ulcers or hemorrhoids) and the use of medicines, such as aspirin, that cause blood loss. Impaired iron absorption due to age-related declines in stomach acid production may also contribute to iron deficiency in older adults. Remember that iron deficiency can be present before any observable signs of anemia. Dietary sources of iron include fortified grains; meat, fish, and poultry; seafood; beans; dark-green leafy vegetables; and peas.

Zinc. Not only is dietary zinc intake less than optimal, diminished stomach acid production impairs zinc absorption as adults age. Poor zinc status may contribute to impairments in the sense of taste, mental lethargy, declines in immune function, and delayed wound healing that many older adults experience. Some dietary sources of zinc include oysters, meats, seafood, fortified grains, yogurt, and chickpeas.

Magnesium. Although the RDA remains constant in adulthood, magnesium tends to be low in the adult dietary pattern. Inadequate magnesium intakes may contribute to the bone loss, muscular weakness, and mental confusion seen in some older adults. It also can lead to sudden death from heart rhythm dysfunction and is linked to the development of cardiovascular disease, osteoporosis, and diabetes. The best source of magnesium comes from food because supplements may cause side effects such as diarrhea. Dietary sources of magnesium include nuts, green leafy vegetables, soy milk, beans, fortified cereals, and peanut butter.

Folate and Vitamins B-6 and B-12. Sufficient folate, because of its role in prevention of neural tube defects, is very important to females during the childbearing years. In later years, folate and vitamins B-6 and B-12 are especially important because they are required to clear the amino acid homocysteine from the bloodstream. Elevated blood concentrations of homocysteine are associated with the increased risk of cardiovascular disease, stroke, bone fracture, and neurological decline seen in some older people. Vitamin B-12 is a particular problem for the older population because a deficiency may exist even when intake appears to be adequate. As people age, the stomach slows its production of acid and intrinsic factor, which leads to poor absorption of vitamin B-12. If vitamin B-12 is depleted, anemia and nerve damage could result. Adults age 51 years and older often must meet vitamin B-12 needs with supplements or fortified foods because synthetic vitamin B-12 is more readily absorbed than natural forms of B-12.

Vitamin E. The dietary intake of most of the population falls short of recommendations for vitamin E. Low vitamin E intake means that the body has a reduced supply of antioxidants, which may increase the degree of cell damage caused by free radicals, promote the progression of chronic diseases and cataracts, and accelerate the aging process. In addition, low vitamin E levels can lead to declines in physical abilities.

Carotenoids. Dietary intakes of certain carotenoids have been shown to have a variety of important antiaging, anticancer, and other protective effects. Specifically, lutein and zeaxanthin have been linked with the prevention of cataracts and age-related macular degeneration.[18] Dietary patterns high in fruits and vegetables, the major sources of carotenoids and other beneficial phytochemicals, are consistently shown to be protective against a wide variety of age-related conditions.

Sodium. The declining sense of taste that typically accompanies aging often contributes to a preference for highly salted foods. The *Dietary Guidelines* advises adults to consume less than 2300 milligrams of sodium per day (about 1 teaspoon of table salt). Yet, the average sodium intakes of American adults are over 3500 milligrams per day. A heavy reliance on highly processed foods and restaurant meals is mostly to blame for the high sodium intakes of Americans. The most widely recognized consequence of high sodium intake is hypertension, but high sodium intake has also been linked to osteoporosis secondary to increased calcium excretion in the urine. Excessive dietary sodium may also overtax poorly functioning kidneys of older adults.

Even though excessive sodium receives most of the attention, low blood sodium (hyponatremia) is also a concern for older adults. Adults older than age 70, especially those who take diuretic medications or who have poor kidney function, are at increased risk for hyponatremia. The consequences of mild hyponatremia include lightheadedness, confusion, and unsteady gait, which can certainly increase the risk for falls among older adults. Other problems include fatigue, muscle cramps, and lack of appetite. There is no reason to severely restrict sodium among older adults who do not have kidney disease, but lowering sodium intakes closer to the AI would improve overall health for most adults.

Dietary Supplements. About half of older adults consume dietary supplements even though there is no solid evidence that dietary supplements provide any health advantages in well-nourished adults. Although a typical multivitamin mineral supplement for older adults (with no more than 100% of the DV of the vitamins and minerals) is likely safe, there is no evidence that dietary supplements prevent chronic diseases.[19]

ARE ADULTS FOLLOWING DIETARY RECOMMENDATIONS?

Since the mid-1950s, adults have consumed less saturated fat as more people substitute fat-free and low-fat milk for cream and whole milk. However, adults still eat more cheese, usually a concentrated form of saturated fat. Since 1963, they have eaten less butter, fewer eggs, less animal fat, and more plant oils and fish. Animal breeders are raising animals leaner than those produced in 1950, which also helps reduce saturated fat intake.

Other aspects of average adult eating patterns are still in need of improvement. The latest nutrition survey data show that the major contributors of calories to the adult dietary pattern are still white bread, beef, doughnuts, cakes and cookies, soft drinks, milk, poultry, cheese, alcoholic beverages, salad dressing, mayonnaise, potatoes, and sugars/syrups/jams. If Americans were truly lowering their intakes of sugar, saturated fat, and sodium while increasing their intakes of fiber, many of these foods would not appear at the top of the list.

✓ CONCEPT CHECK 16.2

1. Describe the changes in metabolism over the life span and changes specific to the aging process after age 60.
2. Identify one nutrient that should be limited in the dietary patterns of most American adults. Suggest three specific dietary changes that would help to reduce intake of this nutrient. (Note: calories are not nutrients.)
3. Name three nutrients that are commonly lacking in dietary patterns of adults. Suggest one rich food source of each of these nutrients.

16.3 Nutritional Status of Adults

Dietary adequacy is influenced by physiological, psychosocial, and economic factors. Figure 16-8 summarizes the nutritional implications of many of the physiological changes that occur during adulthood. Some of the changes listed (e.g., tooth loss and changes in taste and smell) can directly influence dietary intake. Other changes (e.g., loss of lean body tissue) can alter nutrient and/or calorie needs. Some body changes (e.g., reduced stomach acidity, diminished kidney function) can affect nutrient utilization. Furthermore, chronic diseases and the medications used to manage them may influence food intake and nutrient needs. In this section, explore the influences of several of these factors on nutritional status during adulthood.

BODY COMPOSITION

The primary changes in body composition that occur with aging are diminished lean body mass, increased fat stores, and decreased body water. A focus on physical activity can attenuate many of these unwanted changes.

The loss of lean body mass is termed **sarcopenia.** Some muscle cells shrink, others are lost as muscles age, and some muscles lose their elasticity as they accumulate fat and collagen. Loss of muscle mass leads to a decrease in basal metabolism, muscle strength, and energy needs. Less muscle mass also leads to lower fitness performance, which makes the prognosis for maintaining muscle even worse. Clearly, it is best to prevent this downward spiral.

As lean tissue declines with age, body fat often increases, a condition called **sarcopenic obesity.**[20] Much of this increase in body fat results from overconsumption of calories and inadequate physical activity, although even physically fit males and females typically gain some additional body fatness after age 50. A small fat gain in adulthood may

sarcopenia Loss of muscle tissue. Among older adults, this loss of lean mass greatly increases their risk of illness and death.

sarcopenic obesity Advanced muscle loss accompanied by gains in fat mass.

Physiological Changes of Aging

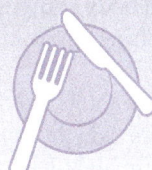
↓ Appetite
- Monitor changes in weight and report unintentional weight loss to your primary care provider.
- Eat small, frequent, calorie- and nutrient-dense meals throughout the day.
- Incorporate nutrient-rich drinks or smoothies between meals.

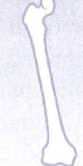
↓ Bone mass
- Meet nutrient needs, especially protein, calcium, and vitamin D (including regular sun exposure).
- Perform regular physical activity, especially weight-bearing activities.
- Aim to maintain a healthy body weight (i.e., BMI between 18.5 and 24.9).

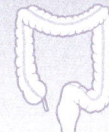
↓ Bowel function
- Emphasize a dietary pattern rich in fruits, vegetables, and whole grains.
- Meet fluid needs and monitor hydration.
- Increase physical activity.

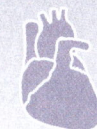
↓ Cardiovascular function
- Achieve and maintain a healthy body weight.
- Choose a dietary pattern rich in fruits, vegetables, whole grains, plant-based protein, and fatty fish.
- Stay physically active.

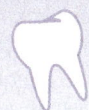
↓ Chewing or swallowing ability
- Work with a dentist or trained therapist to maximize chewing and swallowing ability.
- Modify food consistency as necessary.

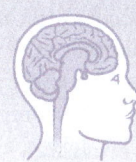
↓ Cognitive function
- Choose a dietary pattern rich in fruits, vegetables, whole grains, and plant sources of protein.
- Consume seafood, a source of omega-3 fatty acids, twice per week.
- Perform regular physical activity.
- Obtain adequate sleep, rest, and relaxation.

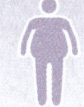
↑ Fat stores
- Avoid overconsumption of calorie-dense foods and beverages.
- Perform regular physical activity.

↓ Immune function
- Meet nutrient needs, especially protein, vitamin A, vitamin C, vitamin E, and zinc.
- Perform regular physical activity.

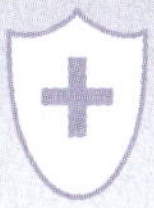

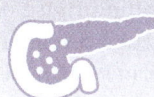
↓ Insulin function
- Maintain a healthy body weight.
- Choose whole grains; limit refined grains and added sugars.
- Perform regular physical activity.

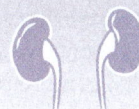
↓ Kidney function
- Consume adequate fluids.
- Maintain normal blood pressure and weight.
- Be cautious about using medications and dietary supplements.

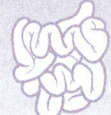
↓ Lactase production
- Reduce serving sizes of milk.
- Substitute yogurt or cheese for milk.
- Use reduced-lactose or lactose-free products and seek nondairy calcium sources.

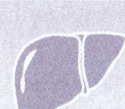
↓ Liver function
- Consume alcohol in moderation, if at all.
- Avoid consuming dietary supplements that contain more than 100% of the Daily Value of nutrients, especially vitamin A.

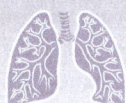
↓ Lung function
- Avoid tobacco.
- Perform regular physical activity.

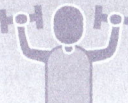
↓ Muscle mass
- Meet nutrient needs, especially protein.
- Perform regular physical activity, including strength training.

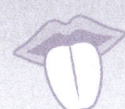
↓ Sense of taste and smell
- Vary the colors and textures of foods.
- Experiment with sodium-free herbs and spices.

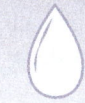
↓ Sense of thirst
- Monitor fluid intake.
- Drink water throughout the day.
- Stay alert for evidence of dehydration (e.g., dark-colored urine).

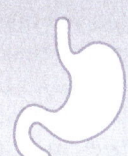
↓ Stomach acidity
- Include lean meats and iron-fortified foods in the dietary pattern.
- Consume vitamin C–rich foods to enhance absorption of nonheme iron from foods.
- Choose foods fortified with vitamin B-12.

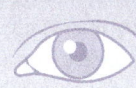
↓ Vision
- Choose a dietary pattern rich in fruits, vegetables, and whole grains.
- Regularly consume fatty fish, a source of omega-3 fatty acids.
- Wear sunglasses in sunny conditions.
- Avoid tobacco.

FIGURE 16-8 Details of the physiological changes of aging.
Source: Adapted from NIH, National Institute on Aging.

not compromise health, but large gains are problematic. Recall that obesity increases risks for hypertension, cardiovascular disease, type 2 diabetes, osteoarthritis, cancers, and many other serious chronic conditions. Ultimately, these changes in body composition may diminish a person's ability to perform daily tasks, such as getting up from a chair and climbing a flight of stairs.

On the other hand, decreases in body weight can also be a problem for adults age 70 and older. Unintended weight loss increases the risk of malnutrition, which alters an individual's ability to cope with illnesses and injuries and could ultimately lead to death. Frailty, or health deficits that result in functional declines and increase injury risk, affects about 15% of older adults in the United States.

BONES AND JOINTS

Recall that some bone loss is an expected consequence of aging. In females, bone loss rapidly occurs after menopause. For males, bone loss is slow and steady from middle age throughout later life. Many older adults have undiagnosed osteomalacia, a condition mainly caused by insufficient vitamin D. Osteoporosis can limit the ability of older people to shop, prepare food, and engage in physical activity. Consuming adequate vitamin D, calcium, and protein; not smoking; avoiding excessive alcohol; and engaging in weight-bearing physical activity can help preserve bone mass.

There are over 100 types of arthritis, a disease that causes the degeneration of the cartilage that covers and cushions the joints. Such changes in the joints cause them to ache and become inflamed and painful to move. Severe arthritis can cause permanent joint changes, and some types of arthritis affect the heart, eyes, lungs, kidneys, and skin in addition to the joints. Over 58 million U.S. adults suffer from some type of arthritis.[21] **Osteoarthritis,** which affects over 32 million U.S. adults, is the leading cause of disability among older persons. **Rheumatoid arthritis,** which affects about 1.5 million U.S. adults, is more prevalent in younger adults. **Gout,** a very painful form of arthritis that comes on suddenly and can be related to changes in eating patterns, affects about 6 million males and 3 million females in the United States. The estimated annual medical costs related to these conditions are over $140 billion.

Although precise causes or cures are unknown, many unproven arthritis remedies have been publicized. Fad diets, food restrictions, and nutrient supplementation are some of the more popular treatments. Maintaining a healthy weight, which reduces stress on painful arthritic joints, is the best strategy to offer relief from arthritis. Although no special diet, food, or nutrient has been proven to reliably prevent, relieve, or cure arthritis, some research shows that a dietary pattern (e.g., Mediterranean diet) that is rich in antioxidant nutrients, anti-inflammatory phytochemicals, and omega-3 fatty acids can help to reduce the inflammation that underlies these conditions.[22] As far as supplements go, results remain controversial. Discuss the pros and cons of supplement use for these conditions with your primary care provider or dietitian.

osteoarthritis A degenerative joint condition caused by a breakdown of cartilage in joints. It often results from wear and tear due to repetitive motions or the pressure of excess body weight.

rheumatoid arthritis A degenerative joint condition resulting from an autoimmune disease that causes inflammation in the joints and other sites of the body.

gout A form of arthritis caused by the buildup of uric acid crystals in the joints.

PHYSICAL ACTIVITY

Many physical changes of aging can be traced back to a sedentary lifestyle. As you might predict, an active lifestyle helps preserve muscle mass and decrease body fat. Physical activity increases muscle strength and mobility; improves balance, which decreases the risk of falling; eases daily tasks that require strength; improves sleep; slows bone loss; and increases joint movement, thus reducing injuries. It also has a positive impact on a person's mental outlook. Ideally, an active lifestyle should be maintained throughout life and include activities to build endurance, strength, balance, and flexibility. The *Physical Activity Guidelines for Americans* provides recommendations specifically for older adults (Table 16-1).

All older adults should avoid inactivity. Having a comprehensive physical activity plan, developed with a health professional to accommodate individual health risks and needs, will enhance success for older adults. Males older than age 40; females older than age 50; those with heart conditions, diabetes, or joint problems; and anyone who has been sedentary should consult a primary care provider before beginning a physical activity program.

TABLE 16-1 ■ Physical Activity Guidelines for Older Adults

Guidelines for all adults

Adults should move more and sit less throughout each day. Any physical activity is better than none and results in health benefits.

For substantial health benefits, adults should engage in at least 150 minutes (2 hours and 30 minutes) to 300 minutes (5 hours) a week of moderate-intensity, or 75 minutes (1 hour and 15 minutes) to 150 minutes (2 hours and 30 minutes) a week of vigorous-intensity, aerobic physical activity, or an equivalent combination of moderate- and vigorous-intensity aerobic activity. Preferably, aerobic activity should be spread throughout the week.

Additional health benefits are gained by engaging in physical activity beyond the equivalent of 300 minutes (5 hours) of moderate-intensity physical activity a week.

Adults should also complete muscle-strengthening activities of moderate or greater intensity that involve all major muscle groups on 2 or more days a week, as these activities provide additional health benefits.

Guidelines for older adults

As part of their weekly physical activity, older adults should engage in multicomponent physical activity that includes balance training as well as aerobic and muscle-strengthening activities.

Older adults should determine their level of effort for physical activity relative to their level of fitness.

Older adults with chronic conditions should understand whether and how their conditions affect their ability to do regular physical activity safely.

When older adults cannot do 150 minutes of moderate-intensity aerobic activity a week because of chronic conditions, they should be as physically active as their abilities and conditions allow.

Source: *Physical Activity Guidelines for Americans*, 2nd ed., available from https://health.gov/paguidelines/secondedition/pdf/Physical_Activity_Guidelines_2nd_edition.pdf

Aerobic Activity. All adults should engage in either moderate-intensity aerobic physical activity for at least 150 to 300 minutes per week or vigorous-intensity aerobic activity for 75 to 150 minutes per week, or an equivalent combination of the two. Moderate-intensity activity requires medium effort. Thinking back to the Rating of Perceived Exertion, moderate activity would be equal to a 4 to 6 (out of 10) and produce increases in breathing rate and heart rate. Vigorous activity might begin at a 7 or 8 (out of 10) and produces larger increases in breathing and heart rate. This amount of aerobic activity improves endurance and aids in prevention of chronic diseases. A longer duration of daily physical activity may be required for weight loss or weight maintenance. Weight-bearing exercises are particularly helpful for preservation of bone mass. For older adults who have not been physically active, it is important to increase the pace gradually. Remember, any amount of physical activity is better than none at all.

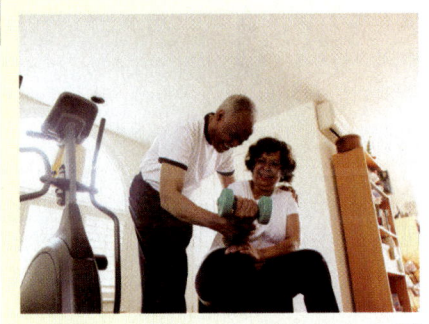
LWA/Dann Tardif/Blend Images LLC

Researchers believe that maintaining lean muscle mass may be the most important strategy for successful aging because doing so:

- Maintains basal metabolic rate, which helps to decrease the risk of obesity
- Keeps body fat within a healthy range, which helps in the management of blood lipids and blood glucose
- Maintains body water, which decreases the risk of dehydration and improves body temperature regulation
- Promotes healthy bones
- Helps to prevent falls
- Helps a person to preserve independence because functional abilities are maintained over time

Muscle-Strengthening Activities. To maintain lean tissue and basal metabolic rate, muscle-strengthening activities should be performed 2 to 3 days per week and involve all major muscle groups (legs, hips, abdomen, chest, back, shoulders, and arms). Specific recommendations for muscle strengthening include performing at least 1 set of 8 to 12 repetitions, although 2 or 3 sets may be more effective. Start slowly, concentrate on breathing and technique, rest between circuits and sets, and stop an activity if it becomes painful.

Balance Activities. For those at risk for falling, activities that improve balance are recommended. Specific guidelines include performing balance activities about three times per week. Examples of safe activities include heel-to-toe walking, repetitive standing from a sitting position, and using a wobble board. Muscle strengthening of the back, abdomen, and legs also improves balance.

Flexibility, Warm-Up, and Cool-Down. Stretching each major muscle group should accompany aerobic or muscle strengthening activities. Improving flexibility can make it easier to perform many simple tasks, such as tying shoes. All fitness programs should

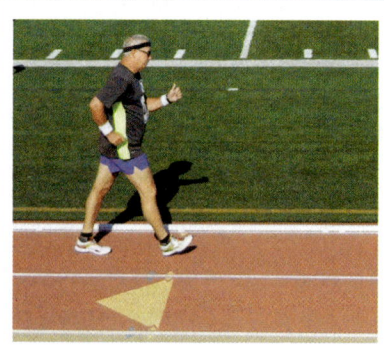

To keep active, adults age 50 and older are eligible to participate in local and national Senior Games (https://nsga.com/), including walking events as shown here. **What activities could you begin now that could be enjoyed throughout adulthood?** Anne Smith

include warm-up and cool-down activities. A safe warm-up before aerobic activities allows a gradual increase in heart rate and breathing. An adequate cool-down after physical activity allows a gradual heart rate decrease at the end of the session.

Multicomponent Physical Activity. These types of activities include incorporating more than one type of physical activity into your physical fitness program. Dancing, tai chi, gardening, or sports are considered multicomponent because they often incorporate several different types of physical activity.

DIGESTIVE SYSTEM

As you will recall from previous chapters, digestion begins in the mouth. Over 25% of older adults have no natural teeth, and many more are missing some teeth.[23] The problem of tooth loss is worse among low-income populations. Even with properly fitting dentures, chewing ability may be limited. Older adults with poor dentition often avoid meats or crunchy fruits and vegetables, thereby missing out on key nutrients such as protein, iron, and zinc (from meat) as well as potassium and fiber (from fruits and vegetables). Ground meats, beans, peas, lentils, and cooked or finely chopped vegetables are easier options for older adults with chewing problems.[24]

Further along the GI tract, the production of hydrochloric acid, intrinsic factor, and some digestive enzymes (e.g., lactase) declines with advancing age.[25] In addition, some medications affect acid production. As a result of low acid production, absorption of some minerals, such as iron, zinc, and calcium, can be impaired. Low levels of acid and intrinsic factor reduce the digestion and absorption of vitamin B-12. Thus, even with adequate intakes of iron and vitamin B-12, older adults may become anemic. Symptoms of lactose intolerance can lead to avoidance of dairy products, which can limit the availability of bone-building nutrients. Again, fortified foods or supplements can help older adults overcome these problems with digestion and absorption of nutrients.

Constipation is also a common problem for older people. To prevent constipation, older people should have a primarily plant-based dietary pattern to meet fiber needs, drink plenty of fluids, and engage in regular physical activity. Fiber supplements may be useful when overall food consumption does not allow for adequate fiber intake. Because some medications can be habit forming, a primary care provider should be consulted to determine if a laxative or stool softener is necessary.

In addition to changes in the GI tract, the functions of the accessory organs decline as we age. For instance, the liver functions less efficiently. A history of significant alcohol consumption or liver disease will intensify existing problems with liver function. As liver efficiency declines, its ability to detoxify substances, including medications, alcohol, and vitamin and mineral supplements, drops. This increases the possibility for vitamin and mineral toxicities.

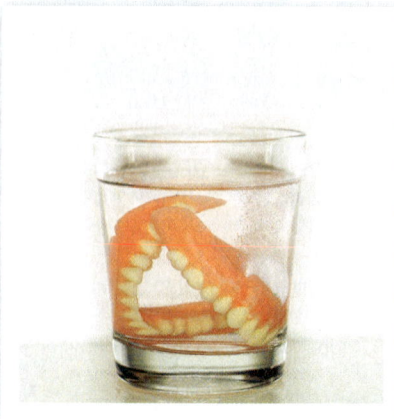

Poor dentition contributes to decreased food intake and digestive problems. **What strategies might be effective in improving the nutritional status of adults who are missing some or all of their natural teeth?** Stockbyte/PunchStock/Getty Images

The gallbladder also functions less efficiently in later years. Gallstones can block the flow of bile out of the gallbladder into the small intestine, thereby interfering with fat digestion. Obesity is a major risk factor for gallbladder disease, especially in older females. Gradual (as opposed to rapid) loss of excess body weight and a low-fat dietary pattern may reduce symptoms.

Although pancreatic function may decline with age, this organ has a large reserve capacity. One sign of a failing pancreas is high blood glucose, although this can occur as the result of several conditions. The pancreas may be secreting less insulin, or cells may be resisting insulin action (as is commonly seen in people with android obesity). Where appropriate, improved nutrient intake, regular physical activity, and loss of excess body weight can improve insulin action and blood glucose regulation.

NERVOUS SYSTEM

A gradual loss of nerve cells may decrease perceptions of taste and smell and impair neuromuscular coordination, reasoning, and memory. Both hearing and vision typically decline with age. Hearing impairment is the greatest in those who have been exposed consistently to loud noises, such as urban traffic, lawnmowers, and loud music.

Declining eyesight, frequently caused by retina degeneration and cataracts, can affect a person's abilities to grocery shop, read labels for nutritional content, and prepare foods safely at home. Vision losses also may cause people to curtail social interactions, reduce physical activity, and have inadequate daily personal health and grooming routines. Age-related macular degeneration, a common cause of failing eyesight, affects about 11 million U.S. adults.[26] A major risk factor is tobacco use. Dietary patterns rich in carotenoids and omega-3 fatty acids help to reduce the risk of certain eye diseases among older adults.[27]

Loss of neuromuscular coordination may also impact food access and preparation for older adults. Physical tasks as simple as opening food packages can become so difficult that individuals restrict dietary intake to foods that require little preparation and depend on others to provide food that is ready to eat. Eating may become difficult, too. Loss of coordination may make it a challenge to grasp cup handles and manipulate eating utensils. As a result, older adults often avoid foods that can be easily spilled (e.g., soups and juices) or that need to be cut (e.g., meats, large vegetables). Some may even withdraw from social activities and eat alone, which often means eating less.

IMMUNE SYSTEM

With age, the immune system often operates less efficiently. Recurrent illnesses and delayed wound healing are warning signs that nutrient deficiencies (especially protein and zinc) may be hindering immune function. On the other hand, overnutrition appears to be equally harmful to the immune system. For example, obesity and excessive fat, iron, and zinc intakes can suppress immune function. Meeting daily requirements for protein, vitamins (especially folate and vitamins A, C, D, and E), iron, and zinc will help to maximize immune function. Increased attention to food safety is crucial to prevent foodborne illness.

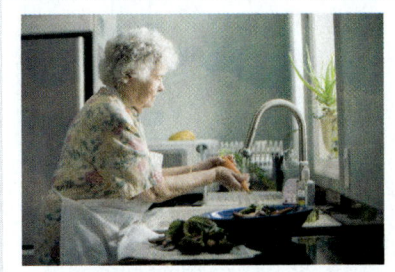

Immune function declines with age, so food safety becomes increasingly important for older adults. **List three simple consumer food safety practices that would help to stave off foodborne illness.** Cade Martin/CDC

ENDOCRINE SYSTEM

As adulthood progresses, the rate of hormone synthesis and release can diminish. Declining thyroid hormone production, for example, can decrease basal metabolic rate, leading to unexpected weight gain. A decrease in insulin release or sensitivity to insulin, for instance, means that it takes longer for blood glucose levels to return to normal after a meal. Maintaining a healthy weight, engaging in regular physical activity, adhering to a dietary pattern that is low in saturated fat and high in fiber, and avoiding highly processed foods can enhance the body's ability to use insulin and restore elevated blood glucose levels to normal after a meal.

CHRONIC DISEASE

The prevalence of obesity, heart disease, osteoporosis, cancers, hypertension, and diabetes rises with age. More than half of older adults have one of these chronic and potentially debilitating diseases. Four out of 10 older adults have at least two chronic conditions contributing to $3.8 trillion in annual health care costs.[28] One small change can trigger a chain of events that results in poor health. Chronic diseases may have a strong impact on dietary patterns. For instance, obesity, heart disease, and osteoporosis may impair physical mobility to the extent that victims are unable to shop for and prepare food. Chronic disease also can influence nutrient requirements. Cancer, for example, boosts nutrient and calorie needs. Hypertension may indicate a need to lower sodium intake. Nutrient utilization can be affected by chronic disease, too. For instance, diabetes alters the body's ability to utilize glucose. Chronic kidney diseases may impair the kidneys' ability to reabsorb glucose, amino acids, and vitamin C.

MEDICATIONS

Older adults are major consumers of medications (both prescription and over-the-counter) and nutritional supplements. The CDC reports that about 90% of older adults take at least one prescription medication daily, and over 41% of all people over age 65 take five or more medicines each day **(polypharmacy)**.[29] Physiological declines that occur during aging (e.g., reduced body water and reduced liver and kidney function) may exaggerate and prolong the effects of medications and dietary supplements in older adults.

Medications can eradicate infections and control chronic diseases, but some also adversely affect nutritional status, particularly of those who are older and/or take many different medications. For instance, some medications depress taste and smell acuity or cause anorexia or nausea that can blunt interest in eating and lead to reduced dietary intake. Some medications alter nutrient needs. Aspirin, for example, increases the likelihood of stomach bleeding, so long-term use may elevate the need for iron, as well as other nutrients. Antibiotics kill beneficial bacteria along with pathogens, so they can limit the amount of vitamin K that is synthesized by bacteria in the large intestine. Some medications may impair nutrient utilization; diuretics and laxatives may cause excessive excretion of water and minerals. Even vitamin and mineral supplements may have unanticipated effects on nutritional status. Iron supplements taken in large doses can interfere with the functioning of zinc and copper. Folate supplements can mask vitamin B-12 deficiencies.

People who must take medications should eat nutrient-dense foods and avoid any specific food or supplement that interferes with the function of their medications. For example, vitamin K can reduce the action of oral anticoagulants, aged cheese can interfere with certain drugs used to treat hypertension and depression, and grapefruit can interfere with medications such as tranquilizers and those that lower cholesterol levels. An RDN can help to plan a dietary pattern that meets nutritional needs while avoiding harmful food/medication interactions.

polypharmacy A term used to describe the use of multiple medicines simultaneously by an individual.

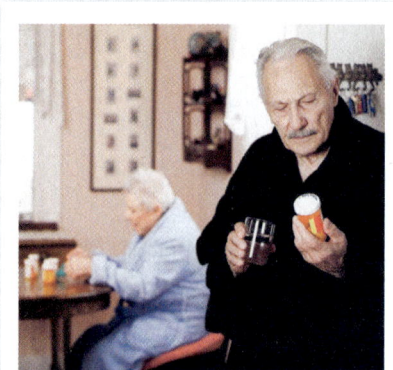

The CDC reports that over 41% of seniors (over 65 years) take five or more medications per day. In some cases, drugs can affect nutrient status. **What are two examples of medications that can directly alter one's nutrient status?** Hill Street Studios/Blend Images LLC

COMPLEMENTARY AND ALTERNATIVE MEDICINE

Approximately 74% of U.S. adults over age 60 use some kind of dietary, botanical, or herbal supplement.[30] Recall that the safety, purity, and effectiveness of dietary supplements are not tightly monitored by the FDA. See the *Ask the RDN* and Table 16-2 for reviews on some popular herbal products used by older adults. Note from the table that these products can pose health risks in certain people. In addition, they may be quite expensive and are not covered by health insurance plans. In recent years, the use of many herbal products has declined because of expense and documented negative effects.

When it comes to herbal products, proceed with caution. Significant health risks—including death—have been associated with the use of many herbal products. The FDA advises anyone who experiences adverse side effects from an herbal product to contact a primary care provider. Clinicians are then encouraged to report adverse events to the FDA, state and local health departments, and consumer protection agencies.

Females who are pregnant or breastfeeding, children under 2 years of age, anyone over the age of 65 years, and anyone with a chronic disease should not take supplements unless under the guidance of a primary care provider. A concern has been raised with regard to patients who abruptly end any alternative medicine at the start of hospital treatments or deny that they are using alternative therapies. Interactions between alternative therapies and pharmaceutical drugs can be drastic and include complications such as delirium, clotting abnormalities, and rapid heartbeat, resulting in the need for intensive care. Full disclosure of all prescription and nonprescription treatments aids in prevention of such complications. Experts recommend that, if time permits, patients stop taking herbal products for about a week before a scheduled surgery or otherwise take all original supplement containers to the hospital so that the anesthesiologist can evaluate what was taken.

TABLE 16-2 ■ Popular Herbal Products

Product	Purported Effects[a]	Side Effects	Use Caution
Black cohosh	Reduce symptoms of menopause (possibly effective)	Nausea Liver damage	Females who have had breast cancer Anyone taking estrogen, or hypertension or blood-thinning medications[b] Anyone with abnormal liver function
Cranberry	Prevent and treat urinary tract infections (possibly effective)	GI upset and diarrhea Kidney stones	People susceptible to kidney stones Anyone taking antidepressants, prescription painkillers, or blood thinners
Echinacea	Prevention or treatment of colds or other infections (possibly effective)	Nausea Skin irritation Allergic reactions GI tract upset Increased urination	Anyone with an autoimmune disease Patients pre- or post-surgery Anyone with allergies to daisies
Garlic	Improve blood sugar, cholesterol, blood pressure (possibly effective)	GI tract upset Unpleasant odor Allergic reactions	Patients pre- or post-surgery Anyone taking blood-thinning medications or AIDS medications
Ginger	Decrease nausea and vomiting (possibly effective) Reduce symptoms of osteoarthritis (possibly effective)	Heartburn Diarrhea Increased menstrual bleeding	Females who are pregnant People with bleeding disorders Anyone with heart conditions People taking blood glucose–lowering or blood-thinning medications
Ginkgo biloba	Reduce symptoms of anxiety and dementia (possibly effective) Improve glaucoma damage (possibly effective)	Mild headache GI tract upset Allergic reactions Irritability Reduced blood clotting Seizures	People with bleeding disorders Patients pre- or post-surgery Concurrent use of feverfew, garlic, ginseng, dong quai, or red clover Anyone taking diabetes medications, blood-thinning medications, vitamin E supplements, antidepressants, or diuretics
Ginseng	Improve symptoms of Alzheimer's and cognition (possibly effective) Prevent influenza (possibly effective) Improve lung disease symptoms (possibly effective)	Hypertension Asthma Irregular heartbeat Hypoglycemia Insomnia Headache Nervousness GI tract upset Reduced blood clotting Menstrual irregularities and breast tenderness	Anyone taking prescription drugs Females who have had breast cancer Anyone with chronic GI tract disease Anyone with uncontrolled hypertension
Glucosamine sulfate	Improve symptoms of osteoarthritis (likely effective)	GI tract upset	People with asthma or shellfish allergies
Milk thistle	Improve blood sugar and indigestion (possibly effective)	GI distress Pain Anorexia	People taking blood glucose–lowering medications People with hormone-sensitive cancers People with allergies to plants in the Asteraceae family

(continued)

TABLE 16-2 ■ *(continued)*

Product	Purported Effects[a]	Side Effects	Use Caution
St. John's wort	Reduce symptoms of depression (likely effective) Improve wound healing (possibly effective) Reduce menopause symptoms (possibly effective)	GI tract upset Rash Fatigue Restlessness Increased sensitivity to sunlight	Anyone who takes a prescription drug People with UV sensitivity[c] People with bipolar disorder, major depression, schizophrenia, or Alzheimer's disease Anyone recovering from a graft or organ transplant
Turmeric	Reduce symptoms of depression and osteoarthritis (possibly effective) Improve cholesterol (possibly effective)	GI tract upset Dizziness	People with gallbladder problems People with GERD Patients pre- or post-surgery

[a] Ratings of effectiveness from Natural Medicines Comprehensive Database
[b] Coumadin®, aspirin, Heparin®, Lovenox®, or Fragmin®
[c] UV sensitivity may be induced by some drugs, such as sulfa medications, anti-inflammatory medications, or acid-reflux medications.

ASK THE RDN: CBD

Dear RDN: *My friend recently began taking CBD. She said it helps her sleep better and manage her anxiety. What are the pros and cons of taking CBD?*

CBD (cannabidiol) is a cannabinoid found in cannabis and hemp. Many people report that CBD helps manage anxiety, as well as pain, inflammation, muscle spasms, insomnia, seizures, inflammatory bowel disease, IBS, migraines, neurodegenerative disorders, and more. CBD is nonintoxicating. THC (tetrahydrocannabinol), another cannabinoid found in cannabis (and in small amounts in hemp), is known for its intoxicating or "high" effect.

The body processes cannabinoids through a neurotransmitter system *(the endocannabinoid system)* whose function is to promote homeostasis in the body. CBD helps to regulate this system. In fact, our body makes its own cannabinoid, called anandamide, also known as the *bliss molecule*. CBD allows our body to keep more of this *feel good* compound, which may explain why many find relief from anxiety using CBD.

There is pronounced synergy between the cannabinoids, terpenes (responsible for the unique aroma in plants), and flavonoids (that contribute antioxidant and anti-inflammatory effects) in cannabis and hemp. Each individual component of the plant may provide therapeutic benefits on its own, but when combined, the so-called entourage effect is dramatic.

CBD comes in many forms, including sublingual tinctures, water-soluble tinctures, edibles/softgels, topicals, and hemp flower/vape cartridges. There are three types of CBD: full spectrum, broad spectrum, and CBD isolate. Full spectrum products contain all the plant's components, including cannabinoids, terpenes, and flavonoids. Broad-spectrum CBD products contain all these synergistic components, minus the THC. CBD isolate is pure CBD, meaning that it does not contain other synergistic plant compounds, which may decrease efficacy and increase side effects.

Dosing of CBD is very individual, depending on the condition being treated and method of administration. Some people find relief with just 2 milligrams and others may require 50 milligrams or more. It's best to *start low and go slow* to find the minimum effective dose.

Today's market is inundated with CBD products, including many of inferior quality. The Food and Drug Administration found that 70% of CBD products sold online are mislabeled, with some containing zero CBD. It's important to buy CBD products from a trusted and safe source. Look for a certificate of analysis (COA) from an independent lab before buying a product.

A word of caution. Taking orally ingested CBD (i.e., edibles/softgels) with other medications that are contraindicated with grapefruit may result in an adverse event, so it's important to talk with a knowledgeable health care professional.

Including CBD in your self-care routine may be effective for managing anxiety, but it's also important to work on other aspects of your life that may promote wellness: engage in regular physical activity, adhere to a healthy eating pattern, get adequate sleep, practice meditation or yoga, and seek professional help from a licensed mental health provider if symptoms of anxiety are severe.

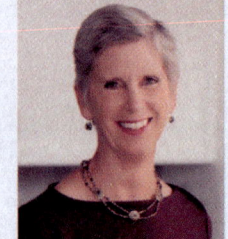

Channing Johnson

Yours in health,

Janice Newell Bissex, MS, RDN, FAND

Holistic Cannabis Practitioner

✓ CONCEPT CHECK 16.3

1. What is *sarcopenia*? What two dietary and lifestyle changes would you suggest to avoid this condition?
2. Describe three ways aging affects the processes of digestion, absorption, and utilization of nutrients.
3. List three risks associated with consuming dietary supplements, herbals, or botanicals.

16.4 Healthful Dietary Patterns for the Adult Years

Recommended dietary practices for later years would be to increase nutrient density and ensure fiber and fluid intakes are adequate. In addition, although plant proteins are always recommended, lean meats can be especially helpful for meeting vitamin B-6, vitamin B-12, iron, and zinc needs. Figure 16-9 outlines healthy U.S.-style dietary patterns at various calorie levels commonly needed by older adults.

Singles of all ages face the following logistical barriers obtaining adequate nutrients: purchasing, preparing, storing, and using food with minimal waste. Value-priced packages of meats and vegetables are normally too large to be useful for a single person. Many singles live in small dwellings, some without kitchens and freezers. Creating an adequate dietary pattern to accommodate a limited budget and a single appetite requires special considerations. Fig. 16-10 provides some practical suggestions for eating healthfully in later years.

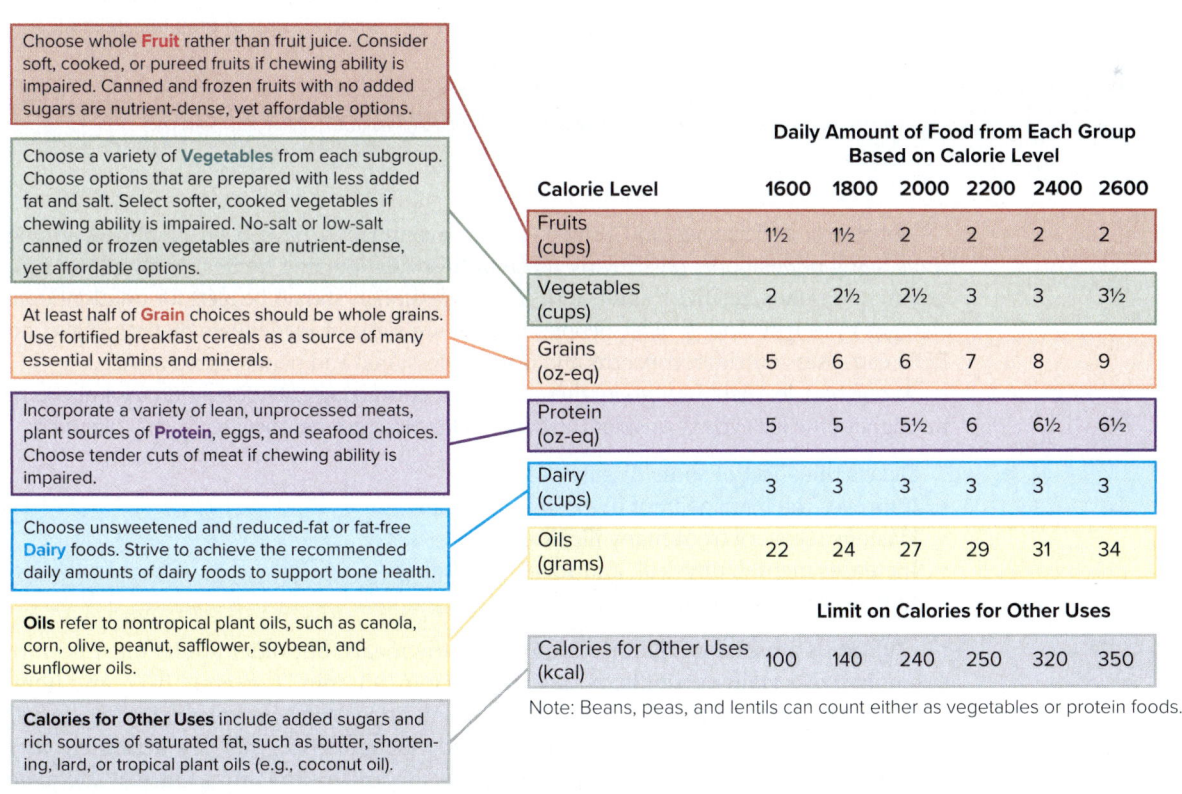

FIGURE 16-9 Healthy U.S.-Style Dietary Patterns for Adults Ages 60 and Older

Source: U.S. Department of Agriculture and U.S. Department of Health and Human Services. *Dietary Guidelines for Americans*, 2020–2025. 9th Edition. Available at DietaryGuidelines.gov

Healthy Eating for Older Adults

Healthy eating is important at every age. Eat a variety of fruits, vegetables, grains, protein foods, and dairy or fortified soy alternatives. When deciding what to eat or drink, choose options that are full of nutrients and limited in added sugars, saturated fat, and sodium. Start with these tips:

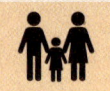
Make eating a social event
Enjoy meals with friends or family members as often as possible. Take advantage of technology to enjoy meals virtually with loved ones in different cities or states.

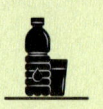
Drink plenty of liquids
You may not always feel thirsty when your body needs fluids, and that's why it's important to drink beverages throughout the day. Enjoy coffee and tea if you like, or some water, milk, or 100% juice.

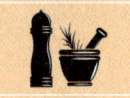
Add a touch of spice
Limiting salt is important as you get older. Fresh and dried herbs and spices, such as basil, oregano, and parsley, add flavor without the salt.

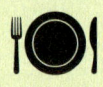
Make the most of your food choices
Older adults need plenty of nutrients but fewer calories, so it's important to make every bite count. Foods that are full of vitamins and minerals are the best way to get what you need.

Be mindful of your nutrient needs
You may not be getting enough nutrients such as calcium, vitamin D, potassium, dietary fiber, vitamin B12, and also protein. Read the **Nutrition Facts Label** on packaged foods and also speak with your healthcare provider about possible supplements.

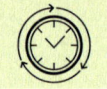
Keep food safe
Discard food if it has an odd odor, flavor, or texture. Refer to the "use by" dates for a guide to freshness. Canned or frozen foods store well when shopping trips are difficult.

FIGURE 16-10 Practical guidance for healthful eating in the later years.
Source: USDA: https://myplate-prod.azureedge.us/sites/default/files/2022-04/TipSheet_21_HealthyEatingForOlderAdults.pdf

Nutritional deficiencies and protein-calorie malnutrition have been identified among some aging populations, particularly those in hospitals, nursing homes, or long-term care facilities.[11] Friends, relatives, and health care professionals should be alert for unintentional changes in weight among older people. If there are signs of inadequate dietary intake, an RDN can assess nutrition concerns and offer professional and personalized advice.

As you have learned throughout these chapters, optimizing nutritional status is important throughout the life cycle. Consider the benefits for older adults, specifically the following:

- Delays the onset of some diseases
- Improves the management of existing diseases
- Hastens recovery from many illnesses
- Increases mental, physical, and social well-being
- Improves quality of life

MyPlate is a useful guide for planning healthy meals, but older adults must be sure to emphasize certain nutrients: potassium, calcium, vitamin D, vitamin B-12, and fiber. MyPlate recommendations for older adults (at https://www.myplate.gov/life-stages/older-adults) illustrates the unique needs and nutrition tips that are accessible and appealing for this population group. This figure also affirms the importance of adequate fluid intake and modified physical activity goals. In some cases, dietary supplementation may be appropriate to address the unique needs of older adults. Discuss this with your primary care provider or dietitian.

Obtaining enough food may be difficult for some older persons, especially if they have a low income, are unable to drive, or do not have social networks that can assist with cooking or shopping. For an older person, a request for help may be equated to a loss of independence. In these cases, family and friends can assist. Special transportation arrangements may also be available through community agencies, local transit companies, or lift services. Indeed, many eligible older people are missing meals and are poorly nourished because they do not realize that programs are available to help them. Irregular meal patterns and weight loss are warning signs that malnutrition may be developing. An effort should be made to identify poorly nourished seniors and inform them of the services available in their communities.

COMMUNITY NUTRITION SERVICES FOR OLDER ADULTS

Health care advice and services for older people can come from clinics, private practitioners, hospitals, and health maintenance organizations. Home health care agencies, adult day care programs, 24-hour-care programs, and **hospice care** (for the terminally ill) also provide daily care for those who qualify.

One in five older adults (about 11 million) are served by the Older Americans Act (OAA).[31] Originally enacted in 1965, the OAA supports a range of home- and community-based services, including Meals on Wheels and other nutrition programs. The OAA nutrition programs serve over 222 million meals each year to approximately 2.4 million U.S. adults over the age of 60. Federal standards mandate that these meals supply at least one-third of adult energy and nutrient requirements.

Some meals, such as Meals on Wheels, are delivered directly to older adults in their homes. Although home-delivered meals can make a valuable contribution to the positive nutritional status of homebound older adults, services are usually limited to one

hospice care A program offering care that emphasizes comfort and dignity at the end of life.

CASE STUDY Dietary Assistance for an Older Adult

Frances is an 82-year-old woman who suffers from macular degeneration, osteoporosis, and arthritis. Since her husband died a year ago, she has moved from their family home to a small one-bedroom apartment. Her eyesight is progressively getting worse, making it difficult to go to the grocery store or even to cook (for fear of burning herself). She is often lonely; her only son lives an hour away and works two jobs, but he visits her as often as he can. Frances has lost her appetite and, as a result, often skips meals during the week. She has resorted to eating mostly cold foods. These are simple to prepare but seriously limit the variety and palatability of her overall intake. Also, she wears dentures and has trouble chewing tough meats and foods with crisp textures. She is slowly losing weight as a result of her eating patterns and loss of appetite.

Her typical dietary intake usually consists of a breakfast that may include 1 slice of wheat toast with margarine, honey, and cinnamon, and 1 cup of hot tea. If she has lunch, she normally has a can of peaches, half of a turkey sandwich, and a glass of water. For dinner, she might have half of a tuna fish sandwich made with mayonnaise and 1 cup of iced tea. She usually includes one or two soft cookies at bedtime.

1. What nutrients are likely to be inadequate in Frances's current dietary pattern?
2. What potential effects might Frances's limited dietary pattern have on her health status?
3. Which physiological changes of aging will add to the effects of her inadequate dietary intake?
4. What services are available in the community that could help Frances improve her dietary pattern?
5. What other convenience foods could be included in her eating pattern to make it more healthful and varied?

Complete the Case Study. Responses to these questions can be provided by your instructor.

Many older adults, like Frances, would benefit from nutritional assessment and counseling. RDNs are the nutrition experts specifically trained to tailor individual recommendations to meet the specific needs of individuals like Frances. Keith Brofsky/Photodisc/Getty Images

or two meals per day. If a recipient has a poor appetite, the food may end up stored for later or simply thrown away. If foods are not eaten immediately upon delivery or not stored properly, risk for foodborne illness could be a concern. Other meals are provided by congregate meal programs, which usually serve lunch at a central location. With congregate meals, the social aspect of eating tends to improve nutritional intake. However, programs generally provide just one meal per day on 5 days per week.

In addition to congregate and home-delivered meals, federal commodity distribution is available in some areas of the United States to low-income older people. Individuals whose incomes are below the poverty level can benefit from the SNAP program. The Senior Farmers Market Nutrition Program provides low-income seniors with coupons that can be exchanged for eligible foods (fruits, vegetables, honey, and fresh-cut herbs) at farmers' markets, roadside stands, and community-supported agriculture programs. Food cooperatives and a variety of clubs and religious and social organizations provide additional aid.

✓ CONCEPT CHECK 16.4

1. Gerald is a 76-year-old male whose wife recently passed away. He now lives alone and is not accustomed to preparing meals for himself. What three recommendations would you give Gerald about eating well?
2. List three nutrition resources for an older adult with limited financial resources.

16.5 Nutrition and Your Health: Lifestyles Linked with Longevity

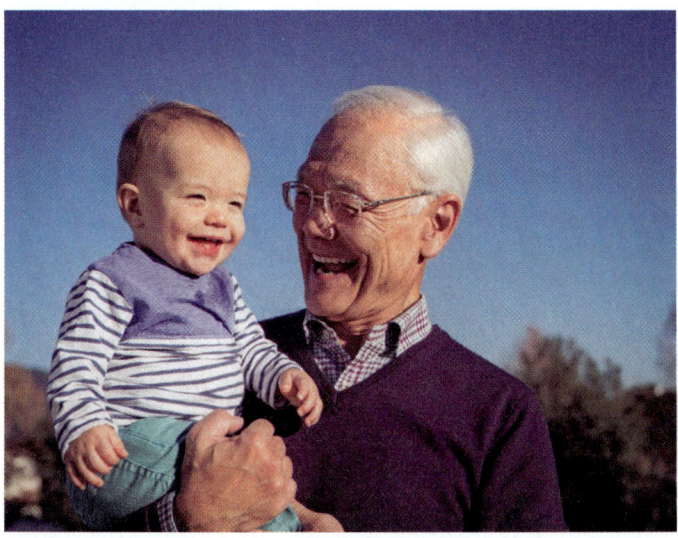
Erik Isakson/Getty Images

However, it would not be desirable to add years to your life without adding life to your years. In other words, we want to know how to extend a healthy life without the burden of chronic diseases. With chronic diseases becoming more and more common in old age, there is increased interest in the behaviors common to people who live exceptionally long lives. Good health and longevity are dependent on numerous factors, including lifestyle and nutrition. Your genetic makeup is also important in determining your lifespan and risk of diseases, but your lifestyle is thought to have an even greater impact.[4]

The Blue Zones

The blue zones are geographic areas whose inhabitants have lived longer and had lower rates of chronic disease than people from other regions of the world. *Blue zones* is a term first used in 2000 by Dan Buettner after leading a *National Geographic* expedition to find the secrets of longevity. The team discovered five regions around the world where people typically live to be over 100 years old.[33,34]

The U.S. Census Bureau indicates that the number of adults in the United States who have reached their 100th birthday grew to over 90,000 in 2020. By 2030, it is estimated that there will be over 130,000 centenarians in the U.S.[32] (Fig. 16-11).

To be considered a certified blue zone, the population lived significantly longer compared to national rates. These populations displayed various behaviors related to their lifestyle, nutrition, genetics, and physical environmental conditions that might be determinants for life quantity and quality. Using epidemiological data, statistics, birth certificates, and other data, five regions on the planet were identified with the highest density of centenarians. These people lived long, healthy, highly active lives and reached age 100 at 10 times greater rates than others in the United States. These regions are described next and in Figure 16-12.[35]

- **Sardinia, Italy:** Some of the oldest men in the world lived in the mountainous Ogliastra region of Sardinia and typically worked on farms and drank one or two glasses of red wine each day.
- **Okinawa, Prefecture of Japan:** The world's oldest females were found in this area, where the dietary pattern was rich in soy-based foods and tai chi, a meditative form of physical activity, was practiced.
- **Ikaria, Greece:** People in this area consumed a Mediterranean diet rich in olive oil, red wine, and homegrown vegetables.
- **Nicoya Peninsula, Costa Rica:** People of this area regularly performed physical jobs into old age. Plant-based foods, such as beans and corn tortillas, formed the base of their dietary pattern.
- **Seventh-day Adventists of Loma Linda, California:** This religious organization followed a strict vegetarian dietary pattern and lived in closely faith-connected communities. In 2020, the Adventist Health system made a commitment to lead the blue zone well-being transformation movement that is the foundation of their 150-year Seventh-day Adventist heritage.

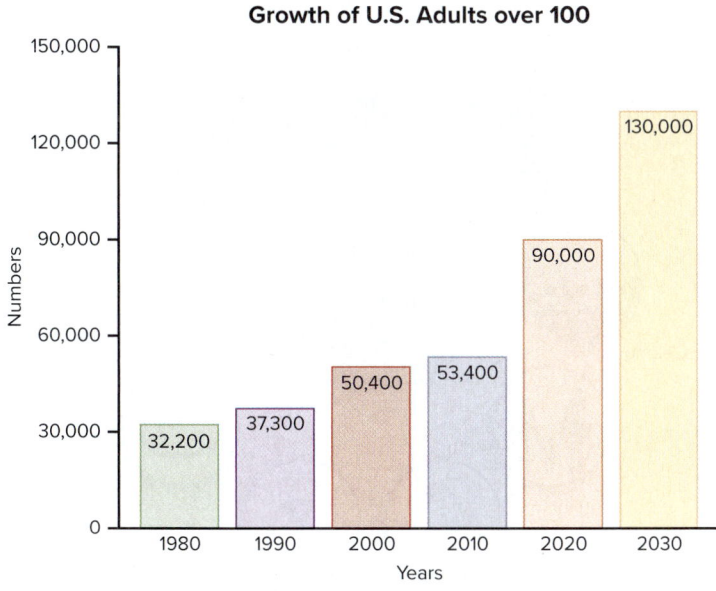

FIGURE 16-11 Estimated growth of U.S. adults living to 100 by the year 2030.
Source: U.S. Census Bureau and Texas A&M.

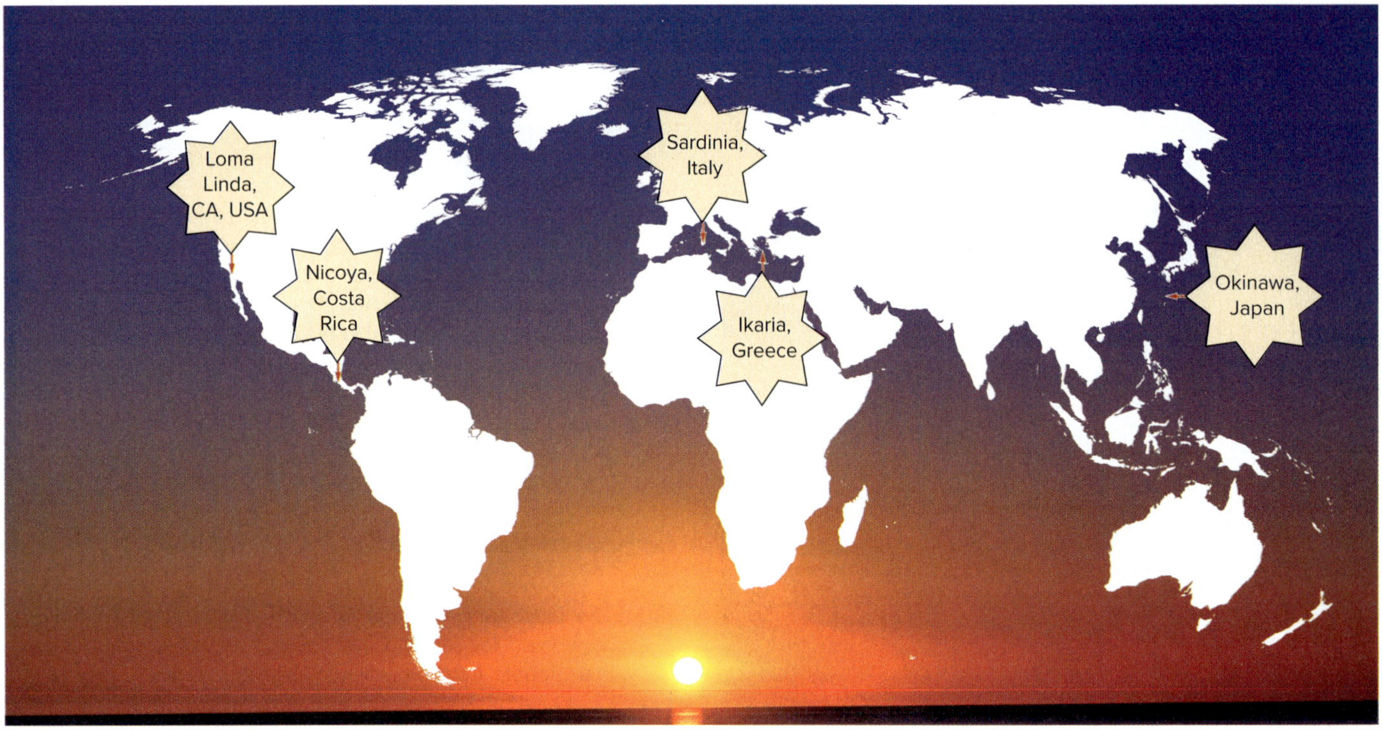

Blue Zone Locations

![Blue Zone world map showing Loma Linda CA USA, Nicoya Costa Rica, Sardinia Italy, Ikaria Greece, and Okinawa Japan]

FIGURE 16-12 World map of the five original blue zone locations.
(1) The Blue Zones, https://blog.insidetracker.com/plan-live-past-100-centenarians; (2) Galyna Andrushko/kamchatka/123RF

There has been recent suggestion that data collected from the blue zones may be misinterpreted or fabricated. Beutner and the Blue Zone team, however, did extensive work to verify age databases, including going to municipal departments and churches in the blue zones to look at birth and baptismal certificates.[36] Buettner does admit that the original blue zones around the world are eroding and predicts that they will all be gone in a generation. He explains that as soon as the standard westernized dietary patterns are accessible in these areas, longevity decreases. Younger people, especially, are not adhering to the eating patterns and lifestyles of the centenarians.[37]

THE POWER 9

In the blue zones, the team of medical researchers, anthropologists, demographers, and epidemiologists found nine evidence-based common lifestyle characteristics called *The Power 9*® (Fig. 16-13). These common denominators are believed to have slowed the aging process among the world's centenarians.

1. **Moving naturally.** In the blue zones, physical activity has been built into daily activities such as gardening, walking, and daily chores completed without mechanical conveniences. A study in the Sardinian blue zone found that the longer life of men was associated with living on steep slopes in the mountains, walking long distances to work, and farming animals.[38] These findings suggest that moderate physical activity, such as walking and climbing stairs, built into daily life improved longevity.
2. **Having a life purpose.** People in the blue zones had a life purpose or a *why I wake up in the morning* philosophy. In Okinawa, it is called *Ikigai* and in Nicoya, it is called *plan de vida*. It is estimated that knowing your sense of purpose added up to 7 years of additional life expectancy.[35] Possessing a high sense of purpose in life was associated with a reduced risk for all-cause mortality and cardiovascular events.[39]

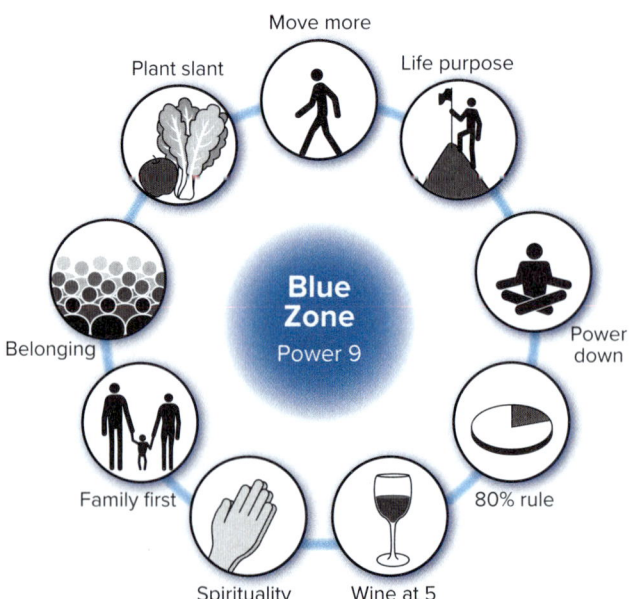

FIGURE 16-13 Lifestyle behaviors shared by individuals of the blue zones who live long lives.

3. **Relieving stress.** Stress impacts longevity by promoting chronic inflammation, associated with every major age-related disease. The world's longest-lived people, however, typically had routines to relieve that stress. For example, Okinawans took time each day to remember their ancestors, Adventists prayed, Ikarians napped, and Sardinians enjoyed a glass of wine. This characteristic is also known as *powering down*.

4. **Fasting and the 80% rule.** Periodic fasting and calorie restriction significantly reduced risk factors for certain diseases and contributed to longer lives in some of the blue zones. For example, fasting for religious holidays throughout the year occured in Ikaria, where residents were typically Greek Orthodox Christians. Okinawans historically maintained a calorie deficit which contributed to their longevity.[40] In Okinawa, a Confucian mantra, the *hara hachi bu,* was recited before meals. This mantra reminded them to stop eating when their stomachs were 80% full.[35] The 20% gap between not being hungry and feeling full prevented the consumption of too many calories.

5. **Consuming alcohol in moderation.** Drinking alcohol moderately and regularly occured in all blue zones except the Loma Linda Adventist population. The evidence was mixed about whether moderate alcohol consumption reduced the risk of death. Whether alcohol consumption was beneficial may depend not only on the amount but also on the type of alcohol consumed. Consumption of one to two glasses of red wine per day was very common in the Ikarian and Sardinian blue zones and seemed to lower the risk of several diseases, including hypertension, heart disease, and type 2 diabetes.[41,42] It made sense that red wine was potentially beneficial because it contains antioxidants. In fact, compared to other wines, extremely high levels of antioxidants were found in Sardinian Cannonau wine made from Grenache grapes.[43] The findings from the blue zones suggested that the key is to drink one to two glasses of red wine per day, with friends and/or with food. This was also known in the blue zones as *wine at 5*.

6. **Being religious or spiritual.** Typically, the blue zones were religious and spiritual communities. All but 5 of the 263 centenarians originally interviewed belonged to a faith-based community. Attending faith-based services four times per month was shown to add 4 to 14 years to life expectancy.[35] This attribute is known as *belonging*. Studies showed that being religious was associated with a lower risk of death, possibly due to social support and reduced rates of depression.[44]

7. **Generations living together.** In many blue zones, younger generations lived together with aging parents and grandparents nearby or in the home. Studies documented that grandparents who care for their grandchildren had a lower risk of death. Grandparents living with their families had also been shown to lower disease and mortality rates of children in the home.[45] Those living in blue zones also typically commited to a life partner, which can added up to 3 years of life expectancy. They invested in their children with time and love, who in turn would be more likely to care for aging parents. This is also known as *loved ones first*.

8. **Choosing a healthy social circle.** Being part of a strong social network, or *right tribe*, that supported healthy behaviors was a common characteristic in the longest living people in the world. Okinawans, for example, created groups of five friends, called *moais*, that commit to each other for life. Research showed that behaviors such as smoking, obesity, happiness, and loneliness were spread person-to-person. If your friends are obese, you have a greater risk of being obese, possibly through social acceptance of weight gain.[46]

9. **Consuming a plant-based dietary pattern.** The blue zone dietary patterns were primarily (95%) plant-based. Legumes, including fava beans, black beans, soy foods, and lentils, were the basis of eating patterns of most centenarians, with fish, eggs, and occasionally dairy making up the remainder. In blue zones, meat (3 to 4 ounces) was eaten on average only five times per month and typically only for celebrations. This dietary pattern was referred to as a *plant slant*.

BLUE ZONE DIETARY PATTERNS

The dietary patterns of the five blue zones differed due to natural variations in culture, history, traditions, and landscape. The nutrients consumed in the regions, however, were quite similar.

The blue zone eating patterns were especially rich in the following:

- *Legumes* including beans, peas, lentils, and chickpeas, which are naturally rich in protein and fiber. A dietary pattern rich in legumes is associated with lower mortality.[47,48]
- *Whole grains* are rich in fiber. Dietary patterns rich in whole grains are linked to a reduction in blood pressure and associated with reduced colorectal cancer and death from heart disease.[49,50,51]
- *Vegetables* are rich sources of vitamins, minerals, and fiber. Consuming more than five servings of fruits and vegetables a day may significantly reduce your risk of death, heart disease, and cancer.[52]
- *Nuts* are great sources of protein, polyunsaturated and monounsaturated fats, and fiber. When part of a healthy dietary pattern, nuts are associated with reduced mortality and can help reverse metabolic syndrome.[53,54,55]

Food sources for each specific blue zone included:[33,34]

- **Sardinia, Italy:** Locally produced wine, sheep's milk, cheese, fennel, fava beans, chickpeas, tomatoes, almonds, and milk thistle tea.
- **Okinawa, Japan:** Bitter melons, tofu, garlic, brown rice, green tea, and shiitake mushrooms.
- **Ikaria, Greece:** Potatoes, goat's milk, honey, beans, wild greens, fruit, feta cheese, lemons, and herbs.
- **Nicoya, Costa Rica:** Beans, corn, squash, tortillas, papayas, yams, bananas, and peach palms.
- **Loma Linda, USA:** Avocados, salmon, nuts, beans, oatmeal, whole wheat bread, and soy milk.

In Sardinia, the current dietary pattern of residents in their 90s included an adequate amount of foods typical of the Mediterranean diet. Some ancient eating behaviors were determined by the local customs of animal farming. The typical intake of locally produced meat and olive oil seemed to be associated with improvement of health indicators, suggesting that a supply of protein, healthy fats, and antioxidants was crucial to maintaining functional capacity among older individuals.[56] The consumption of fish, a good source of omega-3 fats, was also a significant part of the dietary pattern in Sardinia and Ikaria. The consumption of fish was associated with slower brain decline in old age and reduced heart disease.[57,58]

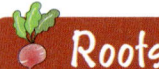

Roots

Bread Intake Across the Blue Zones

Plenty of bread is consumed in the blue zones. Unlike the majority of bread sold in the U.S., which is highly refined, bread in the blue zones are typically homemade from whole grains. The types of breads considered staples in the blue zones and therefore linked to longevity include:

- Sourdough bread, which has prebiotic properties from its fermentation *starter*
- Whole grain breads made from wheat, rye, and barley (popular in Ikaria and Sardinia)
- Pita bread (popular in Ikaria)
- Cornbread, made in Loma Linda with cornmeal and unbleached or spelt flour, flaxseed meal, vegetable oil, soy milk, salt, baking powder, and an unrefined sweetener, like maple syrup

An activity such as baking homemade bread from scratch also employs several of the other Power 9 principles, including reduced stress, an appreciation of food, and gratitude when shared with family and social networks.

Souce: Baum I. The 4 types of bread the longest-living people on the planet eat every day. Well+Good. February 16, 2022. Accessed February 20, 2022. https://www.wellandgood.com/bread-for-longevity/

When it came to meals, centenarians ate *breakfast like a king, lunch like a prince, and dinner like a pauper*. Early in the day, breakfast included protein, complex carbohydrates (beans or vegetables), and plant-based fats (nuts, seeds, oils). Roughly 65% of meals in the blue zones were carbohydrate-based with an emphasis on whole grains, fruits, vegetables, and beans. Lots of fruits and vegetables were eaten at lunch and dinner, with the smallest and last meals of the day eaten in the late afternoon or early evening.

SPREADING OF BLUE ZONE COMMUNITIES®

The blue zone concept started as a way of discovering the healthiest lifestyles that lead to longevity. The founders of Blue Zones® have taken the Power 9® principles into communities across the United States. The *Blue Zones Project*® is designing the healthiest lifestyles possible for individuals and for entire communities. The goal for Blue Zones Project Communities® is to make the healthy choice the easy and unavoidable choice. In Blue Zones Project Communities®, policy makers, local businesses, schools, and individuals work together to transform the environments where people live, work, learn, and play. Through policy and environmental change, these efforts have increased life expectancy, reduced obesity, and made the healthy choice the easier choice for millions of Americans. The changes to the environment are affecting current residents and may impact the lives of future generations.

The first town chosen for the Blue Zones Project® was Albert Lea, Minnesota.[59] With 17,500 residents, Albert Lea transformed in many ways. A 5-mile walking, jogging, and biking route called the *Blue Zones*® *Walkway* was completed around Fountain Lake and connected to another 3.1 miles of sidewalks and trails through neighborhoods, parks, and downtown. Walking groups were formed and served as support groups. These were similar to Okinawa's *moai* concept, which provides physical activity by moving naturally while interacting with the right tribe with a sense of community. Kiosks identifying the *Blue Zones Power 9*® principles will be installed around the walkway.

A *walking school bus* was also created that both parents and children use to walk together to school. This became a popular activity and included older adults volunteering to walk with the walking school bus. This increase in walking programs engaged several factors from the Power 9® principles including greater physical activity by all residents, community spirit, and a sense of purpose for the older adults when helping within their own community. Research also suggests that increasing this type of physical activity in students will have a positive impact on their academic performance.[60]

Grocery stores were also transformed. As part of the transformation, produce was relocated throughout the stores to be at an eye-level and more accessible, sweets at the checkout points were replaced with fruit and nuts, and a specific *Blue Zones*® Checkout Lane was added that offers healthy *grab and go* options.[33,34,59]

Improvements were also made to the school environment, including replacing highly processed chips, cookies, crackers, and carbonated beverages in vending machines with healthier snack options. Farm to school efforts and school gardens were also introduced. By making policy and environmental changes and deepening their social networks to improve their health and well-being, the town of Albert Lea exceeded the expectations of the Blue Zones Project team. Albert Lea residents pledged to begin restocking their own pantries, refrigerators, and freezers with healthier food. Specific positive changes included a 40% reduction in health care costs and 12,000 pounds of weight lost.[33,34,60]

In addition to Albert Lea, Minnesota, other Blue Zone Projects in the U.S. include locations in California (Beach Cities, Lake County, Mendocino County, Tuolumme County, Upper Napa Valley, and Yuba Sutter); Southwest Florida; Hilo and Honolulu, Hawaii; Brevard, North Carolina; Durant and Pottawatomie County, Oklahoma; the State of Oregon; Corry, Pennsylvania; Fort Worth, Texas; and Walla Walla Valley, Washington.[61]

Blue Zones® checklists are available through membership and offer tools to understand your home environment and social network, and provide guidance for improvement.[62] The kitchen checklist recommends the following:[63]

- Placing snacks into small bags
- Moving fruits and vegetables to eye level in your refrigerator
- Reducing the size of plates and glassware
- Creating a specific drawer for junk food to hide them from view
- Removing digital devices, especially televisions, from kitchen and dining room
- Replacing mechanical kitchen appliances with hand-operated ones.
- Placing a longevity food list on your refrigerator.

These recommendations serve as environmental nudges to help you become more conscious of your consumption by eating reasonably sized portions, snacking mindfully, and avoiding distractions while eating.[62]

Food for Thought

If you are looking for the key to a healthy long life, you now know the behaviors of some of the oldest and healthiest people in the world. If you would like to increase your chances of being healthy and physically active into your advanced years (and maybe live to be 100 years old), you may want to follow the Blue Zone Power 9® principles.

If you would like to hear from the team at Blue Zones and test your odds of living to be 100, there is a quiz you can take that addresses how you are doing with regard to the Blue Zone Power 9® principles. It's called the *True Vitality Test* and can be found at apps.bluezones.com/en/vitality/background. After taking the quiz, you will receive advice for making changes to your lifestyle that may add a few years.

✓ CONCEPT CHECK 16.5

1. List the regions of the world where the five blue zones exist and one common food source consumed from each region.
2. Describe the Blue Zone Power 9®.
3. List three community initiatives being implemented to spread the blue zones across the U.S.

16.6 Nutrition and Your Health: Brain Health

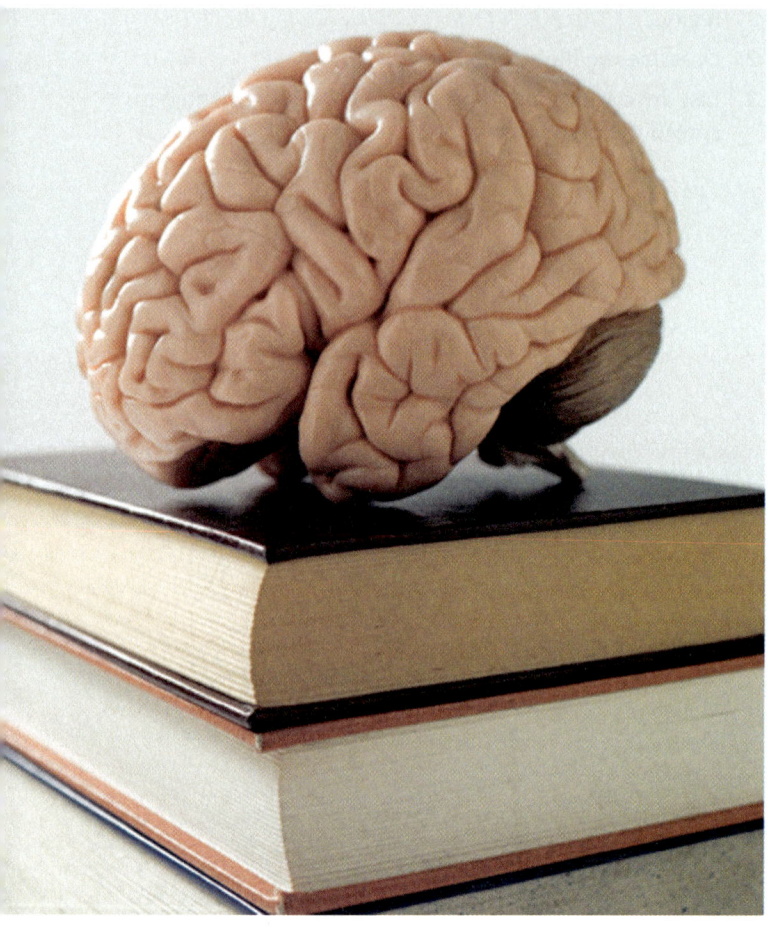

Image Source

The human brain is a metabolically active organ that requires a continual supply of energy—preferably glucose—to meet its energy demands. Even though the average adult brain weighs only 3 pounds (about 2% of body weight), 20% of your blood supply is directed to the brain to supply enough oxygen, glucose, and other nutrients necessary to support proper cognitive function. Indeed, your abilities to speak and understand others, focus on tasks, learn new information, and make decisions, as well as your overall mood, may be significantly impacted by your dietary choices.

So, what does it take to keep your brain's 100 billion neurons alive and functioning optimally? First, let's understand the roles of key nutrients—essential fatty acids, the B vitamins, choline, antioxidant nutrients, and some minerals—in brain function. Then, we'll examine how dietary patterns and other lifestyle choices may influence your risk of developing migraines, depression, and neurodegenerative diseases.

Nutrients That Function in Brain Health

FORMATION OF BRAIN TISSUE

Other than adipose tissue, nervous tissue is the fattiest tissue in the body—the brain is 60% fat by dry weight. Omega-3 and omega-6 fatty acids (including the two essential fatty acids, alpha-linolenic acid and linoleic acid) are used to form phospholipids, which are key players in the formation and maintenance of healthy cell membranes in the brain and nerve cells. Deficiencies of omega-3 or omega-6 fatty acids in the prenatal period or during infancy are detrimental to optimal brain health. Recall that choline is vital for the synthesis of two phospholipids, phosphatidylcholine and sphingomyelin, that are highly concentrated in nervous tissue.

Iodine is a vital nutrient during brain growth and development. Iodine is involved in the synthesis of thyroid hormones, which regulate growth, development, and metabolism. In utero and shortly after birth, iodine participates in the myelination of nerves. Iodine deficiency during early development can result in intellectual disabilities.

Iron is another trace mineral that is vital during brain formation. Iron participates in the pathways that yield energy to fuel the brain, the myelination of nerve tissue, and the formation of neurotransmitters. A deficiency of iron during brain growth and development may result in impaired learning ability and behavioral problems.

FUELING THE BRAIN

The preferred source of fuel for the brain and nervous tissue is glucose, but the brain does not have any way to store appreciable amounts of this carbohydrate. Most of the time, the brain relies on the glucose that is circulating in the blood from your last meal. During times of fasting (e.g., overnight, very-low-carbohydrate diets), glucose can be derived from the breakdown of liver glycogen or the conversion of amino acids to glucose in the liver and kidneys. When the body is in a state of starvation, the brain is able to utilize ketone bodies as a source of fuel. However, ketones are acidic, so high levels of ketones can cause acidosis, which has negative and potentially harmful implications for every body system.

As you learned, the metabolism of glucose for fuel requires many micronutrient cofactors. Thus, deficiencies of thiamin, riboflavin, niacin, pantothenic acid, biotin, iron, magnesium, manganese, and vitamin B-12 can adversely affect brain function.

NERVOUS SYSTEM: COMMUNICATION SUPERHIGHWAY

Communication between the brain and other body tissues occurs via neurons, using a combination of electrical and chemical signals. Recall how sodium and potassium are involved in nerve impulse transmission. Shifts in the concentrations of these electrolyte nutrients across the nerve cell membrane allow for the transmission of an electrical signal along the length of the nerve cell. The speed at which electrical signals move depends on the myelin sheath that surrounds the nerve cell. Thiamin, folate, vitamin B-6, vitamin B-12, and iron are involved in the formation and function of the myelin sheath.

When an electrical signal reaches the end of a nerve cell, the message must be converted into a chemical signal. Neurotransmitters are chemical messengers that are released from nerve cells to transmit a signal to a target cell, such as another nerve cell, an

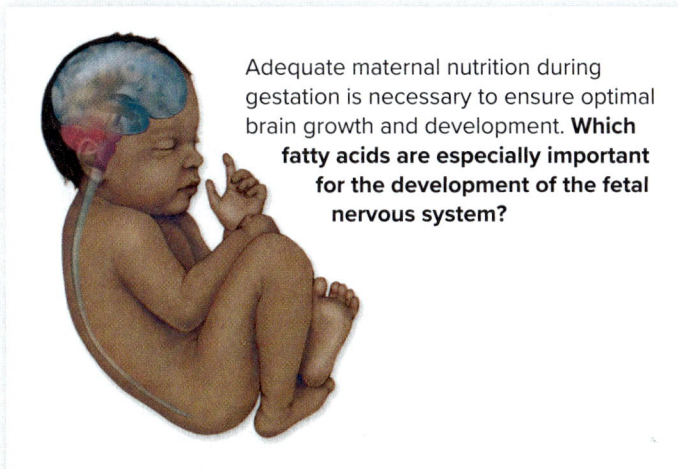

Adequate maternal nutrition during gestation is necessary to ensure optimal brain growth and development. **Which fatty acids are especially important for the development of the fetal nervous system?**

organ, or a gland. **Dopamine, norepinephrine,** and **serotonin** are some examples of neurotransmitters. Amino acids are the building blocks of neurotransmitters. The synthesis and function of these chemical messengers also depends on several B vitamins, including thiamin, riboflavin, niacin, vitamin B-6, folate, and vitamin B-12.

PROTECTING NERVOUS TISSUE

As described, the brain is a metabolically active organ. Energy metabolism naturally generates some damaging free radicals. Recall that free radicals can cause oxidative damage to cell membranes and DNA. With its high concentration of polyunsaturated fatty acids, brain tissue is highly susceptible to the damaging effects of free radicals. Fortunately, the body's antioxidant systems are able to limit this type of cellular damage. An adequate supply of the antioxidant nutrients vitamin C, vitamin E, selenium, and zinc, as well as the phytochemical beta-carotene, help to protect the brain from oxidative damage.

One compound that has been linked to declines in brain health is homocysteine. As you learned, high levels of homocysteine have been identified as a risk factor for poor health outcomes, including heart disease, cancer, stroke, and Alzheimer's disease. Metabolic pathways to convert homocysteine into less harmful amino acids require adequate levels of folate and vitamins B-6 and B-12. Choline may also participate in these metabolic processes.

Evidence clearly shows that in addition to specific dietary choices, the accumulation of excess body fat starting in childhood negatively impacts cognitive function.[64] Insulin resistance appears to be a mediating factor in the relationship between excess body fat and brain health. As you learned in Chapter 7, weight management requires calorie control and physical activity. Independent of body weight, physical activity also improves brain development, cognition, attention, and memory.[65]

dopamine A neurotransmitter involved in memory, concentration, movement, and mood.

norepinephrine A neurotransmitter from nerve endings and a hormone from the adrenal gland. It is released in times of stress and is involved in hunger regulation, blood glucose regulation, and other body processes.

serotonin A neurotransmitter involved in the regulation of mood, sleep, and appetite.

Promoting Brain Health Throughout the Life Cycle

The brain is the body's command center. From brain development in utero until old age, food and lifestyle choices affect brain health. Now that you recognize the importance of nutrients for the growth, development, and function of the nervous system, let us examine how dietary patterns can affect brain health at various stages of the life cycle.

GESTATION AND INFANCY

Gestation and early infancy are critical periods for brain growth and development. Nutrient deficiencies at this stage of the life cycle can profoundly affect neurological health throughout life. At this early phase, it is the biological mother's responsibility to ensure that the developing fetus has optimal nutrients for brain growth and development. Insufficient maternal intakes of folate, vitamin B-12, omega-3 fatty acids, and iron have all been related to reduced cognitive function in offspring.[66] As you saw in Chapter 14, the RDAs for these nutrients increase to as much as 150% for females during pregnancy. A dietary pattern that includes lean meats, plant sources of protein, fatty fish, and fortified breakfast cereals will support proper fetal brain growth and development. While good food sources of these nutrients are important, a female who is pregnant is likely to require a dietary supplement, especially to meet her needs for iron and folic acid.

After birth, breastfeeding is the preferred method to nourish an infant. For brain health, the presence of long-chain polyunsaturated fatty acids (e.g., EPA and DHA) in human milk promotes optimal cognitive development. For a breastfed infant, the adequacy of the mother's dietary pattern will influence the nutrient content of the human milk and impact infant health. However, if breastfeeding is not possible or preferred, iron-fortified infant formula is a safe and healthy alternative. Infant formulas are designed to mimic the nutritional composition of human milk, so most infant formulas contain these fatty acids to promote proper brain development.

CHILDHOOD AND ADOLESCENCE

Throughout childhood and adolescence, iron status is correlated with learning ability and behavior. Children who are deficient in iron experience decreased attention and poor memory, and may display disruptive behavior. In addition, good iron status can help to prevent lead poisoning, which is extremely detrimental to the nervous system. As you learned in Chapter 15, young children are at heightened risk for iron deficiency. Overall intake of iron-rich foods may be insufficient because of low appetite, limited chewing ability, and food selectivity (i.e., picky eating). Caregivers should be sure to offer age-appropriate sources of iron, such as bite-size pieces of lean meat, beans, peas, lentils, and fortified cereals. In addition, they should ensure that excessive intakes of other foods (even nutrient-rich foods, like milk) do not crowd out rich food sources of iron. As children reach puberty, they enter a growth spurt, which increases the demand for iron to build lean tissue and expand blood volume. Adolescent females also require additional iron to compensate for monthly blood loss after menstrual periods begin.

ADULTHOOD

Eating Patterns and Migraines. A migraine is a severe, intense, and recurring throbbing pain affecting one or both sides of the head. Migraines affect about 16% of adults[67] and about 10% of children[68] in the United States and can severely impact quality of life. Depression, anxiety, and sleep disturbances are common for those with chronic migraines. Other potentially debilitating neurological symptoms may include visual disturbances; nausea and vomiting; dizziness; sensitivity to sound, light, touch, and smell; and tingling or numbness in the extremities or face.

Both biologic and lifestyle factors contribute to migraines. Some nonmodifiable risk factors include family history, age, sex, and hormonal changes.[69] Individuals with obesity are at increased risk of migraines, possibly related to higher levels of inflammation.

Dehydration and meal skipping are two often overlooked culprits for migraines. Prolonged fasting can deprive the brain of its go-to fuel source: glucose. Meeting the AI for fluid intake and eating small, frequent meals throughout the day to prevent dehydration and hypoglycemia are simple dietary strategies that may help some people avoid migraines.

There is also a wide range of potential dietary triggers for migraines. The most commonly cited food triggers are aged cheeses, fermented foods, cured meats, alcohol, chocolate, and citrus fruits. These foods contain certain amino acids that may lead to changes in blood flow and neurotransmitter release in the brain.

When it comes to migraines, caffeine is a touchy subject. For some people who ingest caffeine regularly, caffeine withdrawal can precipitate headaches. For others, too much caffeine can trigger symptoms. Most experts recommend that people who have frequent headaches limit caffeine consumption to 200 milligrams (about 2 cups of coffee) per day.

At this time, there is no evidence-based "migraine diet"—individuals vary in their sensitivities to food triggers and, for many people who experience migraines, there may be some underlying pathology that does not involve food at all.[70] Overall, a dietary pattern that complies with the *Dietary Guidelines*—that is, it is high in fruits, vegetables, whole grains, beans, peas, and lentils but low in sodium, solid fats, alcohol, and added sugars—has been linked to fewer complaints of migraines.[71]

Nutrition and Depression. Major depressive disorder affects an estimated 8.4% of adults in the United States.[72] Clinical depression is more than just a *case of the blues*. It is characterized by feelings of sadness, hopelessness, or despair that last for more than 2 weeks and interfere with daily living. Some symptoms of depression include loss of interest in activities that were once enjoyable (e.g., work, hobbies), changes in sleep habits (sleeping either too much or too little), and changes in appetite, which can lead to either weight loss or weight gain.

The causes of depression are varied. Stress, grief, illness, substance abuse, and some medications may certainly lead to depression, but biological changes in the brain are also implicated. For example, people who experience depression may have altered synthesis or activity of hormones (e.g., cortisol) or neurotransmitters (e.g., serotonin).

Does nutrition play a role in the biological basis for depression? Considering the macronutrients, carbohydrates certainly affect mood. Glucose is the brain's primary source of fuel. Nevertheless, studies indicate that dietary patterns high in added sugars may be a risk factor for depression.[73] This may be due to the rapid rises and falls in blood glucose levels that accompany diets high in added sugars. In addition, high sugar intake tends to promote inflammation, which is associated with development of depression. Ensuring an adequate and steady supply of carbohydrates to the brain throughout the day may help to prevent mood swings.

Evidence supports a role of omega-3 fatty acids in the prevention or treatment of depression. The importance of omega-3 fatty acids to brain health is threefold. First, long-chain polyunsaturated fatty acids, particularly DHA, are incorporated into cell membranes throughout the brain. Changes in membrane fluidity may affect how well chemical signals are transmitted by neurotransmitters from nerve cells to target cells. Second, omega-3 fatty acids improve vascular health by reducing the risk of blood clots and atherosclerosis. These changes ensure an adequate blood supply to the brain. Third, omega-3 fatty acids are involved in biochemical pathways that decrease inflammation and are associated with a reduction in depression.[74]

Regarding micronutrients, folic acid, vitamin B-6, and vitamin B-12 are involved in the synthesis and activity of neurotransmitters and have been studied most extensively in relation to depression. Research also suggests that vitamin D and zinc may be particularly important in the prevention or treatment of depressive disorders.

Overall, following a balanced dietary pattern with a slant toward plants, such as the *Dietary Guidelines* or the DASH diet, can benefit the mind as well as the body. Including plenty of fruits, vegetables, and whole grains will supply B vitamins and antioxidant nutrients. Emphasizing healthy sources of fat, such as walnuts, canola oil, flaxseed oil, and fatty fish, will boost levels of omega-3 fatty acids in the body.[75]

Preventing Neurodegenerative Diseases. *Neurodegenerative disease* is a term that encompasses a variety of conditions characterized

---

magnificent *microbiome*

Gut-Brain Axis

For several decades, researchers have been interested in the gut-brain axis. This refers to the communication that occurs along the vagus nerve, transmitting signals back and forth between the central nervous system and the GI tract. Recently, scientists have observed that changes in the gut microbiota may influence brain health. For example, some toxic compounds produced by pathogenic bacteria can be transported via blood and cross the blood–brain barrier. In the brain, these compounds may be promoting inflammation, depression, and neurodegenerative diseases (e.g., Alzheimer's disease and Parkinson's disease). Conversely, metabolic by-products of beneficial gut microbes may be responsible for decreasing inflammation and reducing the risk for these mental health problems. As we learn about the benefits of plant-forward dietary patterns, such as the MIND Diet, let us look beyond how the nutrients nourish our cells and consider how they fuel the microbial cells living within us.

Source: Balan Y, Gaur A, Sakthivadivel V, Kamble B, Sundaramurthy R. Is the gut microbiota a neglected aspect of gut and brain disorders? *Cureus*. 2021 Nov 19;13(11):e19740. doi: 10.7759/cureus.19740

by gradual, progressive deterioration of neurons. Alterations of these cells result in abnormal functioning, plaque formation, and eventual cell death. The most common neurodegenerative diseases in the United States include Alzheimer's disease, Parkinson's disease, and **multiple sclerosis.** In the past, research focused on genetics and aging as the primary risk factors for diseases of the brain. Now, researchers are turning their focus to lifestyle choices, with energy balance and optimal body fatness viewed as very important for optimizing brain health. Research actually links both undernutrition and overnutrition to reduced cognitive function, via mechanisms that involve changes in hormone levels in the body.[66] Compared to adults with a healthy BMI, adults with a BMI in the obese range are three times more likely to suffer impaired cognitive function and dementia.

The most common neurodegenerative disease is Alzheimer's disease, diagnosed in about 6.2 million adults age 65 and older in the United States.[76] It is an irreversible, progressive deterioration of the brain that causes a person to steadily lose the ability to remember, reason, and comprehend. Alzheimer's disease takes a terrible toll on the mental and eventual physical health of people who are older. Scientists have proposed various causes, including alterations in cell development or protein production in the brain, strokes, altered blood lipids, poor blood glucose regulation (e.g., diabetes), high blood pressure, viral infections, and high free radical levels. The 10 warning signs of Alzheimer's disease are listed below.

Ten Warning Signs of Alzheimer's Disease
1. Recent memory loss that affects job performance
2. Difficulty performing familiar tasks
3. Problems with language
4. Faulty or decreased judgment
5. Problems with abstract thinking
6. Tendency to misplace things
7. Changes in mood or behavior
8. Changes in personality
9. Loss of initiative
10. Withdrawal from work or social activities

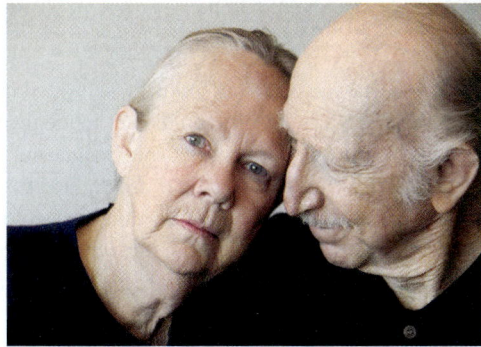

Patients with advanced dementia may be easily distracted during meals, forget to eat, be unable to prepare food safely, and have trouble feeding themselves or swallowing. Caregivers and health care providers need to monitor the patient's weight to ensure maintenance of a healthy weight and nutritional state. CREATISTA/iStock/Getty Images

multiple sclerosis An unpredictable disease of the central nervous system that can range from relatively benign to somewhat disabling to devastating, as communication between the brain and other parts of the body is disrupted.

Early efforts at prevention of Alzheimer's disease should receive the most attention because the process of cognitive decline begins 10 to 20 years before warning signs appear. Preventive measures for Alzheimer's disease focus on engaging in regular physical activity, adhering to a dietary pattern rich in fruits and vegetables, controlling blood pressure, and maintaining brain activity through lifelong learning. Fruits and vegetables provide antioxidant nutrients, such as vitamin C, vitamin E, and selenium, that help to protect the body from the damaging effects of free radicals. In addition, various phytochemicals with antioxidant and anti-inflammatory properties, including polyphenols and carotenoids (e.g., lutein and zeaxanthin), have been shown to protect the brain throughout life.[77] Polyphenols are found in foods such as berries, coffee, green or black tea, and chocolate. Good food sources of lutein and zeaxanthin include green leafy vegetables, yellow-orange fruits and vegetables, and egg yolks.

An elevated blood homocysteine level is a risk factor for neurodegenerative and cardiovascular diseases. Adequate intakes of folate, vitamin B-6, vitamin B-12, and choline are important to decrease the level of homocysteine in the blood. Dietary fats, too, may play a role in keeping Alzheimer's disease at bay. Individuals with dietary patterns rich in omega-3 fatty acids and low in saturated and *trans* fatty acids have a reduced risk of Alzheimer's disease. However, the effects of supplements are not clear.[78] The role of nutrition in preventing or minimizing the risk of this disease continues to be studied.

The MIND Diet is a dietary intervention that shows promising results for protecting the brain against cognitive decline. MIND stands for Mediterranean-DASH Intervention for Neurodegenerative Delay, a hybrid of the nutrient-rich Mediterranean eating pattern with the low-calorie, low-sodium DASH diet. The MIND Diet's 10 *brain-healthy* foods include green leafy vegetables, other vegetables, nuts, berries, beans, whole grains, fish, poultry, olive oil, and wine. The five foods to limit include red meats, butter and stick margarine, cheese, pastries and sweets, and fried or fast food. Each day, followers of the MIND Diet should consume a minimum of three servings of whole grains, a salad plus one other vegetable, and one glass of wine. Nuts, beans, poultry, and berries are recommended regularly, but butter, cheese, and fast food are strictly limited.[79] In population studies, adults who adhered to the MIND Diet had 54% lower rates of Alzheimer's disease. Even more surprising, those that followed the MIND pattern, even periodically, also reduced their risk of the disease by 35%. In 2023, the MIND Diet was ranked among the top five best diets overall in *U.S. News & World Report's* Best Diets Rankings.[80]

Brain Food for Thought. When it comes to studies of individual nutrients and brain health, the results are not that impressive. Recognize, however, that we seldom eat just one nutrient. It is most relevant to examine how overall dietary patterns influence health. Time and time again, we see that dietary patterns rich in fruits, vegetables, beans, peas, lentils, nuts, whole grains, and fish are beneficial for brain health.

Now that you have studied the micronutrients and phytochemicals, you can understand that folate, vitamin B-6, and vitamin B-12 work together to keep homocysteine levels in check. You can describe how vitamins E and C from fruits and vegetables work as antioxidants to prevent damage and decrease inflammation. You understand the importance of polyunsaturated fatty acids in fish oils for brain function. Although a few studies have documented

Newsworthy Nutrition

Mediterranean-style diet linked to reduced Alzheimer's disease

INTRODUCTION: Epidemiological studies estimate that more than 30% of Alzheimer's disease may be attributed to modifiable risk factors and, thus, potentially preventable. A growing body of evidence has linked higher adherence to a Mediterranean-style diet to a lower risk of cognitive decline and dementia. **OBJECTIVE:** To examine the effects of adherence to a Mediterranean diet on biomarkers of Alzheimer's disease in a cohort of adults during their midlife. **METHODS:** Seventy cognitively normal adults, ages 30 to 60 years, were followed over a span of more than 2 years. Based upon food frequency questionnaires, participants were categorized as high or low adherers to a Mediterranean diet. **RESULTS:** At baseline, $\geq$ 90% of the participants reported stability of their eating patterns for $\geq$ 5 years. Of the 70 participants at baseline, 51% were categorized as having low Mediterranean diet adherence and 49% with high adherence. Results showed that higher adherence to the Mediterranean diet was associated with a reduced emergence and progression of Alzheimer's disease. **CONCLUSION:** Higher adherence to a Mediterranean dietary pattern was inversely associated with markers of Alzheimer's disease among middle-aged adults. This study provides support for potential protective effects of a Mediterranean eating pattern in delaying Alzheimer's disease.

Source: Berti V, Walters M, Sterling J, et al. Mediterranean diet and 3-year Alzheimer brain biomarker changes in middle-aged adults. *Neurology*. 2018 May 15;90(20):e1789-e1798. doi: 10.1212/WNL.0000000000005527

that micronutrient supplementation improves mood and psychological well-being, the overall evidence to support use of dietary supplements for brain health remains equivocal. Dietary supplements may seem like a quick fix to fill nutrient gaps to promote optimal brain health, but when we focus on isolated nutrients, we miss out on the synergistic effects of the full complement of brain-healthy nutrients and phytochemicals in whole foods.[81]

✓ CONCEPT CHECK 16.6

1. List four potential triggers for migraines.
2. Name three brain-healthy foods promoted by the MIND Diet.
3. List five early warning signs of Alzheimer's disease.

Summary (Numbers refer to numbered sections in the chapter)

16.1 Although maximum life span has not changed, life expectancy has increased over the past century. For many societies, this means that an increasing proportion of the population is over 65 years of age. As health care costs rise, chronic diseases are a leading concern.

The physiologic changes of aging are the sum of cellular changes, lifestyle behaviors, and environmental influences. Many of these changes can be minimized, prevented, and/or reversed by healthy lifestyles. Usual aging refers to the age-related physical and physiological changes that can be impacted by lifestyle changes. Successful aging describes the declines in physical and physiological function that occur because one grows older. Striving to have the greatest number of healthy years and the fewest years of illness is referred to as compression of morbidity.

16.2 A dietary pattern based on MyPlate and the *Dietary Guidelines* can help one to preserve body function, avoid chronic disease, and age successfully. American adults are fairly well nourished, although common dietary excesses are calories, saturated fat, sodium, and, for some, alcohol. Common dietary inadequacies include vitamins C, D, and E; potassium, folate, magnesium, calcium; zinc; and fiber. The DRIs for adults are divided by sex and age to reflect how nutrient needs change as adults grow older. These changes in nutrient needs take into consideration the aging-related physiological alterations in body composition, metabolism, and organ function. People ages 65 and older, particularly those in long-term care facilities and hospitals, are at risk for malnutrition. How are older adults screened for malnutrition risk?

16.3 Chronic diseases, changes in body composition, and declining function of body systems can influence nutritional status. Of particular concern is sarcopenia, the loss of muscle mass that frequently accompanies aging. Changes in GI tract function can affect nutrient intake and utilization. Some medications and dietary supplements can negatively impact nutritional status. Use of medications and supplements should be guided by a primary care provider.

16.4 Dietary patterns for adults should be based on nutrient-dense foods and need to be individualized for existing health problems, physical abilities, the presence of drug–nutrient interactions, possible depression, and economic constraints. Community nutrition assistance programs, including congregate or home-delivered meal systems, SNAP, and commodity distribution, make wholesome, nutritious foods more accessible for low-income and older adults.

16.5 The blue zones are geographic areas whose inhabitants live longer and have lower rates of chronic disease than people from other regions of the world. These populations display various behaviors related to their lifestyle, nutrition, genetics, and physical environmental conditions that might be determinants for life quantity and quality. In the five blue zones, researchers found nine evidence-based common lifestyles characteristics that they call *The Power 9®*.

16.6 Good nutritional status is essential for proper brain development and function. The brain requires a steady supply of glucose; micronutrient deficiencies adversely affect brain development and function. The key nutrients involved in brain function are the essential fatty acids, B vitamins, choline, antioxidant nutrients, and iron.

Check Your Knowledge (Answers are available at the end of this question set)

1. Among the older population of the United States, the age of the fastest-growing segment is _____ years.
   a. 55 to 65
   b. 65 to 75
   c. 75 to 85
   d. 85+

2. Which of the following accurately portrays a theory about the causes of aging?
   a. Increases in testosterone and estrogen affect cell processes.
   b. Blood sugar decreases, failing to supply adequate energy to brain cells.
   c. Inadequate calorie intake speeds body breakdown.
   d. Excess free radicals damage cell components.

3. Dietary adequacy is influenced by what factor?
   a. Physiological
   b. Psychosocial
   c. Economic
   d. All of the above

4. The immune system becomes less efficient with age, so it is especially important to consume adequate _____ and _____, nutrients that contribute to immune function.
   a. vitamin A, potassium
   b. protein, zinc
   c. zinc, iodine
   d. vitamin A, vitamin K

5. To maintain optimal nutritional status and healthy weight, the dietary pattern of an older person should have a _____ nutrient density and be _____ in energy content.
   a. low, high
   b. low, low
   c. high, moderate
   d. high, high

6. The reason the incidence of obesity increases with aging is that
   a. the basal metabolic rate declines after age 60.
   b. physical activity often decreases with age.
   c. energy intake exceeds energy expenditure.
   d. any of these can occur.

7. Congregate meal programs provide
   a. 100% of nutrient needs.
   b. a social atmosphere for eating.
   c. food stamps.
   d. all of these.

8. One group of centenarians is based in the island nation of Okinawa. They practice a principle called "hara hachi bu." What is the meaning of this term?
   a. Honor and respect the elders in your community.
   b. Stop eating when you are only 80% full.
   c. Rather than planning exercise, incorporate natural movement into each day.
   d. Choose a mostly plant-based diet.

9. Which of the following dietary factors is common among all the blue zone populations?
   a. Avoidance of dairy products
   b. Drinking red wine
   c. Consuming fish daily
   d. Eating a primarily plant-based dietary pattern

10. Each of the blue zones adheres to a vigorous and regimented daily exercise routine.
    a. True
    b. False

11. The preferred energy source for the brain's metabolic activity is
    a. fatty acids.
    b. glucose.
    c. amino acids.
    d. fructose.

12. The MIND Diet is a hybrid of the Mediterranean diet and the
    a. Keto Diet.
    b. Paleo Diet.
    c. DASH Diet.
    d. Diabetes Diet.

Answer Key: 1. d (LO 16.1), 2. d (LO 16.2), 3. d (LO 16.3), 4. b (LO 16.3), 5. c (LO 16.4), 6. d (LO 16.5), 7. b (LO 16.6), 8. b (LO 16.7), 9. d (LO 16.7), 10. b (LO 16.7), 11. b (LO 16.8), 12. c (LO 16.8).

Study Questions (Numbers refer to Learning Outcomes)

1. What is the difference between life span and life expectancy? **(LO 16.1)**
2. Describe two hypotheses proposed to explain the causes of aging, and note evidence for each in your daily life experiences. **(LO 16.2)**
3. List two warning signs of malnutrition in older people. **(LO 16.3)**
4. List four organ systems that can decline in function in later years. Describe the dietary strategies that can help an individual cope with each problem. **(LO 16.3)**
5. List three important points made by the *Dietary Guidelines for Americans* for the general population, and give an example of why each one may be difficult for older adults to implement. What are some suggestions for overcoming these barriers? **(LO 16.4)**
6. Describe two ways the nutritional needs of older people differ from those of younger people. How are their needs similar? Be specific. **(LO 16.4)**
7. Why is it important for older adults to engage in physical activity (especially resistance training)? **(LO 16.5)**
8. List three common herbal remedies. What are the possible benefits and risks of each one? If your grandmother were considering using any of these herbal remedies, what advice would you give her? **(LO 16.5)**
9. What three resources in a community are widely available to aid older adults in maintaining nutritional health? **(LO 16.6)**
10. Describe the blue zone philosophy. What behaviors have these regions adopted to increase their longevity? **(LO 16.7)**
11. Describe at least two ways that nutrients are important for brain development and function. **(LO 16.8)**
12. Identify three key features of a dietary pattern to promote brain health. **(LO 16.8)**

References

1. U.S. Department of Health & Human Services, Administration for Community Living. *2018 Profile of Older Americans.* Accessed December 7, 2023. https://acl.gov/sites/default/files/Aging%20and%20Disability%20in%20America/2018OlderAmericansProfile.pdf
2. NHE fact sheet. Centers for Medicare and Medicaid Service. Accessed December 7, 2023. https://www.cms.gov/Research-Statistics-Data-and-Systems/Statistics-Trends-and-Reports/NationalHealthExpendData/NHE-Fact-Sheet
3. Get the facts on healthy aging. National Council on Aging, Center for Healthy Aging for Professionals. Accessed December 7, 2023. https://www.ncoa.org/article/get-the-facts-on-healthy-aging
4. Passarino G, De Rango F, Montesanto A. Human longevity: genetics or lifestyle? It takes two to tango. *Immun Ageing.* 2016 Apr 5;13:12. https://doi.org/10.1186/s12979-016-0066-z
5. Shephard RJ. Aging and exercise. In: Fahey TD, ed. *Encyclopedia of Sports Medicine and Science.* Internet Society for Sport Science, http://sportsci.org; March 7, 1998.
6. Aging changes in organs, tissues, and cells. U.S. National Library of Medicine, MedlinePlus. Accessed December 7, 2023. https://medlineplus.gov/ency/article/004012.htm
7. Kochanek KD, Anderson RN, Arias E. Changes in life expectancy at birth, 2010–2018. *Health E-Stats.* Accessed December 7, 2023. https://www.cdc.gov/nchs/data/hestat/life-expectancy/life-expectancy-2018.htm
8. Is longevity determined by genetics? U.S. National Library of Medicine, MedlinePlus. Accessed December 7, 2023. https://ghr.nlm.nih.gov/primer/traits/longevity
9. Bernstein M, Munoz N; Academy of Nutrition and Dietetics. Position of the Academy of Nutrition and Dietetics: food and nutrition for older adults: promoting health and wellness. *J Acad Nutr Diet.* 2012 Aug;112(8):1255-1277. doi: 10.1016/j.jand.2012.06.015
10. Thalheimer JC. Nutrition and healthy aging for men. *Today's Dietitian.* 2015 Jun;17(6):44.
11. Fávaro-Moreira NC, Krausch-Hofmann S, Matthys C, et al. Risk factors for malnutrition in older adults: a systematic review of the literature based on longitudinal data. *Adv Nutr.* 2016 May 16;7(3):507-522. doi: 10.3945/an.115.011254
12. Skipper A, Coltman A, Tomesko J, et al. Position of the Academy of Nutrition and Dietetics: malnutrition (undernutrition) screening tools for all adults. *J Acad Nutr Diet.* 2020 Apr;120(4):709-713. doi: 10.1016/j.jand.2019.09.011
13. The RD toolkit: Malnutrition Screening Tool (MST). Abbott Laboratories. Accessed December 1, 2023. https://abbottnutrition.com/tools-for-patient-care/rd-toolkit
14. Pontzer H, Yamada Y, Sagayama H, et al.; IAEA DLW Database Consortium. Daily energy expenditure through the human life course. *Science.* 2021 Aug 13;373(6556):808-812. doi: 10.1126/science.abe5017
15. Deutz NEP, Bauer JM, Barazzoni R, et al. Protein intake and exercise for optimal muscle function with aging: recommendations from the ESPEN Expert Group. *Clin Nutr.* 2014 Dec;33(6):929-936. doi: 10.1016/j.clnu.2014.04.007
16. Paddon-Jones D, Campbell WW, Jacques PF, et al. Protein and healthy aging. *Am J Clin Nutr.* 2015 Jun;101(6):1339S-1345S. doi: 10.3945/ajcn.114.084061
17. U.S. Department of Agriculture, Agricultural Research Service. *What We Eat in America.* NHANES 2015-2018. Table A. Usual nutrient intake from food and beverages, by gender and age. Accessed December 7, 2023. https://www.ars.usda.gov/ARSUserFiles/80400530/pdf/usual/Usual_Intake_gender_WWEIA_2015_2018.pdf
18. Higdon J; updated by Drake VJ, Delage B, Johnson EJ. Carotenoids. Linus Pauling Institute. Accessed December 8, 2023. https://lpi.oregonstate.edu/mic/dietary-factors/phytochemicals/carotenoids
19. Marra MV, Bailey RL. Position of the Academy of Nutrition and Dietetics: micronutrient supplementation [published correction appears in *J Acad Nutr Diet.* 2019 Feb;119(2):344]. *J Acad Nutr Diet.* 2018;118(11):2162-2173. doi:10.1016/j.jand.2018.07.022

20. Buch A, Carmeli E, Boker LK, et al. Muscle function and fat content in relation to sarcopenia, obesity and frailty of old age—an overview. *Exp Gerontol*. 2016 Apr;76:25-32. doi: 10.1016/j.exger.2016.01.008

21. Arthritis. Centers for Disease Control and Prevention, National Center for Chronic Disease Prevention and Health Promotion (NCCDPHP). Accessed December 8, 2023. https://www.cdc.gov/chronicdisease/resources/publications/factsheets/arthritis.htm

22. Oliviero F, Spinella P, Fiocco U, Ramonda R, Sfriso P, Punzi L. How the Mediterranean diet and some of its components modulate inflammatory pathways in arthritis. *Swiss Med Wkly*. 2015 Nov 2;145:w14190. doi: 10.4414/smw.2015.14190

23. Tooth loss in seniors. National Institutes of Health, National Institute of Dental and Craniofacial Research. Accessed December 8, 2023. https://www.nidcr.nih.gov/research/data-statistics/tooth-loss/seniors

24. Touger-Decker R, Mobley C; Academy of Nutrition and Dietetics. Position of the Academy of Nutrition and Dietetics: oral health and nutrition. *J Acad Nutr Diet*. 2013 May;113(5):693-701. doi: 10.1016/j.jand.2013.03.001

25. Scarlata K. Digestive wellness: the link between aging and digestive disorders. *Today's Dietitian*. 2015 July;17(7):12.

26. Eye health data and statistics. National Institutes of Health, National Eye Institute. Accessed December 8, 2023. https://www.nei.nih.gov/learn-about-eye-health/eye-health-data-and-statistics

27. Piazza G. How diet may affect age-related macular degeneration. National Institutes of Health, NIH Research Matters. Accessed December 8, 2023. https://www.nih.gov/news-events/nih-research-matters/how-diet-may-affect-age-related-macular-degeneration

28. Chronic diseases in America. Centers for Disease Control and Prevention, National Center for Chronic Disease Prevention and Health Promotion (NCCDPHP). Accessed December 8, 2023. https://www.cdc.gov/chronicdisease/resources/infographic/chronic-diseases.htm

29. Health, United States, 1018—data finder. Centers for Disease Control and Prevention, National Center for Health Statistics. Table 038. Prescription drug use in the past 30 days, by sex, race and Hispanic origin, and age: United States, selected years 1988–1994 through 2013–2016. Accessed December 8, 2023. https://www.cdc.gov/nchs/hus/contents2018.htm#Table_038

30. Gahche JJ, Bailey RL, Potischman N, Dwyer JT. Dietary supplement use was very high among older adults in the United States in 2011–2014. *J Nutr*. 2017 Oct;147(10):1968-1976. doi: 10.3945/jn.117.255984

31. Bunis D. House approves update of landmark Older Americans Act. AARP. Accessed December 8, 2023. https://www.aarp.org/politics-society/government-elections/info-2019/house-older-americans-act-funding.html

32. Singelmann J, Poston DL Jr, eds. *Developments in Demography in the 21st Century*. Springer; 2020. Demographic Methods and Population Analysis; vol. 48.

33. Buettner D. *The Blue Zones Solution: Eating and Living Like the World's Healthiest People*. Washington, DC: National Geographic Society; 2015.

34. History of Blue Zones. Blue Zones. Accessed December 20, 2023. https://www.bluezones.com/about/history/

35. Buettner D, Skemp S. Blue Zones: lessons from the world's longest lived. *Am J Lifestyle Med*. 2016 Jul 7;10(5):318-321. doi: 10.1177/1559827616637066.

36. Are supercentenarian claims based on age exaggeration? Blue Zones. Accessed December 11, 2023. Available at https://www.bluezones.com/news/are-supercentenarian-claims-based-on-age-exaggeration/

37. Finkelstein P. "Blue zones" have captivated health and longevity experts. But are they real or statistical grift? *Salon*. 2023 Oct 1. https://www.salon.com/2023/10/01/blue-zones-have-captivated-health-and-longevity-experts-but-are-they-real-or-statistical-grift/

38. Pes GM, Tolu F, Poulain M, et al. Lifestyle and nutrition related to male longevity in Sardinia: an ecological study. *Nutr Metab Cardiovasc Dis*. 2013 Mar;23(e):212-219. doi: 10.1016/j.numecd.2011.05.004

39. Cohen R, Bavishi C, Rozanski A. Purpose in life and its relationship to all-cause mortality and cardiovascular events: a meta-analysis. *Psychosom Med*. Feb-Mar 2016;78(2):122-133. doi: 10.1097/PSY.0000000000000274

40. Willcox BJ, Willcox DC, Todoriki H, et al. Caloric restriction, the traditional Okinawan diet, and healthy aging: the diet of the world's longest-lived people and its potential impact on morbidity and life span. *Ann N Y Acad Sci*. 2007 Oct;1114:434-455. doi: 10.1196/annals.1396.037

41. Gepner Y, Golan R, Harman-Boehm I, et al. Effects of initiating moderate alcohol intake on cardiometabolic risk in adults with type 2 diabetes: a 2-year randomized, controlled trial. *Ann Intern Med*. 2015 Oct;163(8):569-579. doi: 10.7326/M14-1650

42. Gepner Y, Henkin Y, Schwarzfuchs D, et al. Differential effect of initiating moderate red wine consumption on 24-h blood pressure by alcohol dehydrogenase genotypes: randomized trial in type 2 diabetes. *Am J Hypertens*. 2016 Apr;29(4):476-483. doi: 10.1093/ajh/hpv126

43. Tuberoso CIG, Boban M, Bifulco E, Budimir D, Pirisi FM. Antioxidant capacity and vasodilatory properties of Mediterranean food: the case of Cannonau wine, myrtle berries liqueur and strawberry-tree honey. *Food Chem*. 2013 Oct 15;140(4):686-691. doi: 10.1016/j.foodchem.2012.09.071

44. Li S, Stampfer MJ, Williams DR, VanderWeele TJ. Association of religious service attendance with mortality among women. *JAMA Intern Med*. 2016 Jun 1;176(6):777-785. doi: 10.1001/jamainternmed.2016.1615

45. Hilbrand S, Coall DA, Gerstorf D, Hertwig R. Caregiving within and beyond the family is associated with lower mortality for the caregiver: a prospective study. *Evol Hum Behav*. 2017 May;38(3):397-403. doi: 10.1016/j.evolhumbehav.2016.11.010

46. Christakis NA, Fowler JH. The spread of obesity in a large social network over 32 years. *N Engl J Med*. 2007 Jul 26;357(4):370-379. doi: 10.1056/NEJMsa066082

47. Darmadi-Blackberry I, Wahlqvist ML, Kouris-Blazos A, st al. Legumes: the most important dietary predictor of survival in older people of different ethnicities. *Asia Pac J Clin Nutr*. 2004;13(2):217-220. PMID: 15228991

48. Nöthlings U, Schulze MB, Weikert C, et al. Intake of vegetables, legumes, and fruit, and risk for all-cause, cardiovascular, and cancer mortality in a European diabetic population. *J Nutr*. 2008 Apr;138(4):775-781. doi: 10.1093/jn/138.4.775

49. Streppel MT, Arends LR, van 't Veer P, Grobbee DE, Geleijnse JM. Dietary fiber and blood pressure: a meta-analysis of randomized placebo-controlled trials. *Arch Intern Med*. 2005 Jan 24;165(2):150-156. doi: 10.1001/archinte.165.2.150

50. Zong G, Gao A, Hu FB, Sun Q. Whole grain intake and mortality from all causes, cardiovascular disease, and cancer: a meta-analysis of prospective cohort studies. *Circulation*. 2016 Jun 14;133(24):2370-2380. doi: 10.1161/CIRCULATIONAHA.115.021101

51. Aune D, Chan DSM, Lau R, et al. Dietary fibre, whole grains, and risk of colorectal cancer: systematic review and dose-response meta-analysis of prospective studies. *BMJ*. 2011 Nov 10;343:d6617. doi: 10.1136/bmj.d6617

52. Wang X, Ouyang Y, Liu J, et al. Fruit and vegetable consumption and mortality from all causes, cardiovascular disease, and cancer: systematic review and dose-response meta-analysis of prospective cohort studies. *BMJ*. 2014 Jul 29;349:g4490. doi: 10.1136/bmj.g4490

53. Luu HN, Blot WJ, Xiang Y-B, et al. Prospective evaluation of the association of nut/peanut consumption with total and cause-specific mortality. *JAMA Intern Med*. 2015 May;175(5):755-766. doi: 10.1001/jamainternmed.2014.8347

54. Luo C, Zhang Y, Ding Y, et al. Nut consumption and risk of type 2 diabetes, cardiovascular disease, and all-cause mortality: a systematic review

54. and meta-analysis. *Am J Clin Nutr.* 2014 July;100(1):256-269. doi: 10.3945/ajcn.113.076109

55. Salas-Salvadó J, Fernández-Ballart J, Ros E, et al. Effect of a Mediterranean diet supplemented with nuts on metabolic syndrome status: one-year results of the PREDIMED randomized trial. *Arch Intern Med.* 2008 Dec 8;168(22):2449-2458. doi: 10.1001/archinte.168.22.2449

56. Pes GM, Poulain M, Errigo A, Dore MP. Evolution of the dietary patterns across nutrition transition in the Sardinian Longevity Blue Zone and association with health indicators in the oldest old. *Nutrients.* 2021 Apr 25;13(5):1495. doi: 10.3390/nu13051495

57. Fotuhi M, Mohassel P, Yaffe K. Fish consumption, long-chain omega-3 fatty acids and risk of cognitive decline or Alzheimer disease: a complex association. *Nat Clin Pract Neurol.* 2009 Mar;5(3):140-152. doi: 10.1038/ncpneuro1044

58. Chowdhury R, Stevens S, Gorman D, et al. Association between fish consumption, long chain omega 3 fatty acids, and risk of cerebrovascular disease: systematic review and meta-analysis. *BMJ.* 2012 Oct 30;345:e6698. doi: 10.1136/bmj.e6698

59. Riddell, B. *Blue Zones: Rethinking the American Landscape.* Thesis: Georgia Institute of Technology, College of Architecture, School of City and Regional Planning. Accessed November 22, 2023. https://smartech.gatech.edu/bitstream/handle/1853/55168/briana_riddell_blue_zones_rethinking_the_american_landscape.pdf

60. Srikanth S, Petrie TA, Greenleaf C, Martin SB. The relationship of physical fitness, self-beliefs, and social support to the academic performance of middle school boys and girls. *J Early Adolesc.* 2015 Apr;35(3):353-377. doi: 10.1177/0272431614530807

61. The Blue Zones Project. Accessed November 21, 2023. https://info.bluezonesproject.com/home

62. Marston HR, Niles-Yokum K, Silva PA. A commentary on Blue Zones®: a critical review of age-friendly environments in the 21st century and beyond. *Int J Environ Res Public Health.* 2021 Jan 19;18(2):837. doi: 10.3390/ijerph18020837

63. Blue Zones checklists: kitchen. Accessed November 20, 2023. https://www.bluezones.com/live-longer-better/checklists/kitchen/

64. Khan NA, Raine LB, Donovan SM, Hillman CH. IV. The cognitive implications of obesity and nutrition in childhood. *Monogr Soc Res Child Dev.* 2014 Dec;79(4):51-71. doi: 10.1111/mono.12130

65. Meeusen R. Exercise, nutrition and the brain. *Sports Med.* 2014 May;44 Suppl 1(Suppl 1):S47-S56. doi: 10.1007/s40279-014-0150-5

66. Dauncey MJ. Nutrition, the brain and cognitive decline: insights from epigenetics. *Eur J Clin Nutr.* 2014 Nov;68(11):1179-1185. doi: 10.1038/ejcn.2014.173

67. Burch R, Rizzoli P, Loder E. The prevalence and impact of migraine and severe headache in the United States: updated age, sex, and socioeconomic-specific estimates from government health surveys. *Headache.* 2021 Jan;61(1):60-68. doi: 10.1111/head.14024

68. Migraine in children. American Migraine Foundation. Published April 8, 2021. Accessed February 22, 2022. https://americanmigrainefoundation.org/resource-library/migraine-children/

69. Andrews L. Integrative nutrition: nutrition for headaches and migraines. *Today's Dietitian.* Nov/Dec 2021;23(9):16.

70. Slavin M, Ailani J. A clinical approach to addressing diet with migraine patients. *Curr Neurol Neurosci Rep.* 2017 Feb;17(2):17. doi: 10.1007/s11910-017-0721-6

71. Evans EW, Lipton RB, Peterlin BL, et al. Dietary intake patterns and diet quality in a nationally representative sample of women with and without severe headache or migraine. *Headache.* 2015 Apr;55(4):550-561. doi: 10.1111/head.12527

72. Major depression. National Institutes of Health, National Institute of Mental Health. Updated January 2022. Accessed February 22, 2022. https://www.nimh.nih.gov/health/statistics/major-depression

73. Gangwisch JE, Hale L, Garcia L, et al. High glycemic index diet as a risk factor for depression: analyses from the Women's Health Initiative. *Am J Clin Nutr.* 2015 Aug;102(2):454-463. doi: 10.3945/ajcn.114.103846

74. Lassale C, Batty GD, Baghdadli A, et al. Healthy dietary indices and risk of depressive outcomes: a systematic review and meta-analysis of observational studies [published correction appears in *Mol Psychiatry.* 2019 Jul;24(7):1094.] [published correction appears in *Mol Psychiatry.* 2021 Jul;26(7):3657]. *Mol Psychiatry.* 2019 Jul;24(7):965-986. doi: 10.1038/s41380-018-0237-8

75. Ljungberg T, Bondza E, Lethin C. Evidence of the importance of dietary habits regarding depressive symptoms and depression. *Int J Environ Res Public Health.* 2020 Mar 2;17(5):1616. doi: 10.3390/ijerph17051616

76. Alzheimer's disease facts and figures. *Alzheimers Dement.* 2021 Mar;17(3):327-406. doi: 10.1002/alz.12328

77. Johnson EJ. Role of lutein and zeaxanthin in visual and cognitive function throughout the lifespan. *Nutr Rev.* 2014 Sep;72(9):605-612. doi: 10.1111/nure.12133

78. Rutjes AW, Denton DA, Di Nisio M, et al. Vitamin and mineral supplementation for maintaining cognitive function in cognitively healthy people in mid and late life. *Cochrane Database Syst Rev.* 2018 Dec 17;12(12):CD011906. doi: 10.1002/14651858.CD011906.pub2

79. Ellis E. Food for thought: can diet prevent Alzheimer's disease? *Food & Nutrition.* Published November 6, 2018. Accessed February 15, 2022. https://foodandnutrition.org/from-the-magazine/food-for-thought-can-diet-prevent-alzheimers-disease/

80. Best diets overall 2023. *U.S. News & World Report.* Accessed November 15, 2023. https://health.usnews.com/best-diet/best-diets-overall

81. Barberger-Gateau P. Nutrition and brain aging: how can we move ahead? *Eur J Clin Nutr.* 2014 Nov;68(11):1245-1249. doi: 10.1038/ejcn.2014.177

Design Element Credits: Fact Check/magnifying glass icon: McGraw Hill; Magnificent Microbiome background image: Alena Ohneva/Shutterstock; Sustainable Solutions icon: McGraw Hill; Roots icon: McGraw Hill; Medicine Cabinet icon: Peter Dazeley/Photographer's Choice/Getty Images

Appendix A
Daily Values Used on Food Labels

TABLE A-1 ■ Daily Values Used on Food Labels in the United States, with a Comparison to the Latest RDAs and Other Nutrient Standards*

Dietary Constituent	Unit of Measure	Current Daily Values for People Over 4 Years of Age	RDA or Other Current Dietary Standard Males 19–30 Years Old	RDA or Other Current Dietary Standard Females 19–30 Years Old
Added sugars	grams (g)	50	—	—
Biotin	micrograms (mcg)	30	30	30
Calcium	milligrams (mg)	1300	1000	1000
Carbohydrate[†]	grams (g)	275	130	130
Chloride[‡]	milligrams (mg)	2300	2300	2300
Cholesterol[§]	milligrams (mg)	300	—	—
Choline	milligrams (mg)	550	550	425
Chromium	micrograms (mcg)	35	35	25
Copper	milligrams (mg)	0.9	0.9	0.9
Dietary fiber	grams (g)	28	38	25
Folate	micrograms (mcg) Dietary Folate Equivalents (DFE)	400	400	400
Iodine	micrograms (mcg)	150	150	150
Iron	milligrams (mg)	18	8	18
Magnesium	milligrams (mg)	420	400	310
Manganese	milligrams (mg)	2.3	2.3	1.8
Molybdenum	micrograms (mcg)	45	45	45
Niacin	milligrams (mg)	16	16	14
Pantothenic acid	milligrams (mg)	5	5	5
Phosphorus	milligrams (mg)	1250	700	700
Potassium[‡]	milligrams (mg)	4700	3400	2600
Protein[†]	grams (g)	50	56	46
Riboflavin	milligrams (mg)	1.3	1.3	1.1
Saturated fatty acids[†]	grams (g)	20	—	—
Selenium	micrograms (mcg)	55	55	55
Sodium[‡]	milligrams (mg)	2300	1500	1500
Thiamin	milligrams (mg)	1.2	1.2	1.1
Total fat[†]	grams (g)	78	—	—
Vitamin A	micrograms (mcg) Retinol Activity Equivalents (RAE)	900	900	700
Vitamin B-6	milligrams (mg)	1.7	1.3	1.3
Vitamin B-12	micrograms (mcg)	2.4	2.4	2.4
Vitamin C	milligrams (mg)	90	90	75
Vitamin D	micrograms (mcg)	20	15	15
Vitamin E	milligrams (mg) alpha tocopherol	15	15	15
Vitamin K	micrograms (mcg)	120	120	90
Zinc	milligrams (mg)	11	11	8

* Daily Values are generally set at the highest nutrient recommendation in a specific age and gender category. Some changes were made in 2016 to the Daily Values and their units as part of the new Nutrition Facts label. Most changes occurred because of the dietary-related diseases that are common in the United States and to more closely match the RDA or AI values for the nutrient.

[†] These Daily Values are based on a 2000 kcal diet, instead of RDAs, with a caloric distribution of 30% from fat (and one-third of this total from saturated fat), 60% from carbohydrate, and 10% from protein.

[‡] The considerably higher Daily Value for sodium is there to allow for more diet flexibility, but the extra amount is not needed to maintain health.

[§] Based on recommendations of U.S. federal agencies.

Appendix B
Diabetes Menu-Planning Tools

The Diabetes Plate, Carb Counting, Food Lists, and Healthy Lifestyles: Dietary Recommendations for Individuals Living with Diabetes

Registered dietitian nutritionists and other diabetes educators work closely with their clients to help them understand how the foods they eat directly impact their day-to-day quality of life. Providing tools, such as the Diabetes Plate, **carbohydrate counting,** and diabetes food lists promote individual choices to help people plan dietary patterns to better manage their blood sugar.

carbohydrate counting Also known as *carb counting*, this process involves counting the number of grams of carbohydrate in a meal and matching it to a prescribed dose of insulin.

DIABETES PLATE

The American Diabetes Association's *Diabetes Plate Method* is a quick and easy way to create healthy meals to help manage blood sugar. Using this method, you can enjoy a healthy dietary pattern without counting, calculating, weighing, or measuring!

This meal represents the diabetes plate method. Half the plate is full of nonstarchy vegetables. About one-fourth of the plate consists of a lean source of protein. Buckwheat, a whole grain, covers one-fourth of the plate supplying grains.

Steps to adopting the Diabetes Plate Method:

1. *Fill half your plate with nonstarchy vegetables*. These include asparagus, broccoli, cabbage, carrots, cucumbers, eggplant, leafy greens, mushrooms, green beans, peppers, and tomatoes.
2. *Fill one quarter of your plate with lean protein foods*. Focus on plant-based protein sources like beans, lentils, nuts, edamame, tofu, and plant-based meat substitutes. If you prefer animal sources of protein, select chicken, turkey, eggs, fish, lean beef, lean pork, cheese, and cottage cheese.
3. *Fill one quarter of your plate with carbohydrate foods*. These include whole grains (like brown rice, oats), starchy vegetables (such as green peas, potatoes, plantains), beans and legumes (like garbanzo, black, kidney, pinto), fruits and dried fruits, and dairy products (such as milk, yogurt, and milk substitutes).
4. *Select water or low-calorie beverages*. Water is the best choice. Other options may include unsweetened tea and coffee, sparkling water or club soda, unsweetened flavored water, and diet soda pop or other diet drinks.

Note that some meals, such as combination meals, do not fit neatly into the diabetes plate. For example, in one slice of a pizza, the crust would count as the carbohydrate food, the cheese and any meat toppings would be the protein foods, and the pizza sauce and vegetable toppings would count as nonstarchy vegetables.

costmo/123RF

CARBOHYDATE (CARB) COUNTING

Recall that carbohydrates are one of the main macronutrients naturally found in a typical dietary pattern (Fig. 4-7). Carbohydrates are broken down into glucose (sugar) in the body, which is then used as a source of energy. Carbohydrates are found in various food sources, including grains, fruits, vegetables, dairy products, and sweets.

The American Diabetes Association (ADA) recommends carbohydrate (or *carb*) counting for people with type 1 diabetes on intensive insulin therapy to improve overall glycemic control. Other individuals with diabetes may benefit from counting carbs to maintain close control of their blood sugar levels throughout the day.

The *Beginner's Guide to Carbohydrate Counting* provides in-depth details on carb counting. In summary, carb counting involves:

1. Identifying and tracking the amount (in grams) of carbohydrates in the foods you eat. This includes reading food labels to determine the total grams of carbohydrates per serving.
2. Setting a carbohydrate goal with your health care team to determine a target daily carbohydrate intake. This goal is based on factors such as age, weight, activity level, and individual insulin sensitivity.
3. Balancing your doses of insulin or other medications to avoid episodes of hyperglycemia or hypoglycemia. For example, rapid-acting insulin doses can be adjusted based on anticipated carbohydrate intake. This helps to maintain stable blood sugar levels.
4. Regular monitoring of your blood glucose levels. Adjustments should be made to the meal plan or medication as needed.

Indeed, carb counting can be a flexible and effective approach to diabetes management, allowing individuals to have better control over their blood sugar levels while still enjoying a variety of foods. The ADA does caution that when consuming a mixed meal that contains carbohydrate or is high in fat and/or protein, insulin dosing should not be based solely on carb counting.[1] Because carb counting can be complex, it is critical that individuals initially work closely with their health care team, including dietitians and diabetes educators, to develop a personalized carb counting plan that meets an individual's specific needs.

FOOD LISTS

Food lists organize the many details of the nutrient composition of foods into a manageable framework based on calorie and macronutrient content. In the *Food Lists for Diabetes*, individual foods are placed into three broad groups: carbohydrates, proteins, and fats. Within these groups are lists that contain foods of similar macronutrient composition: various types of milk and milk substitutes, fruits, vegetables, starches, other carbohydrates, proteins, and fats. There are even lists that show how to account for alcohol, combination foods (e.g., casseroles), and a wide variety of fast foods. These lists are designed so that when the given serving size is observed, each food on a list provides roughly the same amount of carbohydrate, protein, fat, and calories. The patient and a registered dietitian nutritionist first tailor a healthy eating pattern to meet the client's energy and specific macronutrient needs. Then, the client can select choices from each of the various lists that fit into the plan without having to look up or memorize the nutrient values of numerous foods.

Table B-1 summarizes the basic nutrient composition of foods in each food list. The serving sizes of individual foods in a list may vary, but general estimates are given. The protein and milk and milk substitutes lists are divided into subclasses, which vary in fat content and, thus, in the amount of calories they provide. You can see that each food list is unique in the calories and macronutrients it supplies. A healthy meal plan should include foods from each of the lists to ensure nutrient adequacy. Study *Table B-1* to become familiar with the food groupings, the approximate size of choices on each food list, and the amounts of carbohydrate, protein, fat, and calories per choice.

---

1. Evert AB, Dennison M, Gardner CD, et al. Nutrition therapy for adults with diabetes or prediabetes: a consensus report. *Diabetes Care.* 2019;42(5):731-754. doi:10.2337/dci19-0014

FIGURE B-1 Record the *Food Lists for Diabetes* pattern you have chosen in the left-hand column. Then distribute the food choices throughout the day, noting the food to be used and the serving size.

Food List	Total Food Choices to Be Consumed Daily	Food Choices Consumed at Each Meal			
		Breakfast	Lunch	Dinner	Snacks
Milk and milk substitutes					
Nonstarchy vegetables					
Fruits					
Starch					
Proteins					
Fats					

Examples of Food Choices from *Food Lists for Diabetes*

In this section, you will find just a few examples of the many food choices that are included in the most recent edition of *Choose Your Foods: Food Lists for Diabetes*.

Starches

Starches provide 15 grams of carbohydrate, 0 to 3 grams of protein, 0 to 1 gram of fat, and about 80 kcal per serving. Keep in mind that the serving sizes for starch choices on these food lists are usually smaller than those recommended by MyPlate. Typically, 1 starch choice equals ½ cup of cooked cereal, grain, or starchy vegetable; ⅓ cup of cooked rice or pasta; 1 slice (1 oz) of bread; or ¾ to 1 ounce of crackers or grain-based snack foods. Also, some foods with high fat content, such as biscuits or hash browns, may be counted as 1 starch plus 1 or 2 fats. Beans, peas, and lentils count as 1 starch plus 1 lean protein choice.

BREAD

Serving Size	Food
¼ large (1 oz)	Bagel
1 slice (1 oz)	Bread
½	English muffin
½ (¾ oz)	Hamburger bun
1 oz	Naan (3¼-inch square)
1	Pancake (4-inch diameter)
1	Tortilla, flour (6-inch diameter)

STARCHY VEGETABLES

Serving Size	Food
½ cup	Corn, kernel
1 cup	Mixed vegetables (e.g., corn, peas, and carrots)
¼ (3 oz)	Potato, baked with skin
½ cup	Potatoes, mashed with milk and fat (1 starch + 1 fat)
½ cup	Spaghetti sauce
½ cup	Sweet potato
1 cup	Winter squash (e.g., acorn and butternut)

CEREALS

Serving Size	Food
½ cup	Cooked cereal (e.g., oatmeal)
¼ cup	Granola cereal
1½ cups	Puffed cereal (e.g., puffed rice)
½ cup	Sugar-coated cereal (e.g., Frosted Flakes®)
¾ cup	Unsweetened, ready-to-eat cereal (e.g., Cheerios®)

GRAINS

Serving Size	Food
⅓ cup	Pasta, cooked
⅓ cup	Quinoa, cooked
⅓ cup	Rice, cooked (e.g., white and brown)
½ cup	Wild rice, cooked

CRACKERS AND SNACKS

Serving Size	Food
8	Animal crackers
6	Butter crackers (e.g., Ritz®; 1 starch + 1 fat)
3	Graham crackers (2½ inch squares)
3 cups	Popcorn (no fat added)
¾ ounce	Pretzels
13	Tortilla chips (1 starch + 2 fats)

BEANS, PEAS, AND LENTILS
(count as 1 starch and 1 lean protein)

Serving Size	Food
⅓ cup	Baked beans
½ cup	Beans, cooked or canned (e.g., black, garbanzo, and kidney)
½ cup	Lentils, cooked
½ cup	Peas, cooked (e.g., black-eyed and split)

Fruits

One choice from the Fruits list provides 15 grams of carbohydrate, 0 grams of protein, 0 grams of fat, and 60 kcal. Typically, 1 fruit choice is equal to ½ cup of unsweetened canned or frozen fruit, 1 small fresh fruit (about 2½ inch diameter), ½ cup (4 oz) of unsweetened 100% fruit juice, or 2 tablespoons of dried fruit. Recognize that the fruit you buy at the grocery store may amount to more than one fruit choice; a large banana, for example, counts for 2 fruit choices. The serving sizes of fruit juices and dried fruit are small because these are more concentrated sources of carbohydrates and energy.

FRUITS

Serving Size	Food	Serving Size	Food
1 small (4 oz)	Apple, unpeeled	½ cup	Kiwi, sliced
½ cup	Applesauce, unsweetened	1 (6½ oz)	Orange
1 (4 oz)	Banana	½ cup	Pineapple, canned
¾ cup	Blueberries	½ cup	Pomegranate seeds (arils)
12 (3½ oz)	Cherries, fresh	3	Prunes
17 (3 oz)	Grapes	1¼ cup	Strawberries, whole
1 cup	Honeydew melon, diced	1¼ cup	Watermelon, diced

FRUIT JUICE

Serving Size	Food
½ cup (4 oz)	Apple juice or cider
⅓ cup (2.7 oz)	Grape juice
½ cup (4 oz)	Orange juice
⅓ cup (2.7 oz)	Prune juice

Milk and Milk Substitutes

Milk and milk substitutes are divided into subcategories based on their fat content. All milk and yogurt products provide 12 grams of carbohydrate and 8 grams of protein but may vary in fat content from 0 to 8 grams per choice. The subcategory of other milk foods and milk substitutes includes some products that may be used in place of milk in the eating pattern (e.g., soy milk) but have a slightly different nutrient profile than traditional milk and yogurt products. Those foods, as indicated below, are counted as a combination of carbohydrate (15 grams of carbohydrate, 60 kcal) and fat (5 grams of fat, 45 kcal) choices. Please note that other products used as dairy alternatives (e.g., almond milk) are listed with fat choices.

FAT-FREE (SKIM) AND LOW-FAT MILK AND YOGURT
(12 grams of carbohydrate, 8 grams of protein, 0–3 grams of fat, and 100 kcal)

Serving Size	Food
½ cup (4 oz)	Canned, evaporated, fat-free milk
1 cup (8 oz)	Fat-free (skim) milk, low-fat (1%) milk, and buttermilk
⅔ cup (6 oz)	Yogurt (fat-free plain or fat-free Greek, unsweetened) (1 milk + 1 carb)
1 cup (8 oz)	Chocolate milk (1 milk + 1 carb)

REDUCED-FAT (2%) MILK AND YOGURT
(12 grams of carbohydrate, 8 grams of protein, 5 grams of fat, and 120 kcal)

Serving Size	Food
1 cup (8 oz)	Reduced-fat (2%) milk, acidophilus milk, and kefir
⅔ cup (6 oz)	Yogurt, 2% reduced-fat, plain

WHOLE MILK AND YOGURT
(12 grams of carbohydrate, 8 grams of protein, 8 grams of fat, and 160 kcal)

Serving Size	Food
½ cup (4 oz)	Evaporated whole milk
1 cup (8 oz)	Whole milk, buttermilk, and goat's milk
1 cup (8 oz)	Yogurt, whole milk, plain

OTHER MILK FOODS AND MILK SUBSTITUTES

Serving Size	Food	Choices
1 cup (8 oz)	Almond milk, plain	½ carbohydrate + ½ fat
1 cup (8 oz)	Coconut milk, flavored	1 carbohydrate + 1 fat
⅓ cup (2.7 oz)	Eggnog, whole milk	1 carbohydrate + 1 fat
1 cup (8 oz)	Rice milk, flavored, low-fat	2 carbohydrates
1 cup (8 oz)	Soy milk, regular, plain	1 carbohydrate + 1 fat
⅔ cup (6 oz)	Yogurt with fruit, low-fat	1 fat-free milk + 1 carbohydrate

Nonstarchy Vegetables

Nonstarchy vegetables still provide carbohydrates, but not as much as their starchy counterparts. One nonstarchy vegetable provides 5 grams of carbohydrate, 2 grams of protein, 0 grams of fat, and 25 kcal. Typically, a choice is equal to ½ cup of cooked vegetables, 1 cup of raw vegetables, 3 cups of salad or leafy greens, or ½ cup (4 fl oz) vegetable juice. Large servings of nonstarchy vegetables (i.e., three choices) should be counted as one carbohydrate choice (15 grams of carbohydrate, 60 kcal) rather than multiple nonstarchy vegetables. Because of their low carbohydrate content, salad greens (e.g., iceberg, romaine, and endive) actually count as free foods. To comply with advice from the *Dietary Guidelines for Americans*, it is important to select a variety of starchy and nonstarchy vegetables each day because each has a distinct micronutrient and phytochemical profile. Take extra care to select 2 or 3 nonstarchy vegetables with deep colors, such as spinach, carrots, and beets, per day.

Serving Size	Food
½ cup	Asparagus, cooked
½ cup	Beets, cooked
½ cup	Broccoli, cooked
1 cup	Carrots, sliced, raw
½ cup	Collard greens, cooked
1 cup	Cucumber, raw

Serving Size	Food
½ cup	Green beans, cooked
3 cups	Salad greens, raw
½ cup	Summer squash, cooked
½ cup	Tomatoes, stewed
½ cup	Vegetable juice

Sweets, Desserts, and Other Carbohydrates

Foods on this list may not match the nutrient profiles of other starches, but they are commonly consumed and must be accounted for in the eating pattern. Sweetened beverages, desserts, and sweeteners and condiments that we add to foods can be counted as a combination of carbohydrate (15 grams of carbohydrates, 60 kcal) and fat (5 grams of fat, 45 kcal) choices.

BEVERAGES, SODA, AND SPORTS DRINKS

Serving Size	Food	Choices
1 can (8 oz)	Energy drink	2 carbohydrates
1 cup (8 oz)	Fruit drink or lemonade	2 carbohydrates
1 can (12 oz)	Soft drink, regular	2½ carbohydrates
1 cup (8 oz)	Sports drink	1 carbohydrate

BROWNIES, CAKE, COOKIES, GELATIN, PIE, AND PUDDING

Serving Size	Food	Choices
1/12 cake (2 oz)	Angel food cake, unfrosted	2 carbohydrates
1¼-inch square (1 oz)	Brownie, unfrosted	1 carbohydrate + 1 fat
2-inch square (2 oz)	Cake, frosted	2 carbohydrates + 1 fat
2 small	Chocolate chip cookies	1 carbohydrate + 2 fats
½ cup	Gelatin, regular	1 carbohydrate
½ cup	Pudding, regular, 2% milk	2 carbohydrates
1/8 pie	Pumpkin pie	1½ carbohydrates + 1½ fats
5 pieces	Vanilla wafers	1 carbohydrate + 1 fat

CANDY, SPREADS, SWEETS, SWEETENERS, SYRUPS, AND TOPPINGS

Serving Size	Food	Choices
1 tbsp	Agave, syrup	1 carbohydrate
5	Chocolate kisses	1 carbohydrate + 1 fat
1 tbsp	Honey	1 carbohydrate
1 tbsp	Jam or jelly, regular	1 carbohydrate
2 tbsp	Liquid nondairy coffee creamer	1 carbohydrate
1 tbsp	Pancake syrup, regular	1 carbohydrate

CONDIMENTS AND SAUCES

Serving Size	Food	Choices
3 tbsp	Barbecue sauce	1 carbohydrate
½ cup	Gravy	½ carbohydrate + ½ fat
3 tbsp	Ketchup	1 carbohydrate
3 tbsp	Salad dressing, fat-free, cream-based	1 carbohydrate

DOUGHNUTS, MUFFINS, PASTRIES, AND SWEET BREADS

Serving Size	Food	Choices
1 (2½ oz)	Danish	2½ carbohydrates + 2 fats
1 (2 oz)	Glazed doughnut	2 carbohydrates + 2 fats
1 (4 oz)	Muffin, regular	4 carbohydrates + 2½ fats

FROZEN BARS, FROZEN DESSERTS, FROZEN YOGURT, AND ICE CREAM

Serving Size	Food	Choices
1 (3 oz)	Frozen 100% fruit juice bar	1 carbohydrate
½ cup	Greek frozen yogurt, low-fat	1½ carbohydrates
½ cup	Ice cream, no sugar added	1 carbohydrate + 1 fat
½ cup	Ice cream, regular	1 carbohydrate + 2 fats
½ cup	Sherbet, sorbet	2 carbohydrates

Protein

Similar to the choices on the Milk and Milk Substitutes list, protein choices vary in fat and calorie content. Lean protein choices, such as egg whites and skinless poultry, provide 0 grams of carbohydrate, 7 grams of protein, 2 grams of fat, and 45 kcal. Medium-fat protein choices, such as whole eggs and poultry with skin, provide 0 grams of carbohydrate, 7 grams of protein, 5 grams of fat, and 75 kcal. High-fat protein choices, including many types of sausage and bacon, provide 0 grams of carbohydrate, 7 grams of protein, 8 grams of fat, and 100 kcal. Plant-based protein choices usually contain some carbohydrates, so they count as a combination of carbohydrate or starch and protein choices. Note that choices are very small (1-oz portions); a typical hamburger would count as 3 or 4 protein choices.

LEAN PROTEIN (0 grams of carbohydrate, 7 grams of protein, 2 grams of fat, and 45 kcal)

Serving Size	Food
1 oz	Beef with 10% or lower fat (e.g., round and sirloin)
1 oz	Cheese with 3 grams of fat or less (e.g., fat-free mozzarella)
1 oz	Deli meats with 3 grams of fat or less per serving (e.g., turkey and ham)
2	Egg whites
1 oz	Fish, not fried (e.g., catfish, cod, and tuna canned in water)
1 oz	Lean pork (e.g., ham and tenderloin)
1 oz	Poultry, without skin
1 oz	Shellfish (e.g., shrimp and crab)
1 oz	Wild game (e.g., buffalo and venison)

MEDIUM-FAT PROTEIN (0 grams of carbohydrate, 7 grams of protein, 5 grams of fat, and 75 kcal)

Serving Size	Food
1 oz	Beef with 15% or higher (e.g., rib roast and ground beef)
1 oz	Cheese with 4 to 7 grams of fat per ounce (e.g., feta and mozzarella)
1	Egg
1 oz	Fish, fried
1 oz	Pork (e.g., cutlet and shoulder roast)
1 oz	Poultry, with skin

HIGH-FAT PROTEIN (0 grams of carbohydrate, 7 grams of protein, 8 grams of fat, and 100 kcal)

Serving Size	Food
2 slices	Bacon, pork
1 oz	Cheese (e.g., American, Cheddar, Parmesan, and Swiss)
1 oz	Deli meat with 8 grams of fat or more per serving (e.g., bologna and salami)
1	Hot dog
1 oz	Sausage (e.g., bratwurst and summer sausage)

PLANT-BASED PROTEINS

Serving Size	Food	Choices
½ cup	Beans, cooked or canned (e.g., black, kidney, and pinto)	1 starch + 1 lean protein
½ cup	Edamame, shelled	½ carbohydrate + 1 lean protein
⅓ cup	Hummus	1 carbohydrate + 1 medium-fat protein
1 (2½ oz)	Meatless burger, soy-based	½ carbohydrate + 2 lean proteins
1 tbsp	Peanut butter	1 high-fat protein
½ cup	Refried beans, canned	1 carbohydrate + 1 lean protein
½ cup (4 oz)	Tofu	1 medium-fat protein

Fats

One fat choice is 5 grams of fat and 45 kcal. Fats are subdivided into unsaturated fats, which come mainly from plant sources, and saturated fats, which come mainly from animal sources. In line with recommendations from other major health authorities, the *Food Lists for Diabetes* advises people to choose monounsaturated and polyunsaturated fats in place of saturated fats.

UNSATURATED FATS—MONOUNSATURATED FATS (5 grams of fat and 45 kcal)

Serving Size	Food	Serving Size	Food
1 cup	Almond milk, unsweetened	1 tsp	Oil (e.g., canola and olive)
6	Almonds	8	Olives, black
2 tbsp (1 oz)	Avocado	10	Peanuts
1½ tsp	Nut butter (e.g., almond and peanut)	16	Pistachios

UNSATURATED FATS—POLYUNSATURATED FATS (5 grams of fat and 45 kcal)

Serving Size	Food
1½ tbsp	Flaxseed, ground
1 tbsp	Low-fat vegetable oil spread
1 tsp	Margarine, stick and tub
1 tsp	Mayonnaise, regular

Serving Size	Food
1 tsp	Oil (e.g., corn, safflower, and sunflower)
1 tbsp	Reduced-fat mayonnaise
2 tbsp	Salad dressing, reduced-fat (may contain carbohydrate)
1 tbsp	Salad dressing, regular

SATURATED FATS (5 grams of fat and 45 kcal)

Serving Size	Food
1 slice	Bacon, cooked
1 tbsp	Butter, reduced-fat
1½ tsp	Butter, regular

Serving Size	Food
1 tbsp (½ oz)	Cream cheese, regular
2 tbsp	Coconut, shredded
1 tsp	Coconut oil
2 tbsp	Sour cream, regular

Free Foods

A *free food* is any food or drink choice that contains less than 20 kcal or less than 5 grams of carbohydrate per serving. When eaten in small amounts throughout the day, these foods have little impact on blood sugar. Foods with a serving size listed should be limited to 3 servings per day. Foods listed without a serving size (indicated with a *) can be eaten as often as you like. However, many free foods are high in sodium, so moderation is important.

LOW-CARBOHYDRATE FOODS

Serving Size	Food
1 piece	Candy, hard or sugar-free
¼ cup	Cooked nonstarchy vegetables (e.g., carrots, cauliflower, and green beans)
*	Gelatin, sugar-free
2 tsp	Jam or jelly, light or no-sugar-added type

Serving Size	Food
½ cup	Raw nonstarchy vegetables (e.g., broccoli, carrots, cucumber, and tomato)
*	Salad greens (no dressing)
*	Sugar substitutes

REDUCED-FAT OR FAT-FREE FOODS

Serving Size	Food
1 tbsp	Cream cheese, fat-free
4 tsp	Coffee creamer, liquid, sugar-free, flavored
1 tsp	Margarine spread, reduced-fat

Serving Size	Food
1 tbsp	Mayonnaise, fat-free
1 tbsp	Salad dressing, fat-free
2 tbsp	Whipped topping, light or fat-free

CONDIMENTS

Serving Size	Food
2 tsp	Barbecue sauce
1½	Dill pickles (medium)
*	Hot pepper sauce
1 tbsp	Ketchup

Serving Size	Food
*	Mustard (e.g., brown, Dijon, or yellow)
1 tbsp	Parmesan cheese, grated
1 tbsp	Soy sauce

DRINKS/MIXES

Serving Size	Food
*	Bouillon or broth
*	Club soda
*	Coffee, unsweetened or artificially sweetened

Serving Size	Food
*	Diet soft drinks, sugar-free
*	Tea, unsweetened or with sugar substitute
*	Water
*	Water, flavored, sugar-free

SEASONINGS

Serving Size	Food
*	Garlic, fresh or powder
*	Herbs, fresh or dried
*	Spices

Combination Foods

These foods contain a mixture of ingredients and cannot be grouped into one food list. Typical examples of combination foods include casseroles, sandwiches, frozen meals, and fast foods containing multiple ingredients. These foods may be consumed at home, dining out, or after home delivery. Many of these foods are high in sodium.

MAIN DISHES/ENTREES

Serving Size	Food	Choices
1 cup (8 oz)	Casserole-type entrees (e.g., tuna noodle, lasagna, and spaghetti with meatballs)	2 carbohydrates + 2 medium-fat proteins
1 cup (8 oz)	Stews (meat and vegetables)	1 carbohydrate + 1 medium-fat protein + 0 to 3 fats
8 to 10 oz	Vegetarian bowl	3 carbohydrates + 1 lean protein + 1 fat

FROZEN MEALS/ENTREES

Serving Size	Food	Choices
1 (5 oz)	Burrito (beef and bean)	3 carbohydrates + 1 lean protein + 2 fats
9 to 12 oz	Dinner-type healthy meal (< 400 kcal)	2 to 3 carbohydrates + 1 to 2 lean proteins + 1 fat
¼ of a 12-inch (5 oz)	Pizza with thin crust and meat toppings	2 carbohydrates + 2 medium-fat proteins + 1½ fats
1 (4½ oz)	Pocket sandwich	3 carbohydrates + 1 lean protein + 1 to 2 fats

SALADS (DELI-STYLE)

Serving Size	Food	Choices
½ cup	Coleslaw, creamy	1 carbohydrate + 1½ fats
½ cup	Macaroni salad	2 carbohydrates + 3 fats
½ cup (3½ oz)	Tuna salad or chicken salad	½ carbohydrate + 2 lean proteins + 1 fat

SOUPS

Serving Size	Food	Choices
1 cup (8 oz)	Bean, lentil, or split pea soup	2 carbohydrates + 1 lean protein
1 cup (8 oz)	Broth-based soups with vegetables and meat	1 carbohydrate + 1 lean protein
1 cup (8 oz)	Chowder (made with milk)	1 carbohydrate + 1 lean protein + 1½ fats
1 cup (8 oz)	Cream soup (made with water)	1 carbohydrate + 1 fat
1 cup (8 oz)	Ramen noodle soup	2 carbohydrates + 2 fats
1 cup (8 oz)	Tomato soup (made with water)	1 carbohydrate

Fast Foods

Fast foods are high in sodium and fat. These should be consumed in moderation, if at all. It is much easier to control carbohydrate, fat, sodium, and calorie intake when you prepare your own foods at home rather than relying on restaurants.

MAIN DISHES/ENTREES

Serving Size	Food	Choices
1 (7 oz)	Chicken breast, breaded and fried	1 carbohydrate + 6 medium-fat proteins
6 pieces	Chicken nuggets or tenders	1 carbohydrate + 2 medium-fat proteins + 1 fat
1 (2 oz)	Chicken wing, breaded and fried	½ carbohydrate + 2 medium-fat proteins
⅛ of 14-inch	Pizza, thick crust with or without meat toppings	2½ carbohydrates + 1 high-fat protein + 1 fat

ASIAN

Serving Size	Food	Choices
1 (3 oz)	Egg roll with meat filling	1½ carbohydrates + 1 lean protein + 1½ fats
1 cup	Fried rice, meatless	2½ carbohydrates + 2 fats
1 cup (6 oz)	Meat with vegetables in sauce	1 carbohydrate + 2 lean proteins + 1 fat
1 cup	Pad Thai with chicken	3 carbohydrates + 2 lean proteins + 2 fat
1 cup	Sushi, California rolls	1 carbohydrates + 1 fat

MEXICAN

Serving Size	Food	Choices
1 small (6 oz)	Burrito with beans and cheese	3½ carbohydrates + 1 medium-fat protein + 1 fat
1 small (3 oz)	Crisp taco with meat and cheese	1 carbohydrate + 1 medium-fat protein + 1½ fat
8 chips	Nachos with cheese	2½ carbohydrates + 1 high-fat protein + 2 fats
1 salad (1 lb)	Taco salad with chicken and tortilla bowl	3½ carbohydrates + 4 medium-fat proteins + 3 fats

SANDWICHES

Serving Size	Food	Choices
1 small (4 oz)	Breakfast burrito with sausage, egg, and cheese	1½ carbohydrates + 2 high-fat proteins
1 (8½ oz)	Cheeseburger (4 oz) with condiments	3 carbohydrates + 4 medium-fat proteins + 2½ fats
1 (5 oz)	Fried fish fillet sandwich with cheese and tartar sauce	2½ carbohydrates + 2 medium-fat proteins + 1½ fats
1 (7½ oz)	Grilled chicken sandwich with lettuce, tomato, and spread	3 carbohydrates + 4 lean proteins
1 6-inch	Submarine sandwich (no cheese or sauce)	3 carbohydrates + 2 lean proteins + 1 fat

SIDE DISHES

Serving Size	Food	Choices
1 medium (5 oz)	French fries	3½ carbohydrates + 3 fats
8 (4 oz)	Onion rings	3½ carbohydrates + 4 fats
1 small	Side salad (no cheese, croutons, or dressing)	1 nonstarchy vegetable

BEVERAGES AND DESSERTS

Serving Size	Food	Choices
12 fl oz	Coffee, latte, with fat-free milk	1 fat-free milk
1 small	Ice cream cone	2 carbohydrates + ½ fat
16 fl oz	Milk shake	7 carbohydrates + 4 fats

Alcohol

For people with diabetes, up to 1 or 2 drinks per day for females and males, respectively, can fit into a healthy eating plan. Alcohol itself does not raise blood glucose, but alcoholic drinks often contain carbohydrates that must be counted. One alcohol equivalent provides 100 kcal. One carbohydrate choice provides 15 grams of carbohydrate and 60 kcal. Alcohol should be consumed with a meal to lower the risk of hypoglycemia.

Serving Size	Drink	Choices
12 fl oz	Beer, regular	1 alcohol equivalent + 1 carbohydrate
4 fl oz	Champagne	1 alcohol equivalent
3½ fl oz	Dessert wine	1 alcohol equivalent + 1 carbohydrate
1½ fl oz	Distilled spirits (e.g., rum and vodka)	1 alcohol equivalent
5 fl oz	Wine	1 alcohol equivalent

Appendix C
Dietary Assessment

Occasionally tracking and analyzing your dietary pattern can be a good way to make sure you are meeting your nutrient requirements and adhering to public health recommendations. One tip is to record all foods and beverages as soon as possible after consumption. You could record your data on paper (using a form such as that provided in Table C-2) or enter your data directly into your dietary analysis software using an electronic device.

I. **Fill in the food record form that follows.** This appendix contains a blank copy, Table C-2 (see the completed example in Table C-1). Your instructor may ask you to record 1 day or several days. To get a good estimate of your usual nutrient intake, it is best to record several days (e.g., 2 weekdays and 1 weekend day). As you record your intake for use on the nutrient analysis form that follows, consider the following tips:
  - Measure and record the amounts of foods eaten using units of volume (e.g., cups, teaspoons, tablespoons, fluid ounces), weight (e.g., grams, ounces), or units with specific dimensions (e.g., 1 slice of 12-inch pizza, 1 apple—3 inches in diameter, or carrot sticks—4 inches long, ½ inch thick).
  - Record brand names of all food products, such as "Quick Quaker Oats®."
  - Measure and record all those little extras, such as gravies, salad dressings, taco sauces, pickles, jelly, sugar, ketchup, and butter.
  - For beverages:
    - List the type of milk, such as whole, fat-free, 1%, evaporated, chocolate, reconstituted dry, or specific plant-based milk (e.g., soy milk, almond milk).
    - Indicate whether fruit juice is 100%, fresh, frozen, or canned.
    - Indicate type for other beverages, such as fruit drink, smoothie, fruit-flavored drink, Kool-Aid®, and hot chocolate made with water or milk (specify type of milk).
  - For fruits:
    - Indicate whether fresh, frozen, dried, or canned.
    - Indicate the portion eaten (e.g., with or without peel).
    - For canned fruits, indicate whether processed in water, light syrup, or heavy syrup.
  - For vegetables:
    - Indicate whether fresh, frozen, dried, or canned.
    - Record preparation method (e.g., raw, steamed, baked, air-fried).
    - For canned vegetables, include details about sodium content (e.g., regular, low-sodium, or no-salt added).
    - For frozen vegetables, include details about sauces and seasonings.
  - For cereals:
    - If cooked, indicate whether the portion was measured before or after cooking.
    - If butter, milk, sugar, fruit, or something else is added, measure and record amount and type.
  - For bagels, breads, rolls, and biscuits:
    - Indicate whether whole wheat, rye, white, and so on.
    - Include details about the portions (e.g., biscuit—2 inches across, 1 inch thick; slice of homemade rye bread—3 inches by 4 inches, ¼ inch thick).
    - Sandwiches: list all ingredients (lettuce, mayonnaise, tomato, and so on).
  - For meat, meat alternatives, fish, poultry, and cheese:
    - Give size (length, width, and thickness) in inches or weight in ounces after cooking for meat, fish, and poultry (such as cooked hamburger patty—3 inches across, ½ inch thick).

- Record measurements only for the cooked, edible part—without bone or fat left on the plate.
- Describe how meat, poultry, or fish was prepared.
- For eggs:
  - Indicate preparation method (e.g., hard-boiled, fried, scrambled, poached, or omelet).
  - If milk, butter, or drippings are used, specify types and amount.
- For desserts:
  - List commercial brand or "homemade" or "bakery" under brand.
  - Purchased candies, cookies, and cakes: specify kind and size.
  - Measure and record portion size of cakes, pies, and cookies by specifying thickness, diameter, and width or length, depending on the item.

TABLE C-1 ■ Example of a 1-Day Food Record

Time	Minutes Spent Eating	M or S*	H† (0–3)	Activity While Eating	Place of Eating	Food and Quantity	Others Present	Reason for Choice
7:10 A.M.	15	M	2	Standing, fixing lunch	Kitchen	Orange, 1 medium (2.5")	—	Health
						Crispix® cereal, 1 cup		Habit
						Nonfat milk, ½ cup		Health
						Sugar, 2 tsp		Taste
						Regular coffee, 1 cup		Habit
10:00 A.M.	4	S	1	Sitting, taking notes	Classroom	Diet cola, 12 oz	Class	Weight control
12:15 P.M.	40	M	2	Sitting, talking	Student union	Chicken sandwich (3 oz grilled chicken, wheat bun, 1 leaf iceberg lettuce, 1 slice of tomato, and 2 tsp mayonnaise)	Friends	Taste
						Pear, 1 medium		Health
						2% milk, 1 cup		Health
2:30 P.M.	10	S	1	Sitting, studying	Library	Water, 1 cup	Friend	Hunger
6:30 P.M.	35	M	3	Sitting, talking	Kitchen	Pork chop, broiled, 3 oz	Boyfriend	Convenience
						Baked potato, 1 medium		Health
						Butter, 2 tbsp		Taste
						Salad (1 cup of lettuce, 4 cherry tomatoes)		Health
						Ranch dressing, 2 tbsp		Taste
						Peas, steamed from frozen, ½ cup		Health
						2% milk, 1 cup		Habit
						Cherry pie, 1/8 of a 9" pie		Taste
						Water, 1.5 cups		Health
9:10 P.M.	10	S	2	Sitting, studying	Living room	Apple, 1 medium (3")	—	Weight control
						Water, 1 cup		Weight control

*M or S: Meal or snack.

†H: Degree of hunger (0 none; 3 maximum).

TABLE C-2 ■ 1-Day Food Record

Time	Minutes Spent Eating	M or S*	H† (0–3)	Activity While Eating	Place of Eating	Food and Quantity	Others Present	Reason for Choice

*M or S: Meal or snack.

†H: Degree of hunger (0 none; 3 maximum).

II. **Enter all the foods and beverages you consumed into NutritionCalc Plus** (Fig. C-1). As you get started, you will find many useful tutorial videos on the NutritionCalc Plus site. If you have not already done so, you will need to create a profile in NutritionCalc Plus. For each food or drink, select the meal or snack and the appropriate serving size. If you have data for more than 1 day, be sure to enter your foods and beverages on separate days. If the NutritionCalc Plus database does not contain the exact food or drink you consumed, you may need to enter a reasonably close substitute. For example, the grilled chicken sandwich from the student union in the food record example in Table C-1 could be entered as a fast food grilled chicken sandwich. Whenever possible, choose items with "USDA" or "FNDDS" in the name; these database items typically have the most complete nutrient information.

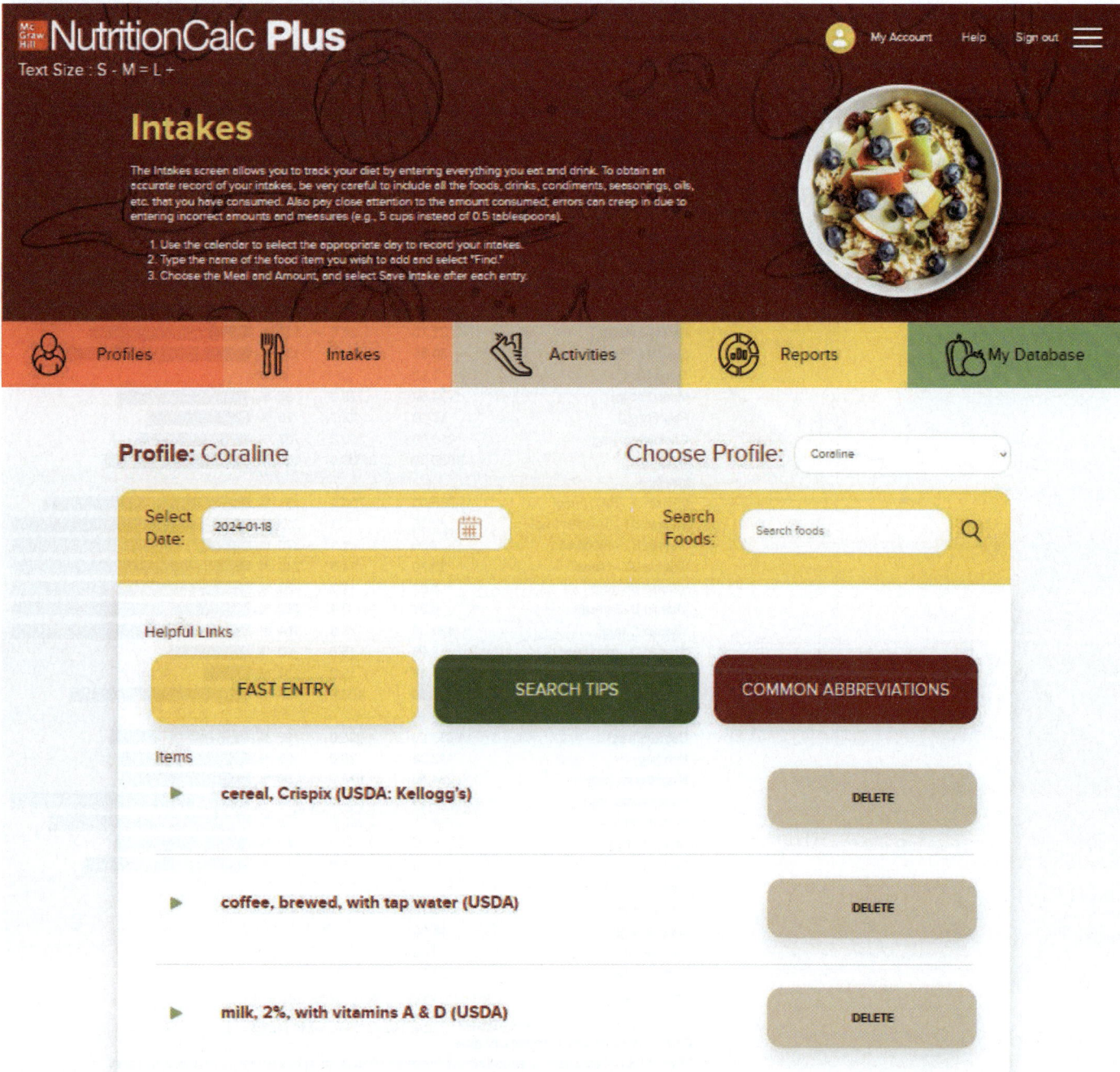

FIGURE C-1 Entering food and beverage intake data using NutritionCalc Plus. NutritionCalc Plus

III. **Use NutritionCalc Plus to generate a report of your nutrient intake** (Fig. C-2). After you have finished entering all the foods and beverages you consumed, save your intake data and click on **Reports.** Select **Bar Graph** to see a report of your nutrient intake for a particular day or several days compared to your nutrient needs. Be sure to enter your student ID information (name, instructor, and course), choose the correct profile for comparison, then select the day(s) and meals(s) you would like to analyze. Then you may save your report as a PDF or Excel spreadsheet or e-mail it as an attachment to yourself or your instructor.

FIGURE C-2 Sample Bar Graph Report from NutritionCalc Plus. NutritionCalc Plus

Bar Graph Report

The Bar Graph Report displays graphically the amount of the nutrient consumed and compares that to the dietary intake recommendations.

Nutrient	Value	DRI Goal	Percent
Basic Components			
Calories	2,123.00	2,272.0	93 %
Calories from Fat	695.00	636.0	109 %
Calories from SatFat	277.00	204.0	136 %
Protein (g)	90.00	50.8*	177 %
Protein (% Calories)	17.00	9.0*	188 %
Carbohydrates (g)	279.00	312.0	89 %
Carbohydrates (% Calories)	52.60	55.0	96 %
Total Sugars (g)	127.00 ^		
Added Sugar (g)	8.38	28.4~	30 %
Dietary Fiber (g)	25.80	31.8	81 %
Soluble Fiber (g)	5.06		
InSoluble Fiber (g)	15.40		
Fat (g)	77.20	70.7	109 %
Fat (% Calories)	32.70	28.0	117 %
Saturated Fat (g)	30.80	22.7~	136 %
Trans Fat (g)	1.62		
Mono Fat (g)	24.50	25.2	97 %
Poly Fat (g)	17.10	22.7	75 %
Cholesterol (mg)	250.00	300.0~	83 %
Water (g)	2,920.00	2,700.0	108 %
Vitamins			
Vitamin A - RAE (mcg)	1,055.00	700.0	151 %
Vitamin B1 - Thiamin (mg)	2.35	1.1	213 %
Vitamin B2 - Riboflavin	3.03	1.1	276 %
Vitamin B3 - Niacin	33.70	14.0	240 %
Vitamin B6 (mg)	3.02	1.3	233 %
Vitamin B12 (mcg)	6.08	2.4	253 %
Vitamin C (mg)	138.00	75.0	184 %
Vitamin D - mcg (mcg)	8.96	15.0	60 %
Vitamin E - a-Toco (mg)	5.11	15.0	34 %
Folate - DFE (mcg)	528.00	400.0	132 %
Minerals			
Calcium (mg)	1,033.00	1,000.0	103 %
Iron (mg)	17.30	18.0	96 %
Magnesium (mg)	294.00	310.0	95 %
Phosphorus (mg)	1,620.00	700.0	231 %
Potassium (mg)	3,851.00	2,600.0	148 %
Sodium (mg)	2,285.00	2,300.0~	99 %
Zinc (mg)	9.71	8.0	121 %
Other			
Omega-3 (g)	2.13 +		
Omega-6 (g)	14.90 +		
Alcohol (g)	0.00		
Caffeine (mg)	137.00		

DRI Goal Key:

Black = Consume at least the DRI goal
Red = Consume less than the DRI goal

* Protein is not adjusted for endurance/strength athletes at an Active or Very Active activity level.
^ Total Sugars includes those naturally occuring in food and added sugars.
+ There is no established recommendation for Omega-3 and Omega-6.

IV. **Use NutritionCalc Plus to compare your dietary pattern to the dietary pattern recommended by the** *Dietary Guidelines for Americans* (Fig. C-3). Click on **Reports** and choose **MyPlate.** Enter your student information, choose the correct profile for comparison, and select the day(s) and meal(s) you would like to analyze. You may save your report, print it, or e-mail it as an attachment to yourself or your instructor.

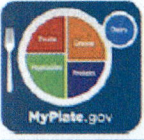

FIGURE C-3 Sample MyPlate report from NutritionCalc Plus.
NutritionCalc Plus; (MyPlate): U.S. Department of Agriculture

MyPlate

The MyPlate Food Guide report displays graphically how close the foodlist compares to the lastest USDA Dietary Guidelines (see MyPlate.gov for more info).

Intake vs. Recommendation
2200 Calorie Pattern

Group	Percent	Amount*
Grains Intake	60 %	4.2 oz equivalent
Grains Recommendation		7.0 oz equivalent
Vegetables Intake	93 %	2.8 cup equivalent
Vegetables Recommendation		3.0 cup equivalent
Fruits Intake	174 %	3.5 cup equivalent
Fruits Recommendation		2.0 cup equivalent
Dairy Intake	79 %	2.4 cup equivalent
Dairy Recommendation		3.0 cup equivalent
Protein Foods Intake	100 %	6.0 oz equivalent
Protein Foods Recommendation		6.0 oz equivalent

Make Half Your Grains Whole
Aim for at least 3.5 oz equivalents whole grains a day

Oils & Empty Calories
Aim for 6.0 teaspoons of oils a day
Limit your extra fats & sugars to 290 Calories

Vary Your Vegetables

Dark Green Vegetables	3.0 cups
Orange Vegetables	2.0 cups
Dry Beans & Peas	3.0 cups
Starchy Vegetables	6.0 cups
Other Vegetables	7.0 cups

* oz equivalent is a 1 ounce estimate, rounded to consumer friendly units. For example, an oz equivalent of Grains is 1 slice of bread, or 1/2 cup of rice. An oz equivalent of Protein Foods 1 oz of meat, 1 egg, or 1/4 cup cooked beans.

V. **Evaluate your dietary pattern.** Answer the following questions about the results of your own dietary assessment and suggest ways that you could improve your dietary pattern.
1. How did your calorie intake compare to the goal recommended by NutritionCalc Plus? If it was much higher or lower than your goal, what specific changes could you make to adjust your energy intake?
2. Do your meals usually resemble MyPlate? If not, what specific changes could you make to improve your meal planning?
3. Use the following worksheet to calculate your fat intake as a percentage of total calories. How does this compare to the Acceptable Macronutrient Distribution Range (AMDR) of 20% to 35% of total kilocalories from fat? If your fat intake does not fall within the AMDR, what specific changes could you make?

> Calculating Percent of Kilocalories from Fat:
>
> _____ grams of fat × 9 kcal per gram = _____ kcal from fat
>
> _____ kcal from fat ÷ _____ total kcal × 100 = _____ % of kcal from fat

4. Use the following worksheet to calculate your saturated fat intake as a percentage of total calories. How does this compare to the *Dietary Guidelines* recommendation to limit saturated fat to 10% of total calories? If your intake of saturated fat was higher than 10% of total calories, what specific dietary changes could you make to lower your intake of saturated fat?

> Calculating Percent of Kilocalories from Saturated Fat:
>
> _____ grams of saturated fat × 9 kcal per gram = _____ kcal from saturated fat
>
> _____ kcal from saturated fat ÷ _____ total kcal × 100 = _____ % of kcal from saturated fat

5. The *Dietary Guidelines* advises Americans to limit their consumption of added sugars. What were some sources of added sugars in your diet on the days you recorded? List several nutrient-dense food choices you could use to replace sources of added sugars in your dietary pattern.
6. What was your average fiber intake for the days you recorded? How close did you come to meeting the AI for fiber? If your intake of fiber was lower than the AI, what specific dietary changes could you make to improve your intake of fiber?
7. How did your average intake of sodium compare to the CDRR for sodium? If your sodium intake was higher than the CDRR, what specific dietary changes could you make to lower your intake of sodium?
8. Are your intakes of any vitamins or minerals less than 75% of the RDA or AI? Choose one of these nutrients and discuss how you could change your *dietary* habits to increase your intake of this nutrient.
9. Besides sodium, do your intakes of any vitamins or minerals exceed the UL? (Also consider any micronutrients consumed in supplement form.) If so, what negative consequences could this have for your health?
10. If you consume alcohol, are your drinking habits consistent with the *Dietary Guidelines* recommendations to limit alcohol to one drink per day (women) or two drinks per day (men)? List one potential benefit of moderate alcohol consumption. List one negative consequence of excessive alcohol consumption.

Appendix D
Chemical Structures Important in Nutrition

Amino Acids

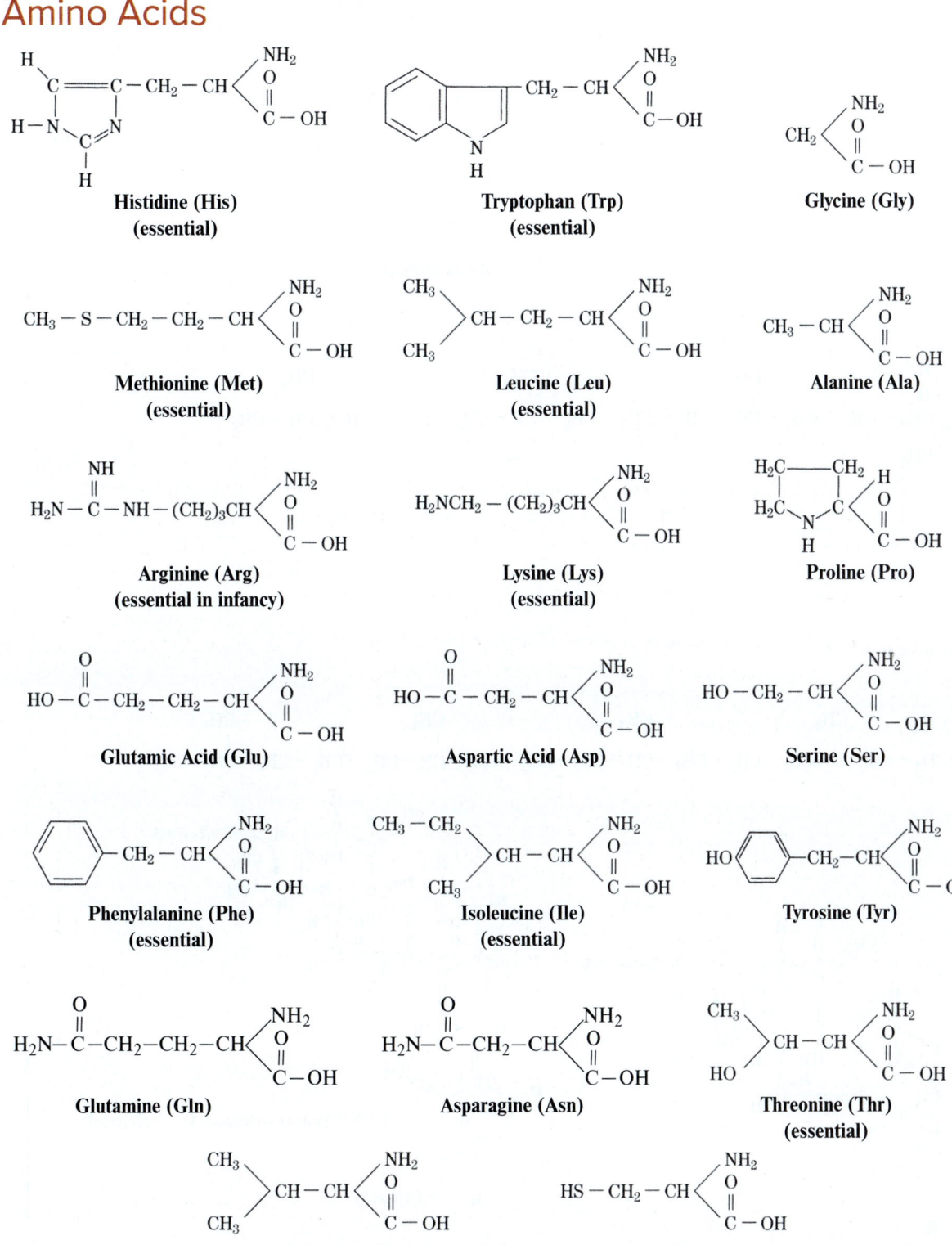

Vitamins

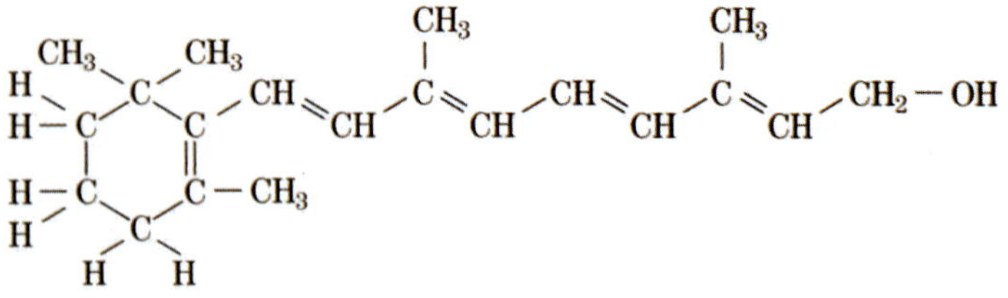

Vitamin A (retinol)

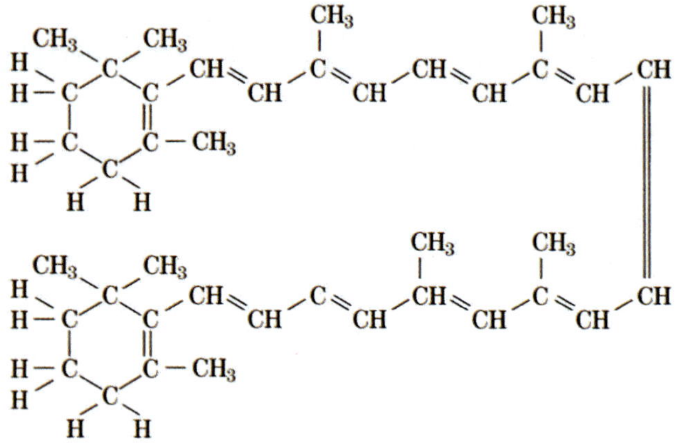

Beta-carotene

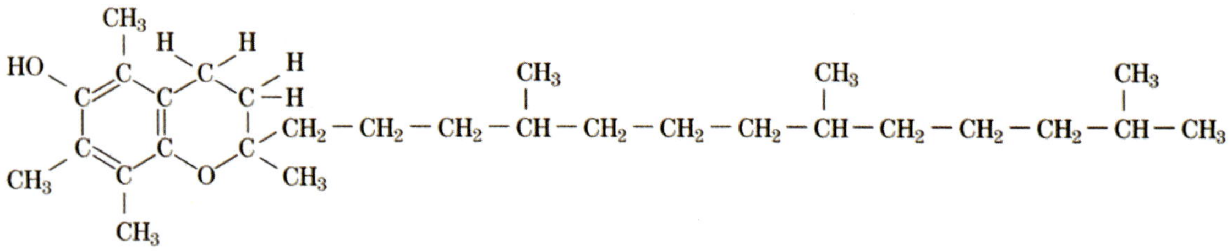

Vitamin E

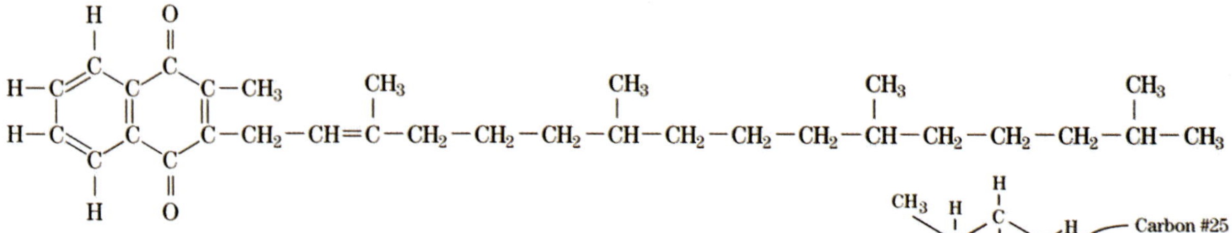

Vitamin K

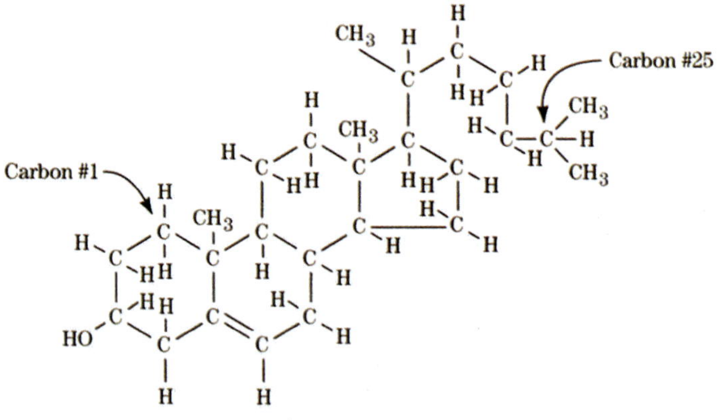

7-Dehydrocholesterol

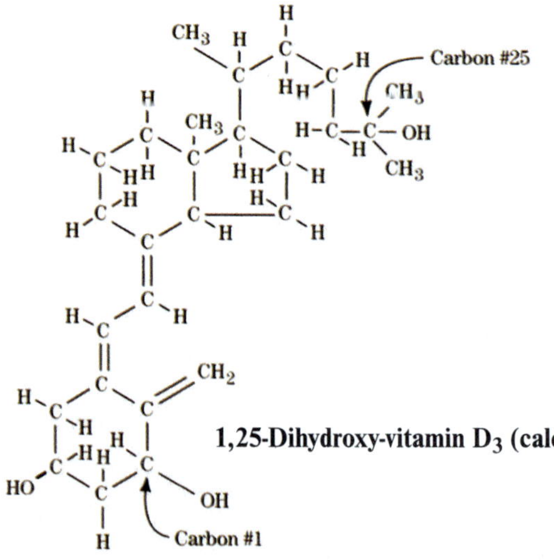

1,25-Dihydroxy-vitamin D_3 (calcitriol)

Active vitamin D (calcitriol) and its precursor 7-dehydrocholesterol

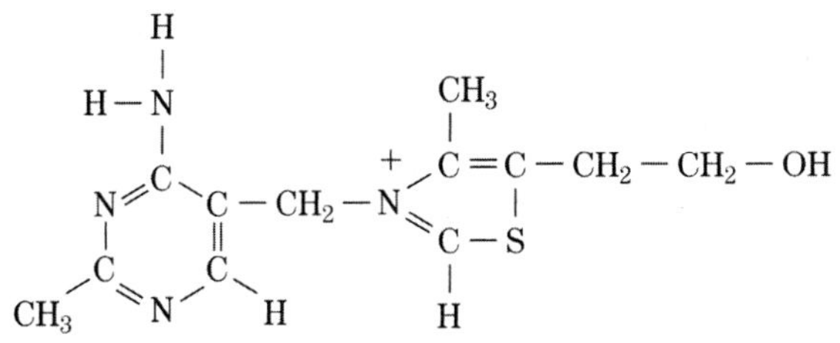

Thiamin

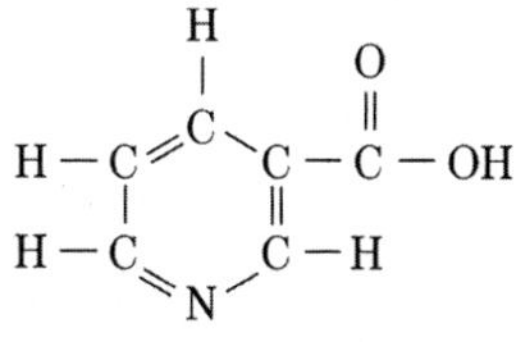

Niacin (nicotinic acid and nicotinamide)

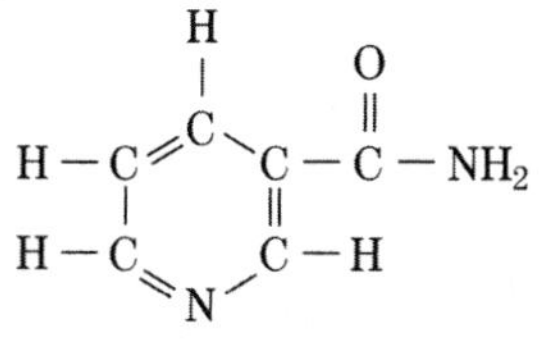

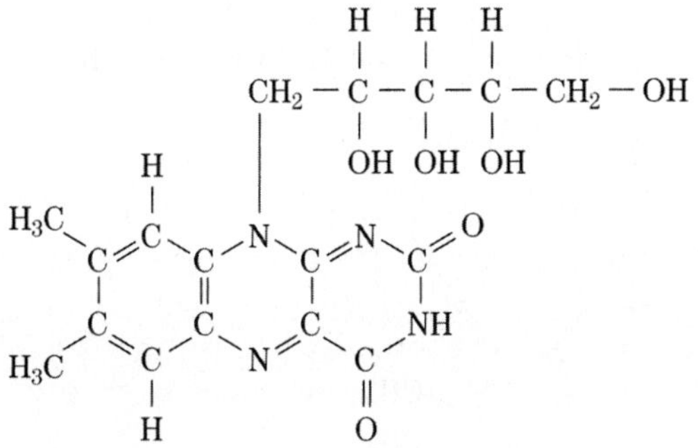

Nicotinic acid

Nicotinamide

Riboflavin

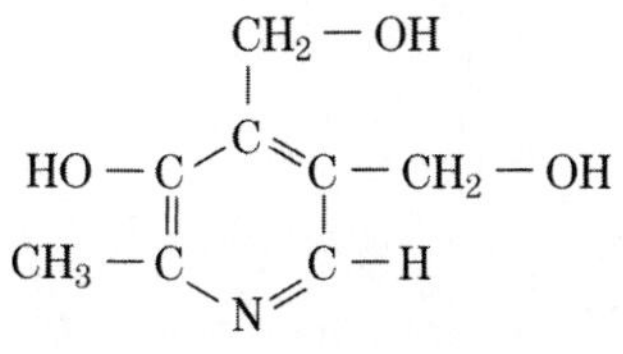

Pyridoxine

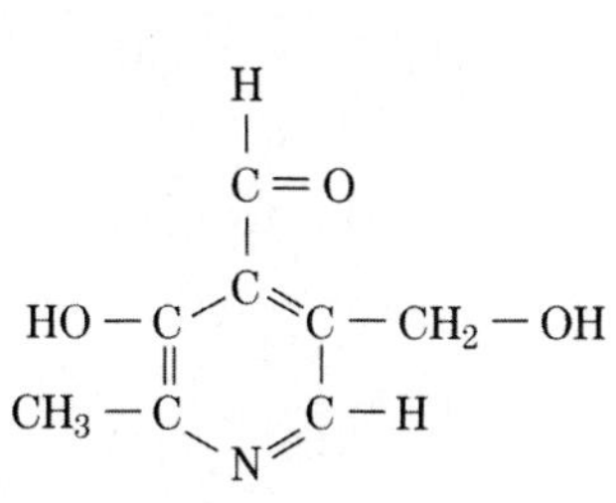

Pyridoxal

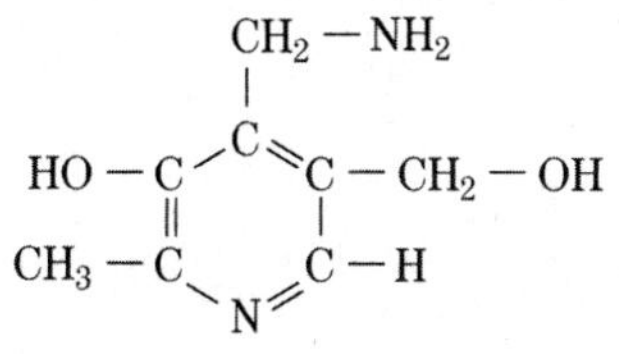

Pyridoxamine

Vitamin B-6 (a general name for three compounds—pyridoxine, pyridoxal, and pyridoxamine)

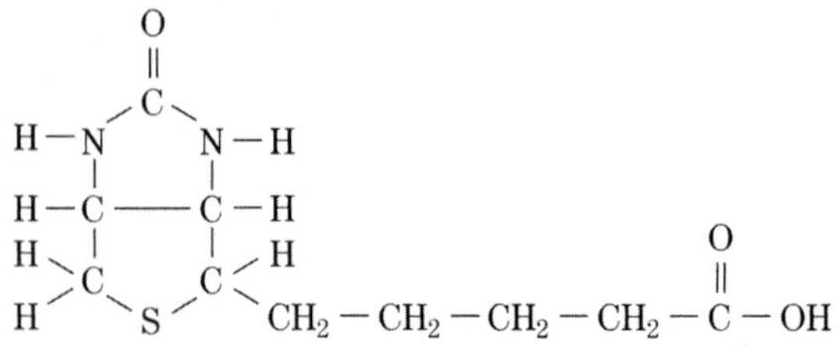

Biotin

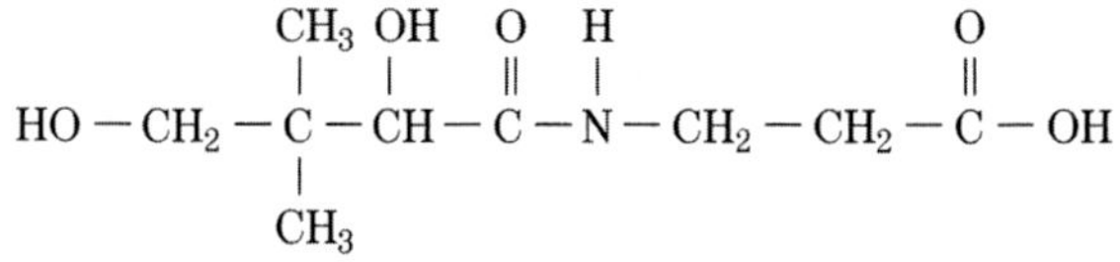

Pantothenic acid

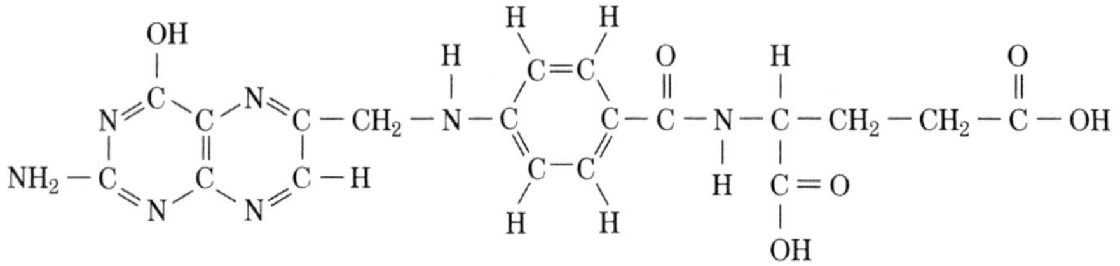

Folate (folic acid form)

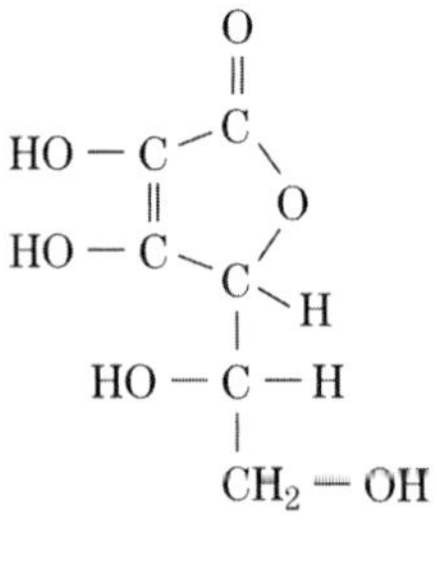

Vitamin C (ascorbic acid)

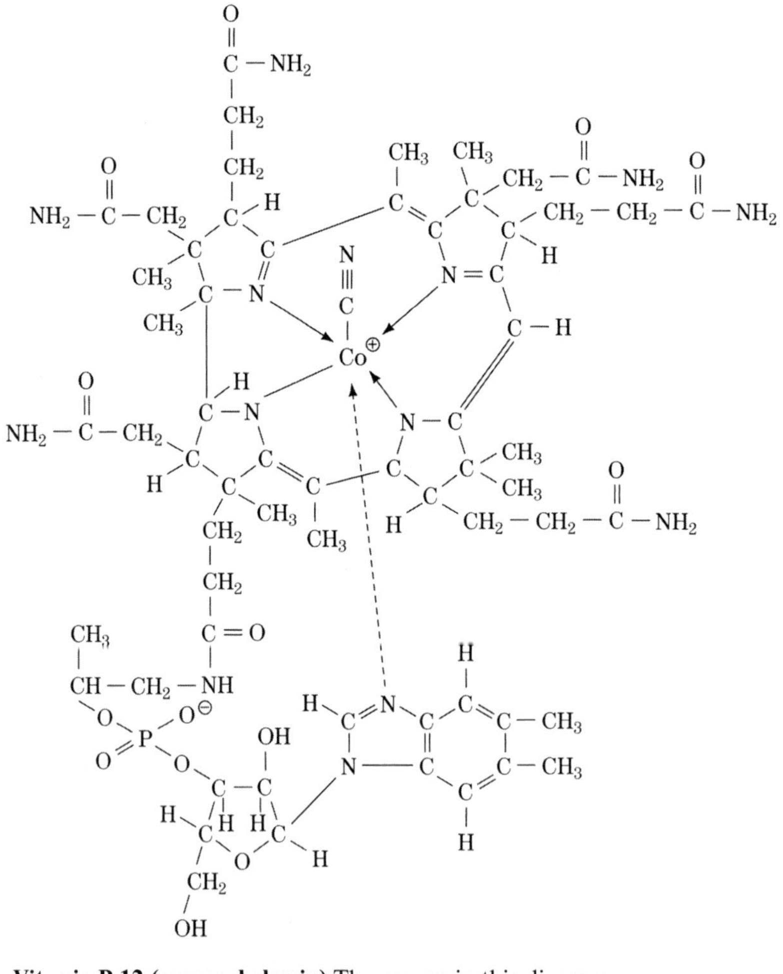

Vitamin B-12 (cyanocobalamin) The arrows in this diagram indicate that the spare electrons on the nitrogens are attracted to the cobalt atom.

Ketone bodies

$$CH_3-\overset{\overset{O}{\|}}{C}-CH_2-\overset{\overset{O}{\|}}{C}-OH$$
Acetoacetic acid

$\xrightarrow{-CO_2}$ $CH_3-\overset{\overset{O}{\|}}{C}-CH_3$ Acetone

$\xrightarrow{2H^+}$ $CH_3-\overset{\overset{OH}{|}}{CH}-CH_2-\overset{\overset{O}{\|}}{C}-OH$ ß-Hydroxybutyric acid

Adenosine triphosphate (ATP)

Triphosphate:
- HO—P(=O)(OH)—O— ← Point of cleavage to yield ADP and energy release
- HO—P(=O)—O—
- HO—P(=O)—O—

Adenine (attached via N to ribose)

Ribose (a sugar): CH₂—O ring with C–H, OH, OH substituents

Appendix E

English-Metric Conversions and Metric Units

Metric-English Conversions

LENGTH

English (USA)	Metric
inch (in)	= 2.54 cm, 25.4 mm
foot (ft)	= 0.30 m, 30.48 cm
yard (yd)	= 0.91 m, 91.4 cm
mile (mi) (statute) (5280 ft)	= 1.61 km, 1609 m
mile (mi) (nautical) (6077 ft, 1.15 statute mi)	= 1.85 km, 1850 m

Metric	English (USA)
millimeter (mm)	= 0.039 in (thickness of a dime)
centimeter (cm)	= 0.39 in
meter (m)	= 3.28 ft, 39.37 in
kilometer (km)	= 0.62 mi, 1091 yd, 3273 ft

WEIGHT

English (USA)	Metric
grain	= 64.80 mg
ounce (oz)	= 28.35 g
pound (lb)	= 453.60 g, 0.45 kg
ton (short—2000 lb)	= 0.91 metric ton (907 kg)

Metric	English (USA)
milligram (mg)	= 0.002 grain (0.000035 oz)
gram (g)	= 0.04 oz (1/28 of an oz)
kilogram (kg)	= 35.27 oz, 2.20 lb
metric ton (1000 kg)	= 1.10 tons

VOLUME

English (USA)	Metric
cubic inch	= 16.39 cc
cubic foot	= 0.03 m^3
cubic yard	= 0.765 m^3
teaspoon (tsp)	= 5 ml
tablespoon (tbsp)	= 15 ml
fluid ounce (fl oz)	= 0.03 liter (30 ml)*
cup (c)	= 237 ml
pint (pt)	= 0.47 liter
quart (qt)	= 0.95 liter
gallon (gal)	= 3.79 liters

Metric	English (USA)
milliliter (ml)	= 0.03 oz
liter (L)	= 2.12 pt
liter	= 1.06 qt
liter	= 0.27 gal

1 liter ÷ 1000 = 1 milliliter or 1 cubic centimeter (10^{-3} liter)
1 liter ÷ 1,000,000 = 1 microliter (10^{-6} liter)

*Note: 1 ml = 1 cc.

Metric and Other Common Units

Unit/Abbreviation	Other Equivalent Measure
milligram (mg)	(1) 1000 of a gram (g)
microgram (mcg)	(1) 1,000,000 of a gram (g)
deciliter (dl)	(1) 10 of a liter (about ½ cup)
milliliter (ml)	(1) 1000 of a liter (5 ml is about 1 tsp)
International Unit (IU)	Crude measure of vitamin activity generally based on growth rate seen in animals

Household Units

3 teaspoons	= 1 tablespoon	= 15 grams
4 tablespoons	= ¼ cup	= 60 grams
5⅓ tablespoons	= ⅓ cup	= 80 grams
8 tablespoons	= ½ cup	= 120 grams
10⅔ tablespoons	= ⅔ cup	= 160 grams
16 tablespoons	= 1 cup	= 240 grams
1 tablespoon	= ½ fluid ounce	= 15 milliliters
1 cup	= 8 fluid ounces	= 237 milliliters
1 cup	= ½ pint	= 240 grams
2 cups	= 1 pint	= 480 grams
4 cups	= 1 quart	= 960 grams = 1 liter
2 pints	= 1 quart	= 960 grams = 1 liter
4 quarts	= 1 gallon	= 3840 grams = 4 liters

Fahrenheit-Celsius Conversion Scale

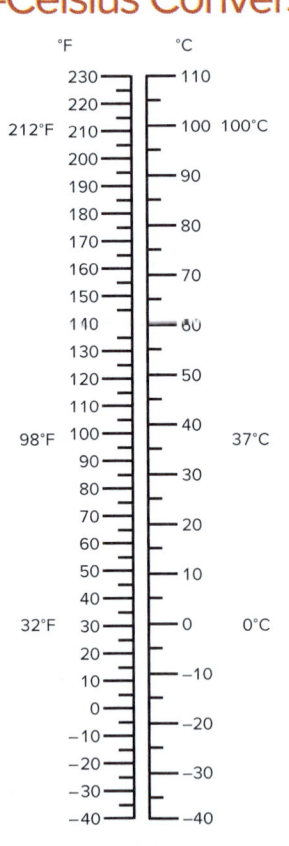

Appendix F
Dietary Reference Intakes

TABLE F-1 ■ Summary Table of EER Equations by Age, Sex, Physical Activity, and Energy Cost of Growth: Children and Adolescents

Age Group	Sex	PAL Category	EER Equation (kcal/day)
0 to 2.99 months	M	—	EER = −716.45 − (1.00 × age) + (17.82 × height) + (15.06 × weight) + 200
	F	—	EER = −69.15 + (80.0 × age) + (2.65 × height) + (54.15 × weight) + 180
3 to 5.99 months	M	—	EER = −716.45 − (1.00 × age) + (17.82 × height) + (15.06 × weight) + 50
	F	—	EER = −69.15 + (80.0 × age) + (2.65 × height) + (54.15 × weight) + 60
6 months to 2.99 years	M	—	EER = −716.45 − (1.00 × age) + (17.82 × height) + (15.06 × weight) + 20
	F	—	EER = −69.15 + (80.0 × age) + (2.65 × height) + (54.15 × weight) + 20/15[a]
3 to 13.99 years	M	Inactive	EER = −447.51 + (3.68 × age) + (13.01 × height) + (13.15 × weight) + 20/15/25[b]
		Low active	EER = 19.12 + (3.68 × age) + (8.62 × height) + (20.28 × weight) + 20/15/25
		Active	EER = −388.19 + (3.68 × age) + (12.66 × height) + (20.46 × weight) + 20/15/25
		Very active	EER = −671.75 + (3.68 × age) + (15.38 × height) + (23.25 × weight) + 20/15/25
	F	Inactive	EER = 55.59 − (22.25 × age) + (8.43 × height) + (17.07 × weight) + 15/30[c]
		Low active	EER = −297.54 − (22.25 × age) + (12.77 × height) + (14.73 × weight) + 15/30
		Active	EER = −189.55 − (22.25 × age) + (11.74 × height) + (18.34 × weight) + 15/30
		Very active	EER = −709.59 − (22.25 × age) + (18.22 × height) + (14.25 × weight) + 15/30
14 to 18.99 years	M	Inactive	EER = −447.51 + (3.68 × age) + (13.01 × height) + (13.15 × weight) + 20
		Low active	EER = 19.12 + (3.68 × age) + (8.62 × height) + (20.28 × weight) + 20
		Active	EER = −388.19 + (3.68 × age) + (12.66 × height) + (20.46 × weight) + 20
		Very active	EER = −671.75 + (3.68 × age) + (15.38 × height) + (23.25 × weight) + 20
	F	Inactive	EER = 55.59 − (22.25 × age) + (8.43 × height) + (17.07 × weight) + 20
		Low active	EER = −297.54 − (22.25 × age) + (12.77 × height) + (14.73 × weight) + 20
		Active	EER = −189.55 − (22.25 × age) + (11.74 × height) + (18.34 × weight) + 20
		Very active	EER = −709.59 − (22.25 × age) + (18.22 × height) + (14.25 × weight) + 20

NOTES: kcal/day = kilocalories per day; PAL = physical activity level; EER = Estimated Energy Requirement. Age is in years, weight is in kilograms, and height is in centimeters.

[a] Energy cost of growth for girls: 6 to 11.99 months: 20 kcal/day; 12 to 35.99 months: 15 kcal/day.

[b] Energy cost of growth for boys: 3 years: 20 kcal/day; 4 to 8 years: 15 kcal/day; 9 to 13 years: 25 kcal/day.

[c] Energy cost of growth for girls: 3 years: 15 kcal/day; 4 to 8 years: 15 kcal/day; 9 to 13 years: 30 kcal/day.

Source: National Academies of Sciences, Engineering, and Medicine. *Dietary Reference Intakes for Energy*. Washington, DC: The National Academies Press; 2023. https://doi.org/10.17226/26818

TABLE F-2 ■ Summary Table of EER Equations Based on TEE Prediction by Age, Sex, and Physical Activity: Adults

Age Group	Sex	PAL Category	EER Equation (kcal/day)
19+ years	M	Inactive	EER = 753.07 − (10.83 × age) + (6.50 × height) + (14.10 × weight)
		Low active	EER = 581.47 − (10.83 × age) + (8.30 × height) + (14.94 × weight)
		Active	EER = 1,004.82 − (10.83 × age) + (6.52 × height) + (15.91 × weight)
		Very active	EER = −517.88 − (10.83 × age) + (15.61 × height) + (19.11 × weight)
	F	Inactive	EER = 584.90 − (7.01 × age) + (5.72 × height) + (11.71 × weight)
		Low active	EER = 575.77 − (7.01 × age) + (6.60 × height) + (12.14 × weight)
		Active	EER = 710.25 − (7.01 × age) + (6.54 × height) + (12.34 × weight)
		Very active	EER = 511.83 − (7.01 × age) + (9.07 × height) + (12.56 × weight)

NOTES: kcal/day = kilocalories per day; PAL = physical activity level; EER = Estimated Energy Requirement; TEE = total energy expenditure. For weight stable adults, EER (kcal/day) = TEE (kcal/day). Age is in years, weight is in kilograms, and height is in centimeters.

Source: National Academies of Sciences, Engineering, and Medicine. *Dietary Reference Intakes for Energy*. Washington, DC: The National Academies Press; 2023. https://doi.org/10.17226/26818

TABLE F-3 ■ Summary Table of EER Equations for Pregnant Women During the Second and Third Trimesters of Pregnancy

Life Stage	PAL Category	EER Equation (kcal/day)
2nd and 3rd trimester of pregnancy[a]	Inactive	EER = 1,131.20 − (2.04 × age) + (0.34 × height) + (12.15 × weight) + (9.16 × gestation) + energy deposition
	Low active	EER = 693.35 − (2.04 × age) + (5.73 × height) + (10.20 × weight) + (9.16 × gestation) + energy deposition
	Active	EER = −223.84 − (2.04 × age) + (13.23 × height) + (8.15 × weight) + (9.16 × gestation) + energy deposition
	Very active	EER = −779.72 − (2.04 × age) + (18.45 × height) + (8.73 × weight) + (9.16 × gestation) + energy deposition

NOTES: For pregnancy: EER (kcal/day) = TEE (kcal/day) + energy deposition (kcal/day). Energy deposition/mobilization (kcal/day) estimated for underweight (UW), normal weight (NW), overweight (OW), and obese (OB) pregnant women during the 2nd and 3rd trimesters of pregnancy: + 300 kcal/day for UW; + 200 kcal/day for NW; + 150 kcal/day for OW; −50 kcal/day for OB. EERs are in kilocalories/day, age is in years, height is in centimeters, weight is in kilograms, gestation is in weeks, energy deposition is in kilocalories/day.

[a] For the 1st trimester of pregnancy, the nonpregnant TEE prediction equation should be used. It is assumed that energy deposition/mobilization is negligible and is therefore ignored.

Source: National Academies of Sciences, Engineering, and Medicine. *Dietary Reference Intakes for Energy*. Washington, DC: The National Academies Press; 2023. https://doi.org/10.17226/26818

TABLE F-4 ■ Summary Table of EER Equations for Women and Girls Exclusively Breastfeeding 0 to 6 Months Postpartum

Age Group	PAL Category	EER Equation (kcal/day)
Females, 19 years and above	Inactive	EER = 584.90 − (7.01 × age) + (5.72 × height) + (11.71 × weight) + energy cost of milk production − energy mobilization
	Low active	EER = 575.77 − (7.01 × age) + (6.60 × height) + (12.14 × weight) + energy cost of milk production − energy mobilization
	Active	EER = 710.25 − (7.01 × age) + (6.54 × height) + (12.34 × weight) + energy cost of milk production − energy mobilization
	Very active	EER = 511.83 − (7.01 × age) + (9.07 × height) + (12.56 × weight) + energy cost of milk production − energy mobilization
Females, < 19 years	Inactive	EER = 55.59 − (22.25 × age) + (8.43 × height) + (17.07 × weight) + energy cost of milk production − energy mobilization
	Low active	EER = −297.54 − (22.25 × age) + (12.77 × height) + (14.73 × weight) + energy cost of milk production − energy mobilization
	Active	EER = −189.55 − (22.25 × age) + (11.74 × height) + (18.34 × weight) + energy cost of milk production − energy mobilization
	Very active	EER = −709.59 − (22.25 × age) + (18.22 × height) + (14.25 × weight) + energy cost of milk production − energy mobilization

NOTES: For exclusively breastfeeding 0 to 6 months postpartum: EER (kcal/day) = TEE (kcal/day) + energy cost of milk production (kcal/day) − energy mobilization (kcal/day). Energy cost of milk production estimated for females exclusively breastfeeding 0 to 6 months postpartum: 540 kcal/day. Energy mobilization estimated for females exclusively breastfeeding 0 to 6 months postpartum: 140 kcal/day. EERs are in kilocalories/day, age is in years, height is in centimeters, weight is in kilograms, energy cost of milk production is in kilocalories/day, and energy mobilization is in kilocalories/day.

Source: National Academies of Sciences, Engineering, and Medicine. *Dietary Reference Intakes for Energy*. Washington, DC: The National Academies Press; 2023. https://doi.org/10.17226/26818

TABLE F-5 ■ **Summary Table of EER Equations for Women and Girls Partially Breastfeeding 7 to 12 Months Postpartum**

Age Group	PAL Category	EER Equation (kcal/day)
Females, 19 years and above	Inactive	EER = 584.90 − (7.01 × age) + (5.72 × height) + (11.71 × weight) + energy cost of milk production
	Low active	EER = 575.77 − (7.01 × age) + (6.60 × height) + (12.14 × weight) + energy cost of milk production
	Active	EER = 710.25 − (7.01 × age) + (6.54 × height) + (12.34 × weight) + energy cost of milk production
	Very active	EER = 511.83 − (7.01 × age) + (9.07 × height) + (12.56 × weight) + energy cost of milk production
Females, < 19 years	Inactive	EER = 55.59 − (22.25 × age) + (8.43 × height) + (17.07 × weight) + energy cost of milk production
	Low active	EER = −297.54 − (22.25 × age) + (12.77 × height) + (14.73 × weight) + energy cost of milk production
	Active	EER = −189.55 − (22.25 × age) + (11.74 × height) + (18.34 × weight) + energy cost of milk production
	Very active	EER = −709.59 − (22.25 × age) + (18.22 × height) + (14.25 × weight) + energy cost of milk production

NOTES: For partially breastfeeding 7 to 12 months postpartum: EER (kcal/day) = TEE (kcal/day) + energy cost of milk production (kcal/day). Energy cost of milk production estimated for females partially breastfeeding 7 to 12 months postpartum: 380 kcal/day. EERs are in kilocalories/day, age is in years, height is in centimeters, weight is in kilograms, and energy cost of milk production is in kilocalories/day.

Source: National Academies of Sciences, Engineering, and Medicine. *Dietary Reference Intakes for Energy*. Washington, DC: The National Academies Press; 2023. https://doi.org/10.17226/26818

TABLE F-6 ■ **Acceptable Macronutrient Distribution Ranges**

	Range (percent of energy)		
Macronutrient	Children, 1–3 y	Children, 4–18 y	Adults
Fat	30–40	25–35	20–35
omega-6 polyunsaturated fats (linoleic acid)	5–10	5–10	5–10
omega-3 polyunsaturated fats[a] (a-linolenic acid)	0.6–1.2	0.6–1.2	0.6–1.2
Carbohydrate	45–65	45–65	45–65
Protein	5–20	10–30	10–35

[a] Approximately 10% of the total can come from longer-chain n-3 fatty acids.

Source: *Dietary Reference Intakes for Energy, Carbohydrate, Fiber, Fat, Fatty Acids, Cholesterol, Protein, and Amino Acids* (2002). The report may be accessed via www.nap.edu.

From the *Dietary Reference Intakes* series, National Academies Press. Copyright 1997, 1998, 2000, 2001, 2011, by the National Academy of Sciences. The full reports are available from the National Academies Press at www.nap.edu.

TABLE F-7 ■ DIETARY REFERENCE INTAKES (DRIS): RECOMMENDED INTAKES FOR INDIVIDUALS, MACRONUTRIENTS
Food and Nutrition Board, Institute of Medicine, National Academies

Life Stage Group	Carbohydrate (g/d)	Total Fiber (g/d)	Fat (g/d)	Linoleic Acid (g/d)	α-Linolenic Acid (g/d)	Protein[a] (g/d)
Infants						
0–6 mo	60*	ND	31*	4.4*	0.5*	9.1*
7–12 mo	95*	ND	30*	4.6*	0.5*	**11.0**
Children						
1–3 y	**130**	19*	ND[b]	7*	0.7*	**13**
4–8 y	**130**	25*	ND	10*	0.9*	**19**
Males						
9–13 y	**130**	31*	ND	12*	1.2*	**34**
14–18 y	**130**	38*	ND	16*	1.6*	**52**
19–30 y	**130**	38*	ND	17*	1.6*	**56**
31–50 y	**130**	38*	ND	17*	1.6*	**56**
51–70 y	**130**	30*	ND	14*	1.6*	**56**
> 70 y	**130**	30*	ND	14*	1.6*	**56**
Females						
9–13 y	**130**	26*	ND	10*	1.0*	**34**
14–18 y	**130**	26*	ND	11*	1.1*	**46**
19–30 y	**130**	25*	ND	12*	1.1*	**46**
31–50 y	**130**	25*	ND	12*	1.1*	**46**
51–70 y	**130**	21*	ND	11*	1.1*	**46**
> 70 y	**130**	21*	ND	11*	1.1*	**46**
Pregnancy						
14–18 y	**175**	28*	ND	13*	1.4*	**71**
19–30 y	**175**	28*	ND	13*	1.4*	**71**
31–50 y	**175**	28*	ND	13*	1.4*	**71**
Lactation						
14–18 y	**210**	29*	ND	13*	1.3*	**71**
19–30 y	**210**	29*	ND	13*	1.3*	**71**
31–50 y	**210**	29*	ND	13*	1.3*	**71**

NOTE: This table presents Recommended Dietary Allowances (RDAs) in **bold type** and Adequate Intakes (AIs) in ordinary type followed by an asterisk (*). RDAs and AIs may both be used as goals for individual intake. RDAs are set to meet the needs of almost all (97% to 98%) individuals in a group. For healthy breastfed infants, the AI is the mean intake. The AI for other life stage and gender groups is believed to cover needs of all individuals in the group, but lack of data or uncertainty in the data prevents being able to specify with confidence the percentage of individuals covered by this intake.

[a] Based on 0.8 g protein/kg body weight for reference body weight.

[b] ND = not determinable at this time.

Sources: *Dietary Reference Intakes for Energy, Carbohydrate, Fiber, Fat, Fatty Acids, Cholesterol, Protein, and Amino Acids* (2002). This report may be accessed via www.nap.edu.

Source: The *Dietary Reference Intake* series, National Academies Press. Copyright 1997, 1998, 2000, 2001, by the National Academy of Sciences. The full reports are available from the National Academies Press at www.nap.edu.

TABLE F-8 ■ DIETARY REFERENCE INTAKES (DRIS): RECOMMENDED INTAKES FOR INDIVIDUALS, ELECTROLYTES AND WATER
Food and Nutrition Board, Health and Medicine Division, National Academies

Life Stage Group	Sodium (mg/d)	Sodium CDRR[a]	Potassium (mg/d)	Chloride (mg/d)	Water (L/d)
Infants					
0–6 mo	110*	ND[b]	400*	180*	0.7*
7–12 mo	370*	ND[b]	860*	570*	0.8*
Children					
1–3 y	800*	Reduce intakes if above 1200 mg/day[c]	2000*	1500*	1.3*
4–8 y	1000*	Reduce intakes if above 1500 mg/day[c]	2300*	1900*	1.7*
Males					
9–13 y	1200*	Reduce intakes if above 1800 mg/day[c]	2500*	2300*	2.4*
14–18 y	1500*	Reduce intakes if above 2300 mg/day[c]	3000*	2300*	3.3*
19–30 y	1500*	Reduce intakes if above 2300 mg/day	3400*	2300*	3.7*
31–50 y	1500*	Reduce intakes if above 2300 mg/day	3400*	2300*	3.7*
51–70 y	1500*	Reduce intakes if above 2300 mg/day	3400*	2000*	3.7*
> 70 y	1500*	Reduce intakes if above 2300 mg/day	3400*	1800*	3.7*
Females					
9–13 y	1200*	Reduce intakes if above 1800 mg/day[c]	2300*	2300*	2.1*
14–18 y	1500*	Reduce intakes if above 2300 mg/day[c]	2300*	2300*	2.3*
19–30 y	1500*	Reduce intakes if above 2300 mg/day	2600*	2300*	2.7*
31–50 y	1500*	Reduce intakes if above 2300 mg/day	2600*	2300*	2.7*
51–70 y	1500*	Reduce intakes if above 2300 mg/day	2600*	2000*	2.7*
> 70 y	1500*	Reduce intakes if above 2300 mg/day	2600*	1800*	2.7*
Pregnancy					
14–18 y	1500*	Reduce intakes if above 2300 mg/day[c]	2600*	2300*	3.0*
19–30 y	1500*	Reduce intakes if above 2300 mg/day	2900*	2300*	3.0*
31–50 y	1500*	Reduce intakes if above 2300 mg/day	2900*	2300*	3.0*
Lactation					
14–18 y	1500*	Reduce intakes if above 2300 mg/day[c]	2500*	2300*	3.8*
19–30 y	1500*	Reduce intakes if above 2300 mg/day	2800*	2300*	3.8*
31–50 y	1500*	Reduce intakes if above 2300 mg/day	2800*	2300*	3.8*

NOTE: This table is adapted from the *DRI reports*. See www.nap.edu. Adequate Intakes (AIs) are followed by an asterisk (*). These may be used as a goal for individual intake. For healthy breastfed infants, the AI is the average intake. The AI for other life stage and gender groups is believed to cover the needs of all individuals in the group, but lack of data prevents being able to specify with confidence the percentage of individuals covered by this intake; therefore, no Recommended Dietary Allowance (RDA) was set.

[a] CDRR = Chronic Disease Risk Reduction Intakes.

[b] Not determined owing to insufficient strength of evidence for causality and intake-response.

[c] Extrapolated from the adult CDRR based on sedentary Estimated Energy Requirements.

Sources: National Academies of Sciences, Engineering, and Medicine. *Dietary Reference Intakes for Sodium and Potassium*. The National Academies Press, Washington, DC, 2019; and *Dietary Reference Intakes for Water, Potassium, Sodium, Chloride, and Sulfate* (2005). These reports may be accessed via www.nap.edu.

TABLE F-9 ■ RECOMMENDED INTAKES FOR INDIVIDUALS, VITAMINS
Food and Nutrition Board, Institute of Medicine, National Academies

Life Stage Group	Vitamin A (μg/d)[a]	Vitamin C (mg/d)	Vitamin D (μg/d)[b,c]	Vitamin E (mg/d)[d]	Vitamin K (μg/d)	Thiamin (mg/d)	Riboflavin (mg/d)	Niacin (mg/d)[e]	Vitamin B-6 (mg/d)	Folate (μg/d)[f]	Vitamin B-12 (μg/d)	Pantothenic Acid (mg/d)	Biotin (μg/d)	Choline (mg/d)[g]
Infants														
0–6 mo	400*	40*	10	4*	2.0*	0.2*	0.3*	2*	0.1*	65*	0.4*	1.7*	5*	125*
7–12 mo	500*	50*	10	5*	2.5*	0.3*	0.4*	4*	0.3*	80*	0.5*	1.8*	6*	150*
Children														
1–3 y	300	15	15	6	30*	0.5	0.5	6	0.5	150	0.9	2*	8*	200*
4–8 y	400	25	15	7	55*	0.6	0.6	8	0.6	200	1.2	3*	12*	250*
Males														
9–13 y	600	45	15	11	60*	0.9	0.9	12	1.0	300	1.8	4*	20*	375*
14–18 y	900	75	15	15	75*	1.2	1.3	16	1.3	400	2.4	5*	25*	550*
19–30 y	900	90	15	15	120*	1.2	1.3	16	1.3	400	2.4	5*	30*	550*
31–50 y	900	90	15	15	120*	1.2	1.3	16	1.3	400	2.4	5*	30*	550*
51–70 y	900	90	15	15	120*	1.2	1.3	16	1.7	400	2.4[h]	5*	30*	550*
>70 y	900	90	20	15	120*	1.2	1.3	16	1.7	400	2.4[h]	5*	30*	550*
Females														
9–13 y	600	45	15	11	60*	0.9	0.9	12	1.0	300	1.8	4*	20*	375*
14–18 y	700	65	15	15	75*	1.0	1.0	14	1.2	400[i]	2.4	5*	25*	400*
19–30 y	700	75	15	15	90*	1.1	1.1	14	1.3	400[i]	2.4	5*	30*	425*
31–50 y	700	75	15	15	90*	1.1	1.1	14	1.3	400[i]	2.4	5*	30*	425*
51–70 y	700	75	15	15	90*	1.1	1.1	14	1.5	400	2.4[h]	5*	30*	425*
>70 y	700	75	20	15	90*	1.1	1.1	14	1.5	400	2.4[h]	5*	30*	425*
Pregnancy														
14–18 y	750	80	15	15	75*	1.4	1.4	18	1.9	600[j]	2.6	6*	30*	450*
19–30 y	770	85	15	15	90*	1.4	1.4	18	1.9	600[j]	2.6	6*	30*	450*
31–50 y	770	85	15	15	90*	1.4	1.4	18	1.9	600[j]	2.6	6*	30*	450*
Lactation														
14–18 y	1200	115	15	19	75*	1.4	1.6	17	2.0	500	2.8	7*	35*	550*
19–30 y	1300	120	15	19	90*	1.4	1.6	17	2.0	500	2.8	7*	35*	550*
31–50 y	1300	120	15	19	90*	1.4	1.6	17	2.0	500	2.8	7*	35*	550*

mg = milligram; μg = microgram

NOTE: This table (taken from the *DRI reports*; see www.nap.edu) presents Recommended Dietary Allowances (RDAs) in **bold type** and Adequate Intakes (AIs) in ordinary type followed by an asterisk (*). RDAs and AIs may both be used as goals for individual intake. RDAs are set to meet the needs of almost all (97 to 98%) individuals in a group. For healthy breastfed infants, the AI is the mean intake. The AI for other life stage and gender groups is believed to cover needs of all individuals in the group, but lack of data or uncertainty in the data prevents being able to specify with confidence the percentage of individuals covered by this intake.

[a] As retinol activity equivalents (RAEs). 1 RAE = 1 μg retinol, 12 μg β-carotene, 24 μg α-carotene, or 24 μg ß-cryptoxanthin. To calculate RAEs from REs of provitamin A carotenoids in foods, divide the REs by 2. For preformed vitamin A in foods or supplements and for provitamin A carotenoids in supplements, 1 RE = 1 RAE.

[b] Cholecalciferol. 1 μg cholecalciferol = 40 IU vitamin D.

[c] In the absence of adequate exposure to sunlight.

[d] As α-tocopherol. α-Tocopherol includes RRR-α-tocopherol, the only form of α-tocopherol that occurs naturally in foods, and the 2R-stereoisomeric forms of α-tocopherol (RRR-, RSR-, RRS-, and RSS-α-tocopherol) that occur in fortified foods and supplements. It does not include the 2S-stereoisomeric forms of α-tocopherol (SRR-, SSR-, SRS-, and SSS-α-tocopherol), also found in fortified foods and supplements.

[e] As niacin equivalents (NE). 1 mg of niacin = 60 mg of tryptophan; 0–6 months = preformed niacin (not NE).

[f] As dietary folate equivalents (DFE). 1 DFE = 1 μg food folate = 0.6 μg of folic acid from fortified food or as a supplement consumed with food = 0.5 μg of a supplement taken on an empty stomach.

[g] Although AIs have been set for choline, there are few data to assess whether a dietary supply of choline is needed at all stages of the life cycle, and it may be that the choline requirement can be met by endogenous synthesis at some of these stages.

[h] Because 10% to 30% of older people may malabsorb food-bound B-12, it is advisable for those older than 50 years to meet their RDA mainly by consuming foods fortified with B-12 or a supplement containing B-12.

[i] In view of evidence linking folate intake with neural tube defects in the fetus, it is recommended that all women capable of becoming pregnant consume 400 μg from supplements or fortified foods in addition to intake of food folate from a varied diet.

[j] It is assumed that women will continue consuming 400 μg from supplements or fortified food until their pregnancy is confirmed and they enter prenatal care, which ordinarily occurs after the end of the periconceptional period—the critical time for formation of the neural tube.

Source: From the *Dietary Reference Intakes* series, National Academies Press. Copyright 1997, 1998, 2000, 2001, 2011, by the National Academy of Sciences. The full reports are available from the National Academies Press at www.nap.edu.

TABLE F-10 ■ DIETARY REFERENCE INTAKES (DRIS): RECOMMENDED INTAKES FOR INDIVIDUALS, ELEMENTS
Food and Nutrition Board, Institute of Medicine, National Academies

Life Stage Group	Calcium (mg/d)	Chromium (μg/d)	Copper (μg/d)	Fluoride (mg/d)	Iodine (μg/d)	Iron (mg/d)	Magnesium (mg/d)	Manganese (mg/d)	Molybdenum (μg/d)	Phosphorus (mg/d)	Selenium (μg/d)	Zinc (mg/d)
Infants												
0–6 mo	200*	0.2*	200*	0.01*	110*	0.27*	30*	0.003*	2*	100*	15*	2*
7–12 mo	260*	5.5*	220*	0.5*	130*	11	75*	0.6*	3*	275*	20*	3
Children												
1–3 y	700	11*	340	0.7*	90	7	80	1.2*	17	460	20	3
4–8 y	1000	15*	440	1*	90	10	130	1.5*	22	500	30	5
Males												
9–13 y	1300	25*	700	2*	120	8	240	1.9*	34	1250	40	8
14–18 y	1300	35*	890	3*	150	11	410	2.2*	43	1250	55	11
19–30 y	1000	35*	900	4*	150	8	400	2.3*	45	700	55	11
31–50 y	1000	35*	900	4*	150	8	420	2.3*	45	700	55	11
51–70 y	1000	30*	900	4*	150	8	420	2.3*	45	700	55	11
> 70 y	1200	30*	900	4*	150	8	420	2.3*	45	700	55	11
Females												
9–13 y	1300	21*	700	2*	120	8	240	1.6*	34	1250	40	8
14–18 y	1300	24*	890	3*	150	15	360	1.6*	43	1250	55	9
19–30 y	1000	25*	900	3*	150	18	310	1.8*	45	700	55	8
31–50 y	1000	25*	900	3*	150	18	320	1.8*	45	700	55	8
51–70 y	1200	20*	900	3*	150	8	320	1.8*	45	700	55	8
> 70 y	1200	20*	900	3*	150	8	320	1.8*	45	700	55	8
Pregnancy												
14–18 y	1300	29*	1000	3*	220	27	400	2.0*	50	1250	60	12
19–30 y	1000	30*	1000	3*	220	27	350	2.0*	50	700	60	11
31–50 y	1000	30*	1000	3*	220	27	360	2.0*	50	700	60	11
Lactation												
14–18 y	1300	44*	1300	3*	290	10	360	2.6*	50	1250	70	13
19–30 y	1000	45*	1300	3*	290	9	310	2.6*	50	700	70	12
31–50 y	1000	45*	1300	3*	290	9	320	2.6*	50	700	70	12

NOTE: This table presents Recommended Dietary Allowances (RDAs) in **bold type** and Adequate Intakes (AIs) in ordinary type followed by an asterisk (*). RDAs and AIs may both be used as goals for individual intake. RDAs are set to meet the needs of almost all (97% to 98%) individuals in a group. For healthy breastfed infants, the AI is the mean intake. The AI for other life stage and gender groups is believed to cover needs of all individuals in the group, but lack of data or uncertainty in the data prevents being able to specify with confidence the percentage of individuals covered by this intake.

Sources: *Dietary Reference Intakes for Calcium, Phosphorus, Magnesium, Vitamin D, and Fluoride* (1997); *Dietary Reference Intakes for Thiamin, Riboflavin, Niacin, Vitamin B-6, Folate, Vitamin B-12, Pantothenic Acid, Biotin, and Choline* (1998); *Dietary Reference Intakes for Vitamin C, Vitamin E, Selenium, and Carotenoids* (2000); *Dietary Reference Intakes for Vitamin A, Vitamin K, Arsenic, Boron, Chromium, Copper, Iodine, Iron, Manganese, Molybdenum, Nickel, Silicon, Vanadium, and Zinc* (2001); and *Dietary Reference Intakes for Calcium and Vitamin D* (2011). These reports may be accessed via www.nap.edu.

Source: *Dietary Reference Intake* series, National Academies Press. Copyright 1997, 1998, 2000, 2001, and 2011 by the National Academy of Sciences. The full reports are available from the National Academies Press at www.nap.edu.

TABLE F-11 ■ DIETARY REFERENCE INTAKES (DRIS): TOLERABLE UPPER INTAKE LEVELS (UL[a]), VITAMINS
Food and Nutrition Board, Institute of Medicine, National Academies

Life Stage Group	Vitamin A (μg/d)[b]	Vitamin C (mg/d)	Vitamin D (μg/d)	Vitamin E (mg/d)[c,d]	Vitamin K	Thiamin	Riboflavin	Niacin (mg/d)[d]	Vitamin B-6 (mg/d)	Folate (μg/d)[d]	Vitamin B-12	Pantothenic Acid	Biotin	Choline (g/d)	Carotenoids[e]
Infants															
0–6 mo	600	ND[f]	25	ND	ND	ND	ND	ND	ND	ND	ND	ND	ND	ND	ND
7–12 mo	600	ND	38	ND	ND	ND	ND	ND	ND	ND	ND	ND	ND	ND	ND
Children															
1–3 y	600	400	63	200	ND	ND	ND	10	30	300	ND	ND	ND	1.0	ND
4–8 y	900	650	75	300	ND	ND	ND	15	40	400	ND	ND	ND	1.0	ND
Males, Females															
9–13 y	1700	1200	100	600	ND	ND	ND	20	60	600	ND	ND	ND	2.0	ND
14–18 y	2800	1800	100	800	ND	ND	ND	30	80	800	ND	ND	ND	3.0	ND
19–70 y	3000	2000	100	1000	ND	ND	ND	35	100	1000	ND	ND	ND	3.5	ND
>70 y	3000	2000	100	1000	ND	ND	ND	35	100	1000	ND	ND	ND	3.5	ND
Pregnancy															
14–18 y	2800	1800	100	800	ND	ND	ND	30	80	800	ND	ND	ND	3.0	ND
19–50 y	3000	2000	100	1000	ND	ND	ND	35	100	1000	ND	ND	ND	3.5	ND
Lactation															
14–18 y	2800	1800	100	800	ND	ND	ND	30	80	800	ND	ND	ND	3.0	ND
19–50 y	3000	2000	100	1000	ND	ND	ND	35	100	1000	ND	ND	ND	3.5	ND

[a] UL = The maximum level of daily nutrient intake likely to pose no risk of adverse effects. Unless otherwise specified, the UL represents total intake from food, water, and supplements. Due to lack of suitable data, ULs could not be established for vitamin K, thiamin, riboflavin, vitamin B-12, pantothenic acid, biotin, or carotenoids. In the absence of ULs, extra caution may be warranted in consuming levels above recommended intakes.

[b] As preformed vitamin A only.

[c] As α-tocopherol; applies to any form of supplemental α-tocopherol.

[d] The ULs for vitamin E, niacin, and folate apply to synthetic forms obtained from supplements, fortified foods, or a combination of the two.

[e] β-Carotene supplements are advised only to serve as a provitamin A source for individuals at risk of vitamin A deficiency.

[f] ND = Not determinable due to lack of data of adverse effects in this age group and concern with regard to lack of ability to handle excess amounts. Source of intake should be from food only to prevent high levels of intake.

Sources: *Dietary Reference Intakes for Calcium and Vitamin D* (2011); *Dietary Reference Intakes for Calcium, Phosphorus, Magnesium, Vitamin D, and Fluoride* (1997); *Dietary Reference Intakes for Thiamin, Riboflavin, Niacin, Vitamin B-6, Folate, Vitamin B-12, Pantothenic Acid, Biotin, and Choline* (1998); *Dietary Reference Intakes for Vitamin C, Vitamin E, Selenium, and Carotenoids* (2000); and *Dietary Reference Intakes for Vitamin A, Vitamin K, Arsenic, Boron, Chromium, Copper, Iodine, Iron, Manganese, Molybdenum, Nickel, Silicon, Vanadium and Zinc* (2001). These reports may be accessed via www.nap.edu.

From the *Dietary Reference Intakes* series, National Academies Press. Copyright 1997, 1998, 2000, 2001, 2011, by the National Academy of Sciences. The full reports are available from the National Academies Press at www.nap.edu.

TABLE F-12 ■ **DIETARY REFERENCE INTAKES (DRIS): TOLERABLE UPPER INTAKE LEVELS (UL[a]), ELEMENTS AND ELECTROLYTES[b]**
Food and Nutrition Board, Institute of Medicine, National Academies

Life Stage Group	Boron (mg/d)	Calcium (g/d)	Copper (µg/d)	Fluoride (mg/d)	Iodine (µg/d)	Iron (mg/d)	Magnesium (mg/d)[c]	Manganese (mg/d)	Molybdenum (µg/d)	Nickel (mg/d)	Phosphorus (g/d)	Selenium (µg/d)	Vanadium (mg/d)[d]	Zinc (mg/d)	Sodium	Potassium	Chloride (mg/d)
Infants																	
0–6 mo	ND[e]	1	ND	0.7	ND	40	ND	ND	ND	ND	ND	45	ND	4	ND	ND	ND
7–12 mo	ND	1.5	ND	0.9	ND	40	ND	ND	ND	ND	ND	60	ND	5	ND	ND	ND
Children																	
1–3 y	3	2.5	1000	1.3	200	40	65	2	300	0.2	3	90	ND	7	ND	ND	2300
4–8 y	6	2.5	3000	2.2	300	40	110	3	600	0.3	3	150	ND	12	ND	ND	2900
Males, Females																	
9–13 y	11	3	5000	10	600	40	350	6	1100	0.6	4	280	ND	23	ND	ND	3400
14–18 y	17	3	8000	10	900	45	350	9	1700	1.0	4	400	ND	34	ND	ND	3600
19–70 y	20	2.5[f]	10000	10	1100	45	350	11	2000	1.0	4	400	1.8	40	ND	ND	3600
>70 y	20	2	10000	10	1100	45	350	11	2000	1.0	3	400	1.8	40	ND	ND	3600
Pregnancy																	
14–18 y	17	3	8000	10	900	45	350	9	1700	1.0	3.5	400	ND	34	ND	ND	3600
19–50 y	20	2.5	10000	10	1100	45	350	11	2000	1.0	3.5	400	ND	40	ND	ND	3600
Lactation																	
14–18 y	17	3	8000	10	900	45	350	9	1700	1.0	4	400	ND	34	ND	ND	3600
19–50 y	20	2.5	10000	10	1100	45	350	11	2000	1.0	4	400	ND	40	ND	ND	3600

[a] UL = The maximum level of daily nutrient intake that is likely to pose no risk of adverse effects. Unless otherwise specified, the UL represents total intake from food, water, and supplements. Due to lack of suitable data, ULs could not be established for arsenic, chromium, and silicon. In the absence of ULs, extra caution may be warranted in consuming levels above recommended intakes.

[b] Although silicon has not been shown to cause adverse effects in humans, there is no justification for adding silicon to supplements.

[c] The ULs for magnesium represent intake from a pharmacological agent only and do not include intake from food and water.

[d] Although vanadium in food has not been shown to cause adverse effects in humans, there is no justification for adding vanadium to food, and vanadium supplements should be used with caution. The UL is based on adverse effects in laboratory animals, and this data could be used to set a UL for adults but not children and adolescents.

[e] ND = Not determinable due to lack of data of adverse effects in this age group and concern with regard to lack of ability to handle excess amounts.

[f] Upper Limit declines to 2 after age 50.

Sources: *Dietary Reference Intakes for Calcium and Vitamin D* (2011); *Dietary Reference Intakes for Calcium, Phosphorus, Magnesium, Vitamin D, and Fluoride* (1997); *Dietary Reference Intakes for Thiamin, Riboflavin, Niacin, Vitamin B-6, Folate, Vitamin B-12, Pantothenic Acid, Biotin, and Choline* (1998); *Dietary Reference Intakes for Vitamin C, Vitamin E, Selenium, and Carotenoids* (2000); *Dietary Reference Intakes for Vitamin A, Vitamin K, Arsenic, Boron, Chromium, Copper, Iodine, Iron, Manganese, Molybdenum, Nickel, Silicon, Vanadium, and Zinc* (2001); *Dietary Reference Intakes for Water, Potassium, Sodium, Chloride, and Sulfate* (2004); and *Dietary Reference Intakes for Sodium and Potassium* (2019). These reports may be accessed via www.nap.edu.

From the *Dietary Reference Intakes* series, National Academies Press. Copyright 1997, 1998, 2000, 2001, 2011, and 2019, by the National Academy of Sciences. The full reports are available from the National Academies Press at www.nap.edu.

Glossary

1,25-dihydroxyvitamin D_3 Biologically active form of vitamin D; also called *calcitriol*; sometimes shortened to *1,25(OH)D_3*.

25-hydroxyvitamin D_3 Intermediate form of vitamin D found in blood; also called *calcidiol* or *calcifediol*; sometimes shortened to *25(OH)D_3*.

7-dehydrocholesterol Precursor of vitamin D found in the skin.

absorption The process by which substances are taken up from the GI tract and enter the bloodstream or the lymph.

absorptive cells The intestinal cells that line the villi and participate in nutrient absorption; also known as *enterocytes*.

Acceptable Macronutrient Distribution Range (AMDR) Range of carbohydrate, protein, or fat intake (as a percentage of total calories) that is associated with reduced risk of chronic disease, yet provides adequate amounts of essential nutrients.

acesulfame-K Artificial sweetener that yields no energy to the body; 200 times sweeter than sucrose.

acetaldehyde dehydrogenase An enzyme used in ethanol metabolism that eventually converts acetaldehyde into carbon dioxide and water.

acid group In chemistry, a functional group that consists of a carbon atom that shares bonds with two oxygen atoms. This is the site where fatty acids are linked to glycerol to form triglycerides.

acquired immunodeficiency syndrome (AIDS) Late stage HIV when the body's immune system is badly damaged because of the virus.

active absorption Movement of a substance across a semipermeable membrane from an area of lower solute concentration to an area of higher solute concentration. This type of transport requires energy and a carrier.

adaptive thermogenesis The ability of humans to regulate body temperature within narrow limits (thermoregulation) in response to changes in dietary patterns or environmental temperatures.

added sugars Nutritive sweeteners (e.g., sugars and syrups) that are not naturally present in foods but are added during processing for the purpose of flavoring and/or preserving foods.

additives Substances added to foods, either intentionally or incidentally.

adenosine diphosphate (ADP) A breakdown product of ATP. ADP is synthesized into ATP using energy from foodstuffs and a phosphate group (abbreviated P_i).

adenosine triphosphate (ATP) The main energy currency for cells. ATP energy is used to promote ion pumping, enzyme activity, and muscular contraction.

Adequate Intake (AI) Nutrient intake amount set for any nutrient for which insufficient research is available to establish an RDA. AIs are based on estimates of intakes that appear to maintain a defined nutritional state in a specific life stage.

adipose cell A cell that is specialized for fat storage; also called an *adipocyte*.

adipose tissue Connective tissue made up of cells that store fat; also cushions and insulates the body.

advantame A sweetener similar in structure to aspartame; 20,000 times sweeter than sucrose.

aerobic Requiring oxygen; with reference to physical activity, all forms of activity that are intense enough and performed long enough to maintain or improve an individual's cardiorespiratory fitness.

aging Time-dependent physical and physiological changes in body structure and function that occur normally and progressively throughout adulthood as humans mature and become older.

air displacement A method for estimating body composition that makes use of the volume of space taken up by a body inside a small chamber (Bod Pod®). This tool is also known as *air displacement plethysmography*.

alcohol Ethyl alcohol or ethanol (CH_3CH_2OH) is the compound in alcoholic beverages.

alcohol dehydrogenase An enzyme used in alcohol (ethanol) metabolism that converts alcohol into acetaldehyde.

alcohol-related birth defects (ARBDs) One or more birth defects (e.g., malformations of the heart, bones, kidneys, eyes, or ears) related to confirmed alcohol exposure during gestation.

alcohol-related neurodevelopmental disorders (ARNDs) One or more abnormalities of the central nervous system (e.g., small head size, impaired motor skills, hearing loss, or poor hand–eye coordination) related to confirmed alcohol exposure during gestation.

alcohol use disorder Problem drinking characterized by a compulsive pattern of alcohol use that leads to significant impairment or distress.

aldosterone A hormone that is produced by the adrenal glands when blood volume is low. It acts on the kidneys to conserve sodium (and therefore water) to increase blood volume.

allergen A foreign protein, or antigen, that induces excess production of certain immune system antibodies; subsequent exposure to the same protein leads to allergic symptoms. Whereas all allergens are antigens, not all antigens are allergens.

allulose Naturally occurring sugar in some food sources that is about 70% as sweet as sugar.

alpha-gal syndrome A food allergy to galactose-α-1,3-galactose, an oligosaccharide found in mammalian meat and milk. Onset of the allergy occurs after a tick bite.

alpha-linolenic acid An essential omega-3 fatty acid with 18 carbons and three double bonds.

alveoli (singular: alveolus). Small, saclike structures. Milk is produced in the alveoli of the breast.

Alzheimer's disease A progressive neurodegenerative disease that gradually impairs memory and thinking skills.

amenorrhea Absence of menstrual periods in a female of reproductive age.

amino acid The building block for proteins containing a central carbon atom with nitrogen and other atoms attached.

amniotic fluid The water-based fluid that surrounds the developing fetus within the amniotic sac during gestation. It cushions the developing fetus, allows for fetal movement, maintains the fetal temperature, and facilitates the development of the lungs and digestive system.

amphipathic Having both hydrophobic (fat-soluble) and hydrophilic (water-soluble) parts. Amphipathic molecules can function as emulsifiers.

amylase Starch-digesting enzyme produced by the salivary glands and the pancreas.

amylopectin A digestible branched-chain type of starch composed of glucose units.

amylose A digestible straight-chain type of starch composed of glucose units.

anabolic Relating to pathways that use small, simple compounds to build larger, more complex compounds.

anaerobic Not requiring oxygen; with reference to physical activity, high intensity activity that exceeds the capacity of the cardiovascular system to provide oxygen to muscle cells for the usual oxygen-consuming metabolic pathways.

anal sphincters A group of two sphincters (inner and outer) that help control expulsion of feces from the body.

anaphylaxis A severe allergic response that results in lowered blood pressure and respiratory distress. This can be fatal.

anemia A decreased oxygen-carrying capacity of the blood. This can be caused by many factors, such as iron deficiency or blood loss.

anencephaly Birth defect characterized by the absence of some or all of the brain and skull.

angiotensin A hormone produced by the liver and activated by enzymes from the kidneys. It signals the adrenal glands to produce aldosterone and also directs the kidneys to conserve sodium (and therefore water). Both of these actions have the effect of increasing blood volume.

angular cheilitis Inflammation of the corners of the mouth with painful cracking; also called *cheilosis* or *angular stomatitis*.

animal experiments Use of animals to study disease to understand more about human disease.

anorexia nervosa An eating disorder characterized by extreme restriction of energy intake relative to requirements, leading to significantly low body weight.

anthropometric assessment Measurement of body weight and the lengths and proportions of parts of the body.

antibody Blood protein that binds foreign proteins found in the body; also called *immunoglobulin*.

antidiuretic hormone (ADH) A hormone that is secreted by the pituitary gland when the blood concentration of solutes is high. It causes the kidneys to decrease water excretion, which increases blood volume.

antigen Any substance that induces a state of sensitivity and/or resistance to microorganisms or toxic substances after a lag period; a foreign substance that stimulates a specific aspect of the immune system.

antioxidant A substance that has the ability to prevent or repair the damage caused by oxidation.

anus Last portion of the GI tract; serves as an outlet for the digestive system.

appetite The primarily psychological (external) influences that encourage us to find and eat food, often in the absence of obvious hunger.

arachidonic acid (ARA) An omega-6 fatty acid made from linoleic acid with 20 carbon atoms and 4 carbon-carbon double bonds.

ariboflavinosis A deficiency disease resulting from a riboflavin deficiency; characterized by mouth sores, dermatitis, glossitis, and/or angular cheilitis.

aril Clear, ruby-colored fruit or seed pod that surrounds a tiny, crisp seed inside a pomegranate.

artery A blood vessel that carries blood away from the heart.

artificial sweetener Synthetic types of sugar substitutes that can be used instead of cane sugar or sucrose.

ascending colon Segment of the large intestine that carries feces from the cecum, up the right side of the abdomen, to the transverse colon.

aseptic processing A method by which food and container are separately and simultaneously sterilized; it allows manufacturers to produce boxes of milk that can be stored at room temperature.

aspartame Artificial sweetener made of two amino acids and methanol; about 200 times sweeter than sucrose.

atherosclerosis A buildup of fatty material (plaque) in the arteries, including those surrounding the heart.

atom Smallest combining unit of an element, such as iron or calcium. Atoms consist of protons, neutrons, and electrons.

atopic disease A condition involving an inappropriate immune response to environmental allergens; examples include asthma, eczema, and seasonal allergies.

atypical anorexia nervosa A subthreshold eating disorder in which a person meets most of the criteria for diagnosis of anorexia nervosa, except BMI is within a normal range.

autism spectrum disorder (ASD) A disorder of neurological development characterized by problems with social interaction, verbal and nonverbal communication, and/or unusual, repetitive, or limited activities and interests.

avidin A protein found in egg whites that binds to and decreases the bioavailability of biotin. Cooking denatures avidin.

avoidant/restrictive food intake disorder (ARFID) Eating disorder characterized by failure to meet energy or nutrient needs, resulting in significant weight loss, nutritional deficiencies, or dependence on tube or intravenous feeding; the eating disturbance is not explained by lack of available food, a medical problem, or another eating disorder.

β-glucan Oats and barley are rich sources of these glucose polymers.

baby-led introduction to solid foods A method of introducing developmentally appropriate complementary foods that allows the infant to have greater control over self-feeding; also called *baby-led weaning*.

bacteria Single-cell microorganisms; some produce poisonous toxins, which cause illness in humans. Bacteria can be carried by water, animals, and people. They survive on skin, clothes, and hair and thrive in foods at room temperature. Some can live without oxygen and survive by means of spore formation.

bariatrics The medical specialty focusing on the treatment of obesity.

basal metabolism The minimal amount of calories the body uses to support itself in a fasting state when resting and awake in a warm, quiet environment. It amounts to roughly 1 kcal per kilogram per hour for males and 0.9 kcal per kilogram per hour for females; these values are often referred to as *basal metabolic rate (BMR)*.

benign Noncancerous; tumors that do not spread.

beriberi The thiamin-deficiency disorder characterized by muscle weakness, loss of appetite, nerve degeneration, and sometimes edema.

beta-carotene The orange-yellow pigment in carrots; beta-carotene is the only carotenoid that can be sufficiently absorbed and converted into retinol in the body.

BHA, BHT Butylated hydroxyanisole and butylated hydroxytoluene: two common synthetic antioxidants added to foods.

bicarbonate Alkaline compound produced as part of the body's buffer systems. For example, the pancreas secretes bicarbonate to neutralize the hydrochloric acid in chyme in the small intestine.

bile A liver secretion stored in the gallbladder and released through the common bile duct into the first segment of the small intestine. It is essential for the digestion and absorption of fat.

bile acid A compound produced by the liver. Bile acids are the main component of bile, which aids in emulsification of fat during digestion in the small intestine.

binge drinking Drinking sufficient alcohol within a 2-hour period to increase blood alcohol content to 0.08% or higher; for males, consuming five or more drinks in a row; for females, consuming four or more drinks in a row.

binge eating Consuming an abnormally large amount of food within a short time period (e.g., 2 hours).

binge eating disorder An eating disorder characterized by recurrent episodes of binge eating that are associated with marked distress and lack of control over behavior, but not followed by inappropriate compensatory behaviors to prevent weight gain.

binge eating disorder of limited duration A subthreshold eating disorder in which a person meets all of the criteria for diagnosis of binge eating disorder, except the duration of the disordered eating behavior is less than 3 months.

binge eating disorder of low frequency A subthreshold eating disorder in which a person meets all of the criteria for diagnosis of binge eating disorder, except the frequency of binges is less than once per week.

biochemical assessment Measurement of biochemical functions (e.g., concentrations of nutrient by-products or biologic activities in the blood, feces, or urine) related to a nutrient's function.

bioelectrical impedance analysis (BIA) The method to estimate total body fat that uses a low-energy electrical current. The more fat storage a person has, the more impedance (resistance) to electrical flow will be exhibited.

biofortification Use of selective breeding or other biotechnology to enhance the nutrient content of crops.

biological pest management Control of agricultural pests by using natural predators, parasites, or pathogens. For example, ladybugs can be used to control an aphid infestation.

biotechnology A collection of processes that involves the use of biological systems for altering and, ideally, improving the characteristics of plants, animals, and other forms of life.

bisphenol A (BPA) An organic compound used in the manufacture of plastics and resins, including some materials used to make food containers. BPA may leach into foods and be ingested by humans.

bisphosphonates Drugs that bind minerals and prevent osteoclast breakdown of bone. Examples are alendronate (Fosamax) and risedronate (Actonel).

Bitot's spots Dry, foamy spots made from an accumulation of keratin (a protein) on the surface of the eye; caused by vitamin A deficiency.

body dissatisfaction Negative thoughts or attitudes about one's own body that may arise from a perceived gap between one's own physical appearance and one's ideal of attractiveness.

body dysmorphic disorder (BDD) A psychiatric condition defined as a preoccupation with a perceived defect or flaw in one's physical appearance that is either not noticeable or only slightly observable by others; formally known as *dysmorphophobia*.

body mass index (BMI) Weight (in kilograms) divided by height (in meters) squared; a value of 25 and above indicates overweight, and a value of 30 and above indicates obesity.

bolus A moistened mass of food swallowed from the oral cavity into the pharynx.

bomb calorimeter An instrument used to determine the calorie content of a food.

bond A linkage between two atoms formed by the sharing of electrons, or attractions.

bone mineral density A measure of the amount of the total mineral contained in a certain volume of bone, generally expressed as grams per cubic centimeter.

bone remodeling The chemical process by which bone is broken down and replaced by new bone.

branched-chain amino acids Amino acids with a branching carbon backbone; these are leucine, isoleucine, and valine. All are essential amino acids.

brown adipose tissue A specialized form of adipose (fat) tissue that produces large amounts of heat by metabolizing energy-yielding nutrients without synthesizing much useful energy for the body. The unused energy is released as heat.

buffer Compounds that cause a solution to resist changes in acid–base conditions.

bulimia nervosa An eating disorder characterized by recurrent episodes of binge eating followed by inappropriate compensatory behaviors to prevent weight gain.

bulimia nervosa of limited duration A subthreshold eating disorder in which a person meets all of the criteria for diagnosis of bulimia nervosa, except the duration of the disordered eating behavior is less than 3 months.

bulimia nervosa of low frequency A subthreshold eating disorder in which a person meets all of the criteria for diagnosis of bulimia nervosa, except the frequency of binge-compensate cycles is less than once per week.

calcitonin A hormone made by the thyroid gland that lowers blood calcium by increasing deposition of calcium in the bones and increasing calcium excretion by the kidneys.

cancer A condition characterized by uncontrolled growth of abnormal cells.

capillary A microscopic blood vessel that connects the smallest arteries and veins; site of nutrient, oxygen, and waste exchange between body cells and the blood.

carbohydrate A compound containing carbon, hydrogen, and oxygen atoms. Most are known as *sugars*, *starches*, and *fibers*.

carbohydrate loading A process in which a high-carbohydrate diet is consumed for several days before an athletic event while tapering exercise duration in an attempt to increase muscle glycogen stores.

carbon footprint The greenhouse gas emissions caused by an organization, event, product, or individual.

cardiovascular disease A general term that refers to any disease of the heart and circulatory system. This disease is generally characterized by the deposition of fatty material in the blood vessels (hardening of the arteries), which in turn can lead to organ damage and death. Also termed *coronary heart disease (CHD)* or simply, *heart disease,* as the vessels of the heart are the primary sites of the disease.

cardiovascular system The body system consisting of the heart, blood vessels, and blood. This system transports nutrients, waste products, gases, and hormones throughout the body and plays an important role in immune responses and regulation of body temperature.

carotenoids Phytochemicals with red, orange, and yellow colors found in squash, tomatoes, and stone fruits; some can be converted to vitamin A in the body.

case-control study A study in which individuals who have a disease or condition, such as lung cancer, are compared with individuals who do not have the condition.

case reports Descriptive studies based on uncontrolled observations of individual patients.

catabolic Relating to pathways that break down large compounds into smaller compounds.

catalase Enzyme that catalyzes the decomposition of hydrogen peroxide into water and oxygen.

cecum A pouch at the first part of the large intestine that houses many bacteria.

celiac disease Chronic, immune-mediated disease precipitated by exposure to dietary gluten in genetically predisposed people.

cell The structural basis of plant and animal organization. In animals it is bounded by a cell membrane. Cells have the ability to take up compounds from and excrete compounds into their surroundings.

cellular differentiation The process of a less-specialized cell becoming a more specialized type. An example is when stem cells in the bone marrow become red and white blood cells.

cellulose An indigestible, insoluble, straight-chain polysaccharide made of glucose molecules and found in plant cell walls.

cerebrospinal fluid The water-based fluid that surrounds the brain and spinal cord. It cushions these structures and allows for the delivery of oxygen and nutrients and the removal of wastes.

ceruloplasmin Copper-containing protein in the blood; functions in the transport of iron.

chemical reaction An interaction between two chemicals that changes both chemicals.

cholecystokinin A hormone produced by the small intestinal cells that stimulates enzyme release from the pancreas and bile release from the gallbladder.

cholesterol A waxy lipid found in all body cells. It has a structure containing multiple chemical rings. Cholesterol is found only in food ingredients of animal origin.

chromosome A single, large DNA molecule and its associated proteins; contains many genes to store and transmit genetic information.

chronic disease The result of a combination of genetic, physiological, environmental, and behavioral factors leading to diseases of long duration. Also referred to as *noncommunicable diseases (NCDs)*.

Chronic Disease Risk Reduction Intake (CDRR) Category of DRIs based upon chronic disease risk.

chronic kidney disease A condition characterized by the gradual loss of kidney function over time, which can lead to the buildup of waste products in the blood.

chylomicron Lipoprotein made of dietary fats surrounded by a shell of cholesterol, phospholipids, and protein. Chylomicrons are formed in the absorptive cells of the small intestine after fat absorption and travel through the lymphatic system to the bloodstream.

chylomicron remnant Lipoprotein that remains after triglycerides have been removed from a chylomicron; composed of protein, phospholipids, and cholesterol.

chyme A mixture of stomach secretions and partially digested food.

chymotrypsin A protein-digesting enzyme secreted by the pancreas to act in the small intestine.

cirrhosis A loss of functioning liver cells, which are replaced by nonfunctioning connective tissue. Any substance that poisons liver cells can lead to cirrhosis. The most common cause is chronic, excessive alcohol intake. Exposure to certain industrial chemicals also can lead to cirrhosis.

***cis* fatty acid** A form of an unsaturated fatty acid that has the hydrogens lying on the same side of the carbon-carbon double bond.

clinical assessment Examination of general appearance of skin, eyes, and tongue; sense of touch; ability to cough and walk; and evidence of rapid hair loss.

coenzyme An organic compound that combines with an inactive enzyme to form a catalytically active form. In this manner, coenzymes aid in enzyme function.

cofactor An inorganic compound (e.g., mineral) that combines with an inactive enzyme to form a catalytically active form.

cognitive behavioral therapy Psychological therapy in which the person's assumptions about dieting, body weight, and related issues are confronted. New ways of thinking are explored and then practiced by the person. In this way, an individual can learn new ways to control disordered eating behaviors and related life stress.

cohort studies Observational studies that look at large groups of people, prospectively or retrospectively, studying their exposure to certain risk factors for disease.

colostrum The first fluid secreted by the breast during late pregnancy and the first few days after birth. This thick fluid is rich in immune factors and protein.

community-supported agriculture (CSA) Farms that are supported by a community of growers and consumers who provide mutual support and share the risks and benefits of food production, usually including a system of weekly delivery or pickup of vegetables and fruit, and sometimes dairy products and meat.

compensatory behaviors Actions taken to rid the body of excess calories and/or to alleviate guilt or anxiety associated with a binge. Examples include purging (i.e., self-induced vomiting or abusing laxatives), fasting, or excessive exercise.

complementary foods Solid or semi solid foods that are introduced to an infant's dietary pattern to complement (not replace) breast milk or infant formula during the latter part of the first year of life. These foods provide energy and essential nutrients to meet the infant's requirements for growth and development.

complementary proteins Two food protein sources that make up for each other's inadequate supply of specific essential amino acids; together, they yield a sufficient amount of all nine essential amino acids and so provide high-quality (complete) protein for the diet.

complex carbohydrate Carbohydrate composed of many monosaccharide molecules. Examples include glycogen, starch, and fiber.

compression of morbidity Delay of the onset of disabilities caused by chronic disease.

concentration The amount of a solute dissolved in a solvent; usually expressed as mass per unit of volume (e.g., milligrams per deciliter).

conditionally essential amino acids Nonessential amino acids that cannot be made in adequate amounts to support the body's increased requirements during conditions of rapid growth, disease, or metabolic stress, and therefore become essential (i.e., must be obtained from food).

congenital hypothyroidism A birth defect that impairs thyroid hormone synthesis. If untreated, this can lead to intellectual disability and stunting of growth.

congenital lactase deficiency A rare birth defect resulting in the inability to produce lactase, such that a lactose-free diet is required from birth.

connective tissue Protein tissue that holds different structures in the body together. Some body structures are made up of connective tissue—notably, tendons and cartilage. Connective tissue also forms part of bone and the nonmuscular structures of arteries and veins.

constipation A condition characterized by difficult and/or infrequent bowel movements (i.e., fewer than three bowel movements per week).

cortical bone The compact or dense bone found on the outer surfaces of bone.

creatine An organic (i.e., carbon-containing) molecule in muscle cells that serves as part of a high-energy compound (termed *creatine phosphate* or *phosphocreatine*) capable of synthesizing ATP from ADP.

cross-contamination Process by which bacteria or other microorganisms are unintentionally transferred from one substance or object to another, with harmful effect.

cross-sectional study Type of observational study that analyzes data from a population group at one specific point in time and based on particular variables of interest.

cytoplasm The fluid and organelles (except the nucleus) in a cell; also called *cytosol*.

Daily Value (DV) Quantity (expressed in percentage) of a specific nutrient that corresponds to the total percentage of the daily requirements for a particular nutrient based on a 2000 kcal diet.

danger zone Temperature range (40°F to 140°F) where bacteria grow most rapidly.

dehydration A harmful condition in which water intake is inadequate to replace losses.

Delaney Clause A clause to the 1958 Food Additives Amendment of the Pure Food and Drug Act in the United States that prevents the intentional (direct) addition to foods of a compound shown to cause cancer in laboratory animals or humans.

dementia A general loss or decrease in mental function.

denaturation Alteration of a protein's three-dimensional structure, usually because of treatment by heat, enzymes, acid or alkaline solutions, or agitation.

dental caries Erosions in the surface of a tooth caused by acids made by bacteria as they metabolize sugars.

deoxyribonucleic acid (DNA) Double strand of nucleic acids that carries hereditary information in cells; DNA directs the synthesis of cell proteins.

depolarization During nerve impulse transmission, the process in which the resting state of the nerve cell membrane (slightly negative charge inside the cell membrane) is temporarily disrupted.

dermatitis Condition that involves itchy, dry skin or a rash on swollen, reddened skin.

descending colon Segment of the large intestine that carries feces from the transverse colon, down the left side of the abdomen, to the sigmoid colon.

diabetes A group of diseases characterized by high blood glucose. Type 1 diabetes involves insufficient or no release of the hormone insulin by the pancreas and therefore requires daily insulin therapy. Type 2 diabetes results from either insufficient release of insulin or general inability of insulin to act on certain body cells, such as muscle cells. Persons with type 2 diabetes may or may not require insulin therapy.

dialysis A medical procedure that removes excess fluid and wastes from the blood when the kidneys are not functioning properly.

diarrhea Increased fluidity, frequency, or amount of bowel movements (i.e., three or more loose stools per day).

diastolic blood pressure The pressure in the arteries when the heart rests between beats and fills with blood and receives oxygen.

dietary assessment Estimation of typical food choices relying mostly on the recounting of one's usual intake or a record of one's previous days' intake.

dietary fiber Indigestible fiber found in food.

dietary pattern The quantity, proportion, variety, or combination of different foods, drinks, and nutrients in diets, and the frequency with which they are habitually consumed.

Dietary Reference Intakes (DRIs) Term used to encompass nutrient recommendations made by the Food and Nutrition Board of the National Academies of Sciences, Engineering, and Medicine. These include RDAs, AIs, EERs, CDRRs, and ULs.

Digestible Indispensable Amino Acid Score (DIAAS) A method of assessing protein quality that compares the amino acid profile of a food protein to human amino acid requirements and also factors in the digestibility of food proteins.

digestion Process by which large ingested molecules are mechanically and chemically broken down to produce basic nutrients that can be absorbed across the wall of the GI tract.

digestive system System consisting of the gastrointestinal tract and accessory structures (liver, gallbladder, and pancreas). This system performs the mechanical and chemical processes of digestion, absorption of nutrients, and elimination of wastes.

diglyceride A breakdown product of a triglyceride consisting of two fatty acids attached to a glycerol backbone.

direct calorimetry A method of determining a body's energy use by measuring heat released from the body. An insulated metabolic chamber is typically used.

direct food additives Additives knowingly (intentionally) incorporated into food products by manufacturers.

disaccharide Class of sugars formed by the chemical bonding of two monosaccharides.

disordered eating Mild and short-term changes in eating patterns that occur in relation to a stressful event, an illness, or a desire to modify one's dietary pattern for a variety of health and personal appearance reasons.

diuretic A substance that increases urinary fluid excretion.

diverticula Pouches that protrude through the exterior wall of the large intestine.

diverticulosis The condition of having many diverticula in the large intestine.

docosahexaenoic acid (DHA) An omega-3 fatty acid with 22 carbons and 6 carbon-carbon double bonds. It is present in large amounts in fatty fish and is slowly synthesized in the body from alpha-linolenic acid. In the human body, high levels of DHA are found in the retina and brain.

dopamine A neurotransmitter involved in memory, concentration, movement, and mood.

double-blind A study or trial in which any information that may influence the behavior of the tester or the subject is withheld until after the test.

dual energy x-ray absorptiometry (DXA) A scientific tool used to measure bone mineral density and body composition.

duodenum First segment of the small intestine that receives chyme from the stomach and digestive juices from the pancreas and gallbladder. This is the site of most chemical digestion of nutrients; approximately 10 inches in length.

dysbiosis A harmful disturbance in the balance of beneficial and pathogenic microorganisms in the microbiota.

early childhood caries Tooth decay that results from formula or juice (and even human milk) bathing the teeth as the child sleeps with a bottle in the mouth. The upper teeth are mostly affected as the lower teeth are protected by the tongue; formerly called *nursing bottle syndrome* or *baby bottle tooth decay.*

eating disorder Severe alterations in eating patterns linked to physiological changes. The alterations are associated with food restriction, binge eating, inappropriate compensatory behaviors, and fluctuations in weight. They also involve a number of emotional and cognitive changes that affect the way a person perceives and experiences their body.

eclampsia A severe form of gestational hypertension accompanied by signs of organ dysfunction and seizures; formerly called *toxemia.*

edema The buildup of excess fluid in extracellular spaces.

eicosanoids A class of signaling compounds, including the prostaglandins, derived from the essential polyunsaturated fatty acids.

eicosapentaenoic acid (EPA) An omega-3 fatty acid with 20 carbons and 5 carbon-carbon double bonds. It is present in large amounts in fatty fish and is slowly synthesized in the body from alpha-linolenic acid.

electrochemical gradient A difference in both the concentration of solutes and the electrical charge across the cell membrane.

electrolyte A mineral that separates into positively or negatively charged ions in water. Electrolytes are able to transmit an electrical current.

elimination diet A restrictive diet that systematically tests foods that may cause an allergic response by first eliminating them for 1 to 2 weeks and then adding them back, one at a time.

embryo In humans, the developing offspring in utero from about the beginning of the third week to the end of the eighth week after conception.

emulsifier A compound that can suspend fat in water by isolating individual fat droplets, using a shell of water molecules or other substances to prevent the fat from coalescing.

endocrine disruptor A natural or synthetic compound that can mimic and interfere with hormones in the body.

endocrine gland A hormone-producing gland.

endocrine system The body system consisting of the various glands and the hormones these glands secrete. This system has major regulatory functions in the body, such as reproduction and cell metabolism.

endoplasmic reticulum (ER) An organelle composed of a network of canals running through the cytoplasm. Part of the endoplasmic reticulum contains ribosomes.

endorphins Natural body tranquilizers that function in pain reduction and may be involved in the feeding response.

energy balance The state in which energy intake, in the form of food and beverages, matches the energy expended, primarily through basal metabolism and physical activity.

energy density A comparison of the calorie (kcal) content of a food with the weight of the food. An energy-dense food is high in calories but weighs very little (e.g., potato chips), whereas a food low in energy density has few calories but weighs a lot (e.g., an orange).

enterohepatic circulation A continual recycling of compounds such as bile acids between the small intestine and the liver.

environmental assessment Includes details about living conditions, education level, and the ability of the person to purchase, transport, and prepare food. The person's weekly budget for food purchases is also a key factor to consider.

enzyme A compound that speeds up the rate of a chemical reaction but is not altered by the reaction. Almost all enzymes are proteins (some are made of genetic material).

epidemiology The study of how disease rates vary among different population groups.

epigenetics The study of heritable changes in gene function that are independent of DNA sequence. For example, malnutrition during pregnancy may modify gene expression in the fetus and affect long-term body weight regulation in the offspring.

epigenome A network of chemical compounds surrounding DNA that modify the genome without altering the DNA sequences and have a role in determining which genes are active (expressed) or inactive (silenced) in a particular cell.

epiglottis The flap that folds down over the trachea during swallowing.

epinephrine A hormone that is released by the adrenal glands (located on each kidney) at times of stress. It acts to increase glycogen breakdown in the liver, among other functions. Also known as *adrenaline*.

epithelial tissue The surface cells that line the outside of the body and all external passages within it.

ergogenic aid A mechanical, nutritional, psychological, pharmacological, or physiological substance or treatment intended to directly improve exercise performance.

esophagus A tube in the GI tract that connects the pharynx with the stomach.

essential amino acids The amino acids that cannot be synthesized by humans in sufficient amounts or at all and therefore must be included in the dietary pattern; there are nine essential amino acids. These are also called *indispensable amino acids*.

essential fatty acids Fatty acids that must be supplied by the diet to maintain health. Currently, only linoleic acid and alpha-linolenic acid are classified as essential.

essential nutrient In nutritional terms, a substance that, when left out of a dietary pattern, leads to signs of poor health. The body either cannot produce this nutrient or cannot produce enough of it to meet its needs. If added back to a dietary pattern before permanent damage occurs, the affected aspects of health are restored.

Estimated Energy Requirement (EER) The average dietary energy intake that is predicted to maintain energy balance in an adult of a defined age, sex, weight, height, and level of physical activity.

ethanol Chemical term for the form of alcohol found in alcoholic beverages.

exercise Physical activities that are planned, repetitive, and intended to improve physical fitness.

extracellular fluid Fluid found outside the cells; it represents about one-third of body fluid.

extracellular space The space outside cells; represents one-third of body fluid.

facilitated diffusion Movement of a substance across a semipermeable membrane from an area of higher solute concentration to an area of lower solute concentration. This type of transport does not require energy, but it does require a carrier.

family-based treatment An intensive outpatient treatment approach for eating disorders that involves the family and teaches the patient how to manage eating and other behaviors in their home environment; also called the *Maudsley method*.

famine An extreme shortage of food, which leads to massive starvation in a population; often associated with crop failures, war, and political unrest.

fat adaptation Manipulating the diet and physical training regimen so that muscles become more efficient at metabolizing fat as fuel during aerobic activity. Also known as *ketoadaptation*.

fat-soluble A group of vitamins that are soluble in dietary fats and are absorbed along with fats in the small intestine. There are four fat-soluble vitamins: Vitamins A, D, E, and K.

fat-soluble vitamins Vitamins that dissolve in fat and some chemical compounds but not readily in water. These vitamins are A, D, E, and K.

fecal impaction The presence of a mass of hard, dry feces that remains in the rectum as a result of chronic constipation.

feces Mass of water, fiber, tough connective tissues, bacterial cells, and sloughed intestinal cells that passes through the large intestine and is excreted through the anus; also called *stool*.

federal poverty level (FPL) An economic measure used to determine if an individual or family qualifies for specific federal benefits and programs; also called *poverty line*.

fermentation The conversion of carbohydrates to alcohols, acids, and carbon dioxide without the use of oxygen.

ferritin A protein that stores iron and releases it in a controlled manner; acts as a buffer against iron deficiency and iron overload.

fetal alcohol spectrum disorders (FASDs) A group of irreversible physical and mental abnormalities in the infant that result from the mother's consumption of alcohol during pregnancy.

fetal alcohol syndrome (FAS) Severe form of FASD that involves abnormal facial features and problems with development of the nervous system and overall growth as a result of maternal alcohol consumption during pregnancy.

fetal macrosomia A condition in which an infant grows excessively large (e.g., birth weight > 4000 grams) in utero, usually as a consequence of maternal hyperglycemia.

fetal origins hypothesis A theory that links nutritional and other environmental factors during gestation to the future health of the offspring.

fetus The developing organism from about the beginning of the ninth week after conception until birth.

fiber Substances in plant foods not digested in the human stomach or small intestine. These add bulk to feces. Fiber naturally found in foods is also called *dietary fiber*.

fibrin An insoluble blood protein that forms a blood clot.

flavonoids Phytochemicals with yellow, red, or blue colors found in citrus fruits, berries, red onion, tea, red wine, and dark chocolate.

fluorosis Discoloration of tooth enamel sometimes accompanied with pitting due to consuming a large amount of fluoride for an extended period.

foam cells Lipid-loaded white blood cells that have surrounded large amounts of a fatty substance, usually cholesterol, on the blood vessel walls.

FODMAPs Fermentable oligosaccharides, disaccharides, monosaccharides, and polyols. These carbohydrates may be poorly digested and lead to GI symptoms such as bloating, gas, and diarrhea in some people.

food allergy An adverse reaction to food that involves an immune response; also called *food hypersensitivity*.

foodborne illness Sickness caused by the ingestion of food containing harmful substances.

food deserts Urban neighborhoods and rural towns without ready access to fresh, healthy, and affordable food. Also referred to as *low-income, low-access areas (LILA)*.

food intolerance An adverse reaction to food that does not involve an immune response.

food jag A period of time (usually a few days or weeks) during which a person will eat only a limited variety of foods.

food security A condition when all people, at all times, have physical and economic access to sufficient safe and nutritious food that meets their dietary needs and food preferences for an active and healthy life.

food waste Food that is edible or fit for consumption which is being discarded as plate waste by consumers and by retailers due to color or appearance.

free radical An unstable atom with an unpaired electron in its outermost shell; also called *reactive oxygen species*.

fructooligosaccharides (FOS) Small, poorly digested carbohydrates made of glucose and fructose; a type of prebiotic found in onion, garlic, leeks, chicory, artichokes, asparagus, and bananas.

fructose A six-carbon monosaccharide that usually exists in a ring form; found in fruits and honey; also known as *fruit sugar*.

fruitarian Referring to a dietary pattern that primarily includes fruits, nuts, honey, and vegetable oils.

functional fiber Indigestible carbohydrates that have beneficial physiological effects in humans.

functional foods Foods that are sources of the chemicals that provide health benefits beyond being essential dietary nutrients.

fungi Simple parasitic life forms, including molds, mildews, yeasts, and mushrooms. They live on dead or decaying organic matter. Fungi can grow as single cells, like yeast, or as a multicellular colony, as seen with molds.

galactooligosaccharides (GOS) Small, poorly digested carbohydrates made of glucose and galactose; a type of prebiotic found in legumes, pistachios, and cashews.

galactose A six-carbon monosaccharide that usually exists in a ring form; closely related to glucose.

galactosemia Inborn error of metabolism in which the enzyme that converts galactose into glucose is missing or deficient.

gallbladder An organ attached to the underside of the liver; site of bile storage, concentration, and eventual secretion.

gastroesophageal reflux disease (GERD) Disease that results from stomach acid backing up into the esophagus. The acid irritates the lining of the esophagus, causing pain.

gastrointestinal (GI) tract The main sites in the body used for digestion and absorption of nutrients. It consists of the mouth, esophagus, stomach, small intestine, large intestine, rectum, and anus. Also called the *digestive tract*.

gene A specific segment on a chromosome. Genes provide the blueprint for the production of cell proteins.

gene expression Use of DNA information on a gene to produce a protein.

generally recognized as safe (GRAS) A list of food additives that in 1958 were considered safe for human consumption. FDA continues to bear responsibility for proving the additives are not safe and can remove unsafe products from the list.

generational poverty Chronic state of poverty lasting for two generations or longer.

gene therapy Altering, replacing, or regulating the expression of genes to prevent or treat disease.

genetically modified organism (GMO) Organisms such as plants, animals, or microorganisms in which the genetic material has been altered by mating or natural recombination.

genetic engineering Manipulation of the genetic makeup of any organism with recombinant DNA technology. This includes DNA insertion, deletion, modification, or replacement. Also referred to as *gene editing* or *genetic editing*.

genome-wide association study (GWAS) Research technique in which the genomes of many human subjects are scanned to identify common genes that are associated with a particular trait or disease.

gestation The period of intrauterine development of offspring, from conception to birth; in humans, normal gestation is 38 to 42 weeks.

gestational diabetes A high blood glucose concentration that develops during pregnancy and returns to normal after birth; one cause is the placental production of hormones that antagonize the regulation of blood glucose by insulin.

gestational hypertension Blood pressure of 140/90 mmHg or higher that is first diagnosed after 20 weeks of gestation. This may evolve into preeclampsia or eclampsia.

ghrelin A hormone produced by stomach cells and the brain that stimulates appetite.

Global Hunger Index (GHI) A tool that tracks the state of hunger worldwide and calls attention to locations where immediate hunger relief is urgently needed.

glossitis Inflammation and swelling of the tongue.

glucagon A hormone made by the pancreas that stimulates the breakdown of glycogen in the liver into glucose; this ends up increasing blood glucose. Glucagon also increases the generation of glucose from noncarbohydrate substances.

glucose A six-carbon sugar that exists in a ring form; found as such in blood and in table sugar bound to fructose; also known as dextrose, it is one of the simple sugars.

glutathione peroxidase An antioxidant enzyme system that requires selenium to convert certain free radicals (peroxides) into less harmful compounds (alcohols and water).

gluten Poorly digested protein found in wheat, barley, and rye.

glycemic index (GI) The blood glucose response of a given food, compared to a standard (typically, glucose or white bread). Glycemic index is influenced by starch structure, fiber content, food processing, physical structure, and macronutrients such as fat in the meal.

glycemic load (GL) A measure of both the quality (GI value) and quantity (grams per serving) of a carbohydrate in a meal.

glycerol A three-carbon alcohol used to form triglycerides.

glycogen A carbohydrate made of multiple units of glucose with a highly branched structure. It is the storage form of glucose in humans and is synthesized (and stored) in the liver and muscles.

goiter An enlargement of the thyroid gland; this is often caused by insufficient iodine in the dietary pattern.

goitrogen A compound that interferes with the uptake or utilization of iodine by the thyroid gland. Food sources of goitrogens include sweet potatoes, broccoli, and soy products.

Golgi complex The cell organelle near the nucleus that packages proteins and lipids for secretion or distribution to other organelles.

gout A form of arthritis caused by the buildup of uric acid crystals in the joints.

green revolution Refers to increases in crop yields that accompanied the introduction of new agricultural technologies in less-developed countries. The key technologies were high-yielding, disease-resistant strains of rice, wheat, and corn; greater use of fertilizer and water; and improved cultivation practices.

growth charts Charts used by health professionals to compare the growth of an individual child to normal patterns of growth in weight, stature, and head circumference over time.

gruel A thin mixture of grains or legumes in milk or water.

gums Polysaccharides occurring naturally that cause an increase in viscosity; used as thickeners, gels, emulsifiers, and stabilizers.

gut-associated lymphoid tissues (GALT) Clusters of lymphoid cells located throughout the gastrointestinal tract that destroy pathogens.

hard water Water that contains high levels of calcium and magnesium.

health disparities Preventable differences in the burden of disease, injury, violence, or opportunities to achieve optimal health that are experienced by socially disadvantaged populations.

Healthy Eating Index (HEI) A measure of diet quality that can be used to assess compliance with the *Dietary Guidelines*.

heart attack Rapid fall in heart function caused by reduced blood flow through the heart's blood vessels. Often part of the heart dies in the process. Technically called a *myocardial infarction*.

heavy drinking Any pattern of alcohol consumption defined as consuming 15 drinks or more per week for males and 8 drinks or more per week for females.

helminth Parasitic worm that can contaminate food, water, feces, animals, and other substances.

hematocrit The percentage of blood made up of red blood cells.

heme iron Iron provided from animal tissues in the form of hemoglobin and myoglobin. Approximately 40% of the iron in meat, fish, and poultry is heme iron; it is readily absorbed.

hemicellulose An insoluble fiber containing xylose, galactose, glucose, and other monosaccharides bonded together.

hemochromatosis A disorder of iron metabolism characterized by increased iron absorption and deposition in the liver and heart. This eventually poisons the cells in those organs.

hemoconcentration Decrease in plasma volume, causing an increase in the concentration of red blood cells and other constituents of the blood.

hemoglobin The iron-containing part of the red blood cell that carries oxygen to the cells and carbon dioxide away from the cells. The heme iron portion is also responsible for the red color of blood.

hemolysis Destruction of red blood cells.

hemolytic uremic syndrome (HUS) Disease characterized by anemia caused by destruction of red blood cells (hemolytic), acute kidney failure (uremic), and a low platelet count.

hemorrhage An escape of blood from blood vessels.

hemorrhagic stroke Damage to part of the brain resulting from rupture of a blood vessel and subsequent bleeding within or over the internal surface of the brain.

hemorrhoid A swollen vein in the rectum or anus.

hepatic portal circulation The portion of the cardiovascular system that uses a large vein (portal vein) to carry nutrient-rich blood from capillaries in the intestines and portions of the stomach to the liver.

hepatic portal vein Large vein that carries absorbed nutrients from the gastrointestinal tract to the liver.

hidden hunger A lack of vitamins and minerals that occurs when the quality of foods people eat does not meet their nutrient requirements.

high-density lipoprotein (HDL) The lipoprotein in the blood that picks up cholesterol from dying cells and other sources and transfers it to the other lipoproteins in the bloodstream or directly to the liver; higher HDL levels are associated with decreased risk for cardiovascular disease, so it is sometimes called *good cholesterol*.

high-fructose corn syrup (HFCS) Corn syrup that has been manufactured to contain between 42% and 55% fructose.

high-quality proteins Dietary proteins that contain ample amounts of all nine essential amino acids; also called *complete proteins*.

homocysteine An amino acid that arises the metabolism of methionine. Vitamin B-6, folate, vitamin B-12, and choline are required for its metabolism. Elevated levels are associated with an increased risk of cardiovascular disease.

hormone A chemical messenger produced by a gland and released into the blood to travel to target tissues at distant sites throughout the body.

hospice care A program offering care that emphasizes comfort and dignity at the end of life.

human immunodeficiency virus (HIV) A virus that attacks cells that fight infection, making a person more susceptible to infections and diseases.

human milk oligosaccharides Small, indigestible carbohydrates made in the human breast from lactose and other simple sugars.

hunger The primarily physiological (internal) drive to find and eat food.

hydrogenation The addition of hydrogen to a carbon-carbon double bond, producing a single carbon-carbon bond with two hydrogens attached to each carbon.

hydrolyzed protein formula Infant formula in which the proteins have been broken down into smaller peptides and amino acids to improve digestibility and reduce exposure to potential food allergens; sometimes called *predigested* or *hypoallergenic infant formula*.

hydroponics This type of agriculture involves growing plants in a nutrient solution root medium in a controlled, soilless environment.

hydroxyapatite Crystalline compound containing calcium, phosphorus, and sometimes fluoride, also known as *bone mineral*.

hygiene hypothesis Assumption that reduced exposure to microorganisms in the environment (e.g., as a result of overuse of antibacterial soaps and antibiotics) impairs proper development of the immune system, making a person more susceptible to allergies and autoimmune diseases.

hyperglycemia High blood glucose, typically defined as above 125 mg/dl while in a fasted state.

hyperkeratosis A condition in which patches of skin become thicker, rougher, or drier than usual; a possible consequence of vitamin A deficiency.

hypertension A condition in which blood pressure remains persistently elevated. Obesity, inactivity, alcohol intake, excess salt intake, and genetics may each contribute to the problem.

hypertonic Having high concentration of solutes.

hypochromic Pale in color (in reference to red blood cells), as could occur with inadequate hemoglobin content.

hypoglycemia A condition caused by low levels of blood sugar that is often related to the treatment of diabetes and often defined by 70 mg/dl or less.

hyponatremia Dangerously low blood sodium level.

hypothalamus A region of the forebrain that controls body temperature, thirst, and hunger.

hypotheses Tentative explanations by a scientist to explain a phenomenon.

hypotonic Having low concentration of solutes.

identical twins Two offspring that develop from a single ovum and sperm and, consequently, are born with the same genetic makeup.

ileocecal sphincter The ring of smooth muscle between the end of the small intestine and the beginning of the large intestine.

ileum Last segment of the small intestine; approximately 5 feet in length.

inborn error of metabolism A genetic condition that affects how specific compounds (e.g., amino acids, fatty acids) are used or broken down in the body.

indirect calorimetry A method to measure energy use by the body by measuring oxygen uptake and carbon dioxide output. Formulas are then used to convert this gas exchange value into energy use, estimating the proportion of energy nutrients that are being oxidized for energy in the fuel mix.

indirect food additives Additives that appear in food products incidentally, from environmental contamination of food ingredients or during the manufacturing process.

infertility Inability of a couple to conceive after 1 year of unprotected intercourse.

inorganic Any substance lacking carbon atoms bonded to hydrogen atoms in the chemical structure.

insoluble fiber A fiber that is not easily metabolized by intestinal bacteria; also called *nonfermentable fiber*.

insulin A hormone produced by the pancreas. Insulin allows for the movement of glucose from the blood into body cells and signals the synthesis of glycogen.

insulin resistance Also known as *impaired insulin sensitivity*, insulin resistance refers to an impaired biological response to insulin that makes it less effective.

intracellular fluid Fluid contained within a cell; it represents about two-thirds of body fluid.

intrinsic factor A protein-like compound produced by the stomach that enhances vitamin B-12 absorption in the ileum.

inulin A mixture of fructose chains that vary in length and occur naturally in plants.

ion A positively or negatively charged atom.

irradiation A process in which radiation energy is applied to foods, creating compounds (free radicals) within the food that destroy cell membranes, break down DNA, link proteins, limit enzyme activity, and alter a variety of other proteins and cell functions of microorganisms that can lead to food spoilage. This process does not make the food radioactive.

ischemic stroke Damage to part of the brain resulting from lack of blood flow to the brain.

isoflavones Phytochemicals produced in legumes; some have hormone-like activities in the body.

isotonic Having equal concentration of solutes.

jejunum Middle segment of the small intestine; approximately 4 feet in length.

ketone bodies Partial breakdown products of fat that contain three or four carbons.

ketosis The condition of having a high concentration of ketone bodies and related breakdown products in the bloodstream and tissues.

kilocalorie (kcal) Heat energy needed to raise the temperature of 1000 grams (1 L) of water 1 degree Celsius.

kwashiorkor A form of protein-calorie malnutrition occurring primarily in young children who have an existing disease and consume a marginal amount of calories and insufficient protein in relation to needs. The child generally suffers from infections and exhibits edema, poor growth, weakness, and an increased susceptibility to further illness.

kyphosis Abnormally increased bending of the spine; commonly known as *dowager's hump*.

lactase An enzyme made by absorptive cells of the small intestine; this enzyme digests lactose to glucose and galactose.

lactate A chemical produced when cells break down carbohydrates for energy; also referred to as *lactic acid*.

lactation The period of milk secretion following pregnancy; typically called *breastfeeding*.

lactation consultant Health care professional (often a registered nurse or RDN) with special training to provide education and support for mothers who are breastfeeding and their infants.

lacteal Lymphatic vessel that absorbs fats from the small intestine.

lactoovovegetarian Referring to a dietary pattern that is primarily plant-based but also includes dairy products and eggs.

lactose A disaccharide consisting of glucose bonded to galactose; also known as *milk sugar*.

lactose intolerance A condition in which symptoms such as abdominal gas and bloating appear as a result of severe lactose maldigestion.

lactovegetarian Referring to a dietary pattern that is primarily plant-based but also includes dairy products.

lanugo Downlike hair that appears after a person has lost much body fat through semistarvation. The hair stands erect and traps air, acting as insulation for the body to compensate for the relative lack of body fat, which usually functions as insulation.

laxative A medication or other substance that stimulates evacuation of the intestinal tract.

lean body mass Body weight minus fat storage weight equals lean body mass. This includes organs such as the brain, muscles, and liver, as well as bone and blood and other body fluids.

lecithin A group of phospholipid compounds that are major components of cell membranes.

lectins Proteins that serve as part of a plant's natural defense system. When ingested intact and in large amounts, they may cause gastrointestinal distress or inflammation or decrease the bioavailability of nutrients.

leptin A hormone made by adipose tissue in proportion to total fat stores in the body that influences long-term regulation of fat mass. Leptin also influences appetite and the release of insulin.

let-down reflex A reflex stimulated by infant suckling that causes the release (ejection) of milk from milk ducts in the mother's breasts; also called *milk ejection reflex*.

life expectancy The average length of life for a given group of people born in a specific year.

life span The potential oldest age a person can reach.

lifetime prevalence The proportion of a population that has had a disease, disorder, or condition at some point during life.

lignin An insoluble noncarbohydrate dietary fiber found in cell walls of woody plants and seeds.

limiting amino acid The essential amino acid in lowest concentration in a food or dietary pattern relative to body needs.

linoleic acid An essential omega-6 fatty acid with 18 carbons and two double bonds.

lipase Fat-digesting enzyme produced by the salivary glands, stomach, and pancreas.

lipid A compound containing much carbon and hydrogen, little oxygen, and sometimes other atoms. Lipids do not dissolve in water and include fats, oils, and cholesterol.

lipoprotein A compound found in the bloodstream containing a core of triglycerides and cholesterol surrounded by a shell of protein and phospholipids.

lipoprotein lipase An enzyme attached to the cells that form the inner lining of blood vessels; it breaks down triglycerides into free fatty acids and glycerol.

lobe A group of several lobules within the human breast; also called a *mammary gland*.

lobule A cluster of alveoli in the human breast.

locavore Someone who eats locally grown food whenever possible.

long-chain fatty acid A fatty acid that contains 12 or more carbons.

low birth weight (LBW) Referring to any infant weighing less than 2.5 kilograms (5.5 pounds) at birth; most commonly results from preterm birth.

low-density lipoprotein (LDL) The lipoprotein in the blood containing primarily cholesterol; elevated LDL is strongly linked to cardiovascular disease risk, so it is sometimes called *bad cholesterol*.

lower-body obesity The type of obesity in which fat storage is primarily located in the buttocks and thigh area. Also known as *gynoid* or *gynecoid obesity*.

lower esophageal sphincter A circular muscle that constricts the opening of the esophagus to the stomach. Also called the *gastroesophageal sphincter* or the *cardiac sphincter*.

lower-quality proteins Dietary proteins that are low in or lack one or more essential amino acids; also called *incomplete proteins*.

lumen The hollow opening inside a tube, such as the GI tract.

luo han guo Extract of the monk fruit, this artificial sweetener is 100 to 250 times sweeter than sucrose.

lymph A clear fluid that flows through lymph vessels; carries most forms of fat after their absorption by the small intestine.

lymphatic system A system of vessels and lymph that accepts fluid surrounding cells and large particles, such as products of fat absorption. Lymph eventually passes into the bloodstream from the lymphatic system.

lymph nodes Clusters of lymphoid tissue, situated along the lymph vessels, that trap and destroy pathogens.

lysosome A cellular organelle that contains digestive enzymes for use inside the cell for turnover of cell parts.

macrocyte A large, immature red blood cell that results from the inability of the cell to divide normally; also called *megaloblast*.

macrocytic anemia Anemia characterized by the presence of abnormally large red blood cells; also called *megaloblastic anemia*.

macronutrient A nutrient needed in gram quantities in a dietary pattern.

macrophages Large white blood cells that arise from monocytes; one of several types of white blood cells that phagocytize pathogens and signal other white blood cells to mount an immune response.

major mineral Vital to health, a mineral that is required in the dietary pattern in amounts greater than 100 milligrams per day.

malignant Malicious; in reference to a tumor, the property of invading surrounding tissues and spreading to distant sites.

malnutrition Failing health that results from chronic eating practices that do not coincide with nutritional needs.

maltase An enzyme made by absorptive cells of the small intestine; this enzyme digests maltose to two glucose molecules.

maltose A disaccharide consisting of glucose bonded to glucose; also known as *malt sugar*.

marasmus A form of protein-calorie malnutrition resulting from consuming a grossly insufficient amount of protein and calories. Victims have little or no fat stores, little muscle mass, and poor strength. Death from infections is common.

medium-chain fatty acid A fatty acid that contains 6 to 10 carbons.

megadose Large intake of a nutrient well beyond estimates of needs or what would be found in a balanced diet; 2 to 10 times above human needs is typically a starting point.

Menkes syndrome An inherited X-linked recessive pattern disorder that affects copper levels in the body.

menopause The cessation of the menstrual cycle in females, usually beginning at about 50 years of age.

messenger RNA (mRNA) A strand of ribonucleic acid that corresponds to a gene to encode a specific protein. In the process of gene expression, mRNA is involved in transcription.

meta-analysis A statistical examination of data from multiple scientific studies of the same subject in order to determine overall trends.

metabolic syndrome A condition in which a person has poor blood glucose regulation, hypertension, increased blood triglycerides, and other health problems. This condition is usually accompanied by obesity, lack of physical activity, and a dietary pattern high in refined carbohydrates. Also called *Syndrome X*.

metabolic water Water formed as a by-product of carbohydrate, lipid, and protein metabolism.

metabolism Chemical processes in the body by which energy is provided in useful forms and vital activities are sustained.

metastasize The spreading of disease from one part of the body to another, even to parts of the body that are remote from the site of the original tumor. Cancer cells can spread via blood vessels, the lymphatic system, or direct growth of the tumor.

methyl group In chemistry, a carbon atom that shares bonds with three hydrogen atoms. The methyl group is the omega end of a fatty acid.

microbiome Entire collection of microorganisms, their genes, and their environment.

microbiota Community of microorganisms living in a particular region; with regard to our discussion of probiotics, the community of microorganisms coexisting on and within the human body.

microcytic Small cell size.

micronutrient A nutrient needed in milligram or microgram quantities in a dietary pattern.

microvilli Extensive folds on the mucosal surface of the absorptive cells.

mineral Element used in the body to promote chemical reactions and to form body structures.

mitochondria (singular: mitochondrion) Organelles that are the main sites of energy production in a cell. They contain the pathway for oxidizing fat for fuel, among other metabolic pathways.

moderate drinking For males, consuming no more than two drinks per day, and for females, consuming no more than one drink per day.

moderate-intensity aerobic physical activity Aerobic activity that increases a person's heart rate and breathing some extent (4–6 on RPE scale). Examples include brisk walking, dancing, swimming, or bicycling on level terrain.

monoglyceride A breakdown product of a triglyceride consisting of one fatty acid attached to a glycerol backbone.

monosaccharide Simple sugar, such as glucose, that is not broken down further during digestion.

monounsaturated fatty acid A fatty acid containing one carbon-carbon double bond.

motility Generally, the ability to move spontaneously. In this context, it refers to movement of food through the GI tract.

mucilage A gelatinous substance of plants that contains protein and polysaccharides and is similar to plant gums.

mucus A thick fluid secreted by many cells throughout the body. It contains a compound that has both carbohydrate and protein parts. It acts as a lubricant and means of protection for cells.

multiple sclerosis An unpredictable disease of the central nervous system that can range from relatively benign to somewhat disabling to devastating, as communication between the brain and other parts of the body is disrupted.

muscle-strengthening activity Physical activity that increases skeletal muscle strength, power, endurance, and mass. Examples include lifting free weights, using weight machines, and calisthenics (e.g., push-ups).

muscle tissue A type of tissue adapted to contract to cause movement.

myelin A combination of lipids and proteins that covers nerve fibers.

myoglobin Iron-containing protein that binds oxygen in muscle tissue.

negative energy balance The state in which energy intake is less than energy expended, resulting in weight loss.

negative protein balance A state in which protein intake is less than related protein losses, such as often seen during acute illness.

neophobia Fear of new things, such as new foods.

neotame General-purpose, nonnutritive sweetener that is approximately 7000 to 13,000 times sweeter than table sugar. It has a chemical structure similar to aspartame.

nephrons The functional units of kidney cells that filter wastes from the bloodstream and deposit them into the urine.

nervous system The body system consisting of the brain, spinal cord, nerves, and sensory receptors. This system detects sensations, directs movements, and controls physiological and intellectual functions.

nervous tissue Tissue composed of highly branched, elongated cells that transport nerve impulses from one part of the body to another.

neural tube defect A defect in the formation of the neural tube occurring during early fetal development. This type of defect results in various nervous system disorders, such as spina bifida. Folate deficiency in a female who is pregnant increases the risk that the fetus will develop this disorder.

neuron The structural and functional unit of the nervous system. Consists of a cell body, dendrites, and an axon.

neurotransmitter A compound made by a nerve cell that allows for communication between it and other cells.

night blindness Vitamin A deficiency disorder that results in loss of the ability to see under low-light conditions.

night eating syndrome An eating disorder characterized by consumption of a large volume of food in the late evening and nocturnal awakenings with ingestion of food.

nitrosamine A carcinogen formed from nitrates and breakdown products of amino acids; associated with cancer risk.

nixtamalization A culinary process in which whole maize (corn) kernels are soaked in a solution of water and calcium hydroxide (lime) or potassium hydroxide (lye) to make hominy and masa.

nonceliac wheat sensitivity (NCWS) One or more of a variety of immune-related conditions with symptoms similar to celiac disease that are precipitated by the ingestion of gluten in people who do not have celiac disease.

nonessential amino acids Amino acids that can be synthesized by a healthy body in sufficient amounts; there are 11 nonessential amino acids. These are also called *dispensable amino acids.*

nonheme iron Iron provided from plant sources, supplements, and animal tissues other than in the forms of hemoglobin and myoglobin. Nonheme iron is less efficiently absorbed than heme iron; absorption is closely dependent on body needs.

nonspecific immunity Defenses that stop the invasion of pathogens; requires no previous encounter with a pathogen; also called *innate immunity.*

nonsteroidal anti-inflammatory drugs (NSAIDs) Medications used to treat painful inflammatory conditions, such as arthritis. Examples: aspirin, ibuprofen (Advil®), and naproxen (Aleve®).

nontropical plant oils Oils derived from plants other than coconut, palm, and palm kernel. Nontropical plant oils are rich in unsaturated fatty acids. Examples: canola oil, grapeseed oil, and olive oil.

norepinephrine A neurotransmitter from nerve endings and a hormone from the adrenal gland. It is released in times of stress and is involved in hunger regulation, blood glucose regulation, and other body processes.

nucleus (plural: nuclei) Membrane-bound organelle that contains the genetic information (DNA) for cell protein synthesis and cell replication.

nutrient density The ratio derived by dividing a food's nutrient content by its calorie content. When the food's overall nutrient contribution exceeds its contribution to our calorie needs, the food is considered to have a favorable nutrient density.

nutrients Chemical substances in food that contribute to health, many of which are essential parts of a dietary pattern. Nutrients nourish us by providing calories to fulfill energy needs, materials for building body parts, and factors to regulate necessary chemical processes in the body.

nutrigenetics A branch of nutritional genomics that studies how genes affect nutritional health, such as variations in nutrient requirements and responsiveness to dietary modifications.

nutrigenomics A branch of nutritional genomics that studies how food impacts health through its interaction with our genes and its subsequent effect on gene expression.

nutritional genomics Study of interactions between nutrition and genetics; includes nutrigenetics and nutrigenomics.

nutritional status The nutritional health of a person as determined by anthropometric measurements (height, weight, circumferences, and so on), biochemical measurements of nutrients or their by-products in blood and urine, a clinical (physical) examination, a dietary analysis, and economic evaluation; also called *nutritional state.*

nutrition literacy Degree to which individuals obtain, process, and understand nutrition information and the skills needed in order to make appropriate nutrition-related decisions.

nutrition security Consistent access, availability, and affordability of foods and beverages that promote well-being, prevent disease, and, if needed, treat disease, particularly among racial/ethnic minority populations, lower income populations, and rural and remote populations.

obesity Ratio of weight to height that is significantly higher than what is associated with optimal health, usually due to excessive body fat. For adults, this is most often defined as BMI of 30 or higher. For children, this is often defined as BMI-for-age at the 95th percentile or higher.

oleogustus A taste for fat. The presence of fatty acids in foods stimulates taste receptors in the mouth; this sensation is unpleasant.

omega-3 (ω-3) fatty acid An unsaturated fatty acid with the first double bond on the third carbon from the methyl end ($-CH_3$).

omega-6 (ω-6) fatty acid An unsaturated fatty acid with the first double bond on the sixth carbon from the methyl end ($-CH_3$).

organ A group of tissues designed to perform a specific function; for example, the heart, which contains muscle tissue, nervous tissue, and so on.

organelles Compartments, particles, or filaments that perform specialized functions within a cell.

organic compounds In chemistry, any chemical compounds that contain carbon.

organic food Food grown without use of pesticides, synthetic fertilizers, sewage sludge, genetically modified organisms, antibiotics, hormones, or ionizing radiation.

organ system A collection of organs that work together to perform an overall function.

orthorexia nervosa A proposed psychological disorder characterized by an obsession with proper or healthful eating.

osmosis The passage of water through a membrane from a less concentrated compartment to a more concentrated compartment.

osteoarthritis A degenerative joint condition caused by a breakdown of cartilage in joints. It often results from wear and tear due to repetitive motions or the pressure of excess body weight.

osteoblast Bone cells that initiate the synthesis of new bone.

osteocalcin Small protein in the organic matrix of bone.

osteoclast Bone cells that break down bone and subsequently release bone minerals into the blood.

osteomalacia Adult form of rickets. The bones have low mineral density and consequently are at risk for fracture.

osteopenia A bone disease defined by low mineral density.

osteoporosis The presence of a stress-induced fracture or a T-score of −2.5 or lower. The bones are porous and fragile due to low mineral density.

overnutrition A state in which nutritional intake greatly exceeds the body's needs.

overweight A ratio of weight to height that is moderately higher than what is associated with optimal health. For adults, this is typically defined as BMI within the range of 25.0 up to 30. For children, this is typically defined as BMI-for-age from the 85th up to the 95th percentile.

ovovegetarian Referring to a dietary pattern that is primarily plant-based but also includes egg products.

ovum The egg cell from which a fetus eventually develops if the egg is fertilized by a sperm cell.

oxalic acid An organic acid found in spinach, rhubarb, and sweet potatoes that can depress the absorption of certain minerals present in the food, such as calcium; also called *oxalate*.

oxidation The process of losing an electron during a chemical reaction.

oxidative stress Imbalance between the production of reactive compounds and the body's ability to protect against their adverse effects.

oxytocin A hormone secreted by the pituitary gland. It causes contraction of the musclelike cells surrounding the ducts of the breasts and the smooth muscle of the uterus.

paraprobiotics Inactivated cells or cell extracts of probiotic microorganisms that may confer health benefits when consumed by humans.

parasite An organism that lives in or on another organism and derives nourishment from it.

parathyroid hormone (PTH) A hormone made by the parathyroid glands that activates the vitamin D hormone and aids calcium release from bone and calcium conservation by the kidneys, among other functions.

Parkinson's disease Disease that belongs to a group of conditions called motor system disorders, which are the result of the loss of dopamine-producing brain cells. The four primary symptoms are tremor, or trembling in hands, arms, legs, jaw, and face; rigidity, or stiffness of the limbs and trunk; bradykinesia, or slowness of movement; and postural instability, or impaired balance and coordination.

passive diffusion Movement of a substance across a semipermeable membrane from an area of higher solute concentration to an area of lower solute concentration. This type of transport does not require a carrier and does not require energy.

pasteurizing The process of heating food products to kill pathogenic microorganisms and reduce the total number of bacteria.

pathogen A microorganism that can cause disease.

pectin A soluble viscous fiber containing chains of monosaccharides and characteristically found between plant cell walls.

pediatric malnutrition An imbalance between nutrient requirements and nutrient intake that results in cumulative deficits of energy, protein, or micronutrients and may negatively impact growth, development, and other physical and mental health outcomes; also called *pediatric undernutrition*.

peer review Evaluation of work by professionals of similar competence (peers) to the producers of the work to maintain standards of quality and credibility. Scholarly peer review is used to determine if a scientific study is suitable for publication.

pellagra Niacin-deficiency disease characterized by dementia, diarrhea, and dermatitis, and possibly leading to death.

People-First Language Linguistic prescription that aims to avoid perceived and subconscious dehumanization when discussing people with disabilities. It can also be applied to any group that is defined by a condition rather than as a people: for example, "those with obesity" rather than "the obese."

pepsin A protein-digesting enzyme produced by the stomach.

peptic ulcer Erosion of the tissue lining, usually in the stomach or the upper small intestine.

peptide bond A chemical bond formed between amino acids in a protein.

percentile With reference to a dataset, the value below which a given percentage of observations fall. For example, a male at the 75th percentile for BMI-for-age has a BMI higher than 74% of other males his age and lower than 25% of other males his age.

perforation A hole made by boring or piercing. With reference to the gastrointestinal tract, the hole is in the wall of the esophagus, stomach, intestine, rectum, or gallbladder. Complications include bleeding and infection.

periodization Cycling the volume, intensity, and activities of workouts throughout the training season.

peristalsis A coordinated muscular contraction used to propel food down the gastrointestinal tract.

pernicious anemia The anemia that results from a lack of vitamin B-12 absorption; it is *pernicious* because of associated nerve degeneration that can result in eventual paralysis and death.

peroxisome A cell organelle that destroys toxic products within the cell.

pescovegetarian Referring to a dietary pattern that is primarily plant-based but also includes fish and other aquatic animal protein. Also called *pescatarian*.

pH A measure of relative acidity or alkalinity of a solution. The pH scale is 0 to 14. A pH of 7 is neutral; a pH below 7 is acidic; a pH above 7 is alkaline.

phagocytosis A process in which a cell forms an indentation, and solid particles enter the indentation and are engulfed by the cell.

pharynx A cavity located at the back of the oral and nasal cavities, commonly known as the throat. It is part of the digestive tract and the respiratory tract.

phenylketonuria (PKU) Disease caused by a defect in the liver's ability to metabolize the amino acid phenylalanine. If left untreated, toxic by-products of phenylalanine build up in the body and lead to brain damage and severe health issues.

phosphocreatine (PCr) A high-energy compound that can be used to reform ATP. It is used primarily during bursts of activity, such as lifting and jumping.

phospholipid Any of a class of fat-related substances that contain phosphorus, fatty acids, and a nitrogen-containing component. Phospholipids are an essential part of every cell.

photosynthesis Process by which plants use energy from the sun to synthesize energy-yielding compounds, such as glucose.

physical activity Any movement of skeletal muscles that requires energy.

physical fitness The ability to perform moderate to vigorous activity without undue fatigue.

physiological anemia The normal decrease in red blood cell concentration in the blood due to increased blood volume during pregnancy; also called *hemodilution*.

phytic acid A constituent of plant fibers that binds positive ions to its multiple phosphate groups; also called *phytate*.

phytochemical A chemical found in plants. Some phytochemicals may contribute to a reduced risk of cancer or cardiovascular disease in people who consume them regularly.

pica A disorder characterized by eating non-food items, such as dirt, laundry starch, or clay.

pinocytosis A process in which a cell forms an indentation, and fluid enters the indentation and is engulfed by the cell.

placebo Generally, an inactive medicine or treatment used to disguise the treatments given to the participants in an experiment.

placenta An organ that forms within the uterus during pregnancy. Through this organ, oxygen and nutrients from the mother's blood are transferred to the fetus, and fetal wastes are removed. The placenta also releases hormones that maintain the state of pregnancy.

plaque A cholesterol-rich substance deposited in the blood vessels; it contains various white blood cells, smooth muscle cells, various proteins, cholesterol and other lipids, and eventually calcium.

plasma The fluid, extracellular portion of blood.

platelets Protoplasmic disks in the blood that promote coagulation; also called *thrombocytes*.

pollovegetarian Referring to a dietary pattern that is primarily plant-based but also includes chicken, turkey, and other poultry.

polycystic ovary syndrome (PCOS) A condition of hormonal imbalance (e.g., elevated testosterone and insulin) in a female that can lead to infertility, weight gain in the abdominal region, excessive growth of body hair, and acne.

polypeptide A group of 10 to 2000 or more amino acids bonded together to form proteins.

polypharmacy A term used to describe the use of multiple medicines simultaneously by an individual.

polysaccharides Complex carbohydrates containing many glucose units, from 10 to 1000 or more. Also called *complex carbohydrates*.

polyunsaturated fatty acid A fatty acid containing two or more carbon-carbon double bonds.

pool The amount of a nutrient stored within the body that can be mobilized when needed.

positive energy balance The state in which energy intake is greater than energy expended, generally resulting in weight gain.

positive protein balance A state in which protein intake exceeds related protein losses, as is needed during times of growth.

postbiotics Metabolic by-products of the microorganisms that colonize the human body.

prebiotic Selectively fermented ingredient that results in specific changes in the composition and/or activity of the gastrointestinal microbiota, thus conferring benefits upon the host.

prediabetes A serious health condition in which blood sugar levels are higher than normal, but not high enough to be diagnosed as type 2 diabetes.

preeclampsia A form of gestational hypertension characterized by signs of organ dysfunction, such as liver or kidney damage and/or blood clotting abnormalities.

preservatives Compounds that extend the shelf life of foods by inhibiting microbial growth or minimizing the destructive effect of oxygen and metals.

preterm Referring to an infant born before 37 weeks of gestation; also referred to as *premature*.

primary hypertension Systolic blood pressure of 130 mmHg or higher and/or diastolic blood pressure of 80 mmHg or higher with no identified cause; also called *essential hypertension*.

primary lactose maldigestion Develops at about age 2 to 5 years when the production of the enzyme lactase decreases. When significant symptoms develop after lactose intake, it is then called *lactose intolerance*.

primary osteoporosis Low bone mineral density that results from changes in bone metabolism caused by aging or imbalances in reproductive hormones.

probiotics Live microorganisms that, when administered in adequate amounts, confer health benefits on the host.

progression Incremental increase in frequency, intensity, and time spent in each type of physical activity over several weeks or months.

prohormone Inactive precursor to a hormone.

prolactin A hormone secreted by the pituitary gland that stimulates the synthesis of milk in the breast.

protein Food and body compounds made of more than 100 amino acids; proteins contain carbon, hydrogen, oxygen, nitrogen, and sometimes other atoms in a specific configuration. Proteins contain the form of nitrogen most easily used by the human body.

protein-calorie malnutrition (PCM) A condition resulting from regularly consuming insufficient amounts of calories and protein. The deficiency eventually results in body wasting, primarily of lean tissue, and an increased susceptibility to infections. Also known as *protein-energy malnutrition (PEM)*.

protein equilibrium A state in which protein intake is equal to related protein losses; the person is said to be in *protein balance*.

protein turnover The process by which cells break down old proteins and resynthesize new proteins. In this way, the cell will have the proteins it needs to function at that time.

proton pump inhibitor (PPI) A medication that inhibits the ability of gastric cells to produce acid.

protozoa (singular, protozoan) One-celled animals that are more complex than bacteria. Disease-causing protozoa can be spread through food and water.

provitamin A A substance that can be converted into vitamin A.

psychiatric genetics The study of the role of genes in the development of mental health disorders.

psyllium Mostly soluble type of dietary fiber found in the seeds of the plantago plant; common ingredient in bulk-forming laxatives, such as Metamucil®.

purging disorder An eating disorder characterized by repeated purging (e.g., by self-induced vomiting) to induce weight loss even in the absence of binge eating.

pyloric sphincter Ring of smooth muscle between the stomach and the small intestine.

pyruvate A three-carbon compound formed during glucose metabolism; also called *pyruvic acid*.

radiation Literally, energy that is emitted from a center in all directions. Various forms of radiation energy include X rays and ultraviolet rays from the sun.

rancidity Production of decomposed fatty acids that have an unpleasant flavor and odor.

randomized controlled trial An experimental design that is double-blind and placebo controlled.

receptor A site in a cell at which compounds (such as hormones) bind. Cells that contain receptors for a specific compound are partially controlled by that compound.

Recommended Dietary Allowance (RDA) Nutrient intake amount sufficient to meet the needs of 97% to 98% of the individuals in a specific life stage.

rectum Terminal section of the large intestine where feces are held prior to expulsion.

red blood cells Cells that transport oxygen and carbon dioxide through the blood; also called *erythrocytes*.

regenerative agriculture A system of farming and grazing practices that aims to reverse climate change by rebuilding soil organic matter and restoring degraded soil biodiversity, resulting in both carbon drawdown and improving the water cycle.

registered dietitian nutritionist (RDN) A person who has completed a degree program approved by the Accreditation Council for Education in Nutrition and Dietetics (ACEND), performed at least 1200 hours of supervised professional practice, passed a national registration examination, and complies with continuing education requirements.

relapse prevention A series of strategies used to help prevent and cope with weight-control lapses, such as recognizing high-risk situations and deciding beforehand on appropriate responses.

relative energy deficiency in sport (RED-S) A syndrome of altered metabolism, immune function, and mental health caused by low energy availability in athletes, which may be due to unintentional failure to meet the high energy demands of sports or intentional restriction of energy intake to control weight.

reserve capacity The extent to which an organ can preserve essentially normal function despite decreasing cell number or cell activity.

resistant starch Indigestible dietary fiber sequestered in plant walls. Bananas and legumes are rich sources.

resorption The process of losing substance. Bone resorption is part of the initial process for remodeling and growth.

responsive feeding A healthy feeding relationship between the caregiver and the child in which the caregiver pays attention to and respects the child's hunger and satiety.

resting metabolism The amount of calories the body uses when the person has not eaten in 4 hours and is resting (e.g., 15 to 30 minutes) and awake in a warm, quiet environment. It is usually slightly higher (~10%) than basal metabolism due to the more flexible testing criteria; often referred to as *resting metabolic rate (RMR)*.

retina A light-sensitive lining in the back of the eye. It contains retinal.

retinal Aldehyde form of vitamin A.

retinoic acid Acid form of vitamin A.

retinoids Chemical forms of preformed vitamin A found in animal foods.

retinol Alcohol form of vitamin A.

retinyl Storage form of vitamin A.

reverse cholesterol transport Process by which HDL picks up cholesterol from the tissues and blood vessels and takes it to the liver for metabolism or excretion.

rheumatoid arthritis A degenerative joint condition resulting from an autoimmune disease that causes inflammation in the joints and other sites of the body.

ribonucleic acid (RNA) The single-stranded nucleic acid involved in the transcription of genetic information and translation of that information into protein structure.

ribosomes Cytoplasmic particles that mediate the linking together of amino acids to form proteins; may exist freely in the cytoplasm or attached to endoplasmic reticulum.

rickets A disease characterized by poor mineralization of newly synthesized bones because of low calcium content. Arising in infants and children, this deficiency is caused by insufficient amounts of vitamin D in the body.

risk factors A term used frequently when discussing the factors contributing to the development of a disease. A risk factor is an aspect of our lives, such as heredity, lifestyle choices (e.g., use of tobacco products), or nutritional habits.

R-proteins Proteins produced by the salivary glands that bind to free vitamin B-12 in the stomach and protect it from stomach acid.

rumination disorder An eating disorder and functional gastrointestinal disorder in which undigested food is regurgitated shortly after a meal, rechewed, then swallowed or spit out; also called *regurgitation syndrome*.

Russell's sign Evidence of abrasion that appears on the knuckles of a person who repeatedly induces vomiting by using the fingers to trigger the gag reflex in the back of the throat; named after the psychiatrist who first identified bulimia nervosa.

saccharin Artificial sweetener that yields no energy to the body; 200 to 700 times sweeter than sucrose.

saliva Watery fluid, produced by the salivary glands in the mouth, which contains lubricants, enzymes, and other substances.

sarcopenia Loss of muscle tissue. Among older adults, this loss of lean mass greatly increases their risk of illness and death.

sarcopenic obesity Advanced muscle loss accompanied by gains in fat mass.

satiety A state in which there is no longer a desire to eat; a feeling of satisfaction.

saturated fatty acid A fatty acid containing no carbon-carbon double bonds.

scavenger cells Specific form of white blood cells that can bury themselves in the artery wall and accumulate LDL. As these cells take up LDL, they contribute to the development of atherosclerosis.

scurvy The vitamin C deficiency disease characterized by weakness, fatigue, slow wound healing, bone pain, fractures, sore and bleeding gums, diarrhea, and pinpoint hemorrhages on the skin.

secondary hypertension Systolic blood pressure of 130 mmHg or higher and/or diastolic blood pressure of 80 mmHg or higher as a result of disease (e.g., kidney dysfunction or sleep apnea) or drug use.

secondary lactose maldigestion Temporary condition in which lactase production is decreased in response to illness or surgery.

secondary osteoporosis Low bone mineral density that results from a chronic condition that accelerates bone loss.

secretory vesicles Membrane-bound vesicles produced by the Golgi complex; contain protein and other compounds to be secreted by the cell.

sequestrants Compounds that bind free metal ions. By so doing, they reduce the ability of ions to cause rancidity in foods containing fat.

serotonin A neurotransmitter involved in the regulation of mood, sleep, and appetite.

set-point theory Theory of weight status that refers to the close regulation of body weight. Although the details remain unclear, there is evidence that complex mechanisms exist that help regulate weight.

short-chain fatty acid A fatty acid with fewer than 6 carbons.

sickle cell disease An illness that results from a malformation of the red blood cell because of an incorrect structure in part of its hemoglobin protein chains; also called *sickle cell anemia*.

sigmoid colon Last segment of the large intestine that carries feces from the descending colon to the rectum.

simple sugar Monosaccharide or disaccharide in the dietary pattern. Also referred to as *sugars* or *simple carbohydrates*.

situational poverty State of poverty caused by specific circumstances such as death, illness, divorce, or catastrophe.

skinfold measurements Skinfold or caliper testing is a common method to determine body fat percentage. This utilizes prediction equations that are population-specific to estimate fat.

small for gestational age (SGA) Referring to infants who weigh less than the expected weight for their length of gestation. This corresponds to less than 2.5 kilograms (5.5 pounds) in a full-term newborn.

soft water Water that contains low levels of calcium and magnesium.

soluble fiber A fiber that is readily fermented by bacteria in the large intestine; also called *viscous fiber*.

solute A substance that dissolves in a solvent to make a solution.

solution Liquid mixture made of a solvent and a solute.

solvent A liquid substance in which other substances dissolve.

sorbitol Alcohol derivative of glucose that yields about 3 kcal/g but is slowly absorbed from the small intestine; used in some sugarless gums and dietetic foods.

specific immunity Function of white blood cells directed at specific antigens; also called *adaptive immunity*.

spina bifida Birth defect resulting from improper closure of the neural tube during embryonic development. The spinal cord or fluid may bulge outside the spinal column.

spontaneous abortion Cessation of pregnancy and expulsion of the embryo or nonviable fetus prior to 20 weeks of gestation. This is the result of natural causes, such as a genetic defect or developmental problem; also called *miscarriage*.

sports anemia Exercise-induced iron-deficiency anemia caused by plasma volume expansion, low hemoglobin synthesis, or increased destruction of red blood cells.

starch A carbohydrate made of multiple units of glucose attached together in a form the body can digest; also known as *complex carbohydrate*.

sterol A compound containing a multi-ring (steroid) structure and a hydroxyl group (–OH). Cholesterol is a typical example.

stevia Artificial sweetener derived from a South American shrub; 200 to 400 times sweeter than sucrose.

stress fracture A fracture that occurs from repeated jarring of a bone. Common sites include bones of the foot and shins.

stroke A decrease or loss in blood flow to the brain that results from a blood clot or other change in arteries in the brain. This in turn causes the death of brain tissue. Also called *cerebrovascular accident*.

stunting Low height (or length) for age, which indicates inadequate growth due to chronic undernutrition.

subclinical Stage of a disease or disorder not severe enough to produce symptoms that can be detected or diagnosed.

subthreshold eating disorder A clinically recognized eating disorder that meets some, but not all, of the criteria for diagnosis of anorexia nervosa, bulimia nervosa, or binge eating disorder.

sucralose Artificial sweetener that has chlorines in place of 3 hydroxyl (–OH) groups on sucrose; 600 times sweeter than sucrose.

sucrase An enzyme made by absorptive cells of the small intestine; this enzyme digests sucrose to glucose and fructose.

sucrose Disaccharide composed of fructose bonded to glucose; also known as *table sugar*.

superoxide dismutase Antioxidant enzyme system that converts certain free radicals (superoxide anions) into less damaging products (oxygen and hydrogen peroxide).

sustainable agriculture Agricultural system that provides a secure living for farm families; maintains the natural environment and resources; supports the rural community; and offers respect and fair treatment to all involved, from farm workers to consumers to the animals raised for food.

sustainable development Economic growth that will simultaneously reduce poverty, protect the environment, and preserve natural capital.

sustainable intensification Agricultural practices that consider whole landscapes, territories, and ecosystems to optimize resource utilization and management.

symptom A change in health status noted by the person with the problem, such as stomach pain.

synapse The space between one neuron and another neuron (or cell).

synbiotic Combination of pro- and prebiotics taken to confer health benefits on the host.

synovial fluid A viscous, water-based fluid that lubricates joints.

systematic review A thorough summary of the results of available carefully designed health care studies (controlled trials) in a particular area.

systolic blood pressure The pressure in blood vessels when the heart beats, squeezing and pushing blood through the arteries to the rest of the body.

teratogen A compound (natural or synthetic) that may cause or increase the risk of a birth defect. Exposure to a teratogen does not always lead to a birth defect; its effects on the fetus depend on the dose, timing, and duration of exposure. Examples: alcohol, some drugs, some industrial or household chemicals, certain infections, and extreme heat.

term Referring to an infant born after a gestational period of 37 weeks up to 42 weeks, counting from the date of the mother's last menstrual period. The American College of Obstetrics and Gynecology further subdivides term pregnancy into *early term* (37 weeks up to 39 weeks), *full term* (39 weeks up to 41 weeks), and *late term* (41 weeks up to 42 weeks).

tetany A body condition marked by sharp contraction of muscles and failure to relax afterward; usually caused by abnormal calcium metabolism.

theory An explanation for a phenomenon that has numerous lines of evidence to support it.

therapeutic phlebotomy Periodic blood removal, as a blood donation, for the purpose of ridding the body of excess iron.

thermic effect of food (TEF) The increase in metabolism that occurs during the digestion, absorption, and metabolism of energy-yielding nutrients. This typically represents 8% to 15% of calories consumed. Also called *diet-induced thermogenesis*.

thyroid hormones Hormones produced by the thyroid gland that regulate growth and metabolic rate.

tissue saturation The limited storage capacity of water-soluble vitamins in the tissues.

tocopherols The chemical name for some forms of vitamin E. The alpha form is the most potent.

Tolerable Upper Intake Level (UL) Maximum chronic daily intake level of a nutrient that is unlikely to cause adverse health effects in almost all people in a specific life stage.

toxicity Capacity of a substance to produce injury or illness at some dosage.

toxins Poisonous compounds produced by an organism that can cause disease.

trabecular bone The less dense, more open structure bone found in the inner layer of bones; also called *cancellous bone*.

trace mineral Vital to health, a mineral that is required in the dietary pattern in amounts less than 100 milligrams per day.

trachea The airway that extends from the throat, down the neck, to the lungs; also called the *windpipe*.

transcription The process by which the code or gene for a protein on a DNA sequence is copied into a single-stranded mRNA molecule that is ready to leave the nucleus.

***trans* fatty acid** A form of an unsaturated fatty acid, usually a monounsaturated one when found in food, in which the hydrogens lie on opposite sides of the carbon-carbon double bond.

transferrin Iron-binding protein; controls the level of free iron in blood.

transfer RNA (tRNA) A type of ribonucleic acid that delivers amino acids to the ribosomes for protein synthesis; tRNA is involved in translation.

translation The process of adding amino acids one at a time to a growing polypeptide chain, according to the instructions on the mRNA.

transverse colon Segment of the large intestine that carries feces from the ascending colon, from right to left across the top of the abdomen, to the descending colon.

triglyceride The major form of lipid in the body and in food. It is composed of three fatty acids attached to glycerol.

trimesters Three 13- to 14-week periods into which the normal pregnancy (on average, 40 weeks) is divided somewhat arbitrarily for purposes of discussion and analysis. Development of the offspring, however, is continuous throughout pregnancy, with no specific physiological markers demarcating the transition from one trimester to the next.

tropical plant oils Oils derived from tropical plants that are high in saturated fatty acids. Examples: coconut oil, palm oil, and palm kernel oil.

trypsin A protein-digesting enzyme secreted by the pancreas to act in the small intestine.

tumor Mass of cells; may be cancerous (malignant) or noncancerous (benign).

type 1 diabetes A form of diabetes characterized by total insulin deficiency due to destruction of insulin-producing cells of the pancreas. Insulin therapy is required.

type 1 osteoporosis Porous trabecular bone characterized by rapid bone demineralization following menopause.

type 2 diabetes A form of diabetes characterized by insulin resistance and often associated with obesity. Insulin therapy may be required in advanced stages of the disease.

type 2 osteoporosis Porous trabecular and cortical bone observed in males and females after the age of 70.

ultra-high temperature (UHT) processing Method of sterilizing food by heating it above 275°F (135°C) for 2 to 5 seconds. Also called *ultra-heat treatment*.

ultraprocessed foods Edible products made with industrial formulations of several ingredients that are derived from whole foods or synthesized by food manufacturers, typically including additives such as flavors, colors, sweeteners, or emulsifiers.

ultratrace mineral A mineral present in the human diet in trace amounts but that has not been shown to be essential to human health.

umami A brothy, meaty, savory flavor in some foods. Monosodium glutamate enhances this flavor when added to foods.

undernutrition Failing health that results from a long-standing dietary intake that is suboptimal and does not meet nutritional needs.

underwater (hydrostatic) weighing This is a method of estimating total body fat by weighing the individual on a standard scale, then weighing the individual again submerged in water. The difference between the two weights is used to estimate total body volume. Also known as *hydrodensitometry*.

underweight Ratio of weight to height that is lower than what is associated with optimal health. For adults, this is defined as BMI less than 18.5. For children, this is defined as BMI-for-age below the 5th percentile.

upper-body obesity The type of obesity in which fat is stored primarily in the abdominal area; defined as a waist circumference more than 40 inches (102 centimeters) in males and more than 35 inches (88 centimeters) in females; closely associated with a high risk for cardiovascular disease, hypertension, and type 2 diabetes. Also known as *android*, *visceral*, or *central obesity*.

urea Nitrogenous waste product of protein metabolism; major source of nitrogen in the urine.

ureter Tube that transports urine from the kidney to the urinary bladder.

urethra Tube that transports urine from the urinary bladder to the outside of the body.

urinary system The body system consisting of the kidneys, urinary bladder, and the ducts that carry urine. This system removes waste products from the blood and regulates blood acid–base balance, overall chemical balance, and water balance in the body.

vegan Referring to a dietary pattern that only includes foods of plant origin.

vein A blood vessel that carries blood to the heart.

very-low-calorie diet (VLCD) This diet allows a person fewer than 800 calories per day, often in liquid form. Of this, 120 to 480 calories are typically from carbohydrate, and the rest are mostly from high-quality protein.

very-low-density lipoprotein (VLDL) The lipoprotein created in the liver that carries cholesterol and lipids that have been taken up or newly synthesized by the liver.

vigorous-intensity aerobic physical activity Aerobic activity that greatly increases a person's heart rate and breathing (7–8 on RPE scale). Examples include jogging, singles tennis, swimming continuous laps, or bicycling uphill.

villi (singular: villus) The fingerlike protrusions into the small intestine that participate in digestion and absorption of food.

virus One of the smallest known types of infectious agents, many of which cause disease in humans. A virus is essentially a piece of genetic material surrounded by a coat of protein. Viruses do not metabolize, grow, or move by themselves. They reproduce only with the aid of a living cellular host.

vitamin An essential organic (carbon-containing) compound needed in small amounts in the dietary pattern to help regulate and support chemical reactions and processes in the body.

vitamin D_2 Form found in nonanimal sources, such as in some mushrooms. Also synthetically produced and included in many supplements; also called *ergocalciferol*.

vitamin D_3 Previtamin form synthesized in the skin and found naturally in some animal sources, including fish and egg yolks; also called *cholecalciferol*.

vitamin K deficiency bleeding Hemorrhage caused by a lack of vitamin K, especially among infants from birth to 6 months of age; also called *hemorrhagic disease of the newborn*.

wasting Low weight for height (thinness) that typically indicates a recent and severe process of weight loss, often associated with acute starvation or severe disease.

water The universal solvent; chemically, H_2O. The body is composed of about 60% water. Water (fluid) needs are about 9 (females) or 13 (males) cups per day; needs are greater if one exercises heavily.

water intoxication Potentially fatal condition that occurs with a high intake of water, which results in a severe dilution of the blood and other fluid compartments.

water-soluble A group of vitamins that dissolve in water and are easily absorbed into the bloodstream. These vitamins are not stored in large amounts in the body and are excreted in the urine. There are nine water-soluble vitamins: vitamin C and eight B vitamins.

water-soluble vitamins Vitamins that dissolve in water. These vitamins are the B vitamins and vitamin C.

weaning The gradual process of switching from breast milk or infant formula to other sources of nutrition for the infant.

weight bias Negative attitudes toward, and beliefs about, others because of their weight that are often manifested by stereotypes or prejudice toward people with overweight and obesity.

wet nursing The practice of breastfeeding (and caring for) another mother's child.

white blood cells Variety of immune cells that circulate in the lymph and blood and work to neutralize, detoxify, and/or destroy pathogens and other foreign proteins; also called *leukocytes*.

whole grains Grains containing the entire seed of the plant, including the bran, germ, and endosperm (starchy interior). Examples are whole wheat bread and brown rice.

Wilson's disease A genetic disorder that results in accumulation of copper in the tissues; characterized by damage to the liver, nervous system, and other organs.

xerophthalmia Hardening of the cornea and drying of the surface of the eye, which can result in blindness as a result of vitamin A deficiency.

xylitol Alcohol derivative of the five-carbon monosaccharide xylose. Absorbed more slowly than sucrose, xylitol supplies 40% fewer calories than table sugar.

zoochemicals Chemicals found in animal products that have health protective actions.

z score A statistical comparison of one measurement to the mean of all measurements. For example, in assessment of child growth, a z score of −1 to −1.9 indicates mild pediatric malnutrition, −2 to −2.9 indicates moderate pediatric malnutrition, and −3 or greater indicates severe pediatric malnutrition.

zygote The fertilized ovum; the cell resulting from the union of an egg cell (ovum) and sperm until it divides.

Index

Note: Page number followed by *f* and *t* indicates figure and table respectively.

A

Abaloparatide (Tymlos), 428
Abortion, spontaneous, 583
Absorption, 94
   active, 100, 102*f*
   of calcium, 390–391, 391*f*
   of carbohydrates, 145
   of chromium, 416
   of copper, 412
   defined, 94
   of fats, 181, 182*f*
   of iron, 400–401
   of minerals, 375
   of phosphorus, 394
   process of, 94, 95*f*, 96
   of proteins, 226–227, 227*f*
   of vitamin B-12, 337, 338*f*
   of vitamin K, 318
   of vitamins, 295–296
   of zinc, 405
Absorptive cells, 100, 101*f*
Accelerometers, 440
Acceptable Daily Intake (ADI), 140
Acceptable Macronutrient Distribution Range (AMDR), 59, 59*t*, 60, 189, A-31
   for proteins, 233
   for total fat intake, 189
Accessory organs, 94, 104–105, 105*f*
ACE (angiotensin-converting enzyme) inhibitors, in hypertension, 420
Acesulfame-K, 140
Acetaldehyde dehydrogenase, 27
Acetylcholine, 344
Acid–base balance
   chloride in, 385
   ketosis and, 147, 287
   kidneys and, 88
   proteins and, 229
Acid group, 166
Acne
   teenagers and, 669
   vitamin A for treatment of, 306
Acquired immunodeficiency syndrome (AIDS), 566
   antiretroviral therapy for, 567
   developing countries and, 566–567
   nutrition and, 567
Active absorption, 100, 102*f*
Adaptive immunity, 93
Adaptive thermogenesis (AT), 252–253
Added sugars, 23, 45, 127, 133, 142, 151
   defined, 139
   infants and, 649
   sources of, 139, 139*f*, 151, 153*f*
   tips for reducing of, 154*t*
Additives, 37, 534–535
   approval for new additive, 538
   defined, 535
   direct, 535, 537
   generally recognized as safe, 536–537
   indirect, 535, 537
   synthetic chemicals, 537
   tests for safety, 537–538
   types of, 535–536*t*
   use of, 535–536
Adenosine diphosphate (ADP), 444, 444*f*
Adenosine triphosphate (ATP), 85, 187, 394, 444, 445, 445*f*
   from aerobic fatty-acid utilization, 447, 447*f*
   aerobic metabolism and, 446
   anaerobic metabolism and, 445, 445*f*
   from carbohydrate, fat, and protein, 446*f*
   chemical structure of, A-27
Adenosine triphosphate-citrate lyase (ACL) inhibitors, 201
Adequate intake (AI), 59–60, 59*t*
   of biotin, 332–333
   of calcium, 387–391
   of carotenoids, 305
   of chloride, 385–386
   of choline, 344–345
   of chromium, 415–416
   of copper, 412
   of essential fatty acids, 189, 189*t*
   of fiber, 151
   of fluoride, 414
   of folate, 335–336
   of iodine, 409–411
   of iron, 401, 402*f*
   of magnesium, 396–397
   of niacin, 327–329
   of pantothenic acid, 329
   of potassium, 383–384
   of riboflavin, 325–326
   of selenium, 406–407
   of sodium, 379–381, 380*f*
   of thiamin, 323
   of vitamin A, 305
   of vitamin B-6, 331
   of vitamin B-12, 339
   of vitamin C, 341–342
   of vitamin D, 309–312
   of vitamin E, 314–315
   of vitamin K, 316, 318
   of water, 369
   of zinc, 404–405
ADH. *See* Antidiuretic hormone
ADI. *See* Acceptable Daily Intake
Adipose cells, 185, 187, 187*f*
Adipose tissue, 111, 187, 251, 582
Adolescence. *See also* Teenagers
   brain health in, 715
   eating disorders during, 479
   EER equation in, A-29
ADP. *See* Adenosine diphosphate
Adrenaline, 90
Adulthood. *See also* Older adults
   aerobic activity in, 699
   arthritis in, 698
   balance activities in, 699
   body composition in, 696–698
   calcium in, 693–694
   calories in, 449, 692
   carbohydrates in, 692–693
   carotenoids in, 695
   chronic disease in, 701
   complementary and alternative medicine in, 702
   dietary recommendations for, 691–696
   dietary supplements in, 695–696
   digestive system in, 700
   EER equation, A-30
   endocrine system in, 701
   fat in, 692
   folate in, 695
   immune system in, 701
   iron in, 694
   magnesium in, 695
   malnutrition risk in, 691, 692*f*

Adulthood. See also Older adults (continued)
  medications in, 702
  minerals and vitamins in, 693–695, 693f
  multicomponent activities in, 700
  muscle-strengthening activities in, 699
  nervous system in, 700–701
  nutrient needs during, 691–696
  nutrient recommendations for, 449–460
  nutritional status in, 696–704
  physical activity in, 698–700
  physiological changes of aging, 697f
  potassium in, 694
  protein in, 692
  sodium in, 695
  vitamin B-6 in, 695
  vitamin B-12 in, 695
  vitamin C in, 694
  vitamin D in, 693–694
  vitamin E in, 695
  warm-up and cool-down activities in, 699–700
  water in, 693
  zinc in, 694
Advantame, 140–141
Advertising, food choices and, 5
Aerobic activity, 48
  in adulthood, 699
  cardiorespiratory fitness and, 441
  components of, 441
  moderate-intensity, 442
  and physical fitness, 441–442
  vigorous-intensity, 442
Aerobic metabolism, 446
  carbohydrates in, 446
  fat in, 447
  protein in, 447–448
Afghan refugee crisis, 564
African Heritage Diet Pyramid, 147f
Agave nectar, 139
Age-related macular degeneration, 302, 303f, 701
Aging
  body composition, changes in, 696, 698
  and bone loss, 698
  causes of, 684–688
  defined, 684
  environmental factors and, 690–691
  extrinsic, 684
  factors affecting rate of, 688–691
  genetics and, 689
  hallmarks of, 686–688, 687f
  healthy, 684–691, 685f
  intrinsic, 684
  lifestyle choices and, 690

  and microbiome diversity, 688
  nutrition on, effects of, 689
  physiological changes of, 697f
  physiological function with, declines in, 686f
  successful, 688
  usual, 688
  WHO on, 684
Agriculture
  biotechnology in, 511–514, 513f
  community-supported, 296, 517
  in developing world, 564–565
  regenerative, 571
  sustainable, 510, 514, 516, 565, 570–572
Agroterrorism, 523–524
AI. See Adequate intake
AIDS. See Acquired immunodeficiency syndrome
Air displacement (Bod Pod), 259, 259f
Albumin, 375
Alcohol, 4, 15, 24, 46
  absorption and metabolism of, 27
  adolescents and, 670
  calories from, 15
  college students and, 72–73
  effects on liver, 28, 29f
  and fertility, 584
  heavy alcohol use, 27–28
  in menu planning for diabetes, A-15
  moderate alcohol use, 27, 46
  production, 26
  signs and symptoms of overdose, 28f
  in standard drink sizes, 26, 27f
  and thiamin deficiency, 322
  use of, guidelines for, 29–30
Alcohol consumption, nutrition implications of, 26–30
Alcohol dehydrogenase, 27
Alcoholics Anonymous, 29
Alcoholimia, 500
Alcohol poisoning, signs and symptoms of, 73
Alcohol-related birth defects (ARBDs), 621
Alcohol-related neurodevelopmental disorders (ARNDs), 621
Alcohol use disorder (AUD), 26, 27, 335, 621
  CAGE Questionnaire for, 28
  college students and, 73
  folate deficiencies and, 335
  magnesium deficiency and, 396
  nutrient deficiencies and, 29
  older adults and, 29
  symptoms of, 29
  and vitamin B-6 deficiency, 331
Aldosterone, 366

Alendronate (Fosamax), 428
Allergens, 69, 635, 672, 673
Allulose, 141
Almond milk, 389
Alpha-gal syndrome, 675
Alpha-linolenic acid, 12, 168, 174, 189, 189t, 597
Alternative sweeteners, 138, 140–142, 140t
  Acceptable Daily Intake (ADI), 140, 140t
  acesulfame-K, 140
  advantame, 140–141
  allulose, 141
  aspartame, 140t, 141
  as food additives, 140
  luo han guo, 141
  neotame, 141
  saccharin, 140t, 141
  stevia, 140t, 141
  sucralose, 140t, 141
Alzheimer's disease, 413, 717, 718
  prevention of, 717
  warning signs of, 717
Amaranth, 136t
AMDR. See Acceptable Macronutrient Distribution Range
Amenorrhea, 483, 484, 582
American Academy of Pediatrics (AAP), 283, 636
American Diabetes Association (ADA), 156
  carbohydrate counting by, A-3
  Diabetes Plate Method, A-2
American Heart Association (AHA), 174, 537
American Institute for Cancer Research, 222
Amino acids, 12, 82, 90, 208, 208t, 227
  branched-chain, 209, 448
  conditionally essential, 209
  defined, 208
  essential, 208, 214
  glucose from, 230–231
  limiting, 214
  metabolism, 229–230, 230f
  nonessential, 208
  peptide bonding of, 209, 209f
  pool of, 214
  structure of, 208, 208f, A-23
  supplements, 218–219
Amniotic fluid, 367, 597
Amphipathic, 169
Amylase, 97, 142
Amylopectin, 129
Amylophagia, 604
Amylose, 129
Anabolic agents, for osteoporosis, 428

Anabolic reaction, 85
Anaerobic activity, 48
Anal sphincters, 104
Anaphylaxis, 671
Android obesity. *See* Upper-body obesity
Anemia, 321, 636
    iron-deficiency, 399–400, 554*t*, 574, 651–652, 668
    macrocytic, 334, 335*f*, 338
    pernicious, 338–339, 639
    in pregnancy, 606–607
    sports, 456
Anencephaly, 334, 618
Angiotensin, 366
Angular cheilitis, 325, 325*f*
Angular stomatitis. *See* Angular cheilitis
Animal experiments, 20
Animal fats, 12, 173
Animal proteins, 216–218
Anorexia nervosa, 477, 481, 502–503, 654
    amenorrhea and, 483
    binge eating/purging type, 481
    cognitive behavioral therapy for, 486
    common behaviors of, 482
    diagnostic criteria for, 481*t*
    extreme dieting and, 482
    family-based treatment for, 486
    low body weight and, 481
    mortality rate, 485
    nutritional therapy for, 485–486
    pharmacological therapy for, 487
    physical effects of, 482–485
    prevention of, 485
    psychological therapy for, 486
    restricting type, 481
    treatment for, 485–487
Antacids, 113
Anthropometric assessment, 57, 58*f*
Antibody, 93, 228, 609
Antidiuretic hormone (ADH), 366
Antigen, 93
Antioxidant-rich foods, 25
Antioxidants, 180, 199, 656
    athletes and, 456
    free radicals and, 313, 456, 619
    in prevention of birth defects, 619
Antiresorptive agents, for osteoporosis, 428
Antiretroviral therapy (ART), 567
Anus, 104
Appearance, in food choices, 5
Appetite, 263
    defined, 7
    food intake and, 7–8
    regulation of, 91
Apples, 501
Aquaculture, 191
Arachidonic acid (ARA), 168

for infant development, 636, 639
Ariboflavinosis, 325
    undernutrition and, 554*t*
Aril, 316, 317
Artery, 86
Artesian water, 370
Arthritis, 698
Artificial sweeteners, 125, 126
Ascending colon, 103, 103*f*
Ascorbic acid. *See* Vitamin C
ASD. *See* Autism spectrum disorder
Aseptic processing, 528, 528*t*, 529
Asian Diet Pyramid, 267*f*
Aspartame, 125, 126, 140*t*, 141, 620
Aspirin, 196
AT. *See* Adaptive thermogenesis
Atenolol (Tenormin), 420
Atherosclerosis, 185, 196, 197*f*, 217, 334
Athletes
    alcohol consumption by, 459
    antioxidants for, 456
    banned/illegal substances for, 470*t*
    B vitamins for, 455–456
    calcium intake for, 457
    calorie needs of, 449–450
    carbohydrates consumption by, 450–453
    commonly used supplements for, 469*t*
    endurance, 461–464
    energy drinks and, 459
    ergogenic aids and, 468–470, 469*t*
    fat recommendations for, 452*f*, 453
    female, 457
    fluid intake of, 368–369, 457–459
    glycogen depletion and, 446
    heat-related illness in, 459, 460*f*
    hyponatremia and, 379
    iron for, 456–457
    muscular fitness, 442
    nutrient recommendations for, 449–460, 452*f*
    protein intakes for, 452*f*, 453–454
    recovery meals for, 466, 466*t*
    sports drinks for, 458–459, 458*f*
    strength and power, 464–466
    vegan diets for, 455
    vitamin D for, 457
    vitamins and minerals for, 454–457
    water intoxication in, 459
    weight loss by, 450
Atkins, Robert, 194
Atoms, 13
Atopic diseases, 615
ATP. *See* Adenosine triphosphate
Atypical anorexia nervosa, 496
AUD. *See* Alcohol use disorder
Autism spectrum disorder (ASD), 496, 658

    nutrition concerns of children with, 658–659
Avidin, 333
Avocados, 173
Avoidant/restrictive food intake disorder (ARFID), 496, 654
Azodicarbonamide, 538

B

Baboumian, Patrik, 454
Baby-Friendly Hospital Initiative, 609
Baby-led introduction to solid foods, 646–647
Baby-led weaning. *See* Baby-led introduction to solid foods
Bacillus cereus, 530
Bacillus thuringiensis, 512
Bacteria, 524
    in GI tract, 109
    lactic acid, 107
Bacteria, foodborne illness by, 530–532
    foodborne infection, 530
    foodborne intoxication, 530
    and gastrointestinal symptoms, 530
    temperature and, 532, 532*f*
    toxin-mediated infection, 530
    types of bacteria and, 530, 531*f*
Bananas, 385
Bariatrics, 282
Bariatric surgery, 282–283, 663
    benefits of, 283
    cost for, 283
    risks of, 282
    types of, 282*f*, 283*t*
    youth and adolescent, 283
Barley, 136*t*
Basal metabolic rate (BMR), 254, 255*f*, 367
Basal metabolism, 254
Basedoxifene + estrogen (Duavee), 428
Beans, 215
Benign tumors, 351
Benzphetamine, 279*t*
Beriberi, 322
    undernutrition and, 554*t*
Beta-blockers, in hypertension, 420
Beta-carotene, 302
β-glucan, 130
Betaine, 343
Beverage choices, tips for, 133*f*
Bicarbonate, 100
Bile, 104, 180
Bile acids, 97, 169
Bile acid sequestrants, 201
Binge drinking, 26, 499, 621
    on college campuses, 72–73
Binge eating, 487

Binge eating disorder, 477, 492
　　behaviors of, 492–493
　　diagnostic criteria for, 492t
　　of limited duration, 497
　　of low frequency, 497
　　negative emotions and, 492
　　nutrition therapy for, 494
　　pharmacological therapy for, 494–495
　　physical effects, 493
　　prevalence of, 492
　　psychological therapy for, 494
　　treatment for, 493–495
Bioavailability, 212, 213, 296
Biochemical assessment, 57, 58f
Bioelectrical impedance analysis (BIA), 260, 260f
Bioengineered labels, on food, 512, 513f
Bioengineering, 512
Biofortification, 304, 305, 573
Biological pest management, 510
Biological Value (BV), 213
Bionic pancreas, 157
Biotechnology, 511
　　in agriculture, 511–514, 513f
Biotin, 319
　　adequate intake of, 332–333
　　avoidance of excess, 333
　　chemical structure of, A-26
　　deficiency, 332
　　food sources of, 332, 333f
　　functions of, 332
Birth defects, 618
　　alcohol-related, 621
　　antioxidants and, 619
　　aspartame and, 620
　　caffeine and, 620
　　causes of, 618
　　chronic health conditions and, 620–621
　　environmental contaminants and, 621–622
　　examples of, 618
　　folic acid and, 618–619
　　iodine and, 619
　　obesity and, 620
　　reducing risk of, 618–622
　　vitamin A and, 620
Bisphenol A (BPA), 371
Bisphosphonates, for osteoporosis, 428
Bitot's spots, 304, 304f
Bitter flavors, 301
Black cohosh, 703t
Blindness, vitamin A deficiency and, 304, 304f
Blood glucose, regulation of, 147–149, 148f
　　glycemic response and, 149
　　insulin and glucagon in, 147–148, 148f

　　lifestyle management and, 148–149
Blood pressure. See also Hypertension
　　control of, 418–420
　　diuretics for, 420
　　guidelines, 418, 418f
　　high, 418, 418f
　　sodium intake and, 381, 382
　　systolic, 418
Blood sugar, 127
Blood thinners, 318
Blueberries, 300, 656
Blue zones, 709–710, 710f
　　bread intake across, 712
　　communities, spread of, 712
　　dietary patterns of, 711–712
　　lifestyle behaviors in, 710–711, 710f
BMI. See Body mass index
BMR. See Basal metabolic rate
Body composition, 259
　　bioelectrical impedance analysis for, 260, 260f
　　densitometry for, 259, 259f
　　dual energy X-ray absorptiometry for, 260–261, 261f
　　estimation of, 259–261
　　skinfold measurements for, 260, 260f
Body dissatisfaction, 479, 653
　　eating disorders and, 479
　　social media use and, 480
Body dysmorphic disorder (BDD), 465
Body fat distribution, 261–262
　　lower-body fat, 261f, 262
　　upper-body fat, 261, 261f
Body mass index (BMI), 258–259, 630
　　body shapes and, 258f
　　calculation of, 258
　　categories, 258t
　　prepregnancy, 591–592
Body weight, 36, 71, 250, 257
　　calorie intake and, 45
　　estimation of, 257
　　healthy, 257
The Body Weight Planner, 276–277
Bolus, 97
Bomb calorimeter, 252, 252f
Bond, defined, 11
Bone
　　biological factors with bone status, 424t
　　cortical, 422
　　growth, 422
　　health assessment, 422–424
　　lifestyle factors and, 424t
　　loss of bone mass, 422, 423f
　　osteoblast, 422
　　osteoclast, 422
　　osteoporotic, 425f
　　remodeling, 422
　　resorption, 422

　　trabecular, 422
　　T-score, 423
Bone mineral, 386
Bone mineral density, 422
Bonking, 446
Borlaug, Norman, 509
Bottled water, 370–371
Botulism, 649
Bovine spongiform encephalopathy, 530
Brain
　　energy source for, 90
　　growth in infancy, 630
Brain health, 714
　　in adolescence, 715
　　in adulthood, 716
　　in children, 715
　　food for, 717–718
　　formation of brain tissue and, 714
　　fuel for brain, 714
　　in gestation, 715
　　homocysteine and, 715
　　in infants, 715
　　nervous tissue, protection of, 715
　　nutrients in, 714–715
　　omega-3 fatty acids in, 716
Branched-chain amino acids (BCAAs), 209, 448
Brazil nuts, 406, 407
Breast. See also Breastfeeding
　　anatomy of, 609, 609f
　　human milk production, 609–611
Breastfeeding, 609, 715. See also Human milk
　　advantages of, 614–615, 614t
　　barriers to, 615–617
　　and body weight regulation, 639
　　cosmetic alterations to breast and, 616–617
　　and dietary supplements, 617
　　EER equation for females, A-30, A-31
　　employment and, 616
　　environmental contaminants and, 617
　　feeding routine, 611
　　and healthy BMI, 639
　　let-down reflex, 610, 610f
　　medical conditions precluding, 616
　　misinformation about, 616
　　nutritional qualities of human milk and, 611–612
　　plans for, 609
　　preterm infant and, 612
　　social concerns and, 616
　　wet nursing, 640
Breast milk, 611–612. See also Human milk
Brown adipose tissue, 253
Brown sugar, 139
Buckwheat, 136t
Buffers, 229

Bulgur, 136*t*
Bulimia nervosa, 477, 487–488, 503
    and anorexia nervosa, difference between, 481
    behaviors of, 488–489
    binge eating in, 487, 488
    debting in, 488
    dental erosion from self-induced vomiting, 490, 490*f*
    diagnostic criteria for, 487*t*
    of limited duration, 497
    of low frequency, 497
    nutrition therapy for, 490–491
    perforations in GI tract in, 490
    pharmacological therapy for, 491
    physical effects of, 490
    prevalence of, 488
    psychological therapy for, 491
    purging after bingeing in, 488
    Russell's sign in, 488, 488*f*
    substance abuse and, 489
    treatment for, 490–491
    vicious cycle of obsession in, 489, 489*f*
B vitamins, 294, 296, 319. *See also specific vitamins*
    athletes and, 455–456
    biotin, 319, 332–333
    as coenzymes, 319–320, 319*f*
    deficiencies of, 320–321
    folate, 319, 333–337
    in grains, 321
    loss during cooking, 320
    niacin, 319, 327–329
    pantothenic acid, 319, 329–330
    riboflavin, 319, 324–326
    thiamin, 319, 322–324
    in typical dietary patterns, 320–321
    vitamin B-6, 319, 330–332
    vitamin B-12, 319, 337–340

C

Caffeine, 539
    adolescents and, 669
    in beverages, 540*f*
    children and, 668–669
    consumption of, 539–541
    harmful effects of, 540
    withdrawal and headaches, 716
CAGE Questionnaire, 28
Calcidiol (25-hydroxyvitamin D_3), 307
Calcifediol, 307
Calcitonin, 307, 387, 428
Calcitriol (1,25-dihydroxyvitamin D_3), 307. *See also* Vitamin D
Calcium, 90, 375
    absorption of, 390–391, 391*f*
    adequate intake of, 387–391
    for adults, 693–694
    athletes and, 457
    avoidance of excess, 391–393
    blood clotting and, 386
    in blood pressure regulation, 386
    in bone health, 386
    in cancer prevention, 386
    deficiency, 58, 387
    food sources of, 387–388, 388*f*
    functions of, 386
    hormonal regulation of, 387, 387*f*
    in muscle and nerve function, 386
    RDA for, 388
    rule of 300s, 391
    supplementation, 391–393, 393*t*
    for teenagers, 667–668
    for toddlers and preschoolers, 652
    Upper Level (UL) for, 391
    vitamin D and, 391
Calcium carbonate, 393, 393*t*
Calcium citrate, 393, 393*t*
Calorie estimation, on fitness machines, 270
Calorie needs
    for females, 265
    for males, 265
    during pregnancy, 593–594
Calories, 15–16, 36, 256
    for adults, 692
    body weight and, 45
    in breast milk, 639
    calculation of, 16
    defined, 15
    eating habits and, 43
    empty/discretionary, 50
    needs, 45, 45*f*
    overnutrition and, 56
    sources of, 15
    weight loss and intake of, 193
Cancer, 351
    body fat and, 353
    defined, 9
    dietary calcium and, 386
    environmental influences on risk of, 242
    foods fighting, 353
    genetics and, 242
    meat consumption and, 217
    metastasis, 351
    nutrition and, 351–354
    nutrition during treatment, 354
    obesity and, 353
    plant-based dietary patterns and risk of, 222
    prevention of, 353–354
    progression of, 351, 351*f*
    red meat and, 363
    risk factors, 352–353
    screening for, 352
    symptoms of, 352, 352*f*
Capillary, 86, 228
Captopril (Capoten), 420
Carb counting. *See* Carbohydrate counting
Carbohydrate counting, A-2, A-3
Carbohydrate gels/chews, 463
Carbohydrate loading, 461, 461*t*
Carbohydrates, 11–12, 111, 125. *See also* Starch; Sugar
    absorption of, 143*f*, 145
    for adults, 692–693
    athletes and, 450–453
    in breast milk, 639
    calories from, 12, 126
    Carbohydrate Concept Map, 131*f*
    complex, 11, 128–131
    defined, 10
    Dietary Guidelines recommendations on, 150–151, 150*f*
    digestion of, 142–144, 143*f*
    for energy needs, 146–147
    in food, 132–142, 132*f*
    forms of, 127–131
    as fuel for muscles, 445, 446
    importance of, 126
    for infants, 635
    needs for, 150–155
    in pregnancy, 597
    RDA for, 150
    regular intake of, 126
    role of, in body, 146–149
    simple, 11, 127–128
    for toddlers and preschoolers, 652
Carbon footprint, 510
Carbon skeletons, of amino acids, 230
Cardiac sphincter. *See* Lower esophageal sphincter
Cardiovascular disease, 165, 191, 196
    AHA Life's Essential 8 and, 199
    animal products and, 217
    calcium supplements and, 392
    defined, 9
    development of, 196–198, 197*f*
    dietary guidance from AHA, 191*t*
    genetics and, 242
    lifestyle modifications for, 199
    lipids and, 196–202
    medications to lower blood lipids, 201–202
    mortality from, 9
    MyPlate and, 201*f*
    physical activity for prevention of, 199
    plant-based dietary patterns and, 221, 222
    reduction of, 191–192
    risk factors for, 198–199, 198*f*
    surgical treatment for, 202

Cardiovascular system, 83f
    defined, 85
    hepatic portal circulation, 87
    structure and function of, 86–87, 86f, 87f
Caries (cavities), 154
Carnitine, 341
Carotenoids, 302. *See also* Vitamin A
    for adults, 695
    in cancer prevention, 304
    in cardiovascular disease prevention, 304
    defined, 299
    food sources of, 305, 306f
    vision and, 302–303
Carrots, 39
    and beets, 453
Case-control study, 20
Case reports, 20
Case study
    anemia, 403
    bone health, 429
    cancer prevention dietary and physical activity recommendations, 355
    choosing weight-management program, 288
    deficiency from vegan and gluten-free diet, 325
    dietary assistance for older adult, 707
    eating disorders, 495
    eating for two, 605
    gastroesophageal reflux disease, 114
    getting most nutrition from food, 350
    heart-healthy dietary pattern, 194
    milk intake, problems with, 144
    planning training diet, 467
    planning vegetarian dietary pattern, 236
    prevention of foodborne illness at gatherings, 545
    undernutrition during childhood, 575
    undernutrition during infancy, 650
Cashews, 398
Catabolic reactions, 85
Catalase, 82
Catalyst, 319
CBD (cannabidiol), 704
Cecum, 103, 103f
Celery, 256
Celiac disease, 118–119, 119f, 239, 316, 615, 632
Celiac sprue, 118
Cell, 11, 80
    defined, 80
    energy for, 111
    structure and function of, 80–82, 80f
Cell membrane, 80–81, 80f, 81f, 377

phospholipids in, 187, 188f
Cellular differentiation, 386
Cellulose, 129
Centers for Disease Control and Prevention (CDC), 524, 630
    National Outbreak Reporting System (NORS), 525, 526f
Central obesity. *See* Upper-body obesity
Cerebrospinal fluid, 367
Cerebrovascular accident. *See* Stroke
Ceruloplasmin, 412
Cheilosis. *See* Angular cheilitis
Chemical digestion, 95, 97
Chemical reaction, 12
Childhood caries, early, 641
Childhood obesity, 660–663, 662f, 667
    body system, effect on, 660, 662f
    causes of, 661–662
    dietary interventions for, 663
    medical and surgical interventions for, 663
    physical activity and, 662–663, 663t
    type 2 diabetes and, 664
    weight bias in management of, 663
Child poverty, 560
Children
    and breakfast, 664
    cardiovascular disease in, 664
    CDRR for sodium for, 664
    EER equation for, A-29
    excess sugar intake by, 151
    fat recommendations for, 189
    food advertisements and obesity in, 5
    food allergies in, 671, 671f
    hyperactivity in, 153
    kwashiorkor in, 237, 237f
    marasmus in, 237–238, 237f
    micronutrient supplementation in, 556
    and obesity, 5 (*See also* Childhood obesity)
    positive energy balance for, 252
    in poverty, 575
    protein-calorie malnutrition in, 236–238, 237f
    rickets in, 308, 308f
    stunted growth, 575
    type 2 diabetes in, 664
    undernutrition in, 575–576
    underweight, 284
    vegetarian dietary pattern and, 225–226
    vitamin A deficiency and blindness in, 304
    weight status classifications for, 633t
Chloride
    in acid–base balance, 385
    adequate intake of, 385–386

    avoidance of excess, 386
    blood pressure and, 385, 386
    deficiency, 385
    in fluid balance, 385
    functions of, 385
Chlorine, 385
Chlorothiazide (Diuril), 420
Cholecystokinin (CCK), 91–92, 91f, 226
Cholesterol, 169, 186–188
    defined, 80
    dietary intake of, 190
    digestion, 181
    from food, 175–176, 176t, 190
    synthesis by body, 190
Cholesterol-lowering medications, 201–202
Choline, 294, 319, 343
    adequate intake of, 344–345
    avoidance of excess, 345
    birth defects and, 343–344
    cardiovascular disease and, 344
    in cell membrane structure, 343
    food sources of, 344, 345f
    functions of, 343–344
    in lipid transport, 344
    in nerve function and brain development, 344
Choose Your Foods: Food Lists for Weight Management, A-5
Chromium
    absorption, 416
    adequate intake of, 415–416
    deficiency, 415
    functions of, 415
    sources of, 415
    toxicity, 416
Chromosomes, 82
Chronic Disease Risk Reduction Intakes (CDRRs), 59–62, 59t, 381
Chronic diseases
    defined, 9
    example of, 9
    lifestyle pattern and, 24
    weight control and, 193
Chronic kidney disease, 238
Chylomicron remnants, 185
Chylomicrons, 181, 183, 184t
    dietary fat transportation by, 183–185
Chyme, 99
Chymotrypsin, 226
Cimetidine (Tagamet), 115
Circulatory system, 85. *See also* Cardiovascular system; Lymphatic system
Cirrhosis, 28
    alcohol intake and, 28–29
Cis fatty acid, 168, 168f
Citrus fruits, 38, 39, 341, 342

Cleft lip/cleft palate, 618
Clinical (physical) assessment, 57, 58f
Closer to Zero, 647
Clostridium botulinum, 139, 530, 649
Cobalamin. *See* Vitamin B-12
Coconut milk, 389
Coconut oil, 173, 179
Coenzyme A (CoA), 329
Coenzymes, 296, 319
    B vitamins as, 319–320, 319f
    defined, 319
Cofactor, 316
Cognitive behavioral therapy, 486
    for anorexia nervosa, 486
    for binge eating disorder, 494
    for bulimia nervosa, 491
Cohort studies, 20
Collagen, 207, 228
Collagen supplements, 207
College food and nutrition security, 562
College students, eating habits of, 72
Colon cancer, dietary patterns and, 146
Colorectal cancer, role of diet and lifestyle in, 22
Colostrum, 611
Combination foods, in menu planning for diabetes, A-13
Community-supported agriculture (CSA), 296, 517
Compensatory behaviors, 481, 482, 487
Complementary and alternative medicine, 702
Complementary foods, 637
Complementary proteins, 214, 215f
Complex carbohydrate. *See also* Starch
    defined, 11
    sources of, 11
Compression of morbidity, 688
Concentration, 377
Conditionally essential amino acids, 209
Congenital hypothyroidism, 409, 600
    due to iodine deficiency, 619, 620f
Congenital lactase deficiency, 143
Congregate meals, 559
Conjugated linoleic acid (CLA), 179
Connective tissue, 82
Constipation, 115–116
    in older adults, 700
    in pregnancy, 605–606
Convenience, food choices and, 5
Copper, 412
    absorption of, 412
    adequate intake of, 412
    avoidance of excess, 412–413
    for blood health, 412
    for brain health, 412
    as cofactor for enzymes, 412
    deficiency, 412

    food sources of, 412, 413f
    functions of, 412
Coprostanol, 202
Corn, 127, 136t
Coronary artery bypass graft (CABG), 202
Coronary artery disease. *See* Cardiovascular disease
Coronary heart disease. *See* Cardiovascular disease
CoroWise, 199
Cortical bone, 422
Cost, in food choices, 6
Coumadin (warfarin), 318
Cow's milk, 218, 293, 389t, 390, 639
    carbohydrate in, 138
    composition of, 635t
    in infant formulas, 639
    for toddlers and preschoolers, 652
Cranberries, 89
Cranberry, 703t
Creatine, 445, 470
CRISPR-Cas9 (Clustered Regulatory Interspaced Short Palindromic Repeats), 513
Critical life stages, malnutrition at, 574–576
Crop rotation, 514
Cross-contamination, 542
Cross-sectional study, 20
Crucifers, 301
CSA. *See* Community-supported agriculture
Cultural foodways, 561
Cultural pica, 604
Cyanocobalamin. *See* Vitamin B-12
Cystic fibrosis, 295
Cytoplasm, 80f, 81

D

Dahi, 107
Daily Value (DV), 59t, 60–61, 65–67
    on food labels, A-1
Dairy, 138
    carbohydrate in, 138
    consumption in U.S., 5, 7f
Dairy alternatives, plant-based, 389
Danger zone, 532
Deficiency
    biotin, 332
    calcium, 387
    chromium, 415
    copper, 412
    essential fatty acids, 189
    folate, 334–335
    iodine, 409
    iron, 399–400

    magnesium, 396
    niacin, 327
    pantothenic acid, 329
    phosphorus, 394
    potassium, 383
    riboflavin, 325
    selenium, 406
    sodium, 379
    thiamin, 322
    vitamin A, 304–305
    vitamin B-6, 331
    vitamin B-12, 224, 338–339
    vitamin C, 341
    vitamin D, 308
    vitamin E, 313–314
    vitamin K, 316
    water, 368–369
Dehydration, 365, 368–369, 378, 450, 458, 500
    effects of, 368, 369f
    heatstroke and, 368
    in infants, 637–638
    mental function and, 368
    and migraines, 716
    during pregnancy, 597
7-dehydrocholesterol, 307
Delaney Clause, 537
Dementia, 327
Denaturation, 211, 212f
Denosumab (Prolia), 428
Densitometry, 259, 259f
Dental caries, 154–155, 658
    causes of, 154–155
    defined, 154
    prevention of, 155, 414
Deoxygenated blood, 86
Deoxyribonucleic acid (DNA), 81–82, 209
Depolarization, 379
Depression
    in adults, 716
    causes of, 716
    nutrition and, 716
    prevention of, 716
Dermatitis, 325
Descending colon, 103, 103f
Detox diets, 323
Developing world
    agriculture in, 564–565
    biotechnology in, role of, 572–573
    food-to-population ratio in, 563–564
    HIV/AIDS in, impact of, 566–567
    improving equality in, 570
    malnutrition in, 563–567, 563f
    micronutrients deficiency in, 554, 556
    natural resources in, 564–565
    political/civil unrest in, 564
    reducing malnutrition in, 568–573

I-8 Index

Developing world (continued)
  sanitation in, 565–566
  shelter in, 565–566
  sustainable agriculture in, 570–572
  undernutrition in, 554
  war in, 564
Dextrose. See Glucose
DHA. See Docosahexaenoic acid
Diabetes, 156, 499
  alcohol in menu planning for, A-15
  carbohydrate counting, A-3
  CDC guide to criteria for, 156, 156f
  combination foods in menu planning for, A-13
  daily menu from food list, A-4–A-5, A-5t
  defined, 9
  Diabetes Plate, A-2
  eating disorders and, 499
  fast foods in menu planning for, A-14
  fats in menu planning for, A-11–A-12
  food choices from food list, A-6–A-15
  food lists for, A-3–A-4, A-4t
  free foods in menu planning for, A-12
  fruits in menu planning for, A-7
  genetics and, 242
  gestational, 157
  menu planning for, A-2–A-15
  milk and milk substitutes in menu planning for, A-8
  nonstarchy vegetables in menu planning for, A-8–A-9
  prediabetes, 156–157
  protein in menu planning for, A-10–A-11
  screening for, 156
  starch in menu planning for, A-6–A-7
  sweets/desserts in menu planning for, A-9–A-10
  type 1, 9, 157–158, 157t, 499
  type 2, 9, 157, 157t, 158–159, 499
Diabetes remission, 156–157
Diabetic hypoglycemia, 159
Diabulimia, 499
Dialysis, 238
Diarrhea, 118
Diastolic blood pressure, 418
Diet and diet plans
  Asian Diet Pyramid, 267f
  assessment of, A-16–A-22
  DASH diet, 420–421, 420t
  detox, 323
  elimination, 288
  fad, 286
  flexitarian, 287, 287t
  gluten-free diet, 119, 120
  guidelines, 41–47
  high-protein, 287

  keto diets, 147
  ketogenic diet, 194–195
  for kidney disease, 238
  Latin American Heritage Diet, 44, 44f
  low-calorie, 287
  low-carbohydrate, 287
  low-fat, 287–288
  low-FODMAP diet, 146
  Mediterranean, 54, 55f
  popular diets, 286–288
  quality of, impact of, 47
  vegan, 287, 287t
  WW (weight watchers), 286–287, 287t
Dietary Approaches to Stop Hypertension (DASH) diet, 420–421, 420t
Dietary assessment, 57, 58f
Dietary fiber, 11, 130
  classification of, 130t
  defined, 130
  fermentable, 130t
  insoluble, 130t
  viscous, 130t
Dietary folate equivalents (DFE), 334, 335
Dietary Guidelines, 38, 41–47
  key guidelines of, 41, 42f
  life-stage approach in, 42f, 43
Dietary patterns
  American, 46, 46f
  cardiovascular health and, 191, 191t
  and deaths in United States, 9, 9f
  defined, 4
  in *Dietary Guidelines,* 43, 45
  evaluation of, A-21–A-22
  global, 22
  globalization on, impact of, 565
  gut microbiota and, 38
  for health promotion and disease prevention, 24, 25
  healthy, 38, 40, 49
  high-fiber, 145
  high-protein, 217
  infant's, 634
  lactoovovegetarian, 603
  lactovegetarian, 603
  mental health and, 25
  noncommunicable diseases risk and, 38
  nutrient density of, 36, 37f
  plant-based, 219–226, 265, 266
  plant-focused, 73
  reduced-salt, 381
  in United States, 21–23
  vegan, 339
  vegetarian, 219, 220
  vitamin A in, 305
  vitamins in, 294

Dietary principles, 36–40
  nutritional needs from foods and beverages, 36–38
  options from food group, 38–39
  portion size, 39–40
Dietary Reference Intakes (DRIs), 59–60, 61f, A-29–A-37
  Acceptable Macronutrient Distribution Ranges (AMDRs), 59t, 60
  Adequate Intakes (AIs), 59–60, 59t
  Chronic Disease Risk Reduction Intakes (CDRRs), 59t, 60
  and Daily Value, 59t
  defined, 59
  development of, 59
  electrolytes and water, A-33
  elements, A-35
  Estimated Energy Requirements (EERs), 59t, 60
  macronutrients, A-32
  Recommended Dietary Allowance (RDA), 59, 59t
  Tolerable Upper Intake Levels (ULs), 59t, 60
  upper intake levels, elements and electrolytes, A-37
  upper intake levels, vitamins, A-36
  vitamins, A-34
Dietary Supplement Health and Education Act of 1994 (DSHEA), 346
Dietary supplements. See also Supplements
  for adults, 695–696
  to infant, 649
Dietary variety, 38
Diethylpropion, 279t
Diet-induced thermogenesis, 255
Diet quackery, 288
Digestible Indispensable Amino Acid Score (DIAAS), 214
Digestion, 94
  of carbohydrates, 142–144, 143f
  chemical, 95, 97
  of fats, 180–181, 181f
  of phospholipids, 180
  of proteins, 226, 227f
  of starch, 142, 143f
  of sugar, 142
  of triglycerides, 180
Digestive enzymes, 95, 96f
Digestive system, 83f, 94–105, 95f, 112
  accessory organs, 94, 104–105
  esophagus, 95f, 97–98, 98f
  gallbladder, 104, 105f
  gastrointestinal tract, 94
  large intestine, 95f, 102–104, 102f

liver, 104, 105f
mouth, 95f, 96–97
pancreas, 105, 105f
rectum, 95f, 104
secretions of, 97t
small intestine, 95f, 100–102, 101f
stomach, 95f, 98–100, 99f
Digestive tract. *See* Gastrointestinal (GI) tract
Diglyceride, 169, 170f
1,25-dihydroxyvitamin D_3 (calcitriol), 92
Dipeptides, 209
Direct calorimetry, 256
Direct food additives, 535
Disaccharides, 127, 128, 142
    defined, 128
    lactose, 128
    maltose, 128
    sucrose, 128, 128f
Discretionary calories, 50
Disordered eating, 73, 476, 653. *See also* Eating disorders
    and binge drinking, 499–500
Dispensable amino acids. *See* Nonessential amino acids
Diuretics, 364, 482, 606
    in hypertension, 420
Diverticula, 116
Diverticulitis, 117
Diverticulosis, 116–117, 116f
DNA testing, 242
Docosahexaenoic acid (DHA), 168, 174, 611
    for infant development, 636, 639
Dopamine, 229, 715
Double-blind study, 19
Dowager's hump. *See* Kyphosis
Down syndrome, 618
Drunkorexia, 499–500
Dual energy X-ray absorptiometry (DXA), 260–261, 261f, 423
Duodenum, 100, 101f, 337
Dysbiosis, 108

E

Early childhood caries, 641
EAT. *See* Exercise-activity thermogenesis
Eating disorders, 476–477, 653. *See also specific disorder*
    during adolescence, 479
    athletes and, 479
    body dissatisfaction and, 479
    changing face of, 478–480
    in children, 479
    college students and, 73
    diabetes and, 499
    extreme dieting and, 479, 482
    females and, 479
    genetics and, 477, 478
    LGBTQ+ individuals and, 479
    males and, 479
    origins of, 477–478
    physical effects of, 483f
    prevalence of, 475, 479
    prevention of, 500–501
    psychological disorders and, 477
    SCOFF questionnaire for, 479–480, 480f
    stressful life events and, 477–478
    subthreshold, 477
    types of, 477
    websites for information on, 500
Eating habits
    calorie balance in, 43
    disordered, 73, 478–480 (*See also* Eating disorders)
    healthy, 47
    for heart health, 191–192
    of students, 72
Eating in moderation, 39, 40
Eating pattern
    animal products, 217
    boosting phytochemical content of, 300t
    chaotic, 476
    for females who breastfeed, 612–613
    lactoovovegetarian, 658
    and migraines, 716
    plant-based, 219–226
    in pregnancy, 601–604
Eating sustainably, 514
Echinacea, 703t
Eclampsia, 608
E. coli O104:H4, 530
E. coli O157:H7, 530
Ecological model assessment, 480
Edema, 228, 229f, 606
    during pregnancy, 606
EER. *See* Estimated Energy Requirement
Eggs, 165
Eicosanoids, 168
Eicosapentaenoic acid (EPA), 168, 174
Einkhorn, 136t
Electrochemical gradient, 379
Electrolytes, 13, 377, 606
    infants and, 637–638
    in sports drinks, 458–459
Electronic benefit transfer (EBT) card, 559, 592
Elimination diets, 288, 672
Embryo, 582
Emotional eating, 267
Empty calories, 50
Emulsifiers, 175, 175f
Endocrine disruptor, 371

Endocrine glands, 91
Endocrine system, 83f, 91–93
Endoplasmic reticulum (ER), 80f, 82
Endorphins, 476
Endurance athletes, 461
    carbohydrate loading, 461, 461t
    fat adaptation by, 462–463
    fuel replenish during event, 463–464, 463t
    glycogen and fluid after physical activity, 464
    goal for, 461
    pre-event meal of, 462, 462t
    strategies to prevent fatigue, 461–464
Energy, 250, 256
    availability, 450
    Estimated Energy Requirement (EER) calculation, 257
    from fatty acids, 187
    need estimates, 256–257
    for physical activity, 255
Energy balance, 582
    defined, 251
    energy expenditure and, 252–253, 253f
    energy intake and, 252, 252f
    and fertility, 582–583
    and health promotion, 250–256
    model for, 251f
    negative, 252, 582
    positive, 252, 582
    throughout life course, 264–269
    variables influencing, 253f
Energy bars, 463–464, 463t
Energy-dense foods, 39, 40
Energy density, 39–40, 40f, 265, 649
Energy drinks, 459, 459t
Energy intake, strategies to reduce, 268, 268t
Energy metabolism, 85
    aerobic, 446–448
    anaerobic, 445
    biotin in, 332
    B vitamins in, 319, 455
    copper in, 412
    manganese in, 416
    niacin in, 327
    pantothenic acid in, 329
    riboflavin in, 324
    thiamin in, 322
    vitamin B-6 in, 330
Energy need, of infants, 634
Energy sources, for active muscles, 444–449
Energy-yielding nutrients, 11, 11f
English-metric conversions, A-28
Enterocytes, 100
Enterohepatic circulation, 104, 180

Entomophagy, 564
Environmental assessment, 57, 58f
Environmental contaminants
　in fish, 523
　in food, 517–524
　pesticide, 519–522
　potential contaminants, 518t
Environmental Protection Agency (EPA), 519–520, 521t
Environmental sustainability, food choices and, 7
Enzymes, 319
　chemical digestion and, 95
　defined, 12, 81
　digestive, 95, 96f
　model of action, 96f
　protein in nature, 12
EPA. See Eicosapentaenoic acid
Epidemiology, 18
Epigenetics, 212, 478
Epigenome, 212
Epiglottis, 97
Epinephrine, 90, 91f, 148
Epithelial tissue, 82
Ergogenic aids, 457, 468
　and athletic performance, 468–470, 469t
　muscle dysmorphia and, 499
Erythrocytes. See Red blood cells
Esomeprazole (Nexium), 115
Esophageal cancer, 113
Esophagus, 95f, 97–98, 98f
Essential amino acids, 208, 214, 603, 635
Essential fatty acids, 12, 168, 169f, 596
　Adequate Intakes (AIs) for, 189, 189t
　deficiency, 189
　food sources of, 174
　for infants, 636
　intake of, 189
　during pregnancy, 597
Essential hypertension. See Primary hypertension
Essential nutrient, 9
Essential oils, 690
Estimated Energy Requirement (EER), 59, 59t, 60, 257, 449, 593, A-29–A-31
Estrogen therapy, 428
Ethanol, 26. See also Alcohol
Exercise, 438. See also Physical activity
　defined, 438
　and gut microbiota, 444
Exercise-activity thermogenesis (EAT), 255
Extracellular fluid, 377
Extracellular spaces, 228
Extrusion reflex, 643
Ezetimibe, 201

F

Facilitated diffusion, 100, 102f
Fad diets, 286
　characteristics of, 286
Fahrenheit-Celsius conversion scale, A-28
Family-based treatment, 486
　for anorexia nervosa, 486
Famine, 557, 563, 582
Famotidine (Pepcid), 115
Farro, 136t
FAS. See Fetal alcohol syndrome
Fast foods, in menu planning for diabetes, A-14
Fat adaptation, 448, 462–463
Fats, 12, 111, 166
　absorption of, 181, 182f
　for adults, 692
　AMDR for, 189
　athletes and, 452f, 453
　digestion of, 180–181, 181f
　flavor and, 176
　on food labels, 176, 177f
　in foods, 171–176
　as fuel for muscles, 447, 447f
　hidden, 176
　hydrogenation, 178
　for infants, 636
　insulating body, 187
　interesterified, 178–179
　in Mediterranean diet, 192
　in menu planning for diabetes, A-11–A-12
　on MyPlate, 172–173, 172f
　in pregnancy, 597
　quality versus quantity, 193
　RDA for, 189
　recommendations for intake, 189–193
　replacement strategies, 177–178
　satiety and, 176
　texture and, 176
　for toddlers and preschoolers, 652
　total intake of, 189
Fat-soluble vitamins, 12, 294, 295. See also Vitamins
Fatty acids, 166
　chain length of, 173, 181
　cis, 168, 168f
　essential, 168, 169f
　as fuel for body, 187
　long-chain, 166, 173
　medium-chain, 166
　monounsaturated, 167, 167f
　nonessential, 168
　omega-3, 168
　omega-6, 168
　omega-9, 168
　polyunsaturated, 167, 167f
　saturated, 166, 167f
　saturation of, 173, 174f
　short-chain, 166
　trans, 168, 168f
　unsaturated, 166–167, 167f
Fatty liver, alcohol and, 28
Fecal impaction, 657
Fecal microbiota transplant (FMT), 109
Feces, 102, 104
Federal poverty level (FPL), 560
Feeding center, 8
Females, empowerment of, 570
Fermentation, 26, 128, 527–528, 528t
Fermented foods, 107, 528
Ferritin, 399, 456
Fertility, 582
　alcohol and, 584
　caffeine intake and, 584
　dietary fat in, 584
　energy balance and, 582–583
　hormonal balance and, 583
　minerals in, 584
　nutrition and, 582–584
　vitamins in, 583–584
Fetal alcohol spectrum disorders (FASDs), 621
Fetal alcohol syndrome (FAS), 621, 621f
Fetal macrosomia, 596
Fetal origins hypothesis, 589
Fetus, 305, 584, 586
Fever, 367
Fiber, 11, 127, 129–131, 130f, 130t. See also Dietary fibers
　Adequate Intake for, 151
　cardiovascular disease risk and, 149
　for children, 657
　Daily Value for, 151
　dietary, 130, 130f, 130t, 149
　in fruits, 138
　functional, 131
　health benefits from, 145, 149
　high-fiber cereal for breakfast, 151, 152f
　for infants, 635, 649
　intake in United States, 151
　and intestinal health, 145–146
　in obesity prevention, 149
Fibrates, 201
Fibrin, 316
Fish
　broiled/baked, 191
　environmental contaminants in, 523
　for heart and brain health, 175
　intake of, 190–191
　mercury in, 175
　omega-3 fatty acids in, 174–175, 174t
Fish oil capsules, 191

Fitness trackers, 270
Flavin adenine dinucleotide (FAD), 324
Flavin mononucleotide (FMN), 324
Flavonoids, 299
Flavor, in food choices, 5
Flaxseeds, 174
Flexibility, 443
Flexitarian, 220
Flexitarian diet, 287, 287t
Fluid intake, in pregnancy, 597–598
Fluoridation of water, 414
Fluoride, 414
    adequate intake of, 414
    avoidance of excess, 414–415
    dental caries prevention by, 414
    food sources of, 414
    functions of, 414
    for infants, 637
    in tap water, 371
    UL for, 414
Fluorosis, 414–415, 415f, 637
Fluoxetine (Prozac), 487, 491
Foam cells, 196
FODMAPs, 117, 146
Folate, 39, 319, 334, 583
    adequate intake of, 335–336
    for adults, 695
    in amino acid metabolism, 334
    avoidance of excess, 337
    in cancer protection, 334
    chemical structure of, A-26
    deficiency, 334–335
    dietary folate equivalents (DFE), 334, 335
    in DNA synthesis, 334
    food sources of, 335, 336f
    functions of, 334
    homocysteine levels and, 334
    leafy green vegetables and, 601
    neural tube defects and, 334–335
    in pregnancy, 334, 335, 598
    recommendations, 334
    red blood cells and, 334
    vitamin B-12 and, 334, 336, 337
    for women of childbearing age, 334
Folic acid, 334
Folic acid supplementation, during pregnancy, 598
Food, 8
    anti-inflammatory properties, 25
    bioengineered, 512, 513f
    carbohydrates in, 132–142, 132f
    environmental contaminants in, 517–524
    fats and oils in, 171–176
    fermented, 528
    functional, 298–299
    high energy density, 39, 40, 40f
    irradiated, 528, 528t, 529
    locally grown, 516–517
    low energy density, 39–40, 40f, 265
    Nova classification, 37
    nutrient density of, 36–38
    and nutrients, difference between, 8
    phytochemicals in, 13–14, 299
    preservation of vitamins in, 296, 298, 298t
    processed, 37
    protein in, 212–219, 213f
    reduced-fat, 177–178
    ultraprocessed, 37
    unprocessed, 37
Food additives, 534
Food Allergen Labeling and Consumer Protection Act (FALCPA), 69, 673
Food allergens, 239f, 673
    labeling of, 69
Food allergy, 238, 635, 671–674
    defined, 118, 671
    diagnosis of, 672–673, 672t
    and elimination diet, 672
    gut microbiota and, 672
    hygiene hypothesis, 672
    living with, 673
    mechanisms of, 671–672
    prevalence of, 671, 671f
    prevention of, 673–674
    symptoms of, 671
Food Allergy Safety, Treatment, Education, and Research (FASTER) Act, 673
Food and Drug Administration (FDA), 65, 125, 221, 512, 520, 521t, 536–537
Food availability, food choices and, 5
Food biotechnology, 511–514
Foodborne illness, 524, 525f
    bacterial causes of, 530–532, 531f
    causes and prevalence of, 530f
    CDC on, 524
    effects of, 524
    microorganisms as cause of, 530–534
    outbreaks of, 526f
    parasitic causes of, 533, 534f
    during pregnancy, 591, 591f
    prevention of, 542–545
    public health and safety, 525, 526f
    risk for, causes of, 525, 527
    steps to food safety, 542–545
    transmission of, 525
    unpasteurized milk and, 529
    viral causes of, 532–533, 532f, 533f
Food choices, 4–8
    advertising and, 5
    appearance in, 5
    convenience and, 5
    cost and, 6
    early influences, 5
    eating behaviors and, 5
    factors influencing, 4f, 5–7
    flavor in, 5
    food availability and, 5
    healthy eaters and, 476
    marketing and, 5
    nutrition and, 7
    restaurant dining and, 5
    students and, 1
    sustainability and, 6–7
    taste in, 5
    texture in, 5
    time and, 5
Food deserts, malnutrition and, 561
Food hypersensitivity. *See* Food allergy
Food intolerances, 671, 674–675
Food irradiation, 528, 528t, 529
Food is Medicine initiative, 25
Food jags, 652
FoodKeeper app, 544
Food labels, 65–70
Food Lists for Diabetes, A-3–A-4
    combination foods in, A-13
    fast foods in, A-14
    fats in, A-11–A-12
    food choices from, A-6–A-15
    free foods in, A-12
    fruits in, A-7
    milk and milk substitutes in, A-8
    nonstarchy vegetables in, A-8–A-9
    nutrient composition of foods in, A-4
    protein in, A-10–A-11
    starches in, A-6–A-7
    sweets/desserts in, A-9–A-10
    use of, to develop daily menu, A-4–A-5
Food packaging, 180
Food philosophy, 36–40
Food preparation, WHO rules for, 545
Food preservation, 524, 527–529
    techniques, 528t
Food processing, 37–38
Food production, 510
Food production chain, 518, 518f
Food quality, 53
Food records, A-16–A-18
Food Safety and Inspection Service (FSIS), 520, 521t
Food Safety Modernization Act (FSMA), 2011, 524
Food safety, steps to, 542–545
    chill, 544
    clean, 542–543
    cook, 543–544
    separate, 543

Food security, 552, 582
  dimensions of, 553f
  integrated food security phase classifications, 552, 553f
  levels of, 553f
Food sources
  of biotin, 332, 333f
  of calcium, 224, 387–388, 388f
  of choline, 344, 345f
  of folate, 335, 336f
  of iodine, 224, 409, 410f
  of iron, 224, 401, 402f
  of magnesium, 396, 397f
  of minerals, 376, 376f
  of niacin, 327, 328f
  of omega-3 fatty acids, 224
  of pantothenic acid, 329, 330f
  of phosphorus, 394, 395f
  of potassium, 383, 384f
  of riboflavin, 325–326, 326f
  of selenium, 406–407, 407f
  of sodium, 380, 380f
  of thiamin, 323, 324f
  of vitamin A, 305, 306f
  of vitamin B-6, 331–332, 331f
  of vitamin B-12, 339, 340f
  of vitamin C, 341, 342f
  of vitamin D, 224, 309–310, 310f
  of vitamin E, 314, 314f
  of vitamin K, 316, 318f
  of water, 369, 370f
  of zinc, 224
Food sterilization, 528, 528t
Food toxins, naturally occurring, 538–539, 539t
Food waste, 510, 515–516
Fortification, 38, 573
Fox, Arthur, 301
Fracture Risk Assessment Tool (FRAX), 424
Freekeh, 136t
Free radicals, 583–584, 621, 695, 715
  antioxidants and, 313, 456, 619
  defined, 313
  in muscle tissue, 456
Fructooligosaccharides (FOS), 107
Fructose, 127, 128f, 145
Fruitarian, 220
Fruit juices
  infants and, 649
  in menu planning for diabetes, A-7
  young children and, 665
Fruits, 271
  carbohydrates in, 138
  commonly consumed, 5, 6f
  consumption of, 38, 53
  low energy-dense, 265
  in menu planning for diabetes, A-7
  vitamins in, 296, 297f, 298t
Fruit sugar. See Fructose
Functional fibers, 136
Functional foods, 298–299
Fungi, 524

G

Galactooligosaccharides (GOS), 107
Galactose, 128, 128f, 145, 610
Galactosemia, 616
Gallbladder, 104, 105f
  removal of, 180
Gallstones, 118, 118f, 700
GALT. See Gut-associated lymphoid tissues
Garlic, 94, 703t
Gastric lipase, 180
Gastrin, 99
Gastroesophageal reflux disease (GERD), 112–113
Gastroesophageal sphincter. See Lower esophageal sphincter
Gastrointestinal health, 108
Gastrointestinal (GI) tract, 94
  absorption along, 103t
  esophagus, 95f, 97–98, 98f
  large intestine, 95f, 102–104, 103f
  lymphatic circulation in, 88
  microbes in, 106, 108
  mouth, 95f, 96–97
  portal circulation in, 87
  rectum, 95f, 104
  small intestine, 95f, 100–102, 101f, 102f
  stomach, 95f, 98–100, 99f
Gene, 82
Gene editing. See Genetic engineering
Gene expression, 82, 210, 210f
Generally recognized as safe (GRAS), 140, 536–537
Generational poverty, 560
Gene therapy, 211
The Genetic Alliance, 243
Genetically modified organisms (GMOs), 512, 572
Genetic editing. See Genetic engineering
Genetic engineering, 211, 512, 572
Genetic Information Nondiscrimination Act, 242
Genetics and nutrition, interactions between, 212. See also Nutritional genomics
Genetic testing, 242
Genogram, 243, 243f
Genome-wide association study (GWAS), 478
Geophagia, 604
GERD. See Gastroesophageal reflux disease
Gestation, 588, 636
Gestational diabetes, 157, 607–608
Gestational hypertension, 608
GHI. See Global Hunger Index
Ghrelin, 91, 91f
GI. See Glycemic index
Ginger, 703t
Ginkgo biloba, 703t
Ginseng, 703t
GL. See Glycemic load
Global dietary patterns, 22
Global Hunger Index (GHI), 564
Glocalization, 516
Glossitis, 325
Glucagon, 91f, 92, 148
  role in blood glucose control, 148, 148f
Glucosamine sulfate, 703t
Glucose, 11, 12, 111, 127, 128f, 145, 146
Glucose breakdown
  aerobic, 446
  anaerobic, 445
Glutathione peroxidase, 324, 408
Gluten, 118, 239
Gluten-free, casein-free (GFCF) diet, 659
Gluten-free diet, 119, 120, 288
Gluten sensitivity/gluten intolerance, 119
Glycemic index (GI), 149
Glycemic load (GL), 149, 583
Glycerol, 166, 169
Glycogen, 111, 126, 129, 147
Glyphosate, 521
GMOs. See Genetically modified organisms
Goat's milk, 649
Goiter, 409, 599
  undernutrition and, 554t
Goitrogens, 410
  and iodine deficiency, 411
Goldberger, Joseph, 327
Golgi complex, 80f, 82
Gooseflesh appearance, 304
Gout, 698
Grains, 137. See also Refined grains; Whole grains
  folic acid enrichment of, 336
Grapes and raisins, 694
GRAS. See Generally recognized as safe
Greenlandic Inuit, 190
Green revolution, 565
Green vegetables, leafy, 601
Growth, assessment of, 630–631
Growth charts, 630–631, 631f, 632f

Gruels, 237
Gums, 129
Gut-associated lymphoid tissues (GALT), 93, 109
Gut-brain axis, 264, 716
Gut microbiota, 25, 106, 108, 108f
    anorexia nervosa and, 486
    and appetite, 264
    autism spectrum disorder and, 659
    bone health and, 427
    cardiovascular disease and, 202
    immune function and, 109–110
    proteins and, 226
    vitamin production and, 295
Gynecoid obesity. *See* Lower-body obesity
Gynoid obesity. *See* Lower-body obesity

H

Hard water, 369
H_2 blockers, 115
HDLs. *See* High-density lipoproteins
Head circumference measurements, 630
Health
    diet quality on, impact of, 47
    nutritional, 55–57
Health and Human Services (HHS), 41
Health at Every Size approach, 501
Health claims, on food labels, 67–68, 69t
Health disparities, 156, 160
Health promotion and disease prevention, 23
    recommendations for, 24
Healthy Drinks. Healthy Kids. campaign, 658
Healthy Eating Index (HEI), 47
Healthy Food Financing Initiative (HFFI), 561
Healthy food priority areas, 561
Healthy, Hunger-Free Kids Act, 2010, 665
Healthy People 2030, 23
    goals of, 23
    nutrition-related objectives, 23
Heart, 86, 86f
Heart attack, 58, 196–197, 197f
Heartburn, 98, 112–113, 112f, 113t
    in pregnancy, 605
Heart defects, 618
Heart disease. *See also* Cardiovascular disease
    processed foods and, 38
Heart health, eating habits for, 191–192
Heavy drinking, 26
Helicobacter pylori, 79, 115
Helminth, 533
Hematocrit, 399

Heme iron, 400, 652
Hemicellulose, 129
Hemochromatosis, 402–403
Hemoconcentration, 368
Hemoglobin, 156, 399, 600
Hemoglobin A1c (HbA1c) test, 156
Hemolysis, 313
Hemolytic uremic syndrome (HUS), 530
Hemorrhage, 315
Hemorrhagic disease of the newborn, 316
Hemorrhagic stroke, 190
Hemorrhoids, 116, 145
    in pregnancy, 606
Hepatic portal circulation, 87
Hepatic portal vein, 87
Herbal products, 702, 703–704t
Hereditary hemochromatosis, 402–403
HFCS. *See* High-fructose corn syrup
Hidden hunger, 56, 552, 554
High-density lipoproteins (HDLs), 184t, 185
High-fructose corn syrup (HFCS), 127, 139
High-protein, low-carbohydrate diets, 287
High-quality proteins, 213
Hitting the wall, 446
HIV. *See* Human immunodeficiency virus
Homelessness
    chronic, 560–561
    and malnutrition, 560–561
    poverty and, 560
Homocysteine, 330
Honey, 139
Hormone, 91, 307
    defined, 7
Hospice care, 707
Household units, A-28
Human immunodeficiency virus (HIV), 524, 566. *See also* Acquired immunodeficiency syndrome
Human Microbiome Action project, 110
Human microbiota, 106–110
Human milk, 634, 635
    colostrum, 611
    composition of, 635t
    expressing and storing, 613–614
    for infants, 638–639
    mature milk, 611–612
    nutritional qualities of, 611–612
    for preterm infants, 612
    production of, 609–611, 610f
Human milk oligosaccharides, 611
Hunger, 552–553, 563
    chronic, 563
    control of, 265, 267–268

    defined, 7
    eating and, 7–8
    Global Hunger Index (GHI), 564
    hidden, 554
    prevalence of, 552, 552f
Hunter-gatherers, health of, 439
Hydrochlorothiazide (Microzide), 420
Hydrogenation, 178
Hydrolyzed protein formula, 640–641
Hydroponics, 517, 571–572
Hydroxyapatite, 386
Hygiene hypothesis, 110
Hypercarotenemia, 305–306
Hyperglycemia, 148, 156, 607
    during gestation, 607
Hyperkeratosis, 304
Hypertension, 418
    aging and, 419
    alcohol intake and, 419
    DASH diet in, 420–421, 420t
    defined, 9, 418
    family history of, 419
    gestational, 608
    medications for, 420, 421
    minerals and, 418–421
    modifiable risk factors for, 419–420
    nonmodifiable risk factors for, 419
    obesity and, 419
    physical inactivity and, 419
    prevention of, 421
    primary, 418
    processed foods and, 38
    salt sensitivity and, 381
    secondary, 418
    as silent disorder, 418
    sodium intake and, 45, 419
    tobacco use and, 420
Hypertensive disorders of pregnancy, 608
Hypertonic, 377
Hypoallergenic infant formula. *See* Hydrolyzed protein formula
Hypochromic, 399
Hypoglycemia, 148, 156, 159
Hypokalemia, 383
Hyponatremia, 371–372, 379, 459
    in infants, 638
Hypothalamus, 8
Hypotheses, 18
Hypotonic, 377

I

Ibandronate (Boniva), 428
Identical twins, 262
Idli, 107
Ileocecal sphincter, 102
Ileum, 100, 101f, 337

Illicit drug use, during pregnancy, 590
Immune function, gut microbiota and, 109–110
Immune system, 93–94
Immunoglobulins, 93
Impaired fasting glucose. See Prediabetes
Inborn errors of metabolism, 239–240, 327
Incomplete proteins. See also Lower-quality proteins
Indirect calorimetry, 256, 256f
Indirect food additives, 535
Indispensable amino acids. See Essential amino acids
Infant formulas
   arachidonic acid in, 636
   composition of, 635t
   docosahexaenoic acid in, 636
   feeding with, 639–641
   forms of, 641
   hydrolyzed protein formula, 640–641
   low-iron infant formula, 637
   preparation and storage of, 641
   soy protein–based formulas, 640
   transition formulas, 641
   typical intake of, 642t
Infants
   baby-led weaning, 646–647
   breast milk for, 638–639
   burp during feeding, 642
   carbohydrate needs of, 635
   complementary foods for, 637, 642, 643
   dehydration in, 637–638
   dietary fat needs of, 636, 647
   dietary supplements for, 617
   energy requirements, 634
   fat recommendations for, 189
   feeding guidelines, 638–649
   fluoride needs of, 637
   food allergies in, signs of, 644
   foods/practices to avoid for, 648–649
   formula feeding for, 639–641
   fortified grain products for, 648
   fruits to, 647
   hyponatremia in, 638
   iron needs of, 637
   low-birth-weight, 589
   mealtime choices for, 642–646
   nutritional needs, 634–638
   Nutrition Facts labels of food for, 645f
   preterm, 588
   protein needs of, 635
   responsive feeding, 642, 647
   rickets in, 308
   sample daily menu, 643t
   self-feeding skills of, 646
   small for gestational age, 589
   solid food intake of, 642–647
   technique for feeding of, 642
   vegetables to, 648
   vitamin B-12 needs of, 636
   vitamin D needs of, 636
   vitamin D supplements for, 312
   vitamin K needs of, 636
   vitamin K supplementation for, 316
   water needs of, 637–638
   weaning from bottle or breast, 647
Infertility, 582
Inflammaging, 687
Innate immunity, 93
Inorganic substance, 13
Input traits, 512
Insect farming, 564
Insoluble fiber, 130
Insulin, 91f, 92, 147, 159
   role in blood glucose control, 147–148, 148f
Insulin infusion pump, 157
Insulin resistance, 159–160, 582, 583
Integrative Human Microbiome Project, 110
Integumentary system, 84f
Intercropping, 514
Interesterified fat, 178–179
Intermittent fasting, 281
International Agency for Research on Cancer (IARC), 125
International Glycemic Index (GI) Database, 149
International Rescue Committee (IRC), 563
Intestinal gas, 145
Intracellular fluid, 377
Intrinsic factor, 100, 337
Inulin, 130
Iodine, 93
   adequate intake of, 409–411
   avoidance of excess, 411
   for brain growth and development, 714
   deficiency, 409
   food sources of, 409, 410f
   functions of, 408
   in pregnancy, 599–600
   RDA for, 409
   UL for, 411
Iodine fortification of salt, 409
Ions, 377
Iron, 375, 399
   absorption of, 400–401
   adequate intake of, 401, 402f
   for adults, 694
   athletes and, 456–457
   avoidance of excess, 402–403
   in brain formation, 714
   deficiency, 399–400, 403
   and fertility, 584
   food sources of, 401, 402f
   functions of, 399
   heme, 400
   for infants, 637
   nonheme, 400–401, 401t
   in pregnancy, 600
   RDA for, 401
   for teenagers, 668
   for toddlers and preschoolers, 651–652
   UL for, 402
Iron-deficiency anemia, 399–400
   in childhood, 651–652
   maternal, 574
   in teenagers, 668
   undernutrition and, 554t
Iron supplements, 400, 402, 404
   for infants, 637
Irradiation, 528, 528t, 529
Irritable bowel syndrome (IBS), 109, 117
Ischemic stroke, 190
Isoflavones, 299
Isotonic, 377
Isotretinoin (Accutane), 306

J

Jaundice, 305
Jejunum, 100, 101f

K

Kamut, 136t
Kañiwa, 136t
Keratin, 304
Ketoacidosis, 194
Ketoadaptation, 448
Ketogenic diet, 194–195
Ketone bodies, 146, 157, 280
   chemical structure of, A-27
Ketosis, 147, 157, 194, 280, 596, 597
Keys, Ansel, 551
Kidney, 88–89
Kidney disease, 238
   protein intake in, 238
Kidney stones, 368
Kilocalorie (kcal), 11, 15
Kosher salt, 381
Kwashiorkor, 237, 237f, 554t
Kyphosis, 425–426, 426f

L

Lactase, 142, 639
Lactase supplements, 144
Lactate (lactic acid), 445

Lactation, 588, 610
    hormonal regulation of, 610
Lactation consultant, 609, 616
Lacteals, 88, 181
Lactic acid bacteria, 107
Lactobacillus bifidus, 611
Lactoovovegetarian, 220, 603, 658
Lactose, 128, 610, 639
    in dairy foods, 139*t*
    in human milk, 610
Lactose intolerance, 143–144, 639, 700
Lactose maldigestion, 142–144
    congenital lactase deficiency, 143
    primary, 142
    secondary, 143
Lactose-reduced milk, 144
Lactovegetarian, 220, 603
La Leche League, 616
Lansoprazole (Prevacid), 115
Lanugo, 484
Large intestine, 95*f*, 102–104, 103*f*
Latin American Diet Pyramid, 44, 44*f*
Laxatives, 116, 482
LBW. *See* Low birth weight
LDL. *See* Low-density lipoprotein
Lead poisoning, children and, 656–657
Leafy green vegetables, 601
Lean body mass (LBM), 254, 255*f*
Lecithin, 169, 175
Lectins, 215
Legumes, 215, 217
Leptin, 91, 91*f*, 263, 582
Let-down reflex, 610, 610*f*
Leukocytes. *See* White blood cells
Life expectancy, 688
Life span, 688
Lifestyle management
    blood glucose control and, 148–149
    cardiovascular disease and, 199
    polycystic ovary syndrome and, 583
Lifetime prevalence, 479
Lignin, 130
Limiting amino acid, 214
Lind, James, 341
Linoleic acid, 12, 168, 173, 174, 189, 189*t*, 597
Lipase, 97
Lipids, 12, 166. *See also* Fats; Oils; Phospholipids; Sterols; Triglycerides
    absorption of, 181, 182*f*
    in cell membranes, 187
    characteristics of, 166
    chemical forms of, 170*f*
    composition of, 166
    concept map, 171*f*
    defined, 10
    digestion of, 180–181, 181*f*
    energy provided by, 187
    fats, 12
    in foods, 171–176
    insulation and protection of body, 187
    oils, 12
    in pregnancy, 597
    in regulation and communication, 187–188
    roles of, in body, 187–189
    storage of energy by, 187
    transportation of, 183–186
Lipoprotein lipase, 184
Lipoproteins, 183
    chylomicrons, 183–185, 184*t*
    classification of, 184*t*
    HDLs, 184*t*, 185
    LDLs, 184*t*, 185
    structure of, 183, 183*f*
    VLDLs, 184*t*, 185
Liraglutide (Saxenda), 279*t*, 280
Lisdexamfetamine (Vyvanse), 491, 494
Lisinopril (Prinivel, Zestril), 420
Listeria monocytogenes, 591
Listeriosis, 532
Liver, 104, 105*f*
Livestock, role of, in health, 218
Lobes, breast, 609, 609*f*
Locally grown foods, 516–517
Locavore, 517
Locavore movement, 516, 517
Long-chain fatty acids, 166, 173
Low birth weight (LBW), 556, 589, 630
Low-calorie diet, 287
Low-carbohydrate diets, 287
Low-density lipoprotein (LDL), 184*t*, 185, 196
Lower-body obesity, 261*f*, 262
Lower esophageal sphincter, 97–98, 113, 605
Lower-quality proteins, 213
Low-fat diets, 287–288
Low FODMAP diet, 288
Low-income, low-access areas (LILA), 561
Lumen, 94
Luo han guo, 141
Lutein, 302, 303*t*
Lycopene, 305
Lymph, 85, 87
Lymphatic system, 83*f*, 85, 87–88, 93
Lymph nodes, 93
Lysosomes, 80*f*, 82

M

Macrocytes, 334
Macrocytic anemia, 334, 335*f*, 338
    undernutrition and, 554*t*

Macronutrients, 11. *See also* Carbohydrates; Lipids; Proteins
    acceptable macronutrient distribution ranges, A-31
    comparison of, 11*f*
    for infants, 636
Macula, 302
Macular degeneration, age-related, 302, 303*f*
Magnesium
    adequate intake of, 396–397
    for adults, 695
    avoidance of excess, 397
    in bone health, 396
    deficiency, 396
    food sources of, 396, 397*f*
    functions of, 396
    RDA for, 396
    in synthesis of DNA and protein, 396
    UL for, 397
Major minerals, 13
Male fertility
    nutritional strategies and, 585
    zinc and, 584
Malignant tumors, 351
Malnutrition, 55, 93, 551, 554, 573, 574
    in adults, 691, 692*f*
    causes of, 553
    in childhood, 575–576
    chronic, 553
    at critical life stages, 574–576
    in developing world, 563–567, 563*f*
    double burden of, 555
    famine and, 563
    during fetal development and infant stage, 575
    food deserts and, 561
    homelessness and, 560–561
    hunger and, 553
    impact of, on health, 555, 555*f*
    medical and societal costs of, 553
    and micronutrient deficiencies, 554–555
    in older adults, 576
    poverty and, 560
    during pregnancy, 574–575
    socioecological factors related to, 560–562
    solutions to, 561–562
    in United States, 556–562
Malnutrition Screening Tool (MST), 691
Maltase, 142
Maltose, 128
Manganese, 416
    AI for, 416
    food sources of, 416
    functions of, 416
    toxicity, 416

Maple syrup, 139
Marasmus, 237–238, 237f, 554t
Marijuana use, during pregnancy, 590
Marine oils and derivatives, 201
Marketing, food choices and, 5
Marshall, Barry, 79
Massive colony collapse disorder (CCD), 520
Maternal age, and pregnancy, 590
Maternal depression and malnutrition in children, 570
Maudsley method, 486
Meatless Monday, 218
Mechanical digestion, 94–95, 97
Mediterranean-DASH Intervention for Neurodegenerative Delay (MIND), 717
Mediterranean diet, 54, 55f, 191–192, 585, 690
Medium-chain fatty acids, 166, 173
Megadose, 63, 295
Megaloblastic anemia. See Macrocytic anemia
Megaloblasts. See Macrocytes
Melons, 523
Menadione, 316. See also Vitamin K
Menaquinone, 316. See also Vitamin K
Menkes syndrome, 412
Menopause, 185
Menstruation, factors affecting, 484
Menu nutrition labeling, 69
Menu planning. See also Diet and diet plans
    basis for, 41–47
    with labels, 69–70
    with MyPlate, 51–52
Messenger RNA, 210
Meta-analysis, 19
Metabolic syndrome, 159–160, 199, 596
Metabolic water, 364
Metabolism, 85. See also Energy metabolism
    alcohol, 27
    defined, 13
Metastasize, 351
Methyl group, 166
Metoprolol tartrate (Lopressor), 420
Metric-English conversions, A-28
Metric system, 17, 17f
Metric units, A-28
Microbial contamination of food, 524. See also Foodborne illness
Microbiome, 29, 106
Microbiota, 29, 104, 639
Microbiota-accessible carbohydrates (MACs), 146
Microcytic, 399
Micronutrient powders (MNP), 555

Micronutrients, 11. See specific micronutrient
    deficiency in developing world, 554
Microorganisms, foodborne illness by, 530–534
    bacteria, 530–532
    parasites, 533, 534f
    viruses, 532–533
Microvilli, 100
Migraines, 716
Milk ejection reflex. See Let-down reflex
Milk siblings, 640
Milk thistle, 703t
Millet, 136t
MIND Diet, 717
Minerals, 13, 90, 373. See also specific mineral
    absorption of, 375
    bioavailability of, 375
    defined, 10
    electrolytes, 13
    and fertility, 584
    food sources of, 376, 376f
    function of, 374, 374f
    in human body, 373, 373f
    and hypertension, 418–421
    for infants, 637
    major, 13, 373–374, 373f
    preservation of, in foods, 376, 376f
    storage of, 111, 375
    in supplement, 376
    toxicities, 376
    trace, 13, 373f, 374–375
    ultratrace, 375
    vitamin–mineral interactions, 375
Mineral water, 370
Minimally processed food, 37
Miscarriage. See Spontaneous abortion
Mitochondria, 80f, 81
Moderate drinking, 26
Moderate-intensity aerobic physical activity, 439
Molybdenum, 417
    food sources of, 417
    RDA for, 417
    UL for, 417
Monoglyceride, 169, 170f
Monosaccharides, 127–128, 145
    chemical structure of, 128f
    defined, 128
    fructose, 127
    galactose, 128
    glucose, 127
Monosodium glutamate (MSG), 674
Monounsaturated fatty acids, 174f
Morning sickness, 606
Motility, 113
Mouth, 95f, 96–97

Mouth sensing, 451
Mucilage, 130
Mucus, 97
Multigrain cereals, 135
Multiple sclerosis, 717
Multivitamin and mineral supplement (MVM). See Supplements
Muscle dysmorphia, 499
Muscles, energy sources for, 444–449, 447t
    aerobic metabolism, 446–448
    anaerobic metabolism, 445, 445f
    physical training and fuel use, 448–449
Muscle-strengthening activities, 439, 442
Muscle tissue, 82
Muscular endurance, 442
Muscular power, 442
Muscular system, 84f
Musculoskeletal fitness, 442–443
Mushrooms, 311
Myelin, 90, 338
Myocardial infarction. See Heart attack
Myoglobin, 399
MyPlate, 38, 49, 348, A-21
    building of healthy plate, 49
    carbohydrates in, 132, 132f
    daily plan, 50
    dietary pattern for adults, 50, 50t
    eating pattern and, healthy, 49
    fat on, 172–173, 172f
    fruit group, 138
    heart-healthy meal, 201f
    limitations of, 54
    meal swaps, 53f
    menu planning with, 51–52
    ratings, 52–54
    for school-age children, 660, 661f
    vitamins in, 297f
MyWW program, 286

N

Naltrexone-bupropion (Contrave), 279t
Namenda, 495
National Bioengineered Food Disclosure Standard (NBFDS), 512
National Collegiate Athletic Association (NCAA), 450, 468
    and nutrition supplements, 468
National Diabetes Prevention Program, 156
National Farm to School Network, 517
National Health and Nutrition Examination Survey (NHANES), 22
National Institute of Alcohol Abuse and Alcoholism (NIAAA), 29

National Weight Control Registry (NWCR), 275f
Nature
　body weight and, 262–264
　nurture and, 262
Nausea and vomiting, of pregnancy, 606
Negative energy balance, 252
Negative protein balance, 232
Neophobia, 653
Neotame, 141
Nephrons, 238
Nerve impulse transmission, 89–90, 90f
Nervous system, 83f, 89–90
Nervous tissue, 82
Neural tube defects, 334–336, 592, 598, 618
Neurodegenerative diseases, 716–717
Neuron, 89, 90f, 338
Neurotransmitters, 90, 90f, 229, 322, 386, 476, 621, 714–715
New breeding techniques (NBTs), 513
New Nordic diet, 192
Niacin, 231, 295, 319
　adequate intake of, 327–329
　avoidance of excess, 329
　chemical structure of, A-25
　deficiency, 327
　food sources of, 327, 328f
　functions of, 327
　tryptophan and, 327
Niacin flush, 329
Nicotinic acid, 327
Night blindness, 302, 304
Night eating syndrome, 497
Nitrosamines, 340
Nixtamalization, 328
Nizatidine (Axid), 115
Nonceliac wheat sensitivity (NCWS), 119
Noncommunicable diseases (NCDs). See Chronic diseases
Nonessential amino acids, 208
Non-Exercise Activity Thermogenesis (NEAT), 255
Non-Exercise Physical Activity (NEPA), 255
Nonheme iron, 400–401, 401t
Nonshivering thermogenesis, 253
Nonspecific immunity, 93
Nonsteroidal antiinflammatory drugs (NSAIDs), 115
Nontropical plant oils, 190
Noom, 288
Nordic diet, 192
Norepinephrine, 90, 91f, 229, 715
Norovirus, 533, 533f
Nova classification, of food, 37
Nucleus, 80f, 81–82
Nursery water, bottled, 641

Nurture
　body weight and, 264
　nature and, 262
Nut butters, 190
Nutrient content claims, on food labels, 67, 68t
Nutrient density, 36–38, 265
　defined, 36
　evaluation of, 36
　food processing and, 37–38
Nutrient recommendations, 59–62, 59t
Nutrients, 8–9, 36
　bone health and, 427
　classes of, 10–14
　defined, 8
　energy-yielding, 11, 11f
　essential, 9
　from food, 8
　functional categories, 11
　for immune system, 94
　macronutrients, 11, 11f
　micronutrients, 11
　in nerve impulse transmission, 89, 90f
　recommendations for active adults and athletes, 449–460
　role in nervous system, 89, 90
　sources of, 14
Nutrient standards, application of, 61–62
Nutrient storage capabilities, 111
Nutrition
　and academic performance, 74
　chemical structures important in, A-23–A-27
　defined, 8
　fitness apps and, 64
　food choices and, 7
　health and, 8–10
　in infancy, 634–638
　math concepts in study of, 14–17
　scientific evidence, 19–20, 19f
　scientific method and knowledge of, 18–19, 18f
　study of, 9
Nutritional assessment, 57–58
　ABCDEs of, 57, 58f
　anthropometric assessment, 57, 58f
　background factors in, 57
　biochemical assessment, 57, 58f
　clinical assessment, 57, 58f
　dietary assessment, 57, 58f
　environmental assessment, 57, 58f
　health history in, 57
　limitations of, 57–58
Nutritional deficiency, 56
Nutritional genomics, 212, 241–244, 241f
　nutrigenetics, 241, 241f
　nutrigenomics, 241–242, 241f

Nutritional health, 55–57
Nutritional ketosis, 194
Nutritional state. See Nutritional status
Nutritional status, 55
　of adults, 696–704
　assessment of (See Nutritional assessment)
　defined, 55
　marginal, 56f
　microbes and, 109
　optimal, 56f
　pregnancy and, 592
NutritionCalc Pl, A-19–A-21
Nutrition education, in schools, 665–666
Nutrition Facts label, 65–67
　calculation, 16
　calories on, 68t
　claims allowed on, 67–68, 68t, 69t
　components listed on, 65, 66f
　Daily Values (DVs) on, 65–67
　dietary fiber on, 130
　exceptions to, 67
　fat on, 68t, 176, 177f
　fiber on, 68t
　health claims on, 67–68, 69t
　for infant foods, 645f
　menu planning with, 69–70
　nutrient content claims on, 67, 68t
　Other Carbohydrates on, 129
　reading of, 265, 266f
　sodium on, 68t
　structure/function claim on, 68
　sugar on, 68t, 127
Nutrition information, evaluation of, 63–64, 64f
Nutrition Labeling and Education Act, 1990, 65
Nutrition literacy, defined, 4
Nutrition security, 552–553, 556–559
　components of, 557f
　health and, 557, 557f
Nutrition therapy
　for anorexia nervosa, 485–486
　for binge eating disorder, 494
　for bulimia nervosa, 490–491
Nutritive sweeteners, 138–140
Nuts, 215–216
　as heart-healthy snack, 221, 222

O

Oatmeal, 298–299
Oats, 136t
Obesity, 9, 21, 24, 56
　anti-obesity drugs/diet pills for, 279–280, 279t
　bariatric surgery in, 282–283, 282f, 283t

Obesity (continued)
  bone health and, 427
  CDC data on, 21, 21f
  chronic diseases and, 24, 56
  conception and, 583
  defined, 5
  genetic contribution to, 262
  genetics and, 242
  management of, 276–278
  nature and nurture and risk of, 262, 263t
  poverty and, 264
  pregnancy and, 595–596
  prevalence of, 21, 21f, 250, 250f
  rate of, rise in, 21
  in school-age children, 660–663, 662f
  severe, 280–283
  societal efforts for, 275–276, 275f
  sodium consumption and, 381
  treatment for, 250
  type 2 diabetes and, 158
  upper-body, 158
  very-low-calorie diet in, 280
Obesity Action Coalition (OAC), 275
Offal, 567
Oils, 12, 166
  in foods, 171–176
  rancidity and, 178–180
Olanzapine (Zyprexa), 487
Older adults. *See also* Adulthood
  blue zones and, 709–710, 710f
  body composition, changes in, 696, 698
  calorie needs of, 43
  community nutrition services for, 707–708
  congregate meals for, 559
  dietary patterns for, 705–707, 705f
  healthy eating for, 706f
  malnutrition in, 576
  medications and, 702
  MyPlate recommendations for, 706
  osteomalacia in, 698
  physical activity guidelines for, 698, 699t
  thiamin deficiency in, 322
  thirst sensation and, 368
  in United States, 684, 684f, 709, 709f
  vitamin D deficiency in, 308
  vitamin D synthesis and, 307
Older Americans Act (OAA), 559, 707
Oleic acid, 173
Oleogustus, 96
Oligopeptides, 209
Olive oil, 200
Olives, 386

Omega-3 fatty acids, 168, 584, 665
  in fish, 174–175, 174t, 191
  intake of, 190–191
  plant sources of, 224
Omega-6 fatty acids, 168
Omeprazole (Prilosec), 115
Onions and garlic, 94
Optifast, 280
Organelles, cell, 80, 80f
Organic compounds, 12
Organic farming, 509
Organic foods, 510–511
  availability and sales of, 510
  defined, 510
  and health, 511
  production of, 510
  USDA organic seal on, 510, 510f
Organ meats, and vitamin B-12, 339
Organs, 82, 84
Organ system, 82–84, 83–84f
Orlistat (Xenical), 279t, 494
Ornish dietary plan, 192
Orthorexia nervosa, 498
Osmosis, 377–378, 378f
Osteoarthritis, 698
Osteoblasts, 422
Osteocalcin, 316
Osteoclasts, 422
Osteomalacia, 308, 698
Osteopenia, 424
Osteoporosis, 58, 387, 422–428, 668, 698
  criteria for diagnosis of, 424
  defined, 9
  definition of, 424
  medications for, 428
  prevalence of, 425
  prevention of, 426–428
  primary, 425
  secondary, 425
  as silent disease, 425
  treatment of, 428
Osteoporotic fractures, 425
Output traits, 512
Overeaters Anonymous, 494
Overnutrition, 56–57, 552, 554
  defined, 55
  excess intake of calories in, 56
  pediatric, 633
  symptoms, 56
Overweight, 21. *See also* Obesity
  management of, 276–278
Ovovegetarian, 220
Ovum, 586
Oxalic acid, 375
Oxidize, 191
Oxygenated blood, 86
Oxytocin, 610

P

Pagophagia, 604
Paleo diet, 439
Palmitic acid, 173
Palm oil, 173
Pancreas, 92, 92f, 105, 105f
Pancreatic amylase, 142
Pancreatic lipase, 180
Pantothenic acid, 319
  adequate intake of, 329
  avoidance of excess, 329
  chemical structure of, A-26
  deficiency, 329
  food sources of, 329, 330f
  functions of, 329
Paraprobiotics, 107
Parasites, 524
  foodborne illness by, 533, 534f
Parathyroid hormone (PTH), 307, 387
Parkinson's disease, 413
Passive diffusion, 27, 100, 102f
Pasteurizing, 524
Pathogen, 93
PCM. *See* Protein-calorie malnutrition
PCOS. *See* Polycystic ovary syndrome
PCr. *See* Phosphocreatine
PCSK9 inhibitors, 201
Peace Corps, 569
Peanut allergy
  early introduction of peanut protein for, 674
  immunotherapy for, 673
Peanuts, 215–216
Pectin, 129
Pediatric malnutrition, 632–633
Pedometers, 270, 440
Peer review, 19, 63
Pellagra, 327
  undernutrition and, 554t
People-First Language Initiative, 275
Pepsin, 226
Peptic ulcer, 113–115, 114f
  H. pylori infection and, 115
  NSAIDs and, 115
  symptoms, 115
  treatment, 115
Peptide bond, 209
Percentages, calculation of, 14–15
Percentile, 630
Percutaneous transluminal coronary angioplasty (PTCA), 202
Perforation, 113, 490
Periodization, 465, 466
Period, normal, 484
  missing, 484
Peripheral artery disease, 196

Peripheral quantitative computed tomography (pQCT), 423–424
Peristalsis, 97, 98f, 116
Pernicious anemia, 338–339, 639
Peroxisomes, 80f, 82
Personalized nutrition, 244
Perspiration, 367, 368f, 379
Pescovegetarian, 220
Pesticides, 519–520
　defined, 519
　personal action and, 522
　reduction of exposure to, 522t
　regulation of, 520, 521t
　safety of, 520–522
　use of, 520
　value of, in crop production, 520
pH, 88
Phagocytosis, 93, 102, 102f
Pharmacological therapy
　for anorexia nervosa, 487
　for binge eating disorder, 494–495
　for bulimia nervosa, 491
Pharynx, 97
Phendimetrazine, 279t
Phentermine, 279t, 494
Phentermine-topiramate (Qsymia), 279t
Phenylalanine, 239, 620
Phenylketonuria (PKU), 141, 239–240, 240f, 620, 621
Phosphatidylcholine, 343
Phosphocreatine (PCr), 445, 445f, 465
Phospholipids, 80, 81f, 166, 169, 170f, 394
　amphipathic property of, 169
　digestion, 180
　food sources of, 175
Phosphorus
　absorption of, 394
　adequate intake of, 394
　avoidance of excess, 395
　deficiency, 394
　food sources of, 394, 395f
　functions of, 394
　kidney diseases and, 395
　RDA for, 394
　UL for, 395
Photosynthesis, 126, 126f
Phylloquinone, 316. See also Vitamin K
Physical activity, 4, 438
　adults and, 47–48, 48t, 698–700
　benefits of, 269, 438, 438f
　and bone health, 426
　calorie costs of, 270t
　calories required for, 449
　CDC recommendations, 269f
　in daily routine, 270
　devices monitoring, 270
　energy for, 255
　exercise and, 438
　getting started, 443–444
　guidelines, 47–48
　levels of, 440
　moderate-intensity aerobic activity, 439
　moderate-intensity, for adults, 47–48
　multicomponent, 443
　muscle-strengthening activities, 439
　during pregnancy, 594, 594f
　progression, 443
　recommendations, 439
　type 1 diabetes and, 158
　type 2 diabetes and, 159
　in United States, 47
　vigorous-intensity aerobic activity, 439
　warm-up and cool-down, 443
　weight loss and, 270, 270t, 272
Physical Activity Guidelines for Americans, 47, 438–439
Physical Activity Readiness Questionnaire (PAR-Q), 440
Physical fitness, 438–439
　achieving and maintaining, 440–444
　aerobic activities and, 441–442
　assessment, 440
　balance activities in, 443
　bone-strengthening activities in, 443
　cardiorespiratory endurance, 441–442
　defined, 438
　FITT-VP principle, 441
　flexibility activities in, 443
　goal setting in, 440–441
　heart rate and, 441, 441f, 442, 442t
　musculoskeletal, 442–443
　program planning, 441–444, 441t, 443f
　RPE scale, 441–442, 442f
　sticking with fitness program, 444
Physiological anemia, 607
Phytic acid, 224, 375
Phytochemical content of eating pattern, boosting of, 300t
Phytochemicals, 12–14, 38, 298–299
　functions, 299–300
　in plant pigment colors, 299f
　recommendations, 300
Phytosterols, 169, 176
Pica, 496, 604
Picky eating, 650, 653–654
Piles. *See* Hemorrhoids
Pineapples, 571
Pinocytosis, 102, 102f
PKU. *See* Phenylketonuria
Placebo, 19
Placenta, 586, 586f
Plant-based dairy alternatives, 389
　cow's milk and, 389t
　infants and, 649
Plant-based dietary patterns, 219–226
　B vitamins and, 224
　calcium and vitamin D in, 224
　and cancer prevention, 222
　cardiovascular disease risk and, 221, 222
　choice of, reasons for, 221
　Dietary Guidelines for Americans on, 220
　food plan for vegetarians, 223t
　health benefits of, 219, 225
　heart health and, 221
　iodine in, 224
　iron in, 224
　MyPlate on, 220
　nutrient adequacy in, 223–224
　nutritional adequacy of, 219
　omega-3 fatty acids in, 224
　type 2 diabetes and, 222–223
　types of, 220, 220f
　zinc in, 224
Plant-based protein powders, 218
Plant-focused dietary patterns, 73
Plant oils, 12
Plant proteins, 215–216, 216f
Plant sterols, 199
Plaque, 196
Plasma, 86
Platelets, 86
Plenity, 280
Pollovegetarian, 220
Polychlorinated biphenyls (PCBs), in fish, 523
Polycystic ovary syndrome (PCOS), 583
　dietary and lifestyle interventions in, 583
　female infertility and, 583
　lifestyle interventions in, 583
Polypeptides, 209
Polypharmacy, 702
Polysaccharides, 127–129
　fiber, 129–131, 130f, 130t
　glycogen, 129, 129f
　starch, 129, 129f
Polyunsaturated fatty acids (PUFA), 174f, 178, 313
Pomegranates, 317
Pool, 214
Popular diets, 286–288
Pork, 322
Portal circulation, in gastrointestinal tract, 87
Portion control, 265
Portion size, 39–40, 40f, 149
Positive energy balance, 252
Positive protein balance, 232

Postbiotics, 107
Postmenopausal osteoporosis, 425
Potassium
    adequate intake of, 383–384
    for adults, 694
    avoidance of excess, 384
    deficiency, 383
    food sources of, 383, 384f
    functions of, 383
    sodium and, 383
Potatoes, 137
Poverty
    federal poverty level (FPL), 560
    generational, 560
    and malnutrition, 560
    situational, 560
    United States and, 556
Prebiotics, 94, 107, 639
Precautionary principle, 538
Precision nutrition, 244
Prediabetes, 148, 156–157
Predigested infant formula. *See* Hydrolyzed protein formula
Preeclampsia, 608
Pregnancy, 588–589
    alcohol intake during, 621
    anemia in, 606–607
    BMI, 591–592
    caffeine during, 620
    calorie needs during, 593–594
    carbohydrate needs in, 597
    choline during, 344, 345
    closely spaced/multiple births and, 590
    constipation in, 605–606
    diabetes during, 607–608
    diet plans in, 601–604, 602f, 603t
    eating patterns in, 601–604
    edema during, 606
    EER equation, A-30
    fluid needs in, 597–598
    folate in, 334, 335, 598
    food cravings during, 602–603
    food safety in, 591, 591f
    goal of, 588
    heartburn in, 605
    hemorrhoids in, 606
    hypertensive disorders of, 608
    iodine in, 409, 599–600, 619
    iron in, 600
    length of, 586
    lipid needs in, 597
    maternal age and, 590
    micronutrient supplementation during, 556
    mineral needs during, 599–600, 599f
    nausea and vomiting of, 606
    nonfood items cravings during, 604
    nutrition and, 592
    nutrition assistance during, 592
    obesity and, 595–596
    physical activity during, 594, 594f
    positive energy balance in, 252
    poverty and, 592
    prenatal supplements and, 600–601
    protein needs in, 596–597
    toxic agents during, 587f, 590–591
    vegetarian dietary patterns during, 603–604
    vitamin A during, 304–306
    vitamin D during, 598–599
    vitamin needs in, 598–599, 598f
    weight gain in, 595–596, 596t
    zinc in, 600
Prenatal care and counseling, 589
Prenatal growth and development, 586–588
    first trimester, 586–588
    second trimester, 588
    third trimester, 588
Prenatal vitamin and mineral supplements, 600–601
Preschoolers. *See* Toddlers and preschoolers
Preservation
    of minerals in foods, 376, 376f
    of vitamins in foods, 296, 298, 298t
Preservatives, 535
Preterm infants, 588, 631
    human milk for, 612
Primary hypertension, 418
Primary lactose maldigestion, 142
Primary osteoporosis, 425
    type 1, 425
    type 2, 425
Probiotics, 29, 107
Processed culinary ingredients, 37
Processed foods, 37
Prohormone, 92
Prolactin, 610
Protein balance, 232–233, 232f
    negative, 232
    positive, 232
Protein-calorie malnutrition (PCM), 236–238, 554
Protein Digestibility Corrected Amino Acid Score (PDCAAS), 213
Protein Efficiency Ratio (PER), 213
Protein equilibrium, 232
Proteins, 12, 146, 208
    absorption of, 226–227, 227f
    in acid–base balance, 229
    for adults, 692
    AMDR for, 233
    amino acids in, 12
    animal, 12, 213, 216–218
    athletes and, 452f, 453–454
    balance, 232–233, 232f
    in bloodstream, 228
    body components by, synthesis of, 228
    at breakfast, 235
    in breast milk, 639
    building blocks of, 208 (*See also* Amino acids)
    complementary, 214, 215f
    complete, 213
    defined, 10
    denaturation of, 211, 212f
    DIAAS score of, 214
    digestion of, 226, 227f
    as energy source, 229–230, 230f
    enzymes as, 229
    feelings of satiety from, 231
    fluid balance by, 228, 229f
    food allergies and, 238
    in foods, 212–219, 213f
    as fuel for muscles, 447–448
    gut microbiota and, 226
    health concerns related to, 236–240
    high-quality, 213
    hormones as, 229
    immune function and, 229
    for infants, 635
    kidney disease and, 238
    lower-quality, 213
    low intake of, 228
    in menu planning for diabetes, A-10–A-11
    needs, 232–235
    organization, 210–211, 211f
    planning dietary pattern with, 235t
    plant, 12, 213, 215–216, 216f
    powders, 218–219
    during pregnancy, 596–597
    Protein Concept Map, 231f
    quality of, 213–214
    RDA for, 233–234
    rebuilding and repairing, 228
    recommendations from *Dietary Guidelines*, 234, 234f
    requirements per meal, 234–235
    role of, in body, 208, 227–231
    synthesis, 209–210, 210f
    for toddlers and preschoolers, 652
Protein supplements, 218–219
Protein turnover, 228
Proton pump inhibitors (PPIs), 113, 115
Protozoa, 533
Provitamin A, 302. *See also* Carotenoids; Vitamin A
Psychiatric genetics, 478
Psychological therapy
    for anorexia nervosa, 486

for binge eating disorder, 494
for bulimia nervosa, 491
Psyllium, 116
Public Health Security and Bioterrorism Preparedness and Response Act, 2001, 523–524
PUFA. *See* Polyunsaturated fatty acids
Purging disorder, 497
Purified water, 370
Pyloric sphincter, 99
Pyridoxal phosphate (PLP), 330
Pyridoxine. *See* Vitamin B-6
Pyruvate, 445

Q

Quantitative ultrasound (QUS) technique, 424
Quinoa, 136*t*
Quinone. *See* Vitamin K

R

Rabeprazole (Aciphex), 115
Radiation, 528, 529
Raloxifene (Evista), 428
Rancidity, 178–180
Randomized controlled trial, 19
Rating of Perceived Exertion (RPE) Scale, 441–442, 442*f*
RDA. *See* Recommended Dietary Allowance
RDN. *See* Registered dietitian nutritionist
Reactive oxygen species. *See* Free radicals
Receptor, 91
Recommended Dietary Allowance (RDA), 59, 59*t*, 61
for proteins, 233–234
for vitamin A, 305
for vitamin D, 309
for vitamin E, 315
Recovery meals for athletes, 466, 466*t*
Rectum, 95*f*, 104
Red and processed meats, consumption of, 217
Red blood cells, 86, 399
Red meat, 363
Red meat allergy. *See* Alpha-gal syndrome
RED-S. *See* Relative energy deficiency in sport
Refined grains, 134, 134*t*
Regenerative agriculture, 571
Registered dietitian nutritionist (RDN), 10, 57, 160
Regurgitation syndrome. *See* Rumination disorder

Relapse prevention
defined, 275
in weight management, 274–275
Relative energy deficiency in sport (RED-S), 450, 451*f*
Reproductive function, energy for, 582
Reproductive system, 84*f*
Reserve capacity, 686
Resistance training, 443
recovery from, 466
Resistant starch, 129
Resorption, 422
Respiratory system, 84*f*
Responsive feeding, 642
Restaurant dining, food choices and, 5
Restaurant menu labeling, 69
Resting metabolic rate (RMR), 254
Resting metabolism, 254
Retina, 302
Retinal, 302
Retinoic acid, 302
Retinoids, 302. *See also* Vitamin A
Retinol, 302
Retinol activity equivalents (RAE), 305
Retinyl, 302
Reverse cholesterol transport, 185
Rheumatoid arthritis, 698
Riboflavin, 319
adequate intake of, 325–326
chemical structure of, A-25
deficiency, 325
in energy metabolism, 324
food sources of, 325–326, 326*f*
functions of, 324
Ribonucleic acid (RNA), 82
Ribosomes, 80*f*, 82
Rice, 136*t*
Rice milk, 389
Rickets, 295, 308, 308*f*, 636
undernutrition and, 554*t*
vitamin D and, 295
Risedronate (Actonel), 428
Risk factors
chronic diseases and, 9
defined, 9
Romosozumab-aqqg (Evenity), 428
Roughage. *See* Insoluble fiber
Roux-en-Y gastric bypass, 663
R-proteins, 337
Rumination disorder, 496
Russell's sign, 488, 488*f*
Rutin, 136*t*
Rye, 136*t*

S

Saccharin, 140*t*, 141
Saccharomyces boulardii, 107

Salatrim (Benefat), 178
Saliva, 97
Salivary amylase, 142
Salivary lipase, 180
Salmon, 12
Salt sensitivity, 381
Salt substitutes, 382
Sanitation, in developing world, 565–566
Sarcopenia, 696
Sarcopenic obesity, 696
Satiety, 7, 263, 639
defined, 8
regulation of, 8
Satiety center, 8
Saturated fats, 45, 50
higher intakes of, 186
intake of, 189–190
tips for cutting back on, 193*t*
Saturated fatty acids, 166, 167*f*, 174*f*
Scavenger cells, 185
School-age children, 660
beverages for, 665
breakfast for, importance of, 664
dietary patterns of, 651*t*, 660, 665
fluid needs of, 665
healthy fats for, 665
MyPlate for meal planning for, 660, 661*f*
nutrition concerns of, 660–666
nutrition education in schools, 665–666
obesity in, 660–663, 662*f*
physical activity guidelines for, 662–663, 663*t*
snacks for, 665
sugar-sweetened beverages and, 665
School breakfast and lunch programs, 559
Scientific evidence, hierarchy of, 19–20, 19*f*
Scientific method, 18–19, 18*f*
Scurvy, 18, 341
undernutrition and, 554*t*
SDGs. *See* Sustainable Development Goals
Seafood, 190, 191
Sea salt, 381
Secondary hypertension, 418
Secondary lactose maldigestion, 143
Secondary osteoporosis, 425
Secretory vesicles, 82
Selective cholesterol absorption inhibitors, 201
Selenium, 408
adequate intake of, 406–407
avoidance of excess, 407
cancer and, 406

Selenium (continued)
    COVID-19 and, 408
    deficiency, 374, 406
    food sources of, 406–407, 407f
    functions of, 406
    RDA for, 407
    UL for, 407
Semaglutide (Wegovy), 279t, 280
Semistarvation, effects of, 555–556
Semivegetarian, 220
Senile osteoporosis, 425
Senior Farmers Market Nutrition Program, 708
Sequestrants, 536, 536t
Serotonin, 90, 229, 715
Sertraline (Zoloft), 497
Serving size, 39
Set-point theory, 263–264
Seventh-day Adventists, vegetarian lifestyle by, 221
SGA. See Small for gestational age
Shivering thermogenesis, 253
Short-chain fatty acids, 166, 173
Sickle cell anemia. See Sickle cell disease
Sickle cell disease, 211, 211f
Sigmoid colon, 103, 103f
Simple sugars, 11, 127, 128
Situational poverty, 560
Skeletal system, 84f
Skinfold measurements, 260, 260f
Sleep-related eating disorder, 497
Slow Food USA, 514
Small for gestational age (SGA), 589
Small intestine, 95, 95f, 100–102, 101f, 102f
Smartphone app accelerometers, 440
Smoking, during pregnancy, 590
SNAP. See Supplemental Nutrition Assistance Program
Sodium, 45, 377
    adequate intake of, 379–381, 380f
    for adults, 695
    avoidance of excess, 381–382
    bone health and, 427–428
    CDRR for, 381, 382
    deficiency, 379
    effects of, on gut microbiota, 420
    in fluid balance, 378–379
    food sources of, 380, 380f
    functions of, 378–379
    in muscle contraction, 379
    in nerve impulse transmission, 379
    sensitive, 381
    from soft water, 370
    in table salt, 377
    for toddlers and preschoolers, 652
Soft drink consumption, decline in, 133
Soft water, 369–370

Soil microbiome, 573
Soluble fibers, 130, 132–133
Solute, 377
Solution, 377
Solvent, 13, 377
Sorbitol, 118, 140
Sorghum, 136t
Soy alternative, 144
Soy milk, 389
Soy products, 221
Soy protein–based infant formulas, 640
Sparkling water, 371
Special Supplemental Nutrition Program for Women, Infants, and Children (WIC), 558t, 559, 592
Specific immunity, 93
Spelt, 136t
Sphingomyelin, 344
Spices, 541
Spicy foods and ulcer, 79
Spina bifida, 334, 618, 619f
Spinach, 375
Spontaneous abortion, 583
Sports anemia, 456
Sports dietitians, 440
Sports drinks, 458–459, 458f, 463
Sports food, 468
Spring water, 370
SSBs. See Sugar-sweetened beverages
Staphylococcus aureus, 530
Starch, 11, 127, 129, 129f
    amylopectin, 129
    amylose, 129
    defined, 129
    digestion of, 142, 143f
    in menu planning for diabetes, A-6–A-7
    in plant-based foods, 132
    resistant, 129
State of Food Security and Nutrition in the World (SOFI) Report, 552
Statins, 201
Step farming, 514
Sterols, 166, 169, 170f
    food sources of, 175–176
Stevia, 140t, 141
St. John's wort, 704t
Stomach, 95f, 98–100, 99f
Stone fruits, 265
Stool, 102
Strength and power athletes, 464–466
Strength training, for weight gain, 284
Stress fractures, 457
Stretching, 443
Stroke, 196
    defined, 9
Students
    alcohol and binge drinking by, 72–73

    athletes, 73, 75
    eating disorders and, 73
    eating habits of, 72
    eating well on budget, 75
    food choices of, 71
    impact of nutrition on academic performance, 74
    vegetarians/vegans, 73
    weight gain by, 71–72
Stunting, 552, 632
Subclinical deficiency, 56
Subthreshold eating disorders, 477, 496–497
Sucralose, 140t, 141
Sucrase, 142
Sucrose, 11, 127, 128, 128f, 138
Sugar, 11, 127, 138, 139. See also Added sugar
    added, 127, 139, 151
    in beverages, 151
    brown, 139
    dietary needs, 151–155
    digestion of, 142
    disaccharides, 127, 128, 128f
    excessive intake of, 151–152
    hyperactivity and, 153
    monosaccharides, 127–128, 128f
    oral health and, 153–155
    reducing intake of, 151–152, 154t
    simple, 127, 128
    sources of, 151, 153f
    turbinado, 139
Sugar alcohol, 139–140
Sugar-sweetened beverages (SSBs), 133, 151, 154
Suicide bags, 82
Superfoods, 13
Superoxide dismutase, 404, 412
Supertasters, 301
Supplemental Nutrition Assistance Program (SNAP), 558–559, 558t
Supplements, 346
    calcium, 391–393, 393t
    emergency department visits and, 348
    fish oil, 191
    of folic acid, 336
    growth of industry, 346f
    immunity and, 353
    ingredients in, 346
    label on, 349, 349f
    needs for, 346–348
    nonessential amino acids, 209
    population groups likely to benefit from, 347t
    protein, 218–219
    reasons for taking of, 346
    selection of, 348–350

use of, and nutrient toxicity, 347
vitamin, 295
vitamin B-12, 339
vitamin C, 343
vitamin D, 312
vitamin E, 313
zinc, 584
Support groups, 272
Sustainability, food choices and, 6–7
Sustainability of dairy, 390
Sustainable agriculture, 510, 514, 516, 565, 570–572
Sustainable development, 570
Sustainable Development Goals (SDGs), 568–569, 568f, 573
SDG Report, 569
Sustainable intensification, 571, 572f
Sustainable living, 514
Sustainable seafood, 514, 516
Swallowing, process of, 97, 98f
Symptoms, 56
Synapse, 90
Synbiotics, 107
Syndrome X, 596. See also Metabolic syndrome
Synovial fluid, 367
Systematic review, 19
Systolic blood pressure, 418

T

Table salt, 381
Table sugar, 11, 127, 138
Tap water, 370–371
Taste, in food choices, 5
Taste sensations, 96, 301
Tears, 367
Teenagers, 666–667
acne and, 669
alcohol abuse among, 670
caffeine consumption of, 668–669
calcium intake of, 667–668
and fast-food habit, 668
fruit and vegetable intake of, 667
growth spurt in, 666
iron for, 668
nutrition concerns for, 666–670
obesity in, 667
vegetarian dietary patterns and, 669–670
vitamin D intake of, 667–668
Teen pregnancy, 590
Teff, 136t
Teratogens, 618
Teriparatide (Forteo), 428
Term infant, 589, 631
Terrace farming, 514
Testosterone, 583

Tetany, 387
Texture, in food choices, 5
Theory, 19
Therapeutic phlebotomy, 402, 403
Thermic effect of food (TEF), 255–256
Thermogenesis, 252
Thiamin, 319, 322
adequate intake of, 323
chemical structure of, A-25
deficiency, 322
in energy metabolism, 322
food sources of, 323, 324f
functions of, 322
Thiamin pyrophosphate (TPP), 322
Thirst, 458
Thirst sensation, 368
Thrifty Food Plan (TFP), 559
Thrifty metabolism, 262
Thrombocytes. See Platelets
Thyroid gland, 408
Thyroid hormones, 91f, 93, 263, 599
synthesis of, 408
Time, food choices and, 5
Tissues, 82
connective, 82
epithelial, 82
muscle, 82
nervous, 82
Tissue saturation, 296
Toadskin appearance, 304
Tocopherols, 312. See also Vitamin E
Toddler drinks, 629
Toddlers and preschoolers, 650
autism spectrum disorder in, 658–659
calcium for, 652
carbohydrates for, 652
constipation in, 657
dietary fat for, 652
dietary patterns for, 651t
dietary supplements for, 656
energy needs of, 650, 651t
fiber for, 657
iron for, 651–652
lead poisoning, protection from, 656–657
nutrition concerns for, 652–659
oral health of, 658
picky eating, 650, 653–654
protein for, 652
snacks for, 655, 655t
sodium for, 652
vegetarian dietary patterns for, 658
Tolerable Upper Intake Level (UL), 59, 59t, 60, 295
Tomatoes, 14
Toxicity, 13
chromium, 416
copper, 412–413

iron, 402
magnesium, 397
manganese, 416
zinc, 406
Toxins, 524
Trabecular bone, 422, 425
Trace minerals, 13
Trachea, 97
Trail mix, 394
Transcription, 210
Trans fat, 178
Trans fatty acids, 168, 168f, 179
Transferrin, 375, 399
Transfer RNA (tRNA), 210
Transgender individuals, nutrition care for, 62
Translation, 210
Transverse colon, 103, 103f
Tretinoin (Retin-A), 306
Triglycerides, 166, 187
composition of, 166
digestion, 180
in foods and body, 169, 170f
food sources of, 171–175
mixtures of fatty acids in, 173
purpose of, 166
Trimesters, 586
Trimethylamine, 226
Trimethylamine oxide (TMAO), 226
Tripeptides, 209
Triticale, 136t
Tropical plant oils, 179
Trypsin, 226
T-score, 423
Tumor, 351
Turbinado sugar, 139
Turmeric, 704t
Type 1 diabetes, 9, 148, 157–158, 157t, 598. See also Diabetes
complications of, 157–158
insulin therapy for, 157
nutrition therapy for, 157
onset of, 157
Type 2 diabetes, 9, 157, 157t, 158–159, 607. See also Diabetes
in children, 158, 664
development of, 158, 158f
medications and insulin in, 159
metabolic syndrome and, 159–160
nutrition therapy for, 159
obesity and, 158–159
onset of, 158
plant-based diet and, 222–223
risk factors for, 158
Type 1 osteoporosis, 425
Type 2 osteoporosis, 425
Tyramine, 674
Tyrosine, 239

U

Ulcer, spicy foods and, 79
Ultra-high temperature (UHT) processing, 528, 528t, 529
Ultraprocessed foods, 37
   defined, 37
   and health outcomes, 38
Ultratrace minerals, 375
Umami, 96
Undernutrition, 55, 56, 552, 554, 564, 582
   in developed countries, 555
   in developing countries, 554
   nutrient-deficiency diseases with, 554t
   pediatric, 632–633
   during pregnancy, 574–575
   protein-calorie malnutrition, 554
   from semistarvation, 555–556
Underwater (hydrostatic) weighing, 259, 259f
Underweight
   causes of, 284
   defined, 284
   energy-dense foods for, consumption of, 284
   health problems with, 284
   lean muscle mass, gain of, 285
   treatment of, 284–285
   weight gain for, 284–285, 285f
UNICEF WASH (water, sanitation, and hygiene) programs, 565
United Nations, 551
United Nations International Children's Emergency Fund (UNICEF), 554, 555
United Nations Sustainable Development Goals (SDGs), 568–569, 568f
United States
   child nutrition programs in, 558t
   Daily Values on food labels, A-1
   death in, causes of, 9, 9f
   eating patterns in, 21–23
   2018 farm bill, 558, 558f
   federal and nonfederal nutrition support programs, 557, 558t
   federal nutrition assistance, 558–559
   fiber intake in, 151
   health objectives for, 23
   malnutrition in, 556–562
   nutrition security, 556–559
   obesity in, 21, 21f
United States Pharmacopeia Convention (USP), 349
Unprocessed food, 37
Upper-body obesity, 158, 261–262, 261f

Urea, 88
Ureter, 88, 88f
Urethra, 88, 88f
Urinary bladder, 88, 88f
Urinary system, 83f, 88–89
   defined, 88
   organs of, 88f
   structure and function of, 88–89
Urine color, hydration status and, 369, 369f
USDA Pesticide Data Program, 520
U.S. Department of Agriculture (USDA), 41, 520, 521t
U.S. Department of Health and Human Services (HHS), 23

V

Vegan, 73, 192, 220, 287, 287t, 339
Vegetables
   carbohydrates in, 135, 137
   commonly consumed, 5, 6f
   consumption of, 38, 52
   lutein and zeaxanthin in, 303t, 305
   in menu planning for diabetes, A-8–A-9
   recommendations for, 137
   subgroups, 137
   vitamins in, 296, 297f, 298t
Vegetarianism, 219
Veins, 87
Vertical sleeve gastrectomy, 663
Very-low-calorie diet (VLCD), 280
Very-low-density lipoproteins (VLDLs), 184t, 185
Vigorous-intensity aerobic physical activity, 439
Viking diet, 192
Villi, 100
Virus, 524
   foodborne illness by, 532–533, 532f, 533f
Visceral obesity. See Upper-body obesity
Vitamin A, 294–295, 302
   for acne treatment, 306
   active forms of, 302
   animal sources, 302
   as anti-infection vitamin, 302
   avoidance of excess, 305–306
   in cancer prevention, 304
   carotenoids and, 302
   chemical structure of, A-24
   deficiency, 304–305, 554
   epithelial cells health and, 302
   excess intake of, 305
   eye health and, 302
   food sources of, 305, 306f
   functions of, 302–304, 303f

   in growth and development, 303–304
   immune system and, 302
   preformed, 302, 304, 305
   during pregnancy, 304–306
   RDA for, 305
   reproduction and, 304
   storage of, 302
   toxicity, 296, 305–306
   vision and, 302–303, 303f, 304
Vitamin B-1. See Thiamin
Vitamin B-2. See Riboflavin
Vitamin B-3. See Niacin
Vitamin B-6, 319
   adequate intake of, 331
   for adults, 695
   in amino acid metabolism, 330
   chemical structure of, A-25
   deficiency, 331
   food sources of, 331–332, 331f
   functions of, 330
   in homocysteine metabolism, 330
   for nausea and vomiting of pregnancy, 606
   toxicity, 332
   UL for, 332
Vitamin B-7. See Biotin
Vitamin B-12, 224, 337
   absorption of, 337, 338f
   adequate intake of, 339
   for adults, 695
   chemical structure of, A-26
   deficiency, 338–339
   folate metabolism and, 334, 337, 338
   food sources of, 339, 340f
   functions of, 338
   for infants, 636
   malabsorption, 339
   synthetic, 339
Vitamin C, 319
   adequate intake of, 341–342
   for adults, 694
   as antioxidant, 340–341
   avoidance of excess, 342–343
   in body defenses, 340–341
   chemical structure of, A-26
   common cold and, 341
   deficiency, 341
   food sources of, 341, 342f
   functions of, 340–341
   immune system and, 341
   iron absorption and, 341, 401
   proteins and, 341
   RDA for, 342
   Upper Level (UL) of, 342
Vitamin D, 92, 295, 307
   adequate intake of, 309–312
   for adults, 693–694
   athletes and, 457

avoidance of excess, 312
in blood calcium and phosphorus regulation, 307–308
in bone health, 308
in cellular differentiation, 308
deficiency, 308
factors impairing, 309t
fat-soluble vitamin, 307
food sources of, 309–310, 310f
forms of, 309
fortified foods, 309–310
functions of, 307–308
as hormone, 307
immune system and, 308
infants and, 636
precursor to, 307, 307f
during pregnancy, 598–599
RDA for, 309
supplementation, 312
synthesis of, 307
for teenagers, 667–668
toxicity, 312
ultraviolet light and production of, 307
whole milk and, 293
Vitamin D_2 (ergocalciferol), 307, 309
Vitamin D_3 (cholecalciferol), 307, 309
Vitamin E, 312
adequate intake of, 314–315
for adults, 695
as antioxidant, 313
avoidance of excess, 315
for cancer prevention, 315
chemical structure of, A-24
chronic diseases and, 313
deficiency, 313–314
as fat-soluble vitamin, 313, 313f
food sources of, 314, 314f
forms of, 312
functions of, 313
RDA of, 315
Vitamin K, 295, 316
absorption of, 318
adequate intake of, 316, 318
blood clotting and, 316
for bone health, 316
cardiovascular disease and, 316
chemical structure of, A-24
deficiency, 316
food sources of, 316, 318f
forms of, 316
functions of, 316
hemorrhage and, 316
infants and, 636
Vitamin K deficiency
bleeding, 316, 636
fat-malabsorption conditions and, 295

Vitamins, 12–13
absorption of, 295–296
chemical structure of, A-23–A-26
criteria for compound as, 295
deficiency, 296
defined, 10, 294
in dietary patterns, 294
excretion of, 296
fat malabsorption and deficiency of, 295
fat-soluble, 12, 294, 295
fertility and, 583–584
function of, 12, 294f
for infants, 636
megadoses of, 295
natural, 295
preservation of, in foods, 296, 298, 298t
production, 295
requirement, 294
storage of, 111, 295–296
synthetic, 295
toxicity, 296
upper intake levels for, A-36
water-soluble, 12–13, 294, 296
VLDLs. See Very-low-density lipoproteins
Vytorin, 201

W

Waist circumference, 262, 262f
Walnuts, 174
Warren, Robert, 79
Wasting, 552, 632
Water, 10, 13, 364
adequate intake for, 369
for adults, 693
avoidance of excess, 371–372
balance, 364–366, 365f
body temperature and, 367, 368f
bottled and tap, 370–372
chemical reactions in, 367
cushioning from, 367
deficiency, 368–369
fluid conservation, 365–366, 366f
food sources of, 369, 370f
functions of, 13, 366–367
hard, 369
human body and, 13, 364, 364f
for infants, 637–638
intake, 364, 365f
intoxication, 459
lubrication from, 367
metabolic, 364
moistening from, 367
nutrient transport by, 367
output, 364–365, 365f
in pregnancy, 597

soft, 369–370
as solvent, 13
sparkling/seltzer, 371
as universal solvent, 366
waste transport by, 367
Water bottles, 371
guidelines for safe use of, 372
Water fluoridation, 414–415
Water intoxication, 371–372
Water loss
insensible, 365
sensible, 365
Water-soluble vitamins, 12–13, 294, 296, 319. See also Vitamins
and fat-soluble vitamins, comparison of, 296, 297f
Weaning, 646
from bottle or breast, 647
Wearable fitness trackers, 440
Weight bias, 249, 250, 275, 275f, 663
Weight control, 193
Weight discrimination. See Weight bias
Weight gain
added sugars and, 127
calorie intake and, 45
during pregnancy, 595–596, 596t
students and, 71–72
Weight loss, 276, 286. See also Weight management
behavioral interventions for, 271
Body Weight Planner and, 276
calorie intake and, 45, 193
daily calorie deficit for, 277
diet plans specific to, 286–287, 287t
energy deficit for, 71, 265
energy intake, strategies to reduce, 268, 268t
healthy eating for, 268
maintenance of, 275, 276
medications for, 279–280, 279t
negative energy balance for, 252
plant-based dietary patterns and, 265, 266
primary determinant of, 265
professional help for, 279–283, 286
success in, 277, 278f
Weight-loss apps, 288
Weight-loss plan
characteristics of, 277, 277f
healthy, 268
Weight-loss plateau, 268–269
Weight management, 286
behavioral strategies for, 271–276
behavior triggers and, 272–274, 272f, 273t
Dietary Guidelines and, 271
non-diet approach to, 501
non-diet strategies for, 274

Weight management (continued)
   in perspective, 278
   physical activity for, 272
   relapse prevention, 274–275
   self-monitoring for, 271
   small plates use for meals, 274, 274f
   SMART goals for, 272, 272t
   social networking and, 272
   support groups and, 272
Weight regain, 280
Weight-restricted athletes, 457
Weight stigma. *See* Weight bias
Wernicke-Korsakoff syndrome, 322
Wet nursing, 640
Wheat, 136t
Wheat bread, 151
Whey protein, 209
White blood cells, 86
White House Conference on Hunger, Nutrition, and Health, 25
Whole30 diet, 288
Whole foods, 39
Whole grains, 130, 130f, 132, 134–135, 137, 150–151
   available, 136t
   benefits of, 134, 136t
   characteristics of, 134t
   Dietary Guidelines on, 134
   examples of, 134
   fiber in, 134
   refined grains and, 134t
Whole Grain Stamp, 135, 135f
Wild rice, 136t
Wilson's disease, 413
Windpipe. *See* Trachea
Women's Health Initiative study, 392
World Health Organization (WHO)
   growth charts, 630
   on healthy aging, 684
World Obesity Federation (WOF), 249
WW (weight watchers), 286–287, 287t

X

Xerophthalmia, 304
   undernutrition and, 554t
Xylitol, 140

Z

Zeaxanthin, 302, 303t
Zinc, 404
   absorption of, 405
   adequate intake of, 404–405
   for adults, 694
   avoidance of excess, 406
   deficiency, 374, 404
   food sources of, 404, 405f
   functions of, 404
   immune function and, 404
   and male fertility, 584
   in pregnancy, 600
   supplementation, 404, 405, 584
Zoledronic acid (Reclast), 428
Zoochemicals, 299
Z score, 630
Zygote, 586